REFERENCE BOOK
NOT TO BE TAKEN
FROM THE LIBRARY

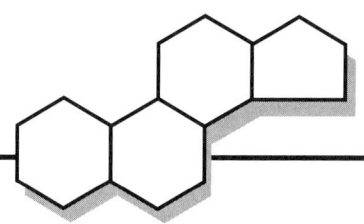

HORMONES, BRAIN and BEHAVIOR

VOLUME TWO

CHAPTERS 16–34

Edited by

Donald W. Pfaff
The Rockefeller University
New York, New York

Arthur P. Arnold
Department of Physiological Science
University of California, Los Angeles
Los Angeles, California

Anne M. Etgen
Department of Neuroscience
Albert Einstein College of Medicine
Bronx, New York

Susan E. Fahrbach
Department of Entomology
University of Illinois at Urbana-Champaign
Urbana, Illinois

Robert T. Rubin
Allegheny General Hospital
Pittsburgh, Pennsylvania

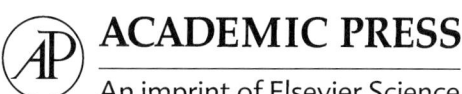

Amsterdam Boston London New York Oxford Paris San Diego San Francisco
Singapore Sydney Tokyo

This book is printed on acid-free paper. ∞

Copyright © 2002, Elsevier Science (USA).

All Rights Reserved.
No part of this publication may be reproduced or transmitted in any form or by any means, electronic or mechanical, including photocopy, recording, or any information storage and retrieval system, without permission in writing from the publisher.

Requests for permission to make copies of any part of the work should be mailed to: Permissions Department, Academic Press, 6277 Sea Harbor Drive, Orlando, Florida 32887-6777

Academic Press
An imprint of Elsevier Science.
525 B Street, Suite 1900, San Diego, California 92101-4495, USA
http://www.academicpress.com

Academic Press
84 Theobalds Road, London WC1X 8RR, UK
http://www.academicpress.com

Library of Congress Catalog Card Number: 2002104386

International Standard Book Number: 0-12-532104-X (set)
International Standard Book Number: 0-12-532105-8 (volume 1)
International Standard Book Number: 0-12-532106-6 (volume 2)
International Standard Book Number: 0-12-532107-4 (volume 3)
International Standard Book Number: 0-12-532108-2 (volume 4)
International Standard Book Number: 0-12-532109-0 (volume 5)

PRINTED IN THE UNITED STATES OF AMERICA
02 03 04 05 06 07 MM 9 8 7 6 5 4 3 2 1

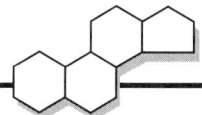

Brief Contents of All Volumes

Contents of Volume One

PART I
MAMMALIAN HORMONE-BEHAVIOR SYSTEMS

CHAPTER 1
Male Sexual Behavior — 1
Elaine M. Hull, Robert L. Meisel, and Benjamin D. Sachs

CHAPTER 2
Feminine Sexual Behavior: Cellular Integration of Hormonal and Afferent Information in the Rodent Brain — 139
Jeffrey D. Blaustein and Mary S. Erskine

CHAPTER 3
Parental Care in Mammals: Immediate Internal and Sensory Factors of Control — 215
Gabriela González-Mariscal and Pascal Poindron

CHAPTER 4
The Neurobiology of Social Affiliation and Pair Bonding — 299
C. S. Carter and E. B. Keverne

CHAPTER 5
Hormonal Processes in the Development and Expression of Aggressive Behavior — 339
Neal G. Simon

CHAPTER 6
Hormonal Basis of Social Conflict and Communication — 393
H. Elliott Albers, Kim L. Huhman, and Robert L. Meisel

CHAPTER 7
Energy Balance, Ingestive Behavior, and Reproductive Success — 435
Jill E. Schneider and Alan G. Watts

CHAPTER 8
Neuroendocrinology of Body Fluid Homeostasis — 525
Steven J. Fluharty

CHAPTER 9
Corticotropin-Releasing Factor, Corticosteroids, Stress, and Sugar: Energy Balance, the Brain, and Behavior — 571
Mary F. Dallman, Victor G. Viau, Seema Bhatnagar, Francisca Gomez, Kevin Laugero, and M. E. Bell

CHAPTER 10
Hormonal Modulation of Central Motivational States — 633
Jay Schulkin

CHAPTER 11
Neurochemical Coding of Adaptive Responses in the Limbic System — 659
Joe Herbert and Jay Schulkin

CHAPTER 12
Stress, Opioid Peptides, and Their Receptors — 691
Ryszard Przewłocki

CHAPTER 13

Effects of Social Stress on Hormones, Brain, and Behavior 735

D. Caroline Blanchard, Christina R. McKittrick, Matthew P. Hardy, and Robert J. Blanchard

CHAPTER 14

Regulation of the Injury-Immune Response in the Central Nervous System: Allostasis and Allostatic Load in Immunity 773

Karen Bulloch and Bruce S. McEwen

CHAPTER 15

Pheromones, Odors, and Vasanas: The Neuroendocrinology of Social Chemosignals in Humans and Animals 797

Martha K. McClintock

Contents of Volume Two

CHAPTER 16

Molecular Recognition and Intracellular Transduction Mechanisms in Olfactory and Vomeronasal Systems 1

Makoto Kashiwayanagi

CHAPTER 17

Pheromonal Signals Access the Medial Extended Amygdala: One Node in a Proposed Social Behavior Network 17

Sarah Winans Newman

CHAPTER 18

Circadian Rhythms in the Endocrine System 33

Lance J. Kriegsfeld, Joseph LeSauter, Toshiyuki Hamada, SiNae M. Pitts, and Rae Silver

CHAPTER 19

Mammalian Seasonal Rhythms: Behavior and Neuroendocrine Substrates 93

Brian J. Prendergast, Randy J. Nelson, and Irving Zucker

CHAPTER 20

Thyroid Hormones in Neural Tissue 157

Ronald M. Lechan and Roberto Toni

CHAPTER 21

Thyroid Hormone, Brain, and Behavior 239

Michael Bauer and Peter C. Whybrow

CHAPTER 22

Gonadal Steroids, Learning, and Memory 265

Gary Dohanich

PART II

NONMAMMALIAN HORMONE-BEHAVIOR SYSTEMS

A. NONMAMMALIAN VERTEBRATES

CHAPTER 23

Life History, Neuroendocrinology, and Behavior in Fish 331

Matthew S. Grober and Andrew H. Bass

CHAPTER 24

Weakly Electric Fish: Behavior, Neurobiology, and Neuroendocrinology 349

Harold H. Zakon and G. Troy Smith

CHAPTER 25

Hormonal Pheromones in Fish 375

Norm Stacey and Peter Sorensen

CHAPTER 26

Social Regulation of the Brain: Status, Sex, and Size 435

Russell D. Fernald

CHAPTER 27

Hormonal Regulation of Motor Output in Amphibians: *Xenopus laevis* Vocalizations as a Model System 445

Darcy B. Kelley

CHAPTER 28

Endocrinology of Complex Life Cycles: Amphibians 469

Robert J. Denver, Karen A. Glennemeier, and Graham C. Boorse

CHAPTER 29
Sensorimotor Processing Model: How Vasotocin and Corticosterone Interact and Control Reproductive Behaviors in an Amphibian — 515
Frank L. Moore and James D. Rose

CHAPTER 30
Hormones, Brain, and Behavior in Reptiles — 545
John Godwin and David Crews

CHAPTER 31
Ecophysiological Studies of Hormone-Behavior Relations in Birds — 587
John C. Wingfield and Bengt Silverin

CHAPTER 32
Neuroendocrine Mechanisms Regulating Reproductive Cycles and Reproductive Behavior in Birds — 649
Gregory F. Ball and Jacques Balthazart

CHAPTER 33
Neural and Hormonal Control of Birdsong — 799
Barney A. Schlinger and Eliot A. Brenowitz

B. INVERTEBRATES

CHAPTER 34
Insect Developmental Hormones and Their Mechanisms of Action — 841
James W. Truman and Lynn M. Riddiford

Contents of Volume Three

CHAPTER 35
Neuropeptide Control of Molting in Insects — 1
John Ewer and Stuart Reynolds

CHAPTER 36
Hormonal Regulation of Sexual Behavior in Insects — 93
John M. Ringo

CHAPTER 37
Hormonal Regulation of Parental Care in Insects — 115
Stephen T. Trumbo

CHAPTER 38
Biogenic Amines as Circulating Hormones in Insects — 141
Wendi S. Neckameyer and Sandra M. Leal

CHAPTER 39
Influence of Juvenile Hormone III on the Development and Plasticity of the Responsiveness of Female Crickets to Calling Males through Control of the Response Properties of Identified Auditory Neurons — 167
John F. Stout, Gordan J. Atkins, Jing Hao, Michael Bronsert, and Randall Walikonis

CHAPTER 40
Endocrine Influences on the Organization of Insect Societies — 195
Guy Bloch, Diana E. Wheeler, and Gene E. Robinson

CHAPTER 41
Hormonal Mediation of Insect Life Histories — 237
Hugh Dingle

CHAPTER 42
Parasite- and Pathogen-Mediated Manipulation of Host Hormones and Behavior — 281
Nancy E. Beckage

CHAPTER 43
Role of Lys-Conopressin in the Control of Male Sexual Behavior in *Lymnaea stagnalis* — 317
Paul F. van Soest and Karel S. Kits

CHAPTER 44
Hormonal Regulation of Neural and Behavioral Plasticity in Insects — 331
Susan E. Fahrbach and Janis C. Weeks

PART III
CELLULAR AND MOLECULAR MECHANISMS OF HORMONE ACTIONS ON BEHAVIOR

CHAPTER 45
Rapid Membrane Effects of Estrogen in the Central Nervous System — 361
Martin J. Kelly and Oline K. Rønnekleiv

CHAPTER 46
Estrogen Regulation of Neurotransmitter and Growth Factor Signaling in the Brain   381
Anne M. Etgen

CHAPTER 47
Genetic Mechanisms in Neural and Hormonal Controls over Female Reproductive Behaviors   441
Donald Pfaff, Sonoko Ogawa, Kami Kia, Nandini Vasudevan, Christopher Krebs, Jonathan Frohlich, and Lee-Ming Kow

CHAPTER 48
Electrophysiological Effects of Androgens   511
Keith M. Kendrick

CHAPTER 49
Model Systems for the Study of Androgen-Regulated Gene Expression in the Central Nervous System   527
Darcy B. Kelley and Donald J. Tindall

CHAPTER 50
Molecular Aspects of Thyroid Hormone–Regulated Behavior   539
Grant W. Anderson and Cary N. Mariash

CHAPTER 51
Rapid Corticosteroid Actions on Behavior: Cellular Mechanisms and Organismal Consequences   567
Miles Orchinik, Paul Gasser, and Creagh Breuner

CHAPTER 52
Corticosteroid Actions on Electrical Activity in the Brain   601
Marian Joëls, Harm J. Krugers, and E. Ronald De Kloet

CHAPTER 53
Mechanisms of Aldosterone Action in Brain and Behavior   627
Randall R. Sakai, James P. Herman, and Steven J. Fluharty

CHAPTER 54
Mechanism of Progesterone Receptor Action in the Brain   643
Shaila K. Mani and Bert W. O'Malley

CHAPTER 55
Progesterone: Synthesis, Metabolism, Mechanisms of Action, and Effects in the Nervous System   683
Michael Schumacher and Françoise Robert

CHAPTER 56
Novel Effects of Neuroactive Steroids in the Central Nervous System   747
Sheryl S. Smith

A. OXYTOCIN AND VASOPRESSIN

CHAPTER 57
Oxytocin   779
Hans H. Zingg

CHAPTER 58
Vasopressin Receptors   803
Mariel Birnbaumer

CHAPTER 59
Cell Biology of Oxytocin and Vasopressin Cells   811
Jeffrey G. Tasker, Cherif Boudaba, Dominique A. Poulain, and Dionysia T. Theodosis

Contents of Volume Four

CHAPTER 60
Electrophysiological and Molecular Properties of the Oxytocin- and Vasopressin-Secreting Systems in Mammals   1
Hiroshi Yamashita, Yoichi Ueta, and Richard E. J. Dyball

B. RELEASING HORMONES

CHAPTER 61
Gonadotropin-Releasing Hormone   51
Lothar Jennes and P. Michael Conn

CHAPTER 62
Corticotropin-Releasing Factor: Putative Neurotransmitter Actions of a Neurohormone   81
Rita J. Valentino and Elisabeth Van Bockstaele

PART IV
DEVELOPMENT OF HORMONE-DEPENDENT NEURONAL SYSTEMS

A. SEXUAL DIFFERENTIATION

CHAPTER 63
Concepts of Genetic and Hormonal Induction of Vertebrate Sexual Differentiation in the Twentieth Century, with Special Reference to the Brain 105
Arthur P. Arnold

CHAPTER 64
Anatomy, Development, and Function of Sexually Dimorphic Neural Circuits in the Mammalian Brain 137
Geert J. De Vries and Richard B. Simerly

CHAPTER 65
What Neuromuscular Systems Tell Us about Hormones and Behavior 193
Stephen Marc Breedlove, Cynthia L. Jordan, and Darcy B. Kelley

CHAPTER 66
Sexual Differentiation of Brain and Behavior in Birds 223
Jacques Balthazart and Elizabeth Adkins-Regan

CHAPTER 67
Differentiation/Maturation of Centers in the Brain Regulating Reproductive Function in Fishes 303
Martin P. Schreibman and Lucia Magliulo-Cepriano

CHAPTER 68
Impact of Environmental Endocrine Disruptors on Sexual Differentiation in Birds and Mammals 325
Mary Ann Ottinger and Frederick S. vom Saal

CHAPTER 69
Masculinization and Defeminization in Altricial and Precocial Mammals: Comparative Aspects of Steroid Hormone Action 385
Kim Wallen and Michael J. Baum

CHAPTER 70
Sexual Differentiation of Human Brain and Behavior 425
Melissa Hines

CHAPTER 71
Sexual Identity and Sexual Orientation 463
Richard Green

B. EARLY STRESS

CHAPTER 72
Glucocorticoids, Stress, and Development 487
Claire-Dominique Walker, Leonie A. M. Welberg, and Paul M. Plotsky

CHAPTER 73
Enduring Effects of Early Experience on Adult Behavior 535
Seymour Levine

CHAPTER 74
Thyroid Hormones and Brain Development 543
Juan Bernal

C. LIFE STAGES

CHAPTER 75
Neuroendocrine Regulation of Puberty 589
Sergio R. Ojeda and Ei Terasawa

CHAPTER 76
Puberty in Boys and Girls 661
Dennis M. Styne and Melvin M. Grumbach

CHAPTER 77
Sex Steroids and Neuronal Growth in Adulthood 717
Catherine S. Woolley and Rochelle S. Cohen

CHAPTER 78
Adult Neurogenesis in the Mammalian Brain 779
Patima Tanapat, Nicholas B. Hastings, and Elizabeth Gould

CHAPTER 79
Evolution and the Plasticity of Aging in the Reproductive Schedules in Long-Lived Animals: The Importance of Genetic Variation in Neuroendocrine Mechanisms 799
Caleb E. Finch

CHAPTER 80
Protective Effects of Estrogen on Aging and Damaged Neural Systems 821
Victor W. Henderson and Donald W. Reynolds

PART V

HORMONE-BEHAVIOR RELATIONS OF CLINICAL IMPORTANCE

A. ENDOCRINE SYSTEMS INTERACTING WITH BRAIN AND BEHAVIOR

CHAPTER 81
Hypothalamic-Pituitary-Adrenal Axis: Introduction to Physiology and Pathophysiology   841
K. Eddie Gabry, Philip W. Gold, and George P. Chrousos

CHAPTER 82
Hypothalamic-Pituitary-Thyroid Axis   867
Russell T. Joffe

Contents of Volume Five

CHAPTER 83
Hypothalamic-Pituitary-Gonadal Axis in Men   1
Ronald S. Swerdloff, Christina Wang, and Amiya P. Sinha Hikim

CHAPTER 84
Gonadal Hormones and Behavior in Women: Concentrations versus Context   37
David R. Rubinow, Peter J. Schmidt, Catherine A. Roca, and Robert C. Daly

CHAPTER 85
Growth Hormone and Insulin-like Growth Factor I: Effects on the Brain   75
Zvi Laron

CHAPTER 86
Brain Prolactin   97
Nira Ben-Jonathan, Sudha Khurana, and Robert Hnasko

CHAPTER 87
Melatonin as a Hormone and as a Marker for Circadian Phase Position in Humans   121
Laurie Hurtado Vessely and Alfred J. Lewy

CHAPTER 88
Cholecystokinin: A Molecular Negative-Feedback Control of Eating   143
Gerard P. Smith

CHAPTER 89
Neuroregulatory Peptides of Central Nervous System Origin: From Bench to Bedside   153
John Kasckow and Thomas D. Geracioti, Jr.

CHAPTER 90
Neuroendocrine–Immune Interactions: Implications for Health and Behavior   209
Charles L. Raison, Jane F. Gumnick, and Andrew H. Miller

B. ENDOCRINOLOGICALLY IMPORTANT BEHAVIORAL SYNDROMES

CHAPTER 91
Genetics of Endocrine–Behavior Interactions   263
Marianne B. Müller, Martin E. Keck, Thomas Steckler, and Florian Holsboer

CHAPTER 92
Gender and Behavior in Subjects with Genetic Defects in Male Sexual Differentiation   303
Julianne Imperato-McGinley and Yuan-Shan Zhu

CHAPTER 93
Consequences of Mutations in Androgen Receptor Genes: Molecular Biology and Behavior   347
Marilyn Y. McGinnis, Marco Marcelli, and Delores J. Lamb

CHAPTER 94
An Evolutionary Psychological Perspective on the Modulation of Competitive Confrontation and Risk-Taking   381
Margo Wilson, Martin Daly, and Nicholas Pound

CHAPTER 95
Pain: Sex/Gender Differences   409
Karen J. Berkley, Gloria E. Hoffman, Anne Z. Murphy, and Anita Holdcroft

CHAPTER 96
Stress and Anxiety Disorders   443
Elizabeth A. Young and Israel Liberzon

CHAPTER 97
The Neuroendocrinology of Affective Disorders   467
Robert T. Rubin, Timothy G. Dinan, and Lucinda V. Scott

CHAPTER 98
Anorexia Nervosa and Bulimia Nervosa   515
André B. Negrão and Julio Licinio

CHAPTER 99
Premenstrual Dysphoric Disorder   531
Barbara L. Parry and Sarah L. Berga

CHAPTER 100
Diabetes Mellitus   553
Christopher M. Ryan

CHAPTER 101
Calcium Metabolism and Psychiatric Disorder   593
Ruth White and David Heath

CHAPTER 102
Hypothalamic Origin of Prevalent Human Disease   607
Per Björntorp

CHAPTER 103
Aging and Alzheimer's Disease   637
Murray A. Raskind, Charles W. Wilkinson, and Elaine R. Peskind

CHAPTER 104
Cocaine, Hormones, and Behavior: Clinical and Preclinical Studies   665
Nancy K. Mello and Jack H. Mendelson

CHAPTER 105
Alcohol Abuse: Endocrine Concomitants   747
Elizabeth S. Ginsburg, Nancy K. Mello, and Jack H. Mendelson

CHAPTER 106
Relationships between Endocrine Functions and Substance Abuse Syndromes: Heroin and Related Short-Acting Opiates in Addiction Contrasted with Methadone and Other Long-Acting Opioid Agonists Used in Pharmacotherapy of Addiction   781
Mary Jeanne Kreek, Lisa Borg, Yan Zhou, and James Schluger

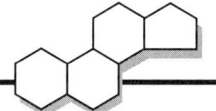

Contents of This Volume

CHAPTER 16

Molecular Recognition and Intracellular Transduction Mechanisms in Olfactory and Vomeronasal Systems   1

Makoto Kashiwayanagi

I. Introduction   1
II. Main Olfactory Organ   2
   A. Olfactory G-Protein-Coupled Receptors   2
   B. Responses of Single Olfactory Receptor Neurons to Multiple Odorants   3
   C. Odor Responses and Olfactory GPCRs during Development   3
   D. Odor Responses Independent on Olfactory GPCR in Adult   4
   E. Does the Specific Projection of Olfactory Receptor Neurons to Mitral Cells Integrate Odor Information?   4
   F. cAMP-Dependent Transduction Pathway   5
   G. Significance of the cAMP-Independent Transduction Pathway   5
   H. cAMP-Independent Aquatic Odor Reception in Vertebrates   6
   I. IP_3-Dependent Transduction Pathway   6
   J. Colocalization of cAMP- and IP_3-Dependent Pathways in Single Olfactory Neurons   6
   K. cAMP- and IP_3-Independent Transduction Pathways   6
   L. cGMP/NO-Mediated Pathway   6
   M. Possible Role of cADP-Ribose in Odor Reception   7
III. Vomeronasal Organ   7
   A. Transduction Pathways in the Reptilian Vomeronasal System   7
   B. Minor Role of cAMP in Mammalian Pheromone Reception   7
   C. Pheromonal Transduction Mediated via IP_3 in the Mammalian Vomeronasal System   8
   D. Selective Pheromone Reception in Vomeronasal Sensory Neurons   8
   E. Putative Receptor for Pheromones   9
   F. Projection of Pheromonal Information to the Accessory Olfactory Bulb   9
   G. Memory Storage in the Accessory Olfactory Bulb   10
   H. Chemical Characterization of Pheromones   10
   References   10

CHAPTER 17

Pheromonal Signals Access the Medial Extended Amygdala: One Node in a Proposed Social Behavior Network   17

Sarah Winans Newman

I. Pheromonal Communication   17
II. Multiple Sensory Systems Innervate the Nasal Cavities   17
III. Importance of the Vomeronasal Organ in Reproductive Neuroendocrine Function and Social Behaviors Varies with Sex and Species   18
IV. Concept of the Medial Extended Amygdala   19
V. Evidence for Anterior and Posterior Circuits in the Medial Extended Amygdala: Connections, Transmitters, Hormone Receptors, and Hormone Action   19
   A. Anatomical Continuity in Parallel Circuits   19
   B. Neurotransmitter or Neuromodulator Continuity in the Posteromedial Extended Amygdala   19
   C. Gonadal Steroid Receptors and Sexual Dimorphism in the Medial Extended Amygdala   20

VI. Continuity of Function in the Medial Extended Amygdala Circuits: Male Sexual Behavior 20
VII. Roles of the Medial Extended Amygdala in Other Social Behaviors 24
References 28

CHAPTER 18

Circadian Rhythms in the Endocrine System 33

Lance J. Kriegsfeld, Joseph LeSauter, Toshiyuki Hamada, SiNae M. Pitts, and Rae Silver

I. Introduction to Circadian Rhythms 33
   A. Characterization of Circadian and Diurnal Rhythms 33
   B. History of the Study of Circadian Rhythms 33
   C. Functions of the Circadian System 34
   D. Circadian Rhythms Orchestrate Internal Physiological Processes 34
   E. Circadian Rhythms Are Entrained to the Environment 35
II. Organization of the Circadian System 38
   A. Finding Circadian Clocks 38
   B. Suprachiasmatic Nucleus Is the Locus of the Body's Circadian Clock in Mammals 38
   C. Anatomy and Physiology of the Suprachiasmatic Nucleus 38
   D. Unique Pacemaker Function of the Suprachiasmatic Nucleus Is Based on Common Mechanisms 39
   E. Circadian Timekeeping Is a Fundamental Property of the Suprachiasmatic Nucleus 40
   F. Cellular Organization of Circadian Systems: Rhythmicity Is a Cell-Autonomous Property 41
III. Genetic and Molecular Basis of Circadian Rhythms: Oscillator Mechanisms Involve Gene Expression 43
   A. *Drosophila melanogaster* 43
   B. Neurospora 44
   C. Mammals 45
IV. Photic Input Pathways to the Suprachiasmatic Nucleus 46
   A. Suprachiasmatic Nucleus Pacemakers Are Reset by External Stimuli 46
   B. Photic Signals Regulate Gene Expression in the Suprachiasmatic Nucleus 47
   C. Circadian System Has Specialized Photoreceptors 48
V. Output Signals of the Suprachiasmatic Nucleus 48
   A. Suprachiasmatic Nucleus Controls the Phase of Rhythmic Responses 48
   B. Neural Efferents 48
   C. Diffusible Signals 50
VI. Suprachiasmatic Nucleus as a Master Oscillator Holds the Circadian System Together: There Are Many Oscillators within Specialized Tissues of Complex Organisms 51
VII. Circadian Regulation of Endocrine Rhythms 52
   A. Circadian Rhythms in Hormone Secretions 52
      1. *Glucocorticoids* 53
      2. *Gonadotropins and Gonadal Steroids* 53
      3. *Prolactin* 54
   B. Interactions between Sleep and Circadian Regulation of Endocrine Rhythms 54
   C. Endocrine Influence on Circadian Rhythms 55
   D. Sex Differences in Circadian Rhythms 56
   E. Suprachiasmatic Nucleus Output and Regulation of Circadian Endocrine Rhythms 57
      1. *Melatonin* 57
      2. *Glucocorticoids* 59
      3. *Sex Steroids and the Estrous Cycle* 60
      4. *Prolactin* 61
   F. Tau Mutation and Endocrine Function 62
VIII. Circadian Regulation of Feeding-Related Hormones 63
   A. Neural Regulation of Feeding 64
   B. Circadian Control of Feeding 64
   C. Feeding Affects Circadian Hormone Rhythms 65
IX. Circadian Effects on Reproduction and Feeding in the Aging Organism 68
   A. Evidence for Suprachiasmatic Nucleus Aging and Rejuvenation 68
   B. Reproduction 68
      1. *Aging in Female Reproductive Rhythms* 68
      2. *Aging in Male Reproductive Rhythms* 70
   C. Aging and Homeostasis 70
      1. *Eating and Metabolism* 71
X. Evolution of the Circadian System 71
References 73

CHAPTER 19

Mammalian Seasonal Rhythms: Behavior and Neuroendocrine Substrates 93

Brian J. Prendergast, Randy J. Nelson, and Irving Zucker

I. Introduction 93
II. Evolution of Seasonal Rhythms—Ecological and Energetic Relations 94

III. Classification of Seasonal Rhythms 96
    A. Brief History of Photoperiodism Research 96
    B. Type I Rhythms: Some Day Lengths Are More Important than Others 96
        1. Induction of Refractoriness to Short Day Lengths and Its Termination by Long Day Lengths 98
        2. Critical Day Lengths 98
        3. Puberty 99
        4. Sexual Behavior and Physiology 100
    C. Type II Rhythms 104
        1. Entrainment of Type II Rhythms: Mediation by Melatonin 105
        2. Phase Response Curves to Hormones 105
        3. Hormones, Seasonal Variation in Locomotor Activity, and Circannual Modulation of Circadian Organization 106
IV. Endocrine Transduction of Photoperiod Signals 107
    A. Duration vs Phase of the Melatonin Signal 107
    B. Decoding of Melatonin Signals 108
    C. Context-Dependent Melatonin Signal Integration 109
V. Neural Bases for Photoperiodism 110
    A. Mechanisms of Photoperiodic Time Measurement: Neural Control of Melatonin Secretion 110
    B. High-Density Melatonin-Binding Sites in the Mammalian Brain 111
    C. Central Sites of Melatonin Action in the Reproductive Neuroendocrine System 112
VI. Maternal–Fetal Communication of Day Length 113
    A. Voles 113
    B. Hamsters 114
VII. Winter Breeding and Photoperiod Nonresponsiveness 115
    A. Definitions 115
    B. Neuroendocrine Mediation of Nonresponsiveness 116
        1. Deer Mice (Peromyscus maniculatus) 117
        2. Siberian Hamsters (Phodopus sungorus) 118
    C. Nonreproductive Traits in Photoperiod Nonresponders 120
    D. Summary 120
VIII. Seasonal Rhythms in Primates 121
    A. Nonhuman Primates 121
    B. Humans 124
        1. Evolution and Human Seasonality 124
        2. Human Seasonal Reproductive Rhythms 125
        3. Melatonin and Human Reproduction 125
        4. What Can Animal Studies Tell Us about Human Seasonality? 126
IX. Seasonal Rhythms in Nonreproductive Traits 126
    A. Food Intake and Body Mass 126
    B. Stress Responses 128
    C. Immune Function 129
        1. Energetics and Immune Function 131
    D. Social Organization: Affiliation and Aggression 133
    E. Brain Development 134
    F. Locomotor Activity 135
        1. Daily Activity Patterns 135
    G. Ultrasonic Vocalizations 136
    H. Odor Preferences 136
    I. Hibernation and Daily Torpor 137
    References 139

CHAPTER 20

Thyroid Hormones in Neural Tissue 157
Ronald M. Lechan and Roberto Toni

I. Introduction 157
    A. Historical Overview 157
    B. Importance of Feedback Regulation by Thyroid Hormone 157
II. Mechanisms of Thyroid Hormone Action in the CNS 158
    A. Thyroid Hormone Transport in the Bloodstream 158
    B. Thyroid Hormone Delivery across the Blood-Brain and Blood-CSF Barriers 160
    C. Thyroid Hormone Transport into the CNS 162
    D. Activation and Inactivation of Thyroid Hormone by Iodothyronine Deiodinases 164
    E. Thyroid Hormone Receptors 167
    F. Nonnuclear Effects of Thyroid Hormone 170
III. Hypothalamic-Pituitary-Thyroid Axis 171
    A. Anatomy of the Hypophysiotrophic TRH Neuroregulatory System 171
        1. TRH Tuberoinfundibular System 171
        2. TRH Gene and Promoter Regulation 173
    B. Biosynthesis and Processing of PreproTRH 174
    C. Feedback Regulation of Hypophysiotrophic TRH by Thyroid Hormone 178
    D. Regulation of Hypophysiotropic TRH by Afferent Inputs 180
    E. Biogenic Amines 182
        1. Norepinephrine and Epinephrine 182
        2. Dopamine 186
        3. Serotonin 187
        4. Histamine 188
    F. Neuropeptides, Proteins, and Amino Acids 188
        1. Neuropeptide Y 188
        2. Agouti-Related Protein 190
        3. α-Melanocortin Stimulating Hormone 191
        4. Cocaine- and Amphetamine-Regulated Transcript 192

5. Thyrotropin-Releasing Hormone 193
6. Somatostatin 194
7. Opioid Peptides 194
8. Neurotensin 195
9. Corticotropin-Releasing Hormone 195
10. Vasoactive Intestinal Peptide (VIP) and Pituitary Adenylate Cyclase Activating Polypeptide (PACAP) 196
11. Gamma Aminobutyric Acid 196
12. Cytokines 197
13. Other Substances 197
G. Steroid Hormones 197
1. Glucocorticoids 197
2. Gonadal Steroids 198
H. Hypothalamic Regulation of TSH 198
1. Molecular Structure and Glycosylation of TSH 198
2. Feedback Regulation of TSH by Thyroid Hormone 199
3. Regulation of TSH by TRH 201
4. TRH Receptor 201
5. Regulation of the TSHβ Subunit Gene by TRH 203
6. Regulation of TSHα Gene by TRH 203
7. Effect of TRH on Glycosylation of TSH 203
8. TRH-Degrading Enzymes 203
9. Mechanism of Action of Other Hypothalamic Hormones on TSH Secretion 204
10. Paracrine/Autocrine Regulation of TSH 205
11. Pulsatility and Circadian Rhythm 205
I. Mechanism of Action of TSH on the Thyroid Gland 207
1. TSH Receptor 207
2. Regulation of Thyroid Follicular Cells by TSH 208
3. Neural Regulation of the Thyroid Gland 208
4. Neuropeptide Y 211
5. Vasoactive Intestinal Polypeptide/Peptide Histidine Isoleucine 211
6. Other Peptides 211
References 211

CHAPTER 21

Thyroid Hormone, Brain, and Behavior 239
Michael Bauer and Peter C. Whybrow

I. Introduction to the Thyroid System and Behavior 239
  A. Historical Perspective 239
  B. Organization and Regulation of the Hypothalamic-Pituitary-Thyroid System 240
  C. Developmental and Metabolic Effects of Thyroid Hormones 240
  D. Molecular and Cellular Effects of Thyroid Hormones in the Brain 241
    1. Thyroid Economy of the Brain 241
    2. Genomic and Extranuclear Effects 242
II. Neuropsychiatric and Behavioral Manifestations in Disorders of the Thyroid Gland 243
  A. Psychiatric and Behavioral Aspects of Thyrotoxicosis 243
    1. Neuropsychiatric Signs and Symptoms in Hyperthyroidism 243
    2. Overt Psychiatric Manifestations 244
    3. Treatment Outcome of Neuropsychiatric Symptoms 244
  B. Psychiatric and Behavioral Aspects of Hypothyroidism 244
    1. Neuropsychiatric Signs and Symptoms in Hypothyroidism 245
    2. Overt Psychiatric Manifestations 246
    3. Treatment Outcome of Neuropsychiatric Symptoms 246
  C. Behavioral Effects of Thyrotropin-Releasing Hormone and Changes in Thyroid Status in Animals 247
III. Hypothalamic-Pituitary-Thyroid Axis Dysfunction in Affective Illness 247
  A. Peripheral Thyroid Hormone in Depression 248
  B. The Thyrotropin-Releasing Hormone Test in Depression 248
  C. Effects of Antidepressant Treatments on Peripheral Thyroid Hormone Levels 248
  D. Thyroid Dysfunction in Bipolar Affective Disorder 249
IV. Thyroid Hormone and Mood Modulation 250
  A. Hormones of the Hypothalamic-Pituitary-Thyroid System in the Treatment of Mood Disorders 250
    1. Historical Perspective 250
    2. Treatment with Thyrotropin-Releasing Hormone and Thyroid-Stimulating Hormone 250
    3. Treatment with Thyroid Hormones Alone 251
    4. Thyroid Hormone Supplementation in Mood Disorders 251
V. Adult Brain—A Site of Thyroid Hormone Action 254
  A. Thyroid-Monoamine Systems Interaction 254
    1. Thyroid–Catecholamine Interaction 254
    2. Thyroid–Serotonin Interaction 255
  B. Modulatory Effects of Thyroid Hormones on the γ-Aminobutyric Acid System 255
  C. Effects of Thyroid Hormones on Postreceptor Mechanisms and Signal Transduction 255
  D. Novel Approaches to Study the Thyroid System and Brain Activity *In Vivo* 256
VI. Summary 256
References 257

CHAPTER 22

Gonadal Steroids, Learning, and Memory 265
Gary P. Dohanich

I. Introduction 265
  A. Steroids, Learning, and Memory 265
    1. Adaptive Value 266
    2. Strength of Effect 266
    3. Neural Substrate 266
    4. Nonmnemonic Processes 266

II. Learning and Memory 267
   A. Study of Learning and Memory 267
   B. Some Basic Elements of Learning and Memory 267
   C. Types of Learning and Memory 268
      1. *Spatial and Nonspatial Learning and Memory* 269
      2. *Conditioning* 270
   D. Study of Learning and Memory in Primates 270
III. Ovarian Hormones and Cognition in Nonhumans 271
   A. Overview 271
      1. *Steroid Mechanisms* 271
      2. *Ovarian Steroids and the Study of Cognition* 273
   B. Working Memory 274
      1. *Working Memory and Radial Arm Maze* 274
      2. *Working Memory and T Maze* 275
      3. *Working Memory and Water Maze* 276
      4. *Working Memory and Object Recognition* 277
      5. *Summary of Ovarian Steroid Effects on Working Memory Performance* 277
   C. Reference Memory 277
      1. *Reference Memory and Radial Arm Maze* 278
      2. *Reference Memory and Water Maze* 278
      3. *Reference Memory and Circular Platform Maze* 280
      4. *Summary of Ovarian Steroid Effects on Reference Memory Performance* 280
   D. Conditioning 280
      1. *Active Avoidance* 280
      2. *Passive Avoidance* 281
      3. *Eye-Blink Conditioning* 282
      4. *Operant Conditioning* 282
      5. *Summary of Ovarian Steroid Effects on Conditioning* 282
   E. Learning Strategies 283
   F. Ovarian Steroids and Nonmnemonic Effects 283
      1. *Pretraining* 283
      2. *Measurement of Nonmnemonic Effects* 284
      3. *Posttraining Treatment* 285
IV. Neuroanatomy and Neuromechanisms of Ovarian Steroid Action 285
   A. Overview 285
   B. Neuroanatomy 286
      1. *Hippocampus* 286
      2. *Basal Forebrain* 289
      3. *Supramammillary Area* 290
      4. *Monoaminergic Nuclei* 291
   C. Regulation of Neurotransmitter Systems by Ovarian Steroids 291
      1. *Acetylcholine* 291
      2. *Glutamate* 292
      3. *γ-Aminobutyric Acid* 292
      4. *Monoamines* 292
   D. Structural Change Associated with Ovarian Steroids 293
   E. Electrical Change Associated with Ovarian Steroids 294
   F. Neuroprotective Effects of Ovarian Hormones 294
      1. *Neuroprotection* 294
      2. *Mechanisms of Neuroprotection* 295
      3. *Alzheimer's Disease* 295
V. Ovarian Hormones and Human Cognition 297
   A. Premenopausal Effects of Ovarian Hormones 297
   B. Postmenopausal Effects of Ovarian Hormones 298
   C. Protective Actions of Ovarian Hormones 299
VI. Androgens and Cognition 301
   A. Overview 301
   B. Androgen and Nonhuman Cognition 301
   C. Androgen and Human Cognition 303
VII. Conclusion 304
   A. Adaptive Value 304
   B. Strength of Effect 304
   C. Neural Substrate 304
   D. Nonmnemonic Factors 305
   E. Final Thought 305
   References 305

PART II
NONMAMMALIAN HORMONE-BEHAVIOR SYSTEMS

A. NONMAMMALIAN VERTEBRATES

CHAPTER 23

Life History, Neuroendocrinology, and Behavior in Fish 331
Matthew S. Grober and Andrew H. Bass

I. Introduction 331
II. Life History 331
III. Correlated Changes in a Suite of Characters 332
IV. Alternative Male Reproductive Morphs in Midshipman Fish 333
   A. Spawning and Vocal Behaviors 333
   B. Somatic and Endocrinological Traits 334
      1. *Vocal Motor Traits* 335
   C. Neuroendocrine Traits 337
      1. *Gonadotrophin-Releasing Hormone* 337
      2. *Arginine Vasotocin* 338
      3. *Gonadal Steroids and Aromatase* 339
   D. Summary Comments 339
V. Primacy of the Behavior—Brain Cascade: Reversible Sex Change in Gobies 340
VI. Temporal Axis for Social Modulation of AVT Phenotype in the Bluehead Wrasse 341
   A. Arginine Vasotocin 342
VII. Summary 343
   References 344

CHAPTER 24

Weakly Electric Fish: Behavior, Neurobiology, and Neuroendocrinology 349

Harold H. Zakon and G. Troy Smith

I. Introduction 349
  A. Electric Organ Discharge as a Communication Signal 350
II. Generation and Reception of Electric Signals 350
  A. Electric-Organ-Discharge Waveform: Pulse or Wave 350
  B. Neural Circuitry Controlling the Electric Organ Discharge 351
  C. Production of Species-Specific Electric-Organ-Discharge Waveforms 352
    1. Pulse Fish 352
    2. Wave Fish 353
    3. Social Signals Are Mediated by Neurotransmission via Glutamate Receptors 354
  D. Reception of the Electric Organ Discharge: The Electroreceptors 355
III. Sex Differences and Individual Variation in Electric-Organ-Discharge Waveform 355
  A. Sexual Dimorphism of the Electric-Organ-Discharge Waveform 355
  B. Individual Differences in Electric-Organ-Discharge Waveform 357
IV. Modulation of Electric Organ Discharges during Social Behavior 357
  A. Aggressive Interactions 358
  B. Courtship and Spawning 360
  C. Parental Care 361
  D. Other Sexually Dimorphic Behaviors 362
V. Steroid Hormones and the Electric-Organ-Discharge Waveform 363
  A. Endogenous Levels of Gonadal Steroids 363
  B. Exogenous Treatment with Steroid Hormones 363
VI. Effects of Hormones on Electric Organ Morphology 365
VII. Influence of Hormones on Ionic Currents of Electromotor System 365
VIII. Rapid Changes in Electric-Organ-Discharge Parameters 367
IX. Hormonal Modulation of Chirping 368
X. Hormonal Plasticity in Electroreceptors 369
XI. Conclusion 370
  References 370

CHAPTER 25

Hormonal Pheromones in Fish 375

Norm Stacey and Peter Sorensen

I. Introduction 375
II. Hormones, Pheromones, Olfaction, and Behavior 378
  A. Olfactory Signals and Pheromones: General Concepts and Definitions 378
  B. Hormonal Pheromones 378
    1. Special Terminology Related to Pheromones and Their Composition 379
    2. Evolution and the Terminology of Pheromone Function 380
  C. Sense of Smell 382
    1. Anatomy of the Olfactory System 382
    2. Olfactory Basis of Hormonal Pheromone Detection 384
  D. Hormones and Reproductive Behavior in Fish 387
    1. Gonadal Steroid Hormones 387
    2. Hormones and Male Behavior 388
    3. Hormones and Female Behavior 388
III. Development of Hormonal Pheromone Studies 390
  A. Fish Reproductive Pheromones 390
  B. Early Studies of Hormonal Pheromones 391
    1. Black Goby (*Gobius niger* = *G. jozo*) 391
    2. Zebrafish (*Danio rerio*) 391
  C. Studies of Pheromone Production, Release, and Detection 392
    1. Hormonal Pheromone Production In Vivo 392
    2. Hormonal Pheromone Release 392
    3. Hormonal Pheromone Detection by the Olfactory Organ 393
IV. Biology of Hormonal Pheromones 394
  A. Phylogenetic Distribution of Hormonal Pheromones in Fishes 394
  B. Lamprey and Hagfish 395
  C. Primitive Fishes (Noneuteleost Actinopterygeans) 396
  D. Order Cypriniformes 396
    1. Goldfish 396
    2. Other Cypriniform Fishes 410
  E. Order Characiformes 412
  F. Order Siluriformes 412
    1. African Catfish (*Clarias gariepinus*) 412
    2. Other Siluriforms 413
  G. Salmonid Fishes (Order Salmoniformes; Family Salmonidae) 413
    1. Genus *Salmo* 413
    2. Genus *Salvelinus* 415
    3. Genus *Oncorhynchus* 416
    4. Conclusions 416
  H. Order Perciformes 416
    1. Round Goby (*Neogobius melanostomus*; Family Gobiidae) 417
    2. Eurasian Ruffe (*Gymnocephalus cernuus*; Family Percidae) 418
  I. Unidentified Pheromones in Other Fish 419

V. Hormonal Modulation of Hormonal
   Pheromone Function 419
VI. Summary 421
   References 422

CHAPTER 26

Social Regulation of the Brain: Status, Sex, and Size 435
Russell D. Fernald

I. Introduction 435
II. Model System 436
III. Differences between Territorial and
     Nonterritorial Males 438
IV. Social Control of Sex and Size 439
   A. Social Regulation of Reproduction 439
   B. Environmental Influences on Social
      Status and Size 442
V. Conclusion 443
   References 443

CHAPTER 27

Hormonal Regulation of Motor Output in Amphibians: *Xenopus laevis* Vocalizations as a Model System 445
Darcy B. Kelley

I. Introduction 445
II. Vocal Repertoire 445
III. Vocal Communication 447
IV. Hormonal Control of Vocal Behaviors
    in Adults 447
V. Mechanisms of Sound Production:
   Cartilaginous and Muscular Elements 448
VI. Sex Differences 449
   A. Laryngeal Muscle 449
      1. Molecules and Physiology 449
      2. Relation to Click Production 453
   B. Laryngeal Motor Neuron: The
      Neuromuscular Synapse 453
   C. Vocal Nerve Activity 455
VII. Progressive Increases in Click Amplitude
     Are Attractive to Females 457
VIII. Generating Vocalizations in Vertebrates 460
   A. Sexually Differentiated Vocal Patterns in
      Xenopus laevis 462
      1. Vocal Effectors 463
IX. Summary and Conclusion 466
   References 467

CHAPTER 28

Endocrinology of Complex Life Cycles: Amphibians 469
Robert J. Denver, Karen A. Glennemeier, and Graham C. Boorse

I. Introduction to Complex Life Cycles 469
II. Evolutionary Ecology of Amphibians 471
   A. Metamorphosis 471
      1. Environmental Factors That Influence the Duration
         of the Larval Period 471
      2. Evolution of the Timing of Metamorphosis 471
   B. Facultative Paedomorphosis 473
III. Endocrinology of Metamorphosis 475
   A. Overview 475
   B. Thyroid Hormone 476
      1. Role in Amphibian Development 476
      2. Thyroid Gland Development and Hormone Production . 476
      3. Control of Thyroid Hormone Secretion, Metabolism,
         and Transport 478
      4. Mechanisms of Thyroid Hormone Action: Thyroid
         Hormone Receptors 483
   C. Corticoids 484
      1. Roles of Corticoids in Amphibian Growth and
         Development 484
      2. Hormones Produced by Amphibian Interrenal Glands . 484
      3. Control of Corticoid Production and Transport 485
      4. Mechanisms of Corticoid Action 486
   D. Prolactin and Growth Hormone 486
   E. Neuroendocrine Control of Amphibian
      Development 488
      1. Neurohormones and the Control of Pituitary Secretion . 488
      2. Thyrotropin-Releasing Hormone (Pyro-
         glutamyl-histidyl-proline-amide) 488
      3. Corticotropin-Releasing Hormone Is a Thyrotropin-
         Releasing Factor 488
      4. Other Neurohormones Regulating Thyroid-
         Stimulating Hormone 490
IV. Endocrinology of Paedomorphosis 491
   A. Overview 491
   B. Thyroid Axis 491
      1. Facultative Paedomorphs 491
      2. Obligate Paedomorphs 491
   C. Reproductive Development 492
V. Integrating Evolution, Ecology, and
   Endocrinology 493
   A. Metamorphosis 493
      1. Limits to the Length of the Larval Period 495
      2. Plasticity in the Timing of Metamorphosis 496
   B. Facultative Paedomorphosis 498
      1. Integrated Organismal Responses to the
         Environment—Metamorphosis vs Paedomorphosis 498
      2. Physiological and Ecological Trade-offs between
         Metamorphosis and Paedomorphosis 499
   References 501

CHAPTER 29

Sensorimotor Processing Model: How Vasotocin and Corticosterone Interact and Control Reproductive Behaviors in an Amphibian 515

Frank L. Moore and James D. Rose

I. Introduction	515
II. Newt Reproductive Behaviors	516
A. Preinsemination Behaviors and Sexual Stimuli	517
B. Neural Control of Clasping in *Taricha*	517
C. Insemination Behaviors	521
D. Postinsemination Behaviors	522
E. Modifying Factors in Reproductive Behaviors	522
III. Activation of Male Reproductive Behaviors: Steroids	522
A. Testicular Steroids in Amphibians	522
B. Seasonal Cycles in Sex Steroids	523
C. Castration and Steroid-Replacement Studies in Amphibians	524
IV. Activation of Male Reproductive Behaviors: Vasotocin	524
A. Behavioral Responses to Vasotocin Injections in Amphibians	524
B. Sex and Seasonal Variations in Vasotocin	525
C. Effects of Sex Steroids on the Vasotocin System	526
D. Effects of Castration and Steroid Replacement on Heterotypical Reproductive Behavior	526
E. Vasotocin as a Regulator of Sensorimotor Processing	527
1. *Vasotocin Effects on Sensory Orientation and Responses to Sex Pheromones*	527
2. *Vasotocin Effects on Visual Sexual Cues*	527
3. *Conclusions about Vasotocin and Sensorimotor Processing Controlling Reproductive Behavior*	528
V. Suppression of Male Reproductive Behaviors: Corticosterone	528
A. Corticosterone Inhibits Courtship Behaviors in *Taricha*	529
B. Membrane Receptor for Corticosterone	530
1. *Behavioral Function for the Membrane Corticosterone Receptor*	530
2. *Evidence That the Membrane Corticosterone Receptor Is a G-Protein-Coupled Receptor*	531
3. *Biochemical Studies of the Membrane Corticosterone Receptor*	531
4. *κ-Selective Ligand Binding to the Membrane Corticosterone Receptor*	532
5. *Membrane Corticosteroid Receptor and Opioid Receptors*	532
C. Neural Mechanisms of mCR-Mediated Corticosterone Effects on Clasping	533
1. *Corticosterone Rapidly Blocks Neuronal Responses to Clasp Trigger Stimuli*	533
2. *Spinal Corticosterone Effect on Clasping*	534
D. Rapid Corticosterone Effects on Forebrain Neurons	534
E. General Conclusions Concerning the Rapid Neural Actions of Corticosterone	534
VI. Neurophysiological Interactions between Corticosterone and the Neuropeptides CRH and Vasotocin	535
A. Rapid Stress Hormone Actions on the Neural Control of Clasping: A Summary Model	537
References	539

CHAPTER 30

Hormones, Brain, and Behavior in Reptiles 545

John Godwin and David P. Crews

I. Introduction	545
A. Advantages as Models	545
B. Pivotal Place in Amniote Evolutionary History	546
C. Reptilian Brain as an Experimentally Tractable Model	546
II. Diversity in Sex Determination, Sexual Differentiation, and Hormone–Behavior Relationships	546
A. Sex Determination and Sexual Differentiation in Reptiles Lacking Sex Chromosomes	547
1. *Molecular Genetics of Temperature-Dependent Sex Determination*	547
2. *Organizing Influence of Incubation Temperature*	549
3. *Parthenogenesis*	552
B. Functional Associations in Hormones, Gamete Production, and Mating Behavior	553
C. Alternative Mating Strategies	554
D. Sex Steroids and Behavior: Other Reptiles	559
1. *Turtles*	559
2. *Crocodilians, Tuatara, and Amphisbaenians*	559
III. Neuroanatomical Substrates of Sexual Behavior in Reptiles	560
A. Integrative Centers for Sexual Behaviors	560
B. Variation in Brain Nuclei and Neuron Soma Sizes	561
IV. Metabolic Indicators of Neural Activity	564
A. Acute Metabolic Activity Associated with Behavioral State: 2-Deoxyglucose Utilization	565
B. Metabolic Capacity Associated with Behavioral Phenotype: Cytochrome Oxidase Histochemistry	566
V. Neurochemical Bases of Sexual and Aggressive Behavior in Reptiles	568
VI. Distribution and Regulation of Sex Steroid Hormone Receptors	570
A. Distribution	570
B. Regulation	573

VII. Conclusion and Future Directions 576
References 577

CHAPTER 31

Ecophysiological Studies of Hormone-Behavior Relations in Birds 587
John C. Wingfield and Bengt Silverin

I. Introduction 587
   A. Temporal Sequence of Life History Stages 588
   B. Expression of Substages That Give State 590
   C. Transitions between Life History Stages 591
   D. Timing of Life History Stages 592
   E. Field Studies in Environmental Endocrinology: Why and How 592
   F. Overview: Ecophysiological Studies of Hormone–Behavior Relations in Birds 594
II. Prealternate Molt 594
   A. A True Life History Stage? 594
   B. Prealternate Molt, Development of Nuptial Plumages, and Their Hormonal Control 595
      1. *Species Showing No Seasonal Change* 595
      2. *Species Showing a Seasonal Change* 597
      3. *Polyandrous Species* 598
      4. *Species Undergoing More Than Two Plumage Changes per Year* 599
      5. *Effects of Estradiol on Plumage* 599
      6. *Effects of Luteinizing Hormone on External Secondary Sex Characteristics* 600
      7. *Is There a Relationship between Hormonal Control and Plumage Type?* 600
   C. Timing Mechanisms 601
III. Vernal Migration 602
   A. Migration Strategies Prebreeding 603
   B. Hormone Control Mechanisms in Vernal Migration 603
   C. Substages of Fat Deposition, Fat Use, and Flight—Fluctuating Extremes of Migration 605
   D. Role of Testosterone in Control of Vernal Fattening and Zugunruhe 605
IV. Breeding Life History Stage 606
   A. Development of Reproductive Function in Ecological Contexts 607
      1. *Effects of Food* 609
      2. *Role of Social Interactions* 609
      3. *Pathways of Action of Environmental Signals* 609
      4. *Periodicity of Reproduction at Low Latitudes* 610
   B. Multiple Brooding 610
   C. Termination of Breeding
      1. *Nonphotoperiodic Regulation of Termination of Reproduction* 612
   D. Mating Systems and Breeding Strategies 613
V. Prebasic Molt 614
   A. Hormonal Bases of Prebasic Molt 615
   B. Molt and the Incompatibility of High Thyroxine and Testosterone Secretion 615
VI. Autumnal Migration 617
   A. Postbreeding Movements 617
   B. Migration Strategies Postbreeding and Their Hormonal Bases 618
      1. *Postjuvenile Dispersal* 618
      2. *Programmed Partial Migration* 618
      3. *Regular Autumnal Migration* 618
VII. Winter (Nonbreeding) Life History Stage 620
   A. Wintering Strategies in Ecological Contexts 620
   B. Hormone–Behavior Interactions in Winter Territoriality (Strategy A) 621
      1. *Hormonal and Gonadal Activities during Winter* 622
      2. *Territoriality in the Nonbreeding Season* 622
   C. Hormone–Behavior Interactions in Social Hierarchies in Flocks (Strategy B) 625
VIII. Emergency Life History Stage 625
   A. Nonstress Components of the Emergency Life History Stage 627
   B. Behavioral and Physiological Responses to the Unpredictable Environment—Mechanisms to Avoid Chronic Stress 627
      1. *Hormonal Changes after Exposure to a Direct Labile Perturbation Factor: The Emergency Life History Stage* 628
      2. *Other Examples of Emergency Stages during Winter* 630
   C. Modulation of the Adrenocortical Response to Stress and Its Ecological Bases 631
   D. Mechanisms Modulating Responses to Stress 632
IX. Conclusion 632
References 633

CHAPTER 32

Neuroendocrine Mechanisms Regulating Reproductive Cycles and Reproductive Behavior in Birds 649
Gregory F. Ball and Jacques Balthazart

I. Introduction: Diversity in Reproductive Strategies in Birds 649
   A. Basic Aspects of Avian Reproduction 650
   B. Avian Species That Have Been Studied in Detail 651
   C. Diversity in Breeding Cycles: Temperate vs Tropical Breeding Cycles 652
   D. Diversity in Mating Systems and Parental Care Patterns 652
   E. Species Diversity and Sexual Dimorphism in Behavior and Morphology 654
   F. Overall Organization of Reproductive Behavior 655
      1. *Male Behavior* 655
      2. *Female Behavior* 655
II. Environmental Control of the Reproductive Cycle 657

A. Photoperiodic Regulation of Breeding 657
  1. Photoperiodic and Extraphotoperiodic Cues 657
  2. Brief Description of the Photoperiodic Response 658
  3. How Is Variation in Day Length Measured? 659
B. Influence of Nonphotoperiodic Cues on the Timing of Breeding 660
  1. Variations in Temperature and Food as Supplementary Factors Influencing Seasonal Gonadal Cycles 660
C. Effects of Social Interactions on Reproductive Physiology 661
  1. Effects of Male Behavior on Female Reproductive Physiology 661
  2. Interaction between Photoperiod and the Effects of Social Stimuli from Male Birds on Female Reproductive Development 663
  3. Effects of Female Behavior on Male Physiology 664

III. Anatomy of the Reproductive Neuroendocrine System in Birds 665
  A. Gonadotropin-Releasing Hormone I and II Neuronal Systems 665
    1. Structure 665
    2. Distribution 666
  B. Distribution of Sex Steroid Hormone Receptors 668
    1. Androgen Receptors 668
    2. Estrogen Receptors, α Subtype 671
    3. Estrogen Receptors, β Subtype 674
    4. Progesterone Receptors 676
  C. Distribution of Steroid-Metabolizing Enzymes 677
    1. Testosterone Metabolism 677
    2. Estradiol Metabolism 687
    3. Progesterone Metabolism 687

IV. Neuroendocrine Mechanisms Mediating the Transduction of Environmental Information 689
  A. Photoperiod 689
    1. Extraretinal Photoreceptor in Birds 690
    2. Suprachiasmatic Nucleus and the Site of the Biological Clock in Birds 690
    3. Steroid Hormone Feedback Effects Are Not Involved in Regulating Response to Photoperiod in Birds 691
    4. Roles of Prolactin and Thyroid Hormones in Regulating Photoperiodic Responses in Birds 692
    5. High Nocturnal Concentrations of Melatonin Code for Day Length in Birds, but Do Not Mediate Physiological Responses to Photoperiod 693
  B. Visual and Auditory Sensory Inputs on the Reproductive Axis 693
    1. Induction by Sexual Behavior of the Immediate Early Genes ZENK and fos 693
    2. Song Induction of ZENK 699
    3. Pathways from Auditory and Visual Areas to the GnRH System 700
  C. Seasonal Plasticity in the Gonadotropin-Releasing-Hormone Neuronal System 701

V. Mechanisms of Steroid Hormone Action on Reproductive Behavior 703

A. Peripheral vs Central Effects of Steroid Hormones 703
B. Male Sexual Behavior: Appetitive and Consummatory Aspects 704
  1. Site of Steroid Hormone Activation 705
  2. Role of Steroid Metabolism in the Regulation of Behavior 712
  3. Control of the Activity of Steroid-Metabolizing Enzymes 727
  4. Steroid–Neurotransmitter Interactions 730
  5. Rapid Actions of Steroids and the Rapid Regulation of Aromatase Activity 744
  6. Effects of Behavior on Endocrine Physiology 750
  7. Is a General Model of the Hormonal Control of Male Sexual Behavior Emerging? 751
C. Female Sexual Behavior 753
  1. Activation of Receptivity and Proceptivity 753
  2. Nest-Building 755
  3. Correlations of Behavioral and Endocrine Changes 756
  4. Sites of Action of Sex Steroid Hormones 757
  5. Steroid–Neurotransmitter Interactions 757
  6. Effects of Behavior Performance on Endocrine State 758
  7. Behavioral Endocrinology of Female Sexual Behavior: Toward a Synthesis 760
D. Parental Behavior 761
  1. Correlations between Hormonal Changes during the Reproductive Cycle and Behavior 761
  2. Prolactin and Parental Care in Pigeons and Doves 761
  3. Experimental Studies of the Role Played by Steroid Hormones and Prolactin in Mediating the Transition from Courtship to Parental Care 761
  4. Hormonal Basis of Parental Care in Brood Parasites and Polyandrous Species 762
  5. Studies of the Neural Basis of Parental Care in Birds 763

VI. Conclusion 763
References 764

CHAPTER 33

Neural and Hormonal Control of Birdsong 799
Barney A. Schlinger and Eliot A. Brenowitz

I. Introduction 799
  A. Avian Systematics 800
  B. Anatomy of the Song System and Mechanism of Song Production 800
  C. Song System of Male and Female Birds 801
  D. Functional Significance of Birdsong 802
  E. Song and the Seasons 802
  F. Song Learning 803
  G. General Anatomy and Function of the Hypothalamic-Pituitary-Gonadal Axis in Adult and Developing Songbirds 803

II. Relationship of Song to Gonadal Hormones 804
  A. Adult Song Expression 804
    1. Studies Relating Reproductive Cycles to the Production of Birdsong 804
    2. Studies Relating Direct Measures of Circulating Hormones with Production of Birdsong 805

3. Experimental Evidence Directly Linking Reproductive Hormones and Birdsong—Gonadectomy or Photoperiod-Induced Gonadal Regression and Steroid Replacement 805
4. Evidence of Gonad-Independent Song Expression 806
B. Development of the Song System 807
1. Studies Relating Sex Steroids to Sexually Dimorphic Development of the Song System 807
2. Measures of Endogenous Gonadal Steroids and Steroid Production and Song-System Development 808
3. Evidence Pointing to Gonad-Independent Sexual Differentiation of the Brain 808
C. Song Learning 809
III. Steroid Sensitivity of the Song System 809
A. Evidence for Steroid Sensitivity of the Song-Control System 809
B. Presence of Androgen Receptors and Estrogen Receptors in Song Nuclei of Adults 810
C. Steroid Sensitivity of Discrete Cell Populations in Song Nuclei 810
D. Development of Steroid Receptors in Song Nuclei 811
E. Colocalization of Steroid Receptors and Neurotransmitters 811
F. Seasonal Changes and Regulation of Steroid Sensitivity 812
G. Comparative Studies of Steroid Receptors in the Song System 815
IV. Evolution of the Song System 816
V. Supply of Active Steroids to Steroid-Sensitive Neural Structures 819
A. Steroid Synthesis by the Gonads 819
B. Alternate Sites of Sex Steroid Synthesis 821
C. Adrenals 822
D. Brain 823
E. Steroid Metabolism in Brain: Evidence for a Role in Song-System Development, Song Learning, and Song Expression 823
F. Aromatase 824
G. 5α-Reductase 826
H. 5β-Reductase 827

VI. Conclusion and Directions for Future Research 827
References 829

B. INVERTEBRATES

CHAPTER 34

Insect Developmental Hormones and Their Mechanism of Action 841
James W. Truman and Lynn M. Riddiford

I. Introduction 841
II. Chemistry and Secretion of Insect Developmental Hormones 841
A. Ecdysteroids—Synthesis and Metabolism 841
B. Juvenile Hormone—Synthesis and Metabolism 843
III. Hormone Titers 844
IV. Hormone Receptors 846
A. Ecdysone Receptor Complex 846
B. JH Receptor 847
V. Molecular Mode of Action of the Hormones 848
A. Mode of Action of the Ecdysones 848
B. Mode of Action of JH 850
VI. Cellular Actions of Hormones on the Nervous System: *Drosophila* and *Manduca* Models 852
A. Overview of Nervous System Changes during Metamorphosis 852
B. Patterns of Steroid Receptor Expression in the Nervous System 854
C. Hormonal Regulation of the Development of Imaginal Neurons 855
D. Remodeling of Larval Neurons 859
E. Steroids and Programmed Cell Death 862
VII. Conclusion and Speculations 862
References 863

16

Molecular Recognition and Intracellular Transduction Mechanisms in Olfactory and Vomeronasal Systems

Makoto Kashiwayanagi
Graduate School of Pharmaceutical Sciences
Hokkaido University
Sapporo 060-0812, Japan

*P*heromones affect gonadal functions and sexual behaviors. They are received by the vomeronasal organ as well as by the main olfactory organ. Binding of chemical stimuli to olfactory G-protein-coupled receptors (GPCRs) has generally been considered to lead to the accumulation of cyclic adenosine monophosphate (cAMP) in olfactory neurons and to the activation of cAMP-gated channels, causing cell depolarization and olfactory nerve responses. This scheme is, however, not fully consistent with experimental data from various olfactory sensory neurons. The results obtained by *in situ* hybridization showing that single neurons have only one type of olfactory GPCR cannot simply explain the observation that single olfactory neurons respond to various species of odorants. I discuss here various pathways in olfactory transduction. In contrast, the mechanism of discrimination and transduction in pheromone reception is simple. Most vomeronasal sensory neurons receive only one kind of pheromone. Pheromonal reception is mediated via the inositol-1,4,5-trisphosphate (IP$_3$)-dependent pathway. In this chapter I describe the mechanisms of pheromonal reception in vomeronasal sensory neurons.

I. INTRODUCTION

Pheromonal signals provide specific information concerning the identity, gender, endocrine, and social status of different members of the population in a variety of mammals (Powers and Winans, 1975; Halpern, 1987; Wysocki and Meredith, 1987). Pheromones have been found in saliva, skin gland secretions, and urine. For example, pheromones in urine excreted from male and female rats induce various changes in gonadal functions such as reflex ovulation in the absence of coitus and mounting (Johns *et al.*, 1978), a reduction in the estrous cycle of female rats from five to four days (Chateau *et al.*, 1976), and estrous synchrony among female rats living together (McClintock, 1978).

Urinary compounds of low volatility stimulate the guinea pig vomeronasal system and provide information that is normally not provided by gustation or olfaction (Wysocki *et al.*, 1980). The vomeronasal system is a chemosensory system organized in parallel with the main olfactory system in most terrestrial vertebrates. The vomeronasal organ, which is the peripheral chemoreceptor organ of the vomeronasal system, forms a tubular structure lying bilaterally in the ventral part of the nasal cavity. Vomeronasal sensory neurons project information to the accessory olfactory bulb located on the dorso-caudal surface of the main olfactory bulb (Barber and Raisman, 1974). Regulation of gonadal functions by urinary pheromones has been well established in the rodent vomeronasal organ. In rodents, removal of the vomeronasal organ attenuates the stimulatory effects of conspecific males on the release of luteinizing hormone (Beltramino and Taleisnik, 1983; Rajendren et al., 1990). The urinary pheromone-induced increase in c-fos messenger RNA (mRNA) levels and Fos-immunoreactivities, an index of neural activity, were eliminated by the removal of the vomeronasal organ in the accessory olfactory bulb of rodents (Guo et al., 1997; Inamura et al., 1999a).

The interaction of a pheromone with the receptive membrane of vomeronasal sensory neurons initiates a sequential molecular event leading to action potential initiation, which transmits pheromonal information to the accessory olfactory bulb. After Luo et al. (1994) showed that a chemical signal excreted from its prey induced inositol-1,4,5-trisphosphate (IP_3) accumulation in the snake vomeronasal organ, the cellular mechanisms of pheromonal reception in reptiles as well as mammalians have become clear. I describe here the mechanism of pheromone reception by the vomeronasal organ in reptiles and mammalians.

Pheromones may stimulate the main olfactory organ as well as the vomeronasal organ. Removal of the vomeronasal organ of mice produces deficits in the patterns of ultrasonic vocalizations elicited by conspecifics or their odors, whereas stimulation of other sensory systems can, to some extent, maintain the male's tendency to vocalize more to females or their odors than to males or their odors in the absence of the vomeronasal organ in heterosexual experienced males (Wysocki et al., 1982). The ability to make gender discrimination by nonvomeronasal chemoreception is contingent upon previous heterosexual experience with the chemical cues of a female in the presence of a functional vomeronasal organ (Wysocki et al., 1982). The main olfactory system is involved in the luteinizing hormone response to chemical stimulation in sexually experienced ewes (Cohen-Tannoudji et al., 1989). Sensitivity and behavior responses of the sow to the boar pheromone (Dorries et al., 1997) and maternal recognition of the newborn lamb by the ewe (Lévy et al., 1995) are mediated by the olfactory organ. There is a sex difference in the role of the vomeronasal organ in the discrimination of individual odors of golden hamsters (Johnston and Peng, 2000). The vomeronasal organ is involved in the discrimination of individual odors by males but not by females (Johnston and Peng, 2000).

The mechanisms of the generation of odor responses and the discrimination of odorants in the main olfactory system have been well explored in the past two decades. It is widely considered that olfactory G-protein-coupled receptors (GPCRs) are receptors for odorants. Binding of an odorant to olfactory GPCRs is considered to stimulate the cyclic adenosine monophosphate (cAMP)-mediated cascade via an olfactory-specific G-protein (G_{olf}), G_s type of GTP-binding proteins (G-proteins), or the IP_3-mediated cascade (Buck and Axel, 1991; Pace et al., 1985; Huque and Bruch, 1986). An increase of intraciliary cAMP and IP_3 level activates cAMP- and IP_3-gated cation channels, respectively (Nakamura and Gold, 1987; Restrepo et al., 1990), causing cell depolarization and triggering the discharge of action potentials. The details of these pathways have been described in many previous reviews (Shepherd, 1994; Ache, 1994; Breer et al., 1994; Ressler et al., 1994b; Ache and Zhainazarov, 1995; Buck, 1996); however, the generation of odor responses by these mechanisms is not completely understood. Here, I will discuss the molecular recognition and multiple transduction pathways in olfactory sensory neurons.

II. MAIN OLFACTORY ORGAN

A. Olfactory G-Protein-Coupled Receptors

Olfactory G-protein-coupled receptors (GPCRs) were initially cloned from the rat olfactory epithelium by Buck and Axel (1991). The function of olfactory GPCR has been investigated mainly by measuring the changes in cytosolic Ca^{2+} concentrations, $[Ca^{2+}]_i$. Nonolfactory cells and olfactory sensory neurons expressing olfactory GPCRs of zebrafish (Wellerdieck et al., 1997), humans (Wetzel et al., 1999), rats (Zhao et al., 1998), and mice (Touhara et al., 1999) showed increases in $[Ca^{2+}]_i$ in response to odorants. To date, however, no convincing evidence that olfactory GPCR couples with G_{olf} and then induces formation of second messengers such as cAMP has been reported. Only one study demonstrated that the application of various odorants to Sf9 cells, which express a member of the olfactory GPCR family (OR5), increased intracellular IP_3 concentration (Raming et al., 1993). Although many odorants induce cAMP accumulation in the olfactory neurons, there has been no report indicating that odorants induce cAMP accumulation via olfactory GPCRs.

The GPCR family is assumed to comprise several hundred molecules. *In situ* hybridization experiments to identify olfactory GPCRs in the rat, mouse, and catfish suggest that a single olfactory GPCR is expressed in only 0.1–2% of olfactory neurons and that each olfactory neuron may have only one type of olfactory GPCR (Ngai et al., 1993; Ressler et al., 1993, 1994a; Kishimoto et al., 1994). The two-step, single-cell reverse transcriptase polymerase chain reaction (RT-PCR) procedure confirms this hypothesis (Malnic et al., 1999).

B. Responses of Single Olfactory Receptor Neurons to Multiple Odorants

Electrophysiological recording of odor responses from single olfactory neurons has shown that single olfactory neurons respond to multiple odorants with quite diverse odor qualities and molecular structures (Mathews, 1972; Gesteland et al., 1982; Sicard and Holley, 1984; Ivanova and Caprio, 1993; Kashiwayanagi and Kurihara, 1994; Kashiwayanagi et al., 1996b). For example, a large portion of bullfrog single olfactory neurons (64% in whole-cell recording and 79% in ciliary recording) responded to many odorants with quite diverse molecular structures (Kashiwayanagi et al., 1996b). A single odorant elicited a response in many bullfrog olfactory cells; e.g., hedione and citralva elicited responses in 100% and 92% of total neurons examined, respectively. The observation that single olfactory neurons respond to multiple odorants may be explained by the broad odor specificity of GPCRs, while olfactory GPCRs have high selectivity to odorants (Zhao et al., 1998; Touhara et al., 1999; Hatt et al., 1999). Individual olfactory neurons may be highly specific for a small number of odorants at concentrations near threshold detection levels, and relatively high concentrations of odorants may induce nonspecific responses. However, the degree of odor discrimination has been shown to be independent of odorant concentration (Duchamp-Viret et al., 1990; Kashiwayanagi et al., 1997), and the degree of cross-adaptation between odorants at high concentrations was similar to that at low concentrations in the turtle olfactory system (Kashiwayanagi et al., 1997).

Cross-adaptation experiments under whole-cell voltage clamp conditions using single bullfrog and turtle olfactory neurons indicated that each neuron has multiple receptors for odorants (Kashiwayanagi and Kurihara, 1994; Kashiwayanagi et al., 1996b). The application of hedione to single bullfrog neurons after the desensitization of an inward current induced by lilial induced a large inward current and vice versa, indicating that pre-application of lilial or hedione did not significantly inhibit the generation of responses to hedione or lilial, respectively (Kashiwayanagi et al., 1996b). The presence of multiple receptors for odorants in single olfactory neurons was also suggested in the catfish (Ivanova and Caprio, 1993). Most single catfish olfactory neurons showed excitatory and suppressive responses to different amino acids (Kang and Caprio, 1995a). These results clearly show that single olfactory neurons have multiple receptors.

C. Odor Responses and Olfactory GPCRs during Development

The responses to various odorants were recorded from the rat olfactory epithelium starting at embryonic day 14 to 16 (Gesteland et al., 1982). The odor selectivity was lower in early immature olfactory neurons than that in mature neurons; each immature olfactory neuron responded to nearly all the odorants applied. These results suggested that the neurons might initially have receptors with broad specificity that are subsequently replaced by specific receptors, or that immature neurons could have a large variety of specific receptors, some of which are lost on maturation (Gesteland et al., 1982). However, olfactory GPCRs that appeared transiently in immature olfactory neurons have not been found. The following results obtained by *in situ* hybridization and quantitative polymerase chain reaction (PCR) were inconsistent with an increase in odor selectivity during development. Strotmann et al. (1995) explored the onset and time course of GPCR expression during the prenatal development of rats by *in situ* hybridization. Olfactory GPCRs (OR5, OR14, OR37, and OR124) were expressed in the early phase of development (embryonic day 14), but the percentage of cells expressing GPCRs was much lower than the percentage in adult olfactory neurons; OR37 and OR14 were expressed in 0.02% and 0.10% of embryonic olfactory neurons and in 0.40% and 0.37% of adult olfactory neurons, respectively (Strotmann et al., 1994). Relative levels of expression of olfactory GPCRs during rat development determined by quantitative PCR showed that olfactory GPCRs were not expressed in early-phase olfactory neurons, and the onset of expression of mRNA for olfactory GPCRs occurred at embryonic day 19 (Margalit and Lancet, 1993). Thus, changes in odor responses in rat olfactory neurons during development are independent of expression of olfactory GPCRs. Margalit and Lancet (1993) suggested that the early odor responses may be generated by nonreceptor protein-mediated mechanisms.

D. Odor Responses Independent of Olfactory GPCR in Adult

Olfactory GPCR-independent odor responses have also been recorded from adult olfactory organs. In *Xenopus laevis,* the olfactory organ is compartmentalized into two independent subregions, the medial diverticulum and the lateral diverticulum. Anatomical observation has indicated that the olfactory sensory epithelium in the medial diverticulum comes into contact with air, while the epithelium in the lateral diverticulum is in contact with water (Altner, 1962). The latter, therefore, is called the water nose. *Xenopus laevis* possesses a gene repertoire encoding two distinct classes of olfactory GPCRs; one class is related to the olfactory GPCRs of fish, and the other is related to the olfactory GPCRs of mammals (Freitag et al., 1995). An *in situ* hybridization study of the fish-like olfactory GPCRs resulted in labeling of the sensory epithelium in the lateral diverticulum, whereas the medial diverticulum was devoid of any hybridization signals. All the probes representing mammalian-like receptor signals yielded results only in the medial diverticulum. On the assumption that these are odor receptors, the results suggest that olfactory neurons in the medial diverticulum are expected to respond to volatile odorants and neurons in the lateral diverticulum should respond to water-soluble odorants (e.g., amino acids). Volatile odorants and amino acids induce inward current responses in the olfactory neurons in the medial and lateral diverticulum of the *Xenopus laevis,* respectively (Lischka and Schild, 1993; Schild and Lischka, 1994; Iida and Kashiwayanagi, 1999a), supporting this idea. Many olfactory neurons in the lateral diverticulum, however, respond not only to amino acids but also to volatile odorants. The sensitivity of the neurons to volatile odorants is similar to that of the olfactory neurons of salamanders (Firestein and Werblin, 1989). It is likely that volatile odorants induce responses in the lateral diverticulum olfactory neurons in an olfactory GPCR-independent manner.

Not only the olfactory system but also various non-olfactory systems respond to odorants. For example, various odorants induced responses in neurons such as the turtle trigeminal nerve (Tucker, 1963), snail neurons (Arvanitaki et al., 1967), and neuroblastoma cells (Kashiwayanagi and Kurihara, 1984). Odorants also induced responses in gustatory cells of the fly (Dethier, 1972), the bullfrog (Kashiwagura et al., 1977), and the rat (Lundy and Contreras, 1993). These systems have the ability to discriminate odor qualities (Kashiwagura et al., 1977; Kashiwayanagi et al., 1994b). Analysis by multidimensional scaling of the results obtained from cross-adaptation experiments on bullfrog gustatory responses to odorants suggested that the ability of the frog gustatory system to discriminate odorants is closely related to that in the human olfactory system (Kashiwayanagi et al., 1994b).

Naim *et al.* (1994) demonstrated that hydrophobic bitter and sweet compounds directly activate GTP-binding proteins in the absence of GPCRs. This mechanism may be applicable to the olfactory system, since volatile odorants are generally hydrophobic. In fact, odorants increased the cAMP concentration in non-olfactory cells such as renal epithelial cells (Friedlander et al., 1987) and melanophores (Lerner et al., 1988).

E. Does the Specific Projection of Olfactory Receptor Neurons to Mitral Cells Integrate Odor Information?

In the mouse, the first olfactory GPCR-positive cells appeared to originate from the central nervous system, suggesting that this receptor serves a functional role in the elaboration of specific pathways between the olfactory bulb and olfactory epithelium during development (Nef et al., 1992). Ressler et al. (1994a) showed that olfactory GPCR probes hybridized in situ to a small subset of olfactory bulb glomeruli, suggesting a highly organized synaptic formation of olfactory neurons expressing the same olfactory GPCR with the mitral cells in the olfactory bulb. In genetically altered strains of mice in which an olfactory GPCR gene P2 is translated along with tau-lac-Z, neurons expressing the P2 receptor projected information to only two glomeruli in the mouse olfactory bulb (Mombaerts et al., 1996). In the rabbit, mitral cells responded to odorants with related molecular structures, suggesting the importance of conformational parameters of odorants (Imamura et al., 1992; Katoh et al., 1993). However, mitral cells of the turtle, monkey, rabbit, frog, and catfish responded to various odorants with diverse molecular structures and odor qualities, which suggests that the specificity of mitral cells to odorants is not remarkably higher than that of olfactory neurons (Mathews, 1972; Tanabe et al., 1975; Kang and Caprio, 1995a). In the catfish, the percentages of the total number of olfactory bulb neurons that responded with excitation and suppression, respectively, to methionine, arginine, and glutamic acid were greater than the percentages of olfactory neurons responding to the same stimuli (Kang and Caprio, 1995a,b). Mouse olfactory sensory neurons labeled in retrograde from a glomeruli in the dorso-lateral region of the olfactory bulb responded to odorants with widely different structures (Bozza and Kauer, 1998). Thus, information regarding odor quality is not clearly integrated in mitral cells.

F. cAMP-Dependent Transduction Pathway

In 1972, Kurihara and Koyama found high adenylyl cyclase activities in the bovine olfactory epithelium. Later, it was shown that various odorants (cAMP-increasing odorants) induced cAMP accumulation in the presence of GTP in olfactory neurons of the frog, bullfrog, rat, sheep, and turtle (Pace et al., 1985; Sklar et al., 1986; Boekhoff et al., 1990; Fabbri et al., 1995; Okamoto et al., 1996). Increases in cAMP concentration activated cyclic nucleotide-gated channels in frog, bullfrog, salamander, newt, and turtle olfactory neurons (Nakamura and Gold, 1987; Suzuki, 1989; Zufall et al., 1991; Kurahashi, 1990; Kashiwayanagi et al., 1994a). Disruption of a cAMP-gated channel (Brunet et al., 1996), G_{olf} (Belluscio et al., 1998) or adenylyl cyclase III gene (Wong et al., 2000) leads to anosmia in transgenic mice. These results suggest that odor responses are generated via cAMP-dependent pathways in the mouse.

G. Significance of the cAMP-Independent Transduction Pathway

In olfactory neurons, cAMP-mediated responses induced by dialysis of cAMP from patch pipettes were desensitized even during the continuous application of cAMP (Suzuki, 1989; Kurahashi, 1990; Kashiwayanagi et al., 1994a; Kashiwayanagi and Kurihara, 1995). After the high concentration of cAMP caused the turtle olfactory receptor neurons to be desensitized, the membrane-permeable cAMP analogue cpt-cAMP did not induce any response in the neurons, thus indicating complete desensitization of the cAMP-dependent pathway (Kashiwayanagi and Kurihara, 1995). However, various odorants induced large odor responses (Kashiwayanagi et al., 1994a; Kashiwayanagi and Kurihara, 1995).

The cAMP-independent odor responses have also been recorded from in vivo systems. The turtle bulbar response to forskolin reached a saturation level around 10 μM. After desensitization of the response to 50 μM forskolin, 11 species of odorants were applied to the olfactory epithelium. The magnitudes of responses to the odorants following forskolin response desensitization were 45–80% of those of the control responses. Thus, cAMP-independent pathways greatly contribute to the in vivo turtle olfactory transduction; at least 45% of the response to all odorants examined, including "cAMP-increasing odorants," was by cAMP-independent components in the turtle.

The cAMP-independent pathway was also examined in rat fetal olfactory cells. Relative levels of expression during rat development determined for olfactory-specific genes by quantitative PCR indicated that the onset of expression for the olfactory cyclic nucleotide-gated channels was at embryonic day 19 (E19) (Margalit and Lancet, 1993), although odor responses were recorded from rat olfactory neurons starting at embryonic days E14–E16 (Gesteland et al., 1982). These results suggested that the odor responses were not elicited via cAMP-gated channels during the early stages of development.

H. cAMP-Independent Aquatic Odor Reception in Vertebrates

Although catfish olfactory sensory neurons possess G-protein-linked adenylyl cyclase (Bruch and Teeter, 1990), rapid kinetic measurements of second messenger formation demonstrated that even a highly concentrated mixture of odorant amino acids did not elicit a change in the cAMP level in the olfactory cilia of the catfish (Restrepo et al., 1993a). Dialysis of a high concentration of cAMP into olfactory sensory neurons of the *Xenopus* water nose did not induce any response (Iida and Kashiwayanagi, 1999b), whereas amino acids induced excitatory responses in these neurons (Iida and Kashiwayanagi, 1999a). These results indicate that amino acids induce olfactory responses via the cAMP-independent pathway.

I. IP_3-Dependent Transduction Pathway

Not all odorants activated adenylyl cyclase in the bullfrog, rat, sheep, and turtle olfactory neurons (Sklar et al., 1986; Breer and Boekhoff, 1991; Fabbri et al., 1995; Okamoto et al., 1996); some ("IP_3-increasing odorants") of these odorants increased IP_3 concentrations in rat and sheep olfactory cilia preparations (Breer and Boekhoff, 1991; Fabbri et al., 1995). Although several investigators have failed to record responses to IP_3 (Firestein et al., 1991; Lowe and Gold, 1993; Nakamura et al., 1994), IP_3 receptors and IP_3-gated ion channels were found in cilia and soma of catfish, rat, cattle, lobster, bullfrog, frog, and turtle olfactory sensory neurons (Kalinoski et al., 1992; Restrepo et al., 1990, 1992; Kahn et al., 1992; Fadool and Ache, 1992; Suzuki, 1992; Kashiwayanagi, 1996; Kashiwayanagi et al., 2000), thereby suggesting that IP_3-dependent pathways may also play roles in the generation of odor responses.

J. Colocalization of cAMP- and IP_3-Dependent Pathways in Single Olfactory Neurons

As shown above, multiple transduction pathways are involved in the generation of odor responses. These transduction pathways are colocalized in single olfactory neurons. In the turtle olfactory neurons, cAMP-dependent and independent pathways are colocalized in single olfactory neurons (Kashiwayanagi et al., 1994a; Kashiwayanagi and Kurihara, 1995). Single olfactory sensory neurons of the turtle, bullfrog, and mouse responded to cAMP-increasing and IP_3-increasing (cAMP-independent) odorants (Kashiwayanagi et al., 1994a; Kashiwayanagi and Kurihara, 1995; Bozza and Kauer, 1998). Colocalization of cAMP- and IP_3-dependent conductances in single olfactory neurons was shown directly in the lobster by measuring single-channel activity of the membrane patches to cAMP and IP_3 (Hatt and Ache, 1994). Single-cell RT-PCR analysis of rat olfactory sensory neurons demonstrated that at least a subpopulation of sensory neurons is equipped with the elements for both active cAMP- and IP_3-dependent pathways (Noé and Breer, 1998).

K. cAMP- and IP_3-Independent Transduction Pathways

Although the odor quality is not dependent on the difference in second messengers (Breer and Boekhoff, 1991; Kashiwayanagi et al., 1996a), cAMP-increasing odorants increase cAMP concentration but have no effect on IP_3 concentration, and IP_3-increasing odorants do not change cAMP concentration in rat olfactory cilia preparations (Breer and Boekhoff, 1991). A similar selectivity to second messengers was observed in sheep and turtle olfactory epithelium preparations (Fabbri et al., 1995; Okamoto et al., 1996), suggesting that there are common transduction mechanisms in vertebrate olfactory reception. Odorants, including cAMP-increasing and IP_3-increasing odorants, induced large odor responses after complete inhibition of the cAMP-dependent pathway (Kashiwayanagi et al., 1994a; Kashiwayanagi and Kurihara, 1995). These results suggest that the cAMP-independent responses to cAMP-increasing odorants are IP_3-independent.

L. cGMP/NO-Mediated Pathway

In general, the sensitivity of cyclic nucleotide-gated channels to cyclic guanosine monophosphate (cGMP) in olfactory neurons is higher than that to cAMP. Strong odor stimulation induced cGMP accumulation in the rat and catfish (Breer *et al.*, 1992; Restrepo *et al.*, 1993a). In rat olfactory cilia preparations, odor-induced cGMP accumulation was inhibited by nitric oxide (NO)-synthetase inhibitors. Although immunoreactivity with neuronal NO synthetase antibody was not found in mature rat olfactory neurons (Roskams *et al.*, 1994), specific staining for nicotinamide adenine dinucleotide phosphate diaphorase was observed in mature olfactory neurons in rat and catfish olfactory epithelia, suggesting the presence of NO synthetase in these cells (Dellacorte *et al.*, 1995). NO activated not only soluble guanylyl cyclase but also cyclic nucleotide-gated channels directly in the olfactory neurons (Broillet and Fierstein, 1996). Therefore, it is possible that cGMP/NO production is involved in the generation of odor responses. However, after complete desensitization of the cyclic nucleotide-dependent pathway, the NO donor sodium nitroprusside did not induce any inward currents in the turtle olfactory neurons, while odorants induced large currents (Inamura *et al.*, 1998), which suggested that cAMP-independent odor responses were not generated via the NO/cGMP pathway.

M. Possible Role of cADP-Ribose in Odor Reception

In many cases, odorant-induced responses are accompanied by increases in $[Ca^{2+}]_i$ (Restrepo *et al.*, 1993b; Sato *et al.*, 1991). Cyclic adenosine diphosphate-ribose (cADP-ribose), which is converted from nicotinamide adenine dinucleotide (NAD^+) by ADP-ribosyl cyclase, has been shown to mobilize Ca^{2+} in various cells, including central and peripheral neurons (Galione *et al.*, 1991; Berridge, 1993; Guse, 1999). It is possible that cADP-ribose responds to odorants by contributing to $[Ca^{2+}]_i$ increases in olfactory cells. In fact, olfactory cells responded to dialysis with cADP-ribose from a pipette with an inward current, an increase in membrane conductance, and an increase in $[Ca^{2+}]_i$ (Sekimoto and Kashiwayanagi, submitted for publication). The magnitudes of the inward current responses to cAMP-increasing odorants were greatly reduced by previous dialyses of a high concentration of cADP-ribose or 8-Br-cADP-ribose, an antagonist, suggesting that the cADP-ribose-dependent pathway greatly contributes to the generation of olfactory responses.

III. VOMERONASAL ORGAN

A. Transduction Pathways in the Reptilian Vomeronasal System

Transduction elements in the reptile sensory neurons of vomeronasal organs are similar to those in olfactory sensory neurons. Functional adenylyl cyclase has been shown biochemically in reptile vomeronasal sensory epithelia; the application of forskolin, GTP, and GTPγS to membrane preparations of snake and the turtle vomeronasal epithelia induced cAMP accumulation (Luo *et al.*, 1994; Okamoto *et al.*, 1996). In the turtle vomeronasal sensory neuron (Taniguchi *et al.*, 1996b), cAMP dialyzed from a patch pipette induced an inward current in a similar dose-dependent manner to that in the turtle olfactory neuron (Kashiwayanagi and Kurihara, 1995), suggesting that the vomeronasal sensory neuron and the olfactory sensory neuron possess similar cyclic nucleotide-mediated transduction pathways in the turtle. Application of forskolin to the turtle vomeronasal sensory epithelium induced an increase in impulse frequency in the vomeronasal sensory neurons and increased brain wave activity at the turtle accessory olfactory bulb (Taniguchi *et al.*, 1996a,b). These results suggest that depolarization mediated via cyclic nucleotide-gated ion channels generates action potentials in the turtle vomeronasal sensory neuron.

G-proteins (G_s, G_i, and G_o) were tentatively identified in the vomeronasal tissue membrane preparations of garter snakes using immunoreactivity and ADP-ribosylation techniques (Luo *et al.*, 1994). Receptors for ES20, a chemoattractant extracted from its prey, coupled with G-proteins in the garter snake (Luo *et al.*, 1994). The binding of ES20 to its receptors resulted in an increase in the basal level of IP_3 (Luo *et al.*, 1994). Dialysis of IP_3 into the turtle and snake vomeronasal receptor neurons induced inward currents (Taniguchi *et al.*, 1995, 2000). These results support the idea that the IP_3-dependent pathway is involved in transduction in reptile vomeronasal sensory neurons.

B. Minor Role of cAMP in Mammalian Pheromone Reception

Application of forskolin, GTP, and GTPγS induced cAMP accumulation in the rat vomeronasal epithelium, and the dose-response relationships of cAMP accumulation induced by forskolin were similar to those in the rat olfactory epithelium (Sasaki et al., 1999). These results suggest that there is a functional cAMP-synthetic pathway in the rat vomeronasal epithelium.

However, none of the three urine preparations containing pheromones, which increased impulse frequency in rat vomeronasal sensory neurons (Inamura et al., 1999a), changed the cAMP levels in the rat vomeronasal epithelium (Sasaki et al., 1999). Exposure to volatile constituents of male mouse urine, 2-(sec-butyl)4,5-dihydrothiazole (SBT) and dehydro-exo-brevicomin (DHB), decreased cAMP levels in mouse vomeronasal tissue preparations (Zhou and Moss, 1997). Application of DHB induced outward currents (inhibitory responses) but not inward currents (excitatory responses) in mouse vomeronasal sensory neurons (Moss et al., 1997). Exposure to DHB and SBT did not induce an increase in the c-fos mRNA level, an index of neuronal excitation, in the mouse accessory olfactory bulb (Guo et al., 1997). Dialysis of concentrations of cAMP as high as 0.5 mM or 1 mM did not induce any response in mouse or rat vomeronasal sensory neurons (Liman and Corey, 1996; Sasaki et al., 1999). These results suggest that cAMP is not a primary second messenger in the excitatory pheromonal responses of rodent vomeronasal sensory neurons.

C. Pheromonal Transduction Mediated via IP$_3$ in the Mammalian Vomeronasal System

Dialysis of IP$_3$ into rat vomeronasal sensory neurons induced inward currents (Inamura et al., 1997a). Increases in the impulse frequency of sensory neurons in response to urine were blocked by ruthenium red, an IP$_3$-dependent channel inhibitor, and U-73122 or neomycin, phospholipase C inhibitors (Inamura et al., 1997b; Holy et al., 2000). Male Wistar urine as well as female Wistar urine and male Donryu urine induced IP$_3$ accumulation in the female Wistar rat (Sasaki et al., 1999). IP$_3$ accumulation in response to pheromones in mammals has also been observed in the hamster and the pig. That is, aphrodisin, a pheromone excreted from the female hamster, and semen fluid from the pig induce IP$_3$ accumulation in preparations of male hamster vomeronasal sensory epithelium (Kroner et al., 1996) and porcine vomeronasal epithelium (Wekesa and Anholt, 1997), respectively. The average reversal potential of urine-induced current was similar to that of the IP$_3$-induced current in rat vomeronasal sensory neurons (Inamura et al., 1997a; Inamura and Kashiwayanagi, 2000). These results indicate that the response of rat vomeronasal sensory neurons to urinary pheromones is generated via the IP$_3$-dependent pathway.

D. Selective Pheromone Reception in Vomeronasal Sensory Neurons

Single vomeronasal sensory neurons of female Wistar rats responded selectively to urine from male and female Wistar rats (Inamura et al., 1999a). Each sensory neuron responded to only one class of urine. The neurons also responded selectively to urine from male Donryu and Sprague-Dawley rats. Thus, vomeronasal sensory neurons discriminate differences in sex and strains in urinary pheromones. High selectivity of vomeronasal sensory neurons to pheromones was also confirmed in mice (Leinders-Zufall et al., 2000). This is in contrast to olfactory neurons, which respond to many odorants with quite diverse molecular structures and odor qualities (Sicard and Holley, 1984; Kang and Caprio, 1995a; Kashiwayanagi et al., 1996b).

The accumulation of IP$_3$ induced by ES20 in the garter snake was enhanced by GTPγS (Luo et al., 1994), while the accumulation of IP$_3$ induced by seminal fluid in the pig was reduced by GDPβS (Wekesa and Anholt, 1997). These results provided evidence that IP$_3$ was generated via the G-protein-linked pathway in the vomeronasal sensory epithelium. In the garter snake, ADP-ribosylation products resulting from pertussis toxin (PTX) was reduced by the binding of ES20 to its receptors (Luo et al., 1994). In the vomeronasal epithelium of female Wistar rats, the accumulation of IP$_3$ induced by the male Wistar urine was enhanced by GTPγS and inhibited by PTX (Sasaki et al., 1999). Immunohistochemical studies have shown the presence of G_i and G_o in opossum, mouse, and rat vomeronasal sensory neurons (Halpern et al., 1995; Jia and Halpern, 1996). These results suggest that receptors to a chemoattractant and those to urinary pheromone(s) in the vomeronasal epithelia are coupled with PTX-sensitive G-proteins such as G_i and G_o. The male Wistar urine and male Donryu urine preferentially decreased ADP-ribosylation of G_i and G_o with PTX in the vomeronasal sensory epithelium of female Wistar rats, respectively, suggesting that pheromones in the male Wistar urine and in the male Donryu urine are received via G_i and G_o, respectively (Sasaki et al., 1999).

Cell bodies of vomeronasal sensory neurons are located at various depths in the cellular layer of sensory epithelium. The sensory neurons at the apical and basal layers of the sensory epithelium of marsupial and rodents are immunoreactive to anti-$G_{i2\alpha}$ and anti-$G_{o\alpha}$ proteins, respectively (Halpern et al., 1995; Jia and Halpern, 1996). Localization of the cell bodies of sensory neurons, which responded to male Wistar and male Donryu urine, was examined using female Wistar rats (Inamura et al., 1999a). The preponderance of neurons responding to conspecific male urine from rats of the same species were found in the $G_{i\alpha}$-positive laminae of the vomeronasal sensory epithelium, and the preponderance of neurons responding to conspecific female rat urine and male urine from a different strain (Donryu or Sprague-Dawley) were found in the G_o-positive laminae of the vomeronasal sensory epithelium. Therefore, it is likely that responses of sensory neurons in the apical portion of the female rat vomeronasal epithelium to the male Wistar urine were mediated via G_i, while responses of neurons in the basal portion to the male Donryu urine were mediated via G_o.

E. Putative Receptor for Pheromones

Two families of vomeronasal GPCRs unrelated to olfactory GPCRs were cloned from the rat and mouse vomeronasal epithelium (Dulac and Axel, 1995; Matsunami and Buck, 1997; Ryba and Tirindelli, 1997; Herrada and Dulac, 1997). The human genome contains a vomeronasal GPCR gene (Rodriguez et al., 2000). Each family comprises about 100 species of vomeronasal GPCR. In situ hybridization studies suggested that a single sensory neuron expressed one type of vomeronasal GPCR. One family consists of the sensory neurons expressing $G_{i2\alpha}$ in the upper layer of the epithelium (Dulac and Axel, 1995), and another family consists of the neurons expressing $G_{o\alpha}$ (Matsunami and Buck, 1997; Ryba and Tirindelli, 1997; Herrada and Dulac, 1997). It is possible that responses to the male Wistar urine are induced via the former type of vomeronasal GPCR, and those to the female Wistar urine and the male Donryu urine are induced via the latter type of vomeronasal GPCR.

F. Projection of Pheromonal Information to the Accessory Olfactory Bulb

Two populations of sensory neurons in the vomeronasal organ project information to different regions of the glomerular layer of the accessory olfactory bulb (Halpern et al., 1995; Jia and Halpern, 1996). The rostral region of the accessory olfactory bulb is innervated by a population of $G_{i2\alpha}$-expressing vomeronasal sensory neurons whose cell bodies are located in the apical layer of the vomeronasal sensory epithelium. The caudal region of the accessory olfactory bulb glomerular layer is innervated by $G_{o\alpha}$-expressing vomeronasal sensory neurons whose cell bodies are located in the basal layer of the vomeronasal sensory epithelium. The two regions of the accessory olfactory bulb have a clear and sharp boundary midway along the rostro-caudal axis of the accessory olfactory bulb that divides the nerve and glomerular layers of the accessory olfactory bulb into rostral and caudal halves. Real-time optical imaging has shown that electrical stimulation of the rostral vomeronasal nerve layer produces neural activity only within the rostral region of the external plexiform layer, and electrical stimulation of the caudal vomeronasal nerve layer produces responses only within the caudal region (Sugai et al., 1997). These observations suggest that there is no anatomical connection between the rostral and caudal regions and that the accessory olfactory bulb is segregated into at least two subdivisions.

These subregions receive different pheromonal information from vomeronasal sensory neurons (Brennan et al., 1999; Inamura et al., 1999b; Matsuoka et al., 1999). As described above, the sensory neurons that respond to the male Wistar urine are localized in the apical layer of the sensory epithelium, where $G_{i2\alpha}$ is selectively expressed (Inamura et al., 1999a). Exposure of the vomeronasal organ of female Wistar rat to male Wistar urine induced the appearance of many more Fos-ir cells in the rostral portion of the accessory olfactory bulb than in the caudal portion (Inamura et al., 1999b). These results suggest that the response to pheromones in the male Wistar rat urine is selectively transmitted to the rostral part of the accessory olfactory bulb of female Wistar rats. It is likely that information from different pheromones is transmitted to the higher brain through the different regions of the accessory olfactory bulb.

G. Memory Storage in the Accessory Olfactory Bulb

Sexually experienced Long-Evans male rats prefer estrous to diestrous urine odor, and diestrous urine odor to distilled water odor (Pfaff and Pfaffmann, 1969; Lydell and Doty, 1972). Sexually inexperienced males do not exhibit these preferences, indicating that there may exist a temporally discrete information source for sexually experienced male rats that may accurately indicate a given female's state of sexual receptivity. Information regarding the females' endocrine state is transmitted to males by means of urinary pheromones. The expression of Fos-ir cells in the accessory olfactory bulb of sexually experienced male rats was compared with that from sexually inexperienced male rats following exposure to oestrous urine (Sakamoto et al., submitted for publication). In the localized region (lateral and rostral regions) of the periglomerular cell layer, many more Fos-ir cells were expressed in the sexually experienced rats than in the inexperienced rats, which suggests that sexual experience promotes the formation of a memory of a pheromone found in estrous urine at the periglomerular cell layer of the accessory olfactory bulb.

H. Chemical Characterization of Pheromones

Pheromones have been found to be proteins and low molecular weight molecules (Brownlee et al., 1969; Melrose et al., 1971; Goodwin et al., 1979; Novotny et al., 1985; Singer et al., 1991, 1997; Mucignat-Caretta et al., 1995). At present, pheromones that induce behavioral and endocrinological changes in rats have not been identified. The activity of the component in male urine to induce expression of Fos-immunoreactivity in the caudal region of the accessory olfactory bulb of female rats was abolished by papain treatment, while that in the rostral region was not (Tsujikawa and Kashiwayanagi, 1999). The pronase treatment of male urine abolished the expression of immunoreactivity in the rostral region as well as in the caudal region, suggesting that at least two urinary peptides (papain-sensitive and -insensitive ones) with the ability to stimulate the vomeronasal organ of female rats are contained in male Wistar rat urine. Exposure of the female rat vomeronasal organ to either the dialyzed urine preparation (<500 Da) or the remaining substances (>500 Da) of male rats did not induce expression of Fos-immunoreactive cells in the accessory olfactory bulb, whereas exposure to a mixture of these preparations did induce expression (Yamaguchi et al., 2000). This suggests that a combination of low and high molecular weight substances is necessary for the increases in Fos-immunoreactivity in the accessory olfactory bulb.

Similar results have been obtained in the mouse. Thus, the application of urine-derived compounds of low molecular weight such as 2,3-dehydro-*exo*-brevicomin induces only hyperpolarizing responses, that is, inhibitory responses, in the mouse vomeronasal sensory neuron (Moss et al., 1997) and does not induce c-fos mRNA expression in the mouse accessory olfactory bulb (Guo et al., 1997). However, 2,3-dehydro-*exo*-brevicomin in combination with major urinary proteins (~ 19 kDa) induced significantly greater c-fos mRNA expression (Guo et al., 1997). The female golden hamster produces a 17-kDa protein (aphrodisin) that is emitted in vaginal discharge and stimulates sexual behavior in the male hamster (Singer, 1991). Gel filtration experiments indicated that a mixture of ligands may be present in the purified aphrodisin (Singer, 1991). Analysis of the crystal structure of aphrodisin revealed the electron density for a small linear ligand in the cavity of the β-barrel (Vincent et al., 2001). At present, it is still not clear whether aphrodisin itself or its combination with a low molecular weight ligand is necessary for pheromonal activity.

References

Ache, B. W. (1994). Towards a common strategy for transducing olfactory information. *Semin. Cell Biol.* **5**, 55–63.

Ache, B. W., and Zhainazarov, A. (1995). Dual second-messenger pathways in olfactory transduction. *Curr. Opin. Neurobiol.* **5**, 461–466.

Altner, H. (1962). Untersuchungen uber Leistungen und bau der Nase des Sudafrikanischen Lrallenfrosches *Xenopus laevis* (Daudin, 1803). *Z. vergl. Physiol.* **45**, 272–306.

Arvanitaki, A., Takeuchi, H., and Chalazonitis, N. (1967). Specific unitary osmereceptor potentials and spiking patterns from giant nerve cells. In "Olfaction and Taste II" (T. Hayashi, ed.), pp. 573–598. Pergamon Press, Oxford.

Barber, P. C., and Raisman, G. (1974). An autoradiographic investigation of the projection of the vomeronasal organ to the accessory olfactory bulb in the mouse. Brain Res. 81, 21–30.

Belluscio, L., Gold, G. H., Nemes, A., and Axel, R. (1998). Mice deficient in G_{olf} are anosmic. Neuron 20, 69–81.

Beltramino, C., and Taleisnik, S. (1983). Release of LH in the female rat by olfactory stimuli. Effect of the removal of the vomeronasal organs or lesioning the accessory olfactory bulbs. Neuroendocrinology 36, 53–58.

Berridge, M. J. (1993). Cell signaling. A tale of two messengers. Nature (London) 365, 388–389.

Boekhoff, I., Tarelius, E., Strotmann, J., and Breer, H. (1990). Rapid activation of alternative second messenger pathways in olfactory cilia from rats by different odorants. EMBO J. 9, 2453–2458.

Bozza, T. C., and Kauer, J. S. (1998). Odorant response properties of convergent olfactory receptor neurons. J. Neurosci. 18, 4560–4569.

Breer, H., and Boekhoff, I. (1991). Odorants of the same odor class activate different second messenger pathways. Chem. Senses 16, 19–29.

Breer, H., Klemm, T., and Boekhoff, I. (1992). Nitric oxide mediated formation of cyclic GMP in the olfactory system. NeuroReport 3, 1030–1032.

Breer, H., Raming, K., and Krieger, J. (1994). Signal recognition and transduction in olfactory neurons. Biochim. Biophys. Acta 1224, 277–287.

Brennan, P. A., Schellinck, H. M., and Keverne, E. B. (1999). Patterns of expression of the immediate-early gene egr-1 in the accessory olfactory bulb of female mice exposed to pheromonal constituents of male urine. Neuroscience 90, 1463–1470.

Broillet, M. C., and Firestein, S. (1996). Direct activation of the olfactory cyclic nucleotide-gated channel through modification of sulfhydryl groups by NO compounds. Neuron 16, 377–385.

Brownlee, R. G., Silverstein, R. M., Müller-Schwarze, D., and Singer, A. G. (1969). Isolation, identification and function of the chief component of the male tarsal scent in black-tailed deer. Nature (London) 221, 284–285.

Bruch, R. C., and Teeter, J. H. (1990). Cyclic AMP links amino acid chemoreception to ion channels in olfactory cilia. Chem. Senses 15, 419–430.

Brunet, L. J., Gold, G. H., and Ngai, J. (1996). General anosmia caused by a targeted disruption of the mouse olfactory cyclic nucleotide-gated cation channel. Neuron 17, 681–693.

Buck, L. B. (1996). Information coding in the vertebrate olfactory system. Annu. Rev. Neurosci. 19, 517–544.

Buck, L., and Axel, R. (1991). A novel multigene family may encode odorant receptors: A molecular basis for odor recognition. Cell (Cambridge, Mass.) 65, 175–187.

Chateau, D., Roos, J., Plas-Roser, S., Roos, M., and Aron, C. (1976). Hormonal mechanisms involved in the control of oestrous cycle duration by the odour of urine in the rat. Acta Endcrinol. (Capenhagen) 82, 426–435.

Cohen-Tannoudji, J., Lavenet, C., Locatelli, A., Tillet, Y., and Signoret, J. P. (1989). Non-involvement of the accessory olfactory system in the LH response of anoestrous ewes to male odour. J. Reprod. Fertil. 86, 135–144.

Dellacorte, C., Kalinoski, D. L., Huque, T., Wysocki, L., and Restrepo, D. (1995). NADPH diaphorase staining suggests localization of nitric oxide synthase within mature vertebrate olfactory neurons. Neuroscience 66, 215–225.

Dethier, V. G. (1972). Sensitivity of the contact chemoreceptor of the blowfly to vapor. Proc. Natl. Acad. Sci. U.S.A. 69, 2189–2192.

Dorries, K. M., Adkins-Regan, E., and Halpern, B. P. (1997). Sensitivity and behavioral responses to the pheromone androstenone are not mediated by the vomeronasal organ in domestic pig. Brain, Behav. Evol. 49, 53–62.

Duchamp-Viret, P., Duchamp, A., and Sicard, G. (1990). Olfactory discrimination over a wide concentration range. Comparison of receptor cell and bulb neuron abilities. Brain Res. 517, 256–262.

Dulac, C., and Axel, R. (1995). A novel family of genes encoding putative pheromone receptors in mammals. Cell (Cambridge, Mass.) 83, 195–206.

Fabbri, E., Ferretti, M. E., Buzzi, M., Cavallaro, R., Vesce, G., and Biondi, C. (1995). Olfactory transduction mechanisms in sheep. Neurochem. Res. 20, 719–725.

Fadool, D. A., and Ache, B. W. (1992). Plasma membrane inositol 1,4,5-trisphosphate-activated channels mediate signal transduction in lobster olfactory receptor neurons. Neuron 9, 907–918.

Firestein, S., and Werblin, F. (1989). Odor-induced membrane currents in vertebrate olfactory receptor neurons. Science 244, 79–82.

Firestein, S., Zufall, F., and Shepherd, G. M. (1991). Single odor-sensitive channels in olfactory receptor neurons are also gated by cyclic nucleotides. J. Neurosci. 11, 3656–3572.

Freitag, J., Krieger, J., Strotmann, J., and Breer, H. (1995). Two classes of olfactory receptors in Xenopus laevis. Neuron 15, 1383–1392.

Friedlander, G., Grimellec, C., Giocondi, M.-C., and Amiel, C. (1987). Benzyl alcohol increases membrane fluidity and modulates cyclic AMP synthesis in intact renal epithelial cells. *Biochim. Biophys. Acta* **903**, 341–348.

Galione, A., Lee, H. C., and Busa, W. B. (1991). Ca^{2+} induced Ca^{2+} release in sea urchin egg homogenates: Modulation by cyclic ADP-ribose. *Science* **253**, 1143–1146.

Gesteland, R. C., Yancey, R. A., and Farbman, A. I. (1982). Development of olfactory receptor neuron selectivity in the rat fetus. *Neuroscience* **7**, 3127–3136.

Goodwin, M., Gooding, K. M., and Regnier, F. (1979). Sex pheromone in the dog. *Science* **203**, 559–561.

Guo, J., Zhou, A., and Moss, R. L. (1997). Urine and urine-derived compounds induce c-*fos* mRNA expression in accessory olfactory bulb. *NeuroReport* **8**, 1679–1683.

Guse, A. H. (1999). Cyclic ADP-ribose: A novel Ca^{2+}-mobilizing second messenger. *Cell. Signal.* **11**, 309–316.

Halpern, M. (1987). The organization and function of the vomeronasal system. *Annu. Rev. Neurosci.* **10**, 325–362.

Halpern, M., Shapiro, L. S., and Jia, C. (1995). Differential localization of G proteins in the opossum vomeronasal system. *Brain Res.* **677**, 157–161.

Hatt, H., and Ache, B. W. (1994). Cyclic nucleotide- and inositol phosphate-gated ion channels in lobster olfactory receptor neurons. *Proc. Natl. Acad. Sci. U.S.A.* **91**, 6264–6268.

Hatt, H., Gisselman, G., and Wetzel, C. (1999). Cloning, functional expression and characterization of a human olfactory receptor. *Cell. Mol. Biol.* **45**, 285–291.

Herrada, G., and Dulac, C. (1997). A novel family of putative pheromone receptors in mammals with a topographically organized and sexually dimorphic distribution. *Cell (Cambridge, Mass.)* **90**, 763–773.

Holy, T. E., Dulac, C., and Meister, M. (2000). Responses of vomeronasal neurons to natural stimuli. *Science* **289**, 1569–1572.

Huque, T., and Bruch, R. C. (1986). Odorant- and guanine nucleotide-stimulated phophoinositide turnover in olfactory cilia. *Biochem. Biophys. Res. Commun.* **137**, 36–42.

Iida, A., and Kashiwayanagi, M. (1999a). Responses of *Xenopus laevis* water nose to water-soluble and volatile odorants. *J. Gen. Physiol.* **114**, 85–92.

Iida, A., and Kashiwayanagi, M. (1999b). Responses to putative second messengers and odorants in water nose olfactory neurons of *Xenopus laevis*. *Chem. Senses* **25**, 55–59.

Imamura, K., Mataga, N., and Mori, K. (1992). Coding of odor molecules by mitral/tufted cells in rabbit olfactory bulb. I. Aliphatic compounds. *J. Neurophysiol.* **68**, 1986–2002.

Inamura, K., and Kashiwayanagi, M. (2000). Inward current responses to urinary substances in rat vomeronasal sensory neurons. *Eur. J. Neurosci.* **12**, 3529–3536.

Inamura, K, Kashiwayanagi, M., and Kurihara, K. (1997a). Inositol-1,4,5-trisphosphate induces responses in receptor neurons in rat vomeronasal sensory slices. *Chem. Senses* **22**, 93–103.

Inamura, K., Kashiwayanagi, M., and Kurihara, K. (1997b). Blockage of urinary responses by inhibitors for IP_3-mediated pathway in rat vomeronasal sensory neurons. *Neurosci. Lett.* **233**, 129–132.

Inamura, K., Kashiwayanagi, M., and Kurihara, K. (1998). Effects of cGMP and sodium nitroprusside on odor responses in turtle olfactory sensory neurons. *Am. J. Physiol.* **275**, C1201–C1206.

Inamura, K., Matsumoto, Y., Kashiwayanagi, M., and Kurihara, K. (1999a). Laminar distribution of pheromone-receptive neurons in rat vomeronasal epithelium. *J. Physiol. (London)* **517**, 731–739.

Inamura, K., Kashiwayanagi, M., and Kurihara, K. (1999b). Regionalization of Fos immunostaining in rat accessory olfactory bulb when the vomeronasal organ was exposed to urine. *Eur. J. Neurosci.* **11**, 2254–2260.

Ivanova, T. T., and Caprio, J. (1993). Odorant receptors activated by amino acids in sensory neurons of the channel catfish *Ictalurus punctatus*. *J. Gen. Physiol.* **102**, 1085–1105.

Jia, C. P., and Halpern, M. (1996). Subclasses of vomeronasal receptor neurons: Differential expression of G proteins ($G_{i\alpha 2}$ and $G_{o\alpha}$) and segregated projections to the accessory olfactory bulb. *Brain Res.* **719**, 117–128.

Johns, M. A., Feder, H. H., Komisaruk, B. R., and Mayer, A. D. (1978). Urine-induced reflex ovulation in anovulatory rats may be a vomeronasal effect. *Nature (London)* **272**, 446–468.

Johnston, R. E., and Peng, M. (2000). The vomeronasal organ is involved in discrimination of individual odors by males but not by females in Golden hamsters. *Physiol. Behav.* **70**, 537–549.

Kahn, A. A., Steiner, J. P., and Snyder, S. H. (1992). Plasma membrane inositol 1,4,5-triphosphate receptor of lymphocytes: Selective enrichment in sialic acid and unique binding specificity. *Proc. Natl. Acad. Sci. U.S.A.* **89**, 2849–2853.

Kalinoski, D. L., Aldinger, S. B., Boil, A. G., Hue, T., Marrakech, J. F., Prestwich, G. D., and Restrepo, D. (1992). Characterization of a novel inositol 1,4,5-trisphosphate receptor in isolated olfactory cilia. *Biochem. J.* **281**, 449–456.

Kang, J., and Caprio, J. (1995a). In vivo responses of single olfactory receptor neurons in the channel catfish, *Ictalurus punctatus*. *J. Neurophysiol.* **73**, 172–177.

Kang, J., and Caprio, J. (1995b). Electrophysiological responses of single olfactory bulb neurons to amino acids in the channel catfish, *Ictalurus punctatus*. *J. Neurophysiol.* **74**, 1421–1434.

Kashiwagura, T., Kamo, N., Kurihara, K., and Kobatake, Y. (1977). Responses of the frog gustatory receptors to various odorants. *Comp. Biochem. Physiol. C* **56C**, 105–108.

Kashiwayanagi, M. (1996). Dialysis of inositol 1,4,5-trisphosphate induces inward currents and Ca^{2+} uptake in frog olfactory receptor cells. *Biochem. Biophys. Res. Commun.* **225**, 666–671.

Kashiwayanagi, M., and Kurihara, K. (1984). Neuroblastoma cell as model for olfactory cell: A mechanism of depolarization in response to various odorants. *Brain Res.* **293**, 251–258.

Kashiwayanagi, M., and Kurihara, K. (1985). Evidence for non-receptor odor discrimination using neuroblastoma cells as a model for olfactory cells. *Brain Res.* **359**, 97–103.

Kashiwayanagi, M., and Kurihara, K. (1994). Odor discrimination in single turtle olfactory receptor neuron. *Neurosci. Lett.* **170**, 233–236.

Kashiwayanagi, M., and Kurihara, K. (1995). Odor responses after complete desensitization of the cAMP-dependent pathway in turtle olfactory cells. *Neurosci. Lett.* **193**, 61–64.

Kashiwayanagi, M., Kawahara, H., Hanada, T., and Kurihara, K. (1994a). A large contribution of cyclic AMP-independent pathway to turtle olfactory transduction. *J. Gen. Physiol.* **103**, 957–974.

Kashiwayanagi, M., Yamada, K., and Kurihara, K. (1994b). Discrimination of odorants in the non-olfactory system: Analysis of responses of the frog gustatory system to odorants by multidimensional scaling. *Comp. Biochem. Physiol. A* **108A**, 479–484.

Kashiwayanagi, M., Nagasawa, F., Inamura, K., and Kurihara, K. (1996a). Odor discrimination of "cAMP-" and "IP$_3$-dependent" odorants at turtle olfactory bulb. *Eur. J. Physiol.* **431**, 786–790.

Kashiwayanagi, M., Shimano, K., and Kurihara, K. (1996b). Responses of single bullfrog olfactory neurons to many odorants including cAMP-dependent and independent odorants: Existence of multiple receptors in single neuron. *Brain Res.* **738**, 222–228.

Kashiwayanagi, M., Sasaki, K., Iida, A., Saito, H., and Kurihara, K. (1997). Concentration and membrane fluidity dependence of odor discrimination in the turtle olfactory system. *Chem. Senses* **22**, 553–563.

Kashiwayanagi, M., Tatani, K., Shuto, S., and Matsuda, A. (2000). Inositol 1,4,5-trisphosphate and adenophostin analogues induce responses in turtle olfactory sensory neurons. *Eur. J. Neurosci.* **12**, 606–612.

Katoh, K., Koshimoto, H., Tani, A., and Mori, K. (1993). Coding of odor molecules by mitral/tufted cells in rabbit olfactory bulb. II. Aromatic compounds. *J. Neurophysiol.* **70**, 2161–2175.

Kishimoto, J., Cox, H., Keverne, E. B., and Emson, P. C. (1994). Cellular localization of putative odorant receptor mRNAs in olfactory and chemosensory neurons: A non radioactive in situ hybridization study. *Mol. Brain Res.* **23**, 33–39.

Kroner, C., Breer, H., Singer, A. G., and O'Connell, R. J. (1996). Pheromone-induced second messenger signaling in the hamster vomeronasal organ. *NeuroReport* **7**, 2989–2992.

Kurahashi, T. (1990). The response induced by intracellular cyclic AMP in isolated olfactory receptor cells of the newt. *J. Physiol. (London)* **430**, 355–371.

Kurihara, K., and Koyama, N. (1972). High activity of adenyl cyclase in olfactory and gustatory organs. *Biochem. Biophys. Res. Commun.* **48**, 30–34.

Leinders-Zufall, T., Lane, A. P., Puche, A. C., Ma, W., Novotny, M. V., Shipley, M. T., and Zufall, F. (2000). Ultrasensitive pheromone detection by mammalian vomeronasal neurons. *Nature (London)* **405**, 792–796.

Lerner, M. R., Reagan, J., Gyorgyi, T., and Roby, A. (1988). Olfaction by melanophores: What does it mean? *Proc. Natl. Acad. Sci. U.S.A.* **85**, 261–264.

Lévy, F., Kendrick, K. M., Goode, J. A., Guevara-Guzman, R., and Keverne, E. B. (1995). Oxytocin and vasopressin release in the olfactory bulb of parturient ewes: Changes with maternal experience and effects on acetylcholine, gamma-aminobutyric acid, glutamate and noradrenaline release. *Brain Res.* **669**, 197–206.

Liman, E. R., and Corey, D. P. (1996). Electrophysiological characterization of chemosensory neurons from the mouse vomeronasal organ. *J. Neurosci.* **16**, 4625–4637.

Lischka, F. W., and Schild, D. (1993). Effects of nitric oxide upon olfactory receptor neurons in *Xenopus laevis*. *NeuroReport* **4**, 582–584.

Lowe, G., and Gold, G. H. (1993). Nonlinear amplification by calcium-dependent chloride channels in olfactory receptor cells. *Nature (London)* **366**, 283–286.

Lundy, R. F., Jr., and Contreras, R. J. (1993). Taste prestimulation increases the chorda tympani nerve response to menthol. *Physiol. Behav.* **54**, 65–70.

Luo, Y., Lu, S., Chen, P., Wang, D., and Halpern, M. (1994). Identification of chemoattractant receptors and G proteins in the vomeronasal system of garter snakes. *J. Biol. Chem.* **269**, 16867–16877.

Lydell, K., and Doty, R. L. (1972). Male rat odor preferences for female urine as a function of sexual experience, urine age, and urine source. *Horm. Behav.* **3**, 205–212.

Malnic, B., Hirono, J., Sato, T., and Buck, L. B. (1999). Combinatorial receptor codes for odors. *Cell (Cambridge, Mass.)* **96**, 713–723.

Margalit, T., and Lancet, D. (1993). Expression of olfactory receptor and transduction genes during rat development. *Dev. Brain Res.* **73**, 7–16.

Mathews, D. F. (1972). Response patterns of single neurons in the tortoise olfactory epithelium and olfactory bulb. *J. Gen. Physiol.* **60**, 166–180.

Matsunami, H., and Buck, L. B. (1997). A multigene family encoding a diverse array of putative pheromone receptors in mammals. *Cell (Cambridge, Mass.)* **90**, 775–784.

Matsuoka, M., Yokosuka, M., Mori, Y., and Ichikawa, M. (1999). Specific expression pattern of Fos in the accessory olfactory bulb of male mice after exposure to soiled bedding of females. *Neurosci. Res.* **35**, 189–195.

McClintock, M. K. (1978). Estrous synchrony and its mediation by airborne chemical communication *(Rattus norvegicus)*. *Horm. Behav.* **10**, 264–276.

Melrose, D. R., Reed, H. C., and Patterson, R. L. (1971). Androgen steroids associated with boar odour as an aid to the detection of oestrus in pig artificial insemination. *Br. Vet. J.* **127**, 497–502.

Mombaerts, P., Wang, F., Dulac, C., Chao, S. K., Nemes, A., Mendelsohn, M., Edmondson, J., and Axel, R. (1996). Visualizing an olfactory sensory map. *Cell (Cambridge, Mass.)* **87**, 675–686.

Moss, R. L., Flynn, R. E., Shen, X. M., Dudley, C., Shi, J. M., and Novotny, M. (1997). Urine-derived compound evokes membrane responses in mouse vomeronasal receptor neurons. *J. Neurophysiol.* **77**, 2856–2862.

Mucignat-Caretta, C., Caretta, A., and Cavaggioni, A. (1995). Acceleration of puberty onset in female mice by male urinary proteins. *J. Physiol. (London)* **486**, 517–522.

Naim, M., Seifert, R., Nürnberg, B., Grünbaum, L., and Schultz, G. (1994). Some taste substances are direct activators of G-proteins. *Biochem. J.* **297**, 451–454.

Nakamura, T., and Gold, G. H. (1987). A cyclic nucleotide-gated conductance in olfactory receptor cilia. *Nature (London)* **325**, 442–444.

Nakamura, T., Tsuru, K., and Miyamoto, S. (1994). Regulation of Ca^{2+} concentration by second messengers in newt olfactory receptor cell. *Neurosci. Lett.* **171**, 197–200.

Nef, P., Hermans-Borgmeyer, I., ArtiŠres-Pin, H., Beasley, L., Dionne, V. E., and Heinemann, S. F. (1992). Spatial pattern of receptor expression in the olfactory epithelium. *Proc. Natl. Acad. Sci. U.S.A.* **89**, 8948–8952.

Ngai, J., Chess, A., Dowling, M. M., Necles, N., Macagno, E. R., and Axel, R. (1993). Coding of olfactory information: Topography of odorant receptor expression in the catfish olfactory epithelium. *Cell (Cambridge, Mass.)* **72**, 667–680.

Noé, J., and Breer, H. (1998). Functional and molecular characterization of individual olfactory neurons. *J. Neurochem.* **71**, 2286–2293.

Novotny, M., Harvey, S., Jemiolo, B., and Alberts, J. (1985). Synthetic pheromones that promote inter-male aggression in mice. *Proc. Natl. Acad. Sci. U.S.A.* **82**, 2059–2061.

Okamoto, K., Tokumitsu, Y., and Kashiwayanagi, M. (1996). Adenylyl cyclase activity in sensory cells of the turtle vomeronasal and olfactory epithelium. *Biochem. Biophys. Res. Commun.* **220**, 98–101.

Pace, U., Hasnski, E., Salomon, Y., and Lancet, D. (1985). Odorant-sensitive adenylate cyclase may mediate olfactory reception. *Nature (London)* **316**, 255–258.

Pfaff, D., and Pfaffmann, C. (1969). Behavioral and electrophysiological responses of male rats to female rat urine odors. In "Olfaction and Taste" (C. Pfaffmann, ed.), Vol. 3, pp. 258–267. Rockefeller University Press, New York.

Powers, J. B., and Winans, S. S. (1975). Vomeronasal organ: Critical role in mediating sexual behavior of the male hamster. *Science* **187**, 961–963.

Rajendren, G., Dudley, C. A., and Moss, R. L. (1990). Role of the vomeronasal organ in the male-induced enhancement of sexual receptivity in female rats. *Neuroendocrinology* **52**, 368–372.

Raming, K., Krieger, J., Strotmann, J., Boekhoff, I., Kubick, S., Baumstark, C., and Breer, H. (1993). Cloning and expression of odorant receptors. *Nature (London)* **361**, 353–356.

Ressler, K. J., Sullivan, S. L., and Buck, L. B. (1993). A zonal organization of odorant receptor gene expression in the olfactory epithelium. *Cell (Cambridge, Mass.)* **73**, 597–609.

Ressler, K. J., Sulivan, S. L., and Buck, L. B. (1994a). A molecular dissection of spatial patterning in the olfactory system. *Curr. Opin. Neurobiol.* **4**, 588–596.

Ressler, K. J., Sullivan, S. L., and Buck, L. B. (1994b). Information coding in the olfactory system: Evidence for a stereotyped and highly organized epitope map in the olfactory bulb. *Cell (Cambridge, Mass.)* **79**, 1245–1255.

Restrepo, D., Miyamoto, T., Bryant, B. P., and Teeter, J. H. (1990). Odor stimuli trigger influx of calcium into olfactory neurons of the channel catfish. *Science* **249**, 1166–1168.

Restrepo, D., Teeter, J. H., Honda, E., Boyle, A. G., Marecek, J. F., Prestwich, G. D., and Kalinoski, D. L. (1992). Evidence for an $InsP_3$-gated channel protein in isolated rat olfactory cilia. *Am. J. Physiol.* **263**, C667–C673.

Restrepo, D., Boekhoff, I., and Breer, H. (1993a). Rapid kinetic measurements of second messenger formation in olfactory cilia from channel catfish. *Am. J. Physiol.* **264**, C906–C911.

Restrepo, D., Okada, Y., and Teeter, J. H. (1993b). Odorant-regulated Ca^{2+} gradients in rat olfactory neurons. *J. Gen. Physiol.* **102**, 907–924.

Rodriguez, I., Greer, C. A., Mok, M. Y., and Mombaerts, P. (2000). A putative pheromone receptor gene expressed in human olfactory mucosa. *Nat. Genet.* **26**, 18–19.

Roskams, A. J., Bredt, D. S., Dawson, T. M., and Ronnett, G. V. (1994). Nitric oxide mediates the formation of synaptic connections in developing and regenerating olfactory receptor neurons. *Neuron* **13**, 289–299.

Ryba, N. J. P., and Tirindelli, R. (1997). A new multigene family of putative pheromone receptors. *Neuron* **19**, 371–379.

Sasaki, K., Okamoto, K., Inamura, K., Tokumitsu, Y., and Kashiwayanagi, M. (1999). Inositol-1,4,5-trisphosphate accumulation induced by urinary pheromones in female rat vomeronasal epithelium. *Brain Res.* **823**, 161–168.

Sato, T., Hirono, J., Tonoike, M., and Takebayashi, M. (1991). Two types of increases in free Ca^{2+} evoked by odor in isolated frog olfactory receptor neurons. *NeuroReport* **2**, 229–232.

Schild, D., and Lischka, F. W. (1994). Amiloride-insensitive cation conductance in *Xenopus laevis* olfactory neurons: A combined patch clamp and calcium imaging analysis. *Biophys. J.* **66**, 299–304.

Shepherd, G. M. (1994). Discrimination of molecular signals by the olfactory receptor neuron. *Neuron* **13**, 771–790.

Sicard, G., and Holley, A. (1984). Receptor cell responses to odorants: Similarities and differences among odorants. *Brain Res.* **292**, 283–296.

Singer, A. G. (1991). A chemistry of mammalian pheromones. *J. Steroid Biochem. Mol. Biol.* **39**, 627–632.

Singer, A. G., Beauchamp, G. K., and Yamazaki, K. (1997). Volatile signals of the major histocompatibility complex in male mouse urine. *Proc. Natl. Acad. Sci. U.S.A.* **94**, 2210–2214.

Sklar, P. B., Anholt, R. H., and Snyder, S. H. (1986). The odorant-sensitive adenylate cyclase of olfactory receptor cells: Differential stimulation by distinct classes of odorants. *J. Biol. Chem.* **261**, 15538–15543.

Strotmann, J., Wanner, I., Helfrich, T., Beck, A., and Breer, H. (1994). Rostro-caudal patterning of receptor-expressing olfactory neurons in the rat nasal cavity. *Cell Tissue Res.* **278**, 11–20.

Strotmann, J., Wanner, I., Helfrich, T., and Breer, H. (1995). Receptor expression in olfactory neurons during rat development: *In situ* hybridization studies. *Eur. J. Neurosci.* **7**, 492–500.

Sugai, T., Sugitani, M., and Onoda, N. (1997). Subdivisions of the guinea-pig accessory olfactory bulb revealed by the combined method with immunohistochemistry, electrophysiological, and optical recordings. *Neuroscience* **79**, 871–885.

Suzuki, N. (1989). Voltage- and cyclic nucleotide-gated currents in isolated olfactory receptor cells. *In* "Chemical Senses" (J. D. Brand, J. H. Teeter, R. H. Cagan, and M. R. Kare, eds.), Vol. 1, pp. 469–494. Dekker, New York and Basel.

Suzuki, N. (1992). IP_3-activated ion channel activity in frog olfactory cell. *Chem. Senses* **17**, 87 (abstr.).

Tanabe, T., Iino, M., and Takagi, S. F. (1975). Discrimination of odors in olfactory bulb, pyriform-amygdaloid area, and orbitofontal cortex of the monkey. *J. Neurophysiol.* **38**, 1284–1296.

Taniguchi, M., Kashiwayanagi, M., and Kurihara, K. (1995). Intracellular injection of inositol 1,4,5-trisphosphate increases a conductance in membranes of turtle vomeronasal receptor neurons in the slice preparation. *Neurosci. Lett.* **188**, 5–8.

Taniguchi, M., Kanaki, K., and Kashiwayanagi, M. (1996a). Difference in behavior between responses to forskolin and general odorants in turtle vomeronasal organ. *Chem. Senses* **21**, 763–771.

Taniguchi, M., Kashiwayanagi, M., and Kurihara, K. (1996b). Intracellular dialysis of cyclic nucleotides induces inward currents in turtle vomeronasal receptor neurons. *J. Neurosci.* **16**, 1239–1246.

Taniguchi, M., Wang, D., and Halpern, M. (2000). Chemosensitive conductance and inositol 1,4,5-trisphosphate-induced conductance in snake vomeronasal receptor neurons. *Chem. Senses* **25**, 67–76.

Touhara, K., Sengoku, S., Inaki, K., Tsuboi, A., Hirono, J., Sato, T., Sakano, H., and Haga, T. (1999). Functional identification and reconstitution of an odorant receptor in single olfactory neurons. *Proc. Natl. Acad. Sci. U.S.A.* **96**, 4040–4045.

Tsujikawa, K., and Kashiwayanagi, M. (1999). Protease-sensitive urinary pheromones induce region-specific fos- expression in rat accessory olfactory bulb. *Biochem. Biophys. Res. Commun.* **260**, 222–224.

Tucker, D. (1963). Olfactory, vomeronasal and trigeminal receptor responses to odorants. *In* "Olfaction and Taste" (Y. Zotterman, ed.), Vol. 1, pp. 45–69. Pergmon Press, Oxford.

Vincent, F., Lobel, D., Brown, K., Spinelli, S., Grote, P., Breer, H., Cambillau, C., and Tegoni, M. (2001). Crystal structure of aphrodisin, a sex pheromone from female hamster. *J. Mol. Biol.* **305**, 459–469.

Wekesa, K. S., and Anholt, R. R. H. (1997). Pheromone regulated production of inositol-(1,4,5)trisphosphate in the mammalian vomeronasal organ. *Endocrinology (Baltimore)* **138**, 3497–3504.

Wellerdieck, C., Oles, M., Pott, L., Korsching, S., Gisselmann, G., and Hatt, H. (1997). Functional expression of odorant receptors of the zebrafish *Danio rerio* and of the nematode *C-elegans* in HEK293 cells. *Chem. Senses* **22**, 467–476.

Wetzel, C. H., Oles, M., Wellerdieck, C., Kuczkowiak, M., Gisselmann, G., and Hatt, H. (1999). Specificity and sensitivity of a human olfactory receptor functionally expressed in human embryonic kidney 293 cells and *Xenopus laevis* oocytes. *J. Neurosci.* **19**, 7426–7433.

Wong, S. T., Trinh, K., Hacker, B., Chan, G. C., Lowe, G., Gaggar, A., Xia, Z., Gold, G. H., and Storm, D. R. (2000).

Disruption of the type III adenylyl cyclase gene leads to peripheral and behavioral anosmia in transgenic mice. *Neuron* **27**, 487–497.

Wysocki, C. J., and Meredith, M. (1987). The vomeronasal System. *In* "Neurobiology of Taste and Smell" (T. E. Finger and W. L. Silver, eds.), pp. 125–150. Wiley, New York.

Wysocki, C. J., Wellington, J. L., and Beauchamp, G. K. (1980). Access of urinary nonvolatiles to the mammalian vomeronasal organ. *Science* **207**, 781–783.

Wysocki, C. J., Nyby, J., Whitney, G., Beauchamp, G. K., and Katz, Y. (1982). The vomeronasal organ primary role in mouse chemosensory gender recognition. *Physiol. Behav.* **29**, 315–327.

Yamaguchi, T., Inamura, K., and Kashiwayanagi, M. (2000). Increases in Fos-immunoreactivity after exposure to a combination of two male urinary components in the accessory olfactory bulb of the female rat. *Brain Res.* **876**, 211–214.

Zhao, H. Q., Ivic, L., Otaki, J. M., Hashimoto, M., Mikoshiba, K., and Firestein, S. (1998). Functional expression of a mammalian odorant receptor. *Science* **279**, 237–242.

Zhou, A. W., and Moss, R. L. (1997). Effect of urine-derived compounds on cAMP accumulation in mouse vomeronasal cells. *NeuroReport* **8**, 2173–2177.

Zufall, F., Shepherd, G. M., and Firestein, S. (1991). Inhibition of the olfactory cyclic nucleotide gated ion channel by intracellular calcium. *Proc. R. Soc. London, Ser. B* **246**, 225–230.

Pheromonal Signals Access the Medial Extended Amygdala: One Node in a Proposed Social Behavior Network[1]

Sarah Winans Newman

Department of Psychology
Cornell University
Ithaca, New York 14853

I. PHEROMONAL COMMUNICATION

Pheromones are the language of social communication among vertebrates, particularly mammals. When broadcast from an animal's body or deposited as a transitory signpost of the animal's passage, pheromones can convey not only sex and reproductive status, but individual identity and thereby familial relationship and social status in the community (Beauchamp *et al.*, 1985; Todrank *et al.*, 1999; Yamazaki *et al.*, 2000). Thus, these signaling molecules serve to attract or separate individuals, and, when individuals interact, to elicit affiliative, agonistic, or defensive behaviors. In addition, pheromones initiate neuroendocrine responses in the receiver, whether male or female, that can have profound effects on the physiological status of the animal, particularly on reproductive status (Clancy *et al.*, 1988; Pfeiffer and Johnston, 1994; Novotny *et al.*, 1997; McClintock, 2000).

Although astute practitioners of animal husbandry have recognized and taken advantage of pheromonal communication for hundreds, perhaps thousands, of years, efforts to discover the neural mechanisms underlying this signaling system did not begin in earnest until the 1960s. By the early 1970s, it was recognized that odors from conspecifics could alter the onset of puberty in females, ovarian cyclicity, and sexual behavior in males and females; and could affect the success of pregnancy in several vertebrate species (see reviews by Wysocki and Meredith, 1987; Vandenberg, 1994). These observations led many investigators to the conclusion that the olfactory receptors and their central nervous system (CNS) connections through the olfactory bulb have a profound effect on reproductive behavior and endocrine function in vertebrates.

II. MULTIPLE SENSORY SYSTEMS INNERVATE THE NASAL CAVITIES

During the 1970s, it also became apparent, however, that not one olfactory system but in fact five different neural systems that innervate the nasal cavities could conceivably contribute to pheromone-mediated functions and that more than one of these were often damaged by experimental manipulations of the

---

[1] The majority of this chapter is reprinted from Newman (1999) with the permission of the New York Academy of Sciences.

nasal cavities and olfactory bulbs (reviewed in Wysocki, 1979). Of these five systems, the olfactory mucosa and vomeronasal organ have received the most experimental attention (Halpern, 1987; Meredith, 1991). Although potential roles for the terminal nerve, including its luteinizing-hormone-releasing-hormone-containing fibers (Wirsig, 1987; Meredith and Fernandez-Fewell, 1994), the organ of Masera (Wysocki, 1979), and the trigeminal nerve (Keverne et al., 1986; Silver, 1987) were acknowledged by most investigators and carefully studied by some, questions remain about the specific roles for these neural systems in pheromonal communication.

Perhaps the largest single factor that focused attention on the vomeronasal system was the concordance of three separate lines of investigation. Anatomical data revealed the projections of the vomeronasal system through the amygdala to the bed nucleus of the stria terminalis (BNST) and medial preoptic area (MPOA) (Krettek and Price, 1978; Kevetter and Winans, 1981). Behavioral data demonstrated that destructive lesions of these CNS targets of the vomeronasal pathway mimicked the effects of olfactory bulbectomy in male rats and hamsters (Larsson and Heimer, 1964; Heimer and Larsson, 1967; Murphy and Schneider, 1970; Harris and Sachs, 1975; Emery and Sachs, 1976; Valcourt and Sachs, 1979; Lehman et al., 1980; Powers et al., 1987). Finally, evidence from steroid autoradiography showed that these same vomeronasal pathway nuclei collectively contained the greatest density of cells that actively accumulate gonadal hormones (Pfaff and Keiner, 1973; Sar and Stumpf, 1977; Rees et al., 1980; Cottingham and Pfaff, 1986), the premier prerequisites for normal reproductive behavior and modulators of other social behaviors.

III. IMPORTANCE OF THE VOMERONASAL ORGAN IN REPRODUCTIVE NEUROENDOCRINE FUNCTION AND SOCIAL BEHAVIORS VARIES WITH SEX AND SPECIES

Evidence supporting an important role for the vomeronasal system in pheromonal modulation of gonadal function and social behavior was strengthened by the development of a surgical technique for removing the vomeronasal organ (Clancy et al., 1988; Wysocki and Lepri, 1991), but extending these investigations clearly demonstrated that the importance of vomeronasal sensory inputs depends on the particular neuroendocrine or behavioral response under consideration and varies significantly across species of mammals and between the sexes. New animal models were investigated and confirmed that tactile, auditory, and visual stimuli could also be important modulators of social behavior, in many cases more important than chemosensory inputs (Silver, 1992). Further, within the realm of pheromonally mediated responses, the relation between olfactory and vomeronasal systems was recognized as complementary at the physiological and behavioral levels. Complementarity of function at the level of the receptors can be seen in the vomeronasal organ's access and response to large molecules of low volatility after direct contact with the source of the molecules (urine, glandular secretions, etc.), as well as its response to small molecules of relatively high volatility that carry information over distances and are the primary stimuli of the olfactory receptors (Wysocki et al., 1985). Complementarity of function at the behavioral level is reflected in the different roles of vomeronasal and olfactory systems in some social behaviors. The expression of these behaviors is heavily dependent on experience (learning or imprinting), which is mediated by the connections of the vomeronasal system (Meredith, 1986; Pfeiffer and Johnston, 1994), but, once learned, the behavior will be unaffected in many animals by removal of the vomeronasal organ and only eliminated if the olfactory system is also destroyed.

The evidence compiled since the 1980s suggests that the vomeronasal system has assumed control over reproductive neuroendocrine function and social behaviors in a variety of vertebrates, not because there is a unique, universal or ancestral role for the vomeronasal organ but rather because this organ has direct and powerful access to a group of structures in the CNS that control these functions. The vomeronasal organ has thus been conveniently adapted for regulation of reproduction and other social behaviors by a large number of vertebrate species. This chapter formulates the hypothesis that a central neural circuit, or network, in the limbic system determines an individual animal's behavioral response to socially relevant stimuli. The vomeronasal system gains direct access to this network via projections from the accessory olfactory bulb to the corticomedial amygdala and the BNST.

IV. CONCEPT OF THE MEDIAL EXTENDED AMYGDALA

During the latter half of the 1980s, de Olmos *et al.* (1985) and Alheid and Heimer (1988) proposed that the medial amygdaloid nucleus and the medial part of the BNST formed one unit in an entity that they called the extended amygdala. In elucidating the organization of the ventral forebrain, these investigators assembled evidence for parallel rings of cells, extending through the medial and central amygdaloid nuclei, supracapsular nucleus of the stria terminalis and BNST, and the substantia innominata, which are related by shared characteristics in cell morphology, reciprocal neuronal connections, and neurochemical or neurotransmitter identity. Whether these discrete rings of cells also share functional identity is less clear. Studies of male rodent sexual behavior are among those that provide support for functional as well as anatomical continuity, especially with regard to the medial extended amygdala.

The medial nucleus of the amygdala is the largest nucleus in the medial extended amygdala. It is a primary target of the vomeronasal system through the efferents of the accessory olfactory bulb. In addition, a small secondary input to the anterior part of the medial nucleus arises in the olfactory bulb (Scalia and Winans, 1975; Davis *et al.*, 1978), and projections from the main olfactory cortex reach its cellular layer (reviewed in Price, 1987). Finally, through relays in the brain stem, somatosensory input also reaches this part of the amygdala (Baum and Everitt, 1992). In the course of studies on mating behavior in the male hamster, Wood and Newman (1995a) have argued that the medial extended amygdala is itself composed of two parallel, functionally different circuits of cells associated with the anterior and posterior divisions of the medial nucleus, respectively, which also can be differentiated on the basis of connections, neurotransmitters, and hormone sensitivity (Fig. 1).

V. EVIDENCE FOR ANTERIOR AND POSTERIOR CIRCUITS IN THE MEDIAL EXTENDED AMYGDALA: CONNECTIONS, TRANSMITTERS, HORMONE RECEPTORS, AND HORMONE ACTION

A. Anatomical Continuity in Parallel Circuits

In both the male rat (Canteras *et al.*, 1995) and male Syrian hamster (Gomez and Newman, 1992; Coolen and Wood, 1998), the efferents of the anterior and posterior regions of the medial amygdala have distinctly different distribution patterns in the BNST. The axons of the anterodorsal part of the medial amygdaloid nucleus (MeAD) project through the ansa peduncularis (ventral amygdalofugal pathway) and the stria terminalis to a lateral territory in the posterior BNST. In the rat, this territory consists of several subgroups of cells for which there is no uniformly accepted terminology (see Alheid *et al.*, 1995). In the hamster, we have designated this region the posterointermediate BNST (BNSTpi). In contrast, the posterodorsal part of the medial nucleus (MePD), and in particular its caudal portion (cMePD), send projections over the same pathways to end in the medial area of the posterior BNST, which we have called the posteromedial subdivision of the BNST (BNSTpm) in the hamster (Gomez and Newman, 1992). Coolen and Wood (1998) have provided evidence that the connections between MeAD and BNSTpi and those between cMePD and BNSTpm in the hamster are not only dense and largely distinct from one another, but that they are also bidirectional. It is important to note, however, that although these two circuits are definably separate entities, they talk to each other via direct connections between MeAD and MePD (Gomez and Newman, 1992).

B. Neurotransmitter or Neuromodulator Continuity in the Posteromedial Extended Amygdala

In the rat, both the MeAD-BNSTpi and cMePD-BNSTpm circuits contain numerous neurons that produce glutamic acid decarboxylase and γ aminobutyric acid (GABA) (Swanson and Petrovich, 1998). A variety of other neurotransmitters and neuromodulators have

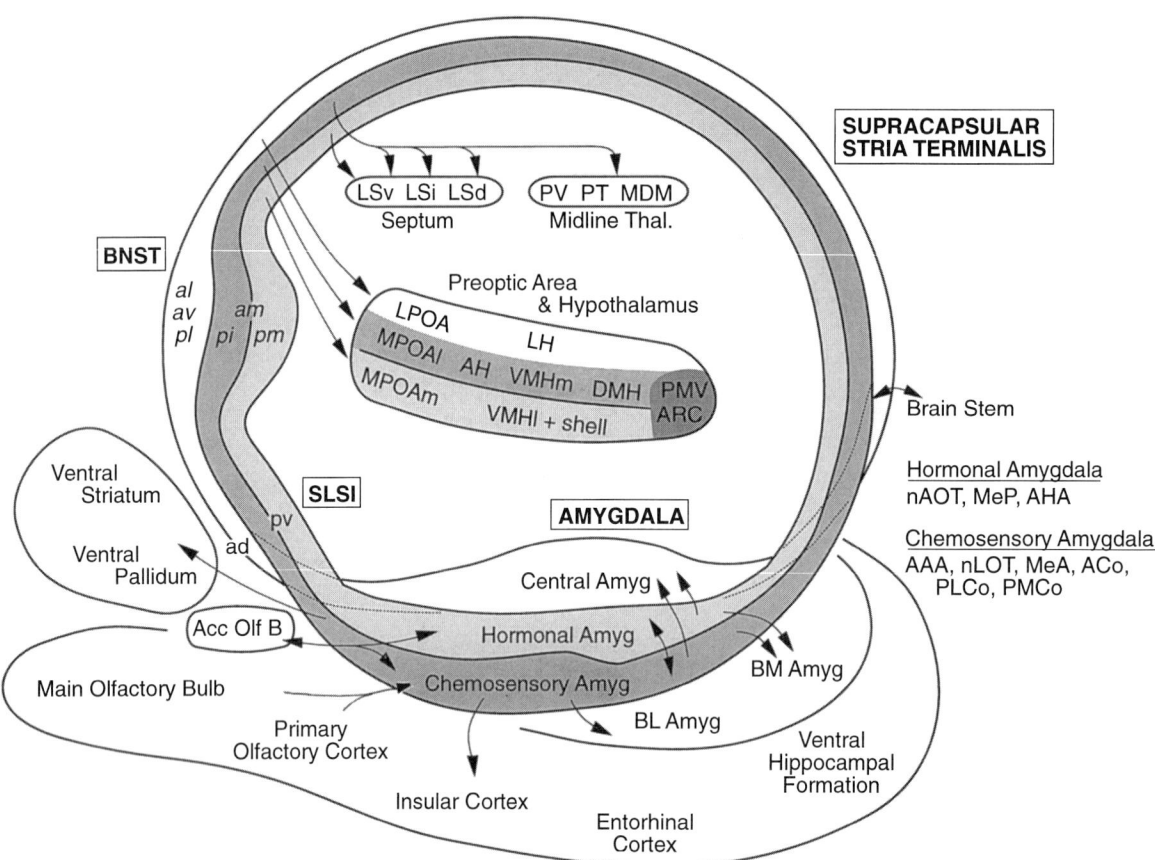

FIGURE 1 Neural circuitry through the central extended amygdala (shown in white) and two separate circuits in the medial extended amygdala: the chemosensory amygdala of the anterior division of the medial nucleus (MeA) (shown in dark shading), and the hormonal amygdala of the posterior division of the medial nucleus (MeP) (shown in light shading). The connections of each of these components of the extended amygdala to the nuclei of the preoptic area and hypothalamus are indicated in the center of the diagram. Common projections of both the anterior and posterior circuits to the ventral premammillary and arcuate nuclei are indicated by dark shading. AAA, anterior amygdaloid area; Acc Olf B, accessory olfactory bulb; Aco, anterior cortical nucleus of the amygdala; AH, anterior hypothalamus; AHA, amygdalo-hippocampal area; ARC, arcuate nucleus of the hypothalamus; BNSTal, BNSTam, BNSTav, BNSTpi, BNSTpl, BNSTpm, bed nucleus of the stria terminalis, anterolateral, anteromedial, anteroventral, posterointermediate, posterolateral, and posteromedial areas; DMH, dorsomedial nucleus of the hypothalamus; LH, lateral hypothalamus; LPOA, lateral preoptic area; LSd, LSi, LSv, lateral septum, dorsal, intermediate, and ventral; MDM, mediodorsal nucleus of the thalamus, medial division; MeA, medial nucleus of the amygdala, anterior division; MeP, medial nucleus of the amygdala, posterior division; MPOAl, MPOAm, medial preoptic area, lateral and medial parts; nAOT, nucleus of the accessory olfactory tract; nLOT, nucleus of the lateral olfactory tract; PLCo, posterolateral cortical nucleus of the amygdala; PMCo, posteromedial cortical nucleus of the amygdala; PMV, ventral premammillary nucleus; PT, paratenial nucleus of the thalamus; PV, paraventricular nucleus of the thalamus; SLSIad, SLSIpv, sublenticular substantia innominata, anterdorsal and posteroventral areas; VMHl, VMHm, ventromedial nucleus of the hypothalamus, lateral and medial parts. From Wood, R. I., and Newman, S. W. (1995). Hormonal influence on neurons of the mating behavior pathway in male hamsters. *In* "Neurobiological Effects of Sex Steroid Hormones" (P. E. Micevych and R. P. Hammer, eds.), p. 11. Copyright © by Cambridge University Press. Reprinted with permission.

been localized predominantly in the cMePD-BNSTpm circuit. This selective distribution of neuroactive substances, particularly neuropeptides, in the posterior circuit is also seen in the Syrian hamster, but there appear to be a number of differences between these two species. In both rat and hamster, the cMePD-BNSTpm system is characterized by numerous substance P neurons (Swann and Newman 1992; Eckersell and Micevych, 1997) and more limited populations of enkephalin-producing cells (Eckersell and Micevych, 1997; Holt, 1997). In the rat, arginine vasopressin (De Vries *et al.*, 1985) and cholecystokinin cells (Micevych *et al.*, 1988; Eckersell and Micevych, 1997) are also abundant in these nuclei, although they have not been localized here in the hamster brain (Albers *et al.*, 1992). In contrast, the hamster has populations of prodynorphin-producing neurons in these nuclei that are not found in the rat (Neal and Newman, 1989) and that overlap by at least 50% with the substance P cell population; that is, at least half of the substance P neurons in cMePD and in BNSTpm also contain prodynorphin and vice versa (Neal *et al.*, 1989). A fourth neurochemically distinctive group of cells localized in cMePD and BNSTpm, also found in the hamster but not in the rat brain, is a population of neurons that are immunoreactive for tyrosine hydroxylase (TH) and dopamine (Asmus *et al.*, 1992). The cells in this caudal MePD circuit differ from TH neurons in MeAD in their dopamine immunoreactivity and in the much larger proportion of the population (75% vs 30%) that contain androgen receptors (Asmus and Newman, 1993).

C. Gonadal Steroid Receptors and Sexual Dimorphism in the Medial Extended Amygdala

The density of gonadal steroid receptors is another important characteristic that distinguishes the cMePD-BNSTpm from the MeAD-BNSTpi circuit. In the rat, Syrian hamster, and gerbil, androgen and estrogen receptors are distributed primarily in the cMePD and BNSTpm (Commins and Yahr, 1985; Simerly *et al.*, 1990; Chen and Tu, 1992; Wood and Newman, 1993, 1995b). In the adult rat, these cell groups are sexually dimorphic with respect to nuclear volume (Mizukami *et al.*, 1983; Hines *et al.*, 1992), synaptic organization (Nishizuka and Arai, 1981, 1983), and neurotransmitters (De Vries *et al.*, 1985; van Leeuwen *et al.*, 1985; Malsbury and McKay, 1987, 1989; Micevych *et al.*, 1988). Furthermore, at least some of these sexually differentiated characteristics can be modulated by hormones in adulthood. Hormone-mediated mRNA or neuropeptide production has been demonstrated in the adult in cholecystokinin cells of this circuit in the rat (Simerly and Swanson, 1987; Oro *et al.*, 1988; Eckersell and Micevych, 1997) and in the substance P neurons in both rat and hamster (Swann and Newman, 1992; Eckersell and Micevych, 1997).

In addition, in both of these species, mounting behavior can be restored in castrated males with an implant of testosterone or its metabolite estradiol, delivered only to the MePD on one side of the brain (Rasia-Fihlo *et al.*, 1991; Wood and Newman, 1995c; Wood, 1996a), whereas similar implants in MeAD are ineffective in the hamster (Wood, 1996a). A testosterone implant that delivers hormone to the BNSTpm also reinstates this behavior (Wood and Newman, 1995c), but in the studies reported the cannulae delivered testosterone to both the BNST and the adjacent medial preoptic nucleus, where hormone delivery has a well-documented role in restoring male copulation (reviewed in Meisel and Sachs, 1994). These data therefore do not prove a role for hormones in the BNSTpm alone.

Taken together, these observations identify neuroanatomical, neurochemical, and neuroendocrine distinctions between the MeAD-BNSTpi circuit and the cMePD-BNSTpm circuit as well as continuity in the cMePD-BNSTpm circuit in these characteristics. They suggest that the caudal circuit may provide a substrate through which hormone fluctuations over diurnal, estrous, and seasonal breeding cycles modulate reproduction. They also demonstrate that limbic nuclei outside the medial preoptic area provide redundancy in the hormone-sensitive network subserving reproduction (Wood, 1996b, 1997).

VI. CONTINUITY OF FUNCTION IN THE MEDIAL EXTENDED AMYGDALA CIRCUITS: MALE SEXUAL BEHAVIOR

Lesions of the corticomedial amygdala produce sexual behavior deficits in male rats (Giantonio *et al.*, 1970;

Harris and Sachs, 1975; McGregor and Herbert, 1992; Kondo, 1992; de Jonge *et al.*, 1992), although the data from these studies do not indicate whether lesions of the anterior and posterior parts of this amygdalar region or of the medial nucleus in particular might have different effects on mating behaviors. Further, only one of the laboratories investigating this system, that of Sachs and his colleagues, examined whether the corticomedial amygdala might have functions in common with the BNST in control of copulation (Emery and Sachs, 1976; Valcourt and Sachs, 1979). After lesions in either the amygdala or BNST, these authors found increased intromission frequencies and ejaculation latencies. Thus, in the male rat we have some evidence for continuity of behavioral function in the medial extended amygdala.

Early lesion data in hamsters indicated that the MeAD and MePD play very different roles in the regulation of male sexual behavior. Males with lesions of the MeAD completely failed to mate and showed essentially no chemoinvestigatory behavior with the female (Lehman *et al.*, 1980; Lehman and Winans, 1982). In contrast, those with corticomedial lesions that included the caudal half of Me mated to ejaculation. However, the temporal pattern of their mating was altered, and they showed some decrement in chemoinvestigatory behavior (Lehman *et al.*, 1983). Over several weeks (and in some cases up to 2 months) of postoperative testing, the latency to ejaculation was consistently increased, primarily as a result of persisting increases in the number of intromissions preceding the first ejaculation and lengthened postejaculatory intervals preceding the second. In addition, these animals showed a decrease of approximately 30% in the rate of anogenital investigation of the female compared to sham-lesioned males. Thus, the contrast between behaviors of males with damage to the anterior vs the posterior medial nucleus was striking. Males with MeAD lesions essentially failed to engage in any chemoinvestigatory or copulatory activities, whereas those with lesions including MePD showed a modest although statistically significant decrease in chemoinvestigation and a lengthening of the copulatory sequence.

Subsequent data from hamsters with lesions of the BNST provided some evidence suggesting that the MeAD-BNSTpi and cMePD-BNSTpm circuits constitute functional as well as anatomical circuits (Powers *et al.*, 1987). The conclusions that can be drawn from these data are limited because in these studies no group of males had lesions entirely confined to either the BNSTpm or BNSTpi. However, histological analysis of behaviorally different groups revealed interesting differences in the brain areas damaged. A group of males with lesions that overlapped only in the BNSTpm, like males with cMePD damage, showed increased ejaculation latencies and decrements of approximately 50% in two different measures of chemoinvestigatory behavior—anogenital investigation of the female and attraction to female hamster vaginal secretions (FHVS) swabbed on the wall of a clean plastic arena. In contrast, a group of males with lesions that included damage to the BNSTpi as well as the BNSTpm at the level of the anterior commissure showed no copulatory behavior, only occasional mounts, or, in one case, ejaculations on one test out of four. Further, these males showed essentially no anogenital investigation in mating tests or response to FHVS in a clean cage. Thus, lesions that included the BNSTpi and BNSTpm, but not BNSTpm alone, produced deficits reminiscent of those seen after lesions of the MeAD, whereas the smaller lesions centered in the BNSTpm produced the same limited behavioral alterations seen after damage to the MePD.

Because all these studies employed electrolytic lesions, they destroyed fibers as well as nuclei and could not provide unambiguous evidence for the function of the cell groups in the damaged area. This was a particular problem with regard to the MePD and the BNSTpi because lesions in either of these areas inevitably damage the stria terminalis, carrying fibers from both the anterior and posterior divisions of the medial amygdala. Additional evidence was needed to test the hypothesis that cell groups in these two circuits of the extended amygdala play different roles in mating behavior.

Subsequent studies from several laboratories, based on *c-fos* gene expression during sexual behavior in male hamsters, have provided important support for this hypothesis. Cells in both MeAD-BNSTpi and cMePD-BNSTpm circuits significantly increase production of Fos protein in response to mating behavior (Kollack and Newman, 1992; Wood and Newman, 1993). However, the behavioral antecedents of this gene expression differ between the two circuits. Whereas selected groups of cells in both cMePD and BNSTpm show increased

Fos-immunoreactivity correlated with either chemoinvestigation or ejaculations (Fiber *et al.*, 1993; Fernandez-Fewell and Meredith, 1994; Kollack-Walker and Newman, 1997), neurons in MeAD and BNSTpi show a generalized and equivalent increase in Fos production after mating and after intermale aggressive encounters (Kollack-Walker and Newman, 1995). No specific motor function or sensory stimulation associated with either mating or agonistic behavior has been correlated with this increase in the MeAD circuit. Furthermore, increased expression of *c-fos* has been observed in MeAD and BNSTpi, not only after mating or aggression in males, but after mating or aggression in female hamsters (Joppa *et al.*, 1995; Potegal *et al.*, 1996). These findings, in conjunction with the observed elimination of sexual behavior after lesions of MeAD and after BNST lesions that include BNSTpi have led us to hypothesize that the MeAD-BNSTpi circuit of the extended amygdala is essential for arousal or nonspecific activation of social behaviors (Newman *et al.*, 1997). This notion is supported by recent observations that tail-pinching male rats, a procedure known to facilitate a variety of social behaviors in the presence of appropriate stimuli, also induces Fos immunoreactivity in this region of the medial amygdala (Smith *et al.*, 1997).

In contrast, cell groups in the MePD-BNSTpm circuit of the hamster appear to be activated selectively in response to discrete stimuli or mating events. Exposure of the male hamster to FHVS in the absence of the female increases Fos production in medial MePD and in the anterodorsal part of BNSTpm [BNSTpm(ad)] (Fiber *et al.*, 1993). This activity may be both olfactory and vomeronasal in origin because bilateral removal of the vomeronasal organs at day 17 significantly reduces but does not eliminate FHVS-mediated activation in these two areas in sexually naive male hamsters (Fernandez-Fewell and Meredith, 1994). In addition, mating to ejaculation produces a significant increase in Fos-ir in the posteroventral continuation of BNSTpm [BNSTpm(pv)] and in cMePD (Kollack-Walker and Newman, 1995). In the cMePD, clusters of labeled cells are apparent with Fos immunocytochemistry when the male nears sexual satiety, regardless of the absolute number of ejaculations exhibited (Parfitt and Newman, 1998). These densely packed Fos-immunoreactive cells in lateral cMePD have also been observed after copulatory behavior in male gerbils (Heeb and Yahr, 1996) and rats (Baum and Everitt, 1992; Coolen *et al.*, 1997b).

The data reviewed here on the functions of interconnected, neurochemically related cell groups in the medial amygdala and BNST of the male hamster and other rodents suggest that both anterior and posterior circuits are processing information important for normal mating behavior, but that they regulate different aspects of this behavior. Olfactory, vomeronasal, and somatosensory stimuli reaching the MeAD-BNSTpi circuit produce a general behavioral arousal, the readiness to respond to specific signals with appropriate action. Through the cMePD-BNSTpm circuit, hormones maintain cell groups that respond to those discrete signals (e.g., odors of male vs female, estrous vs nonestrous, kin vs nonkin) and other cell groups that determine the pattern of the behavioral response. Integration of these functions, as noted earlier, occurs by interconnections between them (Gomez and Newman, 1992).

The evidence reviewed here for functional unity between cell populations in the amygdala and the BNST supports the concept of the extended amygdala. It also expands the distinction between the central extended amygdala and the medial extended amygdala by suggesting that there is more than one functional extended amygdala circuit in the medial extended amygdala.

Canteras *et al.* (1995) and Swanson and Petrovich (1998) have objected to the concept of the extended amygdala on a variety of grounds. Swanson and Petrovich suggest that the amygdala is not an entity but rather an amalgam of dissimilar areas that would more appropriately be reassigned to the cerebral cortex (nuclei of the cortical and basolateral divisions) or to the striatum (the medial and central nuclei). They further suggest that in this framework, the BNST should be recognized as a pallidal element in the forebrain. Heimer *et al.* (1997) argue that the patterns of connections between amygdala and BNST, which are reciprocal and equally heavy in both directions, are unlike the predominantly unidirectional projections from striatal to related pallidal elements. Further study, analysis, and scholarly debate are clearly needed before we reach an agreement on a place for the amygdala and BNST in the organization of the forebrain. Whatever that place, the structural and functional continuity of units in the medial amygdala and the BNST will have to be accommodated.

VII. ROLES OF THE MEDIAL EXTENDED AMYGDALA IN OTHER SOCIAL BEHAVIORS

Ascribing discrete components of behavior to the activity of discrete neuroanatomical units is a basic part of the process of delineating functional pathways in the central nervous system. Since the 1980s, this process has led to the identification of sites in the extended amygdala that play a role in male mating behavior. During this period, the same process has been successfully pursued in delineating neural circuits required for or activated by other social behaviors in rodents, including female sexual behavior (Pfaff et al., 1994; Dudley et al., 1996; Erskine and Hanrahan, 1997), aggression (Kollack-Walker and Newman, 1995; Joppa et al., 1995; Potegal et al., 1996; Albert and Chew, 1980; Kruk et al., 1984; Luiten et al., 1985; Depaulis et al., 1992; Roeling et al., 1994), territorial marking (Ferris et al., 1990; Hennessey et al., 1992), and maternal behavior (Numan and Sheehan, 1997; Rosenblatt et al., 1994; Lonstein and Stern, 1997). Taken together, these studies reveal a significant amount of overlap in the circuitry responsible for the behaviors—a result that was largely unexpected. Thus data from studies employing a wide variety of paradigms, including discrete lesions, electrical stimulation, localized hormonal or neuropharmacological manipulations, and immediate early gene expression, have led investigators studying male and female social behaviors to implicate a common group of limbic areas, including nuclear groups in the medial extended amygdala, the lateral septum (LS), the MPOA, the anterior hypothalamus (AH), the ventromedial nucleus and adjacent ventrolateral hypothalamus, and the midbrain periaqueductal gray and adjacent tegmentum.

Together these brain areas influence not only male and female sexual behavior and maternal behavior, but also the reproductive-related behaviors, such as territorial marking, territorial aggression, and maternal aggression. In fact, the data gathered on neural circuits subserving social behaviors force us to consider the possibility that these structures form an integrated social behavior circuit—a network much like the cortical networks that subserve cognitive functions such as learning and memory or language, but in this case a subcortical limbic network that subserves the entire spectrum of sex-steroid-modulated social behaviors. Obviously not every brain structure that plays a role in any one of these behaviors is a candidate member of such a network; there are important additional areas not mentioned in this particular grouping that subserve specific social behavior reflexes or behavior patterns. Nor does this grouping include all of the sexually dimorphic brain areas that integrate endocrine function with social behaviors (Simerly, 1995). Each of the areas illustrated in Fig. 2 also belongs to other functional circuits through connections that they do not share with all members of this basic network. However, all these areas fulfill several important criteria for nodes in a social behavior network. Each of these six areas is reciprocally interconnected anatomically with all of the others (Simerly and Swanson, 1988; Maragos et al., 1989; Shipley et al., 1991; Rizvi et al., 1992; Canteras et al., 1994, 1995; Risold et al., 1994; Jakab and Leranth, 1995; Simerly, 1995; Coolen and Wood, 1998). Each of these areas is populated with neurons that produce gonadal hormone receptors (Rees et al., 1980; Cottingham and Pfaff, 1986; Commins and Yahr, 1985; Simerly et al., 1990;

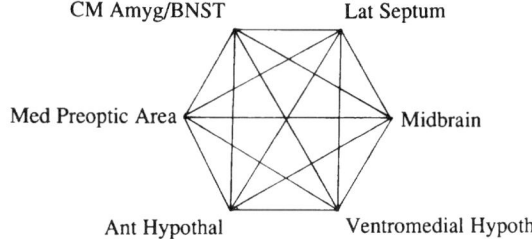

FIGURE 2 Six limbic system areas that are reciprocally interconnected anatomically, each of which is populated with neurons that are sensitive to gonadal steroids and has been implicated in the regulation of more than one mammalian social behavior. Each of these areas is a candidate node for a neuroanatomical network that regulates sexual, aggressive, and parental behaviors in both sexes of mammals. Ant Hypothal, anterior hypothalamus; CM Amyg/BNST, corticomedial amygdala–bed nucleus of the stria terminalis (medial extended amygdala); Lat septum, lateral septum; Med Preoptic Area, medial preoptic area; Midbrain, midbrain periaqueductal gray and tegmentum; Ventromedial Hypothal, ventromedial hypothalamus.

Wood and Newman, 1995b). Finally, each of these areas has been identified as an important site of regulation or activation in more than one social behavior. This last point is most readily documented by enumerating separate experiments, each demonstrating a role for one or several brain areas in social behavior. Collectively these reports indicate that each area participates in more than one behavior—lateral septum (Albert and Chew, 1980; Ferris et al., 1990; Pfaff et al., 1994; Heeb and Yahr, 1996; Kollack-Walker and Newman, 1997), medial extended amygdala (Harris and Sachs, 1975; Emery and Sachs, 1976; Valcourt and Sachs, 1979; Lehman and Winans, 1982; Luiten et al., 1985; Powers et al., 1987; Chateau and Aron, 1988; Potegal et al., 1996; Heeb and Yahr, 1996; Dudley et al., 1996; Erskine and Hanrahan, 1997; Coolen et al., 1997b; Numan and Sheehan, 1997; Parfitt and Newman, 1998), medial preoptic area (Lisk, 1962; Powers and Valenstein, 1972; Baum and Everitt, 1992; reviwed in Meisel and Sachs, 1994; Joppa et al., 1995; Heeb and Yahr, 1996; Numan and Sheehan, 1997), anterior hypothalamus (Ferris et al., 1990; Kollack-Walker and Newman, 1997), ventromedial and ventrolateral hypothalamus (Pfaff et al., 1994; Kollack-Walker and Newman, 1995; Dudley et al., 1996; Heeb and Yahr, 1996; Erskine and Hanrahan, 1997; Numan and Sheehan, 1997), midbrain periaqueductal gray and tegmentum (Baum and Everitt, 1992; Depaulis et al., 1992; Hennessey et al., 1992; Pfaff et al., 1994; Rosenblatt et al., 1994; Kollack-Walker and Newman, 1995, 1997; Heeb and Yahr, 1996; Coolen et al., 1997a; Lonstein and Stern, 1997; Numan and Sheehan, 1997). Only occasionally do these studies analyze the same brain area or areas in the context of more than one type of social behavior (Malsbury et al., 1977; McGregor and Herbert, 1992; Nyby et al., 1992; Rosenblatt et al., 1994; Kollack-Walker and Newman, 1995; Joppa et al., 1995; Lonstein and Stern, 1997) or in both females and males (Leedy and Hart, 1985; Luiten et al., 1985; Coolen et al., 1996), but these approaches are particularly useful in exploring the concept of a network with multiple functions.

In what way could a common neuroanatomical network provide a substrate for the broad behavioral repertoire we must consider under the category of social behaviors? Again, borrowing an important concept from

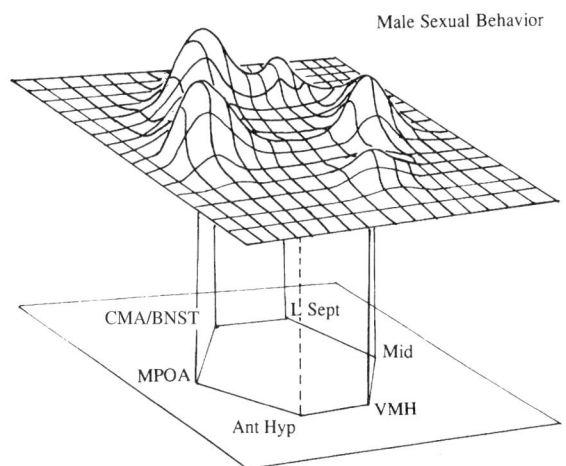

FIGURE 3 An hypothetical representation of the pattern of activity in the mammalian social behavior network at the outset of male sexual behavior. CMA/BNST, corticomedial amygdala–bed nucleus of the stria terminalis (medial extended amygdala); MPOA, medial preoptic area; L Sept, lateral septum; Mid, midbrain periaqueductal gray and tegmentum; VMH, ventromedial hypothalamus; Ant Hyp, anterior hypothalamus.

our colleagues in cognitive neuroscience, we envision that a particular social behavior (e.g., male sexual behavior) is an emergent property of the pattern of activity across the network (Mesulam, 1990) (Fig. 3). It is not an action produced by the on or off state of any one of the nodes such as the MPOA, but a sequence of multiple behaviors (sniffing, mounting, ejaculating, grooming, etc.) that is initiated by and emerges from a temporal pattern, and therefore a dynamic pattern, of activity across the network. The initiation and maintenance of male sexual behavior, then, requires activation of the MPOA, but in conjunction with particular levels of activation of other areas in the network and in the context of a unique temporal pattern of activation across the whole network. It is important to note here that in some of these behaviors a given node in the network appears to play an excitatory role and must be activated (e.g., the MPOA in male sexual behavior and in maternal behavior), whereas in other behaviors this area may play an inhibitory role (e.g., the MPOA in female sexual behavior). Other similar but distinguishable patterns of activity in this same circuit (Fig. 4), arising as a result of changing sensory stimuli or fluctuations

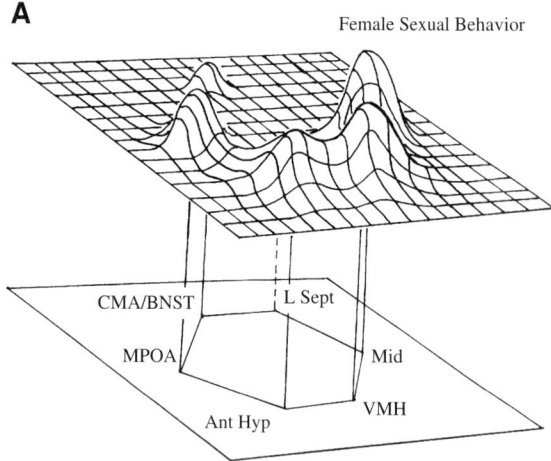

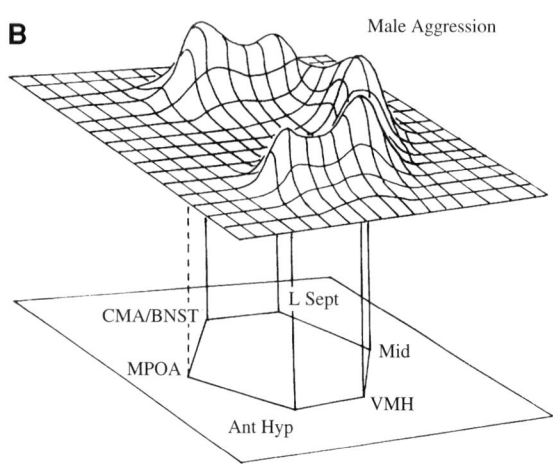

FIGURE 4 Hypothetical representations of the patterns of activity in the mammalian social behavior network at the outset of (A) female sexual behavior and (B) male aggression. CMA/BNST, corticomedial amygdala–bed nucleus of the stria terminalis (medial extended amygdala); MPOA, medial preoptic area; L Sept, lateral septum; Mid, midbrain periaqueductal gray and tegmentum; VMH, ventromedial hypothalamus; Ant Hyp, anterior hypothalamus.

in the hormonal milieu, could result in a progression of behaviors flowing seamlessly from one to another (e.g., territorial marking and aggressive activities interspersed with copulatory acts to produce the full spectrum of mating behavior observed in a variety of species).

Both the social behaviors that arise from activation of this circuit and the neuronal groups that it comprises share a variety of basic developmental and physiological determinants. Clearly, the fundamental developmental determinants are the species and sex of the individual. The species of the animal determines the organization and connections of brain areas and whether they will be responsive to sex steroids, characteristics that are highly conserved in mammals. The species also determines the timing of critical periods for sensitivity to hormones during perinatal development, which is more variable. The genetic sex of the animal determines whether sex steroids will be available to the brain during those critical periods. As a result of steroid action, the network becomes sexually dimorphic with respect to the number of cells and the specific cell types produced in each node. This, in turn, influences the baseline number and types of sex steroid receptors produced by those cells and the strength of connections between nodes in the network. It is these factors that ultimately regulate the predisposition, but not routinely predictable or exclusive function, of the network to produce particular patterns of activity in a given individual, such as male vs female sexual behavior.

These same factors, sex steroid sensitivity and neuronal connections, are of course dynamically modulated throughout life—by sexual maturation, by experience or learning, by reproductive cycles and diurnal cycles, and by disease and aging. Within a shorter time frame, they are modified by sensory stimuli from other animals—by odor, touch, color, motion, and sounds. The pheromones from the female hamster, the flank and vaginal somatosensory stimulation to the female rat, the colorful perineal skin displayed by the female monkey, and the estrous call of the female cat all have short-term effects that modify the functioning of the social behavior network in the receiver. At the very least, these stimuli produce immediate changes in synaptic activity in the nodes of the social behavior network. In some cases, the effects are long-lasting changes in the strength of synaptic connections. In all mammals, all of the sensory systems have access to the sexually dimorphic social behavior network, but all sensory modalities are not equally important in eliciting particular behaviors. Coming full circle, the modalities that are the most salient to an individual animal's social responses are determined, through evolution, by its species and by its sex, in other words, by its genes.

This way of looking at the neural circuits for social behaviors has appealing simplicity. It may appear at first glance to be a useless oversimplification, but it is introduced here as a framework within which to view the data we have collected. It is intended not as an excuse to abandon our efforts to identify behavioral functions attributable to specific cell groups in these areas, but as a way to integrate our findings. It is now clear that male and female courtship behaviors, copulation, attacks, submissiveness, territorial marking, nest building, nursing, guarding of the mate, and protection of the young are regulated by overlapping neural pathways. If we are to sustain the labeled-line point of view, this social behavior network will have to be teased apart at the level of intermingled cell populations in individual limbic nuclei. We will need to demonstrate minicircuits in this network, each one independently regulating a specific aspect of a particular behavior.

This is what I argue in the first part of this chapter. For example, Coolen et al. (1997a), Heeb and Yahr (1996), Kollack-Walker and Newman (1997), and Parfitt and Newman (1998) have indicated that there are small clusters of neurons embedded in the cMePD of male rats, gerbils, and hamsters that are activated when these animals have ejaculated and are reaching sexual satiety. Can we conclude that collectively we have identified a unique minicircuit that is involved in timing and terminating ejaculatory behavior, an exclusively male-typical behavior? Yes and no. We may be forced to abandon the exclusively male-typical point of view when we see the same cell groups activated by vaginocervical stimulation in the female rat, as has been demonstrated clearly by Pfaus et al. (1993), Dudley et al. (1996), and Erskine and Hanrahan (1997). But we are led to what may be a more useful hypothesis—that these cells regulate the timing of both male and female sexual behaviors, an aspect of these behaviors that is critical for the successful end point of copulation, pregnancy (Adler, 1969; Lanier et al., 1975; Huck and Lisk, 1985a,b).

The concept of overlapping functions for a single neuroanatomical network is not an original insight. A number of investigators have noted the duality of function, or multiple functions, of areas in this circuit (Barfield, 1984; de Jonge and van de poll, 1984; Luiten et al., 1985; Nyby et al., 1992; Joppa et al., 1995; Simerly, 1995). However, it clearly will be more difficult to test the hypothesis that individual cell groups have multiple functions than to pursue the more traditional hypothesis that there are intermingled labeled-line minicircuits with separate functions in the same brain areas. A first step might be to actively look for evidence of multiple social behavior functions in studies in which identifiable cells groups (e.g., cells in a specific transmitter circuit) are being manipulated or monitored.

Since the 1970s, we have struggled to dissect the social behaviors of mammals in terms of sensory stimulation, physiological prerequisites, and neuroanatomical substrates. The results of our collective efforts suggest that these behaviors may actually emerge from the activity of a unitary neuroanatomical framework in the CNS. We have learned that this network develops and functions under the influence of gonadal hormones, again with a common denominator, estradiol, across species and sexes. Significant differences in the hormonally influenced behaviors emerging from this network, not only across species and sexes, but over time in individuals, arise primarily from the amount of estrogen available to its neurons during development and by the temporal pattern of estrogen availability in adulthood. All the nodes of this neuroanatomical network are responsive to sex hormones.

A greater diversity in this picture of social behaviors appears to be the sensory stimuli that drive them. Clear species and sex differences in the saliency of various sensory systems have evolved through adaptation to different ecological niches, to nocturnal vs diurnal living and to communal vs noncommunal social systems. However, all sensory systems have access to the limbic network that drives social behaviors in mammals. What we originally viewed as evidence for different social behavior pathways more likely reflects sex and species differences in the weighting of sensory system influences on a common central network. If, in fact, all social behaviors actually emerge from a unitary neuroanatomical framework and shared physiological determinants, our understanding of these behaviors and the neural system that supports them may be greatly advanced by focusing not on the differences but on the common themes arising from our studies of all social behaviors in both sexes and in diverse species.

Acknowledgments

This chapter is gratefully dedicated to my graduate students, postdoctoral fellows, and research associates, who provided the inspiration, insight, and hard work for our studies together. Our research was performed in the Department of Anatomy and Cell Biology, University of Michigan, and was supported by Public Health Service grants from NINDS.

References

Adler, N. T. (1969). Effects of the male's copulatory behavior on successful pregnancy of the female rat. *J. Comp. Physiol. Psychol.* **69**, 613–622.

Albers, H. E., Hennessey, A. C., and Whitman, D. C. (1992). Vasopressin and the regulation of hamster social behavior. *Ann. N. Y. Acad. Sci.* **652**, 227–242.

Albert, D. J., and Chew, G. L. (1980). The septal forebrain and the inhibitory modulation of attack and defense in the rat. A review. *Behav Neural Biol.* **30**, 357–388.

Alheid, G. F., and Heimer, L. (1988). New perspectives in basal forebrain organization of special relevance for neuropsychiatric disorders: The striatopallidal, amygdaloid and corticopetal components of substantia innominata. *Neuroscience* **27**, 1–39.

Alheid, G. F., de Olmos, J. S., and Beltramino, C. A. (1995). Amygdala and extended amygdala. *In* "The Rat Nervous System" (G. Paxinos, ed.), 2nd ed., pp. 495–578. Academic Press, San Diego, CA.

Asmus, S. E., and Newman, S. W. (1993). Tyrosine hydroxylase neurons in the male hamster chemosensory pathway contain androgen receptors and are influenced by gonadal hormones. *J. Comp. Neurol.* **331**, 445–457.

Asmus, S. E., Kincaid, A. E., and Newman, S. W. (1992). A species-specific population of tyrosine hydroxylase-immunoreactive neurons in the medial amygdaloid nucleus of the Syrian hamster brain. *Brain Res.* **575**, 199–207.

Barfield, R. J. (1984). Reproductive hormones and aggressive behavior. *In* "Biological Perspectives on Aggression" (K. J. Flannelly, R. J. Blanchard, and D. C. Blanchard, eds.), pp. 105–134. Liss, New York.

Baum, M. J., and Everitt, B. J. (1992). Increased expression of *c-fos* in the medial preoptic area after mating in male rats: Role of afferent inputs from the medial amygdala and midbrain central tegmental field. *Neuroscience* **50**, 627–646.

Beauchamp, G. K., Yamazaki, K., Wysocki, C. J., Slotnick, B. M., and Boyse, T. (1985). Chemosensory recognition of mouse major histocompatibility types by another species. *Proc. Natl. Acad. Sci. U.S.A.* **82**, 4186–4188.

Canteras, N. S., Simerly, R. B., and Swanson, L. W. (1994). Organization of projections from the ventromedial nucleus of the hypothalamus: A *Phaseolus vulgaris*-leucoagglutinin study in the rat. *J. Comp. Neurol.* **348**, 41–79.

Canteras, N. S., Simerly, R. B., and Swanson, L. W. (1995). Organization of projections from the medial nucleus of the amygdala: A PHAL study in the rat. *J. Comp. Neurol.* **360**, 213–245.

Chateau, D., and Aron, C. (1988). Heterotypic sexual behavior in male rats after lesions in different amygdaloid nuclei. *Horm. Behav.* **22**, 379–388.

Chen, T. J., and Tu, W. W. (1992). Sex differences in estrogen and androgen receptors in hamster brain. *Life Sci.* **50**, 1639–1647.

Clancy, A. N., Singer, A. G., Macrides, F., Bronson, F. H., and Agosta, W. C. (1988). Experiential and Endocrine dependence of gonadotropin responses in male mice to conspecific odors. *Biol. Reprod.* **38**, 183–192.

Commins, D., and Yahr, P. (1985). Autoradiographic localization of estrogen and androgen receptors in the sexually dimorphic area and other regions of the gerbil brain. *J. Comp. Neurol.* **231**, 473–489.

Coolen, L. M., and Wood, R. I. (1998). Bidirectional connections of the medial amygdaloid nucleus in the Syrian hamster brain: Simultaneous anterograde and retrograde tract tracing. *J. Comp. Neurol.* **399**, 189–209.

Coolen, L. M., Peters, H. J. P. W., and Veening, J. G. (1996). Fos immunoreactivity in the rat brain following cosummatory elements of sexual behavior: A sex comparison. *Brain Res.* **738**, 67–82.

Coolen, L. M., Olivier, B., Peters, H. J. P. W., and Veening, J. G. (1997a). Demonstration of ejaculation-induced neural activity in the male rat brain using 5-HT$_{1A}$ agonist 8-OH-DPAT. *Physiol. Behav.* **62**, 881–891.

Coolen, L. M., Peters, H. J. P. W., and Veening, J. G. (1997b). Distribution of Fos immunoreactivity following mating versus anogenital investigation in the male rat brain. *Neuroscience* **77**, 1151–1161.

Cottingham, S. L., and Pfaff, D. W. (1986). Interconnectedness of steroid hormone-binding neurons: existence and implications. *Curr. Top. Neuroendocrinol.* **7**, 223–249.

Davis, B. J., Macrides, F., Young, W. M., Schneider, S. P., and Rosene, D. L. (1978). Efferents and centrifugal afferents of the main and accessory olfactory bulbs in the hamster. *Brain Res. Bull.* **3**, 59–72.

de Jonge, F. H., and van de Poll, N. E. (1984). Relationships between sexual and aggressive behavior in male and female rats: Effects of gonadal hormones. *Prog. Brain Res.* **61**, 283–302.

de Jonge, F. H., Oldenburger, W. P., Louwerse, A. L., and van de Poll, N. E. (1992). Changes in male copulatory behavior after sexual exciting stimuli: Effects of medial amygdala lesions. *Physiol. Behav.* **52**, 327–332.

de Olmos, J. S., Alheid, G. F., and Beltramino, C. A., (1985). Amygdala. *In* "The Rat Nervous System" (G. Paxinos, ed.), 1st ed., pp. 223–334. Academic Press, New York.

Depaulis, A., Keay, K. A., and Bandler, R. (1992). Longitudinal neuronal organization of defensive reactions in the midbrain periaqueductal gray region of the rat. *Exp. Brain Res.* **90**, 307–318.

De Vries, G. J., Buijs, R. M., van Leeuwen, F. W., Caffe, A. R., and Swaab, D. F. (1985). The vasopressinergic innervation of the brain in normal and castrated rats. *J. Comp. Neurol.* **233**, 236–254.

Dudley, C. A., Rajendren, G., and Moss, R. L. (1996). Signal processing in the vomeronasal system: modulation of sexual behavior in the female rat. *Crit. Rev. Neurobiol.* **10**, 265–290.

Eckersell, C. B., and Micevych, P. E. (1997). Opiate receptors modulate estrogen-induced cholecystokinin and tachykinin but not enkephalin messenger RNA levels in the limbic system and hypothalamus. *Neuroscience* **80**, 473–485.

Emery, D. E., and Sachs, B. D. (1976). Copulatory behavior in male rats with lesions in the bed nucleus of the stria terminalis. *Physiol. Behav.* **17**, 803–806.

Erskine, M. S., and Hanrahan, S. B. (1997). Effects of paced mating on c-*fos* gene expression in the female rat brain. *J. Neuroendocrinol.* **9**, 903–912.

Fernandez-Fewell, G. D., and Meredith, M. (1994). c-Fos expression in vomeronasal pathways of mated or pheromone-stimulated male golden hamsters: Contributions from vomeronasal sensory input and expression related to mating performance. *J. Neurosci.* **14**, 3643–3654.

Ferris, C. F., Gold, L., De Vries, G. J., and Potegal, M. (1990). Evidence for a functional and anatomical relationship between the lateral septum and the hypothalamus in the control of flank marking behavior in Golden hamsters. *J. Comp. Neurol.* **293**, 476–485.

Fiber, J. M., Adames, P., and Swann, J. M. (1993). Pheromones induce c-*fos* in limbic areas regulating male hamster mating behavior. *NeuroReport* **4**, 871–874.

Giantonio, G. W., Lund, N. L., and Gerall, A. A. (1970). Effect of diencephalic and rhinencephalic lesions on the male rat's sexual behavior. *J. Comp. Phsyiol. Psychol.* **73**, 38–46.

Gomez, D. M., and Newman, S. W. (1992). Differential projections of the anterior and posterior regions of the medial amygdaloid nucleus in the Syrian hamster. *J. Comp. Neurol.* **317**, 195–218.

Halpern, M. (1987). The organization and function of the vomeronasal system. *Annu. Rev. Neurosci.* **10**, 325–362.

Harris, V. S., and Sachs, B. D. (1975). Copulatory behavior in male rats following amygdaloid lesions. *Brain Res.* **86**, 514–518.

Heeb, M. M., and Yahr, P. (1996). c-*fos* immunoreactivity in the sexually dimorphic area of the hypothalamus and related brain regions of male gerbils after exposure to sex-related stimuli or performance of specific sexual behaviors. *Neuroscience* **72**, 1049–1071.

Heimer, L., and Larsson, K. (1967). Mating behavior of male rats after olfactory bulb lesions. *Physiol. Behav.* **2**, 207–209.

Heimer, L., Harlan, R. E., Alheid, G. F., Garcia, M. M., and de Olmos, J. (1997). Substantia innominata: A notion which impedes clinical-anatomical correlations in neuropsychiatric disorders. *Neuroscience* **76**, 957–1006.

Hennessey, A. C., Whitman, D. C., and Albers, H. E. (1992). Microinjection of arginine vasopressin into the periaqueductal gray stimulates flank marking in Syrian hamsters (*Mesocricetus auratus*). *Brain Res.* **569**, 136–140.

Hines, M., Allen, L. S., and Gorski, R. (1992). Sex differences in subregions of the medial nucleus of the amygdala and the bed nucleus of the stria terminalis of the rat. *Brain Res.* **579**, 321–326.

Holt, A. G. (1997). Immunocytochemical identification of met- and leu-enkephalin positive neurons within mating and agonistic relevant brain nuclei of the male Syrian hamster: Modulation by gonadal steroids and social behaviors. Ph.D. Thesis, University of Michigan, Ann Arbor.

Huck, U., and Lisk, R. (1985a). Determinants of mating success in the golden hamster (*Mesocricetus auratus*): I. Male capacity. *J. Comp. Psychol.* **99**, 98–107.

Huck, U., and Lisk, R. (1985b). Determinants of mating success in the Golden hamster (*Mesocricetus auratus*): II. Pregnancy initiation. *J. Comp. Psychol.* **99**, 231–239.

Jakab, R. L., and Leranth, C. (1995). Septum. In "The Rat Nervous System" (G. Paxinos, ed.), 2nd ed., pp. 405–442. Academic Press, San Diego, CA.

Joppa, M. A., Meisel, R. L., and Garber, M. A. (1995). c-Fos expression in female hamster brain following sexual and aggressive behaviors. *Neuroscience* **68**, 783–792.

Keverne, E. B., Murphy, C. L., Silver, W. L., Wysocki, C. J., and Meredith, M. (1986). Non-olfactory chemoreceptors of the nose: Recent advances in understanding the vomeronasal and trigeminal systems. *Chem. Senses* **11**, 119–134.

Kevetter, G. A., and Winans, S. S. (1981). Efferents of the corticomedial amygdala in the golden hamster. I. Efferents of the 'vomeronasal amygdala.' *J. Comp. Neurol.* **197**, 81–98.

Kollack, S. S., and Newman, S. W. (1992). Mating behavior induces selective expression of Fos protein within the chemosensory pathways of the male Syrian hamster brain. *Neurosci. Lett.* **143**, 223–228.

Kollack-Walker, S., and Newman, S. W. (1995). Mating and agonistic behavior produce different patterns of Fos immunolabeling in the male Syrian hamster. *Neuroscience* **66**, 721–736.

Kollack-Walker, S., and Newman, S. W. (1997). Mating-induced expression of c-*fos* in the male Syrian hamster brain: Role of experience, pheromones, and ejaculations. *J. Neurobiol.* **32**, 481–501.

Kondo, Y. (1992). Lesions of the medial amygdala produce severe impairment of copulatory behavior in sexually inexperienced male rats. *Physiol. Behav.* **51**, 939–943.

Krettek, J. E., and Price, J. L. (1978). Amygdaloid projections to subcortical structures within the basal forebrain and brainstem in the rat and cat. *J. Comp. Neurol.* **178**, 225–254.

Kruk, M. R., Van Der Laan, C. E., Mos, J., van der Poel, A. M., Meelis, W., and Olivier, B. (1984). Comparison of aggressive behavior induced by electrical stimulation in the hypothalamus of male and female rats. *Prog. Brain Res.* **61**, 303–314.

Lanier, D. L., Estep, D. Q., and Dewsbury, D. A. (1975). Copulatory behavior of Golden hamsters: Effects on pregnancy. *Physiol. Behav.* **15**, 209–212.

Larsson, K., and Heimer, L. (1964). Mating behavior of male rats after lesions in the medial preoptic area. *Nature. (London)* **202**, 413–414.

Leedy, M. G., and Hart, B. L. (1985). Female and male sexual responses in female cats with ventromedial hypothalamic lesions. *Behav. Neurosci.* **99**, 936–941.

Lehman, M. N., and Winans, S. S. (1982). Vomeronasal and olfactory pathways to the amygdala controlling male hamster sexual behavior: Autoradiographic and behavioral analyses. *Brain Res.* **240**, 27–41.

Lehman, M. N., Winans, S. S., and Powers, J. B. (1980). Medial nucleus of the amygdala mediates chemosensory control of male hamster sexual behavior. *Science* **210**, 557–560.

Lehman, M. N., Powers, J. B., and Winans, S. S. (1983). Stria terminalis lesions alter the temporal pattern of copulatory behavior in the male Golden hamster. *Behav. Brain Res.* **8**, 109–128.

Lisk, R. D. (1962). Diencephalic placement of estradiol and sexual receptivity in the female rat. *Am. J. Physiol.* **203**, 493–496.

Lonstein, J. S., and Stern, J. M. (1997). Role of the midbrain periaqueductal gray in maternal nurturance and aggression: C-fos and electrolytic lesion studies in lactating rats. *J. Neurosci.* **17**, 3364–3378.

Luiten, P. G. M., Koolhaas, J. M., de Boer, S., and Koopmans, S. J. (1985). The cortico-medial amygdala in the central nervous system organization of agonistic behavior. *Brain Res.* **332**, 283–297.

Malsbury, C. W., and McKay, K. (1987). A sex difference in the pattern of substance P-like immunoreactivity in the bed nucleus of the stria terminalis. *Brain Res.* **420**, 365–370.

Malsbury, C. W., and McKay, K. (1989). Sex difference in the substance P-immunoreactive innervation of the medial nucleus of the amygdala. *Brain Res. Bull.* **23**, 561–567.

Malsbury, C. W., Kow, L.-M., and Pfaff, D. W. (1977). Effects of medial hypothalamic lesions on the lordosis response and other behaviors in female Golden hamsters. *Physiol. Behav.* **19**, 223–237.

Maragos, W. R., Newman, S. W., Lehman, M. N., and Powers, J. B. (1989). Neurons of origin and fiber trajectory of amygdalofugal projections to the medial preoptic area in Syrian hamsters. *J. Comp. Neurol.* **280**, 59–71.

McClintock, M. K. (2000). Human pheromones: Primers, releasers, signalers, or modulators? *In* "Reproduction in Context" (K. Wallen and J. Schneider, eds.), pp. 355–420. MIT Press, Cambridge, MA.

McGregor, A., and Herbert, J. (1992). Differential effects of excitotoxic basolateral and corticomedial lesions of the amygdala on the behavioural and endocrine responses to either sexual or aggression-promoting stimuli in the male rat. *Brain Res.* **574**, 9–20.

Meisel, R. L., and Sachs, B. D. (1994). The physiology of male sexual behavior. *In* "The Physiology of Reproduction" (E. Knobil and J. D. Neill, eds.), 2nd ed., pp. 3–105. Raven Press, New York.

Meredith, M. (1986). Vomeronasal organ removal before sexual experience impairs male hamster mating behavior. *Physiol. Behav.* **36**, 737–743.

Meredith, M. (1991). Sensory processing in the main and accessory olfactory systems: Comparisons and contrasts. *J. Steroid Biochem. Mol. Biol.* **39**, 601–614.

Meredith, M., and Fernandez-Fewell, G. (1994). Vomeronasal system, LHRH, and sex behavior. *Psychoneuroendocrinology* **19**, 657–672.

Mesulam, M.-M. (1990). Large-scale neurocognitive networks and distributed processing for attention, language and memory. *Ann. Neurol.* **28**, 597–613.

Micevych, P., Akesson, T., and Elde, R. (1988). Distribution of cholecystokinin-immunoreactive cell bodies in the male and female rat: II. Bed nucleus of the stria terminalis and amygdala. *J. Comp. Neurol.* **269**, 381–391.

Mizukami, S., Nishizuka, M., and Arai, Y. (1983). Sexual difference in nuclear volume and its ontogeny in the rat amygdala. *Exp. Neurol.* **79**, 569–575.

Murphy, M. R., and Schneider, G. E. (1970). Olfactory bulb removal eliminates mating behavior in the male golden hamster. *Science* **167**, 302–304.

Neal, C. R., Jr., and Newman, S. W. (1989). Prodynorphin peptide distribution in the forebrain of the Syrian hamster and rat: A comparative study with antisera against dynorphin A, dynorphin B and the C-terminus of the prodynorphin precursor molecule. *J. Comp. Neurol.* **288**, 353–386.

Neal, C. R., Jr., Swann, J. M., and Newman, S. W. (1989). The colocalization of substance P and prodynorphin immunoreactivity in neurons of the medial preoptic area, bed nucleus of the stria terminalis and medial nucleus of the amygdala of the Syrian hamster. *Brain Res.* **496**, 1–13.

Newman, S. W. (1999). The medial extended amygdala in male reproductive behavior: A node in the mammalian social behavior network. *Ann. N. Y. Acad. Sci.* **877**, 242–257.

Newman, S. W., Parfitt, D. B., and Kollack-Walker, S. (1997). Mating-induced c-*fos* expression patterns complement and supplement observations after lesions in the male Syrian hamster brain. *Ann. N. Y. Acad. Sci.* **807**, 239–259.

Nishizuka, M., and Arai, Y. (1981). Sexual dimorphism in synaptic organization in the amygdala and its dependence on neonatal hormone environment. *Brain Res.* **212**, 31–38.

Nishizuka, M., and Arai, Y. (1983). Male-female difference in the intra-amygdaloid input to the medial amygdala. *Exp. Brain Res.* **52**, 328–332.

Novotny, M., MA, W., and Zidek, L. (1997). New biochemical insights into puberty acceleration, estrus induction and puberty delay in the house mouse. *In* "Advances in Chemical Signals in Vertebrates" Cornell University Press, Ithaca, NY.

Numan, M., and Sheehan, T. P. (1997). Neuroanatomical circuitry for mammalian maternal behavior. *Ann. N. Y. Acad. Sci.* **807**, 101–125.

Nyby, J., Matochik, J. A., and Barfield, R. J. (1992). Intracranial androgenic and estrogenic stimulation of male-typical behaviors in house mice (*Mus domesticus*). *Horm. Behav.* **26**, 24–45.

Oro, A. E., Simerly, R. B., and Swanson, L. W. (1988). Estrous cycle variations in levels of cholecystokinin immunoreactivity within cells of three interconnected sexually dimorphic forebrain nuclei. Evidence for a regulatory role for estrogen. *Neuroendocrinology* **47**, 225–235.

Parfitt, D. B., and Newman, S. W. (1998). Fos-immunoreactivity within the extended amygdala is correlated with the onset of sexual satiety. *Horm. Behav.* **34**, 17–29.

Pfaff, D. W., and Keiner, M. (1973). Atlas of estradiol-concentrating cells in the central nervous system of the female rat. *J. Comp. Neurol.* **151**, 121–158.

Pfaff, D. W., Schwartz-Giblin, S., McCarthy, M. M., and Kow, L.-M. (1994). Cellular and molecular mechanisms of female reproductive behaviors. *In* "The Physiology of Reproduction" (E. Knobil and J. D. Neill, eds.), 2nd ed., pp. 107–220. Raven Press, New York.

Pfaus, J. G., Kleopoulos, S. P., Mobbs, C. V., Gibbs, R. B., and Pfaff, D. W. (1993). Sexual stimulation activates c-*fos* within estrogen-concentrating regions of the female rat forebrain. *Brain Res.* **624**, 253–267.

Pfeiffer, C. A., and Johnston, R. E. (1994). Hormonal and behavioral responses of male hamster to females and female odors: Roles of olfaction, the vomeronasal system, and sexual experience. *Physiol. Behav.* **55**, 129–138.

Potegal, M., Ferris, C. F., Hebert, M., Meyerhoff, J., and Skaredoff, L. (1996). Attack priming in female Syrian Golden hamsters is associated with a c-*fos*-coupled process within the corticomedial amygdala. *Neuroscience* **75**, 869–880.

Powers, J. B., and Valenstein, E. S. (1972). Sexual receptivity: Facilitation by medial preoptic lesions in female rats. *Science* **175**, 1003–1005.

Powers, J. B., Newman, S. W., and Bergondy, M. L. (1987). MPOA and BNST lesions in male Syrian hamsters: Differential effects on copulatory and chemoinvestigatory behaviors. *Behav. Brain Res.* **23**, 181–195.

Price, J. L. (1987). The central olfactory and accessory olfactory systems. *In* "Neurobiology of Taste and Smell" (T. E. Finger and W. L. Silver, eds.), pp. 179–203. Wiley, New York.

Rasia-Filho, A. A., Peres, T. M. S., Cubilla-Gutierrez, F. H., and Lucion, A. B. (1991). Effect of estradiol implanted in the corticomedial amygdala on the sexual behavior of castrated male rats. *Braz. J. Med. Biol. Res.* **24**, 1041–1049.

Rees, H. D., Switz, G. M., and Michael, R. P. (1980). The estrogen-sensitive neural system in the brain of female cats. *J. Comp. Neurol.* **193**, 789–804.

Risold, P. Y., Canteras, N. S., and Swanson, L. W. (1994). Organization of projections from the anterior hypothalamic nucleus: A *Phaseolus vulgaris*-leucoagglutinin study in the rat. *J. Comp. Neurol.* **348**, 1–40.

Rizvi, T. A., Ennis, M., and Shipley, M. T. (1992). Reciprocal connections between the medial preoptic area and the midbrain periaqueductal gray in rat: A WGA-HRP and PHA-L study. *J. Comp. Neurol.* **315**, 1–15.

Roeling, T. A. P., Veening, J. G., Kruk, M. R., Peters, J. P. W., Vermelis, M. E. J., and Niewenhuys, R. (1994). Efferent connections of the hypothalamic "aggression area" in the rat. *Neuroscience* **59**, 1001–1024.

Rosenblatt, J. S., Factor, E. M., and Mayer, A. D. (1994). Relationship between maternal aggression and maternal care in the rat. *Aggressive Behav.* **20**, 243–255.

Sar, M., and Stumpf, W. E. (1977). Distribution of androgen target cells in rat forebrain and pituitary after [³H]-dihydrotestosterone administration. *J. Steroid Biochem.* **8**, 1131–1135.

Scalia, F., and Winans, S. S. (1975). The differential projections of the olfactory bulb and accessory olfactory bulb in mammals. *J. Comp. Neurol.* **61**, 31–56.

Shipley, M. T., Ennis, M., Rizvi, T. A., and Behbehani, M. M. (1991). Topographic specificity of forebrain inputs to the midbrain periaqueductal gray: Evidence for discrete longitudinally organized input columns. *In* "The Midbrain Periaqueductal Gray Matter: Functional, Anatomical and Neurochemical Organization" (A. Depaulis and R. Bandler, eds.), pp. 417–448. Plenum Press, New York.

Silver, R. A. (1992). Environmental factors influencing hormone secretion. In "Behavioral Endocrinology" (J. Becker, S. Breedlove, and D. Crews, eds.), pp. 401–422. MIT Press, Cambridge, MA.

Silver, W. L. (1987). The common chemical sense. In "Neurobiology of Taste and Smell" (T. E. Finger and W. L. Silver, eds.), pp. 65–87. Wiley, New York.

Simerly, R. B. (1995). Hormonal regulation of limbic and hypothalamic pathways. In "Neurobiological Effects of Sex Steroid Hormones" (P. E. Micevych and R. P. Hammer, eds.), pp. 85–114. Cambridge University Press, Cambridge, UK.

Simerly, R. B., and Swanson, L. W. (1987). Castration reversibly alters levels of cholecystokinin immunoreactivity within cells of three interconnected sexually dimorphic forebrain nuclei in the rat. Proc. Natl. Acad. Sci. U.S.A. **84**, 2087–2091.

Simerly, R. B., and Swanson, L. W. (1988). Projections of the medial preoptic nucleus: A Phaseolus vulgaris leucoagglutinin anterograde tract-tracing study in the rat. J. Comp. Neurol. **270**, 209–242.

Simerly, R. B., Chang, C., Muramatsu, M., and Swanson, L. W. (1990). Distribution of androgen and estrogen receptor mRNA-containing cells in the rat brain: An in situ hybridization study. J. Comp. Neurol. **294**, 76–95.

Smith, W. J., Stewart, J., and Pfaus, J. G. (1997). Tail pinch induces Fos immunoreactivity within several regions of the male rat brain: Effects of age. Physiol. Behav. **61**, 717–723.

Swann, J. M., and Newman, S. W. (1992). Testosterone regulates substance P within neurons of the medial nucleus of the amygdala, the bed nucleus of the stria terminalis and the medal preoptic area of the male golden hamster. Brain Res. **590**, 18–28.

Swanson, L. W., and Petrovich, G. D. (1998). What is the amygdala? Trends Neurosci. **21**, 323–331.

Todrank, J., Heth, G., and Johnston, R. E. (1999). Social interaction is necessary for discrimination between and memory for odours of close relatives in Golden hamsters. Ethology. **105**, 771–782.

Valcourt, R. J., and Sachs, B. D. (1979). Penile reflexes and copulatory behavior in male rats following lesions in the bed nucleus of the stria terminalis. Brain Res. Bull. **4**, 131–133.

Vandenberg, J. G. (1994). Pheromones and mammalian reproduction. In "The Physiology of Reproduction" (E. Knobil and J. D. Neill, eds.), 2nd ed., pp. 343–359. Raven Press, New York.

van Leeuwen, F. W., Caffe, A. R., and De Vries, G. J. (1985). Vasopressin cells in the bed nucleus of the stria terminalis of the rat: Sex differences and the influence of androgens. Brain Res. **325**, 391–394.

Wirsig, C. (1987). Effects of the terminal nerve on mating behavior in the male hamster. Ann. N.Y. Acad. Sci. **519**, 241–251.

Wood, R. I. (1996a). Estradiol, but not dihydrotestosterone, in the medial amygdala facilitates male hamster sex behavior. Physiol. Behav. **59**, 833–341.

Wood, R. I. (1996b). Functions of the steroid-responsive neural network in the control of male hamster sexual behavior. Trends Endocrinol. Metab. **7**, 338–344.

Wood, R. I. (1997). Thinking about networks in the control of male hamster sexual behavior. Horm. Behav. **32**, 40–45.

Wood, R. I., and Newman, S. W. (1993). Mating activates androgen receptor-containing neurons in chemosensory pathways of the male Syrian hamster brain. Brain Res. **614**, 65–77.

Wood, R. I., and Newman, S. W. (1995a). Hormonal influence on neurons of the mating behavior pathway in male hamsters. In "Neurobiological Effects of Sex Steroid Hormones" (P. E. Micevych and R. P. Hammer, eds.), pp. 3–39. Cambridge University Press, Cambridge, UK.

Wood, R. I., and Newman, S. W. (1995b). Androgen and estrogen receptors coexist within individual neurons in the brain of the Syrian hamster. Neuroendocrinology. **62**, 487–497.

Wood, R. I., and Newman, S. W. (1995c). The medial amygdaloid nucleus and medial preoptic area mediate steroidal control of sexual behavior in the male Syrian hamster. Horm. Behav. **29**, 338–353.

Wysocki, C. (1979). Neurobehavioral evidence for the involvement of the vomeronasal system in mammalian reproduction. Neurosci. Biobehav. Rev. **3**, 301–341.

Wysocki, C., and Lepri, J. J. (1991). Consequences of removing the vomeronasal organ. J. Steroid Biochem. Mol. Biol. **39**, 661–669.

Wysocki, C., and Meredith, M. (1987). The vomeronasal system. In "Neurobiology of Taste and Smell" (T. E. Finger and W. L. Silver, eds.), pp. 125–150. Wiley, New York.

Wysocki, C., Beauchamp, G. K., Reidinger, R. R., and Wellington, J. L. (1985). Access of large and nonvolatile molecules to the vomeronasal organ of mammals during social an feeding behaviors. J. Chem. Ecol. **11**, 1147–1159.

Yamazaki, K., Beauchamp, G. K., Curran, M., Bard, J., and Boyse, E. A. (2000) Parent-progeny recognition as a funcion of MHC odortype identity. Proc. Natl. Acad. Sci. U.S.A. **97**, 10500–10502.

18

Circadian Rhythms in the Endocrine System

Lance J. Kriegsfeld
Department of Psychology
Columbia University
New York, New York 10027

Joseph LeSauter
Department of Psychology
Barnard College
New York, New York 10027

Toshiyuki Hamada
Department of Psychology
Columbia University
New York, New York 10027

SiNae M. Pitts
Department of Psychology
Columbia University
New York, New York 10027

Rae Silver
Departments of Psychology
Columbia University and Barnard College
Departments of Anatomy and Cell Biology
College of Physicians and Surgeons
New York, New York 10027

I. INTRODUCTION TO CIRCADIAN RHYTHMS

A. Characterization of Circadian and Diurnal Rhythms

The regular cycles of light and dark are so prominent a cue organizing our lives that we have the impression that daily rhythms in our activities are responses to signals from the environment. Most of these rhythms, however, are endogenously generated by body clocks, and persist in the absence of environmental time cues. Such rhythms are synchronized with the external environment by exposure to periodic cues in the environment termed zeitgebers (German, "time givers"). The process of synchronizing endogenous rhythms with the external environment is called entrainment. The most predictable synchronizing agent for rhythms with a period of approximately 24 hours is light, and most organisms have evolved to use the environmental light:dark (LD) cycle to exquisitely fine-tune the phase of circadian rhythms with respect to the rising and setting of the sun. However, any stimulus that occurs with a period close to 24 hours could act to synchronize circadian rhythms (*circa*, "about"; *diem*, "day") in behavior and physiology. Some daily rhythms are diurnal. Diurnal rhythms are driven by alternating cycles of light and darkness, rather than being internally organized. In contrast to circadian rhythms, diurnal rhythms cease when environmental conditions are constant and no longer provide time cues. (For a summary of definitions, see Table 1.)

B. History of the Study of Circadian Rhythms

The first written evidence of endogenously generated daily cycles in behavior was noted in heliotropic plants by the French astronomer Jean Jacques d'Ortous de Marian in 1729. In order to absorb the sun's rays and promote photosynthesis, the leaves of heliotropic plants open during the day and close at night. De Mairan noted that these rhythms in leaf movement persisted for several days in the darkness of his cellar without

TABLE 1
Definitions and Properties of Circadian Clocks

Endogenous rhythms	Self-sustained rhythms generated within an organism that persist in constant conditions
Driven rhythms	Rhythms requiring exogenous input to be maintained
Circadian rhythm	Biological rhythm with a period of approximately 24 hours
Entrained rhythms	Self-sustained (i.e., endogenous) rhythms that are synchronized to a periodic cue in the environment (typically the light:dark cycle)
Diurnal (nycthemeral) rhythms	Rhythms driven by the light:dark cycle or other entraining agent that occurs with a periodicity of 24 hours
Free-running rhythm	State of a circadian rhythm in constant conditions (i.e., in the absence of an entraining agent), provides the period of the endogenous rhythm
Circadian oscillator	Entity with a 24-hour rhythm that is driven by a pacemaker or zeitgeber
Circadian pacemaker	Self-sustained rhythm generator that synchronizes oscillators
Tau (period)	Time span between recurrences of a defined phase of a rhythm
Zeitgeber	Periodic environmental factor that entrains a biological self-sustaining rhythm or a driven rhythm
Phase response curve	Graphical representation of the amount and direction of a phase shift depending on the point of the phase at which a stimulus is applied
Phase shift	Displacement of an oscillation along the time axis
LL	Constant light conditions
DD	Constant dark conditions
LD	Light:dark cycle

exposure to any time cues or sunlight (of course the plant died after several days without sunlight). Also noteworthy, these rhythms maintained a period of approximately 24 hours. Thus, the leaves of the plant were not opening in response to sunlight, but in anticipation of the rising of the sun (De Marian, 1729). This classic experiment provided the first evidence that biological rhythms could persist in an organism in the absence of environmental cues. This study also highlights the importance of synchronization of circadian rhythms with the environmental LD cycle; organisms can time internal processes so that they occur at an appropriate time during the daily cycle.

C. Functions of the Circadian System

From an evolutionary and adaptive perspective, animals have evolved to synchronize their endogenous circadian rhythms with the environment in order to promote survival (e.g., DeCoursey and Krulas, 1998). Numerous behaviors are restricted to specific times of day in response to a variety of selection pressures. For example, diurnal species (species active during the day) confine behaviors such as feeding, locomotion, foraging, and reproduction to the day in order to avoid predation. Likewise, nocturnal species (species active at night) such as owls are active at night to maximize the availability of nocturnal prey (e.g., small rodents). As described later, the circadian clock that synchronizes rhythms in behavior and physiology is localized to a discrete bilateral nucleus in the anterior hypothalamus. If this nucleus is lesioned, animals in the laboratory (Stephan and Zucker, 1972; Moore and Eichler, 1972) and in the field (e.g., DeCoursey et al., 1997) lose their ability to restrict behaviors to a particular time of day, and this arrhythmicity may compromise survival (DeCoursey and Krulas, 1998). As shown later, temporal variation in behavior is associated with temporal variation in underlying physiology and biochemistry. These underlying processes are modulated by endogenously driven circadian rhythms that are synchronized by environmental time cues. Clearly, a body clock that is not synchronized with the environment is not adaptive.

D. Circadian Rhythms Orchestrate Internal Physiological Processes

Numerous physiological processes occur with a period of approximately 24 hours. Some rhythms, however, exhibit a peak in activity during one time of day, whereas other rhythms are at a nadir at this time. For example, in humans cortisol concentrations peak at dawn, whereas melatonin and prolactin concentrations peak in the middle of the night. The relationship between daily fluctuations in hormones and the environmental LD cycle is different for nocturnal and diurnal species (Fig. 1). Thus, although myriad rhythms have a period of approximately 24 hours, each of these rhythms has a unique phase with respect to one another and to the LD cycle. That is, although bodily rhythms exhibit different phases relative to some objective point in time, the phase relationship among rhythms remains stable, unless a perturbation occurs (e.g., jet lag). Thus, circadian rhythms help to maintain homeostasis in the body.

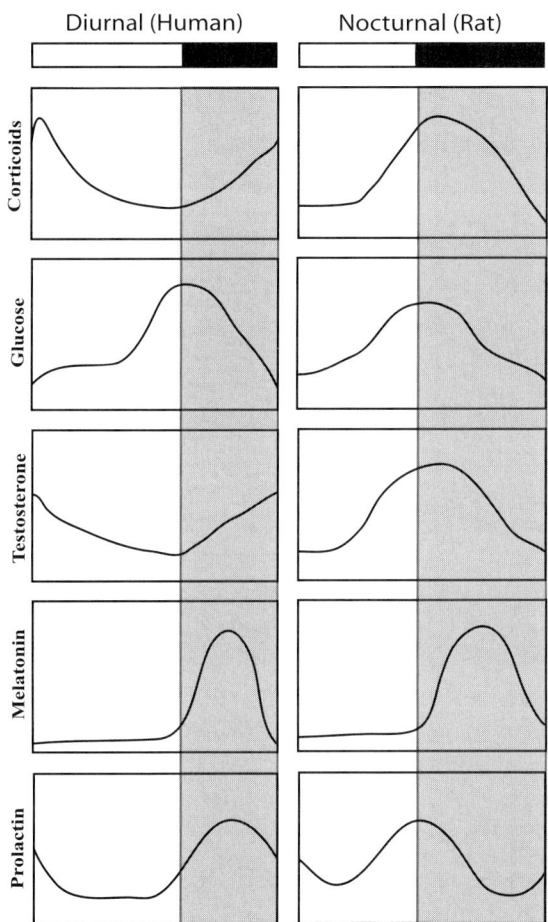

FIGURE 1 Circadian pattern of hormone secretion for humans and nocturnal rodents (e.g., rats). The bar at the top of the page represents approximate periods of light and dark for human and rodent studies. The shaded area represents nighttime on the graphs. Data are replotted from Czeisler and Klerman (1999); La Fleur et al. (2000); Leal and Moreira (1997); Mock et al. (1978); Scharwtz (1993); Selgas et al. (1997); Van Cauter and Refetoff (1985).

In addition, the phase of specific rhythms helps to prepare the body for necessary daily activities in advance of their actual occurrence. For example, cortisol rhythms rise in humans prior to waking in order to facilitate the onset of morning activity (e.g., Weitzman et al., 1971; Van Cauter and Refetoff, 1985).

These two fundamental functions, internal organization and entrainment to the environment, set the stage for the exploration of the role of circadian rhythmicity in the regulation of physiology and behavior in this chapter. For each aspect of physiology and behavior, the circadian system sits upstream of a regulatory system, modulating the timing and synchronization of events. For example, virtually all hormone concentrations show daily variations with a period of approximately 24 hours (see Turek and Van Cauter, 1994). Thus, to measure differences in hormone levels among groups, it is necessary to sample hormones from different experimental subjects at the same time of the day. Likewise, a hormone sample collected at one time of day may not be representative of the mean concentration in an individual if blood samples are collected at the peak or nadir of the hormonal cycle. The neural mechanisms controlling circadian variation in hormonal and other rhythms are the focus of this chapter. An overview of the temporal aspects of circadian and diurnal variations in hormone rhythms is depicted in Fig. 1. The phenomena depicted in this figure set the stage for the regulatory processes that must be understood.

One final caveat regarding the interpretation of circadian rhythm studies is that circadian rhythms may be partly or entirely a consequence of another circadian rhythm. For example, body temperature shows a robust daily rhythm with temperature peaking when human or nonhuman animals are active. Body temperature is partly a function of activity level. Therefore, it is difficult to determine whether daily rhythms in temperature are a result of direct regulation of thermoregulatory brain regions, an indirect result of daily rhythms in activity, or a combination of both processes.

E. Circadian Rhythms Are Entrained to the Environment

The process of entrainment (synchronization) of endogenous rhythms to cyclic environmental stimuli entails daily adjustments in the phase of endogenous rhythms. After the summer solstice, days become shorter, and each passing day incurs a minor delay of sunrise and a small advance in the onset of sunset; the opposite pattern occurs after the winter solstice. Thus, in order to maintain a stable phase relationship with the daily solar cycle, animals must constantly update the phase of circadian processes. For example, daily adjustments (on the order of minutes) in the onset and offset of activity occur in natural populations in order to synchronize this and other rhythms with minor daily changes in sunrise and sunset. This process was elegantly demonstrated in a study of flying squirrels, as shown in Fig. 2.

The means by which organisms achieve this stable entrainment is best represented by phase response curves (Fig. 3). Phase response curves (PRCs) are graphical representations of the effects that light has on the timing of biological rhythms; the effects of light on the phase of circadian rhythms depend on the coincidence of light with particular alternating periods of sensitivity and insensitivity during the circadian cycle. Phase response curves are constructed by maintaining organisms in constant darkness and presenting light at various times during the circadian cycle. For diurnal species, the active portion of the daily cycle has been termed the subjective day, whereas the inactive portion has been termed the subjective night. For nocturnal organisms, subjective night represents the active phase, whereas the inactive phase is the subjective day. Although diurnal and nocturnal organisms have activity patterns 180 degrees out of phase with one another, both are sensitive to the phase-shifting effects of light only during the subjective night. A light pulse presented early in the subjective night produces a phase delay of circadian rhythms, whereas a light pulse presented late in the subjective night produces a phase advance in circadian activity. A phase delay results in setting back the time of the clock, so that the behavior starts later the next day than it did the day before. A phase advance results in setting forward the time of the clock, so that the behavior starts earlier the next day than it did the day before. Thus, light coincident with sensitive portions of the subjective night produces daily minor adjustments in circadian phase. The phase response curve permits predictions about the effects of light presented at different circadian times and provides a means of quantifying and assessing circadian behavior.

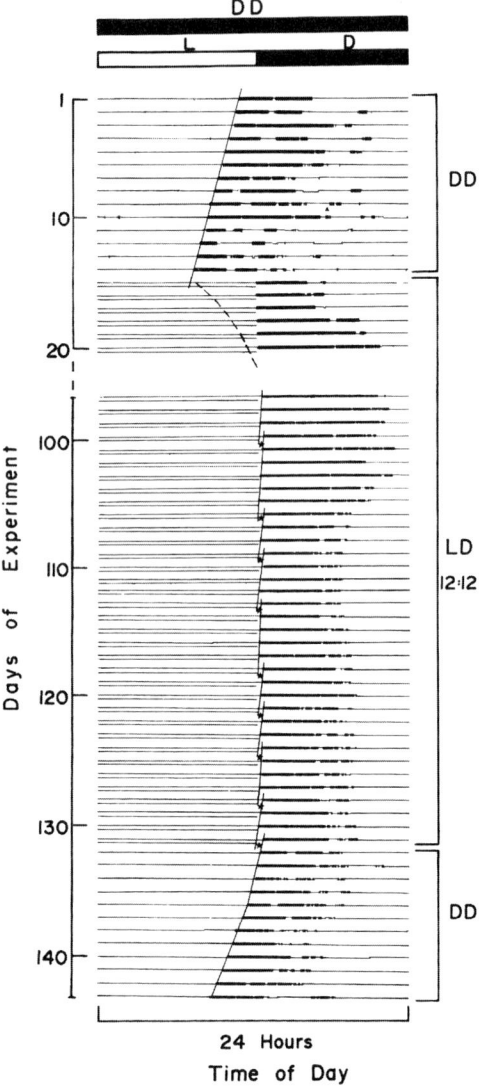

FIGURE 2 Activity pattern and photoentrainment of a flying squirrel. The squirrel was kept in a double cage where the activity wheel was on a programmable light:dark schedule and the nest was in constant darkness. For days 1–14, the activity box was in constant darkness and the animal free-ran. On day 15, the activity box was on a light:dark schedule. It takes a few days for the animal to entrain to the new LD cycle, as can be seen by the timing of activity offset. Masking is seen at onset time. Once the animal had been entrained, a phase shift (∗) could be detected each time the squirrel came into the activity box when the light was still on. Activity onset free-ran the days when the squirrel came out when the light was turned off. This results in a zig-zag pattern of light sampling–phase shifting and dark sampling–free-running. On day 133, the cage was put back in constant darkness and the squirrel free-ran. From DeCoursey (1986).

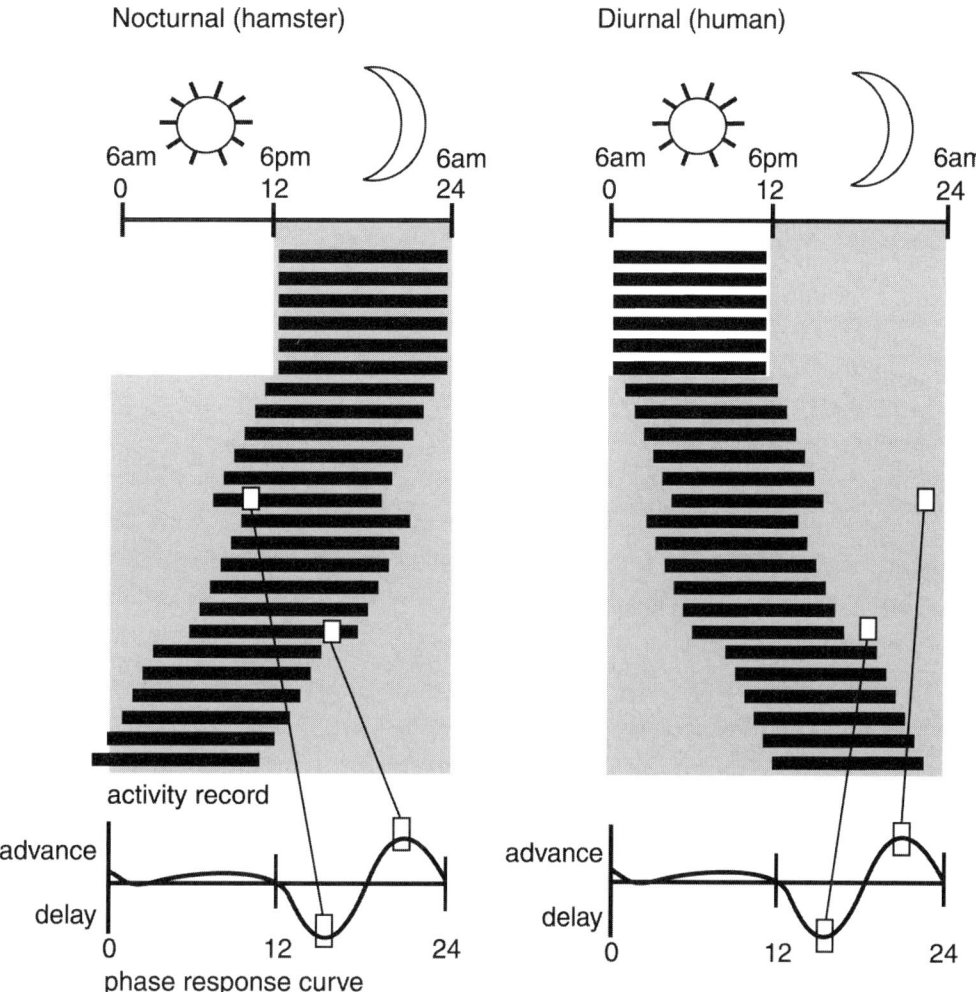

FIGURE 3 Figure representing the activity rhythms and light-induced phase response curve (PRC) of a nocturnal and a diurnal species. The first line indicates the approximate time of day. The second line indicates the conventional circadian time where the beginning of activity is considered as zeitgeber time (ZT) or circadian time (CT) 0 for diurnal, and ZT or CT 12 for nocturnal species. The daily activity is represented by dark horizontal bars. The dark shaded area represents nighttime or constant darkness. The light shaded area represents constant light or isolation from external cues. Nocturnal animals are active during the night and entrain to the day–night cycle. In constant conditions, such as constant darkness, they free-run with a period generally shorter than 24-hr light. A light pulse presented at the beginning of the active phase (or beginning of night) induces a phase delay the next day and a light pulse at the end of the active phase (or end of night) induces a phase advance the next day. Diurnal humans are active during the day and also entrain to the day–night cycle. In constant conditions, such as constant light or without external cues, they free-run with a period longer than 24 hr. A pulse of light given at the end of the rest phase (or end of night) or at the beginning of the rest phase (or beginning of night) induces the same phase shifts as in nocturnal species. When phase shifts obtained by light pulses given at different times of the circadian cycle are plotted on a 24-hr basis, the resulting PRC is obtained. Light given during the day, when nocturnal animals are resting or when diurnal animals are active, does not induce shifts in the clock or in activity. On the other hand, light given at the beginning of the dark (or subjective dark) period produces phase delays, and that given at the end of the dark (or subjective dark) period produces phase advances.

Alternating periods of sensitivity and insensitivity to light, as well as the resultant phase-shifting effects of light, have obvious adaptive significance. Consider a nocturnal rodent that lives in a burrow. Burrowing rodents typically emerge at sunset and return to their burrows prior to dawn. If a nocturnal rodent emerges from its burrow prior to sunset, light will be coincident with the early portion of the animal's active phase, thereby resulting in a phase delay of circadian activity and a delayed emergence the following evening. Alternatively, if a rodent is "late" returning to its burrow, light will be coincident with portion of the circadian cycle that results in phase advances, leading to in an earlier return to its burrow the following day. Thus, this daily process of reentrainment results in precise synchronization between circadian rhythms in physiology and behavior with the daily light:dark cycle. PRCs can also be constructed in response to other zeitgebers such as dark pulses or the effect of hormones or drugs.

II. ORGANIZATION OF THE CIRCADIAN SYSTEM

A. Finding Circadian Clocks

To unravel the neural basis of the circadian system requires a series of studies. The first step is the demonstration of circadian changes under constant environmental conditions. To determine the locus in the body that generates this rhythm, it is necessary to determine whether the measured response is part of the clock or part of an output pathway controlled by clocks lying upstream of that tissue. A good example of the distinction between the clock and the output pathway is the pineal gland in reptiles and birds vs that in mammals. In both groups, the pineal gland produces the hormone melatonin on a circadian basis and has a self-sustained circadian oscillator (e.g., Tosini and Menaker, 1998). Pineal glands isolated *in vitro* continue to produce rhythmic secretion of melatonin. In contrast, the melatonin rhythm in mammals is driven by a pacemaker in the suprachiasmatic nucleus (SCN) from which the pineal receives neuronal input via a multisynaptic pathway (Moore and Klein, 1974). In the absence of a signal from the SCN, the mammalian pineal gland does not produce melatonin in a circadian fashion. Evidence of this type shows that there is an endogenous pacemaker capable of self-sustained oscillations in the pineal gland of reptiles and birds, but not in the same melatonin-synthesizing gland of mammals (Korf *et al.*, 1998).

B. Suprachiasmatic Nucleus Is the Locus of the Body's Circadian Clock in Mammals

Many years of research and converging lines of evidence prove that in mammals the SCN, lying in the anterior hypothalamus, is the necessary and sufficient site of a brain clock regulating all circadian rhythmicity in the body. To understand SCN function it is convenient to visualize the circadian system as having three major components: the pacemaker, its inputs, and its outputs (Fig. 4). The inputs involve a detector that provides temporal information from the environment, allowing the animal to stay in synchrony with local time. The central pacemaker generates the endogenous circadian rhythm. The outputs provide the means whereby the pacemaker phase is communicated to the target tissues in the body. In the case of the SCN, there is evidence for both neural efferents and diffusible neuroendocrine output signals.

The goal of this chapter is to describe how hormone secretions are regulated by the circadian system. Also of interest is the question of how hormonal signals feedback to modulate the circadian system. To bring the available evidence into perspective, we review the evidence for an endogenous timekeeping system in the body, located in the SCN. Next, we examine the pathways by which zeitgeber information reaches the pacemakers in the SCN and how that information is communicated to the rest of the body.

C. Anatomy and Physiology of the Suprachiasmatic Nucleus

In mammals, the pacemakers driving circadian rhythmicity are located in the SCN, which lies above the posterior part of the optic chiasm on both sides of the third ventricle. In birds, there has been uncertainty as to the location of the hypothalamic pacemakers, but evidence indicates a similar organization in avian species (discussed later). Early evidence for the role of the SCN as a mammalian pacemaker was provided by studies demonstrating that bilateral ablation of these nuclei permanently abolishes circadian periodicity of many

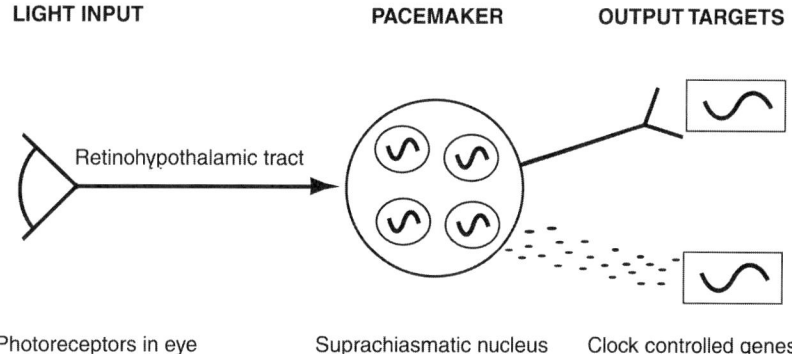

FIGURE 4 Schematic representation of the mammalian circadian system. On the left, the photoreceptors send light information to the clock through the entraining pathways (input pathways). In the center, the SCN contains the pacemaker cells. On the right, the coupling pathways send signals from the pacemakers to the targets in the brain or in peripheral organs (output pathways). Two possible output pathways are represented, a neural pathway and a pathway using a diffusible signal.

physiological and behavioral rhythms even when the lesion is made in very young animals (Stephan and Zucker, 1972; Mosko and Moore, 1979). As far as is known, no other behavioral or physiological functions are altered. Another important line of evidence derives from the fact that the SCN receives direct retinal input via the retinohypothalamic tract (RHT) (Moore and Lenn, 1972). In SCN-ablated animals, vision is not impaired, but these animals do not synchronize their activity to daily LD cycles. If, on the other hand, the primary visual pathway is transected at the level of the optic tract beyond the optic chiasm, then the animal is visually blind, but the circadian system continues to respond to photic cues by entraining to the LD cycle (Johnson et al., 1988; Zucker, 1980). These studies demonstrate the route whereby environmental photic information can reach the pacemakers of the SCN.

In rodents, each SCN contains approximately 8000 neurons (van den Pol, 1980). With regard to its cellular components, the SCN is heterogenous, containing a variety of histochemically distinct neurons. γ-Aminobutyric acid (GABA) appears to be the predominant transmitter (Decavel and van den Pol, 1990; Moore and Speh, 1993). Other intrinsic neurotransmitters include vasopressin (VP), somatostatin (SS), peptide-histidine-isoleucine (PHI), vasoactive intestinal polypeptide (VIP), and gastrin-releasing peptide (GRP) (Moore, 1983; Card and Moore, 1984; van den Pol and Tsujimoto, 1985; Mikkelsen et al., 1991). Similar to the immunocytochemical localization of neuropeptides in the SCN, messenger RNAs encoding VP, GRP, SS, and VIP are localized in the perikarya of SCN neurons (Card et al., 1988; Stopa et al., 1988), indicating that these peptides are synthesized in SCN neurons. The perikarya of these peptide-containing neurons are topographically segregated such that cells containing VP or SS are localized in the dorsomedial aspect of the SCN, whereas perikarya expressing PHI, VIP, or GRP are restricted to the ventrolateral aspect of the nucleus. Circadian variations occur in the structure of VP mRNA in the SCN (Robinson et al., 1988) and in SCN content of VP, SS, and VIP mRNA (Glazer and Gozes, 1994; Inouye and Shibata, 1994; Uhl and Reppert, 1986). The oscillation in VP mRNA parallels changes in the secretory activity of VP neurons in the SCN. For other peptides such as VIP, diurnal variation is observed but there is no circadian rhythm in expression in conditions of constant darkness. The localization of SCN peptides and their diurnal and circadian expression have been extensively reviewed in Inouye and Shibata (1994).

D. Unique Pacemaker Function of the Suprachiasmatic Nucleus Is Based on Common Mechanisms

Many aspects of SCN cell function are common to other regions of the brain. The retinal input to the SCN is mediated by glutamate; and glutamate is a common excitatory transmitter throughout the brain. GABA, the inhibitory transmitter found in most SCN cells, is the most common inhibitory transmitter found in the brain. Peptides that are colocalized with GABA, including VIP, SS, VP, and GRP, are found in other brain regions. The important clock genes, including *Per* and *Clock*, are expressed in many brain sites as well as in peripheral tissues (e.g., Yamazaki *et al.*, 2000). What we know to be truly unique for SCN cells are the constellation of inputs and outputs and the combination of transmitters found in the SCN. We do not know precisely how the SCN is uniquely different from other tissues, but we do know that in mammals only the SCN is competent to coordinate the phase of circadian rhythms in the rest of the body.

The specific roles of different cell types in the circadian pacemaker and entrainment functions of the SCN have long been a puzzle. The distinctions between the ventrolateral and dorsomedial SCN are associated with the distinguishing connections and neurochemical characteristics of these subdivisions. In the ventrolateral SCN, cells displaying PHI-, VIP-, and GRP-immunoreactivity are closely associated with the terminals of fibers of the retina and the intergeniculate leaflet of the thalamus, suggesting that the peptidergic neurons in this subdivision may be involved in the processing of primary and secondary photic information (Moore, 1983; Card and Moore, 1984; van den Pol and Tsujimoto, 1985; Mikkelsen *et al.*, 1991; reviewed in Inouye and Shibata, 1994). This possibility is supported by data indicating that the axon terminals of retinal ganglion cells establish synaptic contacts with VIP-containing neurons in the SCN (Ibata *et al.*, 1989). In contrast, the dorsomedial subdivision of the SCN lacks direct retinal input, but appears to play a more important role in the generation of circadian rhythms than the ventrolateral SCN (Moore, 1996; Shibata *et al.*, 1984; Yan *et al.*, 1999). By examining the expression of genes that are components of the circadian clock mechanism, we have demonstrated that the hypothalamic clock is composed of two compartments (Hamada *et al.*, 2001). One compartment, marked by the presence of calbindin-D28K positive cells, receives photic input but does not have cycling of clock genes. The ability of cells in this compartment to respond to light is gated by a second compartment. This second compartment, marked by VP-containing cells, has endogenous rhythmicity in important circadian clock genes (discussed later). Lesions of the calbindin region of the SCN, which spare large components of the remaining SCN, result in the loss of circadian locomotor rhythmicity (LeSauter and Silver, 1999). The two compartments together constitute the SCN circadian clock.

E. Circadian Timekeeping Is a Fundamental Property of the Suprachiasmatic Nucleus

Consistent with the pacemaker function of the SCN, circadian rhythmicity is an intrinsic property of this tissue. When isolated *in vitro*, the SCN continues to generate circadian rhythms in various measurable indices. In hypothalamic slice preparations, the SCN is intrinsically capable of sustaining circadian rhythms in neuronal firing rate, glucose use, and VP secretion (Gillette and Reppert, 1987; Green and Gillette, 1982; Newman and Hospod, 1986). Primary cultures and organotypic explants of the rat SCN are similarly characterized by the distinctive capacity to generate circadian rhythms in VP and VIP release for multiple cycles (Earnest and Sladek, 1986; Watanabe *et al.*, 1993; Shinohara and Oka, 1994). VP and VIP rhythms in the same SCN explant are independently phased, suggesting that these circadian rhythms are generated by neurons that consist of two distinct populations of oscillators in the SCN (Shinohara *et al.*, 1995).

Neural transplantation studies provide important information with regard to the central role of the SCN in the generation of circadian rhythms (Fig. 5) (Lehman and Silver, 1994; Boer *et al.*, 1998). In all studies, the presence of peptidergic cells and fibers of SCN origin in the grafts has been a requirement for the successful restoration of circadian function. Transplantation of fetal hypothalamic grafts containing the SCN into arrhythmic SCN-lesioned host animals restores circadian rhythms in locomotor activity and activity-dependent responses such as gnawing. Both of these responses recovered simultaneously, suggesting that they are mediated by a common mechanism (LeSauter and Silver, 1994). Important in this, grafting studies using donors and hosts with different circadian genotypes (i.e., having different free-running periods) have provided unequivocal evidence that a specific circadian property, namely period, can be transferred by the graft to the host animal and prove that circadian rhythms are

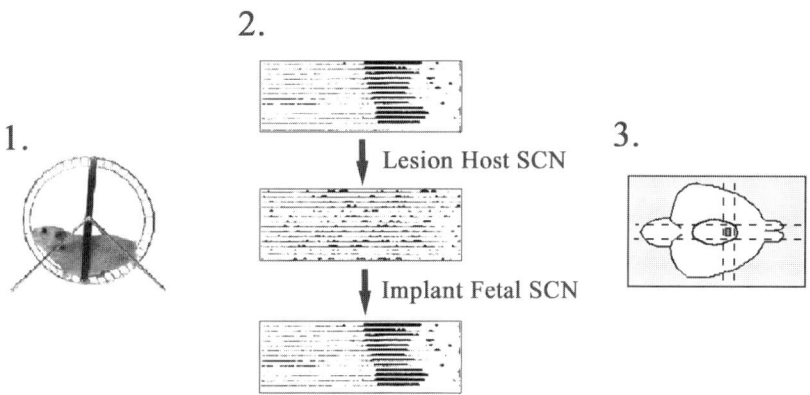

FIGURE 5 Experimental paradigm for the restoration of circadian activity rhythms by neural transplantation. (1) The circadian rhythm of the intact host is determined from wheel-running activity in constant conditions. (2) Subsequently, the host SCN is lesioned and elimination of rhythmicity is confirmed. (3) Tissue from embryonic SCN is taken for transplantation. Restoration of rhythmicty is verified (2 bottom). Courtesy of Dr. Michael Lehman.

generated by pacemaker cells in the graft, and not by any tissue of the host (Ralph *et al.*, 1990; Silver *et al.*, 1990; also see Fig. 9).

Important in the present context, several reports suggest that endocrine rhythms are not restored by SCN grafts. For example, in constant darkness, hamsters undergo regression of the gonads, but such regression is not seen in SCN-lesioned and grafted animals, despite the fact that their circadian system does not entrain to a light:dark cycle (Lehman *et al.*, 1987). Measurements of plasma luteinizing hormone (LH), cortisol, corticosterone, and pineal melatonin also indicate an absence of circadian rhythms (Meyer-Bernstein *et al.*, 1999). The implication of this dissociation of activity-dependent and endocrine-related rhythmicity is that these two types of rhythms are the products of different SCN output systems.

One issue raised by these results is the mechanism whereby the neural graft restores rhythmicity. A number of mediating mechanisms are hypothetically possible, including trophic factors, axon sprouting from the graft to the host, neural growth in the host, paracrine diffusion from the graft, or endocrine release (LeSauter and Silver, 1998). Although the initial assumption was that grafts restored rhythmicity by establishing neural efferent connections to target regions in the host brain (Lehman *et al.*, 1987; Sollars *et al.*, 1995), it has been difficult to prove that successful grafts have made any particular neural connections. Instead, connections appear to be very varied and dependent on the attachment site of the graft (Lehman *et al.*, 1995). Furthermore, as discussed later, there is substantial evidence that the SCN can produce a diffusible signal. These issues are relevant to circadian regulation of the endocrine system, as the various clock-controlled responses do not appear to be uniformly regulated.

F. Cellular Organization of Circadian Systems: Rhythmicity Is a Cell-Autonomous Property

The identification of the SCN as the site of a mammalian circadian pacemaker has stimulated many questions about the relationship between specific cellular components of the SCN and its timekeeping and photoentrainment functions. First, it is important to understand whether a single type of cell or a subset of pacemaker cells controls rhythmic responses, or whether different subnuclei control different rhythms. A related question is whether all the different cell types of the SCN are pacemakers or whether this function is localized to one or few subtypes. Finally, one of the puzzles in understanding circadian rhythmicity has been whether individual, physically isolated cells are capable of generating a circadian oscillation or whether the circadian oscillation is an emergent product of many cells acting together. This last question has been addressed in several models and points to the existence of independent oscillators in individual cells in each circadian system.

Dissociated cells from the chick pineal (Deguchi, 1979; Takahashi *et al.*, 1989), the avian (chicken) retina (Pierce *et al.*, 1993), and the *Xenopus* eye (Cahill *et al.*, 1991) each produce a circadian rhythm of melatonin secretion. Also, single pineal cells of the green anole lizard express a circadian rhythm in melatonin production, as measured by reverse hemolytic plaque assay (Pickard and Tang, 1994). Isolated retinal neurons of a mollusk, *Bulla gouldiana*, maintain a circadian rhythm in membrane conductance (Michel *et al.*, 1993). Such reports indicate that circadian oscillations are cell autonomous.

In studies of the mammalian SCN, the question of whether or not rhythmicity is a cell-autonomous property has been approached in two ways—by the use of dissociated cell-suspension grafts for SCN transplantation and through the direct monitoring of neuronal activity of primary cultures of dissociated SCN cells. Dissociated fetal cells, like whole-tissue SCN grafts, restore locomotor, but not endocrine rhythms, with the period of the donor following implantation into the medial hypothalamus of the lesioned host. This finding suggests that the intrinsic peptidergic organization of the SCN and the network properties this may confer are not necessary for the SCN pacemaker function that regulates locomotor rhythmicity (Silver *et al.*, 1990; Lehman and Silver, 1994).

Although the ability of dissociated hypothalamic cell grafts to restore rhythmicity suggests that pacemaker function is intrinsic to individual SCN cells, it is also possible that the dissociated cells form interconnections after grafting. A more direct demonstration that individual cells can express circadian rhythmicity comes from *in vitro* studies of electrical activity and hormone secretion. Individual SCN neurons grown on multielectrode plates show robust long-term circadian rhythms in their firing rate (Welsh *et al.*, 1995) (Fig. 6). Interestingly, individual SCN neurons in a single culture plate express rhythms with independent circadian periods and phase relationships, even though these cells may be synaptically coupled and sometimes are adjacent to each other. It is important to note that there is a relationship between cellular activity and behavioral

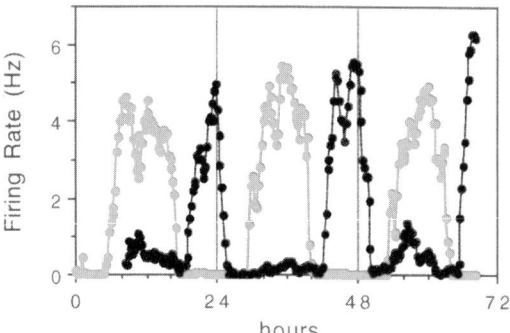

FIGURE 6 Oppositely phased circadian rhythms of two adjacent SCN neurons. Simultaneous recordings of two SCN neurons in the same culture that were known to be very close together because they were recorded from the same electrode and discriminated on the basis of spike amplitude. Each point reflects the mean firing rate for a 5-min record. Despite their proximity, these two cells exhibited circadian firing rhythms of nearly opposite phase, their peaks occurring nearly 12 hr apart. (from Welsh *et al.*, 1995).

rhythmicity, a characteristic revealed in studies of the *tau* mutant hamster and *clock* mutant mice. SCN slices from *tau* mutant hamsters maintain a mean rhythm of spontaneous single-unit neuronal activity that parallels the behavioral free-running period (Davies and Mason, 1994). Also, using the multielectrode plate preparation of dispersed cells (rather than intact tissue sections), *tau* mutant SCN cells and *Clock* mutant SCN cells have a mean period of neuronal activity rhythm that parallels the behavioral activity rhythm of the animal from which it was taken (Liu *et al.*, 1997; Herzog *et al.*, 1998). Together, these *in vitro* reports confirm that the *tau* and *clock* mutations affect circadian function in a cell-autonomous manner. Finally, cultured dissociated SCN cells produce coordinated circadian neurosecretory rhythms in VP and VIP (Murakami *et al.*, 1991; Watanabe *et al.*, 1993; Shinohara *et al.*, 1995).

These results prove that circadian rhythmicity is the property of individual SCN cells. It remains to be determined how these individual cells are normally coupled to produce coherent rhythmicity in the organism. Input from the rest of the brain (integrating environmental and internal cues) contributes to synchronization of the rhythms of the individual pacemaker cells by a variety of pathways and mechanisms, including glia (Shinohara *et al.*, 1995), gap junctions and connexins

(Colwell, 2000; Shinohara *et al.*, 2000a), synaptic communication (Shirakawa *et al.*, 2000), NCAM (Glass *et al.*, 2000), and input from the environment (Meijer *et al.*, 1998). Diffusible substances such as nitric oxide (Yang and Hatton, 1999) or neuropeptides like GABA (Liu and Reppert, 2000; Shinohara *et al.*, 2000b) may mediate synchrony among neighboring cells. These substances provide avenues whereby hormonal cues can influence circadian rhythmcity (see later).

III. GENETIC AND MOLECULAR BASIS OF CIRCADIAN RHYTHMS: OSCILLATOR MECHANISMS INVOLVE GENE EXPRESSION

While classical genetics has been used to investigate the circadian system at the organismal level, molecular genetics has been used to elucidate the genes of "circadian clock" cells. These techniques have been applied in higher plants; the filamentous fungus *Neurospora*; the fruit fly *Drosophila melanogaster*; and mice, hamsters, and rats. The research underlying the discoveries of clock genes and proteins has been amply reviewed, and numerous recent sources can be consulted for details of the studies of cellular clocks (e.g., Allada *et al.*, 2001; Bell-Pedersen, 2001; Harmer *et al.*, 2001; Iwasaki and Dunlap, 2000; King and Takahashi, 2000; Loros and Dunlap, 2001; Reppert and Weaver, 2001; Young and Kay, 2001). The results of studies in diverse organisms give us insights into how a pacemaker can be constructed at the level of gene expression. This work is rapidly developing, with advances from many laboratories around the world. Our aim here is to provide a framework for understanding the molecular basis of common regulatory patterns that can now be discerned among eukaryotic circadian systems, from fungi through mammals, with a view to understanding how the circadian clock can affect hormone regulation. We anticipate that the detailed molecular mechanisms will continue to be rapidly unraveled.

The common theme that has arisen over the past several years is that, across taxa, the molecular mechanisms governing circadian rhythms comprise functionally similar transcription–translation autoregulatory feedback loops, with many conserved sets of genes. The details of each system, mechanisms of entrainment as well as the regulation of pacemaker output, differ among systems.

The conceptualization of this molecular model began with the study of circadian mutants in *Drosophila melanogaster* in the 1970s (Konopka and Benzer, 1971). The universal mechanism modulating circadian rhythms appears to be comprised of complexes of two distinct PER-ARNT-SIM (PAS; PAS is an acronym for the first three genes found to share this dimerization domain) domain-containing transcription activators and suppressors (Fig. 7). PAS domain proteins have been shown to bind DNA at certain E-box recognition sites, as well as mediate protein–protein interactions (Whitmore *et al.*, 1998). The PAS domain activators typically form heterodimers and bind to E-box motifs to positively drive the transcription of "clock" genes. This clock message is translated into clock proteins, which undergo dimerization via their own PAS domains. These PAS domain suppressors translocate back into the nucleus and inhibit their own transcription. Following turnover of these inhibitory components, transcription of clock genes can begin again. This combination of positive and negative regulatory elements produces an oscillatory feedback loop (with a period of approximately 24 hr) that underlies the circadian system. Some of the specific genes and proteins that constitute clock components are discussed briefly later.

A. *Drosophila melanogaster*

Circadian mutations in *Drosophila* that shorten (short period, Per^S), lengthen (long period, Per^L), or abolish (arrhythmic, Per^{01}) daily rhythms have provided significant advances in the understanding of the molecular basis of circadian rhythms (reviewed in Rosbash, 1995; Wilsbacher and Takahashi, 1998; Young and Kay, 2001). Likewise, the identification of *period* (*Per*) and *timeless* (*Tim*) genes, and their subsequent cloning, has provided the foundation for studying regulatory feedback elements of circadian clocks (Crews *et al.*, 1988; Hardin *et al.*, 1990; Myers *et al.*, 1995; Rosato *et al.*, 1997). *Per* and *Tim* gene expression, protein accumulation, and protein localization oscillate with a circadian period, suggesting an important role in circadian function (Hardin *et al.*, 1990; Sehgal *et al.*, 1995). The *Per* and *Tim* genes peak at circadian time (CT) 12–14 (CT 12 being the start of subjective night) and both gene

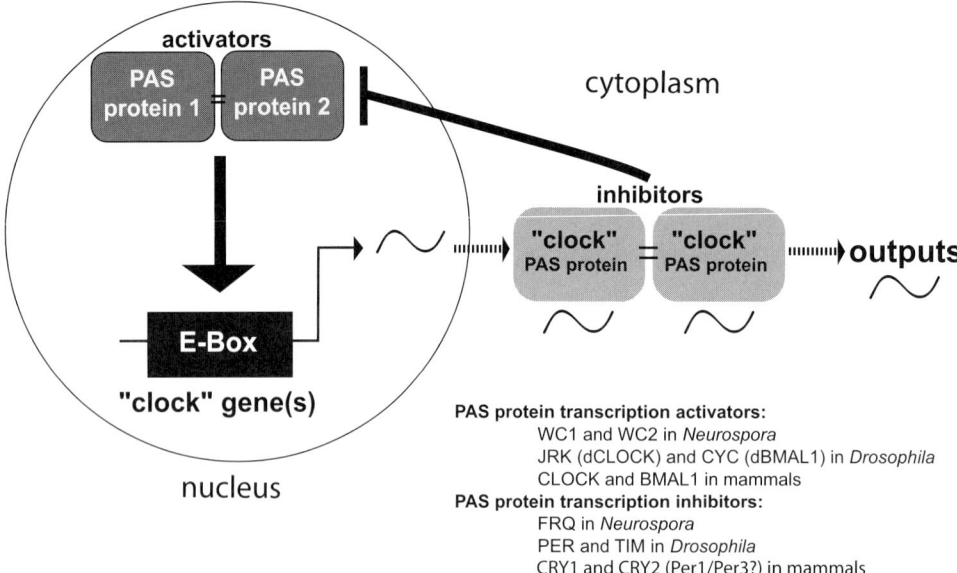

FIGURE 7 Cellular oscillator: transcription and translation feedback loop. This schematic shows the positive and negative regulators in the molecular clock that are common to *Neurospora*, *Drosophila*, and mammals. PAS domain proteins are central elements of both activators and inhibitors in the circadian feedback loop. Activator PAS protein heterodimers initiate transcription by binding to E-box motifs of clock genes. These clock genes are then translated into clock proteins that also undergo dimerization via their own PAS domains. These PAS protein inhibitors translocate back into the nucleus and obstruct their own transcription. The transcription and translation feedback cycle continues when the clock proteins degrade in the cytoplasm, releasing inhibition. The complete cycle has a period of approximately 24 hours. (Adapted from Dunlap, 1998).

products accumulate with a lag of about 6 hours. PER and TIM proteins form heterodimers and enter the cell nucleus at around CT 21, thereby inhibiting transcription of their own genes. In *Drosophila*, light degrades TIM protein, providing a molecular mechanism for circadian entrainment (Hunter-Ensor *et al.*, 1996; Myers *et al.*, 1996; Zeng *et al.*, 1996).

The positive elements in the *Drosophila* clock appear to be two genes and their protein products, namely *dBmal1* (also termed *cyc*) and *dClock* (also termed *Jrk*) (Darlington *et al.*, 1998). According to this model, the proteins encoded by the *Clock* and *Bmal1* genes (CLOCK and BMAL1) heterodimerize to form a transcription factor that binds to an E-box regulatory element on DNA of the *Per* and *Tim* genes, leading to the transcription of these negative components (PER and TIM proteins, discussed above). In turn, PER and TIM proteins accumulate in the cytoplasm and eventually translocate into the cell nucleus to regulate the CLOCK-BMAL1-modulated transcription of their own genes. This process occurs over a period of approximately 24 hours, thereby leading to the generation of circadian oscillations. This model system provides the foundation for understanding circadian rhythms in other systems, described later, and underscores the common mechanisms seen in circadian systems across taxa.

B. *Neurospora*

The molecular mechanisms responsible for generating circadian rhythms in *Neurospora* appear to be analogous to those seen in *Drosophila*. Similar to the PER-TIM dimers, the frequency (FRQ) protein acts to inhibit the transcription of its own gene synthesis (reviewed in Iwasaki and Dunlap, 2000; Loros and Dunlap, 2001). *Frq* RNA and FRQ protein oscillate with a circadian period (Garceau *et al.*, 1997). Similar to the regulatory loop seen in *Drosophila*, FRQ protein appears to inhibit its own transcription by forming a heterodimer with WHITE-COLLAR-1 (WC-1) and WC-2 proteins

(Crosthwaite et al., 1997) before entering the cell nucleus. WC-1 and WC-2, like *Drosophila Clock* (d*Clock*) and d*Bmal1*, act as the positive elements in the feedback loop in *Neurospora* by binding via PAS domains to E-box elements of the *frq* gene (Crosthwaite et al., 1997). Constant *frq* expression abolishes circadian rhythms and alterations in *frq* reset the clock, providing further evidence for a regulatory role for *frq* in *Neurospora* circadian rhythm generation (Aronson et al.,1994). *Frq* gene expression begins to rise at CT 4–6 and peaks approximate 10–12 hours later. FRQ protein peaks approximately 4 hours following peak *frq* transcription. As FRQ accumulates, it enters the cell nucleus and interacts with WC proteins and acts to inhibit its own transcription (reviewed in Dunlap, 1999; Iwasaki and Dunlap, 2000).

In contrast to *Drosophila*, light acts to increase *frq* transcription via WC-1-WC-2-mediated transcription (Aronson et al., 1994; Crosthwaite et al., 1997; Iwasaki and Dunlap, 2000). The effects of this increase in *frq* expression are dependent on the circadian time at which light is coincident. If light is presented when *frq* levels are rising during the late night and early morning, rapid *frq* expression leads to the phase advance of the circadian clock. However, if light is coincident with the time at which *frq* levels are falling, induction of *frq* leads to pronounced phase delays (reviewed in Dunlap, 1999; Crosthwaite et al., 1997). This mechanism accounts for the differential phase advancing and delaying effects of light necessary to entrain circadian rhythms to the environmental light:dark cycle.

C. Mammals

Three *Per* orthologs, *Per1* (Tei et al., 1997; Sun et al., 1997), *Per2* (Shearman et al., 1997; Albrecht et al., 1997), and *Per3* (Zylka et al., 1998) have been identified in humans (h) and mice (m). The finding that *Per* genes are expressed in a circadian fashion in the mammalian SCN has several implications, including the notions that *Per* genes are involved in circadian rhythm generation and that a regulatory feedback loop similar to that identified in *Drosophila* may modulate circadian rhythmicity in vertebrates (Tei et al., 1997; Sun et al., 1997; Shearman et al., 1997; Albrecht et al., 1997; Zylka et al., 1998). Per orthologs are also expressed in the brain outside of the SCN (Sun et al., 1997) in the retina (Sun et al., 1997; Tei et al., 1997), and in peripheral sites including the gonads and skeletal muscle (Balsalobre et al., 1998; Zylka et al., 1998).

Each *Per* ortholog peaks at a different time during the circadian cycle; in the SCN, m*Per1* expression peaks at approximately CT 6, m*Per2* at approximately CT 9, and m*Per3* peaks at approximately CT 6 and remains elevated until CT 9 (reviewed in King and Takahashi, 2000). Light presentation during the subjective night (or during night in an LD cycle) results in increased expression of m*Per1* and m*Per2*, with maximal induction after approximately 1 hour and 3 hours, respectively. m*Per3* does not appear to respond to light (reviewed in King and Takahashi, 2000).

The first "circadian" gene to be cloned in mammals was the *Clock* (Circadian locomotor output cycles kaput) gene in mice (Antoch et al., 1997; King et al., 1997). *Clock* acts as a positive element in the transcription–translation control of circadian function in mammals. CLOCK protein forms a heterodimer with BMAL1 and then binds the promotor of the *Per* and *Cryptochrome* (*Cry*) (discussed later) genes to activate transcription (Gekakis et al., 1998; reviewed in Wilsbacher and Takahashi, 1998; King and Takahashi, 2000). The binding partners for the negative limb of the mammalian clock are still uncertain, but it appears that CRY is an important component (see below). Several findings suggest that, in addition to negative feedback regulation, there is also an interacting positive-feedback loop (reviewed in Reppert and Weaver, 2001). The positive loop in this cycle appears to be PER2 modulated activation of *Bmal1* transcription, with availability of *Bmal1* being the rate-limiting step in *Per/Cry* transcription.

The mammalian cryptochrome genes, namely *Cryptochrome 1* (*Cry1*) and *Cryptochrome 2* (*Cry2*) have been implicated as essential components of the mammalian clock. These genes are interesting in that they are homologous to photolyases (light-activated repair enzymes) and act like blue-light photoreceptors in the retina. Yet they have no photolyase activity in the expressed protein *in vitro* (Hsu et al., 1996). Furthermore, it is clear that the retina is essential for entrainment in mammals, ruling out a photoreceptive role for *Cry* genes in the SCN. Nevertheless, like other clock genes, the mRNA for *Cry* genes is abundant in the SCN, retina, and other tissues of the body (Kobayashi et al., 1998;

Miyamoto and Sancar, 1998), suggesting a role for *Cry* genes in circadian function and entrainment. In support of this, m*Cry2* knockout mice have free-running periods approximately 1-hour longer than wild-type (WT) controls (Thresher *et al.*, 1998). These mice also display dramatically increased phase shifts in response to a light pulse at CT17 compared to WT controls. In contrast to m*Cry2* knockout mice, m*Cry1* knockout mice have a period that is approximately 1 hour shorter than WT controls (van der Horst *et al.*, 1999; Vitaterna *et al.*, 1999). Further evidence that cryptochromes are essential for circadian rhythmicity comes from the fact that mice doubly mutant for both m*Cry1* and m*Cry2* are arrhythmic (van der Horst *et al.*, 1999; Vitaterna *et al.*, 1999). In addition, *Per1* expression is elevated and arrhythmic in these double knockout mice in both light:dark and constant darkness, suggesting an inhibitory role for cryptochromes in the circadian feedback loop (Vitaterna *et al.*, 1999). In contrast, *Per2* expression is rhythmic in a light:dark cycle, yet arrhythmic in constant darkness. mCRY1 and mCRY2 have been found to form heterodimers with PER proteins leading to the nuclear import and inhibition of CLOCK-BMAL1-mediated activation of transcription (Yagita *et al.*, 2000).

Our understanding of the molecular mechanisms regulating clock function has been dramatically advanced by mouse genetic studies. For example, in the 1980s, a circadian mutation name *tau* was identified that resulted in a shortened circadian period in Syrian hamsters (Ralph and Menaker, 1988). It is now known that the *tau* locus is encoded by casein kinase I epsilon (CKIε). CKIε appears to interact with PERIOD to modulate circadian function, and the mutant form of CKIε is unable to phosphorylate PERIOD, suggesting a mechanism by which the *tau* mutation leads to a shortened circadian period (Lowrey *et al.*, 2000; Vielhaber *et al.*, 2000). The importance of this mechanism in organizing circadian rhythmicity and its dependent responses is highlighted in Section VII in the discussion of the endocrine studies of the *tau* mutant hamster. The potential of this line of research is dramatized by the finding of a genetic basis for a sleep abnormality in humans, known as familial advanced sleep-phase syndrome (FASPS). In affected individuals, sleep duration is normal, but sleep onset occurs very early, around 7:30 PM, and wake-up time is advanced to about 4:30 AM. Affected individuals have a serine-to-glycine mutation in the CKIε binding region of the hPER2 gene, leading to hypophosphorylation by CKIε in vitro (Toh *et al.*, 2001).

In summary, the first studies suggested a circadian clock consisting of positively acting transcription factors that produce the transcription of a gene whose protein then fed back to interfere with the action of the positive elements and to inhibit its own transcription. Subsequent studies have shown there are other clock components with the demonstration of two sets of interacting feedback loops (reviewed in Reppert and Weaver, 2001). The specific genes and their interactions that result in circadian timekeeping continue to be explored. At the same time, it is important to bring these results back to the organism and to understand how these molecular oscillations result in the circadian changes in SCN electrical and metabolic activity that regulate circadian time in the rest of the body. We now turn to the ways in which temporal information is communicated to the neural, endocrine, and neuroendocrine systems.

IV. PHOTIC INPUT PATHWAYS TO THE SUPRACHIASMATIC NUCLEUS

A. Suprachiasmatic Nucleus Pacemakers Are Reset by External Stimuli

In addition to its endogenous timekeeping function (measured in constant conditions), a key role of the SCN lies in mediating the entrainment of circadian rhythms to the environment. Because the daily LD cycle provides the most reliable time-locked environmental signal, the route whereby photic information reaches the SCN has been a key to the discovery of not only the general location of the brain clock in the SCN, but also the cellular locus of the oscillator cells and their molecular components. The exclusive role of the retina in the transduction of light information into neural signals subserving circadian entrainment was established through the demonstration that bilateral enucleation and transection of the optic nerves totally abolishes the entrainment of circadian rhythms to light:dark cycles (Rusak and Boulos, 1981). In mammals, all known photoreceptors lie in the retina, and the demonstration of direct retinal input to the SCN via the RHT provided one of the earliest clues to the location of the brain clock

(Moore and Lenn, 1972). Since that time, the existence of an RHT has been demonstrated in every mammalian species investigated (Moore, 1996), even in animals such as the blind mole rat, which has a degenerate retina that is not used for vision (Cooper et al., 1993).

In addition to the RHT, the SCN receives light information via a geniculohypothalamic tract (GHT), an indirect projection arising from neurons in the ventrolateral geniculate nucleus and intergeniculate leaflet of the thalamus (Pickard, 1982; Ribak and Peters, 1975; Swanson et al., 1974). The RHT is necessary for the photoentrainment of mammalian circadian rhythms; transection of RHT fibers (with verification by cholera toxin–horseradish peroxidase histochemistry) eliminates entrainment but not free-running rhythmicity even though projections to thalamic and tectal visual centers are spared (Johnson et al., 1988). The involvement of the RHT, but not the GHT, in the photoentrainment pathway is also supported by the finding that circadian entrainment to light:dark cycles persists following lesions of the primary and secondary optic tracts that spare the former, but not the latter, visual projection to the SCN (Rusak and Boulos, 1981). Visual information transmitted to the SCN via the GHT, although not essential for light:dark entrainment, appears to play a modulatory role in the photic regulation of the SCN pacemaker because the destruction of the intergeniculate leaflet alters the responses of circadian rhythms to light and dark (Harrington and Rusak, 1986).

As an aside, it is worth mentioning that wide attention has been given to a study suggesting that the application of light to the knee may be effective in entraining human circadian rhythms (Campbell and Murphy, 1998). This work is provocative; its broader significance awaits the demonstration of physiological significance, mediating mechanism(s), and replication using other, robust markers of circadian phase (cf. Hebert et al., 1999).

B. Photic Signals Regulate Gene Expression in the Suprachiasmatic Nucleus

Photic input pathways must reach elements of the clock if light is to reset the clock mechanism. Thus, it has been of extreme importance to find which genes and clock components are regulated by light. The heart of this strategy has been to explore how resetting the clock occurs and how such resetting results in an altered circadian phase in clock-controlled genes (CCG) and behaviors. It is now known that a large number of immediate early genes (IEGs), including *c-fos*, *fos-B*, *jun-B*, *zif268* (*NGF1-A*), and *nur77* (*NGF1-B*), are induced by light in a clock-gated fashion. For some of these IEGs (e.g., *c-fos*), there is a correlation between the threshold and magnitude of the light-induced expression of the gene and the amount of behavioral phase shift. How such IEG expression is related to expression of circadian clock genes remains to be elucidated. Light also induces the expression of several clock genes, including *Per1*, *Per2*, and *Clock*. As shown later, by using luciferase reporter gene technology, the responses of such clock genes to phase-resetting cues in various tissues of the body have been used to examine how entrainment occurs.

There has been considerable interest in elucidating the cellular pathway for photic entrainment of the SCN pacemaker. Observations from a number of laboratories have suggested the possible role of transcriptional regulatory factors in the transduction cascade by which light entrains the SCN pacemaker. The immediate-early gene, *c-fos*, provided an initial focus in these investigations because its protein product, Fos, is a component of a DNA-binding complex that (1) regulates gene transcription and (2) may play a role in signaling pathways coupling external stimuli to long-term cellular responses (Sheng and Greenberg, 1990; Morgan and Curran, 1991). Consistent with its putative role in signal transduction, the *c-fos* gene has been implicated in the cellular pathway for circadian photoentrainment by concurrent *in vivo* and *in vitro* studies demonstrating that light induces *c-fos* expression in the SCN (for review, see Takahashi, 1995). Key observations in these studies are related to the fact that the photic regulation of *c-fos* expression and SCN circadian function are gated in the same time domain, such that light has an inductive effect on SCN levels of *c-fos* mRNA and Fos protein(s), but only when photostimulation is capable of phase shifting circadian rhythms (i.e., during the night or subjective night) (Aronin et al., 1990; Kornhauser et al., 1990; Rea, 1992; Rusak et al., 1990). Furthermore, the photic sensitivities to the induction of *c-fos* expression and phase shifts in circadian behavior are quantitatively similar (Kornhauser et al., 1990). Because Fos interacts with the protein products of other

IEGs to form the activating protein-1 (AP-1) transcription factor (Morgan and Curran, 1991), it is noteworthy that light also induces SCN expression of AP-1 activity and the IEGs, *jun-B, NGFI-A,* and *NGFI-B* only at discrete times coinciding with its phase-shifting action (Kornhauser *et al.,* 1992; Rusak *et al.,* 1992; Sutin and Kilduff, 1992). The administration of antisense oligonucleotides against the *c-fos* and *jun-B* genes inhibits the photic induction of proteins encoded by these IEGs and phase shifts in the circadian rhythm of locomotor behavior (Wollnik *et al.,* 1995), suggesting that the induction of IEG expression in the SCN is necessary for the phase-shifting effect of light on circadian behavior.

C. Circadian System Has Specialized Photoreceptors

Photoreceptors providing information to the circadian system have properties that differ from those involved in visual-image formation, as revealed by using the magnitude of the phase shift of locomotor rhythms as a dependent response. Specifically, the reciprocal relationship between intensity and duration holds for unusually long durations of up to 45 minutes (Takahashi *et al.,* 1984). Furthermore, mice lacking rod and cone photoreceptor cells have normal circadian photoentrainment, although they are behaviorally blind (Foster *et al.,* 1991; Provencio *et al.,* 1994; Freedman *et al.,* 1999; von Schantz *et al.,* 2000).

The mammalian eye contains at least two classes of photoactive pigments, the vitamin A–based opsins and the vitamin B(2)–based cryptochromes. Mutant mice lacking either classic photoreceptors or cryptochromes exhibit strongly rhythmic locomotor responses to 10 and 100 lux daily 12:12 light:dark cycles (Selby *et al.,* 2000). Triple mutant mice, however, carrying both cryptochrome and retinal degenerate mutations are nearly arrhythmic under both light:dark cycles and in constant darkness, indicating that classic opsins and cryptochromes serve functionally redundant roles in the transduction of light information to behavioral modulation. The results also suggest that cryptochromes have a role in both photoreception and in the central clock mechanism of the SCN (as discussed previously). More recent evidence indicates that the mammalian photoreceptor important for entrainment is composed of specialized ganglion cells that contain melanopsin, the protein found in amphibian melanophores that causes color changes (Hattar *et al.,* 2002; Provencio *et al.,* 2002). These ganglion cells send axons directly to the suprachiasmatic nucleus (Berson *et al.,* 2002; Hannibal *et al.,* 2002). Importantly, unlike ganglion cells involved in vision, these cells are directly responsive to light, even when input from rods and cones is blocked (Berson *et al.,* 2002). Further developments in understanding circadian photoreceptor and clock function are likely to provide insights into the evolution of the circadian system.

V. OUTPUT SIGNALS OF THE SUPRACHIASMATIC NUCLEUS

A. Suprachiasmatic Nucleus Controls the Phase of Rhythmic Responses

The output pathways of the SCN are of direct interest to the understanding of circadian oscillation of hormones. There is evidence for a redundant output signal from the SCN. Neural efferents of the SCN have been well characterized. Substantial evidence supports a role for diffusible signals in coordinating circadian rhythms. At target sites, some dependent responses are likely to be nonoscillating and driven. Other targets may themselves oscillate, and SCN pacemakers drive the phase of this oscillation. Understanding the mediating mechanisms in diverse tissues of the body has been the focus of intense interest.

B. Neural Efferents

As suggested by the neural-tissue-transplant studies, discussed later, there are both neural efferents and diffusible neuroendocrine signals produced by SCN cells. That SCN efferent projections reach nearby intra- and extrahypothalamic targets has long been known (Watts, 1991; Morin *et al.,* 1994). Outputs can generally be divided into those that regulate motivated behavior (e.g., general activity, drinking, feeding, and estrous behavior) and homeostatic behavior (e.g., body temperature and plasma hormone concentrations). Theoretically, these rhythms in behavior and physiology can be regulated by neural efferents from the SCN, diffusible signals, or a combination of both.

Hypothalamic-releasing hormones such as gonadotropin-releasing hormone (GnRH) act on the anterior pituitary by releasing their contents into the fenestrated portal capillaries in the external layer of the median eminence. There is no evidence for direct SCN projections to either the median eminence or the organum vasculosum of the lamina terminalis (OVLT), suggesting that the SCN does not directly regulate hypophyseal function (Horvath, 1997; Watts et al., 1987). Instead, projections from the SCN contact many brain areas rich in neuroendocrine cells and releasing factors, thereby providing a means for indirect neural regulation of neuroendocrine rhythms (Fig. 8).

The most dense efferent pathway from the SCN projects to the area beneath the paraventricular nucleus, termed the subparaventricular zone (sPVZ) (Watts and Swanson, 1987). Numerous other neural targets of the SCN have been identified in rats and Syrian hamsters (Kalsbeek et al., 1993; Moore, 1995; Stephan et al., 1981; Watts and Swanson, 1987). As previously suggested, many of these targets contain neuroendocrine cells and hypothalamic-releasing factors. Among others, there are direct projections to the medial preoptic area (MPOA), supraoptic nucleus (SON), anteroventral periventricular nucleus (AVPV), paraventricular nucleus (PVN), the dorsomedial nucleus of the hypothalamus (DMH), the lateral septum (LS) and the arcuate (ARH). These projections suggest that the SCN may indirectly regulate neuroendocrine function by acting on hypophysiotropic neuroendocrine cells. Indeed, there is evidence for direct projections from the SCN to neuroendocrine cells containing releasing factors such as corticotropin-releasing hormone (CRH) and GnRH (Buijs et al., 1998; Horvath, 1997; Horvath et al., 1998; Kalsbeek et al., 1996a; van der Beek et al., 1993, 1997a; Vrang et al., 1995).

In addition to direct SCN regulation of brain areas controlling hormone release, the SCN has polysynaptic projections to endocrine glands and peripheral organs. The best-characterized pathway involves the polysynaptic pathway from the SCN to the pineal gland, which is involved in the regulation of melatonin production (reviewed in Pevet, 2000; Card, 2000). In addition, the use of retrograde transneuronal tracers has allowed the identification of brain targets innervating peripheral organs via the sympathetic nervous system. Using this technique, projections from the SCN to peripheral organs such as the liver, adrenals, and thyroid have been identified (Buijs et al., 1999; Kalsbeek et al., 2000; La Fleur et al., 2000; Teclemariam-Mesbah et al., 1999). These findings suggest that the SCN can regulate endocrine rhythms by acting directly on the target gland in addition to acting indirectly via hypothalamic neuroendocrine cells. These issues are discussed in further detail later.

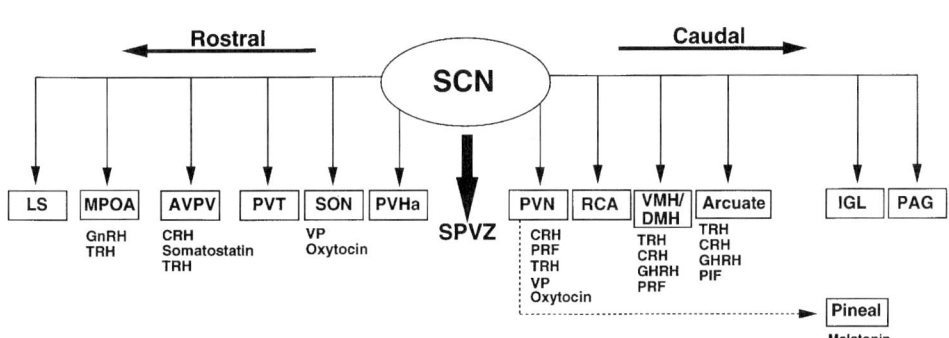

FIGURE 8 Efferent projections of the rodent SCN to its targets in the brain. Below each target area is a list of neuroendocrine cells that lie in that region of the brain and could potentially be regulated by direct projections from the SCN. Solid lines represent monosynaptic projections; the dotted line represents a polysynaptic projection to the pineal gland. The pronounced overlap between neuroendocrine cells and SCN efferent terminals, combined with reports demonstrating direct neuronal projections from the SCN to neuroendocrine cells (e.g., GnRH and corticotropin-releasing hormone, CRH, cells), provides suggestive evidence for a global mechanism of circadian hormonal regulation.

C. Diffusible Signals

The SCN has a circadian rhythm of arginine VP expression, and SCN neurons are the source of the circadian rhythm of VP in the cerebrospinal fluid (CSF) (for review, see Majzoub et al., 1991). VP exhibits a prominent daily rhythm in the CSF. A circadian rhythm of VP release is seen in SCN explants *in vitro* (Earnest and Sladek, 1986), and transplantation of fetal SCN into VP-deficient Brattleboro rats that normally lack this peptide results in a normal diurnal rhythm in VP levels in the CSF (Earnest et al., 1989). The rhythm is abolished following SCN lesions, but survives transection of most SCN efferents, with a damped amplitude (Reppert et al., 1987). It should be noted that the precise function of VP secretion by the SCN is unknown. It is not thought, however, to generate the expression of circadian rhythmicity because Brattleboro rats lack VP, yet express normal circadian rhythms (for review, see Majzoub et al., 1991; Reppert et al., 1987).

Several lines of evidence suggest indirectly that a diffusible signal from the SCN can sustain locomotor rhythmicity in hamsters. SCN-lesioned hamsters recover locomotor rhythmicity following the grafting of anterior hypothalamic tissue containing the SCN into the third ventricle (reviewed in Lehman et al., 1994). In such grafts, there are often few neural connections between graft and host, and the precise locus of these connections seems variable among animals (Lehman et al., 1987; Aguilar-Roblero et al., 1994). SCN grafts are functional irrespective of their precise attachment sites at various loci in the third ventricle or in the lateral ventricle near the foramen of Monro. This fact is important because the grafted SCN makes local connections with brain regions that lie near the attachment site of the graft, but no single graft reestablishes all normal efferent connections (Canbeyli et al., 1991a,b; Wiegand and Gash, 1988). Furthermore, hamsters bearing an "SCN island" created with a Halasz knife recover free-running rhythms, often at the phase seen prior to the transection of SCN efferents. Although it is possible that efferent fibers may have grown across the knife cut to form the correct synaptic connections, there is no evidence of such plasticity in the mammalian brain.

Direct proof of the existence of a diffusible signal comes from a study of encapsulated SCN grafts transplanted into SCN-lesioned adults (Silver et al., 1996) (Fig. 9). These capsules prevented neural outgrowth while allowing the diffusion of signals between graft and host. Donor tissue taken from WT animals and placed in SCN-lesioned *tau* mutant hosts is viable, expresses SCN neuropeptide cells, and restores circadian locomotor rhythmicity with the period of the donor animal, even though these grafts are isolated from the rest of the brain. The results of these studies demonstrate that the transplanted biological clock of mammals, like the pacemakers described in *Drosophila* and silk moth nervous tissue, and in avian pineal gland, regulates rhythmicity by means of a diffusible signal.

The definitive identification of a physiologically significant endogenous diffusible signal is a wonderfully complex task because the SCN has both diffusible and neural outputs. This makes it difficult to distinguish the unique contribution of each output pathway because these may be redundant for some rhythmic responses. The necessary and sufficient criteria that must be met to confirm the existence of a diffusible signal in a fluid volume have been summarized by Nicholson (1999). First, there should be evidence that the removal or replacement of the signaling substance results in a change in the response being controlled and an assay of the substance should indicate that it is present or increases, or both, in a well-defined temporal relationship to the response (and similarly declines when the response disappears). In addition, evidence must be obtained that a fluid compartment is the conduit for a diffusible or transported signal. The signal must have access to and enter the compartment where the fluid dynamics and turnover in the compartment should allow appropriate movement of the signal. One candidate diffusible signal for controlling circadian locomotor rhythms has been identified as transforming growth factor-alpha (TGF-α) (Kramer et al., 2001). TGF-α is expressed rhythmically in the SCN, and when infused into the third ventricle it reversibly inhibits locomotor activity. This finding suggests that TGF-α may be an important SCN signal in the regulation of locomotor rhythms. Nonetheless, most evidence suggests that circadian rhythmicity is the result of multiple regulatory mechanisms, involving both neural efferents that reach specific targets in the brain, diffusible signals that reach widespread regions perhaps via the CSF, and feedback mechanisms to the SCN.

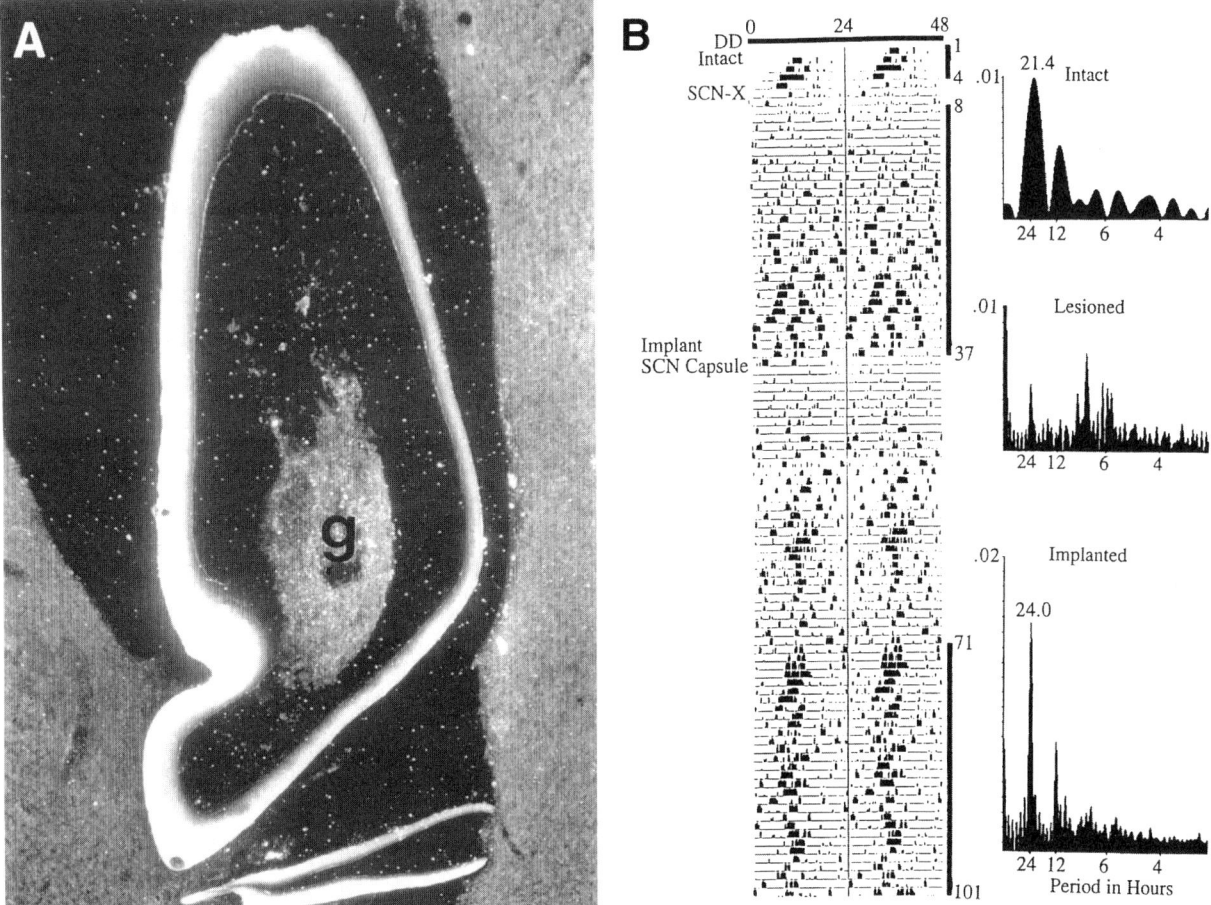

FIGURE 9 A. Microphotograph of an encapsulated graft (g) that restored locomotor rhythmicity in a SCN-lesioned host with the donor period. The capsule lies in the third ventricle of the host brain. B. Actogram of a *tau* mutant hamster with a circadian rhythm of 21.4-hr. The animal received an SCN lesion and then an encapsulated graft containing the SCN at the point indicated on the left of the actogram. Recovery of locomotor rhythmicity with the period (24-hr) of the donor (wild-type) hamster is seen. A spectral analysis of the data is shown on the right of the actogram. The black vertical bar indicates the days analyzed (intact, lesioned, and transplanted). From Silver *et al.* (1996).

In *Drosophilia*, the output signal(s) controlling circadian behavior seem to be humoral because a WT brain transplanted into the abdomen restores circadian rhythms of activity in arrhythmic flies (Handler and Konopka, 1979). A pigment-dispersing factor (PDF) has been proposed as a candidate humoral factor because it is necessary for the free-running activity rhythms. PDF is expressed in the ventrolateral neurons, and the majority of *Drosophila* lacking ventrolateral neurons or PDF become arrhythmic in constant darkness (Renn *et al.*, 1999).

VI. SUPRACHIASMATIC NUCLEUS AS A MASTER OSCILLATOR HOLDS THE CIRCADIAN SYSTEM TOGETHER: THERE ARE MANY OSCILLATORS WITHIN SPECIALIZED TISSUES OF COMPLEX ORGANISMS

Once circadian pacemakers have been localized to a specialized tissue such as the SCN, a new set of questions emerges. In the context of hormone secretions, it is important to know whether all rhythms are controlled by this unified oscillator or whether the circadian system is constructed of several pacemakers, each controlling different sets of rhythms? At least two substantially different mechanisms may be imagined to regulate the wide range of circadian responses that have been described. In one view, SCN pacemakers drive rhythms in passive nonoscillating cells. In second view, SCN pacemakers coordinate cell-autonomous "slave" oscillators in other tissues. Also, we can ask whether the inputs and outputs of the system are unidirectional or whether they constitute feedback loops. Is the sensitivity of input pathways controlled by the pacemaker, and can the outputs of the system affect its own properties? The number of oscillators in the circadian system at the level of whole organisms has long been a point of discussion because different output rhythms can run with different periods under constant conditions. Historically, numerous lines of evidence have pointed to the existence of multiple oscillators. These include the internal desynchronization of circadian rhythms, involving the uncoupling of the temperature rhythm and the sleep–wake cycle in humans (Aschoff and Wever, 1965; Aschoff et al., 1967); a phenomenon called splitting, in which a given response splits into two components that can be expressed with different circadian phases (Schardt et al., 1989; Meijer et al., 1990); and the occurrence of food-entrainable rhythms, in which food can entrain circadian rhythms following ablation of the SCN (e.g., Stephan et al., 1979). Direct evidence for peripheral oscillators in mammals derives from the use of reporter gene technology (Yamazaki et al., 2000; see later). Taken together, the evidence indicates several mechanisms whereby SCN output signals can regulate rhythmic responses of the endocrine system.

VII. CIRCADIAN REGULATION OF ENDOCRINE RHYTHMS

A. Circadian Rhythms in Hormone Secretions

Circadian rhythmicity can be measured in a vast array of behavioral and physiological responses, including such varied responses as latency to tap a key in response to a cue and daily rhythms of urinary pH. The most widely used index of circadian rhythmicity involves measures of activity. Activity-based measures are useful because they are easy to monitor at very short intervals (or continuously) without perturbing the animal. Under stable environmental circumstances, all the various rhythms in the body are phase-locked; hence, measuring one response is a reasonable predictor of the phase of other responses.

In travel across time zones (jet lag) or an unusual sleep–wake cycle (shift work), the phase of various rhythms in the body can be shifted with respect to one another. In this section, we review circadian control of endocrine rhythms and their relation to other homeostatic systems such as sleeping and eating. We also examine the changes in the circadian control of endocrine secretions with age.

Most hormones are released episodically, typically at intervals ranging from 1 to 4 hours (i.e., ultradian rhythm; reviewed in Turek and Van Cauter, 1994). In addition to these ultradian rhythms in hormone production and secretion, there are also circadian variations in circulating hormone concentrations. These alterations are achieved by the modulation of pulse amplitude (i.e., amount of hormone released), pulse frequency (i.e., rate of hormone release), or by a combination of these processes. The fact that hormones are released episodically complicates the study of circadian endocrine rhythms because circulating concentrations of hormones can vary dramatically within a period as short as 30 minutes. This property of hormone secretion requires that numerous samples be taken at equal intervals over a 24-hour period to assay the blood concentration of hormones. The interpretation of studies of circadian endocrine rhythms are limited by the fact that samples are often collected from animals held in a LD cycle. This method does not allow for the determination of endogenous circadian control vs environmentally driven daily rhythms (i.e., diurnal rhythms). Despite these complications, numerous studies reveal clear daily patterns of hormone secretion that are endogenously driven and are under the direct control of the SCN.

Virtually every endocrine factor measured shows a circadian or diurnal rhythm. For example, studies in male rhesus macaques, in which animals were sampled at 20-min intervals in a LD cycle, revealed clear diurnal rhythms in LH, testosterone, prolactin, and cortisol (Plant, 1981). Likewise, studies in rats, Syrian hamsters, and humans show clear circadian variation in gonadotropins and gonadal steroids around the onset of puberty (Blomquist and Holt, 1992;

Boyar *et al.*, 1976; Smith and Stetson, 1980; Andrews and Ojeda, 1981; Jakacki *et al.*, 1982; Keating and Tcholakian, 1979). There have been suggestions that diurnal variation in hormone concentrations may simply be modulated by sleep. However, sleep-reversal and sleep-interruption experiments confirm that regulation is, at least in part, controlled by an endogenous circadian clock (Desir *et al.*, 1982; Kapen *et al.*, 1974; Van Cauter and Refetoff, 1985; Van Cauter, 1988; Wehr *et al.*, 1993), although interactions between sleep and the circadian system exist (see later). Taken together, these findings provide clear evidence for robust circadian rhythms in endocrine function that are generated by an endogenous time-keeping mechanism. Several systems that have been well characterized are discussed in more detail later.

1. Glucocorticoids

Serum cortisol concentrations exhibit a robust diurnal rhythm in both human and nonhuman primates (Weitzman *et al.*, 1971; Van Cauter and Refetoff, 1985; Gallagher *et al.*, 1973). In humans, cortisol concentrations begin to rise late in the night (during sleep) and peak in the early morning. In rats and other nocturnal rodents, the pattern or glucocorticoid production and secretion is approximately 180 degrees out of phase with humans, with a peak occurring during the night when these animals are active (e.g., Albers *et al.*, 1985; Ottenweller *et al.*, 1987; Wong *et al.*, 1983). The rhythm in cortisol secretion continues in constant conditions in both human and nonhuman primates (Dubey *et al.*, 1983; Czeisler *et al.*, 1999) and rodents (e.g., Moore and Eichler, 1972). Research in humans suggests that the daily pattern of cortisol secretion is the result of a change in pulse amplitude rather than a change in pulse frequency (Follenius *et al.*, 1992).

In 1972, the first evidence for SCN regulation of hormone secretion was reported, demonstrating that bilateral SCN lesions abolished circadian corticosterone rhythms in rats (Moore and Eichler, 1972), providing the first evidence of SCN control over circadian rhythms in endocrine function. Since the 1970s, numerous studies have confirmed the SCN regulation of various circadian hormone rhythms.

2. Gonadotropins and Gonadal Steroids

One of the first studies to demonstrate a robust daily pattern in testosterone secretion was conducted in male rhesus monkeys (Plant, 1981). This study showed a clear diurnal rhythm with a peak when blood was collected at night. Prior to this time, most studies had failed to collect blood at frequent enough intervals to detect a clear diurnal rhythm (Turek and Van Cauter, 1994). A subsequent study in male monkeys revealed that the rhythm in testosterone persists in constant environmental conditions (Dubey *et al.*, 1983).

Gonadal steroid secretion is regulated by gonadotropin release from the anterior pituitary. In humans and rodents, the general consensus is that gonadotropins are released in a diurnal pattern around the time of puberty (e.g., Andrews and Ojeda, 1981; Smith and Stetson, 1980). Among peripubertal boys and girls, the diurnal pattern of LH and follicle-stimulating hormone (FSH) are associated with a nighttime increase in both factors (Dunkel *et al.*, 1992; Apter *et al.*, 1993). As peripubertal children enter adulthood, the pulse amplitude of the gonadotropins during the daytime increases, thereby reducing the diurnal pattern; most studies in adults do not show circadian patterns of gonadotropins (Krieger *et al.*, 1972; Veldhuis *et al.*, 1986). The diurnal (or circadian) pattern of the gonadotropins is, in part, regulated by sleep (see later).

In contrast to the gonadotropins, it is generally accepted that there is a robust circadian rhythm in testosterone concentrations in adult males, with concentrations being lowest in late evening, rising throughout the night, and being highest in the early morning (Clair *et al.*, 1985; Miyatake *et al.*, 1980; Mock *et al.*, 1978; Spratt *et al.*, 1988; Veldhuis *et al.*, 1987). The disparity between a lack of adult male gonadotropin rhythms and the robust rhythm in testosterone suggests that regulation of the testosterone rhythm is downstream from LH, possibly via diurnal variation in testicular blood flow or LH receptor density or affinity, or diurnal variation in hormonal (or other) systems that interact with the hypothalamic-pituitary-gonadal (HPG) axis.

In human females, major hormonal changes associated with the menstrual cycle have been well characterized. However, diurnal or circadian changes in estradiol and progesterone in females have not received substantial attention. Nonhuman primates show diurnal variation in estrogen and progesterone during the luteal, but not the follicular, stage of the menstrual cycle (Spies *et al.*, 1974). The results in humans have been equivocal, with some studies showing no diurnal variation in progesterone or estradiol (Aedo *et al.*, 1981;

Rossmanith *et al.*, 1990) and others show circadian changes during some phases of the menstrual cycle [early follicular phase (Rebar and Yen, 1979), and estradiol in the late luteal phase and progesterone during all phases (Carandente *et al.*, 1989)]. However, the degree to which the menstrual cycle is a function of the circadian timing system in humans remains to be examined.

3. Prolactin

A pronounced daily rhythm in prolactin secretion has been reported for a number of species, including both human and nonhuman primates (Dunn *et al.*, 1980; Spies *et al.*, 1979; Van Cauter *et al.*, 1981). Prolactin has a robust diurnal rhythm, with plasma concentrations being highest during sleep and lowest during the waking hours in humans (reviewed in Freeman *et al.*, 2000; Parker *et al.*, 1974; Sassin *et al.*, 1973). Evidence in humans maintained in constant conditions demonstrates that this rhythm is circadian and persists independent of sleep (Waldstreicher *et al.*, 1996). Likewise, in rats prolactin secretion has a robust circadian pattern that persists in constant conditions (Bethea and Neill, 1979; Kizer *et al.*, 1975) and is abolished after lesions of the SCN (Bethea and Neill, 1979).

B. Interactions between Sleep and Circadian Regulation of Endocrine Rhythms

Circadian studies in humans and animals are typically conducted by placing subjects in constant conditions and allowing them to sleep either whenever desired or during scheduled sleep periods. These studies do not allow the dissociation of circadian control from sleep regulation of hormones. However, sleep can have a marked effect on the endocrine system. Studies in humans, in which sleep bouts can be more readily controlled, have been helpful in parsing the circadian and sleep effects on daily fluctuations of hormone concentrations. One protocol that has been developed to dissociate the effects of sleep and circadian influences on human rhythms is termed the constant routine (CR) technique (Mills *et al.*, 1978; Czeisler *et al.*, 1989). In these CR studies, humans remain awake in a semirecumbent position, receiving frequent small meals for approximately 1 or 2 days. Other study designs used with humans have employed sleep deprivation, but have not controlled for posture throughout the testing period. Another technique that has been applied has been abrupt shifts in the sleep–wake cycle. In these studies, the effects of the circadian system vs those of sleep can be seen independently on the day of the shift. These studies have found that some endocrine oscillations are driven primarily by the circadian system, some by sleep, and others by an interaction between sleep and the circadian timing system (Fig. 10) (reviewed in Czeisler and Klerman, 1999).

In general, melatonin and cortisol levels are primarily driven by the circadian system and are relatively unaffected by sleep (Wehr, 1998; Czeisler and Kleman, 1999). For some hormones, such as LH, thyroid-stimulating hormone (TSH), prolactin (PRL), and parathyroid hormone (PTH), the circadian pattern is a function of an interaction between the sleep and circadian systems (Allan and Czeisler, 1994; Kapen *et al.*, 1974; El-Hajj Fuleihan *et al.*, 1997; Rossmanith, 1998; Van Cauter and Refetoff, 1985). For example, the regulation of LH was shown in a study in which the sleep–wake cycle was abruptly shifted (Kapen *et al.*, 1974). On the day following the shift, LH shows a pronounced peak in peripubertal children during the new time at which sleep occurred. However, a small peak is also seen at the time during which sleep occurred the previous night. This finding suggests the modulation of LH by sleep with a modest circadian regulation contributing to the daily rhythm. Similar findings have been found with PRL and phase-shifting studies in humans (Van Cauter and Refetoff, 1985). For TSH, a CR study demonstrated an interaction between the circadian and sleep systems (Allan and Czeisler, 1994). TSH normally shows a peak following the onset of sleep, with a slow decline throughout the night. Human subjects on a CR schedule still exhibited a robust circadian pattern of TSH concentrations, but there was a steady rise as night approached, with a peak in the middle of the night and a decline not beginning until morning. This finding suggests that the circadian peak of TSH occurs in the middle of the night, but that under normal conditions sleep acts to suppress TSH, and the interaction between sleep and the circadian system leads to the pattern observed.

In contrast to the hormones already mentioned that are either solely regulated by the circadian system or regulated by an interaction between the sleep and circadian systems, some hormones appear to be markedly

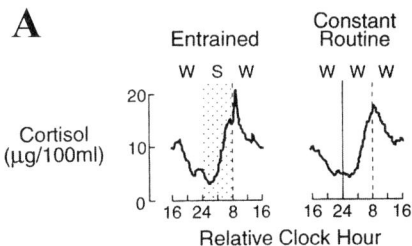
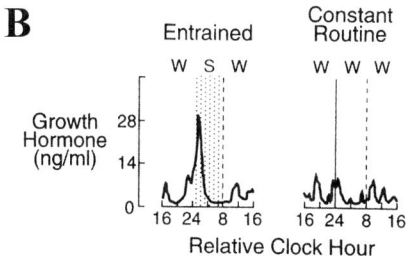
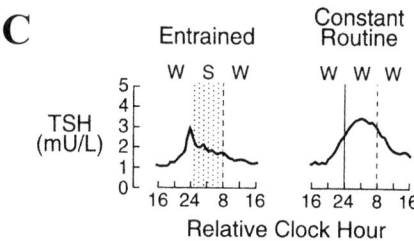

FIGURE 10 Relationship between the sleep and circadian systems. A. Daily pattern of cortisol concentrations in healthy males studied under baseline conditions while maintaining a regular schedule of nocturnal sleep (left panel, shaded area), compared with the cortisol profile of subjects under constant routine (CR) conditions (right panel). Note that cortisol concentrations throughout the day are relatively unaffected by sleep B. Daily patterns of growth hormone concentrations under baseline (left panel) and CR conditions (right panel). Note that sleep significantly drives the daily rhythm in growth hormone secretion. C. Daily patterns of thyroid-stimulating hormone (TSH) concentrations under baseline (left panel) and CR conditions (right panel). Note the interaction between sleep and the circadian system. Vertical dashed lines in all graphs indicate habitual wake times during the week prior to the study. From Czeisler and Klerman (1999).

affected by sleep. For example, growth hormone (GH) exhibits a pronounced peak at the time of sleep onset (Czeisler and Kleman, 1999; Weibel et al., 1997; Van Cauter and Refetoff, 1985). During a CR experiment, GH still shows a small peak at the time during which sleep onset would have occurred, but this pulse is small in amplitude and similar to pulses seen throughout the day (Czeisler and Kleman, 1999). This finding suggests that GH is primarily regulated by sleep rather than by the circadian system. This sleep-regulated diurnal fluctuation in GH may be a function of altered pituitary sensitivity to growth-hormone-releasing hormone (GHRH); the amount of GH produced in response to administration of GHRH is a function of the stage of sleep during which the GHRH is administered (Van Cauter et al., 1992).

Taken together, these findings suggest that there are pronounced interactions between the sleep and circadian timing system in the regulation of daily endocrine cycles. These findings underscore the importance of considering the effects of sleep on circadian parameters. They also have implications for shift work, jet lag, and sleep disturbances, and they suggest a need for further study of these interactions.

C. Endocrine Influence on Circadian Rhythms

Not only does the SCN regulate hormonal rhythms, but these hormonal systems also feed back to the SCN, presumably to regulate their own production and to fine-tune circadian rhythmicity. For example, high-affinity melatonin receptors have been localized to the SCN and the administration of melatonin can alter SCN phase (Dubocovich et al., 1996; Hastings et al., 1997; Lewy et al., 1992; Slotten et al., 2000; Vanecek and Watanabe, 1999). In addition, exogenous melatonin has been shown to alter the phase of electrical activity *in vitro*, in a manner predictable by the PRC (McArthur et al., 1991). The sensitivity of the SCN to melatonin may be a function of daily variation in the density of melatonin binding sites in the SCN (Anis et al., 1989). In humans, melatonin administration causes phase delays when it is taken late at night or early in the morning and phase advances when it is administered in the late morning to early afternoon (Lewy and Sack, 1997). This finding has obvious implications for shift work, jet lag, and the blind.

Evidence indicates that cells that express estrogen receptor-α (ER-α) in the preoptic area and amygdala, as well as the bed nucleus of the stria terminalis (BNST) and arcuate, provide input to the SCN (de la Iglesia et al., 1999). In the same study, using combined anterograde and retrograde tract tracers simultaneously injected into the SCN, there was little evidence of reciprocal connections between ER-α immunoreactive (ir) neurons and the SCN. Although the SCN does not communicate directly with these ER-α-containing cells, these results indicate that projections from ER-α-ir neurons may represent a means by which gonadal steroids modulate SCN function.

In accord with the observation that ER-α-ir neurons project to the SCN, gonadal steroids can affect circadian activity rhythms, suggesting that estradiol may act indirectly to modulate the circadian rhythms. However, there are some reports that estrogen receptors are present in the SCN, although at low levels (Gundlah et al., 2000; Hileman et al., 1999; Shughrue et al., 1997). Regardless of mode of action, estrogen has pronounced effects on circadian rhythms. Cycling female hamsters and rats show a phase advance in locomotor activity on the day of estrus (scalloping), when estradiol levels are highest (Morin et al., 1977), and, indeed, the continuous administration of estradiol in silastic capsules shortens the free-running period of ovariectomized hamsters (Morin et al., 1977). In addition to regulating circadian period, estradiol is thought to consolidate rhythms of locomotor activity. When hamsters are maintained in constant light, the normally stable activity phase frequently splits and desynchronizes, and the continuous administration of estradiol in silastic capsules to ovariectomized hamsters prevents splitting and desynchrony of locomotor rhythms (Morin, 1980).

In males, testosterone also seems to have a role in the consolidation of locomotor activity rhythms. Extended exposure to a short day lengths induces a decrease in testicular size and in testosterone levels in male hamsters (Ellis and Turek, 1983). Following testicular regression (or after castration) there is an increase in lability of activity onset, an expansion of the daily activity duration, and a decrease in wheel revolutions per cycle; testosterone replacement prevents these changes (Morin and Cummings, 1981). However testosterone and photoperiod interact in their regulation of activity. In animals kept in a long photoperiod before castration, testosterone replacement first reduces, but then increases wheel-running activity. In addition, testosterone is incapable of reversing the effects of short day lengths on running activity if it is administered to castrates following extended short-day exposure (Ellis and Turek, 1983). These findings suggest that short day lengths lead to an insensitivity to testosterone administration, presumably due to a down-regulation or reduced sensitivity of androgen receptors in short-day animals.

Testosterone may feed back to the SCN to act on androgen receptors. Receptors for testosterone in the SCN have only been identified in adult ferrets (Kashon et al., 1996). Alternatively, testosterone may exert its effects through conversion to estradiol, which may act either directly on the receptors in the SCN (e.g., Shughrue et al., 1997) or indirectly in ER-containing cells in other brain areas that, in turn, communicate with the SCN (e.g., de la Iglesia et al., 1999). In rats, the conversion of testosterone to estradiol may be important for the activity-stimulating effects of testosterone (Roy and Wade, 1975). Estradiol is nearly 100 times as effective at increasing activity than testosterone. In addition, dihydrotesosterone (a nonaromatizable androgen) has no effect on wheel-running activity (Roy and Wade, 1975). Taken together, these findings suggest that the conversion of testosterone to estrogen by aromatase may be important for the effects of testosterone on circadian rhythms.

One study suggests a novel means by which estrogen may affect circadian function. As already mentioned, single SCN cells can act as autonomous oscillators, and intercellular communication is necessary to maintain synchrony in a population of oscillators (e.g., Welsh et al., 1995). One of the means by which this synchrony may occur is through the formation and maintenance of gap junctions (Jiang et al., 1997; Shinohara et al., 2000a). Gap junctions are formed from transmembrane proteins called connexins. One study found that estrogen administration increased connexin32 mRNA in the SCN of ovariectomized rats (Shinohara et al., 2000b). This finding suggests that estrogen (and testosterone through the conversion to estradiol) may act on the SCN to strengthen the coupling among oscillators by the formation of gap junctions.

D. Sex Differences in Circadian Rhythms

The fact that hormones affect various aspects of circadian function suggests that, under normal conditions, sex differences in circadian rhythms may be observed.

Indeed, studies of circadian rhythms have revealed a variety of sex differences in numerous species, including hamsters, mice, rats, and humans. For example, female rats have a shorter free-running period than males and they have higher activity levels (Schull *et al.*, 1989). In addition, female rats have a greater circadian fluctuation of plasma corticosterone than males (Critchlow *et al.*, 1963). Like rats, female Syrian hamsters also have a shorter free-running period than male hamsters and have greater difficulty than males in entraining to photoperiods greater than 24 hr (Davis *et al.*, 1983). Similarly, female humans exhibit a shorter free-running period than males (Wever, 1984). In addition, there are pronounced sex differences in temperature rhythms, sleep patterns, and timing of glucocorticoid peaks in humans (Wever, 1984).

Octodon degus, diurnal precocial South American rodents, display pronounced sex differences in several circadian parameters that may be regulated by gonadal steroids. Unlike rats, Syrian hamsters, and humans, female degus have a longer free-running period than males (Labyak and Lee, 1995, 1997). Males reentrain to a phase shift of the LD cycle 15–20% faster than female degus (Goel and Lee, 1995). Interestingly, circadian patterns of phase angle, activity level, and free-running period are unaltered in female degus ovariectomized in adulthood. This finding suggests that sex differences in degus are the result of ontogenetic differences (organizational effects of sex steroid hormones) or a result of testosterone affecting male circadian function. The castration of adult degus does not affect the free-running period or phase shifting in response to light pulses, although phase angle of entrainment is affected by adult castration (Jechura *et al.*, 2000). Taken together, these findings suggest that pronounced sex differences in circadian rhythms in degus are either a function of ontogenetic differences or the organizational actions of sex steroid hormones.

E. Suprachiasmatic Nucleus Output and Regulation of Circadian Endocrine Rhythms

Efferent connections from the SCN appear to be necessary for circadian endocrine regulation. The transplantation of the SCN into an SCN-lesioned animal restores circadian behavioral rhythms, but does not restore the gonadal regression that normally occurs in Syrian hamsters and other reproductively photoperiodic species after prolonged exposure to short day lengths or constant darkness (Silver *et al.*, 1996). Gonadal regression requires particular daily patterns of melatonin for several weeks, a rhythm that is controlled by the SCN (Bartness *et al.*, 1993; Goldman and Nelson, 1993).

As previously mentioned, additional evidence for this differential SCN regulation of behavior and endocrine function comes from one study in which transplanted SCN tissue was encapsulated in a semipermeable membrane allowing humoral signals to pass through, but not allowing neural outgrowth (Silver *et al.*, 1996). These encapsulated grafts restored locomotor rhythms to SCN-lesioned hamsters, yet failed to restore the photoperiodic response of gonadal regression. This finding suggests that a humoral signal may act to regulate locomotor rhythms, whereas endocrine rhythms require neural output from the SCN. SCN transplants that restore circadian behavioral rhythms fail to restore circadian rhythms in neuroendocrine function (Meyer-Bernstein *et al.*, 1999).

Additional evidence for the regulation of circadian endocrine rhythms by neural SCN outputs comes from knife-cut studies in which SCN efferents are severed while the SCN remains intact (reviewed in LeSauter and Silver, 1998). For example, semicircular knife cuts posterior to the SCN abolish estrous cycles, yet spare circadian rhythms in drinking behavior (Nunez and Stephan, 1977). In addition, horizontal knife cuts abolish short-day-induced gonadal regression in males, and estradiol-induced daily surges in LH in females, yet leave locomotor behavior intact (Watts *et al.*, 1989; Badura *et al.*, 1987). Taken together, these findings suggest that neural efferents from the SCN are required to drive circadian endocrine rhythms, although these neural connections may not be required for circadian behavioral rhythms.

1. Melatonin

Although there are several studies suggesting that circadian fluctuations in hormone concentrations require neural efferents from the SCN, there is little known about the specific mechanisms by which the SCN regulates neuroendocrine rhythms. Perhaps the best-studied hormonal system that exhibits circadian patterns of production and secretion is pineal melatonin. Melatonin is secreted in a circadian pattern, with peak concentrations occurring during the dark phase or subjective night (Klein, 1985; Arendt et al., 1999; Pevet, 2000). Daily variation in hormone secretion is controlled by an endogenous mechanism and is relatively unaffected by sleep disturbances and dietary alterations. Likewise, circadian variation in melatonin concentrations persist during exposure to constant dim light or dark (Cassone, 1990; Vaughn et al., 1976; Wehr, 1998). Although melatonin production is regulated by an endogenous circadian system, environmental modulation of melatonin secretion is observed in both humans and nonhumans. Thus, light exposure during the night (or dark phase) rapidly inhibits melatonin secretion (Lewy et al., 1980).

The function of melatonin has been a subject of substantial investigation in animals. In general, melatonin codes day length (reviewed in Goldman and Nelson, 1993). Because melatonin is only secreted at night (or during darkness), the duration of the melatonin peak is inversely proportional to day length (or amount of light per day). In nature, the melatonin signal provides information needed to phase seasonal breeding and other adaptions (e.g., changes in fur density, adipose tissue content and distribution, and immune function) with the correct time of year. Thus, numerous behavioral and physiological alterations occur seasonally in animals inhabiting temperate environments in response to a melatonin signal. There is also evidence suggesting that melatonin duration may act as a signal to regulate reproduction and other physiological parameters in humans, including sleep, immune function, and affective disorders (Arendt, 2000; Pevet, 2000).

The neural mechanisms regulating circadian changes in melatonin secretion have been well characterized (Fig. 11). Circadian rhythms in melatonin secretion in most mammals depend on neural efferents from the SCN to the PVN. This projection continues through the medial forebrain bundle to the superior cervical ganglion (SCG) of the spinal cord. From the SCG, sympathetic neurons drive pineal melatonin secretion during the dark, whereas melatonin production and secretion are inhibited during the light portion of the LD cycle (Cassone, 1990; Badura et al., 1987). This multisynaptic pathway has been confirmed using the transneuronal retrograde tracer, pseudorabies virus, injected into the pineal (Card, 2000; Larsen et al., 1998; Larsen, 1999; Teclemariam-Mesbah et al., 1999). This technique confirmed the links in the pathway from the SCN to pineal and also suggested that two parallel circuits from the SCN (one dorsomedial and one ventrolateral) probably drive melatonin secretion. This day–night regulation of melatonin is regulated by the SCN

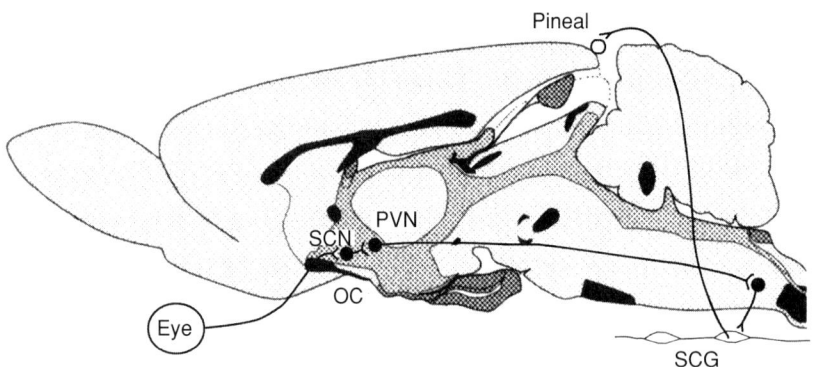

FIGURE 11 Input pathway from the retina to the pineal gland in mammals. Light information is transduced into a neural signal in the retina and transmitted via a direct RHT to the SCN. From the SCN, fibers synapse in the PVN. From the PVN, fibers travel through the medial forebrain bundle to the SCG. Postganglionic fibers from the SCG then project to the pineal gland to modulate melatonin production and secretion. OC, optic chiasm; PVN, paraventricular nuclens of the hypothalamus; RHT, retinohypothalamic tract; SCN, suprachiasmatic nucleus; SCG, superior cervical ganglion.

(reviewed in Cassone, 1990), and, as with other hormonal systems already mentioned, lesions of the SCN abolish circadian rhythms in melatonin production and secretion (Scott *et al.*, 1995; Tessonneaud *et al.*, 1995).

Some aspects by which melatonin, in turn, affects physiology and behavior are well understood. With regard to seasonal changes in reproductive function, melatonin is thought to initiate gonadal regression in short days by acting on membrane-bound receptors located in a region of the dorsomedial hypothalamus (DMH) that binds both melatonin and androgen with high affinity (Maywood *et al.*, 1996). Presumably melatonin acts to enhance the negative feedback effects of androgen on the GnRH system. In addition to acting on the DMH, feedback to the SCN is necessary to modulate melatonin-induced seasonal alterations in several physiological parameters. Lesions of the SCN block the effects of daily long-duration melatonin infusions (i.e., short-day pattern) on body mass, fat-pad distribution, and reproductive function (Bartness *et al.*, 1991). This finding suggests that the circuit beginning with the SCN also requires the SCN as a target. In addition to acting on the DMH, melatonin binding is largely seen in the pars tuberalis of seasonally breeding mammals (Bittman and Weaver, 1990; Weaver and Reppert, 1990). In hypothalamic-pituitary-transected sheep, melatonin implants in the region of the pars tuberalis reduce PRL secretion in a manner similar to short day lengths (Lincoln and Clarke, 1997). However, melatonin implants in this region do not affect gonadotropin secretion, suggesting that this region may be important for the regulation of the lactotropic, but not gonadotropic, effects of photoperiod (Lincoln and Clarke, 1997). Research on the means by which melatonin regulates other parameters is still in its infancy.

2. Glucocorticoids

Adrenal corticoid rhythms are thought to be regulated, in part, by direct projections from the SCN to neuroendocrine cells (Saeb-Parsy *et al.*, 2000) (Fig. 12). For example, projections from the SCN to the CRH neurons in the PVN are thought to directly regulate adrenocorticotropic hormone (ACTH), which, in turn, regulates rhythms in corticosterone secretion (Buijs *et al.*, 1998; Vrang *et al.*, 1995). In addition to acting on CRH neurons in the PVN, a multisynaptic pathway

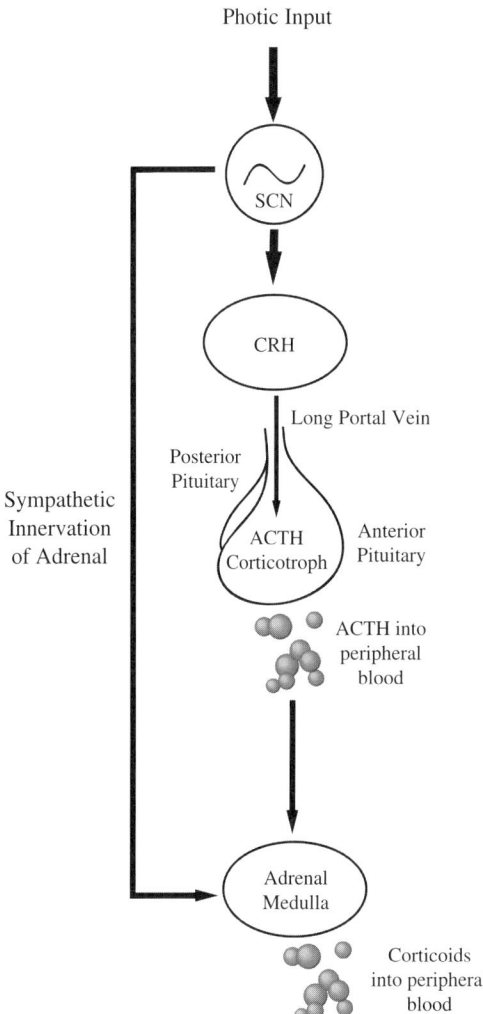

FIGURE 12 Circadian regulation of adrenal steroid production by the SCN. The SCN drives circadian rhythms in glucocorticoid secretion by direct projections from the SCN to CRH cells in the PVN (and potentially other brain regions). In turn, these CRH neurons project to the median eminence to regulate adrenocorticotropic hormone (ACTH) secretion from the anterior pituitary. ACTH is then released into the systemic circulation to regulate glucocorticoid production. A polysynaptic projection from the SCN to the adrenal represents a second mechanism whereby the SCN could drive rhythms in glucocorticoid secretion.

from the SCN to the adrenal gland has been identified (Buijs *et al.*, 1999). These neurons appear to be both VIP- and VP-containing cells in the SCN. In the same study, light exposure during the dark phase led to a rapid drop in corticosterone that was not associated with a change in ACTH concentrations; this response was abolished in SCN-lesioned animals (Buijs *et al.*, 1998). This finding underscores the importance of direct SCN innervation of the adrenal gland in the regulation of glucocorticoids.

The remaining question is: what specific SCN peptides regulate glucocorticoid production? Studies in which either VP or VP antagonists were delivered to the DMH by reverse microdialysis provide evidence for an inhibitory role of SCN-derived VP in the modulation of corticosterone rhythms (Kalsbeek *et al.*, 1996a,b). However, the stimulatory factor regulating glucocorticoid production has not been identified. Taken together, these findings suggest that the SCN can modulate circadian rhythms in hormone secretion via neural connections to the target endocrine gland in addition to acting on releasing hormones in the brain and suggest an important role for SCN-derived VP in this regulation.

3. Sex Steroids and the Estrous Cycle

In rodents, there is abundant evidence indicating that the circadian timing system regulates the female reproductive cycle. The normal duration of the estrous cycle in Syrian hamsters is 4 days (4×24 hr). In constant conditions (e.g., dim illumination), the estrous cycle in hamsters is quadruple the free-running period of locomotor activity (approximately 4×24.05 hr) (Fitzgerald and Zucker, 1976; Hoffmann, 1968). Animals in constant conditions whose period of free-running activity is lengthened by the addition of deuterium oxide to their drinking water, exhibit the predicted increase in estrus onset (Fitzgerald and Zucker, 1976). Finally, under entrained conditions of different day lengths (T cycles of 23.5–21.5 hr), the estrous cycle remains a quadruple of the day length in which the animals are housed (Carmichael *et al.*, 1981). For example, if the LD cycle is changed to a 22-hr day, the estrous cycle length is approximately 88 hr.

As with estrous behavior, the preovulatory LH surge occurs at regular 4- or 5-day intervals in rats, on the day of proestrus, and at a specific time of day coupled to the LD cycle (Colombo *et al.*, 1974). It has long been known that the LH surge requires a neuronal signal that is only present at a specific critical period of the day (Everett *et al.*, 1947; Everett and Sawyer, 1950). In fact, if this neuronal signal is blocked (by barbiturate administration) the LH surge is delayed by 24 hr (Everett and Sawyer, 1950), presumably due to the blocking of the time-specific neuronal signal initiating the LH surge and its recurrence the next day. This daily signal to the female reproductive axis can be unmasked in animals that are ovariectomized and treated with estradiol. In this case, daily LH surges occur (Legan and Karsch, 1975; Legan *et al.*, 1975). Lesions studies confirm that this daily signal is generated by the SCN (e.g., Gray *et al.*, 1978).

The estrous cycle is thought to be modulated by direct projections from the SCN to GnRH neurons (Fig. 13) (Horvath *et al.*, 1998; van der Beek *et al.*, 1993, 1997b). SCN cells projecting on GnRH neurons appear to contain VIP (van der Beek *et al.*, 1993), and these VIPergic neurons from the SCN synapse in a sex-specific way in the MPOA (Horvath *et al.*, 1998). More specifically, VIP-IR axons regularly contact GnRH neurons in both males and females. However, more GnRH cells receive VIP contact in females, and more contacts per neuron are seen in females than in males (Horvath *et al.*, 1998). These projections are thought to modulate the timing of the preovulatory surge in female rodents as well as daily rhythms in androgens in males. In addition, GnRH neurons in the female rat contain VIP$_2$ receptors (Smith *et al.*, 2000), providing further evidence for direct modulation of GnRH neurons.

Theoretically, those GnRH neurons particularly important for the regulation of the estrous cycle would be activated at the time of proestrus. In accord with this hypothesis, it has been shown that GnRH neurons receiving innervation from VIP cells in the SCN are preferentially activated (i.e., express Fos) during the LH surge (van der Beek *et al.*, 1994). Also, sex differences in the daily expression of VIP mRNA, but not VP mRNA, are seen in rats (Krajnak *et al.*, 1998a). Presumably, the signal regulating the estrous cycle is sexually dimorphic, thereby lending further support for VIP regulation of estrus. However, results from studies of VIP effects on the LH surge have been equivocal, with VIP having both stimulatory and inhibitory effects on LH (van der Beek *et al.*, 1999; Weick and Stobie, 1995). Likewise, the blockade of VIP by either VIP antisense or an antibody directed against VIP, leads to an attenuation of the LH surge (Harney *et al.*, 1996; van der Beek *et al.*, 1999). This attenuation is strikingly similar to the attenuation of the LH surge seen in aged rats (Harney *et al.*, 1996; Wise *et al.*, 1997).

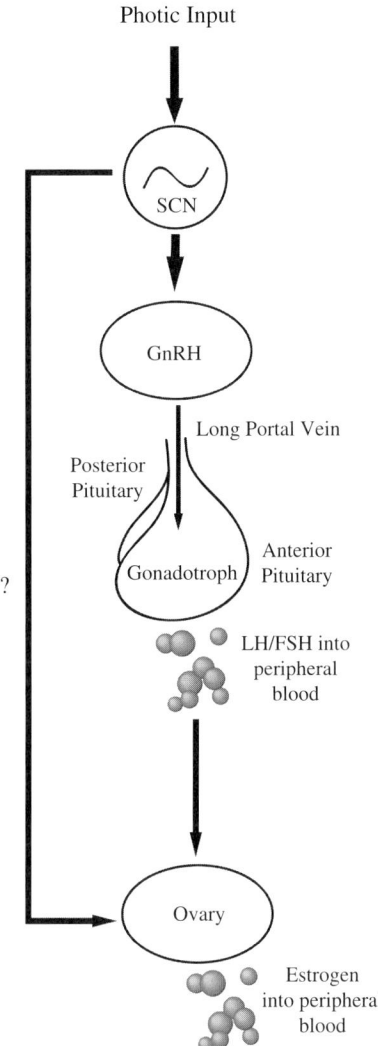

FIGURE 13 Circadian regulation of gonadal steroid production, important for the regulation of the estrus cycle. Gonadal steroid (e.g., estrogen) production is modulated by direct projection from the SCN to GnRH neuroendocrine cells in the hypothalamus. These GnRH neurons project to the median eminence to regulate the secretion of LH into the peripheral blood. In turn, LH modulates gonadal production and secretion of gonadal sex steroids.

Another SCN peptide thought to be important in the regulation of the estrous cycle is VP that is synthesized and released in a circadian pattern, with a peak during the sensitive time window prior to the LH surge (Kalsbeek et al., 1995). Vasopressin administration into the MPOA induces an LH surge in SCN-lesioned ovariectomized rats treated with estradiol (Palm et al., 1999). It is important to note that only electrical stimulation of the MPOA and VP administration into the MPOA have been able to induce LH surges in SCN-lesioned rats (Coen and MacKinnon, 1980; Palm et al., 1999). Finally, in cocultures of POA and SCN tissue, the rhythm of GnRH release is in phase with the rhythm of VP release, but not VIP release (Funabashi et al., 2000). Taken together, these data indicate the importance of VP in inducing the LH surge. It has been suggested that VP may be more important for the initiation of the LH surge, whereas VIP may modulate the exact timing and amplitude of the surge (Palm et al., 1999).

4. Prolactin

Circadian regulation of PRL may be achieved via SCN projections to prolactin-inhibiting factors (PIF) such as dopamine (DA), SS, or GABA, in addition to projections to prolactin-releasing factors (PRF) such as thyrotropin-releasing hormone (TRH), oxytocin (OT), and neurotensin (NT) (Fig. 14). For example, dopaminergic activity in the median eminence shows daily changes, strongly suggesting a daily rhythm of DA levels in the long portal vessels reaching the anterior lobe of the pituitary gland (Mai et al., 1994; Shieh et al., 1997). In addition, direct projections from the SCN to dopamine neurons have been identified (Horvath, 1997). DA has been shown to be the primary modulator of PRL (reviewed in Freeman et al., 2000). This tuberoinfundibular dopaminergic (TIDA) rhythm is endogenously generated, persists in constant conditions, and is abolished after SCN lesions (Mai et al., 1994). In addition to abolishing the DA rhythm, SCN lesions result in an abolition of the PRL rhythm (Mai et al., 1994). One finding suggests that this TIDA rhythm is regulated, in part, by serotonin acting on serotonin 2A (5-HT_{2A}) receptors, presumably on dopaminergic neurons (Liang and Pan, 2000). Taken together, these data suggest that the SCN may regulate the circadian PRL rhythm via neural projections from the SCN to TIDA neurons, which, in turn, regulate PRL.

During the estrous cycle, rising levels of estradiol eventually trigger the release of PRL on the day of proestrus. This release of PRL is dependent on the estradiol-induced increase in TIDA (Neill et al., 1971). Estrogen is required for this response and the administration of an antiserum to estradiol on the morning of diestrus 2 blocks the proestrous surge of PRL (Neill

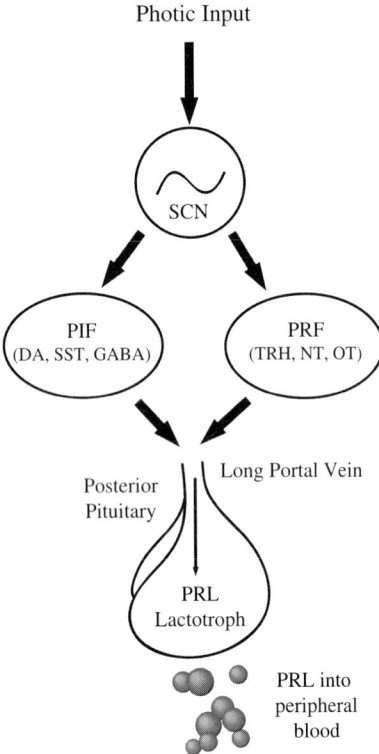

FIGURE 14 Circadian regulation of prolactin production by the SCN. The circadian rhythm of prolactin is driven by direct (or indirect) projections to prolactin-inhibitory factors (PIF; e.g., DA, SS, and GABA) and prolactin-releasing factors (PRF; e.g., TRH, NT, and OT). In turn, PIF and PRF from neuroendocrine cells act on the anterior pituitary to regulate prolactin secretion.

et al., 1971). Likewise, a single injection of estradiol given to ovariectomized rats results in PRL release that is temporally similar to that of the proestrous surge of PRL (Neill, 1972). These data suggest the existence of a circadian hypothalamic timing mechanism that is enhanced by estradiol.

Several lines of evidence suggest that the preoptic area of the hypothalamus is crucial for the expression of this proestrous surge of PRL. First, ER-IR is seen in neurons of the preoptic area in rodents (e.g., Li et al., 1993; Pasterkamp et al., 1997). In addition, caudal transection of preoptic efferents (Kimura and Kawakami, 1978) or lesions of the preoptic area (Pan and Gala, 1985) block the estradiol-stimulated surge of PRL secretion, whereas implantation of estradiol in the preoptic area stimulates the surge (Pan and Gala, 1985). Combined with the previous data, these findings suggest that the circadian timing system modulates the estrus-related surge in prolactin by the modulation of estradiol, which, in turn, affects dopamine to finally regulate PRL.

The data suggest that the timing of the PRL surge associated with the estrous cycle is generated by interactions between the reproductive axis and the circadian timing system. In addition to these endogenous mechanisms, environmental factors act to fine-tune this endogenous regulation of the reproductive cycle. For example, the timing of the PRL surge is regulated by phase shifts in the LD cycle, such that a change in the LD cycle leads to predictable changes in the timing of the estrogen-induced PRL surge and the mating-induced PRL surge (Blake, 1976; Pieper and Gala, 1979). In conditions of constant darkness or constant dim light, proestrus-like PRL surges have a free-running cycle in ovariectomized estradiol-treated rats that is abolished after ablation of the SCN (Bethea and Neill, 1980; Blake, 1976). Together, these findings further suggest the SCN regulates PRL secretion and that this rhythm is modified by exogenous factors.

F. *Tau* Mutation and Endocrine Function

The discovery of the circadian *tau* mutation in hamsters was not only important for the study of the molecular basis of circadian rhythms, but was also important for demonstrating the circadian regulation of endocrine function. The *tau* mutant provides a unique opportunity to study the mechanisms responsible for modulating circadian endocrine rhythms. As alluded to previously, the homozygous *tau* mutant has a shortened (~20 hr) free-running period of locomotor activity (Ralph and Menaker, 1988). A discrepancy between the period of the circadian locomotor rhythm and hormonal rhythms would suggest hormonal control by separate or by multiple oscillators.

Refinetti and Menaker (1992) examined the relationship between circadian periodicity and estrous cycle length by comparing free-running rhythms in locomotor activity and several estrus-related measures, such as body temperature, vaginal secretion, and sexual receptivity in both WT and *tau* mutant hamsters. The records for each of these measures under constant light indicated an estrous cycle of approximately 96 hours for both circadian genotypes. The estrous period measured in number of circadian cycles was approximately 4 cycles for wild types and approximately 5 cycles for homozygous *tau* mutants. The fact that the estrous period measured in absolute hours was indistinguishable between animals with different circadian periods supports the existence of separate mechanisms in the control of circadian and estrous periodicity. However, behavioral measures and vaginal cell cytology may not be sensitive enough to detect subtle alterations in the timing of estrus.

A more sensitive assay of the estrous cycle can be accomplished by measuring the timing of the LH surge in ovariectomized animals treated with estradiol. When this was done in hamsters bearing the *tau* mutation, the period of consecutive daily LH surges was 24 hr for WT animals and 20.5 hr for *tau* homozygotes, consistent with the free-running locomotor period for these animals (Fig. 15; Lucas *et al.*, 1999). Taken together, these findings suggest that behavioral and endocrine circadian rhythms are probably generated by a common molecular mechanism residing in the SCN.

Consistent with the regulation of the LH surge in female hamsters, free-running rhythms of cortisol and melatonin each have a circadian period that is synchronized with the period of activity rhythms in both WT and *tau* mutant hamsters (Lucas *et al.*, 1999). However, the rise in plasma melatonin concentrations occurs significantly earlier in homozygous *tau* mutants than in WT animals. In the same study, pineal glands maintained *in vitro* exhibited equal responsiveness to norepinephrine (NE), suggesting that the cause of this delayed response is not related to an inability of the pineal to respond to sympathetic innervation, but is probably the result of alterations in the SCN signal driving melatonin production.

The shortened circadian period seen in *tau* mutants also alters the timing of gonadal regression after exposure to short day lengths. Gonadal regression occurs more rapidly in *tau* mutants than in WT animals, with a nadir occurring earlier in mutant hamsters (Loudon *et al.*, 1998). Although this regression is more rapid in mutant hamsters, correction for total circadian cycles revealed that regression occurs after a similar number of circadian cycles in both *tau* mutants and WT hamsters. In contrast to these data, no differences were seen in gonadal response to timed melatonin infusions in pinealectomized WT and *tau* mutant animals (Stirland *et al.*, 1995, 1996). Thus, it appears that the reproductive system may respond to the frequency of melatonin signals generated by the circadian timing system. In pinealectomized WT hamsters, inhibitory melatonin signals given every 20 hr led to greater gonadal regression and lower gonadotropin concentrations at 8 wk, compared to hamsters receiving infusions at 24-hr intervals (Maywood *et al.*, 1990). Taken together, these findings suggest that alterations in the circadian timing system also alter the regulation and timing of seasonal reproductive cycles. This adjustment in the timing of gonadal regression probably represents the increased frequency of the melatonin signal in *tau* mutants, due to the shorter period of SCN activity driving the pineal gland.

VIII. CIRCADIAN REGULATION OF FEEDING-RELATED HORMONES

Food intake is controlled by a multitude of factors (see also Schneider and Watts, Chapter 7). These include long-term regulatory factors and external influences that interact with physiological signals related to the ingestion, digestion, absorption, and metabolism

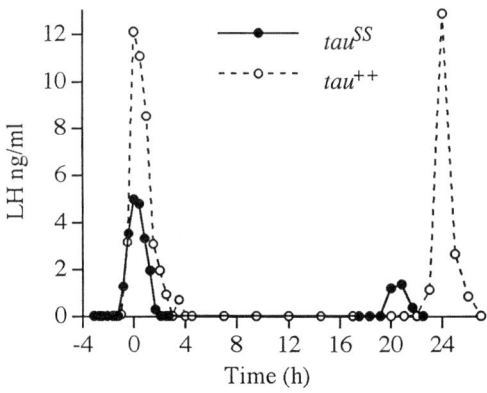

FIGURE 15 LH surges on consecutive circadian cycles in a WT (*tau*++; ~24-hr free-running period) and a *tau* mutant (*tau*ss; ~20-hr free-running period) hamster. The data are plotted with respect to the time of peak LH concentration on the first day of sampling (time zero). The period between peak LH concentrations on consecutive days is ~20 hr (*tau*ss) and 24-hr (*tau*++), indicating that the circadian system regulates the timing of LH. From Lucas *et al.* (1999).

of food. The circadian timing system is one of the regulatory factors that controls the temporal pattern of food intake. This has been shown by studies in which circadian rhythms in eating are maintained under constant conditions in rats (Boulos et al., 1980) and in humans (Green et al., 1987). In animals, these feeding rhythms are abolished by SCN lesions so that food intake is about equal during the day and night, without changes in total intake (Nagai et al., 1978; Rusak and Zucker, 1979; van den Pol and Powley, 1979).

A. Neural Regulation of Feeding

The temporal regulation of food intake, like the regulation of eating itself, occurs at many different hypothalamic and extrahypothalamic loci, several of which are affected by the circadian system. Historically, a few hypothalamic sites were shown to be crucial in the regulation of food intake. Specifically, the ventromedial hypothalamic nuclei (VMH) were regarded as a satiety center because VMH lesions produced obesity. The lateral hypothalamic nuclei were regarded as a feeding center because lesions of the lateral hypothalamus produced aphagia (Anand and Brobeck, 1951). Subsequent discoveries of a multitude of neurotransmitters and neuropeptides as candidates for the enhancement or inhibition of food intake and of their pathways have led to the understanding of hypothalamic circuitry controlling appetite (for review, see Kalra et al., 1999). The ARH-PVN axis forms an important part of that circuitry and includes many hypothalamic nuclei (Kalra et al., 1999). The ARH contains neurons that produce the orexigenic petides NPY, galanin, the opioids dynorphin and β-endorphin and the anorexigenics α-melanocortin-stimulating hormone (α-MSH) and agouti-related transcript (ART; also called AGRP). The terminal fields of these orexigenics and anorexigenics are found in hypothalamic sites such as the VMH, DMH, PVN, and preoptic area where the administration of these substances affect food intake. The lateral hypothalamus is also part of the ARH-PVN axis. Neurons of the lateral hypothalamus produce orexins and glutamate, and they project to the DMN. Electrical stimulation as well as the administration of orexin (Dube et al., 1998) and glutamate agonists (Stanley et al., 1993) in the lateral hypothalamus stimulate eating, whereas lesions of the lateral hypothalamus severely reduce food intake (as already noted). In addition, these appetite-regulating areas are interconnected. VMN efferents project to the DMN and the PVN; DMN efferents project to the VMN and the PVN. Finally, the PVN is recognized as one of the most important sites of action of many orexigenic and anorexigenics substances (Weingarten et al., 1985). The administration of orexigenic agents into the PVN stimulates eating (Dube et al., 1998; Grandison and Guidotti, 1977; Kelly and Grossman, 1980; Schick et al., 1993; Stanley et al., 1985), whereas some anorexigenics agents such as CRH (Monnikes et al., 1992) and leptin (Satoh et al., 1997) attenuate fasting-induced eating.

In addition to studies of the foregoing peptides, the regulation of eating by other substances such as DA, noradrenaline, 5-HT, opioids, and cholecystokinin have been extensively studied (see Cooper and Clifton, 1996). 5-HT is implicated in the inhibitory control of eating (Simansky, 1996) and acts at many sites, including the PVN. Noradrenaline enhances food intake when administered into the brain (Currie and Wilson, 1993). Cholecystokinin inhibits food intake in the periphery (Gibbs et al., 1973) as well as in the brain (Della-Fera and Baile, 1979). Opioids and dopamine can have differential effects depending on the sites of administration and on their interactions with other substances (Vaccarino, 1996).

B. Circadian Control of Feeding

The SCN probably influences the timing of food intake at a variety of sites. The SCN sends efferents to all the hypothalamic nuclei and the disruption of the ARH-PVN axis perturbs the temporal pattern of eating. For example, the SCN directly innervates NPY, galanin and proopiomelanocortin (POMC, a β-endorphin precursor) neurons in the ARH, and although lesions of the mediobasal ARH do not change 24-hr food intake, they reduce its LD ratio. VMH lesions that include the VMN or fibers transections between the lateral hypothalamus and the VMN result in the loss of rhythmicity of food intake and in hyperphagia (Anand and Brobeck, 1951; Powley et al., 1980). VMH lesions also increase levels of adipocyte leptin during the day, abolishing the day–night difference seen in control animals (Dube et al., 1999). Lesions of the DMN do not affect food intake or body weight but do disrupt the circadian blood levels of corticosterone (Bernardis and Bellinger, 1998), a feeding-associated response (see later). The SCN sends projections to the lateral hypothalamus that affect eating patterns. Rats with lateral hypothalamic lesions have an exaggerated nocturnal pattern of eating (Kissileff, 1970) and SCN lesions abolish food intake rhythms in lateral hypothalamic-lesioned rats (Rowland, 1976). Lesions of the PVN that also result in hyperphagia disrupt the day–night pattern of food intake (Aravich and Sclafani, 1983) and blunt the diurnal rhythm of corticosterone (Tokunaga et al., 1986).

Lesions to any site in the ARH-PVN axis may perturb the timely release of the orexigenic and anorexigenic substances, thereby changing the daily patterns of food intake. The orexigenics, such as NPY, galanin and POMC, have a daily rhythm in their blood levels and in the brain (Xu et al., 1999). These substances increase at the beginning of the dark phase in nocturnal animals when food intake is highest (Kalra et al., 1999). The SCN may regulate the day–night pattern of eating by coordinating the release of orexigenics to stimulate eating at night in nocturnal animals (see Kalra et al., 1999, for review).

For the hormone leptin, there is an apparent discrepancy between the timing of its expression and its effect on food intake. Leptin exerts a tonic restraint on food intake. The administration of leptin, either peripherally or in the ARH, VMH, or LH, inhibits eating (Satoh et al., 1997). Leptin may suppress feeding by regulating the orexigenic effect of NPY. The leptin receptor and NPY are coexpressed in the ARH. Leptin inhibits NPY mRNA in the ARH and reduces levels of NPY in the ARH, DMN, and PVN. Finally, leptin suppresses NPY-induced feeding. Surprisingly, the blood levels of the anorexigenic agent leptin are higher at night, when animals eat more, than during daytime (Kalra et al., 1999). This also suggests that leptin exerts tonic control on food intake rather than serving as a satiety signal acting on meal size. Leptin mRNA in adipocytes is regulated by the availability of food (see later). It increases before the onset of eating during the dark phase or when food is restricted to daytime (Fig. 16A).

The circadian modulation of other regulatory factors such as adrenaline or 5-HT has also been described. For example, exogenous noradrenaline is more effective in disinhibiting eating at the beginning of the dark phase than at other times (Currie and Wilson, 1993). 5-HT may decrease feeding during early night by stimulating satiety neurons in the PVN and VMN (Leibowitz, 1990) and neurons in the SCN (Mason, 1986). However, to the best of our knowledge, the transmitters or neuromodulators whereby the SCN regulates food intake have not been directly demonstrated.

In addition to influencing neurotransmitters and ARH-PVN peptides, the SCN also regulates circadian rhythms of insulin and glucagon, which modulate food intake. Plasma concentrations of insulin and glucagon both show diurnal rhythms, and these rhythms are abolished by SCN lesions (Yamamoto et al., 1987), suggesting a role for the SCN in the control of glucagon and insulin homeostasis (reviewed in Nagai et al., 1994). In fact, electrical stimulation of the SCN causes an increase in blood glucagon and a decrease in blood insulin levels (Nagai et al., 1982). Insulin infusion into the SCN increases food intake during the day and decreases food intake at night with no effect on total intake (Mori et al., 1985; Nagai et al., 1982). SCN lesions abolish this response to insulin administration (Mori et al., 1985). The SCN may stimulate glucagon and inhibit insulin secretion. Consistent with this suggestion, the levels of plasma glucagon are much lower in SCN-lesioned rats than in sham-operated food-deprived rats or rats fed *ad libitum,* and levels of insulin are higher in SCN-lesioned rats than in sham-operated food-deprived rats (Yamamoto et al., 1987). Thus, the SCN modulates the interactions between insulin and glucagon homeostasis, thereby affecting food intake.

C. Feeding Affects Circadian Hormone Rhythms

In natural conditions, the temporal aspect of sleep–wake cycles, activity cycles, feeding rhythms, and internal hormonal and physiological rhythms are maintained. This harmony can be altered by changing entraining cues (zeitgebers). LD cycles are an important zeitgeber of circadian rhythms, especially for sleep–wake and activity rhythms, but so is food availability. For example, the rhythms of corticosterone readily entrain to the time of eating. The peak of plasma corticosterone occurs at the beginning of the activity phase in both diurnal and nocturnal animals, just prior to the onset of food intake. Restriction of food access shifts

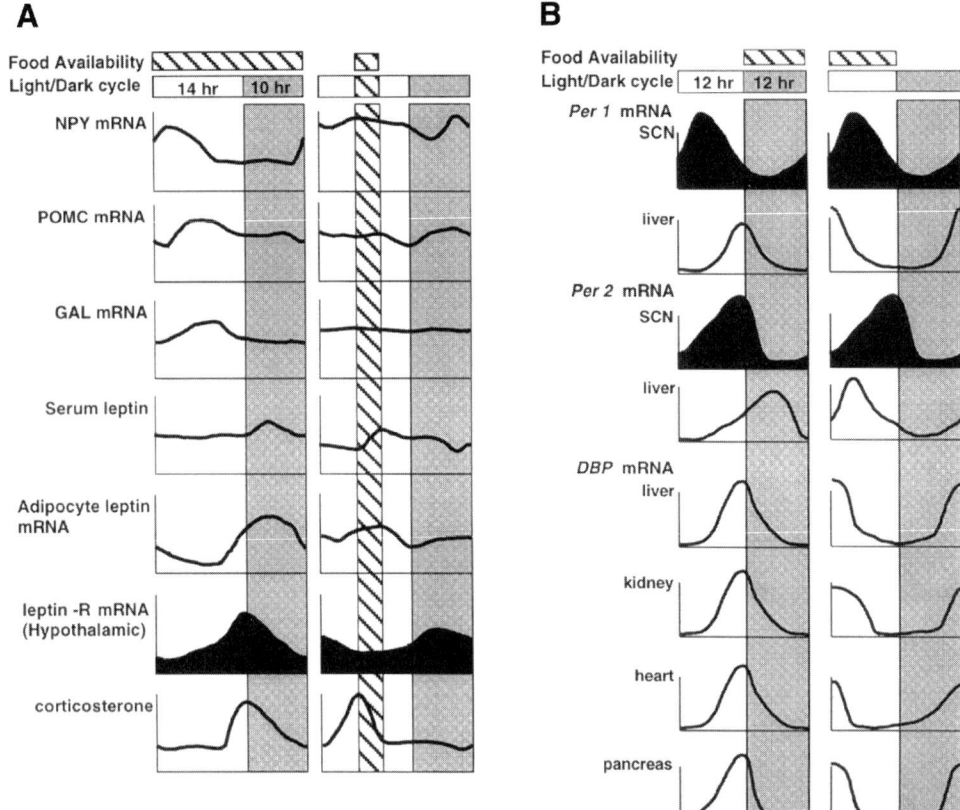

FIGURE 16 Changes in various rhythmic responses induced by changes in feeding time. A. Left panel shows the rhythms in hormones known to control feeding and in corticosterone when animals are fed *ad libitum* (most of the eating occurs at night). Right panel shows the changes in the rhythms of the same hormones when food intake is restricted to 4 hr during the day. Adapted from Xu *et al.* (1999). B. Left panel shows the rhythms of various clock genes in the SCN and in peripheral organs when animals are fed during the night. Right panels show the rhythms in the same clock genes when food intake is restricted to 12 hr during the daytime. The rhythms that do not shift in response to changes in feeding time are shown by the black-filled curves. Adapted from Damiola *et al.* (2000).

the peak of plasma corticosterone to the new prefeeding time (Krieger, 1974; Fig. 16A).

Hormones and other signals associated with the control of food intake can also be entrained by food availability. The diurnal rhythm of plasma leptin is shifted by a shift in meal time (Schoeller *et al.*, 1997) or when food intake is restricted to 4 hours within the light portion (Ahima *et al.*, 1998; Xu *et al.*, 1999). The same is true for the rhythms of hypothalamic NPY mRNA, POMC mRNA, galanin mRNA, serum leptin levels, and adipocytes leptin mRNA (Xu *et al.*, 1999). As can be seen in Fig. 16A, under *ad libitum* feeding conditions (left panel), when most of food is consumed at night, the hypothalamic expressions of NPY mRNA, POMC mRNA, and galanin mRNA are higher during the day than at night. The restriction of feeding to 4 hours during daytime (right panel) prevents the daytime decreases of NPY mRNA and decreases daytime levels of POMC and galanin mRNA. It also reverses the rhythm of adipocyte leptin mRNA and of serum leptin. Although it blunts the early night increase in hypothalamic leptin mRNA, the shape of the rhythm is not affected.

Food availability is a stronger zeitgeber for the rhythms of expression of the orexigenic substances than is the LD cycle. With food restriction, these rhythms become uncoupled from other circadian rhythms, except for the rhythm in hypothalamic leptin mRNA (Xu et al., 1999; Fig. 16A).

As previously described, circadian oscillators have been demonstrated in peripheral organs such as the liver, muscle, heart, and pancreas. These organs contain clock genes such as the Period genes (Per1, Per2, and Per3), the cryptochrome gene Cry1, the transcription factors DBP (D-site binding protein), which are rhythmically expressed. Under normal conditions, the rhythms of these peripheral clock genes phase-lag the rhythms in the SCN by several hours (Lopez-Molina et al., 1997; Yamazaki et al., 2000). Using a transgenic rat model in which the Per1 gene promoter is linked to a luciferase reporter, Yamazaki et al. (2000) observed the phase of Per1 gene expression by measuring the light emitted by cultured tissue explants. Peak light expression in the lung lagged that in the SCN by 7 hr, and in the muscle and liver, by 10–11 hr. A 6-hr shift in the LD cycle fully shifted the peak luciferase expression in the SCN after 1 day. Lung and muscle had shifted 4 hr after day 1 and had fully shifted after 6 days. Liver, on the other hand, was very slow to shift. Especially when exposed to a phase delay, some liver tissue transiently lost rhythmicity and had shifted by only 4 hr after 16 days. Therefore, a change in the LD cycle, such as when a person flies to another continent, may result in a rapid shift in the circadian clock, but a slower shift in the peripheral organs.

Changes in other zeitgebers, such as the restriction of food availability to the daytime or to the subjective day, also induce phase resetting of the peripheral clock genes. Damiola et al. (2000) measured the expression of clock genes in the SCN, liver, kidney, heart, and pancreas in LD or constant dark conditions, with food available for 12 hr during the night or subjective night and with the feeding schedule shifted to daytime feeding. As can be seen in Fig. 16B, the expression of Per1, Per2, Per3, DBP, Cry1, Rev-erbα, and Cryp2a5 had all shifted in the liver after 1 week, but Per1 and Per2 did not shift in the SCN. DBP, Cry1, and Rev-erbα in the liver, or DBP in the kidney, heart, and pancreas completely shifted after 7 days, but hand only partially shifted after 3 days, and the shift was more rapid in liver than in the pancreas and heart, and slower in the kidneys. This shows that the response of peripheral organs to food entrainment is progressive and different tissues shift at different rates. Overall, the LD cycle is a strong zeitgeber for the circadian clock, whereas food availability is important for peripheral oscillators, especially at sites involved in food metabolism. Changes in food availability, however, do not affect the phase of the SCN as measured by clock genes expression.

In parallel with daily rhythms in feeding behavior and peripheral organs, there are also pronounced daily rhythms in tissues of the digestive system. For example, intestinal expression of the high-affinity Na^+/glucose cotransporter (SGLT1), responsible for the absorption of dietary glucose and galactose, exhibits daily variation in its activity and displays gated induction by dietary carbohydrates (Rhoads et al., 1998). Two transcription factors, hepatocyte nuclear factor (HNF)1-α and HNF-1-β, have been shown to regulate SGLT1 daily activity (Rhoads et al., 1998). Although this SGLT1 rhythm can be established by feeding schedule, the rhythm persists in food-deprived animals, suggesting that this rhythm is endogenously regulated (Saito et al., 1976). As with daily variation in SGLT1, uroguanylin (UGN) and guanylin (GN), intestinal ligands for guanylyl cyclase (GC), express daily variation (Scheving and Jin, 1999). Taken together these findings suggest that, like other peripheral organs, the digestive system has clock-controlled genes. Whether the digestive system is directly driven by the SCN or expresses clock genes and/or the ability to independently oscillate requires further investigation.

In Drosophila, a novel gene has been implicated in the circadian control of feeding. The takeout gene (to) and its protein are expressed in the brain and in structures related to feeding and olfaction, including the alimentary canal in the cardia, the crop, and the antennae (Sarov-Blat et al., 2000). It is expressed in a circadian fashion, lagging the expression of Per and Tim. It is undetectable in several strains of arrhythmic clock-mutant flies. Its expression is induced by starvation and reduced by refeeding. Finally, takeout mutant flies become less active more quickly and die sooner when food deprived. Whether such regulation by a homologous gene occurs in mammals remains to be assessed.

In summary, the temporal control of food intake and of the rhythmic secretion of hormones that regulate food intake are under the control of the circadian clock. Under normal circumstances, the master circadian clock in the SCN synchronizes these rhythms in peripheral oscillators. In perturbed conditions, such as restriction of feeding to daytime hours in nocturnal animals, plasticity in the circadian system allows for the desynchronization of the peripheral clocks from the master circadian clock. Feeding then acts as a zeitgeber that overrides the synchronization of the peripheral oscillators by the SCN.

IX. CIRCADIAN EFFECTS ON REPRODUCTION AND FEEDING IN THE AGING ORGANISM

Aging is accompanied by changes in every major endocrine system (reviewed in Lamberts *et al.*, 1997). The most prominent changes associated with aging with respect to circadian rhythms are decreased amplitude of rhythms, altered phase, and diminished ability to synchronize with periodic cues in the environment. Aging affects the period and the amplitude of various neuroendocrine systems, each to a different degree, leading to a loss of temporal organization. It is beyond the scope of this chapter to document all age-related changes associated with rhythmic hormone secretion. The goal here is to provide insight into the mechanisms mediating age-related changes in circadian rhythms by focusing on a few best-understood representative examples. In this context, it is interesting to determine whether age-related changes are due to a gradual lack of organization in the master clock, its coupling to outputs, an inability of the clock to respond rapidly to afferent environmental signals, or to changes in the target-tissue responses to SCN signals that are necessary to promote normal physiology.

A. Evidence for Suprachiasmatic Nucleus in Aging and Rejuvenation

The examination of rhythmicity in the brain clock, achieved by monitoring single-unit firing rates in SCN brain slices, indicate aberrant SCN firing patterns and a decrease in amplitude in aged rats. The results imply that aging disrupts either coupling among SCN pacemaker cells or their output, or causes a deterioration of the pacemaking properties of SCN cells (Satinoff *et al.*, 1993). Similarly, local cerebral glucose utilization (LCGU) is a direct measure of the level of neural activity (Sokoloff, 1979). Both young and middle-age rats demonstrate a diurnal rhythm in LCGU in the SCN, but this rhythm is phase advanced and attenuated in middle-age rats (Wise *et al.*, 1988). These changes occur as rats enter the transition to irregular cycles. That the degeneration of circadian organization in aging rats contributes to the diminished circadian rhythms is supported by evidence that fetal SCN tissue transplanted into aging animals restores the deteriorated circadian responses of the aging animals (Li and Satinoff, 1998).

In young animals, light exposure during the dark results in a strong expression of Fos. By the time rats reach middle age light-induced Fos expression is decreased and delayed. Transplantation of fetal SCN tissue into the third cerebral ventricle of middle-age rats restores light-induced Fos expression to a level similar to those observed in young animals in the host SCN (Cai *et al.*, 1997a). Young rats exhibit a rhythm of hypothalamic CRH (which controls the ACTH-glucocorticoid rhythm) and anterior pituitary POMC mRNA. It is noteworthy that aging abolishes both rhythms and SCN transplants restore both rhythms (Cai *et al.*, 1997b).

However, as previously noted, some neuroendocrine functions abolished by SCN lesions or diminished by age are not restored by SCN transplants (Meyer-Bernstein *et al.*, 1999; Lehman *et al.*, 1987; Wise *et al.*, 1997). Most notably, reproductive responses are not reinstated, which may suggest that the GnRH-LH axis may require more precisely timed neurochemical signals than the CRH-POMC axis or that the former requires more complex neural connections than the latter, which may rely on a humoral signal released from the SCN transplant. Taken together, these data show that the aging host SCN declines in function; however, it remains capable of expressing diurnal rhythmicity when fetal SCN donor transplants confer the appropriate signals.

B. Reproduction

1. Aging in Female Reproductive Rhythms

The female reproductive system and the effects of aging on this system have attracted much attention from neuroendocrinologists because the menstrual cycle requires a very complex regulation that is tightly linked to the circadian system. As pointed out by Wise *et al.*

(1997), studies of the hypothalamic-pituitary-ovarian axis implicate the central circadian clock as a key pacemaker of reproductive senescence. An important role for the circadian system in the regulation of ovulation in the rat has been known since the classic studies of Everett and Sawyer (1950), already discussed. In both rodents and humans, alterations in hormone patterns are seen prior to cycle shortening or complete follicular loss.

The maintenance of consistently timed cyclic LH surges requires extremely precise synchrony of an ordered array of neurochemical signals. The temporal complexity of the female reproductive system combined with the finite and nonrenewable supply of germ cells, make females particularly vulnerable to changes in the master pacemaker. Aging of the pacemaker could lead to desynchrony in the dynamics of gonadotropin secretion and ovarian follicular development, which can result in reduced fertility. This drop in reproductive function seen in middle-age females occurs much earlier than the decline seen in the males of most mammalian species (reviewed in Wise, 2000).

For many years, the exhaustion of the ovarian follicular supply was accepted as the single, most important cause of the transition from fertility to menopause (vom Saal *et al.*, 1994). The developing follicle is the primary source of estrogens, and its depletion has far-reaching consequences in terms of normal physiology and cognitive function. Hypothalamic and pituitary changes seen during menopause were believed to be a consequence of this depletion. It is now clear that both the ovary and the brain are key pacemakers in menopause (Wise *et al.*, 1996). According to this view, the aging SCN, with the dampening and destabilization of either the central pacemaker or its output oscillations, leads to a decline of regular cyclicity and an accelerated rate of follicular loss. The evidence for such a mechanism is especially strong in rats.

There is evidence of increasing imprecision in the timing of the preovulatory LH surges during middle-age (van der Schoot, 1976). The critical period during which barbiturates can block the LH is extended 1–2 hours longer in middle-age rats than in young rats. Furthermore, middle-age rats show both delayed and attenuated LH surges (Cooper *et al.*, 1980; Wise, 1982; Nass *et al.*, 1984). Significantly, these changes precede any overt changes in the length or regularity of the LH surge and can be used to predict the transition to irregularity up to 6 months later (Nass *et al.*, 1984). Parallel changes are seen at the ultradian level in the frequency of LH pulses, a marker for the GnRH pulse generator, and a broadening of the duration of LH pulses, prior to the transition from regular to irregular cycling in both middle-age female humans and rats (10–12 months old) (Matt *et al.*, 1998; Cooper *et al.*, 1980; Wise, 1982; Nass *et al.*, 1984). In a similar vein, although in the opposite direction, normally cycling middle-age humans have increased plasma FSH concentrations, which are not distributed uniformly across the cycle but confined predominantly to the midfollicular and postovulatory phases (Lee *et al.*, 1988). These data strongly suggest a desynchronization of hypothalamic signaling before the initiation of perimenopausal transition.

This breakdown in hypothalamic organization is associated with many of the hallmarks of menopause, such as hot flashes, sleep disturbances, and changes in the pulsatile pattern of gonadotropin secretion. These symptoms become evident in humans when they are 35–40 years old, concomitant with the acceleration of follicular loss (Gougeon *et al.*, 1994). Hot flashes indicate a deterioration of the hypothalamic thermoregulatory centers. In postmenopausal humans, hot flashes are temporally correlated with pulses of LH, suggesting that a common higher brain center regulating both body temperature and GnRH is altered during aging (Meldrum *et al.*, 1980).

In middle-age rats, GnRH neurons express reduced activity, as indexed by both GnRH brain perfusates (Rubin and Bridges, 1989) and by protooncogene products (Rubin *et al.*, 1994) as compared to younger rats. The mean proportion of GnRH neurons containing Fos is lower, the time course for activation is delayed in the brains of aging females, and double-labeled Fos cells are less likely to remain elevated during peak LH release, compared to younger brains. These data suggest a causal relationship between the uncoupling of neurotransmitter signals that regulate GnRH secretion and the initial expression of gonadotropin secretion. The overriding theme emerging from the data is that reproductive decline is accompanied and often predicted by the dampening or advancement of a broad spectrum of circadian rhythms in activity, neurotransmitter level, receptor density, and the level of gene expression in the SCN (Wise *et al.*, 1997).

VIP from the SCN, which has a robust daily rhythm, may communicate time-of-day information to GnRH cells of the preoptic area (van der Beek et al., 1993, 1994). The number of VIP-IR cells in the SCN decreases with age (Chee et al., 1988). Injecting VIP antisense in the peri-SCN region delays and attenuates peak LH levels in a manner similar to the LH pattern seen in middle-age rats, thereby mimicking the effect of age on estradiol-induced LH surge (Harney et al., 1996). VIP mRNA levels in the SCN exhibit a 24-hr rhythm in young female rats, but by the time animals are middle-age, this rhythm disappears (Krajnak et al., 1998a). Finally, as previously noted, VIP neurons in the SCN communicate directly with GnRH neurons; triple-label immunofluorescence studies indicate that approximately 40% of all GnRH neurons analyzed contain the VIP_2 receptor and that VIP-containing processes occur in close apposition to the VIP_2 receptor–positive GnRH neurons (Smith et al., 2000).

The mechanisms associated with the decreased amplitude and precision of circadian regulation are likely to be numerous. Some have been well characterized. In proestrous and estradiol-treated young rats, norepinephrine (NE) exhibits a diurnal rhythm that is characterized by elevated turnover stimulating the LH surge (reviewed in Wise et al., 1997). The suppression of the afternoon rise in NE prevents the expected LH surge (Kalra and McCann, 1974), and the administration of NE agonists induces preovulatory-like LH surges (Krieg and Sawyer, 1976). Middle-age proestrous rats fail to show a daily rhythm in NE turnover in the SCN (Wise, 1982), and the peak in NE release is markedly attenuated, although the average NE release is increased compared to that in the young proestrous animals (Mohankumar et al., 1994). No age-related differences were observed in DA turnover rates (Wise, 1984) or pattern of release (Mohankumar et al., 1994). The stimulatory effects of NE on the LH surge are thought to be mediated through α1-adrenergic receptors (Drouva et al., 1982; Ojeda et al., 1982). Young rats display a daily rhythm in the SCN and other anterior regions of the hypothalamus, with the density of receptors peaking during the evening (Weiland and Wise, 1990). There is a progressive disappearance in this rhythm with age, even though the average density of receptors is maintained until very old age.

2. Aging in Male Reproductive Rhythms

The relatively rapid and irreversible changes that characterize female reproductive aging are among the most dramatic of any neuroendocrine axis. In males, there is a more gradual and subtle decline in reproductive function. Testosterone levels decrease in the morning, and the nocturnal rise of testosterone is markedly attenuated or absent in healthy elderly (>50 years old) male humans, even though afternoon levels are comparable (Bremner et al., 1983). The flattening of the circadian rhythm in testosterone results in lower mean testosterone concentrations for the entire 24-hr day in healthy older male humans than in young (23–25 years old) male humans. The number and capacity of Leydig cells that produce testosterone is reduced in older men (Zirkin and Chen, 2000). Older males also secrete LH more irregularly, and when evaluated against the joint release of testosterone, LH is secreted more asynchronously than in younger males (Pincus et al., 1996). Inhibin secretion also demonstrates circadian and chronological changes in normal adult humans. Inhibin usually peaks in the morning, with the highest values observed in men in their twenties and a lowering of this peak value with age (Yamaguchi et al., 1991). This relationship suggests that increased FSH in elderly humans might be due to the reduced amount of basal inhibin. As in females, alterations in the hypothalamus and possibly the SCN, apparently drive these testicular and hormonal events. These changes are accompanied by changes in reproductive behaviors, including frequency of intercourse and impotence. Similarly and probably under common central pacemaker control, phase advances with respect to the LD cycle have been recorded in the plasma levels of cortisol, TSH, melatonin, PRL, and GH in older male humans (van Coevorden et al., 1991). The reader is referred to Hermann et al. (2000) for a review of aging and the male reproductive system.

C. Aging and Homeostasis

GH secretion decreases with age in daily mean pulse amplitude, duration, quantity, and, possibly, frequency (Corpas et al., 1992, 1993; Veldhuis et al., 1995). This disruption has important clinical implications because muscle mass, lean body mass, muscle strength, and bone density, all GH-regulated physiological functions, decline in old age. In parallel, there is a progressive fall in circulating insulin-like growth factor I (IGF-I) levels in both sexes (Corpas et al., 1993). The triggering pacemaker seems localized mainly in the hypothalamus because pituitary somatotrops, even in the elderly, can be restored to their normal secretory capacity with treatment with GH-releasing peptides (Lamberts et al., 1997).

The circadian rhythm of adrenal corticosterone secretion shows some blunting with age, although this is less dramatic than changes seen in the other neuroendocrine system (Weiland et al., 1992). Although baseline levels are not much altered, there are important alterations in responsiveness to stimulation and stress in this system. Glucocorticoids exert major effects on metabolic homeostasis, and disruptions in the feedback mechanism are implicated in the reduced ability of older animals to recover from stress. For example, the initial response to stress and the return to baseline levels is much faster in young animals (Sapolsky et al., 1984).

In young animals, estradiol treatment induces a diurnal rhythm and suppressed mean levels of POMC mRNA. In the middle-age and aged rats, the ability of estradiol to suppress POMC mRNA levels and to allow the expression of a diurnal rhythm of POMC mRNA was abolished, but the expression is not correlated with other age-related changes in the serum concentrations of LH, PRL, and corticosterone. This finding suggests that fundamental changes in diurnal function or in the biological clock underlie and differentially regulate the age-related changes in POMC gene expression and LH, PRL, and corticosterone secretion (Weiland et al., 1992). As previously noted, SCN transplants restore CRH level and POMC mRNA rhythms.

1. Eating and Metabolism

Age-related changes in circadian rhythms in a variety of enzymes associated with metabolism and in behaviors related to eating have been characterized (Duffy and Feuers, 1991; Mistlberger et al., 1990). Insulin is secreted in a pulsatile fashion, and its rate and pattern of release are important for inhibiting hepatic glucose output and for stimulating peripheral glucose disposal. With age, humans show increased variability and attenuated release of insulin, leading to a blunted circadian pattern (Meneilly et al., 1997). Aging also affects food-entrained circadian rhythms, measured as behavioral anticipation of a 1-hr daily mealtime (during the day), and the persistence of this anticipation rhythm during food deprivation. Following a long duration of restricted diurnal food access, elderly rats, like young rats, rapidly return to nocturnal activity when transferred to *ad libitum* feeding. When restricted diurnal feeding is reinstated after an interval of *ad libitum* feeding, elderly animals require more time for a food-anticipation pattern to emerge and have a lower-amplitude food-anticipation rhythm compared to young adult rats (Mistlberger et al., 1990).

It has long been known that restricting food intake to 50–70% of *ad libitum* intake markedly increases longevity in rats (McCay et al., 1935). In fact, it is the only intervention known to extend the lifespan in mammalian species (Rogina et al., 2000). The antiaging effects of caloric restriction has been shown in a wide variety of species, from rodents to fish to flies (reviewed in Weindruch and Walford, 1988; see also Carlson and Riley, 1998) and preliminary studies suggest that caloric restriction may have a life-extending action in nonhuman primates, as well (reviewed in Roth et al., 1999). Related to increasing longevity, caloric restriction maintains many physiological processes in a youthful state, including hormonal rhythms (Masoro et al., 1992; Masoro, 1996, 2000). One means by which caloric restriction has been proposed to produce antiaging effects is hormesis, the beneficial action(s) resulting from the response of an organism to a low-intensity stressor (Masoro, 2000). Rats on a caloric-restriction regimen have moderately elevated afternoon peak concentrations of plasma free corticosterone (Sabatino et al., 1991). This moderate increase in afternoon glucocorticoid concentrations may increase the ability of animals to cope with more acute stressors, thereby reducing stressed-related alterations and disease (Masoro, 1998, 2000).

X. EVOLUTION OF THE CIRCADIAN SYSTEM

Rhythms are advantageous for survival of the organism. There is an optimal time of day for animals to forage for food. Likewise, the safest time to be active is when predators are not active. A biological mechanism that synchronizes and coordinates internal physiological events with the external environment prepares the organism for predictable environmental changes, especially when an animal is removed from direct external cues, as when it is sleeping in its burrow. Furthermore, all of the energetic requirements of the body cannot be simultaneously fulfilled, and peaks in energetic processes must be partitioned throughout the day. Circadian rhythms permit bodily functions to assume an appropriate temporal niche.

From an evolutionary and adaptive perspective, animals have evolved to synchronize circadian rhythms with the environment in order to promote survival (cf. DeCoursey and Krulas, 1998). Organisms have evolved to restrict numerous behaviors to specific times of day in response to a variety of selection pressures. For example, nocturnal species have evolved to confine behaviors such as feeding, locomotion, foraging, and reproduction to the night in order to avoid predation. Likewise, diurnal species, such as birds, that rely on vision for foraging have evolved to be active during the day.

At the level of the organism, there are impressive differences among vertebrate classes in the presence of circadian pacemakers in various tissues. As previously noted, the mammalian SCN regulates the phase of all circadian pacemakers in the body under normal physiological conditions. In the absence of the SCN, mammals are arrhythmic. There is, however, evidence of an extra-SCN pacemaker function in the retina in mammals, demonstrated by measuring retinal melatonin *in vitro* (Cahill *et al.*, 1991; Tosini and Menaker, 1996). Retinal pacemakers are thought to govern a wide array of intraretinal rhythms, including melatonin synthesis (reviewed in Cahill and Besharse, 1991), iodopsin production (Pierce *et al.*, 1993), tryptophan hydroxylase production (Green *et al.*, 1996), and retinal activities such as photoreceptor outer-segment disk shedding (LaVail, 1976), retinomotor movements (Levinson and Burnside, 1981), visual pigment synthesis (von Schantz *et al.*, 1999), the relative expression of rod and cone signals in the electroretinogram (Manglapus *et al.*, 1998), and circadian rhythms of visual detection (Bassi and Powers, 1986, 1987). Other cyclic retinal functions may be driven by daily LD cues (e.g., ocular length; Nickla *et al.*, 1998). Retinal pacemakers do not affect rhythmicity in extra-SCN sites, in contrast to SCN pacemakers.

In birds and other nonmammalian vertebrates, the characterization of the precise role of SCN pacemakers has been more difficult to achieve. On the one hand, there has been uncertainty as to the location of the avian SCN. This has been clarified with the demonstration of rhythmic and light-induced *Per* and *Clock* mRNA in the quail medial SCN, adjacent to the third ventricle—a location similar to that in mammals (Yoshimura *et al.*, 2001). It is important to note that in nonmammalian vertebrates extra-SCN photoreceptors and oscillators lying in the pineal or retina or in extra-SCN neural sites are capable of sustaining behavioral rhythmicity in the absence of the SCN (reviewed in Menaker *et al.*, 1997). To account for the differences in circadian organization between mammals and nonmammalian vertebrates Menaker *et al.* have hypothesized that mammals passed through a nocturnal bottleneck, which resulted in loss of photoreceptor function in all but the most sensitive photoreceptors of the retina. The circadian system differs among vertebrates, with no organizational pattern apparent at this time. Nevertheless, it appears that light and darkness have been important in shaping the circadian system and that the examination of the photic niche of animals will provide insight into their evolution. Edery (2000) suggests that primitive cells probably had spontaneous oscillations in levels of macromolecules, driven by changing rates of synthesis and destruction. He suggests that circadian organization evolved from random biochemical oscillations that had an intrinsic period of approximately 24 hr and a photosensitive entity. As these authors have suggested, the circadian organization is very old, ubiquitous, and, makes an important contribution to fitness. A dramatic direct test of the adaptiveness of circadian rhythms derives from studies of cyanobacteria—a group of prokaryotes. Impressively, these organisms track circadian time, even when the cells are dividing more rapidly than once a day. Analysis of the relative fitness of different strains of cyanobacteria shows that strains with a circadian period similar to the LD cycle of the environment have greater reproductive success (Ouyang *et al.*, 1998; Johnson and Golden, 1999). This finding highlights the adaptive significance of endogenously generated rhythms that are entrained by the environment.

Circadian biologists are generally impressed with the ubiquity of circadian rhythmicity, with most behavioral, biochemical, and physiological responses of organisms showing daily variation that persists in constant environmental conditions. It is interesting to explore the circadian regulation of rhythmicity at the genetic level in order to investigate the origins and phylogeny of circadian regulation. As already noted, circadian controlled genes occur in most of the major tissues of the body, including the heart, lung, liver, muscle, and testes (Johnson and Golden, 1999). The first approximation at understanding the evolution of circadian influences involves estimating what proportion of the genome is under circadian control across taxa. In the plant *Arabidopsis*, approximately 6% of the estimated 8000 genes studied are rhythmic (Harmer *et al.*, 2000). In contrast, in the retina of *Xenopus* perhaps only a few critical proteins are directly under the control of the circadian clock—Green and Besharse (1996) found that only 4 of 2000 (0.2%) retinal mRNAs examined showed a circadian rhythm of expression. The determination of clock-controlled genes and the signals that set their phase will be important in understanding both the mechanisms and the evolution and adaptations of the circadian system.

Acknowledgments

The authors are grateful to Dr. David Crews and Dr. Nori Geary for providing valuable comments on an earlier version of this chapter. We also thank Ani Aydin, Honor Kirwan, Ruslan Korets, and Daan van der Veen for bibliographic and editorial assistance. Our research is supported by NIH grants NS-37919 (R.S.) and DK-07328 (L.J.K.).

References

Aedo, A. R., Landgren, B. M., and Diczfalusy, E. (1981). Studies on ovarian and adrenal steroids at different phases of the menstrual cycle: II. A comparative assessment of the circadian variation in steroid and lutropin levels during the follicular, periovulatory and luteal phases. *Contraception* **23**, 407–424.

Aguilar-Roblero, R. A., Morin, L. P., and Moore, R. Y. (1994). Morphological correlates of circadian rhythm restoration induced by transplantation of the suprachiasmatic nucleus in hamsters. *Exp. Neurol.* **130**, 250–260.

Ahima, R. S., Prabakaran, D., and Flier, J. S. (1998). Postnatal leptin surge and regulation of circadian rhythm of leptin by feeding. Implications for energy homeostasis and neuroendocrine function. *J. Clin. Invest.* **101**, 1020–1027.

Albers, H. E., Yogev, L., Todd, R. B., and Goldman, B. D. (1985). Adrenal corticoids in hamsters: Role in circadian timing. *Am. J. Physiol.* **248**, R434–R438.

Albrecht, U., Sun, Z. S., Eichele, G., and Lee, C. C. (1997). A differential response of two putative mammalian circadian regulators, mPer1 and mper2, to light. *Cell (Cambridge, Mass.)* **91**, 1055–1064.

Allada, R., Emery, P., Takahashi, J. S., and Rosbash, M. (2001). Stopping time: The genetics of fly and mouse circadian clocks. *Annu. Rev. Neurosci.* **24**, 1091–1119.

Allan, J. S., and Czeisler, C. A. (1994). Persistence of the circadian thyrotropin rhythm under constant conditions and after light-induced shifts of circadian phase. *J. Clin. Endocrinol. Metab.* **79**, 508–512.

Anand, B. K., and Brobeck, J. R. (1951). Hypothalamic control of food intake in rats and cats. *Yale J. Biol. Med.* **24**, 123–146.

Andrews, W. W., and Ojeda, S. R. (1981). A detailed analysis of the serum luteinizing hormone secretory profile in conscious, free-moving female rats during the time of puberty. *Endocrinology (Baltimore)* **109**, 2032–2039.

Anis, Y., Nir, I., and Zisapel, N. (1989). Diurnal variations in melatonin binding sites in the hamster brain: Impact of melatonin. *Mol. Cell. Endocrinol.* **67**, 121–129.

Antoch, M. P., Song, E. J., Chang, A. M., Vitaterna, M. H., Zhao, Y., Wilsbacher, L. D., Sangoram, A. M., King, D. P., Pinto, L. H., and Takahashi, J. S. (1997). Functional identification of the mouse circadian Clock gene by transgenic BAC rescue. *Cell (Cambridge, Mass.)* **89**, 655–667.

Apter, D., Butzow, T. L., Laughlin, G. A., and Yen, S. S. (1993). Gonadotropin-releasing hormone pulse generator activity during pubertal transition in girls: Pulsatile and diurnal patterns of circulating gonadotropins. *J. Clin. Endocrinol. Metab.* **76**, 940–949.

Aravich P. F., and Sclafani, A. (1983). Paraventricular hypothalamic lesions and medial hypothalamic knife cuts produce similar hyperphagia syndromes. *Behav. Neurosci.* **97**, 970–983.

Arendt, J. (2000). Melatonin, circadian rhythms, and sleep. *N. Engl. J. Med.* **343**, 1114–1116.

Arendt, J., Middleton, B., Stone, B., and Skene, D. (1999). Complex effects of melatonin: Evidence for photoperiodic responses in humans? *Sleep* **22**, 625–635.

Aronin, N., Sagar, S. M., Sharp, F. R., and Schwartz, W. J. (1990). Light regulates expression of a Fos-related protein in rat suprachiasmatic nuclei. *Proc. Natl. Acad. Sci. U.S.A.* **87**, 5959–5962.

Aronson, B. D., Bell-Pedersen, D., Block, G. D., Bos, N. P., Dunlap, J. C., Eskin, A., Garceau, N. Y., Geusz, M. E., Johnson, K. A., Khalsa, S. B. *et al.* (1993). Circadian rhythms. *Brain Res. Brain Res. Rev.* **18**, 315–333.

Aronson, B. D., Johnson, K. A., and Dunlap, J. C. (1994). Circadian clock locus frequency: Protein encoded by a single open reading frame defines period length and temperature compensation. *Proc. Natl. Acad. Sci. U.S.A.* **91**, 7683–7687.

Aschoff, J., and Wever, R. (1965). Circadian rhythms of finches in light:dark cycles with interposed twilights. *Comp. Biochem. Physiol.* **16**, 507–514.

Aschoff, J., Gerecke, U., and Wever, R. (1967). Desynchronization of human circadian rhythms. *Jpn. J. Physiol.* **17**, 450–457.

Badura, L. L., Sisk, C. L., and Nunez, A. A. (1987). Neural pathways involved in the photoperiodic control of reproductive physiology and behavior in female hamsters (*Mesocricetus auratus*). *Neuroendocrinology* **46**, 339–344.

Balsalobre, A., Damiola, F., and Schibler, U. (1998). A serum shock induces circadian gene expression in mammalian tissue culture cells. *Cell (Cambridge, Mass.)* **93**, 929–937.

Barraclough, C. A., and Wise, P. M. (1982). The role of catecholamines in the regulation of pituitary luteinizing hormone and follicle-stimulating hormone secretion. *Endocr. Rev.* **3**, 91–119.

Barraclough, C. A., Wise, P. M., and Selmanoff, M. K. (1984). A role for hypothalamic catecholamines in the regulation of gonadotropin secretion. *Recent Prog. Horm. Res.* **40**, 487–529.

Bartness, T. J., Goldman, B. D., and Bittman, E. L. (1991). SCN lesions block responses to systemic melatonin infusions in Siberian hamsters. *Am. J. Physiol.* **260**, R102–R112.

Bartness, T. J., Powers, J. B., Hastings, M. H., Bittman, E. L., and Goldman, B. D. (1993). The timed infusion paradigm for melatonin delivery: What has it taught us about the melatonin signal, its reception, and the photoperiodic control of seasonal responses? *J. Pineal Res.* **15**, 161–190.

Bassi, C. J., and Powers, M. K. (1986). Daily fluctuations in the detectability of dim lights by humans. *Physiol. Behav.* **38**, 871–877.

Bassi, C. J., and Powers, M. K. (1987). Circadian rhythm in goldfish visual sensitivity. *Invest. Ophthalmol. Visual. Sci.* **28**, 1811–1815.

Bell-Pedersen, D. (2000). Understanding circadian rhythmicity in *Neurospora crassa*: From behavior to genes and back again. *Fungal. Genet. Biol.* **29**, 1–18

Bell-Pedersen, D., Crosthwaite, S. K., Lakin-Thomas, P. L., Merrow, M., and Kland, M. (2001). The Neurospora circadian clock: Simple or complex? *Philos. Trans. R. Soc. Lond. B Biol. Sci.* **356**, 1697–1709.

Bernardis, L. L., and Bellinger, L. L. (1998). The dorsomedial hypothalamic nucleus revisited: 1998 update. *Proc. Soc. Exp. Biol. Med.* **218**, 284–306.

Berson, D. M., Dunn, F. A., and Takao, M. (2002). Phototransduction by retinal ganglion cells that set the circadian clock. *Science* **295**, 1070–1073.

Bethea, C. L., and Neill, J. D. (1979). Prolactin secretion after cervical stimulation of rats maintained in constant dark or constant light. *Endocrinology (Baltimore)* **104**, 870–876.

Bethea, C. L., and Neill, J. D. (1980). Lesions of the suprachiasmatic nuclei abolish the cervically stimulated prolactin surges in the rat. *Endocrinology (Baltimore)* **107**, 1–5.

Bittman, E. L., and Weaver, D. R. (1990). The distribution of melatonin binding sites in neuroendocrine tissues of the ewe. *Biol. Reprod.* **43**, 986–993.

Blake, C. (1976). Effects of pinealectomy on the rat oestrus cycle and pituitary gonadotrophin release. *J. Endocrinol.* **69**, 67–75.

Blomquist, C. H., and Holt, J. P. J. (1992). Chronobiology of the hypothalamic-pituitary-gonadal axis in men and women. In "Biological Rhythms in Clinical and Laboratory Medicine" (Y. Touitou and E. Haus, eds.), pp. 315–329. Springer-Verlag, Berlin.

Boer, G. J., van Esseveldt, L. E., and Rietveld, W. J. (1998). Cellular requirements of suprachiasmatic nucleus transplants for restoration of circadian rhythm. *Chronobiol. Int.* **15**, 551–566.

Boulos, Z., Rosenwasser, A. M., and Terman, M. (1980). Feeding schedules and the circadian organization of behavior in the rat. *Behav. Brain Res.* **1**, 39–65.

Boyar, R. M., Wu, R. H., Kapen, S., Hellman, L., Weitzman, E. D., and Finkelstein, J. W. (1976). Clinical and laboratory heterogeneity in idiopathic hypogonadotropic hypogonadism. *Clin. Endocrinol. Metab.* **43**, 1268–1275.

Bremner, W. J., Vitiello, M. V., and Prinz, P. N. (1983). Loss of circadian rhythmicity in blood testosterone levels with aging in normal men. *Clin. Endocrinol. Metab.* **56**, 1278–1281.

Buijs, R. M., Hermes, M. H., and Kalsbeek, A. (1998). The suprachiasmatic nucleus-paraventricular nucleus interactions: A bridge to the neuroendocrine and autonomic nervous system. *Prog. Brain Res.* **119**, 365–382.

Buijs, R. M., Wortel, J., Van Heerikhuize, J. J., Feenstra, M. G., Ter Horst, G. J., Romijn, H. J., and Kalsbeek, A. (1999). Anatomical and functional demonstration of a multisynaptic suprachiasmatic nucleus adrenal (cortex) pathway. *Eur. J. Neurosci.* **11**, 1535–1544.

Cahill, G. M., and Besharse, J. C. (1991). Resetting the circadian clock in cultured Xenopus eyecups: Regulation of retinal melatonin rhythms by light and D2 Dopamine receptors. *J. Neurosci.* **11**, 2959–2971.

Cahill, G. M., Grace, M. S., and Besharse, J. C. (1991). Rhythmic regulation of retinal melatonin: Metabolic pathways, neurochemical mechanisms, and the ocular circadian clock. *Cell. Mol. Neurobiol.* **11,** 529–560.

Cai, A., Lehman, M. N., Lloyd, J. M., and Wise, P. M. (1997a). Transplantation of fetal suprachiasmatic nuclei into middle-aged rats restores diurnal Fos expression in host. *Am. J. Physiol.* **272,** R422–R428.

Cai, A., Scarbrough, K., Hinkle, D. A., and Wise, P. M. (1997b). Fetal grafts containing suprachiasmatic nuclei restore the diurnal rhythm of CRH and POMC mRNA in aging rats. *Am. J. Physiol.* **273,** R1764–R1770.

Campbell, S. S., and Murphy, P. J. (1998). Extraocular circadian phototransduction in humans. *Science* **279,** 396–399.

Canbeyli, R., Lehman, M. N., and Silver, R. (1991a). Tracing SCN graft efferents with DiI. *Brain Res.* **554,** 15–21.

Canbeyli, R. S., Romero, M. T., and Silver, R. (1991b). Neither triazolam nor activity phase advance circadian locomotor activity in SCN-lesioned hamsters bearing fetal SCN transplants. *Brain Res.* **566,** 40–45.

Carandente, F., Angeli, A., Candiani, G. B., Crosignani, P. G., Dammacco, F., De Cecco, L., Marrama, P., Massobrio, M., and Martini, L. (1989). Rhythms in the ovulatory cycle. 2nd: LH, FSH, estradiol and progesterone. *Chronobiologia* **16,** 353–363.

Card, J. P. (2000). Pseudorabies virus and the functional architecture of the circadian timing system. *J. Biol. Rhythm* **15,** 453–461.

Card, J. P., and Moore, R. Y. (1984). The suprachiasmatic nucleus of the Golden hamster: Immunohistochemical analysis of cell and fiber distribution. *Neuroscience* **1,** 415–431.

Card, J. P., Fitzpatrick-McElligott, S., Gozes, I., and Baldino, F., Jr. (1988). Localization of vasopressin-, vasoactive intestinal polypeptide-, peptide histidine isoleucine- and somatostatin-mRNA in rat suprachiasmatic nucleus. *Cell. Tissue Res.* **252,** 307–315.

Carlson, J. C., and Riley, J. C. (1998). A consideration of some notable aging theories. *Exp. Gerontol.* **33,** 127–134.

Carmichael, M. S., Nelson, R. J., and Zucker, I. (1981). Hamster activity and estrous cycles: Control by a single versus multiple circadian oscillator(s). *Proc. Natl. Acad. Sci. U.S.A.* **78,** 7830–7834.

Cassone, V. M. (1990). Melatonin: Time in a bottle. *Oxfford Rev. Reprod. Biol.* **12,** 319–367.

Chee, C. A., Roozendaal, B., Swaab, D. F., Goudsmit, E., and Mirmiran, M. (1988). Vasoactive intestinal polypeptide neuron changes in the senile rat suprachiasmatic nucleus. *Neurobiol. Aging* **9,** 307–312.

Clair, P., Claustrat, B., Jordan, D., Dechaud, H., and Sassolas, G. (1985). Daily variations of plasma sex hormone-binding globulin binding capacity, testosterone and luteinizing hormone concentrations in healthy rested adult males. *Horm. Res.* **21,** 220–223.

Coen, C. W., and MacKinnon, P. C. (1980). Lesions of the suprachiasmatic nuclei and the serotonin-dependent phasic release of luteinizing hormone in the rat: Effects on drinking rhythmicity and on the consequences of preoptic area stimulation. *J. Endocrinol.* **84,** 231–236.

Colombo, J. A., Baldwin, D. M., and Sawyer, C. H. (1974). Timing of the estrogen-induced release of LH in ovariectomized rats under an altered lighting schedule. *Proc. Soc. Exp. Biol. Med.* **145,** 1125–1127.

Colwell, C. S. (2000). Circadian modulation of calcium levels in cells in the suprachiasmatic nucleus. *Eur. J. Neurosci.* **12,** 571–576.

Cooper, H. M., Herbin, M., and Nevo, E. (1993). Visual system of a naturally microphthalmic mammal: The blind mole rat, Spalax ehrenbergi. *J. Comp. Neurol.* **328,** 313–350.

Cooper, R. L., Conn, P. M., and Walker, R. F. (1980). Characterization of the LH surge in middle-aged female rats. *Biol. Reprod.* **23,** 611–615.

Cooper, S. J., and Clifton, P. G. (1996). "Drug Receptor Subtypes and Ingestive Behavior." Academic Press, San Diego, CA.

Corpas, E., Harman, S. M., Pineyro, M. A., Roberson, R., and Blackman, M. R. (1992). Growth hormone (GH)-releasing hormone-(1–29) twice daily reverses the decreased GH and insulin-like growth factor-I levels in old men. *J. Clin. Endocrinol. Metab.* **75,** 530–535.

Corpas, E., Harman, S. M., Pineyro, M. A., Roberson, R., and Blackman, M. R. (1993). Continuous subcutaneous infusions of growth hormone (GH) releasing hormone 1–44 for 14 days increase GH and insulin-like growth factor-I levels in old men. *J. Clin. Endocrinol. Metab.* **76,** 134–138.

Crews, S. T., Thomas, J. B., and Goodman, C. S. (1988). The Drosophila single-minded gene encodes a nuclear protein with sequence similarity to the per gene product. *Cell (Cambridge, Mass.)* **52,** 143–151.

Critchlow, V., Liebelt, R. A., Bar-Sela, M., Mountcastle, W., and Lipscomb, H. S. (1963). Sex difference in resting pituitary-adrenal function in the rat. *Am. J. Physiol.* **205,** 807–815.

Crosthwaite, S. K., Dunlap, J. C., and Loros, J. J. (1997). Neurospora wc-1 and wc-2: Transcription, photoresponses, and the origins of circadian rhythmicity. *Science* **276,** 763–769.

Currie, P. J., and Wilson, L. M. (1993). Potentiation of dark onset feeding in obese mice (genotype ob/ob) following central injection of norepinephrine and clonidine. *Eur. J. Pharmacol.* **232,** 227–234.

Czeisler, C. A., and Klerman, E. B. (1999). Circadian and sleep-dependent regulation of hormone release in humans. *Recent Prog. Horm. Res.* **54,** 97–130.

Czeisler, C. A., Kronauer, R. E., Allan, J. S., Duffy, J. F., Jewett, M. E., Brown, E. N., and Ronda, J. M. (1989). Bright light induction of strong (type 0) resetting of the human circadian pacemaker. *Science* **244**, 1328–1333.

Czeisler, C. A., Duffy, J. F., Shanahan, T. L., Brown, E. N., Mitchell, J. F., Rimmer, D. W., Ronda, J. M., Silva, E. J., Allan, J. S., Emens, J. S., Dijk, D. J., and Kronauer, R. E. (1999). Stability, precision, and near-24-hour period of the human circadian pacemaker. *Science,* **284**(5423), 2177–2181.

Damiola, F., Le Minh, N., Preitner, N., Kornmann, B., Fleury-Olela, F., and Schibler, U. (2000). Restricted feeding uncouples circadian oscillators in peripheral tissues from the central pacemaker in the suprachiasmatic nucleus. *Genes Dev.* **14**, 2950–2961.

Darlington, T. K., Wager-Smith, K., Ceriani, M. F., Staknis, D., Gekakis, N., Steeves, T. D. L., Weitz, C. J., Takahashi, J. S., and Kay, S. A. (1998). Closing the circadian loop: CLOCK-induced transcription of its own inhibitors per and tim. *Science* **280**, 1599–1603.

Davies, I. R., and Mason, R. (1994). Tau-mutant hamster SCN clock neurones express a 20 hr firing rate rhythm *in vitro*. *NeuroReport* **5**, 2165–2168.

Davis, F. C., Darrow, J. M., and Menaker, M. (1983). Sex differences in the circadian control of hamster wheel-running activity. *Am. J. Physiol.* **244**, R93–R105.

Decavel, C., and van den Pol, A. N. (1990). GABA: A dominant neurotransmitter in the hypothalamus. *J. Comp. Neurol.* **302**, 1019–1037.

DeCoursey, P. J. (1986). Light-sampling behavior in photoentrainment of a rodent circadian rhythm. *J. Comp. Physiol. A* **159**, 161–169.

DeCoursey, P. J., and Krulas, J. R. (1998). Behavior of SCN-lesioned chipmunks in natural habitat: A pilot study. *J. Biol. Rhythms* **13**, 229–244.

DeCoursey, P. J., Krulas, J. R., Mele, G., and Holley, D.C. (1997). Circadian performance of suprachiasmatic nuclei (SCN)-lesioned antelope ground squirrels in a desert enclosure. *Physiol. Behav.* **62**, 1099–1108.

Deguchi, T. (1979). A circadian oscillator in cultured cells of chicken pineal gland. *Nature (London)* **282**, 94–96.

de la Iglesia, H. O., Blaustein, J. D., and Bittman, E. L. (1999). Oestrogen receptor-alpha-immunoreactive neurones project to the suprachiasmatic nucleus of the female Syrian hamster. *J. Neuroendocrinol.* **11**, 481–490.

Della-Fera, M. A., and Baile, C. A. (1979) Cholecystokinin octapeptide: Continuous picomole injections into the cerebral ventricles of sheep suppress feeding. *Science* **206**, 471–473.

De Marian, J. J. (1729). "Observation Botanique," pp. 35–36. Academie Royale des Sciences, Paris.

Desir, D., Van Cauter, E., L'Hermite, M., Refetoff, S., Jadot, C., Caufriez, A., Copinschi, G., and Robyn, C. (1982). Effects of jet lag on hormonal patterns. III. Demonstration of an intrinsic circadian rhythmicity in plasma prolactin. *J. Clin. Endocrinol. Metab.* **55**, 849–857.

Drouva, S. V., Laplante, E., and Kordon, C. (1982). Alpha 1-adrenergic receptor involvement in the LH surge in ovariectomized estrogen-primed rats. *Eur. J. Pharmacol.* **81**, 341–344.

Dube, M. G., Kalra, S. P., and Kalra, P. S. (1998). Food intake elicited by central administration of orexins: Identification of hypothalamic sites of action. *Program 28th Annu. Meet. Soc. Neurosci.* Los Angeles, CA, Vol. 24, p. 448 (Abstr. 175.8).

Dube, M. G., Xu, B., Kalra, P. S., Sninsky, C. A., and Kalra, S. P. (1999). Disruption in neuropeptide Y and leptin signaling in obese ventromedial hypothalamic-lesioned rats. *Brain Res.* **816**, 38–46.

Dubey, A. K., Puri, C. P., Puri, V., and Anand Kumar, T. C. (1983). Day and night levels of hormones in male rhesus monkeys kept under controlled or constant environmental light. *Experientia* **39**, 207–209.

Dubocovich, M. L., Benloucif, S., and Masana, M. I. (1996). Melatonin receptors in the mammalian suprachiasmatic nucleus. *Behav. Brain Res.* **73**, 141–147.

Duffy, P. H., and Feuers, R. J. (1991). Biomarkers of aging: Changes in circadian rhythms related to the modulation of metabolic output. *Biomed. Environ. Sci.* **4**, 182–191.

Dunkel, L., Alfthan, H., Stenman, U. H., Selstam, G., Rosberg, S., and Albertsson-Wikland, K. (1992). Developmental changes in 24-hour profiles of luteinizing hormone and follicle-stimulating hormone from prepuberty to midstages of puberty in boys. *J. Clin. Endocrinol. Metab.* **74**, 890–897.

Dunlap, 1988.

Dunlap, J. C. (1999). Molecular bases for circadian clocks. *Cell (Cambridge, Mass.)* **96**, 271–290.

Dunlap, J. C., Loros, J. J., Merrow, M., Crosthwaite, S., Bell-Pedersen, D., Garceau, N., Shinohara, M., Cho, H., and Luo, C. (1996). The genetic and molecular dissection of a prototypic circadian system. *Prog. Brain Res.* **111**, 11–27.

Dunn, J. D., Johnson, D. C., Castro, A. J., and Swenson, R. (1980). Twenty-four hour pattern of prolactin levels in female rats subjected to transection of the mesencephalic raphe or ablation of the suprachiasmatic nuclei. *Neuroendocrinology* **31**, 85–91.

Earnest, D. J., and Sladek, C. D. (1986). Circadian rhythms of vasopressin release from individual rat suprachiasmatic explants *in vitro*. *Brain Res.* **382**, 129–133.

Earnest, D. J., Sladek, C. D., Gash, D. M., and Wiegand, S. J. (1989). Specificity of circadian function in transplants of the fetal suprachiasmatic nucleus. *J. Neurosci.* **9**, 2671–2677.

Ebihara, S., Adachi, A., Hasegawa, M., Nogi, T., Yoshimura, T., and Hirunagi, K. (1997). *In vivo* microdialysis studies of pineal and ocular melatonin rhythms in birds. *Biol. Signals* **6**, 233–240.

Edery, I. (2000). Circadian rhythms in a nutshell. *Physiol. Genom.* **3**, 59–74.

El-Hajj Fuleihan, G., Klerman, E. B., Brown, E. N., Choe, Y., Brown, E. M., and Czeisler, C. A. (1997). The parathyroid hormone circadian rhythm is truly endogenous. a. general clinical research center study. *J. Clin. Endocrinol. Metab.* **82**, 281–286.

Ellis, G. B., and Turek, F. W. (1983). Testosterone and photoperiod interact to regulate locomotor activity in male hamsters. *Horm. Behav.* **17**, 66–75.

Eskin, A. (1979). Identification and physiology of circadian pacemakers. Introduction. *Fed. Proc., Fed. Am. Soc. Exp. Biol.* **38**, 2570–2572.

Everett, J. W., and Sawyer, C. H. (1950). A 24-hour periodicity in the LH-release apparatus of female rat disclosed by barbiturate administration. *Endocrinology (Baltimore)* **47**, 198–218.

Everett, J. W., Sawyer, C. H., and Markee, J. E. (1949). A neurogenic timing factor in control of the ovulatory discharge of luteinizing hormone in the cyclic rat. *Endocrinology (Baltimore)* **44**, 234–250.

Fantl, J. A. (1994). The lower urinary tract in women—effect of aging and menopause on continence. *Exp. Gerontol.* **29**, 417–422.

Fitzgerald, K., and Zucker, I. (1976). Circadian organization of the estrous cycle of the Golden hamster. *Proc. Natl. Acad. Sci. U.S.A.* **73**, 2923–2927.

Follenius, M., Brandenberger, G., Bandesapt, J. J., Libert, J. P., and Ehrhart, J. (1992). Nocturnal cortisol release in relation to sleep structure. *Sleep* **15**, 21–27.

Foster, R. G., Provencio, I., Hudson, D., Fiske, S., De Grip, W., and Menaker, M. (1991). Circadian photoreception in the retinally degenerate mouse (rd/rd). *J. Comp. Physiol.* **169**, 39–50.

Freedman, M. S., Lucas, R. J., Soni, B., von Schantz, M., Munoz, M., David-Gray, Z., and Foster, R. (1999). Regulation of mammalian circadian behavior by non-rod, non-cone, ocular photoreceptors. *Science* **284**, 502–504.

Freeman, M. E., Kanyicska, B., Lerant, A., and Nagy, G. (2000). Prolactin: Structure, function, and regulation of secretion. *Physiol. Rev.* **80**, 1523–1631.

Funabashi, T., Shinohara, K., Mitsushima, D., and Kimura, F. (2000). Gonadotropin-releasing hormone exhibits circadian rhythm in phase with arginine-vasopressin in co-cultures of the female rat preoptic area and suprachiasmatic nucleus. *J. Neuroendocrinol.* **12**, 521–528.

Gallagher, T. F., Yoshida, K., Roffwarg, H. D., Fukushima, D. K., Weitzman, E. D., and Hellman, L. (1973). ACTH and cortisol secretory patterns in man. *J. Clin. Endocrinol. Metab.* **36**, 1058–1068.

Garceau, N. Y., Liu, Y., Loros, J. J., and Dunlap, J. C. (1997). Alternative initiation of translation and time-specific phosphorylation yield multiple forms of the essential clock protein FREQUENCY. *Cell (Cambridge, Mass.)* **89**, 469–476.

Gaston, S., and Menaker, M. (1968). Pineal function: The biological clock in the sparrow? *Science* **160**, 1125–1127.

Gekakis, N., Staknis, D., Nguyen, H. B., Davis, F. C., Wilsbacher, L. D., King, D. P., Takahashi, J. S., and Weitz, C. J. (1998). Role of the CLOCK protein in the mammalian circadian mechanism. *Science* **280**, 1564–1569.

Gibbs, J., Young, R. C., and Smith, G. P. (1973). Cholecystokinin decreases food intake in rats. *J. Comp. Physiol. Psychol.* **84**, 488–495.

Gillette, M. U., and Reppert, S. M. (1987). The hypothalamic suprachiasmatic nuclei: Circadian patterns of vasopressin secretion and neuronal activity *in vitro*. *Brain Res. Bull.* **19**, 135–139.

Glass, J. D., Shen, H., Fedorkova, L., Chen, L., Tomasiewicz, H., and Watanabe, M. (2000). Polysialylated neural cell adhesion molecule modulates photic signaling in the mouse suprachiasmatic nucleus. *Neurosci. Lett.* **280**, 207–210.

Glazer, R., and Gozes, I. (1994). Diurnal oscillation in vasoactive intestinal peptide gene expression independent of environmental light entraining. *Brain Res.* **644**, 164–167.

Goel, N., and Lee, T. M. (1995). Sex differences and effects of social cues on daily rhythms following phase advances in *Octodon degus*. *Physiol. Behav.* **58**, 205–213.

Golden, S. S., Johnson, C. H., and Kondo, T. (1998). The cyanobacterial circadian system: A clock apart. *Curr. Opin. Microbiol.* **1**, 669–673.

Goldman, B. D., and Nelson, R. J. (1993). Melatonin and seasonality in mammals. *In* "Melatonin: Biosynthesis, Physiological Effects and Clinical Applications" (H. S. Yu and R. J. Reiter, eds.), pp. 225–252. CRC Press, New York.

Gougeon, A., Ecochard, R., and Thalabard, J. C. (1994). Age-related changes of the population of human ovarian follicles: Increase in the disappearance rate of non-growing and early-growing follicles in aging women. *Biol. Reprod.* **50**, 653–663.

Grandison, L., and Guidotti, A. (1977). Stimulation of food intake by muscimol and beta endorphin. *Neuropharmacology* **16**, 533–536.

Gray, G. D., Soderstein, P., Tallentire, D., and Davidson, J. M. (1978). Effects of lesions in various structures of the suprachiasmatic-preoptic region on LH regulation and sexual behavior in female rats. *Neuroendocrinology* **25**, 174–191.

Green, C. B., and Besharse, J. C. (1996). Use of a high stringency differential display screen for identification of retinal mRNAs that are regulated by a circadian clock. *Brain Res. Mol. Brain Res.* **37**, 157–165.

Green, C. B., Besharse, J. C., and Zatz, M. (1996). Tryptophan hydroxylase mRNA levels are regulated by the circadian clock, temperature, and amp in chick pineal cells. *Brain Res.* **738**, 1–7.

Green, D. J., and Gillette, R. (1982). Circadian rhythm of firing rate recorded from single cells in the rat suprachiasmatic brain slice. *Brain Res.* **245**, 198–200.

Green, J., Pollak, C. P., and Smith, G. P. (1987). Meal size and intermeal interval in human subjects in time isolation. *Physiol. Behav.* **41**, 141–147.

Gundlah, C., Kohama, S. G., Mirkes, S. J., Garyfallou, V. T., Urbanski, H. F., and Bethea, C. L. (2000). Distribution of estrogen receptor beta (Erbeta) mRNA in hypothalamus, midbrain and temporal lobe of spayed macaque: Continued expression with hormone replacement. *Brain Res. Mol. Brain Res.* **76**, 191–204.

Hall, J. C. (1995). Tripping along the trail to the molecular mechanisms of biological clocks. *Trends Neurosci.* **18**, 230–240.

Hamada, T., LeSauter, J., Venuti, J. M., and Silver, R. (2000). The role of calbindin-D28K on the photoentrainment mechanism of hamster suprachiasmaatic nucleus. *Soc. Res. Biol. Rhythms, Bienn. Meet. Abstr.* No. 160.

Hamada, T., LeSauter, J., Venuti, J. M., and Silver, R. (2001). Expression of Period genes: Rhythmic and nonrhythmic compartments of the suprachiasmatic nucleus pacemaker. *J. Neurosci.* **21**, 7742–7750.

Handler, A. M., and Konopka, R. J. (1979). Transplantation of a circadian pacemaker in *Drosophila*. *Nature (London)* **279**, 236–238.

Hannibal, J., Hindersson, P., Knudsen, S. M., Georg, B., and Fahrenkrug, J. (2002). The photopigment melanopsin is exclusively present in pituitary adenylate cyclase-activating polypeptide-containing retinal ganglion cells of the retinohypothalamic tract. *J. Neurosci.* **22**, RC191.

Hardin, P. E., and Glossop, N. R. (1999). Perspectives: Neurobiology. The CRYs fo flies and mice. *Science* **286**, 2460–2461.

Hardin, P. E., Hall, J. C., and Rosbash, M. (1990). Feedback of the *Drosophila* period gene product on circadian cycling of its messenger RNA levels. *Nature (London)* **343**, 536–540.

Harmer, S. L., Hogenesch, J. B., Straume, M., Chang, H. S., Han, B., Zhu, T., Wang, X., Kreps, J. A., and Kay, S. A. (2000). Orchestrated transcription of key pathways in arabidopsis by the circadian clock. *Science* **290**, 2110–2113.

Harmer, S. L., Panda, S., and Kay, S. A. (2001). Molecular bases of circadian rhythms. *Annu. Rev. Cell. Dev. Biol.* **17**, 215–253.

Harney, J. P., Scarbrough, K., Rosewell, K. L., and Wise, P. M. (1996). *In vivo* antisense antagonism of vasoactive intestinal peptide in the suprachiasmatic nuclei causesaging-like changes in the estradiol-induced luteinizing hormone and prolactin surges. *Endocrinology (Baltimore)* **137**, 3696–3701.

Harrington, M. E., and Rusak, B. (1986). Lesions of the thalamic intergeniculate leaflet alter hamster circadian rhythms. *J. Biol. Rhythms* **1**, 309–325.

Hastings, M. H., Duffield, G. E., Ebling, F. J., Kidd, A., Maywood, E. S., and Schurov, I. (1997). Non-photic amp dian in the suprachiasmatic nucleus. *Biol. Cell* **89**, 495–503.

Hattar, S., Liao, H. W., Takao, M., Berson, D. M., and Yau, K. W. (2002). Melanopsin-containing retinal ganglion cells: architecture, projections, and intrinsic photosensitivity. *Science* **295**, 955–957.

Hebert, M., Martin, S. K., and Eastman, C. I. (1999). Nocturnal melatonin secretion is not suppressed by light exposure behind the knee in humans. *Neurosci. Lett.* **274**, 127–130.

Herbert, J. (1995). The age of dehydroepiandrosterone. *Lancet* **345**, 1193–1194.

Hermann, M., Untergasser, G., Rumpold, H., and Berger, P. (2000). Aging of the male reproductive system. *Exp. Gerontol.* **35**, 1267–1279.

Herzog, E. D., Takahashi, J. S., and Block, G. D. (1998). Clock controls circadian period in isolated suprachiasmatic nucleus neurons. *Nat. Neurosci.* **1**, 708–713.

Heymsfield, S. B., Gallagher, D., Poehlman, E. T., Wolper, C., Nonas, K., Nelson, D., and Wang, Z. M. (1994). Menopausal changes in body composition and energy expenditure. *Exp. Gerontol.* **29**, 377–389.

Hileman, S. M., Handa, R. J., and Jackson, G. L. (1999). Distribution of estrogen receptor-beta messenger ribonucleic acid in the male sheep hypothalamus. *Biol. Reprod.* **60**, 1279–1284.

Hoffmann, J. C. (1968). Effect of photoperiod on estrous cycle length in the rat. *Endocrinology (Baltimore)* **83**, 1355–1357.

Honma, S., Honma K., and Hiroshige, T. (1986). Circadian locomotor rhythms in SCN lesioned rats: Effects of metamphetamine, *J. Physiol. Soc. Jpn.* **48**, 415.

Honma, S., Honma, K., and Hiroshige, T. (1991). Methamphetamine effects on rat circadian clock depend on actograph. *Physiol. Behav.* **49**, 787–795.

Horvath, T. L. (1997). Suprachiasmatic efferents avoid phenestrated capillaries but innervate neuroendocrine cells, including those producing dopamine. *Endocrinology (Baltimore)* **138**, 1312–1320.

Horvath, T. L., Cela, V., and van der Beek, E. M. (1998). Gender-specific apposition between vasoactive intestinal peptide-containing axons and gonadotrophin-releasing hormone-producing neurons in the rat. *Brain Res.* **795**, 277–281.

Hsu, D. S., Zhao, X., Zhao, S., Kazantsev, A., Wang, R. P., Todo, T., Wei, Y. F., and Sancar, A. (1996). Putative human blue-light photoreceptors hCRY1 and hCRY2 are flavoproteins. *Biochemistry* **35**, 13871–13877.

Hunter-Ensor, M., Ousley, A., and Sehgal, A. (1996). Regulation of the *Drosophila* protein timeless suggests a mechanism for resetting the circadian clock by light. *Cell (Cambridge, Mass.)* **84**, 77–85.

Ibata, Y., Takahashi, Y., Okamura, H., Kawakami, F., Terubayashi, H., Kubo, T., and Yanaihara, N. (1989). Vasoactive intestinal peptide (VIP)-like immunoreactive neurons located in the rat suprachiasmatic nucleus receive a direct retinal projection. *Neurosci. Lett.* **97**, 1–5.

Inouye, S. T., and Shibata, S. (1994). Neurochemical organization of circadian rhythm in the suprachiasmatic nucleus. *Neurosci. Res.* **20**, 109–130.

Iwasaki, H., and Dunlap, J. C. (2000). Microbial circadian oscillatory systems in *Neurospora* and *Synechococcus*: Models for cellular clocks. *Curr. Opin. Microbiol.* **3**, 189–196.

Jakacki, R. I., Kelch, R. P., Sauder, S. E., Lloyd, J. S., Hopwood, N. J., and Marshall, J. C. (1982). Pulsatile secretion of luteinizing hormone in children. *J. Clin. Endocrinol. Metab.* **55**, 453–458.

Jechura, T. J., Walsh, J. M., and Lee, T. M. (2000). Testicular hormones modulate circadian rhythms of the diurnal rodent, *Octodon degus*. *Horm. Behav.* **38**, 243–249.

Jiang, Z. G., Yang ,Y., Liu, Z. P., and Allen, C. N. (1997). Membrane properties and synaptic inputs of suprachiasmatic nucleus neurons in rat brain slices. *J. Physiol. (London)* **499**, 141–159.

Jin, X., Shearman, L. P., Weaver, D. R., Zylka, M. J., De Vries, G. J., and Reppert, S. M. (1999). A molecular mechanism regulating rhythmic output from the suprachiasmatic circadian clock. *Cell (Cambridge, Mass.)* **96**, 57–68.

Johnson, C. H., and Golden, S. S. (1999). Circadian programs in cyanobacteria: Adaptiveness and mechanism. *Annu. Rev. Microbiol.* **53**, 389–409.

Johnson, R. F., Morin, L. P., and Moore, R. Y. (1988). Retinohypothalamic projections in the hamster and rat using cholera toxin. *Brain Res.* **462**, 301–312.

Kalra, S. P., and McCann, S. M. (1974). Effects of drugs modifying catecholamine synthesis on plasma LH and ovulation in the rat. Neuroendocrinology **15**, 79–91.

Kalra, S. P., Dube, M. G., Pu, S., Xu, B., Horvath, T. L., and Kalra, P. S. (1999). Interacting appetite-regulating pathways in the hypothalamic regulation of body weight. *Endocr. Rev.* **20**, 68–100.

Kalsbeek, A., Teclemariam-Mesbah, R., and Pevet, P. (1993). Efferent projections of the suprachiasmatic nucleus in the Golden hamster (*Mesocricetus auratus*). *J. Comp. Neurol.* **332**, 293–314.

Kalsbeek, A., Buijs, R. M., Engelmann, M., Wotjak, C. T., and Landgraf, R. (1995). *In vivo* measurement of a diurnal variation in vasopressin release in the rat suprachiasmatic nucleus. *Brain Res.* **682**, 75–82.

Kalsbeek, A., van der Vliet, J., and Buijs, R. M. (1996a). Decrease of endogenous vasopressin release necessary for expression of the circadian rise in plasma corticosterone: A reverse microdialysis study. *J. Neuroendocrinol.* **8**, 299–307.

Kalsbeek, A., van Heerikhuize, J. J., Wortel, J., and Buijs, R. M. (1996b). A diurnal rhythm of stimulatory input to the hypothalamo-pituitary-adrenal system as revealed by timed intrahypothalamic administration of the vasopressin V1 antagonist. *J. Neurosci.* **16**, 5555–5565.

Kalsbeek, A., Fliers, E., Franke, A. N., Wortel, J., and Buijs, R. M. (2000). Functional connections between the suprachiasmatic nucleus and the thyroid gland as revealed by lesioning and viral tracing techniques in the rat. *Endocrinology (Baltimore)* **141**, 3832–3841.

Kaneko, M., Helfrich-Forster, C., and Hall, J. C. (1997). Spatial and temporal expression of the period and timeless genes in the developing nervous system of *Drosophila*: Newly identified pacemaker candidates and novel features of clock gene product cycling. *J. Neurosci.* **17**, 6745–6760.

Kapen, S., Boyar, R. M., Finkelstein, J. W., Hellman, L., and Weitzman, E. D. (1974). Effect of sleep-wake cycle reversal on luteinizing hormone secretory pattern in puberty. *J. Clin. Endocrinol. Metab.* **39**, 293–299.

Kashon, M. L., Arbogast, J. A., and Sisk, C. L. (1996). Distribution and hormonal regulation of androgen receptor immunoreactivity in the forebrain of the male European ferret. *J. Comp. Neurol.* **376**, 567–586.

Keating, R. J., and Tcholakian, R. K. (1979). *In vivo* patterns of circulating steroids in adult male rats. II. Effect of total parenteral nutrition. *J. Surg. Res.* **27**, 23–28.

Kelly, J., and Grossman, S. P. (1980). GABA and hypothalamic feeding systems. *Brain Res. Bull.* **5**, 237–244.

Kimura, F., and Kawakami, M. (1978). Reanalysis of the preoptic afferents and efferents involved in the surge of LH, FSH and prolactin release in the proestrous rat. *Neuroendocrinology* **27**, 74–85.

King, D. P., and Takahashi, J. S. (2000). Molecular genetics of circadian rhythms in mammals. *Annu. Rev. Neurosci.* **23**, 713–742.

King, D. P., Vitaterna, M. H., Chang, A. M., Dove, W. F., Pinto, L. H., Turek, F. W., and Takahashi, J. S. (1997). The mouse Clock mutation behaves as an antimorph and maps within the W19H deletion, distal of Kit. *Genetics* **146**, 1049–1060.

Kissileff, H. R. (1970). Free feeding in normal and recovered lateral rats monitored by a pellet-detecting eatometer. *Physiol. Behav.* **5**, 163–173.

Kizer, J. S., Zivin, J. A., Jacobowitz, D. M., and Kopin, I. J. (1975). The nyctohemeral rhythm of plasma prolactin: Effects of ganglionectomy, pinealectomy, constant light, constant darkness or 6-OH-dopamine administration. *Endocrinology (Baltimore)* **96**, 1230–1240.

Klein, D. C. (1985). Photoneural regulation of the mammalian pineal gland. *Ciba Found. Symp.* **117**, 38–56.

Kobayashi, K., Kanno, S., Smit, B., van der Horst, G. T., Takao, M., and Yasui, A. (1998). Protein, nucleotide, OMIM characterization of photolyase/blue-light receptor homologs in mouse and human cells. *Nucleic Acids Res.* **26**, 5086–5092.

Konopka, R. J., and Benzer, S. (1971). Clock mutants of *Drosophila melanogaster. Proc. Natl. Acad. Sci. U.S.A.* **68**, 2112–2116.

Korf, H. W., Schomerus, C., and Stehle, J. H. (1998). The pineal organ, its hormone melatonin, and the photoneuroendocrine system. *Adv. Anat. Embryol. Cell. Biol.* **146**, 1–100.

Kornhauser, J. M., Nelson, D. E., Mayo, K. E., and Takahashi, J. S. (1990). Photic and circadian regulation of c-fos gene expression in the hamster suprachiasmatic nucleus. *Neuron* **5**, 127–134.

Kornhauser, J. M., Nelson, D. E., Mayo, K. E., and Takahashi, J. S. (1992). Regulation of jun-B messenger RNA and AP-1 activity by light and a circadian clock. *Science* **255**, 1581–1584.

Krajnak, K., Kashon, M. L., Rosewell, K. L., and Wise, P. M. (1998a). Sex differences in the daily rhythm of vasoactive intestinal polypeptide but not arginine vasopressin messenger ribonucleic acid in the suprachiasmatic nuclei. *Endocrinology (Baltimore)* **139**, 4189–4196.

Krajnak, K., Kashon, M. L., Rosewell, K. L., and Wise, P. M. (1998b). Aging alters the rhythmic expression of vasoactive intestinal polypeptide mRNA but not arginine vasopressin mRNA in the suprachiasmatic nuclei of female rats. *J. Neurosci.* **18**, 4767–4774.

Kramer, A., Yang, F. C., Snodgrass, P., Li, X., Scammell, T. E., Davis, F. C., and Weitz, C. J. (2001). Regulation of daily locomotor activity and sleep by hypothalamic EGF receptor signaling. *Science* **294**, 2511–2515.

Krieg, R. J., and Sawyer, C. H. (1976). Effects of intraventricular catecholamines on luteinizing hormone release in ovariectomized-steroid-primed rats. *Endocrinology (Baltimore)* **99**, 411–419.

Krieger, D. T. (1974). Food and water restriction shifts corticosterone, temperature, activity and brain amine periodicity. *Endocrinology (Baltimore)* **95**, 1195–1201.

Krieger, D. T., Ossowski, R., Fogel, M., and Allen, W. (1972). Lack of amp dian periodicity of human serum FSH and LH levels. *J. Clin. Endocrinol. Metab.* **35**, 619–623.

Kume, K., Zylka, M. J., Sriram, S., Shearman, L. P., Weaver, D. R., Jin, X., Maywood, E. S., Hastings, M. H., and Reppert, S. M. (1999). MCRY1 and MCRY2 are essential components of the negative limb of the circadian clock feedback loop. *Cell (Cambridge, Mass.)* **98**, 193–205.

Labrie, F., Bélanger, A., Simard, J., Van, L.-T., and Labrie, C. (1995). DHEA and peripheral androgen and estrogen formation: Intracrinology. *Ann. N. Y. Acad. Sci.* **774**, 16–28.

Labyak, S. E., and Lee, T. M. (1995). Estrus- and steroid-induced changes in circadian rhythms in a diurnal rodent, *Octodon degus. Physiol. Behav.* **58**, 573–585.

Labyak, S. E., and Lee, T. M. (1997). Individual variation in reentrainment after phase shifts of light-dark cycle in a diurnal rodent *Octodon degus. Am. J. Physiol.* **273**, R739–R746.

La Fleur, S. E., Kalsbeek, A., Wortel, J., and Buijs, R. M. (2000). Polysynaptic neural pathways between the hypothalamus, including the suprachiasmatic nucleus, and the liver. *Brain Res.* **87**, 50–56.

Lamberts, S. W., van den Beld, A. W., and van der Lely, A. J. (1997). The endocrinology of aging. *Science* **278**, 419–424.

Larsen, P. J. (1999). Tracing autonomic innervation of the rat pineal gland using viral transneuronal tracing. *Microsc. Res. Tech.* **46**, 296–304.

Larsen, P. J., Enquist, L. W., and Card, J. P. (1998). Characterization of the multisynaptic neuronal control of the rat pineal gland using viral transneuronal tracing. *Eur. J. Neurosci.* **10**, 128–145.

LaVail, M. M. (1976). Rod outer segment disk shedding in rat retina: Relationship to cyclic lighting. *Science* **194**, 1071–1074.

Leal, A. M., and Moreira, A. C. (1997). Food and the circadian activity of the hypothalamic-pituitary-adrenal axis. *Braz. J. Med. Biol. Res.* **30**, 1391–1405.

Lee, S. J., Lenton, E. A., Sexton, L., and Cooke, I. D. (1988). The effect of age on the cyclical patterns of plasma LH, FSH, oestradiol and progesterone in women with regular menstrual cycles. *Hum. Reprod.* **3**, 851–855.

Lee, W. S., Smith, M. S., and Hoffman, G. E. (1990). Luteinizing hormone-releasing hormone neurons express Fos protein during the proestrous surge of luteinizing hormone. *Proc. Natl. Acad. Sci. U.S.A.* **87**, 5163–5167.

Lee, W. S., Abbud, R., Smith, M. S., and Hoffman, G. E. (1992). LHRH neurons express cJun protein during the proestrous surge of luteinizing hormone. *Endocrinology (Baltimore)* **130**, 3101–3103.

Legan, S. J., and Karsch, F. J. (1975). A daily signal for the LH surge in the rat. *Endocrinology (Baltimore)* **96**, 57–62.

Legan S. J., Coon, G. A., and Karsch, F. J. (1975). Role of estrogen as initiator of daily LH surges in the ovariectomized rat. *Endocrinology (Baltimore)* **96**, 50–56.

Lehman, M. N., and Silver, R. (1994). Restoration of circadian rhythms by neural transplants. In "Neuronal Transplantation, CNS Neuronal Injury and Regeneration" (J. Marwah, ed.), pp. 141–160. CRC Press, Boca Raton, FL.

Lehman, M. N., Silver, R., Gladstone, W. R., Kahn, R. M., Gibson, M., and Bittman, E. L. (1987). Circadian rhythmicity restored by neural transplant. Immunocytochemical characterization of the graft and its integration with the host brain. *J. Neurosci.* **7**, 1626–1638.

Lehman, M. N., LeSauter, J., Kim, C., Berriman, S. J., Tresco, P. A., and Silver, R. (1995). How do fetal grafts of the suprachiasmatic nucleus communicate with the host brain? *Cell Transplant.* **4**, 75–81.

Lehman M. N., LeSauter, J., and Silver, R. (1998). Fiber outgrowth from anterior hypothalamic and cortical xenografts in the third ventricle. *J. Comp. Neurol.* **391**(2), 133–145.

Leibowitz, S. F. (1990). The role of serotonin in eating disorders. *Drugs* **39**(Suppl. 3), 33–48.

LeSauter, J., and Silver, R. (1998). Output signals of the SCN. *Chronobiol. Int.* **15**, 535–550.

LeSauter, J., and Silver, R. (1994). Suprachiasmatic nucleus lesions abolish and fetal SCN grafts restore circadian gnawing rhythms in hamsters. *Restorative Neurol. Neurosci.* **6**, 135–143.

LeSauter J., and Silver, R. (1999). Localization of a suprachiasmatic nucleus subregion regulating locomotor rhythmicity. *J. Neurosci.* **19**, 5574–5585.

Levinson, G., and Burnside, B. (1981). Circadian rhythms in teleost retinomotor movement. A comparison of the effects of circadian rhythm and light condition on cone length. *Invest. Ophthalmol. Visual Sci.* **20**, 294–303.

Lewy, A. J., and Sack, R. L. (1997). Exogenous melatonin's phase-shifting effects on the endogenous melatonin profile in sighted humans: A brief review and critique of the literature. *J. Biol. Rhythms* **12**, 588–594.

Lewy, A. J., Wehr, T. A., Goodwin, F. K., Newsome, D. A., and Markey, S. P. (1980). Light suppresses melatonin secretion in humans. *Science* **210**, 1267–1269.

Lewy, A. J., Ahmed, S., Jackson, J. M., and Sack, R. L. (1992). Melatonin shifts human circadian rhythms according to a phase-response curve. *Chronobiol. Int.* **9**, 380–392.

Li, H. Y., and Satinoff, E. (1998). Fetal tissue containing the suprachiasmatic nucleus restores multiple circadian rhythms in old rats. *Am. J. Physiol.* **275**, R1735–R1744.

Li, H. Y., Blaustein, J. D., De Vries, G. J., and Wade, G. N. (1993). Estrogen-receptor immunoreactivity in hamster brain: Preoptic area, hypothalamus and amygdala. *Brain Res.* **631**, 304–312.

Liang, S. L., and Pan, J. T. (2000). An endogenous serotonergic rhythm acting on 5- HT(2A) receptors may be involved in the diurnal changes in tuberoinfundibular dopaminergic neuronal activity and prolactin secretion in female rats. *Neuroendocrinology* **72**, 11–19.

Lincoln, G. A., and Clarke, I. J. (1997). Refractoriness to a static melatonin signal develops in the pituitary gland for the control of prolactin secretion in the ram. *Biol. Reprod.* **57**, 460–467.

Liu, C., and Reppert, S. M. (2000). GABA synchronizes clock cells within the suprachiasmatic circadian clock. *Neuron* **25**, 123–128.

Liu, C., Weaver, D. R., Strogatz, S. H., and Reppert, S. M. (1997). Cellular construction of a circadian clock: Period determination in the suprachiasmatic nuclei. *Cell (Cambridge, Mass.)* **91**, 855–860.

Lloyd, J. M., Hoffman, G. E., and Wise, P. M. (1994). Decline in immediate early gene expression in gonadotropin-releasing hormone neurons during proestrus in regularly cycling, middle-aged rats. *Endocrinology (Baltimore)* **134**, 1800–1805.

Lopez-Molina, L., Conquet, F., Dubois-Dauphin, M., and Schibler, U. (1997). The DBP gene is expressed according to a circadian rhythm in the suprachiasmatic nucleus and influences circadian behavior. *EMBO, J.* **16**, 6762–6771.

Loros, J. J., and Dunlap, J. C. (2001). Genetic and molecular analysis or circadian rhythms in Neurospora. *Annu. Rev. Physiol.* **63**, 757–794.

Loudon, A. S., Wayne, N. L., Krieg, R., Iranmanesh, A., Veldhuis, J. D., and Menaker, M. (1994). Ultradian endocrine rhythms are altered by a circadian mutation in the Syrian hamster. *Endocrinology (Baltimore)* **135**, 712–718.

Loudon, A. S., Ihara, N., and Menaker, M. (1998). Effects of a circadian mutation on seasonality in Syrian hamsters (*Mesocricetus auratus*). *Proc. R. Soc. London, Ser. B* **265**, 517–521.

Lowrey, P. L., and Takahashi, J. S. (2000). Genetics of the mammalian circadian system: Photic entrainment, circadian pacemaker mechanisms, and posttranslational regulation. *Annu. Rev. Genet.* **34**, 533–562.

Lowrey, P. L., Shimomura, K., Antoch, M. P., Yamazaki, S., Zemenides, P. D., Ralph, M. R., Menaker, M., and Takahashi, J. S. (2000). Positional syntenic cloning and functional characterization of the mammalian circadian mutation tau. *Science* **288**, 483–492.

Lucas, R. J., Stirland, J. A., Darrow, J. M., Menaker, M., and Loudon, A. S. (1999). Free running circadian rhythms of melatonin, luteinizing hormone, and cortisol in Syrian hamsters bearing the circadian tau mutation. *Endocrinology (Baltimore)* **140**, 758–764.

Mai, L. M., Shieh, K. R., and Pan, J. T. (1994). Circadian changes of serum prolactin levels and tuberoinfundibular dopaminergic neuron activities in ovariectomized rats treated with or without estrogen: The role of the suprachiasmatic nuclei. *Neuroendocrinology* **60**, 520–526.

Majzoub, J. A., Robinson, B. C., and Emanuel, R. L. (1991). Suprachiasmatic nuclear rhythms of vasopressin mRNA *in vivo*. In "The Suprachiasmatic Nucleus: The Mind's Clock" (D. C. Klein, R. Y. Moore, and S. M. Reppert, eds.), pp. 177–190. Oxford University Press, New York.

Manglapus, M. K., Uchiyama, H., Buelow, N. F., and Barlow, R. B. (1998). Circadian rhythms of rod-cone dominance in the Japanese quail retina. *J. Neurosci.* **18**, 4775–4784.

Mason, R. (1986). Circadian variation in sensitivity of suprachiasmatic and lateral geniculate neurones to 5-hydroxytryptamine in the rat. *J. Physiol. (London)* **377**, 1–13.

Masoro, E. J. (1992). Retardation of aging processes by nutritional means. *Ann. N. Y. Acad. Sci.* **673**, 29–35.

Masoro, E. J. (1996). Possible mechanisms underlying the antiaging actions of caloric restriction. *Toxicol. Pathol.* **24**, 738–741.

Masoro, E. J. (1998). Hormesis and the antiaging action of dietary restriction. *Exp. Gerontol.* **33**, 61–66.

Masoro, E. J. (2000). Caloric restriction and aging: An update. *Exp. Gerontol.* **35**, 299–305.

Masoro, E. J., McCarter, R. J., Katz, M. S., and McMahan, C. A. (1992). Dietary restriction alters characteristics of glucose fuel use. *J. Gerontol.* **47**, B202–B208.

Masoro, E. J., Shimokawa, I., Higami, Y., McMahan, C. A., and Yu, B. P. (1995). Temporal pattern of food intake not a factor in the retardation of aging processes by dietary restriction. *J. Gerontol. A* **50A**, B48–B53.

Matt, D. W., Veldhuis, J. D., and Evans, W. S. (1995). *Gerontol. Soc. Am.* **35**, 146 (abstr.).

Matt, D. W., Kauma, S. W., Pincus, S. M., Veldhuis, J. D., and Evans, W. S. (1998). Characteristics of luteinizing hormone secretion in younger versus older premenopausal women. *Am. J. Obstet. Gynecol.* **178**, 504–510.

Maywood E. S., Buttery R. C., Vance G. H., Herbert J., and Hastings M. H. (1990). Gonadal responses of the male Syrian hamster to programmed infusions of melatonin are sensitive to signal duration and frequency but not to signal phase nor to lesions of the suprachiasmatic nuclei. *Biol. Reprod.* **43**, 174–182.

Maywood, E. S., Bittman, E. L., and Hastings, M. H. (1996). Lesions of the melatonin- and androgen-responsive tissue of the dorsomedial nucleus of the hypothalamus block the gonadal response of male Syrian hamsters to programmed infusions of melatonin. *Biol. Reprod.* **54**, 470–477.

McArthur, A. J., Gillette, M. U., and Prosser, R. A. (1991). Melatonin directly resets the rat suprachiasmatic circadian clock *in vitro*. *Brain Res.* **565**, 6158–6161.

McCay, C. M., Crowell, M. F., and Manard, L. A. (1935). The effect of retarded growth upon the length of life and upon ultimate size. *J. Nutr.* **10**, 63–79.

McShane, T. M., and Wise, P. M. (1996). Life-long moderate caloric restriction prolongs reproductive life span in rats without interrupting estrous cyclicity: Effects on the gonadotropin-releasing hormone/luteinizing hormone axis. *Biol. Reprod.* **54**, 70–75.

Meijer, J. H., Daan, S., Overkamp, G. J., and Hermann, P. M. (1990). The two-oscillator circadian system of tree shrews (Tupaia belangeri) and its response to light and dark pulses. *J. Biol. Rhythms* **5**, 1–16.

Meijer, J. H., Watanabe, K., Schaap, J., Albus, H., and Detari, L. J. (1998). Light responsiveness of the suprachiasmatic nucleus: Long-term multiunit and single-unit recordings in freely moving rats. *Neuroscience* **18**, 9078–9087.

Meldrum, D. R., Tataryn, I. V., Frumar, A. M., Erlik, Y., Lu, K. H., and Judd, H. L. (1980). Gonadotropins, estrogens, and adrenal steroids during the menopausal hot flash. *J. Clin. Endocrinol. Metab.* **50**, 685–689.

Menaker, M., Moreira, L. F., and Tosini, G. (1997). Evolution of circadian organization in vertebrates. *Braz. J. Med. Biol. Res.* **30**, 305–313.

Meneilly, G. S., Ryan, A. S., Veldhuis, J. D., and Elahi, D. (1997). Increased disorderliness of basal insulin release, attenuated insulin secretory burst mass, and reduced ultradian rhythmicity of insulin secretion in older individuals. *J. Clin. Endocrinol. Metab.* **82**, 4088–4093.

Meyer-Bernstein, E. L., Jetton, A. E., Matsumoto, S. I., Markuns, J. F., Lehman, M. N., and Bittman, E. L. (1999). Effects of suprachiasmatic transplants on circadian rhythms of neuroendocrine function in goldenhamsters. *Endocrinology (Baltimore)* **140**, 207–218.

Michel, S., Geusz, M. E., Zaritsky, J. J., and Block, G. D. (1993). Circadian rhythm in membrane conductance expressed in isolated neurons. *Science* **259**, 239–241.

Mikkelsen, J. D., Larsen, P. J., O. Hare, M. M., and Wiegand, S. J. (1991). Gastrin-releasing peptide in the rat suprachiasmatic nucleus: An immunohistochemical, chromatographic and radioimmunological study. *Neuroscience* **40**, 55–66.

Mills, J. N., Minors, D. S., and Waterhouse, J. M. (1978). The effect of sleep upon human circadian rhythms. *Chronobiologia* **5**, 14–27.

Mistlberger, R. E., Houpt, T. A., and Moore-Ede, M. C. (1990). Effects of aging on food-entrained circadian rhythms in the rat. *Neurobiol. Aging* **11**, 619–624.

Miyamoto, Y., and Sancar, A. (1998). Vitamin B2-based blue-light photoreceptors in the retinohypothalamic tract as the photoactive pigments for setting the circadian clock in mammals. *Proc. Natl. Acad. Sci. U.S.A.* **95**, 6097–6102.

Miyamoto, Y., and Sancar, A. (1999). Circadian regulation of cryptochrome genes in the mouse. *Brain Res. Mol. Brain Res.* **71**, 238–243.

Miyatake, A., Morimoto, Y., Oishi, T., Hanasaki, N., Sugita, Y., Iijima, S., Teshima, Y., Hishikawa, Y., and Yamamura, Y. (1980). Circadian rhythm of serum testosterone and its relation to sleep: Comparison with the variation in serum luteinizing hormone, prolactin, and cortisol in normal men. *J. Clin. Endocrinol. Metab.* **51**, 1365–1371.

Mock, E. J., Norton, H. W., and Frankel, A. I. (1978). Daily rhythmicity of serum testosterone concentration in the male laboratory rat. *Endocrinology (Baltimore)* **103**, 1111–1121.

Moenter, S. M., Caraty, A., Locatelli, A., and Karsch, F. J. (1991). Pattern of gonadotropin-releasing hormone (GnRH) secretion leading up to ovulation in the ewe: Existence of a preovulatory GnRH surge. *Endocrinology (Baltimore)* **129**, 1175–1182.

Mohankumar, P. S., Thyagarajan, S., and Quadri, S. K. (1994). Correlations of catecholamine release in the medial preoptic area with proestrous surges of luteinizing hormone and prolactin: Effects of aging. *Endocrinology (Baltimore)* **135**, 119–126.

Monnikes, H., Heymann-Monnikes, I., and Tache, Y. (1992). CRF in the paraventricular nucleus of the hypothalamus induces dose-related behavioral profile in rats. *Brain Res.* **574**, 70–76.

Moore, R. Y. (1983). Organization and function of a central nervous system circadian oscillator: The suprachiasmatic hypothalamic nucleus. *Fed. Proc., Fed. Am. Soc. Exp. Biol.* **42**, 2783–2789.

Moore, R. Y. (1995). Organization of the mammalian circadian system. *Ciba Found.* **183**, 88–99; discussion, pp. 100–106.

Moore, R. Y. (1996). Entrainment pathways and the functional organization of the circadian system. *Prog. Brain Res.* **111**, 103–119.

Moore, R. Y., and Eichler, V. B. (1972). Loss of a circadian adrenal corticosterone rhythm following suprachiasmatic lesions in the rat. *Brain Res.* **42**, 201–206.

Moore, R. Y., and Klein, D. C. (1974). Visual pathways and the central neural control of a circadian rhythm in pineal serotonin N-acetyltransferase activity. *Brain Res* **71**, 17–33.

Moore, R. Y., and Lenn, N. J. (1972). A retinohypothalamic projection in the rat. *J. Comp. Neurol.* **146**, 1–14.

Moore, R. Y., and Speh, J. C. (1993). GABA is the principal neurotransmitter of the circadian system. *Neurosci. Lett.* **150**, 112–116.

Morgan, J. I., and Curran, T. (1991). Proto-oncogene transcription factors and epilepsy. *Trends Pharmacol. Sci.* **12**, 343–349.

Mori, T., Nagai, K., Hara, M., and Nakagawa, H. (1985). Time-dependent effect of insulin in suprachiasmatic nucleus on blood glucose. *Am. J. Physiol.* **249**, R23–R30.

Morin, L. P. (1980). Effect of ovarian hormones on synchrony of hamster circadian rhythms. *Physiol. Behav.* **24**, 741–749.

Morin, L. P., and Cummings, L. A. (1981). Effect of surgical or photoperiodic castration, testosterone replacement or pinealectomy on male hamster running rhythmicity. *Physiol. Behav.* **26**, 825–838.

Morin, L. P., Fitzgerald, K. M., and Zucker, I. (1977). Estradiol shortens the period of hamster circadian rhythms. *Science* **196**, 305–307.

Morin, L. P., Goodless-Sanchez, N., Smale, L., and Moore, R. Y. (1994). Projections of the suprachiasmatic nuclei subparaventricular zone and retrochiasmatic area in the golden hamster. *Neuroscience* **61**, 391–410.

Mosko, S. S., and Moore, R. Y. (1979). Neonatal suprachiasmatic nucleus lesions: Effects on the development of circadian rhythms in the rat. *Brain Res.* **164**, 17–38.

Murakami, N., Takamure, M., Takahashi, K., Utunomiya, K., Kuroda, H., and Etoh, T. (1991). Long-term cultured neurons from rat suprachiasmatic nucleus retain the capacity for circadian oscillation of vasopressin release. *Brain Res.* **545**, 347–350.

Myers, M. P., Wager-Smith, K., Wesley, C. S., Young, M. W., and Sehgal, A. (1995). Positional cloning and sequence analysis of the *Drosophila* clock gene, timeless. *Science* **270**, 805–808.

Myers, M. P., Wager-Smith, K., Rothenfluh-Hilfiker, A., and Young, M. W. (1996). Light-induced degradation of TIMELESS and entrainment of the *Drosophila* circadian clock. *Science* **271**, 1736–1740.

Nagai, K., Nishio, T., Nakagawa, H., Nakamura, S., and Fukuda, Y. (1978). Effect of bilateral lesions of the suprachiasmatic nuclei on the circadian rhythm of food intake. *Brain Res.* **142**, 384–389.

Nagai, K., Mori, T., and Nakagawa, H. (1982). Effects of intracranial insulin infusion on the circadian feeding rhythm of rats. *Biomed. Res.* **3**, 175–180.

Nagai, K., Nagai, N., Sugahara, K., Niijima, A., and Nakagawa, H. (1994). Circadian rhythms and energy metabolism with special reference to the suprachiasmatic nucleus. *Neurosci. Biobehav. Rev.* **18**, 579–584.

Nass, T. E., LaPolt, P. S., Judd, H. L., and Lu, J. K. (1984). Alterations in ovarian steroid and gonadotrophin secretion preceding the cessation of regular oestrous cycles in ageing female rats. *J. Endocrinol.* **100**, 43–50.

Neill, J. D. (1972). Sexual differences in the hypothalamic regulation of prolactin secretion. *Endocrinology (Baltimore)* **90**, 1154–1159.

Neill, J. D., Freeman, M. E., and Tillson, S. A. (1971). Control of the proestrus surge of prolactin and luteinizing hormone secretion by estrogens in the rat. *Endocrinology (Baltimore)* **89**, 1448–1453.

Newman, G. C., and Hospod, F. E. (1986). Rhythm of suprachiasmatic nucleus 2-deoxyglucose uptake *in vitro*. *Brain Res.* **381**, 345–350.

Nicholson, C. (1999). Signals that go with the flow. *Trends Neurosci.* **22**, 143–145.

Nickla, D. L., Wildsoet, C., and Wallman J. (1998). Visual influences on diurnal rhythms in ocular length and choroidal thickness in chick eyes. *Exp. Eye Res.* **66**, 163–181.

Nikaido, S. S., and Takahashi, J. S. (1989). Twenty-four hour oscillation of amp in chick pineal cells: Role of amp in the acute and circadian regulation of melatonin production. *Neuron* **3**, 609–619.

Nunez, A. A., and Stephan, R. K. (1977). The effects of hypothalamic knife cuts on drinking rhythms and the estrous cycle of the rat. *Behav. Biol.* **20**, 224–234.

Ojeda, S. R., Negro-Vilar, A., and McCann, S. M. (1982). Evidence for involvement of alpha-adrenergic receptors in norepinephrine-induced prostaglandin E2 and luteinizing hormone-releasing hormone release from the median eminence. *Endocrinology (Baltimore)* **110**, 409–412.

Okano, T., Yoshizawa, T., and Fukada, Y. (1994). Pinopsin is a chicken pineal photoreceptive molecule. *Nature (London)* **372**, 94–97.

Oren, D. A., and Terman, M. (1998). Tweaking the human circadian clock with light. *Science* **279**, 333–334.

Ottenweller, J. E., Tapp, W. N., Pitman, D. L., and Natelson, B. H. (1987). Adrenal, thyroid, and testicular hormone rhythms in male Golden hamsters on long and short days. *Am. J. Physiol.* **253**, R321–R328.

Ouyang, Y., Andersson, C. R., Kondo, T., Golden, S. S., and Johnson, C. H. (1998). Free in PMC Resonating circadian clocks enhance fitness in cyanobacteria. *Proc. Natl. Acad. Sci. U.S.A.* **95**, 8660–8664.

Paganini-Hill, A., and Henderson, V. W. (1994). Estrogen deficiency and risk of Alzheimer's disease in women. *Am. J. Epidemiol.* **140**, 256–261.

Palm, I. F., van der Beek, E. M., Wiegant, V. M., Buijs, R. M., and Kalsbeek, A. (1999). Vasopressin induces a luteinizing hormone surge in ovariectomized, estradiol-treated rats with lesions of the suprachiasmatic nucleus. *Neuroscience* **93**, 659–666.

Pan, J. T., and Gala, R. R. (1985). Central nervous system regions involved in the estrogen-induced afternoon prolactin surge. II. Implantation studies. *Endocrinology (Baltimore)* **117**, 388–395.

Parker, D. C., Rossman, L. G., and Vanderlaan, E. F. (1974). Relation of sleep-entrained human prolactin release to REM-nonREM cycles. *J. Clin. Endocrinol. Metab.* **38**, 646–651.

Pasterkamp, R. J., Yuri, K., Morita, N., and Kawata, M. (1997). Differential expression of estrogen receptor mRNA and protein in the female rat preoptic area. *Neurosci. Lett.* **239**, 81–84.

Pau, K. Y., Berria, M., Hess, D. L., and Spies, H. G. (1993). Preovulatory gonadotropin-releasing hormone surge in ovarian-intact rhesus macaques. *Endocrinology (Baltimore)* **133**, 1650–1656.

Pevet, P. (2000). Melatonin and biological rhythms. *Biol. Signals Recept.* **9**, 203–212.

Pickard, G. E. (1982). The afferent connections of the suprachiasmatic nucleus of the Golden hamster with emphasis on the retinohypothalamic projection. *J. Comp. Neurol.* **211**, 65–83.

Pickard, G. E., and Tang, W. X. (1993). Individual pineal cells exhibit a circadian rhythm in melatonin secretion. *Brain Res.* **627**, 141–146.

Pickard, G. E., and Tang, W. X. (1994). Pineal photoreceptors rhythmically secrete melatonin. *Neurosci. Lett.* **171**, 109–112.

Pieper, D. R., and Gala, R. R. (1979). The effect of light on the prolactin surges of pseudopregnant and ovariectomized, estrogenized rats. *Biol. Reprod.* **20**, 727–732.

Pierce, M. E., Sheshberadaran, H., Zhang, Z., Fox, L. E., Applebury, M. L., and Takahashi, J. S. (1993). Circadian regulation of iodopsin gene expression in embryonic photoreceptors in retinal cell culture. *Neuron* **10**, 579–584.

Pincus, S. M., Mulligan, T., Iranmanesh, A., Gheorghiu, S., Godschalk, M., and Veldhuis, J. D. (1996). Older males secrete luteinizing hormone and testosterone more irregularly, and jointly more asynchronously, than younger males. *Proc. Natl. Acad. Sci. U.S.A.* **93**, 14100–14105.

Plant, J. M. (1981). Time course of concentrations of circulating gonadotropin, prolactin, testosterone, and cortisol in male rhesus macaque monkeys (*Macaca mulatta*) through the 24-hour light-dark cycle. *Biol. Reprod.* **25**, 244–252.

Plautz, J. D., Kaneko, M., Hall, J. C., and Kay, S. A. (1997a). Independent photoreceptive circadian clocks throughout *Drosophila*. *Science* **278**, 1632–1635.

Plautz, J. D., Straume, M., Stanewsky, R., Jamison, C. F., Brandes C., Dowse, H. B., Hall, J. C., and Kay, S. A. (1997b). Quantitative analysis of *Drosophila* period gene transcription in living animals. *J. Biol. Rhythms* **12**, 204–217.

Powley, T. L., Opsahl, C. H., Cox, J. E., and Weingarten, H. P. (1980). The role of the hypothalamus in energy homeostasis. *In* "Handbook of the Hypothalamus" (P. J. Morgane and J. Panksepp, eds.), Part A, Vol. 3, pp. 211–298. Dekker, New York.

Provencio, I., Wong, S., Lederman, A. B., Argamaso, S. M., and Foster, R. G. (1994). Visual and circadian responses to light in aged retinally degenerate mice. *Vision Res.* **34**, 1799–1806.

Provencio, I., Rollag, M. D., and Castrucci, A. M. (2002). Photoreceptive net in the mammalian retina. This mesh of cells may explain how some blind mice can still tell day from night. *Nature* **415**, 493.

Ralph, M. R., and Menaker, M. (1988). A mutation of the circadian system in Golden hamsters. *Science* **241**, 1225–1227.

Ralph, M. R., Foster, R. G., Davis, F. C., and Menaker, M. (1990). Transplanted suprachiasmatic nucleus determines circadian period. *Science* **247**, 975–978.

Rance, N., Wise, P. M., Selmanoff, M. K., and Barraclough, C. A. (1981). Catecholamine turnover rates in discrete hypothalamic areas and associated changes in median eminence luteinizing hormone-releasing hormone and serum gonadotropins on proestrus and diestrous day 1. *Endocrinology (Baltimore)* **108**, 1795–1802.

Ravaglia, G., Forti, P., Maioli, F., Boschi, F., Bernardi, M., Pratelli, L., Pizzoferrato, A., and Gasbarrini, G. (1996). The relationship of dehydroepiandrosterone sulfate (DHEAS) to endocrine-metabolic parameters and functional status in the oldest-old. Results from an Italian study on healthy free-living over-ninety-year-olds. *J. Clin. Endocrinol. Metab.* **81**, 1173–1178.

Rea, M. A. (1992). Different populations of cells in the suprachiasmatic nuclei express c-fos in association with light-induced phase delays and advances of the free-running activity rhythm in hamsters. *Brain Res.* **579**, 107–112.

Rebar, R. W., and Yen, S. S. (1979). Endocrine rhythms in gonadotropins and ovarian steroids with reference to reproductive success. *In* "Endocrine Rhythms" (D. T. Krieger, ed.), pp. 259–298. Raven Press, New York.

Redlin, U., and Mrosovsky, N. (1997). Exercise and human circadian rhythms: What we know and what we need to know. *Chronobiol. Int.* **14**, 221–229.

Refinetti, R., and Menaker, M. (1992). Evidence for separate control of estrous and circadian periodicity in the Golden hamster. *Behav. Neural Biol.* **58**, 27–36.

Renn, S. C., Park, J. H., Rosbash, M., Hall, J. C., and Taghert, P. H. (1999). A pdf neuropeptide gene mutation and ablation of PDF neurons each cause severe abnormalities of behavioral circadian rhythms in *Drosophila*. *Cell (Cambridge, Mass.)* **99**, 791–802.

Reppert, S. M. (2000). Cellular and molecular basis of circadian timing in mammals. *Semin. Perinatol.* **24**, 243–246.

Reppert, S. M., and Weaver, D. R. (2000). Comparing clockworks: Mouse versus fly. *J. Biol. Rhythms* **15**, 357–364.

Reppert, S. M., and Weaver, D. R. (2001). Molecular analysis of mammalian circadian rhythms. *Annu. Rev. Physiol.* **63**, 647–676.

Reppert, S. M., Schwartz, W. J., and Uhl, G. R. (1987). Arginine vasopressin: A novel peptide rhythm in cerebrospinal fluid. *Trends Neurosci.* **10**, 76–80.

Rhoads, D. B., Rosenbaum, D. H., Unsal, H., Isselbacher, K. J., and Levitsky, L. L. (1998). Circadian periodicity of intestinal Na^+/glucose cotransporter 1 mRNA levels is transcriptionally regulated. *J. Biol. Chem.* **273**, 9510–9516.

Ribak, C. E., and Peters, A. (1975). An autoradiographic study of the projections from the lateral geniculate body of the rat. *Brain Res.* **92**, 341–368.

Robinson, B. G., Frim, D. M., Schwartz, W. J., and Majzoub J. A. (1988). Vasopressin mRNA in the suprachiasmatic nuclei: Daily regulation of polyadenylate tail length. *Science* **241**, 342–344.

Rogina, B., Reenan, R. A., Nilsen, S. P., and Helfand, S. L. (2000). Extended life-span conferred by cotransporter gene mutations in drosophila. *Science* **290**, 2137–2140.

Rosato, E., Peixoto, A. A., Costa, R., and Kyriacou, C. P. (1997). Linkage disequilibrium, mutational analysis and natural selection in the repetitive region of the clock gene, period, in *Drosophila melanogaster*. *Genet. Res.* **69**, 89–99.

Rosbash, M. (1995). Molecular control of circadian rhythms. *Curr. Opin. Genet. Dev.* **5**, 662–668.

Rossmanith, W. G. (1998). The impact of sleep on gonadotropin secretion. *Gynecol. Endocrinol.* **12**, 381–389.

Rossmanith, W. G., Liu, C. H., Laughlin, G. A., Mortola, J. F., Suh, B. Y., and Yen, S. S. (1990). Relative changes in LH pulsatility during the menstrual cycle: Using data from hypogonadal women as a reference point. *Clin. Endocrinol. (Oxford)* **32**, 647–660.

Roth, G. S., Ingram, D. K., and Lane, M. A. (1999). Calorie restriction in primates: Will it work and how will we know? *J. Am. Geriatr. Soc.* **47**, 896–903.

Rowland, N. (1976). Endogenous circadian rhythms in rats recovered from lateral hypothalamic lesions. *Physiol. Behav.* **16**, 257–266.

Roy, E. J., and Wade, G. N. (1975). Role of estrogens in androgen-induced spontaneous activity in male rats. *J. Comp. Physiol. Psychol.* **89**, 573–579.

Rubin, B. S., and Bridges, R. S. (1989). Alterations in luteinizing hormone-releasing hormone release from the mediobasal hypothalamus of ovariectomized, steroid-primed middle-aged rats as measured by push-pull perfusion. *Neuroendocrinology* **49**, 225–232.

Rubin, B. S., Lee, C. E., and King, J. C. (1994). A reduced proportion of luteinizing hormone (LH)-releasing hormone neurons express Fos protein during the preovulatory or steroid-induced LH surge in middle-aged rats. *Biol. Reprod.* **51**, 1264–1272.

Rusak, B., and Boulos, Z. (1981). Pathways for photic entrainment of mammalian circadian rhythms. *Photochem. Photobiol.* **34**, 267–273.

Rusak, B., and Zucker, I. (1979). Neural regulation of circadian rhythms. *Physiol. Rev.* **59**, 449–526.

Rusak, B., Robertson, H. A., Wisden, W., and Hunt, S. P. (1990). Light pulses that shift rhythms induce gene expression in the suprachiasmatic nucleus. *Science* **248**, 1237–1240.

Rusak, B., McNaughton, L., Robertson, H. A., and Hunt, S. P. (1992). Circadian variation in photic regulation of immediate-early gene mRNAs in rat suprachiasmaticnucleus cells. *Brain Res. Mol. Brain Res.* **14**, 124–130.

Sabatino, F., Masoro, E. J., McMahan, C. A., and Kuhn, R. W. (1991). Assessment of the role of the glucocorticoid system in aging processes and in the action of food restriction. *J. Gerontol.* **46**, B171–B179.

Saeb-Parsy, K., Lombardelli, S., Khan, F. Z., McDowall, K., Au-Yong, I. T., and Dyball, R. E. (2000). Neural connections of hypothalamic neuroendocrine nuclei in the rat. *J. Neuroendocrinol.* **12**, 635–648.

Saito, M., Murakami, E., Nishida, T., Fujisawa, Y., and Suda, M. (1976). Circadian rhythms of digestive enzymes in the small intestine of the rat. II. Effects of fasting and refeeding. *J. Biochem. (Tokyo)* **80**, 563–568.

Sapolsky, R. M., Krey, L. C., and McEwen, B. S. (1984). Glucocorticoid-sensitive hippocampal neurons are involved in terminating the adrenocortical stress response. *Proc. Natl. Acad. Sci. U.S.A.* **81**, 6174–6177.

Sarkar, D. K., Chiappa, S. A., Fink, G., and Sherwood, N. M. (1976). Gonadotropin-releasing hormone surge in pro-oestrous rats. *Nature (London)* **264**, 461–463.

Sarov-Blat, L., So, W. V., Liu, L., and Rosbash, M. (2000). The *Drosophila* takeout gene is a novel molecular link between circadian rhythms and feeding behavior. *Cell (Cambridge, Mass.)* **101**, 647–656.

Sassin, J. F., Frantz, A. G., Kapen, S., and Weitzman, E. D. (1973). The nocturnal rise of human prolactin is dependent on sleep. *J. Clin. Endocrinol. Metab.* **37**, 436–440.

Satinoff, E., Li, H., Tcheng, T. K., Liu, C., McArthur, A. J., Medanic, M., and Gillette, M. U. (1993). Do the suprachiasmatic nuclei oscillate in old rats as they do in young ones? *Am. J. Physiol.* **265**, R1216–R1222.

Satoh, N., Ogawa, Y., Katsuura, G., Hayase, M., Tsuji, T., Imagawa, K., Yoshimasa, Y., Nishi, S., Hosoda, K., and Nakao, K. (1997). The arcuate nucleus as a primary site of satiety effect of leptin in rats. *Neurosci. Lett.* **224**, 149–152.

Scarbrough, K., and Wise, P. M. (1990). Age-related changes in pulsatile luteinizing hormone release precede the transition to estrous acyclicity and depend upon estrous cycle history. *Endocrinology (Baltimore)* **126**, 884–890.

Schardt, U., Wilhelm, I., and Erkert, H. G. (1989). Splitting of the circadian activity rhythm in common marmosets (*Callithrix j. jacchus*; primates). *Experientia* **45**, 1112–1115.

Scheving, L. A., and Jin, W.-H. (1999). Circadian regulation of uroguanylin and guanylin in the rat intenstine. *Am. J. Physiol.* **277**, C1177–C1183.

Schick, R. R., Samsami, S., Zimmermann, J. P., Eberl, T., Endres, C., Schusdziarra, V., and Classen, M. (1993). Effect of galanin on food intake in rats: Involvement of lateral and ventromedial hypothalamic sites. *Am. J. Physiol.* **264**, R355–R361.

Schoeller, D. A., Cella, L. K., Sinha, M. K., and Caro, J. F. (1997). Entrainment of the diurnal rhythm of plasma leptin to meal timing. *J. Clin. Invest.* **100**, 1882–1887.

Schull, J., Walker, J., Fitzgerald, K., Hiilivirta, L., Ruckdeschel, J., Schumacher, D., Stanger, D., and McEachron, D. L. (1989). Effects of sex, thyro-parathyroidectomy, and light regime on levels and circadian rhythms of wheel-running in rats. *Physiol. Behav.* **46**, 341–346.

Schwartz, J., Freeman, R., and Frishman, W. (1995). Clinical pharmacology of estrogens: Cardiovascular actions and cardioprotective benefits of replacement therapy in postmenopausal women [corrected and republished article originally printed in *J. Clin. Pharmacol.* **35**(1), 1–16 (1995)]. *J. Clin. Pharmacol.* **35**, 314–329.

Schwartz, W. J. (1993). A clinician's primer on the circadian clock: Its localization, function, and resetting. *Adv. Intern. Med.* **38**, 81–106.

Scott, C. J., Jansen, H. T., Kao, C. C., Kuehl, D. E., and Jackson, G. L. (1995). Disruption of reproductive rhythms and patterns of melatonin and prolactin secretion following bilateral lesions of the suprachiasmatic. *J. Neuroendocrinol.* **7**, 429–443.

Sehgal, A., Rothenfluh-Hilfiker, A., Hunter-Ensor, M., Chen, Y., Myers, M. P., and Young, M. W. (1995). Rhythmic expression of timeless: A basis for promoting circadian cycles in period gene autoregulation. *Science* **270**, 808–810.

Selby, C. P., Thompson, C., Schmitz, T. M., Van Gelder, R. N., and Sancar, A. (2000). Functional redundancy of cryptochromes and classical photoreceptors for nonvisual ocular photoreception in mice. *Proc. Natl. Acad. Sci. U.S.A.* **97**, 14697–14702.

Selgas, L., Arce, A., Esquifino, A. I., and Cardinali, D. P. (1997). Twenty-four-hour rhythms of serum ACTH, prolactin, growth hormone, and thyroid-stimulating hormone, and of median-eminence norepinephrine, dopamine, and serotonin, in rats injected with Freund's adjuvant. *Chronobiol. Int.* **14**, 253–265.

Shearman, L. P., Zylka, M. J., Weaver, D. R., Kolakowski, L. F., Jr., and Reppert, S. M. (1997). Two period homologs: Circadian expression and photic regulation in the suprachiasmatic nuclei. *Neuron* **19**, 1261–1269.

Shearman, L. P., Sriram, S., Weaver, D. R., Maywood, E. S., Chaves, I., Zheng, B., Kume, K., Lee, C. C., van der Horst, G. T., Hastings, M. H., and Reppert, S. M. (2000). Interacting molecular loops in the mammalian circadian clock. *Science* **288**, 1013–1019.

Sheng, M., and Greenberg, M. E. (1990). The regulation and function of c-fos and other immediate early genes in the nervous system. *Neuron* **4**, 477–485.

Sherwin, B. B. (1994). Estrogenic effects on memory in women. *Ann. N.Y. Acad. Sci.* **743**, 213–230; discussion: pp. 230–231.

Sherwin, B. B. (1996). Hormones, mood, and cognitive functioning in postmenopausal women. *Obstet. Gynecol.* **87**, 20S–26S.

Shibata, S., Oomura, Y., Kita, H., Liou, S. Y., and Ueki, S. (1984). Field potentials in the suprachiasmatic nucleus of rat hypothalamic slice produced by optic nerve stimulation. *Brain Res. Bull.* **12**, 377–379.

Shieh, G. J., Ravis, W. R., and Walters, D. E. (1997). Up-regulation of dopamine D1-receptors in the brain of 28-day-old rats exposed to the delta (delta) opioid agonist SNC80 during the preweaning period. *Brain Res. Dev. Brain Res.* **103**, 209–211.

Shinohara, K., and Oka, T. (1994). Protein synthesis inhibitor phase shifts vasopressin rhythms in long-term suprachiasmatic cultures. *NeuroReport* **5**, 2201–2204.

Shinohara, K., Honma, S., Katsuno, Y., Abe, H., and Honma, K. (1995). Two distinct oscillators in the rat suprachiasmatic nucleus in vitro. *Proc. Natl. Acad. Sci. U.S.A.* **92**, 7396–7400.

Shinohara, K., Funabashi, T., Mitushima, D., and Kimura, F. (2000a). Effects of estrogen on the expression of connexin32 and connexin43 mRNAs in the suprachiasmatic nucleus of female rats. *Neurosci. Lett.* **286**, 107–110.

Shinohara, K., Hiruma, H., Funabashi, T., and Kimura, F. (2000b). GABAergic modulation of gap junction communication in slice cultures of the rat suprachiasmatic nucleus.

Shirakawa, T., Honma, S., Katsuno, Y., Oguchi, H., and Honma, K. I. (2000). Synchronization of circadian firing rhythms in cultured rat suprachiasmatic neurons. *Eur. J. Neurosci.* **12**, 2833–2838.

Shughrue, P. J., Lane, M. V., and Merchenthaler, I. (1997). Comparative distribution of estrogen receptor-alpha and beta mRNA in the rat central nervous system. *J. Comp. Neurol.* **388**, 507–525.

Silver, R., and LeSauter, J. (1993). Efferent signals of the suprachiasmatic nucleus. *J. Biol. Rhythms* **8**, S89–S92.

Silver, R., Lehman, M. N., Gibson, M., Gladstone, W. R., and Bittman, E. L. (1990). Dispersed cell suspension of fetal SCN restore circadian rhythmicity in SCN-lesioned adult hamsters. *Brain Res.* **525**, 45–58.

Silver, R., LeSauter, J., Tresco, P. A., and Lehman, M. N. (1996). A diffusible coupling signal from the transplanted suprachiasmatic nucleus controlling circadian locomotor rhythms. *Nature (London)* **382**, 810–813.

Silver, R., Sookhoo, A. I., LeSauter, J., Stevens, P., Jansen, H. T., and Lehman, M. N. (1999). Multiple regulatory elements result in regional specificity in circadian rhythms of neuropeptide expression in mouse SCN. *NeuroReport* **10**, 3165–3174.

Simansky, K. J. (1996). Serotonergic control of the organization of feeding and satiety. *Behav. Brain Res.* **73**, 37–42.

Slotten, H. A., Pitrosky, B., and Pevet, P. (2000). Entrainment of rat circadian rhythms by melatonin does not depend on the serotonergic afferents to the suprachiasmatic nuclei. *Brain Res.* **876**, 10–16.

Smith, M. J., Jiennes, L., and Wise, P. M. (2000). Localization of the VIP2 receptor protein on GnRH neurons in the female rat. *Endocrinology (Baltimore)* **141**, 4317–4320.

Smith, S. G., 3rd, and Stetson, M. H. (1980). Maturation of the clock-timed gonadotropin release mechanism in hamsters: A key event in the pubertal process? *Endocrinology (Baltimore)* **107**, 1334–1337.

Sokoloff, L. (1979). Mapping of local cerebral functional activity by measurement of local cerebral glucose utilization with [14C]deoxyglucose. *Brain* **102**, 653–668.

Sollars, P. J., Kimble, D. P., and Pickard, G. E. (1995). Restoration of circadian behavior by anterior hypothalamic heterografts. *J. Neurosci.* **15**, 2109–2122.

Spies, H. G., Mahoney, C. J., Norman, R. L., Clifton, D. K., and Resko, J. A. (1974). Evidence for a diurnal rhythm in ovarian steroid secretion in the rhesus monkey. *J. Clin. Endocrinol. Metab.* **39**, 347–351.

Spies, H. G., Norman, R. L., and Buhl, A. E. (1979). Twenty-four-hour patterns in serum prolactin and cortisol after partial and complete isolation of the hypothalamic-pituitary unit in rhesus monkeys. *Endocrinology (Baltimore)* **105**, 1361–1368.

Spratt, D. I., O'Dea, L. S., Schoenfeld, D., Butler, J., Rao, P. N., and Crowley, W. F., Jr. (1988). Neuroendocrine-gonadal axis in men: Frequent sampling of LH, FSH, and testosterone. *Am. J. Physiol.* **254**, E658–E666.

Stanewsky, R., Kaneko, M., Emery, P., Beretta, B., Wager-Smith, K., Kay, S. A., Rosbash, M., and Hall, J. C. (1998). The cryb mutation identifies cryptochrome as a circadian photoreceptor in *Drosophila*. *Cell (Cambridge, Mass.)* **95**, 681–692.

Stanley, B. G., Chin, A. S., and Leibowitz, S. F. (1985). Feeding and drinking elicited by central injection of neuropeptide Y: Evidence for a hypothalamic site(s) of action. *Brain Res. Bull.* **14**, 521–524.

Stanley, B. G., Magdalin, W., Seirafi, A., Thomas, W. J., and Leibowitz, S. F. (1993). The perifornical area: The major focus of (a) patchily distributed hypothalamic neuropeptide Y-sensitive feeding system (s). *Brain Res.* **604**, 304–317.

Stephan, F. K. (1986). Interaction between light- and feeding-entrainable circadian rhythms in the rat. *Physiol. Behav.* **38**, 127–133.

Stephan, F. K., and Zucker, I. (1972). Circadian rhythms in behavior and locomotor activity of rats are eliminated by hypothalamic lesions. *Proc. Natl. Acad. Sci. U.S.A.* **69**, 1583–1586.

Stephan, F. K., Swann, J. M., and Sisk, C. L. (1979). Entrainment of circadian rhythms by feeding schedules in rats with suprachiasmatic lesions. *Behav. Neural. Biol.* **25**, 545–554.

Stephan, F. K., Berkley, K. J., and Moss, R. L. (1981). Efferent connections of the rat suprachiasmatic nucleus. *Neuroscience* **6**, 2625–2641.

Stirland, J. A., Grosse, J., Loudon, A. S., Hastings, M. H., and Maywood, E.S. (1995). Gonadal responses of the male tau mutant Syrian hamster to short-day-like programmed infusions of melatonin. *Biol. Reprod.* **53**, 361–367.

Stirland, J. A., Hastings, M. H., Loudon, A. S., and Maywood, E. S. (1996). The tau mutation in the Syrian hamster alters the photoperiodic responsiveness of the gonadal axis to melatonin signal frequency. *Endocrinology (Baltimore)* **137**, 2183–2186.

Stopa, E. G., Minamitani, N., Jonassen, J. A., King, J. C., Wolfe, H., Mobtaker, H., and Albers, H. E. (1988). Localization of vasoactive intestinal peptide and peptide histidine isoleucine immunoreactivity and mRNA within the rat suprachiasmatic nucleus. *Brain Res.* **464**, 319–325.

Strayer, C. A., and Kay, S. A. (1999). The ins and outs of circadian regulated gene expression. *Curr. Opin. Plant Biol.* **2**, 114–120.

Sullivan, J. M., and Fowlkes, L. P. (1996). The clinical aspects of estrogen and the cardiovascular system. *Obstet. Gynecol.* **87**, 36S–43S.

Sun, Z. S., Albrecht, U., Zhuchenko, O., Bailey, J., Eichele, G., and Lee, C. C. (1997). Protein, nucleotide, OMIM RIGUI, a putative mammalian ortholog of the *Drosophila* period gene. *Cell (Cambridge, Mass.)* **90**, 1003–1011.

Sutin, E. L., and Kilduff, T. S. (1992). Circadian and light-induced expression of immediate early gene mRNAs in the rat suprachiasmaticnucleus. *Brain Res. Mol. Brain Res.* **15**, 281–290.

Swanson, L. W., Cowan, W. M., and Jones, E. G. (1974). An autoradiographic study of the efferent connections of the ventral lateral geniculate nucleus in the albino rat and the cat. *Comp. Neurol.* **156**, 143–163.

Takahashi, J. S. (1995). Molecular neurobiology and genetics of circadian rhythms in mammals. *Annu. Rev. Neurosci.* **18**, 531–553.

Takahashi, J. S., and Zatz, M. (1982). Regulation of circadian rhythmicity. *Science* **217**, 1104–1111.

Takahashi, J. S., DeCoursey, P. J., Bauman, L., and Menaker, M. (1984). Spectral sensitivity of a novel photoreceptive system mediating entrainment of mammalian circadian rhythms. *Nature (London)* **308**, 186–188.

Takahashi, J. S., Murakami, N., Nikaido, S. S., Pratt, B. L., and Robertson, L. M. (1989). The avian pineal, a vertebrate model system of the circadian oscillator: Cellular regulation of circadian rhythms by light, second messengers, and macromolecular synthesis. *Recent Prog. Horm. Res.* **45**, 279–348.

Teclemariam-Mesbah, R., Ter Horst, G. J., Postema, F., Wortel, J., and Buijs, R. M. (1999). Anatomical demonstration of the suprachiasmatic nucleus-pineal pathway. *J. Comp. Neurol.* **406**, 171–182.

Tei, H., Okamura, H., Shigeyoshi, Y., Fukuhara, C., Ozawa, R., Hirose, M., and Sakaki, Y. (1997). Circadian oscillation of a mammalian homologue of the *Drosophila* period gene. *Nature (London)* **389**, 512–516.

Tessonneaud, A., Locatelli, A., Caldani, M., and Viguier-Martinez, M. C. (1995). Bilateral lesions of the suprachiasmatic nuclei alter the nocturnal melatonin secretion in sheep. *J. Neuroendocrinol.* **7**, 145–152.

Thresher, R. J., Vitaterna, M. H., Miyamoto, Y., Kazantsev, A., Hsu, D. S., Petit, C., Selby, C. P., Dawut, L., Smithies, O., Takahashi, J. S., and Sancar, A. (1998). Role of mouse cryptochrome blue-light photoreceptor in circadian photoresponses. *Science* **282**, 1490–1494.

Toh, K. L., Jones, C. R., He, Y., Eide, E. J., Hinz, W. A., Virshup, D. M., Ptacek, L. J., and Fu, Y.-H. (2001). An hPer2 phosphorylation site mutation in familial advanced sleep-phase syndrome. *Science* **291**, 1040–1043.

Tokunaga, K., Fukushima, M., Kemnitz, J. W., and Bray, G. A. (1986). Comparison of ventromedial and paraventricular lesions in rats that become obese. *Am. J. Physiol.* **251**, R1221–R1227.

Tosini, G., and Menaker, M. (1996). Circadian rhythms in cultured mammalian retina. *Science* **272**, 419–421.

Tosini, G., and Menaker, M. (1998). Multioscillatory circadian organization in a vertebrate, iguana iguana. *J. Neurosci.* **18**, 1105–1114.

Truman, J. W., and Riddiford, L. M. (1970). Neuroendocrine control of ecdysis in silkmoths. *Science* **167**, 1624–1626.

Turek, F. W. (1994). Circadian rhythms. *Recent Prog. Horm. Res.* **49**, 43–90.

Turek, F. W., and Van Cauter, E. (1994). Rhythms in reproduction. *In* "The Physiology of Reproduction" (E. Knobil and J. D. Neill, eds.), 2nd ed., pp. 487–540. Raven Press, New York.

Uhl, G. R., and Reppert, S. M. (1986). Suprachiasmatic nucleus vasopressin messenger RNA: Circadian variation in normal and Brattleboro rats. *Science* **232**, 390–393.

Vaccarino, F. J. (1996). Dopamine-opioid mechanisms in ingestion. *In* "Drug Receptor Subtypes and Ingestive Behavior" (S. J. Cooper and P. G. Clifton, eds.), pp. 219–232. Academic Press, San Diego, CA.

Van Cauter, E. (1988). Estimating false-positive and false-negative errors in analyses of hormonal pulsatility *Am. J. Physiol.* **254**, E786–E794.

Van Cauter, E., and Refetoff, S. (1985). Multifactorial control of the 24-hour secretory profiles of pituitary hormones. *Endocrinol. Invest.* **8**, 381–391.

Van Cauter, E., L'Hermite, M., Copinschi, G., Refetoff, S., Desir, D., and Robyn, C. (1981). Quantitative analysis of spontaneous variations of plasma prolactin in normal man. *Am. J. Physiol.* **241**, E355–E363.

Van Cauter, E., Caufriez, A., Kerkhofs, M., Van Onderbergen, A., Thorner, M. O., and Copinschi, G. (1992). Sleep, awakenings, and insulin-like growth factor-I modulate the growth hormone (GH) secretory response to GH-releasing hormone. *J. Clin. Endocrinol. Metab.* **74**, 1451–1459.

van Coevorden, A., Mockel, J., Laurent, E., Kerkhofs, M., L'Hermite-Baleriaux, M., Decoster, C., Neve, P., and Van Cauter, E. (1991). Neuroendocrine rhythms and sleep in aging men. *Am. J. Physiol.* **260**, E651–E661.

van den Pol, A. N. (1980). The hypothalamic suprachiasmatic nucleus of rat: Intrinsic anatomy. *J. Comp. Neurol.* **191**, 661–702.

van den Pol, A. N., and Powley, T. (1979). A fine-grained anatomical analysis of the role of the rat suprachiasmatic nucleus in circadian rhythms of feeding and drinking. *Brain Res.* **160**, 307–326.

van den Pol, A. N., and Tsujimoto, K. L. (1985). Neurotransmitters of the hypothalamic suprachiasmatic nucleus: Immunocytochemical analysis of 25 neuronal antigens. *Neuroscience* **15**, 1049–1086.

van der Beek, E. M., Wiegant, V. M., van der Donk, H. A., van den Hurk, R., and Buijs, R. M. (1993). Lesions of the suprachiasmatic nucleus indicate the presence of a direct vasoactive intestinal polypeptide-containing projection to gonadotrophin-releasing hormone neurons in the female rat. *J. Neuroendocrinol.* **5**, 137–144.

van der Beek, E. M., van Oudheusden, H. J., Buijs, R. M., van der Donk, H. A., van den Hurk, R., and Wiegant, V. M. (1994). Preferential induction of c-fos immunoreactivity in vasoactive intestinal polypeptide-innervated gonadotropin-releasing hormone neurons during a steroid-induced luteinizing hormone surge in the female rat. *Endocrinology (Baltimore)* **134**, 2636–2644.

van der Beek, E. M., Horvath, T. L., Wiegant, V. M., van den Hurk, R., and Buijs, R. M. (1997a). Evidence for a direct neuronal pathway from the suprachiasmatic nucleus to the gonadotropin-releasing hormone system: Combined tracing and light and electron microscopic immunocytochemical studies. *J. Comp. Neurol.* **384**, 569–579.

van der Beek, E. M., Wiegant, V. M., van Oudheusden, H. J., van der Donk, H. A., van den Hurk, R., and Buijs, R. M. (1997b). Synaptic contacts between gonadotropin-releasing hormone-containing fibers and neurons in the suprachiasmatic nucleus and perichiasmatic area: An anatomical substrate for feedback regulation? *Brain Res.* **755**, 101–111.

van der Beek, E. M., Swarts, H. J., and Wiegant, V. M. (1999). Central administration of antiserum to vasoactive intestinal peptide delays and reduces luteinizing hormone and prolactin surges in ovariectomized, estrogen-treated rats. *Neuroendocrinology* **69**, 227–237.

van der Horst, G. T., Muijtjens, M., Kobayashi, K., Takano, R., Kanno, S., Takao, M., de Wit, J., Verkerk, A., Eker, A. P., van Leenen, D., Buijs, R., Bootsma, D., Hoeijmakers, J. H., and Yasui, A. (1999). Mammalian Cry1 and Cry2 are essential for maintenance of circadian rhythms. *Nature (London)* **398**, 627–630.

van der Schoot, P. (1976). Changing pro-oestrous surges of luteinizing hormone in ageing 5-day cyclic rats. *J. Endocrinol.* **2**, 287–288.

Vanecek, J., and Watanabe, K. (1999). Mechanisms of melatonin action in the pituitary and SCN. *Adv. Exp. Med. Biol.* **460**, 191–198.

Vaughan, G. M., Pelham, R. W., Pang, S. F., Loughlin, L. L., Wilson, K. M., Sandock, K. L., and Vaughan, M. K. (1976). Nocturnal elevation of plasma melatonin and urinary 5-hydroxyindoleacetic acid in young men: Attempts at modification by brief changes in environmental lighting and sleep and by autonomic drugs. *J. Clin. Endocrinol. Metab.* **42**, 752–764.

Veldhuis, J. D., Rogol, A. D., Evans, W. S., Iranmanesh, A., Lizarralde, G., and Johnson, M. L. (1986). Spectrum of the pulsatile characteristics of LH release in normal men. *J. Androl.* **7**, 83–92.

Veldhuis, J. D., King, J. C., Urban, R. J., Rogol, A. D., Evans, W. S., Kolp, L. A., and Johnson, M. L. (1987). Operating characteristics of the male hypothalamo-pituitary-gonadal axis: Pulsatile release of testosterone and follicle-stimulating hormone and their temporal coupling with luteinizing hormone. *J. Clin. Endocrinol. Metab.* **65**, 929–941.

Veldhuis, J. D., Liem, A. Y., South, S., Weltman, A., Weltman, J., Clemmons, D. A., Abbott, R., Mulligan, T., Johnson, M. L., Pincus, S. *et al.* (1995). Differential impact of age, sex steroid hormones, and obesity on basal versus pulsatile growth hormone secretion in men as assessed in an ultrasensitive chemiluminescence assay. *J. Clin. Endocrinol. Metab.* **80**, 3209–3222.

Vielhaber, E., Eide, E., Rivers, A., Gao, Z. H., and Virshup, D. M. (2000). Nuclear entry of the circadian regulator mPer1 is controlled by mammalian casein kinase I epsilon. *Mol. Cell. Biol.* **20**, 4888–4899.

Vitaterna, M. H., Selby, C. P., Todo, T., Niwa, H., Thompson, C., Fruechte, E. M., Hitomi, K., Thresher, R. J., Ishikawa, T., Miyazaki, J., Takahashi, J. S., and Sancar, A. (1999). Differential regulation of mammalian period genes and circadian rhythmicity by cryptochromes 1 and 2. *Proc. Natl. Acad. Sci. U.S.A.* **96**, 12114–12119.

vom Saal, F. S., Finch, C. E., and Nelson, J. F. (1994). Natural history and mechanisms of aging in humans, laboratory rodents and other selected vertebrates. *In* "The Physiology of Reproduction" (E. Knobil and J. D. Neill, eds.), Vol. 2, pp. 1213–1314. Raven Press, New York.

von Schantz, M., Lucas, R. J., and Foster, R. G. (1999). Circadian oscillation of photopigment transcript levels in the mouse retina. *Brain Res. Mol. Brain Res.* **72**, 108–114.

von Schantz, M., Provencio, I., and Foster, R. G. (2000). Recent developments in circadian photoreception: More than meets the eye. *Invest. Ophthalmol. Visual Sci.* **41**, 1605–1607.

Vrang, N., Larsen, P. J., Moller, M., and Mikkelsen, J. D. (1995). Topographical organization of the rat suprachiasmatic-paraventricular projection. *J. Comp. Neurol.* **353**, 585–603.

Waldstreicher, J., Duffy, J. F., Brown, E. N., Rogacz, S., Allan, J. S., and Czeisler, C. A. (1996). Gender differences in the temporal organization of proclactin (PRL) secretion: Evidence for a sleep-independent circadian rhythm of circulating PRL levels—a clinical research center study. *J. Clin. Endocrinol. Metab.* **81**, 1483–1487.

Watanabe, K., Koibuchi, N., Ohtake, H., and Yamaoka, S. (1993). Circadian rhythms of vasopressin release in primary cultures of rat suprachiasmatic nucleus. *Brain Res.* **624**, 115–120.

Watson, R. E., Jr., Langub, M. C., Jr., Engle, M. G., and Maley, B. E. (1995). Estrogen-receptive neurons in the anteroventral periventricular nucleus are synaptic targets of the suprachiasmatic nucleus and peri-suprachiasmatic region. *Brain Res.* **689**, 254–264.

Watts, A. G. (1991). The efferent projections of the suprachiasmatic nucleus: Anatomical insights into the control of circadian rhythms. *In* "The Suprachiasmatic Nucleus: The Mind's Clock" (D. C. Klein, R. Y. Moore, and S. M. Reppert, eds.), pp. 77–106. Oxford University Press, New York.

Watts, A. G., and Swanson, L. W. (1987). Efferent projections of the suprachiasmatic nucleus: II. Studies using retrograde transport of fluorescent dyes and simultaneous peptide immunohistochemistry in the rat. *J. Comp. Neurol.* **258**, 230–252.

Watts, A. G., Swanson, L. W., and Sanchez-Watts, G. (1987). Efferent projections of the suprachiasmatic nucleus: I. Studies using anterograde transport of *Phaseolus vulgaris* leucoagglutinin in the rat. *J. Comp. Neurol.* **258**, 204–229.

Watts, A. G., Sheward, W. J., Whale, D., and Fink, G. (1989). The effects of knife cuts in the sub-paraventricular zone of the female rat hypothalamus on oestrogen-induced diurnal surges of plasma prolactin and LH, and circadian wheel-running activity. *J. Endocrinol.* **122**, 593–604.

Weaver, D. R., and Reppert, S. M. (1990). Melatonin receptors are present in the ferret pars tuberalis and pars distalis, but not in brain. *Endocrinology (Baltimore)* **127**, 2607–2609.

Wehr, T. A. (1998). Effect of seasonal changes in daylength on human neuroendocrine function. *Horm. Res.* **49**, 118–124.

Wehr, T. A., Moul, D. E., Barbato, G., Giesen, H. A., Seidel, J. A., Barker, C., and Bender, C. (1993). Conservation of photoperiod-responsive mechanisms in humans. *Am. J. Physiol.* **265**, R846–R857.

Weibel, L., Follenius, M., Spiegel, K., Gronfier, C., and Brandenberger, G. (1997). Growth hormone secretion in night workers. *Chronobiol. Int.* **14**, 49–60.

Weick, R. F., and Stobie, K. M. (1995). Role of VIP in the regulation of LH secretion in the female rat. *Neurosci. Biobehav. Rev.* **19**, 251–259.

Weiland, N. G., and Wise, P. M. (1990). Aging progressively decreases the densities and alters the diurnal rhythms of alpha 1-adrenergic receptors in selected hypothalamic regions. *Endocrinology (Baltimore)* **126**, 2392–2397.

Weiland, N. G., Scarbrough, K., and Wise, P. M. (1992). Aging abolishes the estradiol-induced suppression and diurnal rhythm of proopiomelanocortin gene expression in the arcuate nucleus. *Endocrinology (Baltimore)* **131**, 2959–2964.

Weindruch, R., and Walford, R. (1988). "The Retardation of Aging and Disease by Dietary Restriction." Thomas, Springfield, IL.

Weingarten, H. P., Chang, P. K., and McDonald, T. J. (1985). Comparison of the metabolic and behavioral disturbances following paraventricular- and ventromedial-hypothalamic lesions. *Brain Res. Bull.* **14**, 551–559.

Weitzman, E. D., Fukushima, D., Nogeire, C., Roffwarg, H., Gallagher, T. F., and Hellman, L. (1971). Twenty-four hour pattern of the episodic secretion of cortisol in normal subjects. *J. Clin. Endocrinol. Metab.* **33**, 14–22.

Welsh, D. K., Logothetis, D. E., Meister, M., and Reppert, S. M. (1995). Individual neurons dissociated from rat suprachiasmatic nucleus express independently phased circadian firing rhythms. *Neuron* **14**, 697–706.

Wever, R. A. (1984). Sex differences in human circadian rhythms: Intrinsic periods and sleep fractions. *Experientia* **40**, 1226–1234.

Whitmore, D., Sassone-Corsi, P., and Foulkes, N. S. (1998). PASting together the mammalian clock. *Curr. Opin. Neurobiol.* **8**, 635–641.

Wiegand, S. J., and Gash, D. M. (1988). Organization and efferent connections of transplanted suprachiasmatic nuclei. *J. Comp. Neurol.* **267**, 562–579.

Wild, R. A. (1996). Estrogen: Effects on the cardiovascular tree. *Obstet. Gynecol.* **87**, 27S–35S.

Wilsbacher, L. D., and Takahashi, J. S. (1998). Circadian rhythms: Molecular basis of the clock. *Curr. Opin. Genet. Dev.* **8**, 595–602.

Wise, P. M. (1982). Alterations in proestrous LH, FSH, and prolactin surges in middle-age rats. *Proc. Soc. Exp. Biol. Med.* **169**, 348–354.

Wise, P. M. (1984). Estradiol-induced daily luteinizing hormone and prolactin surges in young and middle-aged rats: Correlations with age-related changes in pituitary responsiveness and catecholamine turnover rates in microdissected brain areas. *Endocrinology (Baltimore)* **115**, 801–809.

Wise, P. M. (2000). Neuroendocrine correlates of aging. In "Neuroendocrinology in Physiology and Medicine" (P. M. Conn and M. E. Freeman, eds.), pp. 371–387. Humana Press, Totowa, NJ.

Wise, P. M., Rance, N., and Barraclough, C. A. (1981). Effects of estradiol and progesterone on catecholamine turnover rates in discrete hypothalamic regions in ovariectomized rats. *Endocrinology (Baltimore)* **108**, 2186–2193.

Wise, P. M., Cohen, I. R., Weiland, N. G., and London, E. D. (1988). Aging alters the circadian rhythm of glucose utilization in the suprachiasmatic nucleus. *Proc. Natl. Acad. Sci. U.S.A.* **85**, 5305–5309.

Wise, P. M., Krajnak, K. M., and Kashon, M. L. (1996). Menopause: The aging of multiple pacemakers. *Science* **273**, 67–70.

Wise, P. M., Kashon, M. L., Krajnak, K. M., Rosewell, K. L., Cai, A., Scarbrough, K., Harney, J. P., McShane, T., Lloyd, J. M., and Weiland, N. G. (1997). Aging of the female reproductive system: A window into brain aging. *Recent Prog. Horm. Res.* **52**, 279–303.

Wollnik, F., Brysch, W., Uhlmann, E., Gillardon, F., Bravo, R., Zimmermann, M., Schlingensiepen, K. H., and Herdegen, T. (1995). Block of c-Fos and JunB expression by antisense oligonucleotides inhibits light-induced phase shifts of the mammalian circadian clock. *Eur. J. Neurosci.* **7**, 388–393.

Wong, C. C., Dohler, K. D., Geerlings, H., and von zur Muhlen, A. (1983). Influence of age, strain and season on circadian periodicity of pituitary, gonadal and adrenal hormones in the serum of male laboratory rats. *Horm. Res.* **17**, 202–215.

Xu, B., Kalra, P. S., Farmerie, W. G., and Kalra, S. P. (1999). Daily changes in hypothalamic gene expression of neuropeptide Y, galanin, proopiomelanocortin, and adipocyte leptin gene expression and secretion: Effects of food restriction. *Endocrinology (Baltimore)* **140**, 2868–2875.

Yagita, K., Yamaguchi, S., Tamanini, F., van der Horst, G. T., Hoeijmakers, J. H., Yasui, A., Loros, J. J., Dunlap J. C., and Okamura, H. (2000). Dimerization and nuclear entry of mPER proteins in mammalian cells. *Genes* **14**, 1353–1363.

Yamaguchi, M., Mizunuma, H., Miyamoto, K., Hasegawa, Y., Ibuki, Y., and Igarashi, M. (1991). Immunoreactive inhibin concentrations in adult men: Presence of a circadian rhythm. *J. Clin. Endocrinol. Metab.* **72**, 554–559.

Yamamoto, H., Nagai, K., and Nakagawa, H. (1987). Role of SCN in daily rhythms of plasma glucose, FFA, insulin and glucagon. *Chronobiol. Int.* **4**, 483–491.

Yamazaki, S., Numano, R., Abe, M., Hida, A., Takahashi, R., Ueda, M., Block, G. D., Sakaki, Y., Menaker, M., and Tei, H. (2000). Resetting central and peripheral circadian oscillators in transgenic rats. *Science* **288**, 682–685.

Yan, L., Takekida, S., Shigeyoshi, Y., and Okamura, H. (1999). Per1 and Per2 gene expression in the rat suprachiasmatic nucleus: Circadian profile and the compartment-specific response to light. *Neuroscience* **94**, 141–150.

Yang, Q. Z., and Hatton, G. I. (1999). Nitric oxide via cGMP-dependent mechanisms increases dye coupling and excitability of rat supraoptic nucleus neurons. *J. Neurosci.* **19**, 4270–4279.

Yoshimura, T., Yasuo, S., Suzuki, Y., Makino, E., Yokota, Y., and Ebihara, S. (2001). Identification of the suprachiasmatic nucleus in birds. *Am. J. Physiol. Regul. Integr. Comp. Physiol.* **280**, R1185–R1189.

Young, M. W., and Kay, S. A. (2001). Time zones: A comparative genetics of circadian clocks. *Natl. Rev. Genet.* **2**(9), 702–715.

Yu, B. P. (1994). How diet influences the aging process of the rat. *Proc. Soc. Exp. Biol. Med.* **205**, 97–105.

Zeng, H., Qian, Z., Myers, M. P., and Rosbash, M. (1996). A light-entrainment mechanism for the *Drosophila* circadian clock. *Nature (London)* **380**, 129–135.

Zheng, B., Larkin, D. W., Albrecht, U., Sun, Z. S., Sage, M., Eichele, G., Lee, C. C., and Bradley, A. (1999). The mPer2 gene encodes a functional component of the mammalian circadian clock. *Nature (London)* **400**, 169–173.

Zirkin, B. R., and Chen, H. (2000). Regulation of leydig cell steroidogenic function during aging. *Biol. Reprod.* **63**, 977–981.

Zucker, I. (1980). Light, behavior, and biological rhythms. In "Neuroendocrinology" (D. T. Krieger and J. C. Hughs, eds.), pp. 93–101. Sinauer, Assoc., Sunderland, MA.

Zylka, M. J., Shearman, L. P., Weaver, D. R., and Reppert, S. M. (1998). Three period homologs in mammals: Differential light responses in the suprachiasmatic circadian clock and oscillating transcripts outside of brain. *Neuron* **20**, 1103–1110.

19

Mammalian Seasonal Rhythms: Behavior and Neuroendocrine Substrates

Brian J. Prendergast, Randy J. Nelson
Department of Psychology
The Ohio State University
Columbus, Ohio 43210

Irving Zucker
Departments of Psychology and Integrative Biology
University of California at Berkeley
Berkeley, California 94720

"Environmental seasonality... a basic component of the ecosystem within which our ancestors evolved... left its mark indelibly upon the makeup of our biology and our behaviour."

(Johnston, 1993)

"the ability to perceive changes in daylength indicated by changes in the duration of melatonin secretion... is the only essential function attributable to melatonin in mammals to date."

(Arendt, 2000)

I. INTRODUCTION

Seasonal phenotypes in behavior and physiology are legion; many reflect adaptations to matching environmental periodicities and presumably have their highest fitness in the seasons in which they occur (Brakefield, 1996). The imprimatur of seasonality is appropriately conferred only on traits that recur during a relatively limited time in the same months in successive years. Peaks or troughs that occur at divergent times of the year during successive cycles do not define seasonal rhythms; nor can seasonality be inferred or distinguished from mere synchrony when only a single cycle has been tracked. Strong seasonality generally implies interanimal synchrony within a population, but the converse is not necessarily true (Di Bitetti and Janson, 2000).

Pronounced seasonal variations in day length, temperature, and humidity derive from the yearly orbit of Earth about the Sun. The amount and intensity of solar radiation varies with latitude; the greater the distance from the equator, the more pronounced the interseasonal differences in ambient temperature and solar radiation. Plant growth, which is also affected by other abiotic factors such as seasonal winds and patterns of rain and snowfall determines food availability and reproduction in herbivores and, consequently, in carnivores.

The climatological shaping of animal structure and function is rarely considered in analyses of mammalian neuroendocrinology; this is not a minor limitation, considering that "the seasonal... change in temperatures over North America from winter to summer is far greater than glacial-interglacial changes in mean annual temperatures of the Pleistocene" (p. 113; Potts, 1998). Nonclimatological factors also contribute to the evolution of seasonality, not least in humans, in which social customs, religious practices, and legal regulations account for some seasonal rhythms (Farrell and Pease, 1994; Brewis *et al.*, 1996)—the reliable increase in births in the United States during the last week of December, for example, reflects a year-end surge in induced deliveries implemented for convenience and increased tax rebates (Dickert-Conlin and Chandra, 1999).

The approach taken in this chapter is selective rather than inclusive. Because the subject has been well reviewed previously, we do not consider formal models of photoperiodism. We also do not consider the literatures on nonmammalian vertebrates and invertebrates, each of which informs analyses of mammalian seasonality. Nor do we, except incidentally, consider the extensive literature on endocrine changes unrelated to behavior. The emphasis on reproductive rhythms and rodents reflects our own research interests; it is not intended to diminish the importance of nonreproductive rhythms in the overall economy of mammals or the significance of other mammalian orders. Where information is available, conclusions derived from the consideration of reproduction generalize well to nonreproductive traits.

II. EVOLUTION OF SEASONAL RHYTHMS—ECOLOGICAL AND ENERGETIC RELATIONS

Successful reproduction is profoundly influenced by food availability. Distances traveled, ambient temperatures experienced, predators encountered, and quality and quantity of food located during above-ground foraging by mammals presumably determine whether or not reproduction will succeed or fail (Bronson, 1989). Natural selection is thought to favor individual females who produce offspring coincident with an abundance of high-quality food (Fig. 1A). The latter stage of lactation is an extreme energetic bottleneck for small mammals and the time of weaning a corresponding challenge for large mammals (Bronson, 1985).

Animals resident in highly seasonal environments with short growing seasons are more likely to evolve seasonal phenotypes than conspecifics whose niches provide more evenly distributed food resources throughout the year. Food generalists that exploit diverse diets tend to be less subject to seasonal pressures than specialists reliant on a few seasonally variable foods.

Small mammals have higher metabolic rates, higher costs of thermoregulation, reduced fat stores with which to bridge intervals of food scarcity, and shorter life spans than do larger animals. They tend to breed more opportunistically than larger species, with greater year-to-year and locale-to-locale variability. Although seasonal timing of food availability is usually reasonably constant from year to year, animals that rigidly commit to reproduction at a specified calendar date regardless of local temperature variations, time of the first frost, or snow melt are disadvantaged (Lee and Gorman, 2000). Because day length is by far the most accurate predictor of phase in the geophysical cycle and is sufficient to synchronize most seasonal rhythms, it is often overlooked that mammalian reproduction in the wild is typically controlled by multiple cues (Bronson, 1989). The neglect of interactions among the several proximate determinants of seasonal rhythms is a serious shortcoming in all but a handful of laboratory investigations.

The period during which mating and conception occur is often remote from the time of peak food availability, particularly in mammals with gestations that endure for 3 or more months. In such species, individuals that evolve a restricted mating season may be greatly advantaged over those that mate indiscriminately at any time of year. Despite the plausibility of this argument, very few empirical studies have documented disadvantages of out-of-season breeding (e.g., Di Bitetti and Janson, 2000).

The degree to which reproduction is constrained seasonally must also depend on the extent to which the decrease in offspring production imposed by seasonal reproductive quiescence is countered by the enhanced survival of young born in times of plenty. The strain on females that undertake unsuccessful reproduction presumably decreases their subsequent fitness. Gestation length, the interval between successive conceptions, and investment in individual offspring are also relevant (Kiltie, 1988). Seasonal breeding may be abandoned or relaxed in animals that are approaching the ends of their lives; their residual reproductive value is reduced (Kiltie, 1988), and they presumably have less to lose by out-of-season breeding.

Interannual variability in food availability and costs of reproduction may favor animals that breed at different times of year, thereby accounting for the persistence of different seasonal morphs in a single population or litter (cf. Kiltie, 1988).

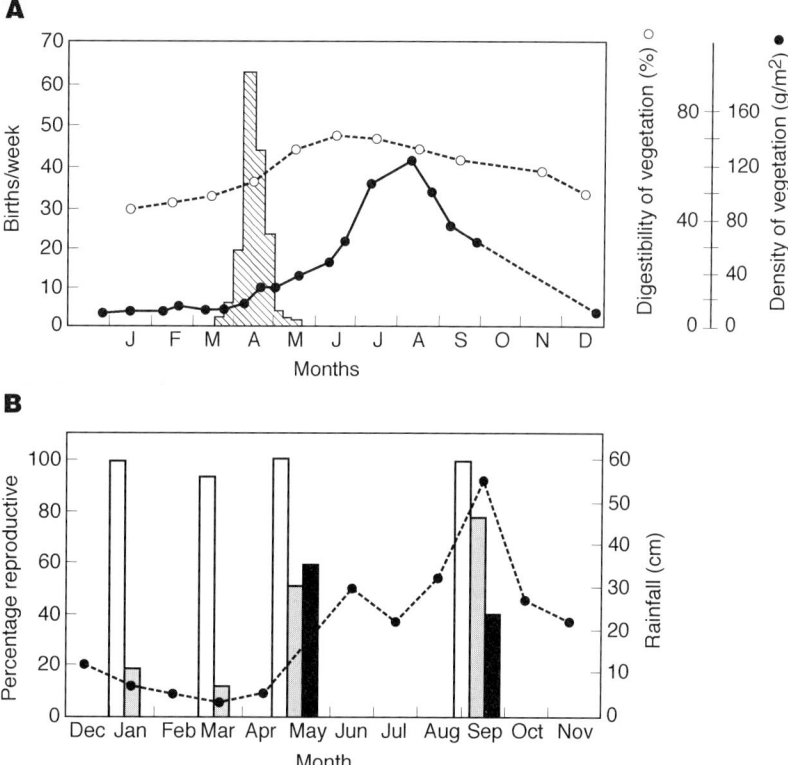

FIGURE 1 (A) Timing of births among Soay sheep on the island of St. Kilda in relation to availability and digestibility of food. Births are restricted to a period early enough for the ewe and lambs to capitalize on abundant food of the spring pasture. From Lincoln and Short (1980). (B) Seasonal reproduction in wild-caught female cloud-forest mice (*Peromyscus nudipes*) in relation to rainfall. Open bars, females with evidence of recent corporea lutea; hatched bars, females with implanted embryos; dark bars, lactating females. The dotted line indicates seasonal changes in rainfall. From Heideman and Bronson (1992); Heideman et al. (1992).

These views of seasonality emphasize post hoc adaptive scenarios of considerable surface plausibility, but suffer from the liability that, in principle, it is impossible to directly measure natural selection in the past (Sinervo and Basolo, 1996). The adaptive hypothesis approach has been justly criticized because it stops short of direct field validation (Huey and Berrigan, 1996) and assumes, perhaps unjustifiably, that physiological adjustments to the immediate environment must increase fitness. In so doing, this approach ignores the caution that natural selection yields adequacy, not perfection (Bartholemew, 1987). A given seasonal phenotype can reflect random drift, factors other than natural selection, and adaptation to past rather than present environmental conditions (Huey and Berrigan, 1996).

Some of these issues are illustrated by a study of cloud-forest mice (*Peromyscus nudipes*) in Costa Rica. Adult females produce no offspring during the 4- to 5-month dry season (December–March; Fig. 1B), but do mate and ovulate during this time; their embryos either fail to implant successfully or are absorbed postimplantation (Heideman and Bronson, 1992). Year-round breeding, concurrent with striking seasonal production of young, even if a relatively rare pattern among mammals, nevertheless challenges the notion that ovulation and early pregnancy are energetically expensive and to be avoided. Year-round ovulation may be a vestigial pattern in this species, previously effective in a different environment and en route to elimination in the current setting.

III. CLASSIFICATION OF SEASONAL RHYTHMS

Three forms of seasonal rhythms have been distinguished (Zucker *et al.*, 1991). Type I rhythms, although based on an endogenous interval timer, do not persist for more than a single cycle in the absence of environmental resetting, which usually is accomplished by seasonal changes in day length (Fig. 2A). Common among many short-lived temperate and boreal mammals, this may be the ancestral form of mammalian seasonality from which Type II rhythms evolved (Farner, 1985). Type II rhythms are fully endogenous and persist for two or more cycles even when day length, temperature, humidity, and food availability are held constant throughout the year (Fig. 2B) (Pengelley and Asmundson, 1974; Gwinner, 1986). These circannual rhythms are characteristic of long-lived mammals from several orders, including primates, bats, carnivores, ungulates, and rodents; the period of Type II rhythms is usually shorter than 12 months and generated by endogenous oscillators that have eluded localization (Zucker, 2001). Both Type I and II rhythms are entrained to a period of 12 months by the seasonal change in day length. Syrian hamsters (*Mesocricetus auratus*) and golden-mantled ground squirrels (*Spermophilus lateralis*) are the most thoroughly studied species with Type I and II rhythms, respectively.

Type III rhythms (Zucker *et al.*, 1991), which have been neglected by chronobiologists, are based on a strict stimulus–response system. Typically, environmental signals present at a particular time of year control effector systems with little or no modulation from time-keeping mechanisms (Fig. 2C). Allergic reactions that induce runny noses and red eyes triggered by airborne vectors during the hay fever season exemplify such rhythms (von Mutius, 2000).

A. Brief History of Photoperiodism Research

Hard upon the discovery of photoperiodism in plants and birds in the 1920s, both rodents and carnivores were reported to control seasonal reproduction by measuring day length. Not until the 1970s, however, was the circadian basis of photoperiodic time measurement established for mammals (reviewed in Elliott and Goldman, 1981). Resonance and interrupted night protocols documented that rodents discriminate long from short days without reference to an hourglass mechanism that measures the duration of the light or dark phases; nor is the ratio of light to darkness (LD) of significance (Elliott *et al.*, 1972). Two 10-minute light pulses, positioned to simulate dusk and dawn on a daily basis for several weeks, replicate many of the stimulatory effects of 14-hour day lengths on the reproductive system (Milette and Turek, 1986); by contrast, a regimen of 10 hr uninterrupted light each day induces complete gonadal involution (Hoffmann, 1982). Such findings yielded the insight that timing rather than duration of light was paramount. Implication of the circadian system was followed by the formulation of external and internal coincidence models for photoperiodism (Pittendrigh, 1974). The first of these specifies that light entrains a circadian rhythm of photosensitivity and induces a photoperiodic response when the daily light signal coincides with the hypothesized photosensitive phase; this only occurs at certain times of year, within a specified range of day lengths. The internal coincidence model posits that the sole role of seasonal changes in day length is to alter patterns of entrainment of two separate circadian oscillators whose phase relation determines whether a long- or short-day response occurs (Follett *et al.*, 1981).

The circadian basis of photoperiodic time measurement has been confirmed and extended in studies of *tau* mutant Syrian hamsters. Unlike wild-type hamsters, whose free-running circadian period in constant darkness is approximately 24.1 hr, hamsters homozygous for the *tau* mutation have free-running circadian periods of approximately 20 hr and fail to undergo gonadal regression in 24-hr day lengths even when the photophase is as short as 1 hr (Menaker and Refinetti, 1993). Regression does ensue in *tau* mutants maintained on 20-hr days and provided with photophases between 10 and 11.5 hr; in circadian hours this value is proportionately similar to the minimum day length of 12.5 hr required to induce gonadal collapse in wild-type hamsters (Stirland *et al.*, 1996).

B. Type I Rhythms: Some Day Lengths Are More Important Than Others

Many temperate-zone female rodents restrict reproduction to the months of April–August, during which

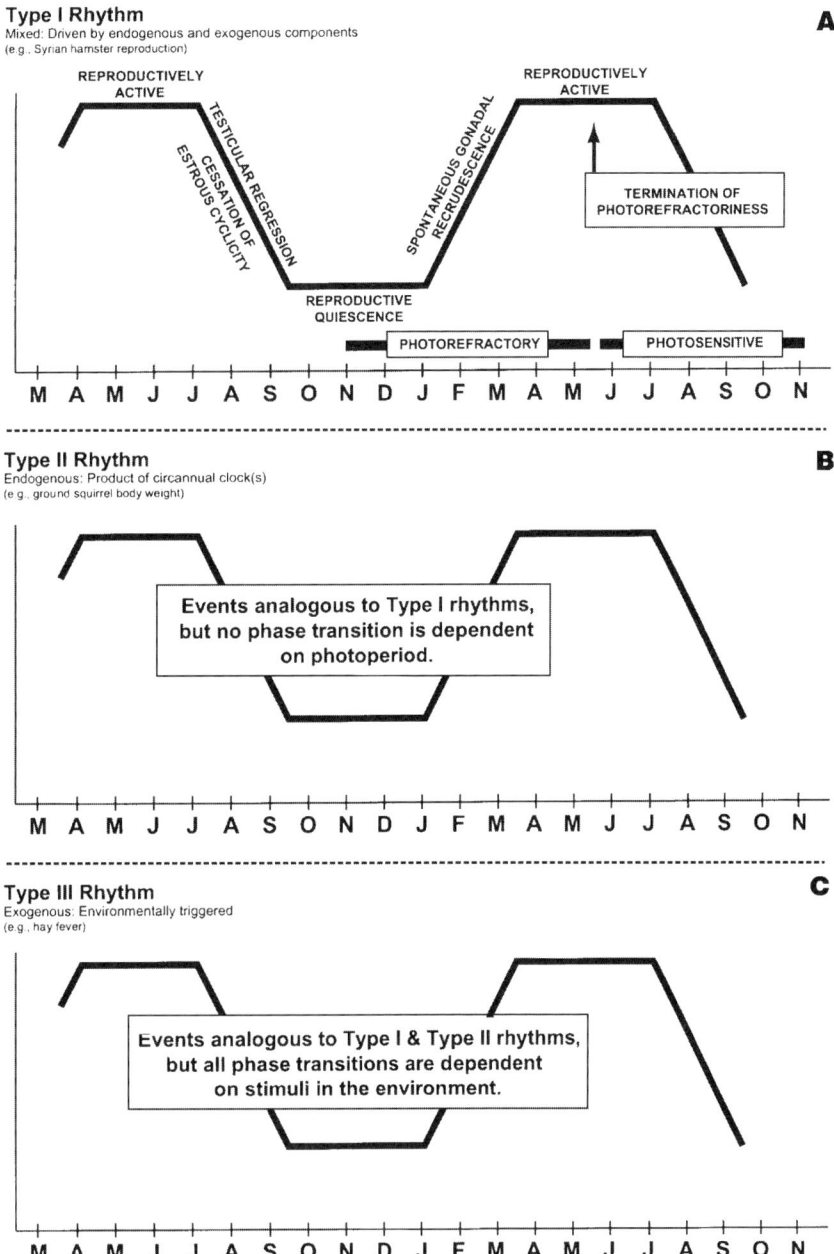

FIGURE 2 Schematic representation of seasonal rhythms. (A) Type I (mixed) rhythms involve exogenous (photoperiod) and endogenous (interval timer) components. Decreasing day lengths: (1) initiate gonadal regression in the late summer and (2) trigger an interval timer that eventually renders animals refractory to short days 20 weeks later, leading to gonadal recrudescence. Exposure to long day lengths in the spring and summer breaks refractoriness and resensitizes the neuroendocrine axis to short days. (B) Type II (circannual) rhythms are entirely endogenous and typically have a period less than 12 months. Seasonal changes in day length synchronize Type II rhythms to a period of exactly 1 year. (C) Type III rhythms are entirely exogenous and driven by environmental stimuli.

they produce one or more litters. The seasonal rhythm for such long-day breeders can be replicated by exposing animals to natural photocycles, even as all other factors are held constant throughout the year. For sexually mature individuals, the decreasing day lengths of mid- to late summer trigger the onset of gonadal involution, eventually eliminating spermatogenesis, ovulation, and mating behavior. Reproductive quiescence endures for 5 months, yielding in mid-winter to gonadal recrudescence; approximately 6 weeks later animals mate.

1. Induction of Refractoriness to Short Day Lengths and Its Termination by Long Day Lengths

Late-winter to early-spring gonadal recrudescence reflects the development of refractoriness to short day lengths and is independent from the small increases in day length between the winter solstice and the resumption of gonadal growth in early February. Thus, hamsters transferred from long to short days and held in the reduced photoperiod thereafter undergo gonadal recrudescence at the same time as hamsters exposed from late December through early March to increasing simulated natural photoperiods (Gorman and Zucker, 1995). Mid-winter gonadal rejuvenation is termed spontaneous recrudescence because it occurs in the absence of long day lengths; it defines the onset of the refractory state in which reproduction no longer depends on the presence of long day lengths (Fig. 2A). Synchrony in timing of gonadal recrudescence is quite precise in hamsters held in fixed short day lengths (Hoffmann, 1979). An interval timer, triggered by the first few weeks of short day lengths, mediates the development of refractoriness (Prendergast et al., 2000), which persists until animals are exposed for several weeks to the increasing or absolutely long day lengths of spring and summer. The long photoperiods that break refractoriness to short day lengths permit overwintered animals to undergo a second gonadal regression when day lengths again decrease in late summer. The foregoing description applies to virtually all Type I photoperiodic traits, including seasonal changes in locomotor activity, body mass, pelage molts, and thermoregulatory adaptations (e.g., Ellis and Turek, 1983; Wade et al., 1986).

To date all long-day photoperiodic rodent species develop refractoriness to short day lengths, and the winter state cannot be maintained indefinitely. Refractoriness is almost surely neurally mediated and not dependent on feedback from peripheral structures (e.g., Watson-Whitmyre and Stetson, 1988; Freeman and Zucker, 2001). In contrast, most long-day species can sustain the summer phenotype indefinitely when housed continuously in an unchanging long photoperiod. The summer phenotype appears to be the default condition.

2. Critical Day Lengths

In an influential study, Elliott (1974) transferred groups of male Syrian hamsters from 14 hr light/day (14L) to photoperiods that provided from 24 to 0 hr/light per day. The transition from 14L to shorter or longer days, accomplished in a single day, established 12.5 hr as the critical day length for testicular regression; day lengths shorter than this value promoted gonadal regression and those longer than it sustained reproduction (Fig. 3). The critical day length varies between species and intraspecifically as a function of latitude of origin (Dark et al., 1983a; Heath and Lynch, 1982); individual traits in a single animal can have different critical day lengths (Duncan et al., 1985).

The conception of the critical day length as a fixed value above and below which traits adopt the summer and winter phenotypes, requires revision; it does not accommodate observations that an animal's photoperiodic history determines how it responds to a particular

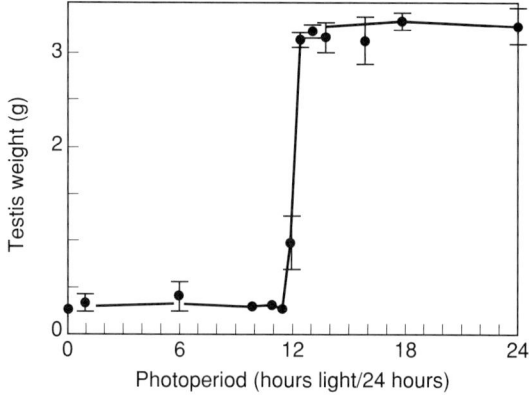

FIGURE 3 Testicular responses of Syrian hamsters after exposure to different fixed photoperiods for 85–96 days. Only photoperiods that provided ≥12.5 hr light/day resulted in maintenance of large, functional testes; the critical day length in this species lies between 12L and 12.5L. [From Elliott (1976).]

day length (Duncan *et al.*, 1985; Darrow and Goldman, 1985; Hoffmann *et al.*, 1986), nor does it explain the different rates of gonadal involution among animals housed in different short day lengths shorter than the critical day length (Donham *et al.*, 1994; Niklowitz *et al.*, 1994; Powers *et al.*, 1997) or the more rapid gonadal growth in Siberian hamsters transferred from 8 hr light/day to either 16 or 14 hr days (Niklowitz *et al.*, 1994). In its simple form, the critical day length concept is incompatible with the observation that Syrian hamsters that receive daily subcutaneous infusions of melatonin for 12 or 8.5 hr/day, each infusion schedule representing a different day length below the critical value, undergo gonadal regression at different rates (Powers *et al.*, 1997).

Critical day length values were originally established with an unnatural protocol. Typically, animals housed for the preceding months in a constant day length were abruptly transferred to a second constant photoperiod that was 4 or 6 hours shorter or longer (e.g., from a 16L to a 10L photophase). These conditions bear little resemblance to the continuous and gradual changes in day length experienced by nonequatorial mammals in nature, where the daily light fraction changes by at most 5–6 minutes per day. The simplified photoperiodic regimens used in laboratory studies discard the predictive information inherent in natural photocycles and the verisimilitude of neuroendocrine relations elaborated with such protocols is questionable. In fact, interindividual synchrony in testicular regression is reduced in Syrian hamsters presented with gradual rather than abrupt changes in day length (Heideman and Bronson, 1993), and the range of day lengths that affects reproduction in Siberian hamsters is significantly extended when transitions are gradual rather than abrupt (Gorman and Zucker, 1995; Rivkees *et al.*, 1988). Shorter but increasing day lengths accelerate somatic and gonadal growth compared to fixed day lengths of absolutely longer duration. None of these results is accommodated by critical day length models that posit equivalence of all day lengths on either side of the threshold value (Gorman and Zucker, 1998). The pattern of change in day length codes information that animals abstract to phase seasonal traits; in some instances changes in day length are more salient than the absolute length of the day (Nicholls *et al.*, 1988; Gorman and Zucker, 1998). A second difficulty is that the standard housing conditions for nocturnal rodents lack a dark nest box to which animals can retreat during the daylight hours. Hamsters provided with such refuges have later activity onsets and earlier offsets and overall abbreviated active periods (Boulos *et al.*, 1996). The extent to which housing conditions affect the generation of critical day lengths and photoperiodic time measurement remains to be explored. The critical day length concept, as generally employed, refers to a single value at which a trait reverts from the summer to the winter phenotype, or vice versa, under conditions of thermoneutrality, access to unlimited free food, absence of conspecifics, and other salient conditions that prevail in nature. Although useful as an analytic tool, its value in the exegesis of seasonality in photoperiodic rodents has been overemphasized.

3. Puberty

Animals born at the beginning of the breeding season face different environmental challenges than those born several months later. In temperate latitudes, rodents weaned in May encounter relatively plentiful food; those born at the end of the breeding season, circa mid-September, are less fortunate and must contend with lower ambient temperatures and a less abundant food supply. Rates of somatic and reproductive development differ markedly in beginning- vs end-of-season cohorts—rapid somatic growth and puberty by 1.5 months of age are the rule for early-born offspring of several species (Worth *et al.*, 1973; Lincoln and MacKinnon, 1976), whereas those born later forgo reproduction in the season of birth, overwinter, and first attain reproductive competence and adult body mass at approximately 6 months of age. Variations in day length proximately control timing of puberty—rodents provisioned with excess food and exposed to increasing or absolutely long day lengths undergo accelerated reproductive and somatic development compared to those housed in decreasing or absolutely short photoperiods. After approximately 4 months of exposure to short day lengths, young voles and hamsters, in common with their elders, develop refractoriness to short days and undergo spontaneous gonadal development and body mass increases. The subset of individuals born several weeks after the summer solstice does not breed in the summer or fall, but instead forms the main breeding nucleus the following spring. Individuals born before the summer solstice generally do not survive for more than a single breeding season (Sadleir, 1969).

4. Sexual Behavior and Physiology

Mating can place animals at increased risk from predation; males of some species also incur heavy costs in establishing and defending territories. According to adaptationist dogma, a species with a short gestation should prudently curtail mating with the approach of winter. Because copulation in most mammals is strictly tied to gonadal hormones, this end could be achieved by a reduction in hormone secretion several weeks before conditions become unfavorable for offspring survival. Alternatively, substrates that mediate mating activity could become unresponsive to steroid hormones several weeks before the decline of gonadal steroidogenesis eliminates copulatory behavior. There is little indication that a steroid-independent decrease in motivation to mate contributes to seasonal reproductive quiescence. In principle, only one sex need terminate reproductive activity to prevent out-of-season breeding.

a) Males Mating behavior declines in Syrian hamsters transferred from long to short days (Morin and Zucker, 1978; Campbell *et al.*, 1978). Male hamsters undergo gonadal regression after 6–10 weeks of exposure to short photoperiods; gonadal production of testosterone (T) declines precipitously over this interval (Reiter, 1980). Deficits in male sexual behavior are apparent after several weeks of exposure to short days, evidenced by a reduction in the number of intromissions and ejaculations (Powers *et al.*, 1989). Ejaculations were eliminated in almost all males after 9 weeks of short-day exposure, as compared to a 3-week latency to eliminate this behavior in males that were surgically castrated. The difference is attributable to gradual vs abrupt withdrawal of gonadal steroids (Morin and Zucker, 1978). Castrated hamsters held in short days for 17 weeks copulated much less than their long-day counterparts during replacement therapy with testosterone (Fig. 4A). Reduced behavioral responsiveness to testosterone in short-day males contrasts with increased responsiveness of gonadotropin secretion to feedback inhibition by testosterone (reviewed in Turek and van Cauter, 1994). Short-day behavioral deficits were no longer detectable by week 19, presumably because the neural substrates that mediate male copula-

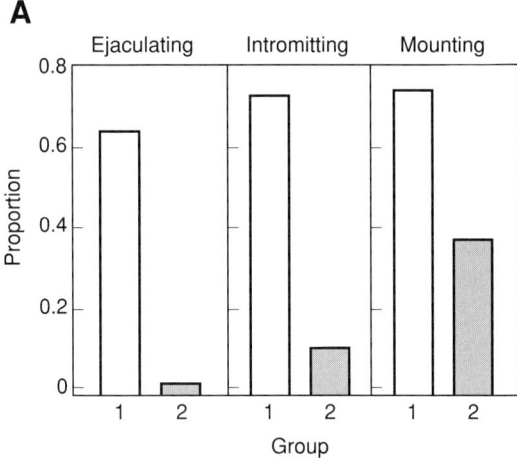

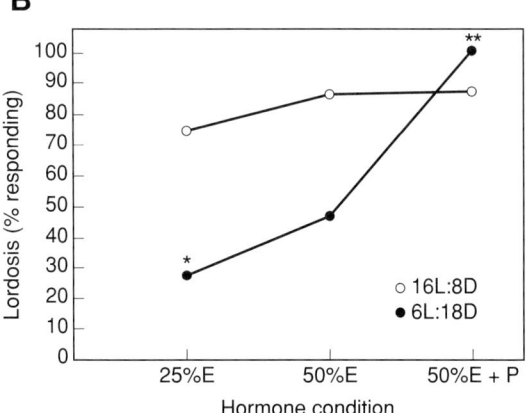

FIGURE 4 Short day lengths decrease responsiveness to hormones in Syrian hamsters. A. Incidences of mounting, intromission, and ejaculation in castrated males bearing testosterone implants. Hamsters were treated with testosterone after 12 weeks in either long (open bars) or short (dark bars) day lengths, and behavior was assessed 5 weeks later. [From Morin and Zucker (1978), reproduced by permission of the Society for Endocrinology.] B. Incidences of lordosis in ovariectomized females bearing implants of 25% or 50% estradiol (E) and in females implanted with 50% E and injected with 0.25 mg progesterone (P). Implants of E were less effective in short- than in long-day females as indicated by a single asterisk. Treatment with E + P restored lordosis equally well in both day lengths (double asterisk). [From Badura *et al.* (1987). *Physiol. Behav.* **40**, 551–554, copyright 1987, with permission of Elsevier Science.]

tion became refractory to short days (Morin and Zucker, 1978). Honrado *et al.* (1991) noted that sex behavior of short-day males recovered to long-day values several weeks in advance of full recovery of spermatogenesis. Behavioral differences attributable to day length are more pronounced as testosterone concentrations decline (Pospichal et al., 1991); short photoperiods may elevate thresholds for hormonal activation of copulation. The conclusions derived from the foregoing replacement studies can be questioned on the grounds that these regimens deliver hormones continuously and fail to replicate the episodic pattern of testicular androgen secretion.

It is hardly surprising that reductions in gonadal steroidogenesis in short day lengths are accompanied by deficits in sex behavior. But changes in behavior are not simply a result of declining concentrations of circulating steroids. After exposure to short days for 15 weeks, male Syrian hamsters intromitted and ejaculated much less than did long-day hamsters; castrated short-day males bearing T implants were as likely as long-day hamsters to achieve intromissions and ejaculations, but the several components of the sexual repertoire that were still impaired in these individuals included latency to first intromission, number of intromissions immediately preceding ejaculation, inter-intromission interval, and overall copulatory efficiency (Powers et al., 1989). In agreement with earlier studies (Morin and Zucker, 1978), short day lengths apparently reduce the responsiveness to hormones in neural substrates that activate copulatory behavior.

Part of the decline of mating in short-day male hamsters may be caused by altered perception or reduced attention to vaginal chemoattractants (Miernicki et al., 1990), but in some studies, investigation of estrous females was greater in short- than in long-day males (Honrado et al., 1991). The authors argued that this change in short days is a consequence not a cause of the decline in male copulation; that is, estrous females that contend with sexually indifferent short-day males apparently increase solicitation behavior, thereby eliciting more investigation by males. The discrepancy may be procedural because the two studies employed different measures of male proceptivity.

Social stimuli interact with seasonal changes in day length to influence gonadal status. In short-day deer mice (*Peromyscus maniculatus*) the growth of the testes and seminal vesicles, indicators of increased androgen secretion, was stimulated by the presence of a long-day female in each male's cage (Whitsett and Lawton, 1982). The trophic effect of long-day females fell short of that produced by exposing males to long day lengths.

The recovery of sexual behavior in short-days was also accelerated in male Syrian hamsters that were provided with opportunities to interact with long-day females (Honrado and Fleming, 1996). Three weeks of direct access to a female was more effective than distal visual or auditory cues or volatile pheromones from estrous females. Testicular regression was ameliorated in Siberian hamsters transferred to short days in tandem with summer-phenotype females (Hegstrom and Breedlove, 1999b). Cues from estrous females are more likely to override effects of short day lengths by direct stimulation of gonadotropin-releasing hormone (GnRH) and gonadotropin secretion pathways than by interfering with melatonin secretion or photoperiodism. GnRH neurons that are inhibited by long nightly melatonin signals presumably are stimulated by cues from females. The extent to which interactions with estrous females prevent males in the field from undergoing gonadal involution as the end of the breeding season approaches is unknown.

In many behavioral studies, rodents are provided with activity wheels that they use avidly. Notwithstanding the lack of agreement on which natural behavioral analogs, if any, are tapped by wheel-running activity (Mather, 1981; Sherwin, 1998), this behavior interacts with day length to control reproduction. Testicular regression in short days was delayed in Syrian hamsters given access to running wheels (Elliott, 1974); among meadow voles with photoregressed gonads, males given activity wheels recovered reproductive function much more rapidly than those not so provisioned (Kerbeshian and Bronson, 1996). Although wheel-running activity overrides the inhibitory effects of short day lengths, it is ineffective in countering reproductive suppression induced by pheromones in house mice or testosterone treatment in laboratory rats (Kerbeshian et al., 1994). The neuroendocrine pathway by which day length and melatonin (see later) restrain androgen secretion appears particularly susceptible to masking influences from other stimuli that impinge on the GnRH-gonadotropin axis.

An intact pineal gland is essential for the inhibition of sexual behavior in short day lengths (Miernicki et al., 1990). Male Syrian hamsters housed in short or long days for 2 weeks prior to castration all developed copulatory deficits, but this occurred less rapidly in pinealectomized animals. Conversely, sex behavior was restored more rapidly in pinealectomized than pineal-intact castrates treated with testosterone. Pinealectomized male–female pairs of Syrian hamsters, unlike intact controls, produced offspring during the winter months when housed in a natural photocyle (Reiter, 1974), again pointing to the essential role of the pineal gland in transducing the effects of short day lengths on the reproductive axis.

The activation of male sex behavior in Syrian hamsters involves the conversion of testosterone to estradiol via aromatization in neural tissue (Wood, 1996). Aromatase activity in the preoptic area was not affected by day length or castration, but was decreased in the anterior hypothalamus of short-day males and may contribute to behavioral deficits (Hutchison et al., 1991). Callard et al. (1986) previously documented decreased aromatase activity in the whole hypothalamus of both intact and castrated males housed in short days; androstenedione and testosterone replacement therapy in castrates not only were associated with lowered aromatase activity, but also induced fewer estradiol receptors in short than long days. The suggestion that aromatase activity is an important rate-limiting step that determines the number of estrogen receptors in diencephalic tissues is a plausible mechanism by which changes in day length control androgen-dependent processes.

Low ambient temperature does not by itself induce winter responses in some photoperiodic rodents; Syrian hamsters held at 5°C in long days maintain the typical summer reproductive phenotype (Desjardins and Lopez, 1980). In conjunction with shorter day lengths, however, decreases in ambient temperature markedly accelerate the appearance of the winter phenotype in several hamster species (Pevet et al., 1989; Steinlechner et al., 1991; Ruf, 1993; Stieglitz et al., 1994; Larkin et al., 2001) and in deer mice (Millar and Gyug, 1981); high ambient temperatures can delay the appearance of short-day gonadal responses (Li et al., 1987). The day length at which testicular regression occurs in Siberian hamsters is 2 hours longer at 5° than at 22°C (~15 hr vs 13 hr) (Steinlechner et al., 1991). At a latitude of 50°N, well within the home range of this species, a 2-hr increase in the critical day length accelerates gonadal regression by approximately 5 weeks at the lower temperature (Steinlechner et al., 1991). We are unaware of studies of mating behavior of photoperiodic rodents under conditions of elevated or reduced ambient temperature. It also remains unknown whether modulatory effects of temperature on reproductive behavior are mediated exclusively by changes in steroid hormone secretion.

b) Females Female Syrian hamsters cease to undergo estrous cycles and are rendered anovulatory within 6 weeks of transfer from long to short days (Reiter et al., 1977; Seegal and Goldman, 1975). They also cease to display lordosis behavior (Badura and Nunez, 1989); recovery of behavioral receptivity during prolonged maintenance in short days occurs several weeks before physiological measures of reproductive competence are restored to long-day values (Honrado et al., 1991). In Siberian hamsters, estrous cyclicity is eliminated for 20 weeks beginning after 7 weeks of short-day exposure; full recovery occurs many weeks later (Schlatt et al., 1993).

Short day lengths reduced behavioral responsiveness to estradiol and progesterone in female Syrian hamsters (Elliott and Nunez, 1992; Karp and Powers, 1993; Bittman et al., 1990; Honrado et al., 1991; Badura and Nunez, 1989; Mangels et al., 1998). This effect was only observed at relatively low doses of estradiol (Badura et al., 1987; Karp and Powers, 1993). In one instance, sexual receptivity was attenuated in response to treatment with estradiol but not to estradiol followed by progesterone (Fig. 4B) (Badura et al., 1987). Hormone replacement studies suggest that substrate responsiveness to steroids is reduced but not eliminated in short day lengths and may reflect an elevation of the threshold for the activation of specific behavioral components (Morin and Zucker, 1978). By simultaneously suppressing hormone secretion and decreasing the responsiveness of target tissues to hormones, short photoperiods appear to activate parallel mechanisms, thus ensuring seasonal reproductive quiescence. The restoration of behavioral responsiveness to estradiol in short-day females follows a time course similar to that for the recovery of behavioral responsiveness to testosterone in males (Morin and Zucker, 1978).

Diminished responsiveness to low doses of estradiol has also been documented in acutely ovariectomized ewes; decreases in estrous behavior did not precede the end of other reproductive functions and were not the primary proximate cause of reproductive quiescence

(Goodman et al., 1981). Whether behavioral changes precede, follow, or occur concurrently with changes in ovulation is not known for many photoperiodic species.

There is disagreement about whether photoperiodic inhibition of female sex behavior in Syrian hamsters is mediated by the pineal gland. Karp and Powers (1993) implicated the pineal gland, whereas Badura and Nunez (1989) did not. In the former study, females were pinealectomized many weeks before steroid hormone treatments were initiated; only 2 weeks intervened between pinealectomy and initial hormone treatment in the experiment of Badura and Nunez. The residual effects of pineal hormones can persist for as long as 1 month (Ruby et al., 1989), perhaps accounting for the diminished responsiveness to steroid hormones in the recently pinealectomized females and the complete restoration of behavioral responsiveness in the long-term pinealectomized animals. Pinealectomy accelerated the resumption of estrous cycles in anestrus Siberian hamsters housed in short days (Schlatt et al., 1993). Additional evidence that the pineal gland mediates the effects of day length on sociosexual behavior was provided in a study of intrasexual aggressive behavior of female hamsters (Fleming et al., 1989).

Reduced behavioral responsiveness to estradiol in short-day female hamsters is accompanied by reduced estrogen receptor immunoreactivity (ER-ir) in the medial preoptic area (MPOA) and by an increase in the number of ER-ir cells in part of the medial nucleus of the amygdala. The induction of progesterone receptors by estradiol is significantly reduced in the ventromedial nucleus of the hypothalamus (Mangels et al., 1998), a critical target tissue for induction of lordosis by hormones (Pleim et al., 1990). An earlier less refined analysis did not detect photoperiodic differences in the concentration of nuclear estrogen or cytoplasmic progesterone receptors in a single block of tissue that contained the hypothalamus and preoptic area (POA) (Bittman et al., 1990).

In some rodents and ungulates, day length may affect female fecundity indirectly, via changes in male physiology and behavior. Weanling female *Peromyscus* caged together with adult males in short days sustained greater uterine weights than singly housed females (Garcia and Whitsett, 1983). Seasonally anovulatory goats ovulated, displayed estrous behavior, and became pregnant in the first 11 days after exposure to sexually active males. Female sexual responsiveness appeared to be retained year-round in this species, and insufficient stimulation from males accounted for the failure to reproduce during the nonbreeding season (Flores et al., 2000). This is another instance in which masking effects of pheromones and the behavior of one sex may override the inhibitory effects of short day lengths on the other sex (reviewed by Walkden-Brown et al., 1999).

Almost all female meadow voles (*Microtus pennsylvanicus*) are pregnant during the summer, but fewer than 50% are pregnant during the winter (reviewed in Meek and Lee, 1993a). Behavioral changes contribute to the decreased incidence of winter pregnancy. Virgin female meadow voles maintained in long or short days for 8 weeks all mated when paired with long-day males, but significantly fewer short-day females produced litters (Meek and Lee, 1993a). The latency to onset of mating was substantially longer in short- than long-day females; many of the latter mated within hours, whereas a substantial proportion of short-day females first mated after several days of cohabitation with males. Long latencies to initiate mating were associated with large decreases in fertility; 100% of females that mated within 48 hr of pairing ovulated, whereas approximately 40% of females with intermediate or long mating latencies failed to do so. Females with short-latency mating onsets received fewer intromissions from males prior to ejaculation and the interval between successive intromissions was increased compared to females with delayed estrous onsets (Meek and Lee, 1993b). The female's responsiveness to male pheromones and the male's responsiveness to the female interact to affect winter pregnancy rates in this species. Additional complexity is indicated by the finding that all primiparous females, whether housed in long or short days, mated within 48 hr of pairing with a long-day male and had similarly high birth rates (Meek and Lee, 1993b). Parity may permanently decrease responsiveness to short days, or more likely, sensitize females to male pheromones, thereby resulting in early male-induced estrus. Parous females in the field also continue to breed during short day lengths (reviewed by Meek and Lee, 1993a), in accord with the proposed reduction in residual reproductive potential in this short-lived species. In congeneric female prairie voles (*M. ochrogaster*) day length does not affect fecundity (Moffatt and Nelson, 1994).

C. Type II Rhythms

Endogenous annual rhythms have been documented in a wide variety of organisms, ranging from primitive plants to primates (Gwinner et al., 2001). In the golden-mantled ground squirrel, these rhythms persist for many cycles irrespective of environmental lighting conditions (short or long days, constant light or constant darkness; it matters not; Zucker 2001) (Fig. 5A); in others, only certain photoperiodic or temperature conditions are compatible with rhythm expression (Goss, 1984; Gwinner, 1986), and in still others the rhythm fades after several years (Fig. 5B).

The annual sequence of gonadal growth, a restricted breeding season, and gonadal involution are superficially similar in Type I and II cycles; closer examination reveals significant differences—reproduction in

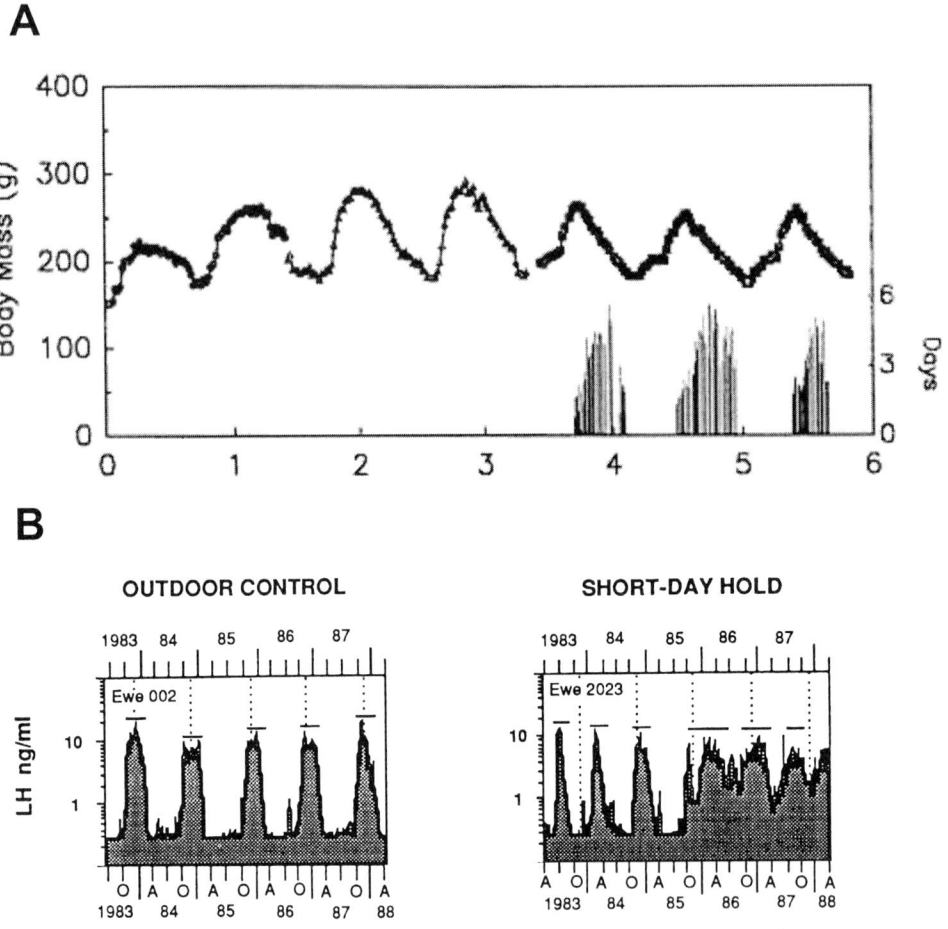

FIGURE 5 Examples of circannual rhythms in physiology and behavior. A. Circannual changes in body weight and hibernation of a squirrel kept in a fixed 12L:12D photoperiod, then held in constant light for the last 11 months of testing. The body weight rhythm persisted with a period of <12 months for 6 consecutive years. Beginning in year 3, squirrels were housed at 5°C. The ordinate axis on the right side indicates the duration of each hibernation bout. Hibernation occurred during 4–6 month intervals for 3 consecutive years, and this rhythm persisted with a period of <12 months. [From Ruby et al. (1998). *Brain Res.* **782**, 63–72, copyright 1998, with permission of Elsevier Science.] B. Circannual rhythms in plasma LH concentrations in ewes maintained outdoors and exposed to natural variations in day length (left) or kept indoors and exposed to a fixed short day of 8L:16D (right) for 5 years. From Karsch et al. (1989).

Type II species is not maintained indefinitely during exposure to any sequence of constant or variable day lengths; gonadal recrudescence either is not accompanied by refractoriness or if refractoriness occurs it terminates spontaneously. This feature permits a self-sustaining annual rhythm (Fig. 2B).

An alternative view is that Type II rhythms emerge from sequential refractoriness to short and long days. Ferrets initiate reproductive activity in the spring as they become refractory to winter day lengths and maintain stimulated reproductive systems in long days for several months; subsequently, gonadotropin secretion diminishes and reproductive quiescence develops in long day lengths (Herbert and Klinowska, 1978). Sheep similarly appear to develop refractoriness to both prolonged long and short day lengths (Almeida and Lincoln, 1984; Robinson et al., 1985). This feature may be characteristic of many Type II rhythms, but it is not universally present; golden-mantled ground squirrels repeatedly make transitions from winter to summer phenotypes spontaneously, even when housed continuously in an unvarying day length (Zucker, 2001).

1. Entrainment of Type II Rhythms: Mediation by Melatonin

The period of Type II rhythms deviates from 12 months in the absence of entraining signals—free-running periods of the rhythms of body mass, hibernation, and reproduction of golden-mantled squirrels are approximately 10.5 months, necessitating a phase delay of 1.5 months each year to synchronize with the annual geophysical cycle. Simulated annual variations in day length effect this correction (Lee and Zucker, 1991). Seasonal differences in the duration of nightly melatonin secretion transduce the effects of day length on the neuroendocrine axis. Pinealectomy eliminates melatonin from the peripheral circulation and obliterates Type I rhythms, which invariably revert to the summer or long-day phenotype (Reiter, 1980). Type II rhythms, in contrast, persist after pinealectomy (Zucker, 1985; Woodfill et al., 1994), but the ability to entrain to a simulated natural photoperiod is lost (Hiebert et al., 2000). Infusions of melatonin that mimic durations of nocturnal melatonin secretion in natural day lengths entrain the luteinizing hormone (LH) rhythm of pinealectomized ewes to a period of 12 months; the endogenous pattern of melatonin secreted in the 3 months between the summer solstice and the autumnal equinox entrains the annual rhythm of LH in pinealectomized females with phase and period similar to those of intact ewes held outdoors (Fig. 6) (Woodfill et al., 1994; Barrell et al., 2000). The absolute duration of day length and the direction of day length change, both transduced by melatonin secretion, influence entrainment of Type II sheep reproductive rhythms (Woodfill et al., 1991, 1994).

2. Phase Response Curves to Hormones

The responsiveness to hormones varies over the course of the annual cycle. In golden-mantled ground squirrels, body mass almost doubles in the spring and then declines during the fall and winter months, reflecting first accretion and then depletion of white adipose tissue (Dark et al., 1992). Estradiol treatments restricted to mass gain and loss phases, respectively, produce substantial phase delays and advances in the rhythms of body mass of ovariectomized squirrels (Lee and Zucker, 1992); similar effects are observed in gonadectomized males (Hiebert et al., 1998). It is unusual that sexual differentiation does not eliminate the responsiveness of males to phase-shifting actions of estradiol; in Syrian hamsters, the circadian rhythms of males, unlike those of females, are completely unresponsive to phase-shifting actions of estradiol (Zucker et al., 1980a,b).

Melatonin treatments initiated in late summer produced durable phase shifts of Type II reproductive and body mass rhythms of juvenile female ground squirrels; identical treatments in the spring were ineffective (reviewed in Zucker, 2001). Circannual oscillators in squirrels and sheep (Woodfill et al., 1994) evidently respond differently to melatonin at discrete phases of the annual cycle.

Although hormones influence the phasing of rhythms, they are not essential for rhythm generation. The ablation of several endocrine organs (testes, ovaries, and pineal gland) of ground squirrels did not interfere with rhythm expression (Zucker, 2001). Thyroidectomy, on the other hand, extended the breeding season of rams and ewes (Parkinson and Follett, 1994; Karsch et al., 1995). It is unlikely that a circannual oscillator in the thyroid gland mediates this effect. The normal annual rhythm in blood prolactin concentrations persists in thyroidectomized sheep and damage to the anterior hypothalamus produces an extension of

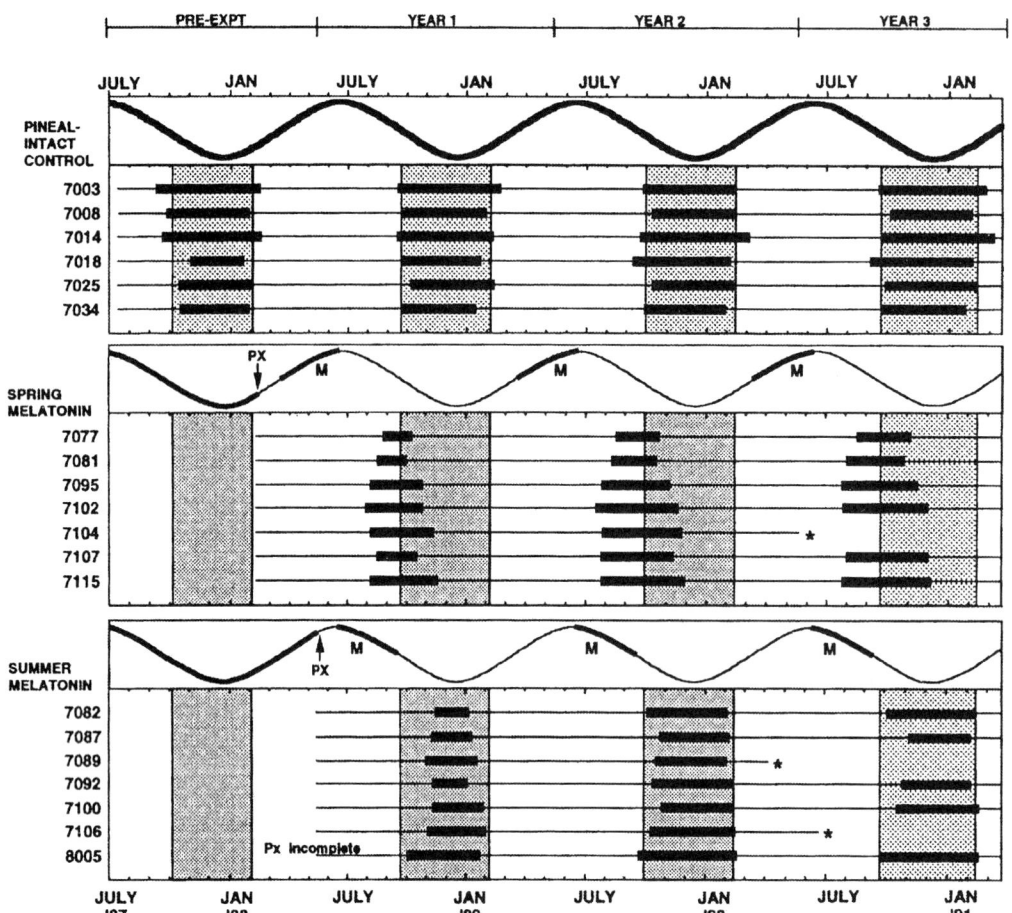

FIGURE 6 Hormone secretion at different phases of the year synchronizes circannual rhythms. Summary of timing of high and low LH stages in pineal-intact control ewes (top panel) and in pinealectomized ewes treated with melatonin (M) for 3 consecutive months each year for 4 years. Thick curved lines indicate when melatonin was present and its changing pattern. The timing of the high LH stage of each cycle relative to the calendar year (abscissa) is plotted as a thick horizontal bar, with the high LH stage of the first observed cycle depicted by the leftmost horizontal bar for each animal. Asterisks indicate that an animal died before observations were completed. [From Woodfill et al. (1994).]

reproduction similar to that resulting from thyroidectomy (Hileman et al., 1994), together implicating a specialized thyroid-brain system that modulates photoperiodic influences on the neuroendocrine axis.

3. Hormones, Seasonal Variation in Locomotor Activity, and Circannual Modulation of Circadian Organization

Home range size and the amount of wheel-running activity vary seasonally in several rodents. In voles, locomotor activity reverts from a predominantly nocturnal pattern in spring to a diurnal pattern in winter (Erkinaro, 1961; Rowesmitt et al., 1982). In Type I species, these transitions in activity are driven by seasonal changes in day length, temperature, and food availability; in Type II species, however, similar seasonal variations in locomotor activity are evident in the absence of environmental change. In golden-mantled ground squirrels housed in constant light at 22°C for several years, the period of the free-running circadian locomotor rhythm is less than 24 hr during the subjective summer and greater than 24 hr during subjective winter (Mrosovsky et al., 1976; Zucker et al., 1983). Among squirrels kept in invariant 14-hr day lengths, locomotor activity begins earlier and ends later in the day during subjective spring and summer than in autumn and winter (Lee et al., 1986, 1990a; Lee and Zucker, 1995; Freeman and Zucker, 2000). The interval between successive recurrences of the summer or winter patterns of activity is 10.5 months. An endogenous circannual mechanism modulates the amount and daily timing of locomotion. Although increases in the duration and distribution of activity are correlated with the reproductive cycle and with striking seasonal changes in body temperature, the circannual locomotor rhythms nevertheless persist unaltered in gonadectomized individuals (Lee and Zucker, 1995) and those in which large body-temperature fluctuations are eliminated (Freeman and Zucker, 2000).

IV. ENDOCRINE TRANSDUCTION OF PHOTOPERIOD SIGNALS

Postulated as the seat of the soul by Descartes, the pineal gland remained a biological enigma until Lerner and colleagues (1958) isolated and characterized melatonin from the bovine pineal gland and demonstrated a physiological action in lightening amphibian melanocytes. Primarily through the impetus of work by Reiter and co-workers (e.g., Hoffman and Reiter, 1965), the pineal gland came to be recognized as a mediator of seasonal changes in day length in mammals. The proliferation of research and speculation that ensued established the physiological significance of the pineal gland and its principal indolamine hormone, melatonin (Arendt, 1995).

In 1964, surgical excision of the pineal gland was found to be associated with a reduction in the rate and magnitude of seasonal gonadal regression in male Syrian hamsters (Czyba et al., 1964). This outcome anticipated results obtained under more controlled laboratory conditions by Hoffman and Reiter (1965), who reported that gonadal regression in response to blinding or exposure to short photoperiods was absent in pinealectomized hamsters. Reiter and colleagues' work during this decade was largely responsible for describing in detail "[t]he sensitivity of the hamster to manipulations of the environment, in this case light…" (p. 1610), and establishing, "the concept that the pineal gland has the important function of regulating gonadal activity so that it is compatible with certain changing environmental conditions" (Hoffman and Reiter, 1965). A search for the antigonadal pineal factor turned squarely to melatonin, which is secreted by the pineal gland in a circadian pattern, with peak gland and blood concentrations occurring during subjective night. The light-entrainable circadian clock in the suprachiasmatic nuclei (SCN) drives the melatonin secretory rhythm; separate circadian oscillators, entrained to lights off (dusk) and lights on (dawn), are proposed to regulate the onset and offset of nocturnal hormone secretion, respectively (Illnerova et al., 1984; Illnerova, 1991). Consequently, over the annual cycle, the duration of nocturnal melatonin secretion varies inversely with day length (Fig. 7) (Sumova et al., 1995).

A. Duration vs Phase of the Melatonin Signal

The circadian phase during which melatonin is elevated and the duration of nocturnal elevation are two features that could account for its gonadotrophic effects. In the 1970s, Syrian hamsters housed in 14L were shown to undergo gonadal regression when injected with melatonin during late afternoon (i.e., shortly before the onset of darkness), but not when treated in early to mid-day (Reiter et al., 1977; Tamarkin et al., 1977). This temporal coding of melatonin's antigonadal effects suggested a circadian rhythm in tissue responsiveness to melatonin (Tamarkin et al., 1977). Subsequent experiments in hamsters and sheep indicated, however, that for control of seasonal traits, the duration of the nocturnal melatonin peak is paramount (Carter and Goldman, 1983a,b; Bittman and Karsch, 1984; Goldman et al., 1984). Thus, melatonin infusions induced gonadal regression in pinealectomized Siberian hamsters irrespective of the stage in the circadian cycle of its administration; only the duration of the melatonin signal was critical to its antigonadotrophic effects (Goldman et al., 1984). Melatonin infusions ≥ 8 hr per day suppressed serum gonadotropin and prolactin concentrations and provoked gonadal regression, whereas infusions ≤ 6 hr per day stimulated the reproductive axis. Moreover, two melatonin infusions separated by <1 hr summated as a single longer signal (Goldman et al., 1984; Goldman, 1991). As few as 4 consecutive weeks of daily long-duration melatonin signals are sufficient to

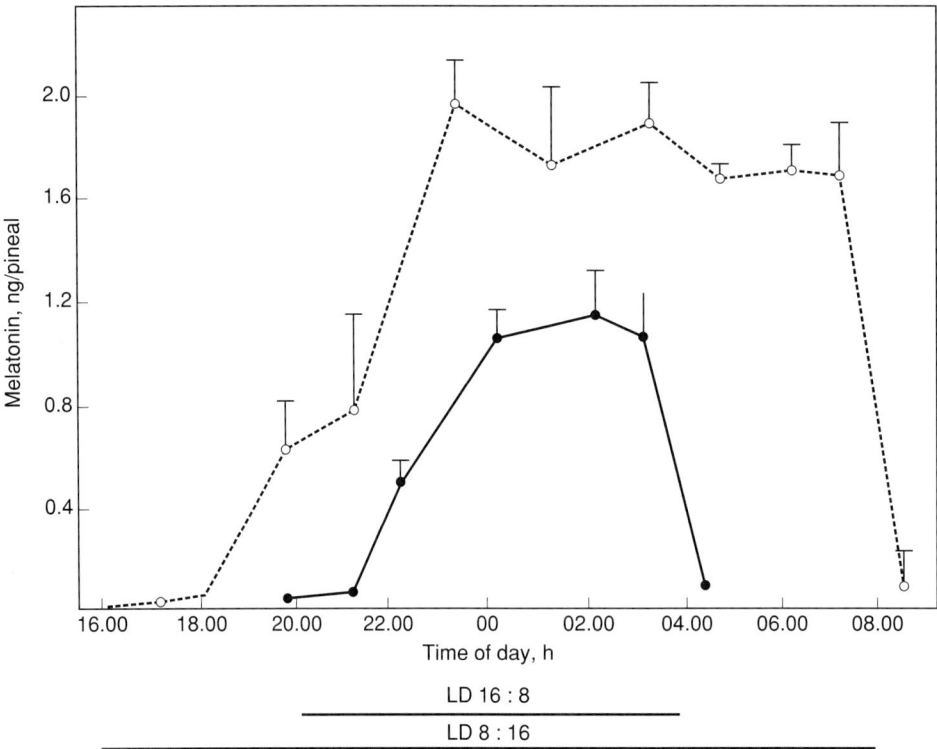

FIGURE 7 Pineal melatonin content in female Siberian hamsters housed in long day lengths of 16L:8D (filled circles) and short day lengths of 8L:16D (open circles). Lines below the abscissa indicate the timing and duration of darkness. The duration of nocturnal melatonin synthesis and secretion varies inversely with day length. [From Illnerova et al. (1984).]

induce gonadal regression in adult Siberian hamsters, and 6 weeks of such treatments suffices in Syrian hamsters (Prendergast et al., 2000; Maywood and Hastings, 1995). From this and other work, the duration hypothesis has emerged. The apparent rhythm in responsiveness of the reproductive system to melatonin injections in pineal-intact animals was explained as follows. Exogenous melatonin delivered a few hours before the natural onset of melatonin secretion transforms the endogenous long-day signal to the longer one characteristic of short days. Treatments given at other times produce transient melatonin elevations that do not summate with endogenous melatonin secretion to produce an extended signal. The viability of the duration hypothesis has been established in several rodent and ungulate species and at present best accounts for the way in which melatonin mediates photoperiodism (Arendt, 1995). Pitrosky and colleagues (1995; Pitrosky and Pevet, 1997) resurrected a version of the circadian sensitivity hypothesis to account for their observation that Syrian hamsters undergo gonadal regression when provided with two 2.5-hr melatonin infusions per day separated by a 5-hr melatonin-free interval. Their interpretations have been challenged (Hastings, 1996; Loudon, 1996).

B. Decoding of Melatonin Signals

How the neuroendocrine system extracts information from melatonin signals remains of great interest. In nature, melatonin signals corresponding to changing day lengths are generated on a nightly basis. Given that the duration of a melatonin signal on any given night is highly predictive of signal duration on subsequent nights, work has probed the optimality of nightly melatonin signals in communicating seasonal information. At issue is whether nightly melatonin signals are necessary to activate or inhibit the reproductive system or whether a lesser number of signals is sufficient. Short-duration melatonin signals provided on a daily basis provoked gonadal growth in Siberian hamsters, but failed to do so when delivered less frequently (Prendergast and Hugenberger, 1999) and elicited no additional growth when provided more frequently (Flynn et al., 2000). Similarly, long-duration melatonin infusions induced gonadal regression if given at 24-hr, but not less frequent, intervals (Elliott et al., 1989). In Syrian hamsters, long-duration melatonin infusions elicited gonadal regression when provided at 20- or 24-hr intervals; higher or lower infusion frequencies were ineffective. Long-duration melatonin pulses infused at lower (16-hr) frequencies induced gonadal regression in tau mutant hamsters (Stirland et al., 1996). Neuroendocrine responsiveness to melatonin thus appears to be frequency-tuned—only signals that recur at frequencies that approximate the organism's endogenous frequency (in most cases ~24 hr) elicit duration-appropriate physiological responses. Whether the inability to extract information from signals that deviate from one per circadian day is restricted to the gonadal axis or is characteristic of the processing of melatonin signals throughout the nervous system awaits further investigation.

C. Context-Dependent Melatonin Signal Integration

The delivery of unnatural melatonin signals has unveiled formal properties of the melatonin signal-processing system. The context in which melatonin signals are generated influences whether or not they activate the hypothalamic-pituitary-gonadal axis. For example, short-duration (5-hr) melatonin infusions delivered every other day against a background of no melatonin to pinealectomized hamsters did not elicit gonadal growth (Prendergast and Hugenberger, 1999), but similar short melatonin signals given every other day sustained gonadal growth when interposed with long-duration (10-hr) signals on intervening days (Prendergast et al., 1998). Short-duration melatonin signals delivered every 72 hours, however, did not sustain gonadal development even against a background of long-duration signals (Prendergast et al., 1998). Melatonin-responsive elements thus appear capable of bridging a gap of approximately 48 hours between short signals, provided a melatonin signal, even a long-duration signal that normally inhibits gonadal growth, is received on the intervening day.

A small number of consecutive daily melatonin signals is required to impart photoperiod information. During days 13 to 16 of gestation, Siberian hamsters communicate day length information (photoperiod history) to their fetuses; maternal melatonin secretion thereby influences pups' postnatal development and responsiveness to intermediate day lengths (Weaver and Reppert, 1986; Weaver et al., 1987; Elliott et al., 1989; Stetson et al., 1989). Pregnant pinealectomized females that received at least two consecutive long-duration melatonin infusions during the latter part of gestation communicated photoperiod information to their fetuses; those receiving only one infusion did not (Weaver et al., 1989). Two, rather than one, long-duration melatonin infusions much more effectively inhibited gonadal development in juvenile Siberian hamsters (Goldman et al., 1984). In adult Siberian hamsters, gonadal growth was provoked by short-duration melatonin signals delivered on 2 consecutive days when followed by 2 days of long-duration infusions (Flynn et al., 2000); in the latter study, two successive signals extended the interval over which short signals could sustain gonadal growth, but the 72-hr gap between short signals was not bridged in the absence of melatonin on intervening days. The neuroendocrine system requires the presence of some melatonin at approximately daily intervals to maintain responsiveness to short melatonin signals.

In nature, the duration of nightly melatonin secretion neither varies markedly nor remains static from night-to-night; rather, melatonin signals either gradually increase or decrease as days get shorter and longer, respectively. Just as photoperiod information is contained in the direction of change in day length, independently of absolute day length (Gorman and Zucker, 1995), the direction of change in melatonin secretion conveys seasonal information to the neuroendocrine system. Melatonin infusions gradually decreasing in duration from 10 to 7.5 hours per night elicited gonadal growth in Siberian hamsters, whereas those gradually increasing from 5 to 7.5 hours per night induced regression (Gorman and Zucker, 1997).

Prior photoperiod history modifies the critical day length for reproductive stimulation and inhibition. Siberian hamsters previously housed in 16L:8D and 8L:16D undergo gonadal regression and growth, respectively, when exposed to a 14L:10D photocycle; such intermediate-duration photoperiods are regarded as long or short days, depending on an individual's photoperiodic history (Fig. 8) (Duncan et al., 1985; Hoffmann and Illnerova, 1986). The range of photoperiods that elicit gonadal stimulation or regression as a function of photoperiodic history is considerable; day lengths as short as 12L:12D and as long as 16L:8D may be regarded as long and short days, respectively, by hamsters previously exposed to shorter (6L:18D) and longer (20L:4D) day lengths (Rivkees et al., 1988). An individual's photoperiod history likewise determines whether melatonin signals of intermediate duration are regarded as long- or short-day cues. For example, 7-hr melatonin infusions elicited gonadal growth in hamsters previously housed in short days, but caused gonadal regression in hamsters from long days (Prendergast et al., 2000). Photoperiodic mammals encode a representation of prior day lengths that affects the interpretation of subsequent melatonin signals. Two or more weeks of exposure to a long day length (15 hr light/day) was sufficient to encode such a photoperiodic memory, permitting gonadal regression in response to a subsequent intermediate day length (13.5 hr light/day). Photoperiodic memories encoded by 15-hr days persisted for approximately 13 weeks (Prendergast et al., 2000). The photoperiodic memory system provides a constantly changing context for the interpretation of intermediate day lengths. In nature, the encoding and eventual decay of photoperiodic memories may ensure that hamsters' responses to ambiguous photoperiod cues are influenced only by relatively recent day lengths.

V. NEURAL BASES FOR PHOTOPERIODISM

A. Mechanisms of Photoperiodic Time Measurement: Neural Control of Melatonin Secretion

Pineal melatonin, the principal endocrine mediator of day length in mammals, provides photoperiod information essential for the generation (Type I) and entrainment (Types I and II) of seasonal rhythms. Most investigations have assessed reproductive end points in probing actions of melatonin. The GnRH-pituitary-gonadal system is well-suited for physiological analyses of the processing of day-length information.

Seasonal changes in day length impinge on the neuroendocrine axis via a retinal-hypothalamic-pineal pathway (Moore 1996). Briefly, light entrains circadian oscillators in the SCN, which via a polysynaptic pathway control melatonin synthesis in the pineal gland (Fig. 9) (Illnerova et al., 1984; Elliott and Tamarkin 1994). Circadian output from the SCN is transmitted to the parvocellular autonomic component of the hypothalamic paraventricular nucleus (PVN), which

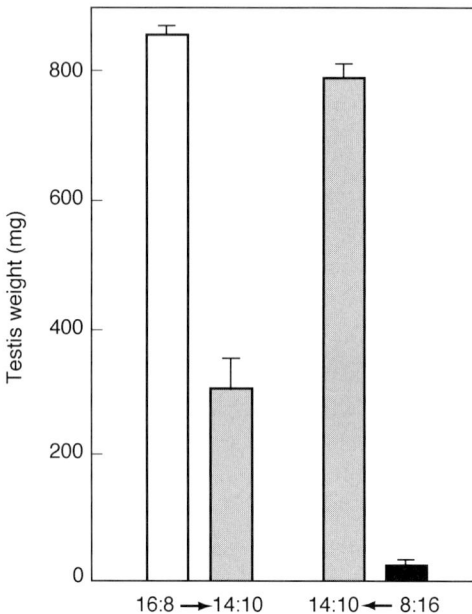

FIGURE 8 Photoperiodic history determines the reproductive response to intermediate day lengths. Siberian hamsters previously housed in long days of 16L:8D undergo gonadal regression when exposed to intermediate-duration photoperiods of 14L:10D for 10 weeks (left side), whereas hamsters previously housed in short days of 8L:16D respond to the intermediate-duration photoperiod with gonadal development (right side). [From Hoffmann et al. (1986). Neurosci. Lett. **67**, 68–72, copyright 1986, with permission of Elsevier Science.]

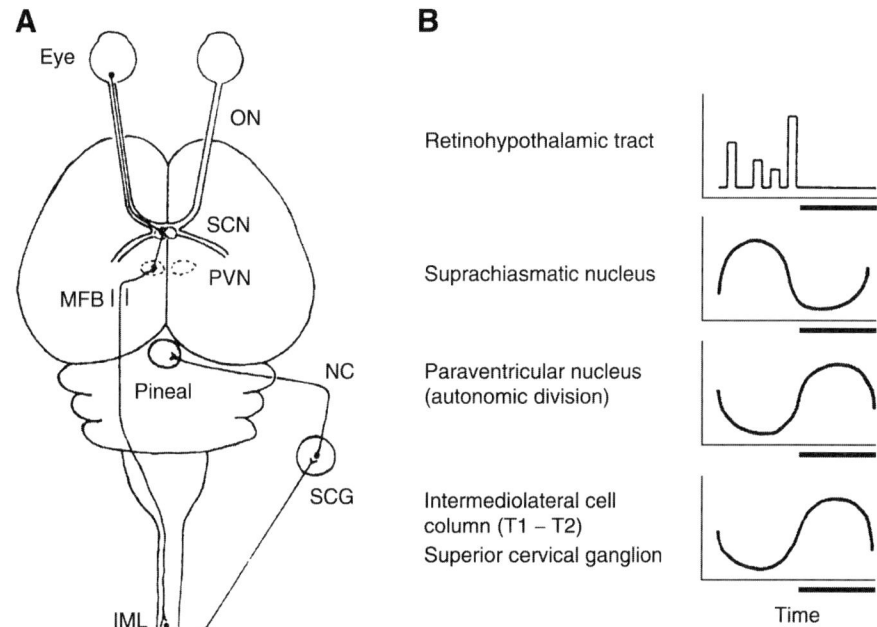

FIGURE 9 A. Neural pathway that controls the circadian rhythm in pineal melatonin secretion. IML, intermediolateral spinal cord cell column; MFB, medial forebrain bundle; NC, nervi conarii; ON, optic nerve; PVN paraventricular nucleus; SCG, superior cervical ganglion; SCN, suprachiasmatic nucleus. B. Schematic illustration of rhythms of neuronal activity in sequential components of the neural pathway that mediates the effects of light on pineal secretory activity. [From Moore (1996). *Behav. Brain Res.* **73**, 125–130, copyright 1966, with permission of Elsevier Science.]

projects to the upper thoracic intermediolateral cell column via the medial forebrain bundle (MFB). MFB neurons innervate the superior cervical ganglion (SCG), which project β-noradrenergic sympathetic fibers to pinealocytes (Moore, 1996). Information that originates in the SCN drives a circadian rhythm of synthesis of N-acetyltransferase (NAT), the rate-limiting enzyme in the conversion of N-acetyl-serotonin to melatonin. Pineal melatonin is secreted exclusively at night, in proportion to the duration of the scotophase. The ablation of the SCN eliminates the diurnal pineal NAT rhythm (Moore and Klein, 1974), as do lesions of the PVN (Klein et al., 1983), MFB (Moore, 1996), and SCG (Reiter et al., 1979) or damage to the ICNs (Bowers et al., 1984). Consistent with the essential role of melatonin in mammalian photoperiodism, lesions along this pathway eliminate the reproductive response to day length in hamsters (Rusak and Morin, 1976; Pickard and Turek, 1983; Eskes et al., 1984; Lehman et al., 1984; Bittman and Lehman, 1987).

B. High-Density Melatonin-Binding Sites in the Mammalian Brain

Autoradiographic analyses indicate high-density binding of ^{125}I melatonin in the SCN of several rodent species (Weaver et al., 1989); in Siberian hamsters, the thalamic paraventricular nucleus (PVt) and the reuniens nuclei exhibit a high degree of melatonin uptake (Duncan et al., 1989). In rats, Syrian hamsters, and Siberian hamsters, the SCN and median eminence display significant melatonin binding, as do several areas of the thalamus, hypothalamus, subiculum, and area postrema (Weaver et al., 1989). Interestingly, little ^{125}I melatonin binding was detected in the anterior pituitary gland of adult photoperiodic rodents, despite the profound influence of melatonin on the secretion of gonadotropins (Vanecek, 1988; Carlson et al., 1991). Among three suborders of Rodentia, there is considerable interspecific variability in sites of high-affinity melatonin binding (Bittman et al., 1994). Among orders of mammals, variability in melatonin binding sites is noteworthy; for example, in sheep numerous telencephalic, diencephalic, hypothalamic, and midbrain structures bind melatonin, whereas in ferrets only the pars tuberalis and pars distalis of the pituitary bind ^{125}I melatonin, despite the fact that both species are highly reproductively photoperiodic (Bittman and Weaver, 1990; Weaver and Reppert, 1990). The pars tuberalis is the only structure that binds melatonin in all mammals and appears to feature prominently in the transduction of photoperiod information for control of prolactin (PRL) secretion (Morgan and Williams, 1989).

C. Central Sites of Melatonin Action in the Reproductive Neuroendocrine System

As described in Section IV, the nightly duration of melatonin secretion is the critical parameter for transducing the effects of light on the neuroendocrine axis. A series of long-duration melatonin signals suppresses anterior pituitary gonadotropin secretion (Bartness et al., 1993; Goldman and Nelson, 1993). Melatonin must either suppress GnRH secretion in the hypothalamus, attenuate its ability to stimulate pituitary follicle-stimulating hormone (FSH) and LH release, or reduce gonadal responsiveness to gonadotropins (in any combination). There is no consistent evidence from in vivo or in vitro studies of rodents that day length or melatonin alters pituitary responsiveness to GnRH (e.g., Martin et al., 1977; Jetton et al., 1994), but in ruminants a significant modulatory role for photoperiod signals has been documented (Fowler et al., 1992; Xu et al., 1992). In some studies of Syrian and Siberian hamsters, the number of hypothalamic GnRH immunoreactive (GnRH-ir) neurons was increased in short day lengths (Ronchi et al., 1992; Bernard et al., 1999), but in others no differences were detected between long- and short-day animals (e.g., Urbanski et al., 1991; Bittman et al., 1991, 1996; Yellon, 1994). It is not known whether melatonin affects GnRH neurons directly or indirectly, although some overlap exists between brain nuclei that bind melatonin and those that contain GnRH neurons (Glass, 1986; Glass and Dolan, 1988; Korytko et al., 1995).

The reproductive effects of melatonin have been characterized most extensively in Syrian and Siberian hamsters. Among hypothalamic nuclei with high densities of ^{125}I-iodomelatonin binding, those in the mediobasal hypothalamus (MBH), specifically in the dorsomedial nucleus of the hypothalamus (DMH) appear to be essential for decoding photoperiod signals. The ablation of the DMH eliminated the gonadal response to long-duration melatonin infusions in male Syrian hamsters (Maywood and Hastings, 1995; Maywood et al., 1996), and destruction of tissue in the adjacent ventromedial nucleus of the hypothalamus (VMH) DMH region resulted in the premature recovery of testicular function in photoregressed Syrian hamsters (Bae et al., 1999). The ablation of the SCN eliminated the antigonadal effects of long-duration melatonin signals in Siberian hamsters (Bartness et al., 1991) but not Syrian hamsters (Bittman et al., 1979, 1989). Interestingly, the ablation of the DMH spared the lactotropic PRL response to long melatonin signals and short day lengths in Syrian hamsters, even though the responsiveness of gonadotropins to these signals was lost (Maywood and Hastings, 1995). This suggests that melatonin signals are transduced into the hypothalamic-pituitary axis via multiple parallel pathways that may be trait-specific (Maywood and Hastings, 1995; Lincoln, 1990, 1999). In support of this conjecture, the ablation of the SCN, which eliminated nocturnal melatonin secretion, abolished the gonadal response to short day lengths, yet spared the PRL response (Bartness et al., 1991; Bittman et al., 1991). Microinfusions of melatonin into the SCN, reunions nuclei, or the PVt each induced testicular regression in juvenile Siberian hamsters, but only infusions of the SCN yielded short-day-like PRL concentrations (Badura and Goldman, 1992).

Brain regions that transduce photoperiod signals into changes in gonadotropin secretion are concentrated in the medial basal hypothalamic region in rodents, but in other orders (e.g., carnivores), reproductive responses to photoperiod may not involve a direct action of melatonin in the brain at all (e.g., ferrets; Weaver and Reppert, 1990), although the possibility of neural melatonin receptors that have not been detected by procedures remains a possibility. Melatonin binding sites outside the brain play a significant role in photoperiodic regulation of reproductive hormone secretion. Indeed, in hypothalamic-pituitary disconnected sheep, melatonin implants in the pars tuberalis inhibited PRL secretion in a manner that mimicked the effects of photoperiod (Lincoln and Clarke, 1997). Melatonin treatments restricted to the pars tuberalis were sufficient to drive the entire cycle of responsiveness and refractoriness of PRL to melatonin, mimicking, in part, the response to short days even as gonadal responses to melatonin were absent in this preparation (Lincoln and Clarke, 1997). In hamsters, both short days and melatonin treatments decreased the amplitude of *per1* (an early-immediate gene) and ICER (an inducible cyclic adenosine monophosphate (cAMP) early repressor) rhythms in the pars tuberalis. Such changes in gene expression covaried with decreases in pituitary PRL secretion and suggest an internal representation of short days in the reproductive neuroendocrine axis (Messager *et al.*, 1999). GnRH fibers traverse the median eminence and pars tuberalis, areas of dense melatonin binding where melatonin could potentially influence peptide release from synaptic terminals, although in sheep melatonin implants in the pars tuberalis did not alter pituitary gonadotropin secretion (Lincoln and Clarke, 1997). Little is known about the extent to which the sites of melatonin binding interact in the induction, maintenance, or termination of gonadal regression under short days.

VI. MATERNAL–FETAL COMMUNICATION OF DAY LENGTH

Long-day breeding rodents typically begin issuing offspring in March–April and stop producing litters in September–October. If the length of a given breeding season permits, litters may be born as many as 6 months apart (Millar *et al.*, 1979). Upon weaning, young born in the spring months encounter increasing day lengths, moderate ambient temperatures, and relatively plentiful food, whereas those born late in the breeding season face decreasing day lengths and food scarcity (Iverson and Turner, 1974). In several photoperiodic rodent species, somatic growth and sexual maturation are delayed in fall-born offspring; animals born in late summer and autumn typically do not reach sexual maturity until spring of the following year. In contrast, spring-born pups mature rapidly and reach sexual maturity within 1–3 months (Martinet and Spitz, 1971; Worth *et al.*, 1973; Petterborg, 1978; Pistole and Cranford, 1982; Spears and Clarke, 1986).

Day length is the main proximate cue triggering puberty in small temperate-zone rodents. Very young pups do not generate pineal melatonin rhythms, and thus do not transduce day length information during early-postnatal life. Nocturnal pineal melatonin rhythms typically emerge between 11 and 25 days of age in various species (Yellon and Goldman, 1984; Stetson *et al.*, 1986; Sato *et al.*, 1989; Kaufman and Menaker, 1991), and only then can juveniles directly encode the ambient photoperiod. Prevailing day lengths around the time of weaning arrest or accelerate somatic and reproductive growth in several photoperiodic rodents (Hoffmann, 1979; Johnston and Zucker, 1980; Horton, 1984; Stetson *et al.*, 1989; Gower *et al.*, 1994). Postnatal photoperiods alone, however, do not determine these developmental trajectories. In all rodent species that have been studied, day lengths that prevail prenatally (and even those experiencxed by dams prior to conception) influence the weanling's prepubertal development.

In spring and fall, newly weaned offspring encounter comparable intermediate day lengths (12–14 hr light per day). By communicating day-length information to their fetuses during gestation, dams remove much of the seasonal ambiguity inherent in intermediate day lengths. Comparison of pre- and postnatal day lengths provides pups with directional information regarding changes in photoperiod duration and thereby either promotes or retards growth and development.

A. Voles

Pregnant montane voles (*Microtus montanus*) communicate day-length information to their fetuses. Fetuses maintained in a short photoperiod of 8L during gestation grew faster than those gestated in 14L when exposed to 8L, 10L, or 14L photoperiods after birth (Horton, 1984). Day length during lactation had no effect on the somatic or reproductive development of juveniles (Horton, 1985). The photoperiodic information communicated to fetuses *in utero* encodes a reference day length that is accessed postnatally to initiate or inhibit somatic and reproductive development; which developmental trajectory is followed depends on whether current day lengths are longer or shorter, respectively, than those during gestation.

The winter phenotype (inhibition of reproduction, decreased food intake, and increased fur thickness) in weanling meadow voles depends on day lengths experienced by their dams prior to conception as well as those present during gestation and lactation. Pups born to dams housed in short days prior to conception and housed in short days postnatally manifested reduced rates of somatic and reproductive development and thicker pelages than the offspring of dams housed in long days prior to conception (Lee et al., 1987; Lee and Zucker, 1988). A prenatal short-day photoperiod signal mimicked by treating long-day pregnant voles with melatonin also affected rates of postnatal development; this suggests that changes in the duration of maternal melatonin secretion during gestation provide the requisite signals to fetuses (Lee et al., 1989). Maternal signals during lactation also influenced the food intake and somatic growth of pups (Lee and Zucker, 1988; Lee, 1993). Postnatal exposure to short days did not, however, inhibit reproductive development or body mass in pups born to photorefractory dams housed in short days for 26 weeks prior to mating (Lee and Zucker, 1988). Seasonal information—regarding both the ambient day length during gestation and the number of weeks dams have been exposed to short days prior to mating—is communicated to fetal meadow voles and probably facilitates physiological adjustments to the environmental conditions pups encounter after weaning.

B. Hamsters

Gestational day lengths can have enduring effects on reproductive development in the absence of postnatal photoperiod signals (i.e., in animals that are functionally pinealectomized); effects generated by pre- and postnatal day lengths also interact to regulate postnatal growth and reproductive development (Stetson et al., 1989; Prendergast et al., 1996). Developmental trajectories of Siberian hamsters differ depending on whether postnatal photoperiods are longer or shorter than those in force prenatally. Hamsters gestated in 12L, but not those gestated in 16L, underwent rapid testicular growth when housed in 14L beginning at 15 days of age (Fig. 10A) (Stetson et al., 1986). Similar to montane voles but unlike in meadow voles, mothers trans-

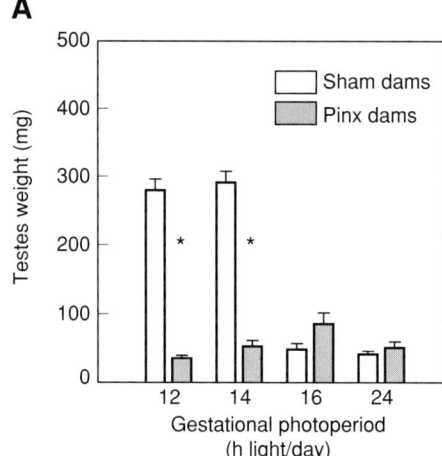

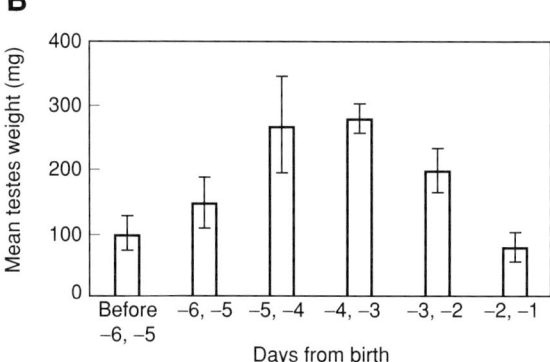

FIGURE 10 (A) Testes weights of 28-day-old offspring of Siberian hamster dams kept in different photoperiods during gestation and from birth in a 14L:10D photoperiod. Exposure to intermediate-duration day lengths postnatally stimulated reproductive development in pups gestated in equivalent or shorter day lengths, but inhibited development in pups gestated in longer day lengths. Intact, but not pinealectomized, dams communicated day-length information to their fetuses. (Asterisks indicate values that differ significantly from those of sham-operated animals in a given gestational day length.) (B) Testicular weights of 34-day-old Siberian hamsters born to pinealectomized dams that received two consecutive 10-hr melatonin infusions during gestation. Abscissa indicates timing of infusions relative to day of birth. Pups were maintained from birth in 14L:10D. Long-duration melatonin infusions (mimicking short day lengths) delivered between days 6 and 3 prior to birth provoked significant gonadal growth in pups postnatally. From Horton et al. (1990); Weaver et al. (1987).

fer photoperiod information during gestation, but not during lactation (Stetson et al., 1989).

Only dams with intact intact pineal glands transfer photoperiod information to their fetuses (Weaver and

Reppert, 1986; Weaver et al., 1987); the duration of maternal nocturnal melatonin secretion communicated to fetuses during the latter stage of gestation is the relevant signal (Weaver and Reppert, 1986; Weaver et al., 1987; Horton et al., 1989; Stetson et al., 1989; Prendergast et al., 1996). Juvenile *Phodopus* born to pinealectomized dams that received long-duration melatonin infusions on two or more consecutive days between days 6 and 3 before parturition underwent gonadal growth when housed in 14L postnatally (Fig. 10B); that is, this intermediate-duration day length was perceived as relatively longer than the day length communicated by the melatonin signals provided *in utero*. In contrast, pups born to dams that received either multiple consecutive daily melatonin infusions at other gestational stages or only a single melatonin infusion during the appropriate interval did not exhibit rapid gonadal development (Weaver and Reppert, 1986; Weaver et al., 1987). A mechanism—formally similar to that operative in adult hamsters (Prendergast et al., 2000)—encodes a reference photoperiod *in utero* that permits pups to measure the directional change in day length postnatally over an interval of several weeks.

VII. WINTER BREEDING AND PHOTOPERIOD NONRESPONSIVENESS

A variable and in some cases substantial proportion of individuals in many long-day-breeding photoperiodic species remains reproductively active in winter. In the laboratory, this presents as a failure to undergo involution of the reproductive apparatus in short day lengths (Fig. 11). This phenomenon has also been observed in the field, where some individuals produce offspring in mid-winter (Christian, 1980). Thus, despite inhabiting a seasonally variable environment, these individuals sustain reproductive activity during the short days of winter. The dogma that seasonal curtailment of reproduction is an adaptive response to the energetic challenges of autumn and winter is challenged by the existence of nonphotoperiodic individuals. Why and how these animals are unresponsive to decreasing day lengths requires explanation. Here we examine the existence of nonresponsiveness to day length in nominally photoperiodic species.

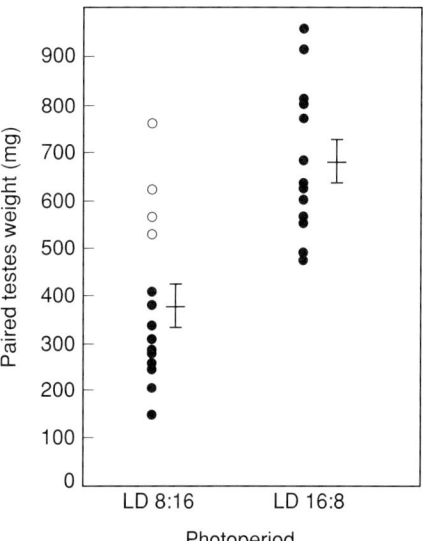

FIGURE 11 Paired testes weights for individual prairie voles maintained from birth until 35 days of age in long (16L:8D) or short (8L:16D) day lengths. Horizontal bars, group means; vertical bars, standard errors; filled circles, individual values for paired testis mass; open circles, values for voles that underwent testicular development during exposure to short day lengths. From Nelson (1985).

A. Definitions

Individuals are reproductively photoperiodic if changes in day length (or their neuroendocrine sequelae) alter traits directly involved in successful reproduction. As described in Section V, short days alter the synthesis and storage of brain peptides that regulate reproduction, resulting in reduced blood concentrations of gonadotropins and steroids, diminished reproductive organ weights, and elimination of reproductive behavior. Photoperiodic rodents also commonly decrease body mass in preparation for winter, thereby conserving energy (Iverson and Turner, 1974; Wunder et al., 1977; Wolff and Lidicker, 1980; Pistole and Cranford, 1982; Dark et al., 1983b; Dark and Zucker, 1984a,b; Wunder, 1984); steroid-dependent behaviors such as mating, territorial defense, dispersal, and aggressive and agonistic interactions all decline in winter as well (Jannett, 1984; Madison et al., 1984).

Divergent mechanisms mediate photoperiod nonresponsiveness in mice (*Peromyscus maniculatus* and *P. leucopus*), voles (*Microtus* sp.), and hamsters (*Phodopus sungorus*)—genera in which the majority of research on nonresponsiveness has been conducted. Intrinsic

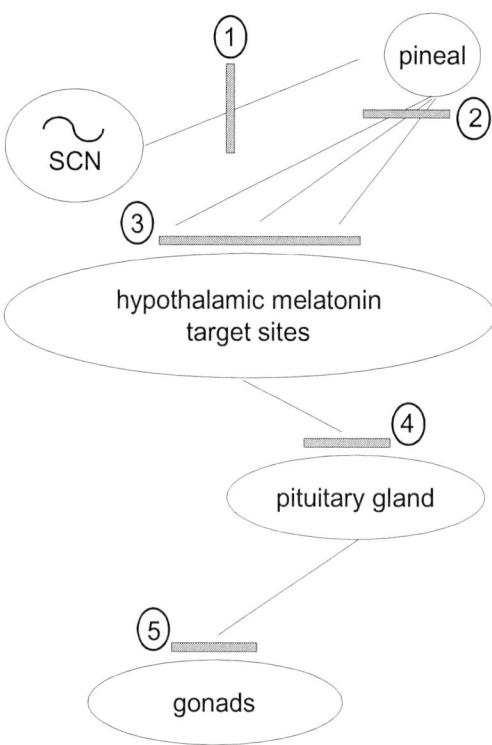

1. Pre-pineal (circadian control of pineal activity)
2. Pineal depletion
3. Post-pineal (hypothalamic target tissue insensitivity)
4. Post-hypothalamic (pituitary target tissue insensitivity)
5. Post-pituitary (gonadal insensitivity)

FIGURE 12 Schematic representation of neuroendocrine levels at which impairments in short-day signal processing could result in reproductive nonresponsiveness to short day lengths.

and extrinsic factors that influence the reproductive response to short day lengths include age, genetic predisposition, latitude of origin, activity level, ambient temperature, social factors, and photoperiodic history. A more limited body of data documents reproductive and behavioral nonresponsiveness to other winter cues (e.g., inanition and low temperatures; Eskes, 1983; Larkin et al., 2001).

B. Neuroendocrine Mediation of Nonresponsiveness

Photoperiod influences reproduction via an information-processing pathway in which a light signal is converted into a gonadotrophic signal that ultimately controls the gonads (Fig. 12). Failure to undergo gonadal involution in short days can reflect degradation or loss of the short-day signal at any stage of this pathway. For example, the circadian clock that discriminates long from short days (a pre-pineal stage of the pathway) may differ between photoresponsive and nonresponsive individuals; alternatively, modification in the pineal gland or in post-pineal hypothalamic, pituitary, or gonadal tissues might form the basis for nonresponsiveness to short days.

Nonresponsiveness to day length has been examined most thoroughly in Siberian hamsters (*Phodopus sungorus*), prairie voles (*Microtus ochrogaster*), white-footed mice (*Peromyscus leucopus*), and deer mice (*P. maniculatus*). The extent to which neural and endocrine differences between the two phenotypes are intrinsic (genetic) or extrinsic (experiential) varies between species. Siberian hamsters and deer mice exemplify two distinct neuroendocrine mechanisms that mediate the loss of responsiveness to short day lengths.

1. Deer Mice (Peromyscus maniculatus)

The extent to which deer mice undergo gonadal regression when exposed to winter conditions or short day lengths (<12.5 hr light/day) (Stebbins, 1977; Whitsett and Miller, 1982; Ruf *et al.*, 1997) depends on latitude of origin (Gram *et al.*, 1982; Dark *et al.*, 1983a), ambient temperature and availability of food (Demas and Nelson, 1998), and a genetic polymorphism that renders animals nonresponsive to inhibitory patterns of melatonin secretion (Desjardins *et al.*, 1986). Approximately one-third of North American deer mice responds to short days with gonadal regression, another third maintain gonadal function, and the remaining animals exhibit an intermediate response to short days, characterized by a moderate (35–45%) reduction in testis size and intermediate levels of testicular activity (Blank and Desjardins, 1986; Ruf *et al.*, 1997). Differences in reproductive responsiveness to photoperiod are also reflected in changes in sperm number, weight of accessory glands, plasma concentrations of gonadotropins, and features of the GnRH neuronal system (Blank, 1992; Korytko *et al.*, 1995). Though capable of breeding under laboratory conditions, it is unknown whether intermediate responders or nonresponders are fertile under simulated winter conditions.

Photoperiodism in this species has a strong genetic basis. As few as two generations of directional selection on photoperiod nonresponsiveness yielded strains of deer mice in which >80% or <20% of individuals are short-day nonresponders (Desjardins *et al.*, 1986). The proportion of nonresponders in wild populations of deer mice may undergo rapid changes in years when environmental conditions permit successful autumn or winter breeding.

Experiential factors also influence photoresponsiveness. Gonadal development was delayed by 5–6 months in male deer mice maintained in short days from birth; however, cohabitation with an adult female resulted in a substantial maturation of the testes and seminal vesicles (Whitsett and Lawton, 1982). The neuroendocrine mechanisms that mediate positive masking by cues from conspecifics have not been investigated.

Nocturnal melatonin rhythms were comparable in photoperiod-responsive and nonresponsive deer mice. It is therefore unlikely that differences in pineal melatonin synthesis or secretion acount for differences in reproductive responsiveness to short days (Blank *et al.*, 1988; Ruf *et al.*, 1997). Deer mice that vary in reproductive responsiveness to short days do, however, differ in responsiveness to melatonin. Spermatogenesis was suppressed by melatonin implants in photoresponsive deer mice, but the same treatment was ineffective in photoperiod nonresponders (Blank and Freeman, 1991). Identical patterns of pineal melatonin secretion in short days produce different effects in the two types of animals; this suggests that target tissues downstream from the pineal gland respond differently to melatonin signals in responsive and nonresponsive individuals (Blank and Freeman, 1991).

Differences in the GnRH-ir neuronal system are also associated with divergent reproductive responses to short days (Korytko *et al.*, 1995). Deer mice that undergo gonadal regression in short days exhibited increases in the number, area, or optical density of GnRH-ir neurons in the anterior hypothalamus (AH), diagonal band of Broca (DBB), lateral hypothalamus, POA, and MBH. In nonresponders, some brain regions (e.g., the lateral POA) adopted a short-day GnRH-ir phenotype, whereas others (e.g., the lateral hypothalamus) remained unaffected by short photoperiods and maintained the long-day GnRH-ir phenotype; still other regions (e.g., DBB and MPOA) manifested a GnRH-ir pattern that resembled neither the long-day nor short-day pattern (Korytko *et al.*, 1995). Furthermore, increases in GnRH accumulation under short days were steroid-dependent in some brain regions (Korytko *et al.*, 1997, 1998). In nonresponder deer mice some short-day information apparently is lost at the level of hypothalamic GnRH neurons and may reflect failure to respond to normally inhibitory melatonin signals; other GnRH neurons adopt a normal short-day phenotype in reproductively nonresponsive deer mice (Korytko *et al.*, 1995), pointing to a complex interaction between melatonin and GnRH subpopulations.

The pattern of GnRH-ir in nonresponders suggests that subpopulations of GnRH neurons in the AH, lateral hypothalamus, and MBH mediate short-day reproductive responses; the phenotype of these GnRH neurons was comparable in short-day nonresponders and long-day mice (Korytko et al., 1995). Because the response of these GnRH neurons differs between short-day responders and nonresponders, some short-day information either is lost or has deteriorated prior to or at the level of GnRH neurons; whether these changes are sufficient to mediate reproductive nonresponsiveness to day length or signals downstream in the hypothalamic-pituitary-gonadal axis are also implicated awaits further analyses.

Photoperiod nonresponsiveness in deer mice is trait-specific. In short days, decreases in plasma PRL concentrations are comparable in reproductively responsive and nonresponsive mice (Blank and Desjardins, 1986); this is also the case in female prairie voles (Smale et al., 1985). Thus, short-day signals sufficient to modulate some photoperiodic traits are transmitted to the pituitary gland, even as others retain the long-day phenotype. It is therefore more appropriate to designate specific traits, rather than individual animals, as nonresponsive to short day lengths (Nelson, 1987; Zucker, 1988).

2. Siberian Hamsters (Phodopus sungorus)

Genetic factors strongly influence responsiveness to day length in Siberian hamsters. The first bidirectional selection experiments conducted by Lynch and colleagues yielded inbred strains of nonresponder Siberian hamsters in which four generations of selection against responsiveness to short days resulted in >90% nonresponsiveness to short days (Lynch et al., 1989; Kliman and Lynch, 1992). Across several experiments, estimates of heritability ranged from $h^2 = 0.20$ to $h^2 = 0.52$ (moderate to strong; Lynch et al., 1989; Kliman and Lynch, 1992). It appeared that selection acted primarily on the period (τ) of the circadian pacemaker (Puchalski and Lynch, 1994; Freeman and Goldman, 1997a,b). Nocturnal photoperiodic rodents typically expand the duration of nightly locomotor activity (α) on transfer from long to short days. The duration of α is proportional to the duration of nightly melatonin secretion, both consequences of the entrained phase of the circadian pacemaker (Elliott and Tamarkin, 1994). Hamsters with large (>24 hr) values of τ were reproductively nonresponsive to short days; their pattern of circadian entrainment was characterized by a compressed α under short photoperiods (Fig. 13) (Puchalski and Lynch, 1986; Freeman and Goldman, 1997a). The short-duration (6 hr/night) melatonin secretory pattern associated with a compressed α is incompatible with testicular regression in this species (Goldman et al., 1984; Bartness et al., 1993).

The short-day signal transduction pathway is altered at the level of the circadian clock in the SCN of genetic nonresponders (Margraf et al., 1991). Consequently, these animals do not exhibit the normal short-day pattern of entrainment of circadian rhythms (Puchalski and Lynch, 1988). Unlike photoresponsive conspecifics, they generate a melatonin signal in short day lengths that differs little from the normal long-day pattern. In terms of circadian time (CT), the onset of subjective night (CT12) is phase delayed by at least 4–6 hr, and circadian α and the duration of melatonin secretion are consequently truncated; these animals never register or encode their presence in short days. Nonresponsiveness is reversed either by manipulations of the circadian system early in life (Freeman and Goldman, 1997b) or by prolonged exposure to continuous darkness in adulthood (Freeman and Goldman, 1997a). Each of these treatments recalibrates the circadian system and results in an expansion of α and a corresponding expansion of nightly melatonin secretion (Freeman and Goldman, 1997a). Photoperiod-nonresponsive Siberian hamsters were reproductively responsive to exogenous short-day-like melatonin treatments; this suggests that components of the reproductive axis downstream of the pineal gland function normally in these morphs (Puchalski and Lynch, 1988).

Nonresponsiveness to short days can also be induced in otherwise responsive individuals by appropriately timed photoperiod manipulations. In >85% of hamsters, exposure to long day lengths (e.g., 18L) for 10 weeks prevented α from expanding on subsequent exposure to short days (Fig. 13). It was inferred that a compressed pattern of nocturnal melatonin secretion in these animals is incompatible with the regression of the reproductive apparatus under short photoperiods (Gorman and Zucker, 1997; Prendergast and Freeman, 1999). Environmentally induced nonresponsiveness is qualitatively similar to genetic nonresponsiveness

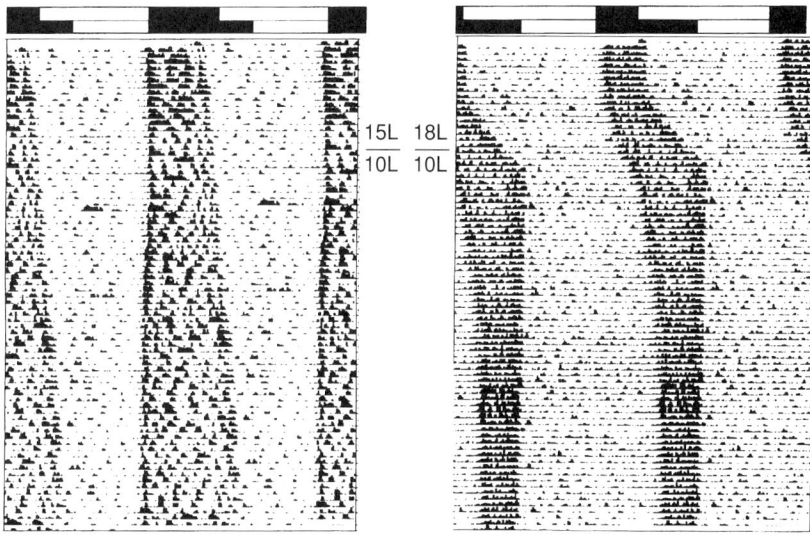

FIGURE 13 Double-plotted circadian locomotor activity rhythms of a photoresponsive (left) and nonresponsive (right) male Siberian hamster housed in a short day photoperiod (10L:14D) beginning on the day 7 of the record. The responsive hamster was previously housed in 15L:9D, whereas the nonresponsive hamster had been kept in 18L:6D. Black and white bars at the top of the figures indicate times of dark and light phases, respectively. The upper and lower bars represent the initial and final photoperiod conditions, respectively. From Prendergast and Freeman (1999).

in that α remains compressed in short day lengths. The mechanisms by which the circadian system is transformed by an episode of 18L so as to render hamsters unresponsive to short days remain unknown. Environmental induction of nonresponsiveness may reflect changes in coupling strength among circadian oscillators induced during the 18L treatment (Gorman and Zucker, 1997).

Environmental induction of nonresponsiveness by very long day lengths may be functionally significant in the wild. Siberian hamsters that attain reproductive competence prior to the summer solstice are unlikely to survive the winter or live to breed again in the following summer. A failure to respond to short days with reproductive inhibition may constitute a go-for-broke strategy that sometimes permits successful breeding during milder than normal winters or if animals have access to adequate food resources (Gorman and Zucker, 1997). The existence of long-day-induced nonresponsiveness in other short-lived photoperiodic rodent species (e.g., *Peromyscus* sp.) would buttress such a functional account, as would data on successful rearing of winter-born young during mild winters.

In several rodent species, social cues influence reproductive responses to short days (Whitsett and Lawton, 1982). Long-day male hamsters failed to undergo gonadal regression when paired with a reproductively active long-day female on the day of transfer to short days (Hegstrom and Breedlove, 1999a). On the assumption that these males have normal short-day patterns of melatonin secretion, it appears that contact with fecund heterosexual conspecifics masks the inhibitory effects of long-duration melatonin signals. This form of nonresponsiveness operates differently from the one previously described in that responsiveness to an otherwise inhibitory melatonin signal is changed.

Advanced age also may increase the likelihood of nonresponsiveness to short days. After approximately 1 year of age, most male hamsters failed to undergo gonadal regression when exposed to short days (Bernard *et al.*, 1997). In this study, hamsters were housed in alternating cycles of 16L and 6L; thus, advanced age was conflated with increased duration of exposure to long photoperiods, as well as intermittent episodes of exposure to short days, both of which are known to induce nonresponsiveness to short days (Gorman and Zucker, 1997; Prendergast et al., 2000).

C. Nonreproductive Traits in Photoperiod Nonresponders

Short-day responses of photoperiodic Siberian hamsters include several energy-saving adaptations such as decreased body weight (Hoffmann, 1982), fur molt (Duncan and Goldman, 1984), increased nest construction, daily torpor (Puchalski et al., 1988; Ruf and Heldmaier, 1992), and decreased food intake and burrowing activity (Puchalski et al., 1988; Fine and Bartness, 1996). Siberian hamsters, in common with other daily heterotherms, continue to forage throughout the winter; bouts of torpor permit a savings of approximately 20% in daily energy expenditure (Ruf and Heldmaier, 1992). Few studies have assessed the status of nonreproductive traits in animals that failed to undergo regression of the reproductive apparatus in short days. Exposure to low ambient temperatures (T_a; 10°C) and short days suppressed burrowing and increased nest-building activity in reproductively responsive Siberian hamsters, but nonresponder hamsters did not exhibit these thermoregulatory adaptations (Puchalski et al., 1988). Concomitant exposure to low T_a (5°C), however, decreased the incidence of reproductive nonresponsiveness to short days (Larkin et al., 2001).

Reproductive nonresponder prairie voles maintained in short days at 22°C did not differ from responders in food intake, basal metabolic rate (BMR), capacity for nonshivering thermogenesis, or collection of nesting material (Moffatt et al., 1993). Thus, energetic traits and reproduction responded differently to short day lengths. A similar pattern of results was observed in responder and nonresponder deer mice, except that nonresponder deer mice exhibited a long-day pattern of nest building in short days (Moffatt et al., 1993). The maintenance of long-day reproductive function and short-day metabolic adaptations are not incompatible. The coexistence of several short-day traits with reproductive nonresponsiveness suggests that the former may be controlled by photoperiodic signals other than melatonin; alternatively, if such traits are indeed controlled by melatonin, then the melatonin signal transduction pathways that are disabled or overridden in the reproductive axis of nonresponders remain functional in other physiological systems.

When nonresponders are exposed to challenging environmental conditions, the energetic costs associated with reproductive nonresponsiveness become apparent. Nonresponder deer mice did not decrease their body weight in short days (Ruf et al., 1997), an adaptation that normally lowers the cost of thermoregulation (Dark and Zucker, 1985, 1986b); consequently, nonresponder deer mice ate more food under simulated winter conditions. Unlike prairie voles, nonresponder deer mice failed to develop a short-day behavioral-energetic phenotype. This is energetically costly—in short days at 5°C, daily energy requirements were reduced by 13% in photoresponsive males, compared to an increase of 8% in nonresponsive animals (Ruf et al., 1997). Under simulated winter conditions, individuals with a propensity for reproductive nonresponsiveness to short day lengths may become responsive when additional winter cues (decreased food availability and low ambient temperature) are present (Kriegsfeld et al., 2000; Larkin et al., 2001).

D. Summary

Photoperiod, which by itself confers no fitness benefits, serves as a nearly noise-free proximate cue that is highly predictive of seasonal changes in biotic and abiotic factors that impinge on reproduction (Goldman and Nelson, 1993). Photoperiodic control of reproduction is thus an adaptive response to the challenges of a seasonally changing environment. Populations of photoperiodic rodents contain a substantial proportion of individuals that do not adopt a photoperiodic breeding strategy and instead ignore inhibitory day-length signals. Presumably, in nature these individuals mate and attempt to rear young during the energetically unfavorable winter months. Although animals that breed continuously may have higher direct fitness than those that only breed seasonally, animals whose offspring do not survive to maturity achieve no reproductive success and may even lose residual reproductive value (Clutton-Brock, 1991). Maternal energetic constraints in female nonresponders have yet to receive experimental attention, but may ultimately dictate the fitness associated with winter breeding on a year-to-year basis.

The mechanisms by which the reproductive neuroendocrine system fails to respond to short-day signals vary substantially among rodent species. Comparative studies of nonresponsiveness indicate that pre- vs postpineal-based mechanisms are critical to understanding species differences in the mediation of nonresponsiveness. In deer mice, a global short-day signal emanates from the pineal gland and is subsequently disregarded by some behavioral and physiological effector systems; short-day responses can occur or not occur independently in the same organism. In Siberian hamsters, no such signal escapes the pineal.

VIII. SEASONAL RHYTHMS IN PRIMATES

A. Nonhuman Primates

With few exceptions, the proximate mechanisms for seasonal rhythms in nonhuman primates remain uncharted. Lindburg (1987) noted that discrete birth seasons have been conclusively established or are probable for some two dozen species of nonhuman primates. Other species, although they have birth peaks, produce some young at all times of year, and lorises, mangabeys, and Asian colobines have births evenly distributed throughout the year. This pattern reflects the dependence of primate reproduction on food availability in tropical forests. Van Schaik and colleagues (1993) noted that "tropical plants display nearly every possible phenological behavior from near continuous activity to repeated brief bursts, and from complete intraspecific synchrony to complete asynchrony" (p. 355) in leafing, flowering, and fruiting.

Prosimians are among the most seasonal of primates. In southwest Madagascar, lemurs (*Propithecus verreauxi*) give birth mainly between June and August. Although there is a lack of sexual dimorphism in body mass during most of the year, females undergo significantly greater reductions in body mass than males during the dry season of low food availability. This is critical because the female's body mass determines whether she will give birth the following season (Richard *et al.*, 2000).

The lesser mouse lemur (*Microcebus murinus*), a small nocturnal prosimian, generates robust seasonal variations in blood testosterone concentrations reminiscent of those of many nocturnal rodents—blood values are high in males kept in long day lengths and low in those kept in short days (Perret, 1992). The timing of puberty also is controlled by day length. The social environment alters the sexual activity of males housed in heterosexual groups such that behavioral and physiological indices of reproductive competence are depressed in all but the dominant male by cues emanating from the urine of this individual (Perret, 1992). A masking effect of hormones, linked to adrenocortical activity, overrides the photoperiodic mechanism that otherwise controls reproduction (Perret, 1992).

After 14 weeks in long day lengths, during which male mouse lemurs sustain high testosterone concentrations, androgen secretion diminishes and gonadal regression is completed 6 weeks later. Transfer to short days or maintenance in long days at this time sustains reproductive quiescence for several weeks, but after a fixed interval testicular recrudescence ensues in either photoperiod (Perret and Schilling, 1993). This sequence of events is suggestive of a Type II reproductive cycle.

The longevity of lesser mouse lemurs may be determined by the number of seasonal cycles. Lemurs exposed to an accelerated annual photoregimen that alternated 5 months of long days with 3 months of short days (i.e., an 8-month year) had a life span of 45.5 months compared to 63.2 months for lemurs kept in a 12-month photocycle. Maximum life span also was reduced in the first group (Perret, 1997). The 30% reduction in longevity is not due to desynchronization of reproductive rhythms or time spent in the active mode; the expression of a fixed number of seasonal cycles rather than chronological age per se may determine longevity (Perret, 1997).

Among new world primates, squirrel monkeys (*Saimiri sciureus*) are highly seasonal, with births restricted to a 3–5 month interval each year. In a captive colony exposed to natural day length variations in California, 87% of births were recorded between May and September (Kaplan, 1977). Squirrel monkeys housed indoors for 3 years in a 14L photoperiod sustained marked annual rhythms; full-term pregnancies usually terminated in the months of August–October. Striking annual body mass rhythms and variations in testicular size also persisted under constant conditions (Clewe, 1969). These rhythms may be generated by a

Type II circannual mechanism, but a firm conclusion is not possible in the absence of data from individual animals.

The presence of multiple females in a captive colony of squirrel monkeys facilitated reproduction in both sexes (Schiml et al., 1996), but the suggestion that seasonality in male primates is contingent on exposure to females is not supported by other studies of squirrel monkeys (Schiml et al., 1999) and rhesus monkeys (Herndon et al., 1996). Other New World primates, such as howler and spider monkeys, breed throughout the year (Lindburg, 1987).

The rhesus macaque (*Macaca mulatta*) is perhaps the best exemplar of seasonality among Old World monkeys. Long the monkey of choice in laboratory studies of behavior and endocrinology, this species has contributed disproportionately to assessments of seasonality in Old World primates. In the field in India at latitudes between 24 and 31°N, approximately 80% of rhesus births occur between March and May and none between November and March (reviewed by Lindburg, 1987). The endogenous nature of rhesus reproductive rhythms was suggested by the observation that clear seasonal rhythms in plasma testosterone secretion persisted in males housed in a 14L photoperiod for up to 3 years (Fig. 14) (Plant et al., 1974; Michael and Bonsall, 1977). The rhythm appears to free-run with a period of approximately 13 months (Michael and Bonsall, 1977). Individually housed male rhesus monkeys that were maintained in a 13-hr day length for 14 months generated clear rhythms in serum concentrations of PRL, LH, and testosterone, but not FSH (Beck and Wuttke, 1979). The absence of interindividual synchrony in the timing of PRL peaks suggests that the rhythms were free-running, each with its characteristic endogenous period; this again suggests a Type II circannual organization. In the most comprehensive study, males were kept for up to 4 years in a constant laboratory environment with no apparent changes in the LD cycle, humidity, or temperature. Marked circannual variations in spermatogenesis, testicular volume, spontaneous and provoked ejaculations, and sperm output were noted, with maximal values in the autumn and winter, corresponding to the time of the mating season in the natural habitat (Wicklings and Nieschlag, 1980). Comparable data are lacking for females maintained for several years in unvarying environmental conditions, although Riesen and colleagues (1971) established that female rhesus monkeys sustain seasonal anovulatory rhythms when housed for several years in a fixed 13-hr day length.

Changes in day length are sufficient to entrain the annual rhythms of rhesus monkeys. Males housed indoors and exposed to alternating 16-week cycles of 16L and 8L, manifested reproductive rhythms with a period of 31 ± 1.3 weeks; there was no evidence of 52-week periodicity in testis growth, plasma testosterone, or PRL concentrations. Day-length variation is also posited as the proximate synchronizer of rhythms of testosterone, dihydrotestosterone, frequencies of mounts and ejaculations, number of female partners, courtship displays, and aggression in Japanese macaques (*Macaca fuscata*) (Rostal et al., 1986). On the other hand, there was no systematic evidence of seasonal rhythms in testis size,

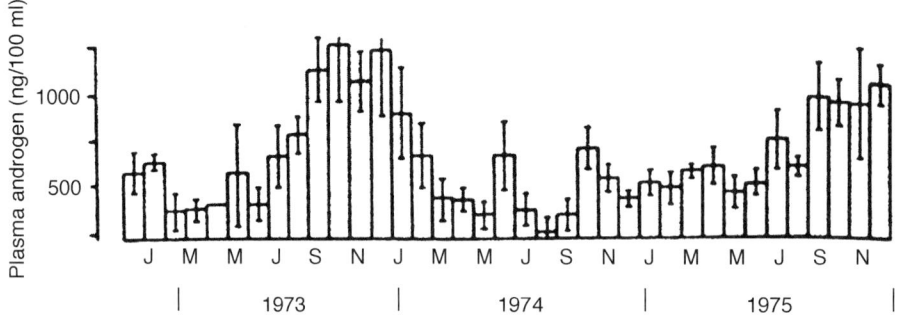

FIGURE 14 Annual changes in plasma androgen concentrations in a male rhesus monkeys maintained in the laboratory in constant photoperiod and temperature. From Michael and Bonsall (1977).

plasma testosterone concentrations, copulation, masturbation, aggression, or body mass, although seasonality in grooming and branch shaking were evident among a mixed-sex group of stump-tailed macaques (*Macaca arctoides*) exposed to natural variations of day length in the Netherlands (Nieuwenhuijsen *et al.*, 1987).

The physiological mechanisms that mediate seasonality in female primates have been assessed most thoroughly in rhesus monkeys. Analyses by Wilson, Gordon, and colleagues, confirmed that ovulation was restricted to the months of August–March in a group housed outdoors in Atlanta, GA (cf. Riesen *et al.*, 1971) and that estradiol failed to induce gonadotropin surges during the summer months at a time when endogenous concentrations of gonadotropins and ovarian steroids are low (Riesen *et al.*, 1971). Estradiol lowered basal LH concentrations to a greater extent in ovariectomized females treated during the summer anovulatory season than during the fall–winter season, during which ovulation ordinarily occurs. As in hamsters and sheep, the negative feedback sensitivity of gonadotropin secretion to steroid hormones increases during the nonbreeding season. As is also true for hamsters, squirrels, and sheep, steroid-independent seasonal regulation of gonadotropin secretion operates in rhesus females— untreated ovariectomized females generated LH pulses with a lower frequency in summer than fall (Wilson *et al.*, 1987).

Behavioral responsiveness to estradiol also varies seasonally in rhesus macaques. Ovariectomized females treated with estradiol engaged in heterosexual behavior during the breeding season but not during the nonbreeding season (Fig. 15). Estradiol treatment did provoke homosexual behavior in females during both treatment intervals (Pope *et al.*, 1987). The duration of female proximity to males was influenced by season, but not by estradiol, and the percentage of time spent with non-kin was increased by estradiol, regardless of the time of year. Females were not attracted to males during the nonbreeding season, as indicated by an absence of proceptive behavior; nor were males interested in females during this time of year, despite the induction of high out-of season testosterone secretion. Males as well as females may be refractory to behavioral actions of steroids during the nonbreeding season, as previously established for rodents (see Section III).

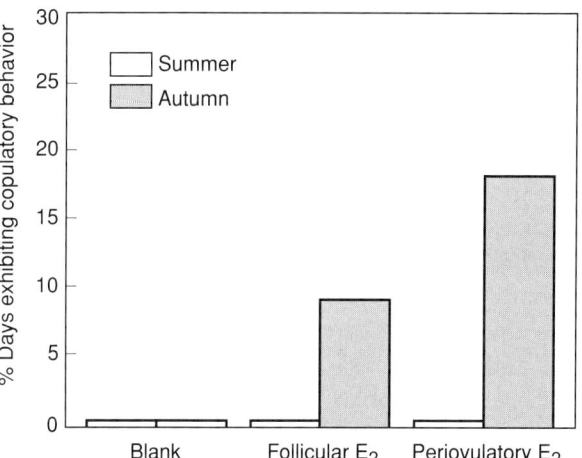

FIGURE 15 Percentage of observation days during the summer (May–July) and autumn (September–November) on which ovariectomized female rhesus monkeys treated with empty or estradiol-filled capsules engaged in copulatory behavior. Implants that mimicked late-follicular (100 pg/ml) and periovulatory (190 pg/ml) estradiol concentrations elicited copulatory behavior only during the autumn months. From Pope *et al.* (1987).

The females' reproductive state and history influence seasonality of ovulation. Young nulliparous and lactating female rhesus monkeys have a later onset and earlier termination of ovulatory cycles and thus a shorter ovulatory season than adult nonlactating females (Pope *et al.*, 1986). Lactation delays ovulation by 2–3 months in this species. Age and reproductive history interact to affect seasonality in female Japanese macaques. Three-year-old prepubertal females have low LH concentrations throughout the breeding season; 4 to 17-year-old females have elevated LH from September to January during exposure to natural day lengths in Japan. The most marked seasonal LH rhythms are observed in postmenopausal females and reflect decreased sensitivity to negative feedback inhibition by estradiol during the breeding season (Nozaki *et al.*, 1995).

There is little evidence for seasonality of reproduction among the apes (Lindburg, 1987; Watts, 1998). Savanna baboons at the equator in Kenya experience two rainy seasons with two intervening dry seasons each year, but display no significant birth seasonality; nor is the number of births per year significantly correlated with rainfall (Bercovitch and Harding, 1993). Birth seasonality has not been reported for this species at any locale in Africa. A month by month analysis of free-ranging chimpanzees in Tanzania at 5°S reveals a random distribution of conceptions throughout the year for the years 1967–1978, whereas for the interval 1979–1990, 78% of conceptions occurred during the dry season. The reasons for the change over time are unknown and may simply reflect stochastic processes associated with small sample size or variations in food availability (Wallis, 1997).

Among mountain gorillas in Rwanda, the mean number of births per female varies little across months and conception is not dependent on monthly rainfall (Watts, 1998). Gorillas at this site feed on perennially available herbaceous vegetation, so seasonal shortages in food availability are not a factor; rainfall, however, is thought to contribute to seasonal patterns of mortality and respiratory infections (Watts, 1998).

Dietary diversity, the extent to which primates rely on specific food types and the readiness with which they switch between food items, may contribute to the evolution of seasonal rhythms in reproduction (e.g., Bercovitch and Harding, 1993; Jablonski et al., 2000). Dietary diversity ameliorates seasonal variations in the availability of particular food and may be a necessary but not sufficient condition for nonseasonal reproduction (Bercovitch and Harding, 1993; van Schaik et al., 1993).

As the foregoing analysis indicates, no single pattern of seasonality is discernable among the many nonhuman primates. Thus, noninvasive fecal hormone analysis of individual female hanuman langurs (*Presbytis entellus*) in Nepal indicated that ovulatory cycles and estrous behavior were restricted to the period July–October, during which most conceptions occurred (Ziegler et al., 2000). In contrast, Struhsaker (1997) found no evidence of a restricted birth season in any of five monkey species in a tropical rainforest in Kimbale. In some species, conception is associated with the presence of abundant food, and at the time of parturition both food availability and quality are at their worst (Ziegler et al., 2000). In other species, the opposite relation obtains (Struhsaker, 1997). The prevalence and usefulness of seasonality depends on local conditions.

B. Humans

Given humans' ability to buffer themselves from the environment, the number and diversity of human traits that vary seasonally is impressive. Depression, stroke, suicide, sudden infant death, cardiac arrest, infections, homicides, battering of women, rape, hip fractures among the newborn, multiple sclerosis, intracerebral hemorrhage, autism, and nonpathological functions such as breastfeeding, hormone secretion, food consumption, and energy expenditure are but a subset of human traits that vary seasonally. It is not unlikely that sensory and motor capacity and perhaps even cognitive function change on a seasonal basis. Given the prevalence of and interest in human seasonal rhythms, it is disappointing and surprising that the underlying mechanisms are essentially unknown.

The discussion that follows neglects descriptive accounts of human seasonal rhythms and focuses on historical and evolutionary trends that contribute to the amelioration of seasonality in our species. The perspective gained thereby may facilitate the understanding of contemporary human seasonal rhythms.

1. Evolution and Human Seasonality

Early hominids originated in Africa. The development of human-like attributes, such as increased bipedalism and hunting, coincided with a decline in global temperatures during the middle Pliocene and the emergence of mosaic habitats far more seasonal than previously (Foley, 1993). Earliest human-like fossils are found in a region that today is characterized by 4- to 10-month dry seasons, which may also have prevailed during the Pleistocene (Speth, 1987). The ability to contend with drought and the associated nutritional stress are considered key features in hominid evolution (Foley, 1993). The savanna occupied by our early ancestors was marked by striking seasonal variation in plant and animal resources. For extended periods each year, hunting and scavenging were unlikely to have provided adequate sustenance, in part because deterioration of grazing and browsing matter during drought renders the meat of game animals marginally nutritious (Stewart, 1994). Evidence from the late Pleistocene suggests that hominids relied heavily on fish when other foods were scarce or of low quality (Stewart, 1994). They may also have built up fat reserves to ameliorate seasonal food shortages (Speth, 1987).

Thermoregulatory stress from extreme winter conditions is thought to have limited the expansion of African hominids from tropical and warmer mid-latitudes to more temperate and boreal regions (Foley, 1993). Foley suggests that mid-Pleistocene hominids colonized warmer latitudes during times of relative warmth and probably went locally extinct with advent of colder climatic conditions. The European Neanderthals of approximately 200,000 years ago permanently occupied sites with temperature minima equivalent to those at present-day latitudes of 50–60°N. The nasal and facial morphology and changed limb-bone proportions of Neanderthals promoted cold tolerance. By contrast, the modern humans who subsequently displaced Neanderthals in these regions lacked such structural specializations (Potts, 1998). Modern humans, dating from 40,000–50,000 years ago, were able to colonize the entire Earth not by habitat-specific adaptations but by relying on increased cognitive and behavioral capacity, which necessarily presupposes increased brain development or cognitive function. The increased use of fire, improved weapons for hunting, language for communication, and animals skins for warmth all contributed to this development (Foley, 1993; Potts, 1998).

The past 18,000 years have seen some of the largest climatic changes in Earth's history (Webb, 1993) with large temperature changes in mid- to high latitudes accompanied by significant alterations in atmospheric circulation and moisture balance. The two principal causes are seasonal variations in insulation and the melting of the ice sheets. The heightened seasonality of northern hemispheric solar radiation from 12,000–6000 years ago increased the seasonality of northern hemispheric climates, bringing warmer summers and cooler winters (Kutzback and Webb, 1993). The development of agriculture some 12,000 years ago led to the eventual wordwide settlement of agrarian societies 8000–3000 years before present. During this time, the climate of Earth was highly variable compared to preceding and succeeding millennia (Sandweiss et al., 1999).

2. Human Seasonal Reproductive Rhythms

Environmental factors, not the least being food availability, contribute to seasonal variations in human births (Roenneberg and Aschoff, 1990a,b; Bronson, 1995). With rare exceptions, these rhythms pale in comparison to those of most mammals; peak to trough variations usually are in the range of 10–20%. Thus, reproduction occurs throughout the year and is not truly seasonal unless driven by food shortages or religious and cultural customs. Bronson (1995) concludes that there is little evidence that such rhythms that exist are generated by a circannual mechanism or are subject to photoperiodic regulation. The contention that cultural factors are more important than direct environmental signals (Bronson, 1995) is borne out by reports that the seasonality of first coitus is more pronounced among adolescents, 13–18 years old, than among those 19–25 years of age (Rodgers et al., 1992), that tax laws influence human birth times (Dickert-Conlin and Chandra, 1999), and that a taboo on sexual relations during the yam-growing season in one New Guinea society is associated with pronounced birth seasonality (Brewis et al., 1996).

Much evidence suggests that shortages in metabolic energy are sufficient to suppress reproduction in all mammals, with females far more sensitive than males and puberty the most sensitive part of the life cycle (Bronson, 1989; Bronson and Heideman, 1994). Shortages in energy impact the neuroendocrine mechanism that controls ovulation. Specifically, the GnRH pulse generator stops functioning when energy supplies are restricted or expenditures are very great, as in anorectic women or athletes (Bronson, 1995). Studies of subsistence foragers, agriculturists, and pastoralists suggest this mechanism impacts human reproduction (Bronson, 1995; Bentley, 1999). For example, the Ache people, contemporary hunter-gatherers in eastern Paraguay, do not practice horticulture and have little contact with outsiders. The scarce food period for these people is associated with lowest conception rates (Hill and Hurtado, 1996). Given that seasonal food shortages are common among rural populations throughout the world, it is little wonder that there are associated fluctuations in conception and birth peaks.

3. Melatonin and Human Reproduction

Humans, in common with all other mammals, secrete melatonin nearly exclusively at night, and exposure to light at night interrupts melatonin secretion (Wehr, 1997). In urban environments with artificial lighting, people differ in the extent to which the duration of nocturnal melatonin secretion corresponds to seasonal changes in day length (Wehr, 1997; Vondrasova et al.,

1997). For example, at latitudes of 35°, 39°, and 50°N, there were no seasonal differences in the duration of nocturnal melatonin secretion, even though day length varied from 8 to 16 hr (Vondrasova *et al.*, 1997). When exposure to artificial lighting was eliminated, nocturnal melatonin duration was 6 hours in summer and 8 hours in winter. Vondrasova and colleagues (1997) suggest that during the Middle Ages, when people worked the fields from dawn to dusk, summer vs winter melatonin durations may have differed by as many as 4 hours at 50°N. If this was so, then an uncoupling of melatonin secretion from gonadotropin regulatory mechanisms must have been in place for many centuries in *Homo sapiens*. Otherwise seasonal rhythms in human reproduction would be far more pronounced in preindustrial societies than is indicated by the historical record (Lummaa *et al.*, 1998). There is no convincing evidence for a functional relation of human reproduction and melatonin (Reiter, 1998).

Most human seasonal rhythms appear to be of the Type III variety and represent direct responses to environmental signals. Seasonal variations in viruses present at birth may account for the greater incidence of early adult onset of schizophrenia in individuals born in winter (Pulver *et al.*, 1983), just as changes in weather contribute to increased mortality from coronary disease (Kloner *et al.*, 1999). The consideration of these many rhythms is beyond our scope (see, e.g., Johnston, 1993).

4. What Can Animal Studies Tell Us about Human Seasonality?

Animal research provides a conceptual framework for the exegesis and manipulation of human seasonal rhythms. Lessons learned from research on rodents and monkeys raise the possibility that hormone treatments will be effective in modifying behavior at one but not another stage of the annual cycle. The demonstration that drugs and hormones phase-shift annual rhythms at some but not other stages of the annual cycle can open the way for rational drug treatments for human rhythm dysfunction. Limits to the usefulness of animal models are apparent, however, when we consider that the many social, religious, and cultural customs that influence human seasonality have no parallels in the animal kingdom.

IX. SEASONAL RHYTHMS IN NONREPRODUCTIVE TRAITS

A. Food Intake and Body Mass

Annual changes in day length regulate several components of energy balance, including adjustments in food intake and body mass, traditionally central in studies of hormone-brain-behavior interactions (Mercer, 1998). Individuals of several species of rodents undergo seasonal shifts in body mass. Sciurid rodents (e.g., squirrels and woodchucks) undergo a summer fattening prior to entering hibernation; increased adiposity provides a convenient energy store, as well as insulation (Davis, 1976; Dark *et al.*, 1992). During hibernation, fat stores are slowly oxidized to provide the energy essential for overwinter survival. The annual fluctuations of body mass in sciurid rodents are controlled by an endogenous circannual biological clock and persist for years, even when the animals are maintained in laboratories under constant environmental conditions (Barnes and York, 1990; Heller and Poulson, 1970; Mrosovsky, 1985). Synchronization of this cycle between individuals and entrainment to a period of 12 months is effected by changes in day length (Lee and Zucker, 1991).

In muroid rodents (e.g., deer mice, *Peromyscus* spp.; hamsters, *Mesocricetus* and *Phodopus* spp.; voles, *Microtus* spp.; and lemmings, *Dicrostonyx*, *Lemmus* spp.), body mass and food intake change during late summer and autumn in response to decreasing day lengths (Fig. 16) (Bartness and Wade, 1985; Loudon, 1994; Kriegsfeld and Nelson, 1996). Short days trigger an increase in body fat stores in Syrian hamsters without corresponding changes in food intake, suggesting that photoperiod affects metabolic pathways (Bartness and Wade, 1984). This does not exclude metabolic changes independent of changes in the activity of the gonadal axis. Collared lemmings (*Dicrostonyx groenlandicus*) also may increase body mass by as much as 50% when transferred from long to short photoperiods (Nagy, 1993).

Prairie voles (*M. ochrogaster*) increase body mass in short days (Kriegsfeld and Nelson, 1996), the increase being greater in gonadectomized than intact males. Body mass also increased at a greater rate in short than in long day lengths in intact and ovariectomized females. Thus in both sexes, photoperiod affects body

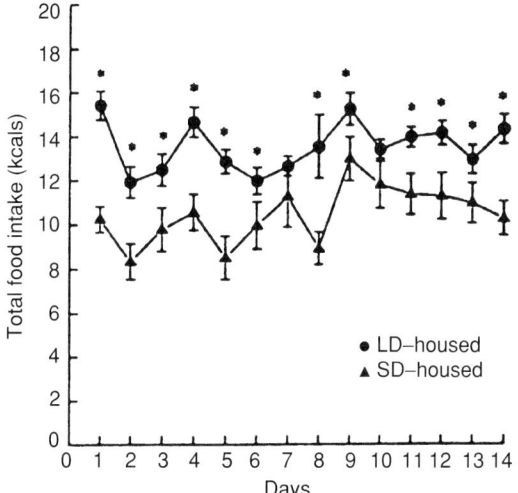

FIGURE 16 Daily food intake in adult male Siberian hamsters over the course of 14 days beginning 10 weeks after transfer to long or short days. Asterisks indicate values that differ from those of SD-housed animals. From Fine and Bartness (1996).

mass via both steroid-dependent and -independent mechanisms (Kriegsfeld and Nelson, 1996).

Other muroid species undergo a regulated decrease in body mass in anticipation of winter. Lowered body mass results in a greater surface-to-volume ratio, increased heat loss to the environment, and decreased insulation, but these effects apparently are more than compensated for by the reduced energy requirements of a smaller body mass (Dark and Zucker, 1985). Reductions in foraging time and concomitant exposure to unfavorable climatic conditions presumably enhance survival. Meadow voles are representative of several species that decrease their food intake before body mass declines in short day lengths; in contrast, the decrease in body mass precedes the reduction in food intake in Siberian hamsters (Bartness and Wade, 1985; Dark and Zucker, 1983; Dark et al., 1983b). Short day lengths also reduce body mass in Siberian and Djungarian hamsters (Phodopus sp.) (Bartness and Wade, 1985; Mercer et al., 1994), deer mice (Ruf et al., 1997), European hamsters (Cricetus cricetus), and several vole species (Dark and Zucker, 1985).

Part of the loss in body mass is a consequence of reductions in circulating blood plasma concentrations of gonadal steroid hormones, but a steroid-independent influence of day length on metabolism, mediated by melatonin, has been implicated in Siberian hamsters (Bartness and Wade, 1985). Male meadow voles (M. pennsylvanicus) typically eat less food and reduce body mass after castration (Dark and Zucker, 1984a), but individual voles vary markedly and lawfully in response to hormone withdrawal. Males of identical age vary in body mass from 35 g to >60 g, with virtually all of the variation due to differences in the amounts of white adipose tissue. Voles weighing >47 g lost mass, whereas those weighing <47 g gained mass after castration (Dark et al., 1987). Testosterone replacement reversed the effects of castration in the appropriate direction for the heavy and light males. The individual differences in body-fat content were not correlated with blood plasma testosterone concentrations but, rather, appeared to reflect differences in target tissue responsiveness to androgens (Dark et al., 1987).

The hormone leptin, produced by adipose tissue, influences seasonal body mass regulation as well as reproductive and immune function (Campfield et al., 1995; Finck et al., 1998; Schneider et al., 2000; Takahashi et al., 1999). Leptin gene expression in white adipose tissue (WAT) and brown adipose tissue (BAT) of Siberian hamsters was markedly decreased with acclimatization during winter, independently of changes in ambient temperature, and largely in response to shorter day lengths (Klingenspor et al., 1996). Siberian hamsters treated with murine recombinant leptin for 10 days decreased food intake and body mass, the latter due to the depletion of body fat. The reduction in body-fat mass in response to leptin treatments was greater in short- than long-day animals, despite similar reductions in food intake (Klingenspor et al., 2000). Leptin may mediate seasonal changes in body mass that occur independently of changes in food intake (Klingenspor et al., 1996).

The relations among photoperiod, leptin, and steroid hormones are complex. Body mass, body-fat content, and serum leptin concentrations were correlated with reproductive responsiveness to photoperiod in Siberian hamsters; short-day animals with regressed gonads had reduced body-fat content and serum leptin concentrations, whereas short-day nonresponders resembled long-day animals with relatively high body-fat content and serum leptin concentrations (Drazen et al., 2000).

Body mass, percentage of body fat, and circulating leptin concentrations are higher during the summer than winter in both young and mature mares (Fitzgerald and McManus, 2000). The reproductive response to short photoperiods or an inhibitory melatonin signal is modified by energy availability, which may be signaled by leptin (Fitzgerald and McManus, 2000). Leptin may also mediate seasonal changes in body mass of rhesus monkeys (Mann *et al.*, 2000), sheep (Bocquier *et al.*, 1998), and little brown bats (*Myotis lucifugus*) (Widmaier *et al.*, 1997).

B. Stress Responses

Reduced food availability, in common with many other energetic challenges, is a potent stressor. The number and types of stressors vary seasonally (Breuner *et al.*, 1999). Many energetic adaptations apparently evolved to attenuate the stress response during winter; at this time energy shortages may limit animals' abilities to cope with stress. A comprehensive view of the mechanisms underlying the stress response requires the consideration of its temporal organization. The role of circadian fluctuations is outside the scope of this chapter; the subject has been well reviewed elsewhere (e.g., Wetterberg, 1999; Chrousos, 1998; Dallman *et al.*, 1993).

The primary endocrine components of the stress response involve epinepherine and the glucocorticoids, hormones that suppress energy storage and promote energy use from adipose and liver stores (Sapolsky *et al.*, 2000). Although a relatively steady supply of energy is required to sustain biological functions, daily and seasonal fluctuations occur in response to challenges animals face. Most animals eat discontinuously, storing and accessing energy to maintain cellular function while engaged in nonfeeding activities. Eventually, however, the depletion of energy stores requires replacement. In most habitats, food availability fluctuates on a daily and seasonal basis. For example, outside the tropics, food availability is generally low during the winter, whereas thermogenic energy demands are typically high. Consequently, energy intake and energy expenditures are often out of balance. A stress response in the form of secreted glucocorticoids ensues whenever a significant imbalance of energy is detected. The high energy demands associated with reproduction usually elicit stress responses (Nelson and Drazen, 1999). Thus, glucocorticoids are released during territorial defense or courtship behaviors. When energy is insufficient to support both reproduction and thermoregulation, a prolonged stress response can have pathological consequences (Sapolsky, 1998).

Glucocorticoids released in response to stressful stimuli can compromise cellular and humoral immune function, reproduction, digestion, growth, and virtually any process that consumes significant energy (Sapolsky *et al.*, 2000). A direct link between melatonin and glucocorticoid biology has been established (Gupta, 1990; Maestroni, 1993, 1995; Maestroni and Conti, 1990; Maier *et al.*, 1994). Generally, melatonin and glucocorticosteroids enhance and compromise, respectively, immune function (Aoyama *et al.*, 1986, 1987). Melatonin can ameliorate the immunocompromising effects of glucocorticosteroids (Persengiev *et al.*, 1991a,b), and glucocorticosteroids can reduce the immunoenhancing actions of melatonin (e.g., Poon *et al.*, 1994).

Environmental stressors elevate blood glucocorticoid concentrations, which in turn suppress immune function (Ader and Cohen, 1993; Baxter and Forsham, 1972; Besedovsky *et al.*, 1986; Black, 1994). As previously noted, low ambient temperatures are often stressful and can potentially compromise immune function (Claman, 1972; MacMurray *et al.*, 1983; Monjan, 1981). A positive balance between short-day enhanced immune status and glucocorticoid-induced immunosuppression may be essential for winter survival in small mammals (Nelson and Drazen, 1999; Sinclair and Lochmiller, 2000). Overcrowding, increased competition for scarce resources, low temperatures, reduced food availability, increased predator pressure, and lack of shelter may each contribute to immunosuppression. Each of these potential stressors may elevate blood concentrations of glucocorticoids. Winter breeding and the concomitant increase in sex-steroid-hormone secretion may also result in immunocompromise (Nelson and Demas, 1996; Lochmiller *et al.*, 1994; Sinclair and Lochmiller, 2000). Presumably, winter breeding occurs when normal challenges from environmental stressors such as low temperature and reduced food availability are ameliorated. The advantages of winter reproduction must be balanced against the increased risks of autoimmune disease and susceptibility to opportunistic pathogens and parasites associated with winter steroidogenesis. Thus, reproductive and immune function seem intertwined.

In general, studies of captive animals reveal an inverse relation between dominance and glucocorticoid concentrations. However, this may not be the case in the wild. After capture, animals generally increase the secretion of epinephrine and glucocorticoids, and blood concentrations of steroids are generally much higher at this time than several hours later (e.g., Licht *et al.*, 1983; Mahmoud and Licht, 1997; Mendonca and Licht, 1986; Orchinik *et al.*, 1988). The assay of glucocorticoid by-products in the urine or feces of freely behaving dwarf mongooses (*Helogale parvula*) and African wild dogs (*Lycos pictus*) suggests that high-ranking animals may be under high levels of social stress (Creel and Creel, 1996).

Seasonal variations in glucocorticoids are influenced by day length. Among Syrian hamsters, blood concentrations of glucocorticoids are lower in short than long day lengths (De Souza and Meier, 1987; Ottenweiler *et al.*, 1987). Decreased glucocorticoid concentrations in short days can derive from the suppression of adrenal corticosteroid synthesis (e.g., Mehdi and Sandor, 1976) or enhanced negative feedback inhibition of glucocorticoid secretion (Motta *et al.*, 1967, 1969). Glucocorticoid-sensitive hippocampal receptors, especially Type I, have been implicated in the negative feedback control of adrenal glucocorticoid secretion (e.g., Sapolsky *et al.*, 1984; Herman *et al.*, 1993; Fischette *et al.*, 1980). Changes in circulating glucocorticoid concentrations in short-day hamsters may be caused by alterations in hippocampal Type I binding, glucocorticoid receptor mRNA expression, or both (Ronchi *et al.*, 1998). Total hippocampal receptor binding was significantly elevated in short-day hamsters, compared to long-day hamsters, after 8 weeks of treatment regardless of gonadal-steroid status, primarily due to a significant increase in Type I receptor numbers in the former group. Type I receptor levels were also significantly elevated in the hypothalamus, but not in cortical tissues, of short-day animals (Ronchi *et al.*, 1998). Basal corticosterone and cortisol concentrations, gonadal mass, and testosterone concentrations did not differ between hamsters housed for 4 weeks in long days vs short days (Ronchi *et al.*, 1998). Corticosteroid concentrations were similarly elevated in both long- and short-day animals after 10 minutes of ether stress, but returned to baseline values after 60 minutes in short-day, but not long-day, hamsters (Fig. 17) (Ronchi *et al.*, 1998). Short day lengths reduce hypothalamo-pituitary-adrenal (HPA) reactivity to the ether stress; this effect is evident after 2 months of short-day exposure (Ronchi *et al.*, 1998). Short-day exposure likewise reduces the magnitude of the stress response elicited by exposure to low ambient temperatures (Fig. 17) (Demas and Nelson, 1996).

Indeed, after only 18 days of exposure, hippocampal mineralocorticoid-receptor mRNA expression was increased in short- compared to long-day hamsters (Lance *et al.*, 1998). Up-regulation of mRNA expression was associated with increased adrenal-gland mass in short days. The absence of changes in reproductive organ function or circulating glucocorticoid concentrations, suggests that the brain-adrenal axis responds relatively rapidly to changes in day length and may mediate short-day responses (Lance *et al.*, 1998).

There is a marked circadian rhythm in glucocorticoid secretion. Increased glucocorticoid release just prior to awakening each day elevates blood glucose concentrations in anticipation of the increased energy demands associated with wakefulness. On this basis, we might expect increased glucocorticoid secretion during the energetically demanding phases of the annual cycle that encompass territorial defense, migration, low temperatures, or food scarcity. Low ambient temperatures and decreased food availability indeed evoke stress responses in mammals (reviewed in Nelson and Demas, 1996). Individual differences in stress responses are common, however, and whether individuals are stressed by a change in a specific environmental variable is probably a complex function of individual and species differences (Mason, 1975).

C. Immune Function

Seasonal cycles of illness and death as well as birth are common among many mammalian populations (e.g., Bolinger *et al.*, 1996; Bradley *et al.*, 1980; Lochmiller *et al.*, 1994). Many stressful environmental conditions are seasonally recurrent, and animals may have evolved mechanisms to combat seasonal stress-induced reductions in immune function (Nelson and Drazen, 1999; Yellon *et al.*, 1999; Sinclair and Lochmiller, 2000). From evolutionary and ecological perspectives, it is plausible that fitness would be increased in individuals that

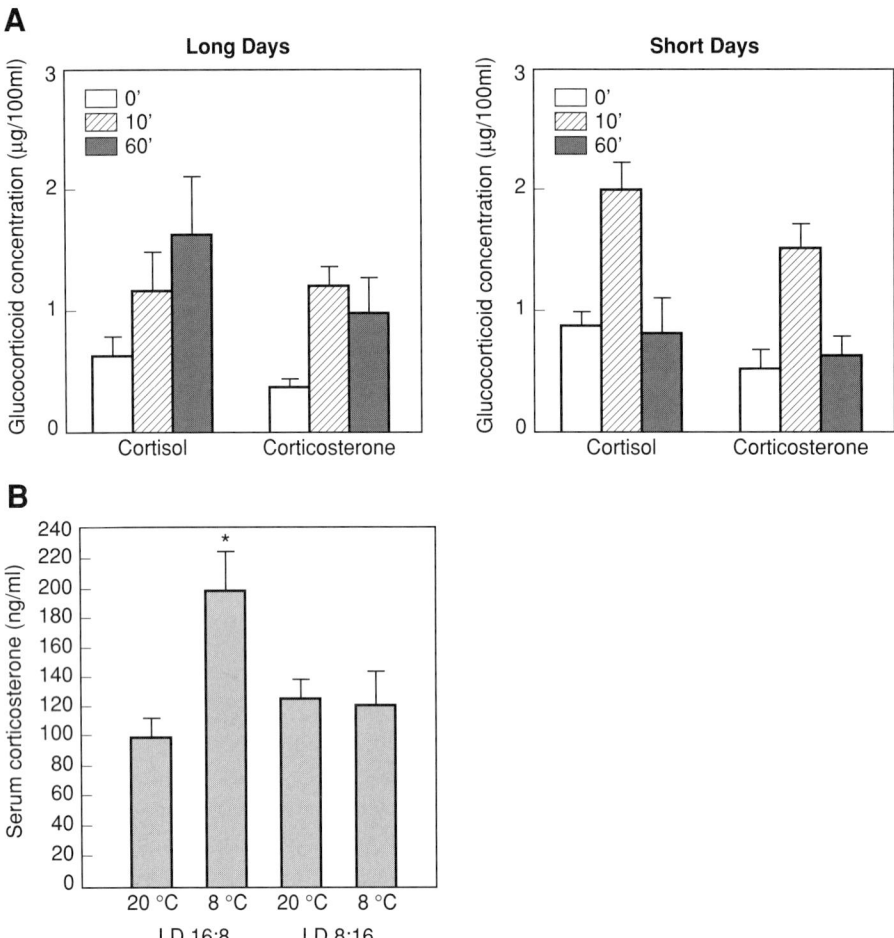

FIGURE 17 (A) Concentrations of serum cortisol before and 10 or 60 min after exposure to ether stress in long-term castrated male Syrian hamsters bearing testosterone implants and kept in either long or short days. One hour after exposure, circulating cortisol concentrations were still significantly elevated in long-day, but not short-day, hamsters. [From Ronchi et al. (1998), Brain Res. **780**, 348–351, copyright 1998, with permission from Elsevier Science.] (B) Corticosterone concentrations of male deer mice housed in long (16L:8D) or short (8L:16D) days at 20°C or 8°C for 10 weeks. Asterisk indicates value differs from that for all other groups. Short days ameliorated the glucocorticoid response to thermal stressors. [From Demas and Nelson (1996). J. Biol. Rhythms **11**, 94–102, ©1996 by Sage Publications. Reprinted by permission of Sage Publications, Inc.]

bolstered immune function in advance of seasonally recurring immunosuppression.

Several studies of laboratory-housed rodents document enhanced immune function in short day lengths (reviewed in Nelson and Demas, 1996; Nelson et al., 1995, 1998); many field studies also are consistent with enhanced immune function and decreased disease prevalence during winter as compared to summer. Several studies have, however, recorded the opposite pattern of results (Nelson and Demas, 1996; Nelson et al., 1995, 1998)—immune function compromised during the short days of winter. Additional environmental factors, not usually manipulated in laboratory studies, may account for the discrepancy. For example, winter-associated stressors such as restricted food availability and low ambient temperatures counteract the short-day enhancement of immune function in the laboratory (reviewed in Demas and Nelson, 1996). Thus, immune function should be enhanced and compromised during mild and severe winters, respectively.

Long-term field studies are required to test this hypothesis (see, e.g., Sinclair and Lochmiller, 2000). Although the effects of melatonin on immunity are well established (Caroleo et al., 1992; Giordano et al., 1993; Persengiev et al., 1991b; Pioli et al., 1993; Nelson et al., 2001), an understanding of how the ecological context affects immune function is necessary to appreciate that these actions of melatonin may be adaptive, rather than merely physiological oddities. Understanding seasonal fluctuations in immune function may help define the potential, as well as the constraints, of melatonin immunotherapy.

Mounting an immune response requires energy. The cascade of cellular events during the acute phase immune response and inflammation and the elevation of body temperature in response to cytokine activation presumably require substantial energy, although precise quantification is lacking (Henken and Brandsma, 1982; Maier et al., 1994; see later). Cytokine activation elevates body temperature and the energy requirements of inflammation and acute phase immune responses may increase metabolic rates by more than 10% for each degree of increase in body temperature (reviewed in Grimble, 1994). In house mice (*Mus musculus*), the injection of Keyhole Limpet Hemocyanin (KLH), a specific antigen that evokes an antibody response without inducing fever or symptoms of illness, resulted in increased oxygen consumption and metabolic heat production. Risk of infection and mortality increase in animals whose energy deficits impair the ability to sustain immunity.

Stress compromises immune function (see reviews by Ader and Cohen, 1993; Dunn, 1989; O'Leary, 1990; Maier and Watkins, 1999). Prolonged or severe food shortages may evoke the secretion of glucocorticoid hormones (Nakano et al., 1987); glucocorticosteroids actively compromise aspects of immune function (Kelley, 1985; Maier et al., 1994; Munck and Guyre, 1991; see later), possibly by shunting energy from immunological processes to other systems needed for coping with stress (Sapolsky, 1992).

1. Energetics and Immune Function

Maintaining optimal immune function is energetically expensive; the cascades of dividing immune cells, the onset and maintenance of inflamation and fever, and the production of humoral immune factors all require substantial energy (Demas et al., 1997b; Spurlock, 1997). Mounting an immune response probably requires resources that could otherwise be allocated to other functions (Sheldon and Verhulst, 1996). Thus, it is reasonable to consider immune function from an ultimate perspective of energetic trade-offs. Individuals may optimize immune function, and allocate energetic resources among the costs of immune function and other maintenance or reproductive functions. Seasonal changes in immune function are consistent with this energetic perspective and are probably driven by seasonal changes in energy requirements and availability (Nelson and Demas, 1996). According to this hypothesis, animals maintain the highest level of immune function that is energetically possible (without evoking autoimmune diseases) given the constraints of other survival needs, growth, and reproduction in an environment where energy needs and demands continuously fluctuate. A complete understanding of seasonal cycles in human immune function requires the consideration of how energetic and other stressors impinge on immunocompetence. Animal models illustrate these relations.

Among domesticated animals reduced food intake is associated with compromised immune function (reviewed in Spurlock, 1997). For example, pro-inflammatory cytokines, particularly interleukin-1 (IL-1), IL-6, and tumor necrosis factor (TNF), interrupt anabolic processes and alter nutrient uptake and use (e.g., Grimble, 1994; Johnson, 1997). These cytokines may also cause the release of glucocorticoids, catecholamines, and prostaglandins, each of which can modulate metabolism and immune function. Although pro-inflammatory cytokines are critical in the responses to infection, an excess of cytokines can damage tissue and even lead to death. Excess or inappropriate secretion of cytokines has been linked to morbidity in malaria, sepsis, meningitis, inflammatory bowel disease, and rheumatoid arthritis (Beutler and Cerami, 1988; Waage et al., 1989; Kelley and Dantzer, 1990). Consequently, a balanced release of cytokines must be achieved for maximal effectiveness in protecting the host from infection.

Decreases in ambient temperature impinge on an individual's energy budget. Day length and ambient temperature interact to affect immune function. In deer mice maintained in long or short photoperiods

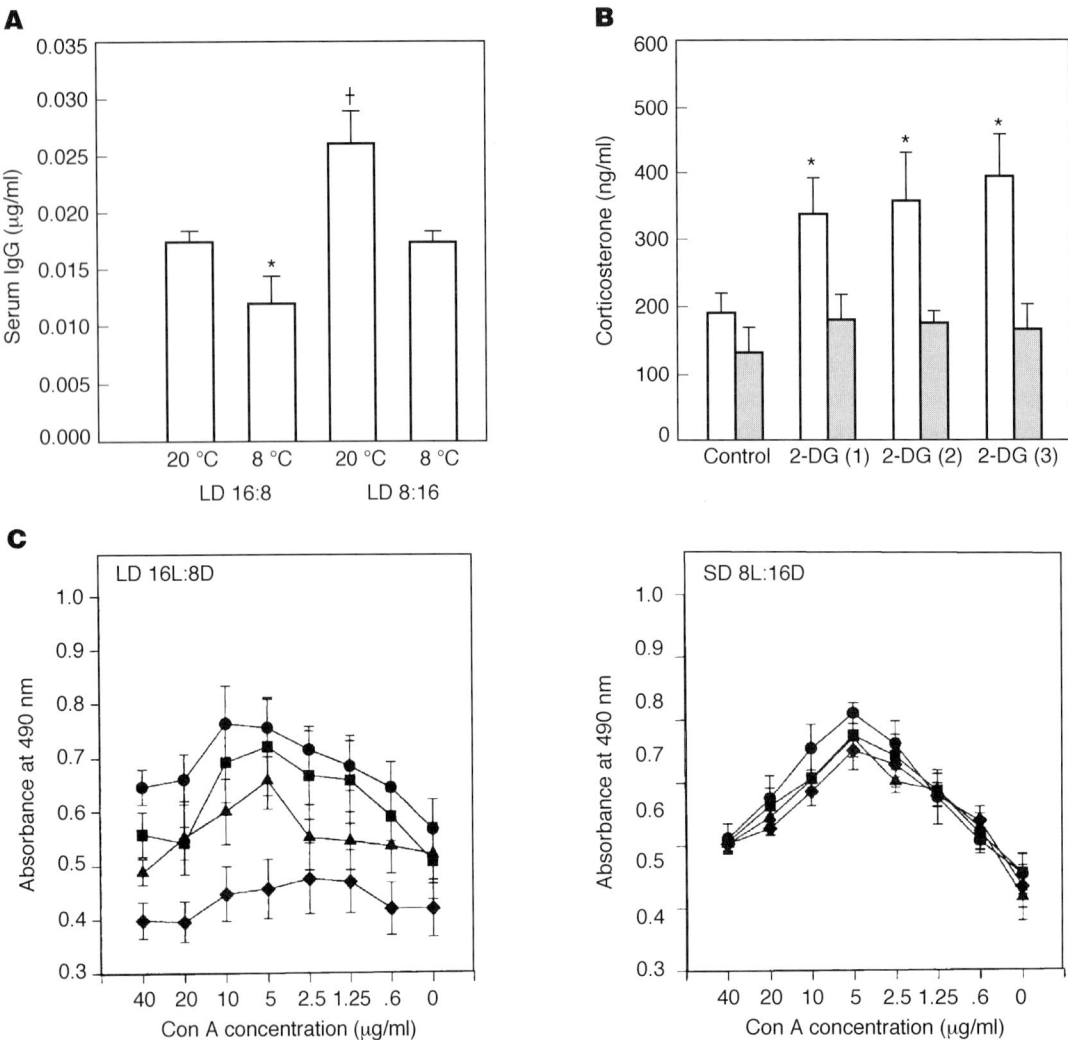

FIGURE 18 Effects of photoperiod on stress and immune responses. (A) Mean total serum IgG of male deer mice housed in long (16L:8D) or short (8L:16D) days at 20°C or 8°C for 10 weeks. Humoral immunity (antibody production) was impaired by low temperatures in both long- and short-day deer mice, but this effect was ameliorated by enhanced baseline (20°C) immunity in short-day deer mice. Symbols indicate values that differ from the long-day 20°C group. (B) Corticosterone concentrations of male deer mice housed in long (open bars) or short (dark bars) days 24 hr after treatment with 0 (control), 1, 2, or 3 consecutive daily injections of 2-deoxy-D-glucose (2-DG; 750 mg/kg). Short-day deer mice ameliorated the glucocorticoid response to glucoprivic stress. Asterisk indicates value differs from that for corresponding short-day group. (C) Splenic lymphocyte proliferative responses to a T-cell mitogen, concanavalin A (ConA; in absorbance units) of male deer mice housed in either long (left panel) or short (right panel) day lengths and treated with saline (diamonds) or 2-DG for 1 (triangles), 2 (squares), or 3 (circles) consecutive days. From Demas and Nelson (1996); Demas et al. (1997a).

at 20°C temperatures, serum immunoglobulin G (IgG) concentrations were elevated in short-day, as compared to long-day, mice (Fig. 18A). The increased nonspecific IgG concentrations may indicate increased infection or could reflect increased immunosurveillance. Because sentinel mice housed in the same rooms were pathogen-free, it was surmised that increased IgG concentrations reflected increased immunosurveillance, not infection (Demas and Nelson, 1996). At 8°C, long-day deer mice had reduced IgG concentrations and short-day animals had IgG concentrations comparable to those of long-day mice at 20°C; IgG concentrations were higher in short-day than in long-day mice, and low temperatures significantly reduced IgG concentrations. Short day lengths and low temperatures produce the opposite effects on IgG concentrations, in essence restoring the values to those of long-day animals, which may help animals cope with the seasonal stress of winter and ultimately increase reproductive fitness (Fig. 18A) (Demas and Nelson, 1996).

The role of energy availability in seasonal changes in immune function was assessed in deer mice administered 2-deoxy-D-glucose (2-DG), a glucose analog that inhibits cellular use of glucose, thus inducing a state of glucoprivation (Wick *et al.*, 1957). 2-DG is a metabolic stressor, increasing serum corticosterone concentrations in male rats (Weidenfeld *et al.*, 1984). The administration of 2-DG inhibits murine splenic T-lymphocyte proliferation in a dose-dependent fashion in laboratory mice (Miller *et al.*, 1994). Short day lengths buffered deer mice against glucoprivic stress. In long day lengths, corticosterone concentrations were elevated in mice injected with 2-DG vs saline; this effect was not evident in short days (Fig. 18B) (Demas *et al.*, 1997a). The muted response in short days may reflect an adjustment in the negative feedback of glucocorticoids on the HPA axis, an action analogous to the enhancement of negative feedback of the hypothalamic-pituitary-gonadal (HPG) axis of rodents housed in short days (Ellis and Turek, 1980). In terms of immune function, 2-DG was associated with reduced splenocyte proliferation to ConA in long-day mice. Splenocyte proliferation did not differ among short-day deer mice regardless of experimental treatment; short-day animals exhibited enhanced immune function and, in response to 2-DG treatment, splenocyte proliferation was higher in short- than long-day mice (Fig. 18C; Demas *et al.*, 1997a).

These data suggest that short day lengths buffer animals against metabolic stress. Reduced corticosterone concentrations in animals maintained on short days or treated with melatonin are probably a consequence of improved metabolic function (Nelson and Demas, 1996; Sinclair and Lochmiller, 2000). Accordingly, enhanced immune function in short days is one component of the winter adaptation mediated by melatonin. The expectation is that natural perturbations of energy associated with pregnancy, lactation, torpor, and hibernation affect immune function in predictable directions (Lochmiller and Deerenberg, 2000).

D. Social Organization: Affiliation and Aggression

In many rodent species, there is a shift from highly territorial asocial behavior during the breeding season to a social, highly interactive existence during winter. These species typically undergo reproductive quiescence at the end of the breeding season in response to short days; the resulting decrease in androgen secretion may be necessary for and permissive of the seasonal shift in sociality, but in wood rats (*Neotoma fuscipes*) nonsteroidal mechanisms mediate the seasonal change in social behavior (Caldwell *et al.*, 1984). The seasonal change in social organization confers several advantages. During the breeding season, rodents control resources that promote their own survival and that of their offspring, and they often aggressively exclude non-kin from access to resources. During the winter, however, this strategy is abandoned in favor of group living that conserves energy and enhances survival in the face of low temperatures and reduced food availability. Many species of rodents conserve energy during the winter by forming aggregations of huddling animals (West and Dublin, 1984). In these aggregations, different sexes and even different species commingle (Madison *et al.*, 1984).

Even in the absence of huddling behavior, animals may tolerate one another better in close quarters during the winter than during the breeding season. For example, male meadow voles are highly territorial in the spring and summer and occupy open meadows, whereas red-backed voles (*Clethrionomys gapperi*) breed in forest habitats. During the winter months, meadow voles move into the spruce forest habitats occupied by the red-backed voles, presumably to take advantage of the protective cover provided by the trees. In some cases, they share nests with other rodent species (Madison *et al.*, 1984). Individual meadow voles trapped during the winter and tested in paired encounters in a small neutral arena exhibited less interspecific aggression than voles trapped in summer (Turner *et al.*, 1975). The winter reduction in aggressiveness permits energy-saving habitat sharing. As the animals enter breeding condition in the spring, they reestablish mutually exclusive territories.

As discussed in Section VII, some males do not undergo reproductive regression, maintaining testicular function and producing sperm and androgens during simulated winter conditions (Nelson, 1987; Prendergast et al., 2001). The advantages of continuous breeding capability evidently incur substantial hidden costs because only a minority of each population adopts this strategy. One such cost may be that reproductively competent males, because of unusual aggressiveness during the winter, are unable to participate in communal huddling and thus incur greater energetic costs in overwintering. High behavioral and energetic costs associated with the maintenance of the reproductive system in winter may explain why nonregressive types do not normally predominate in temperate- or boreal-zone populations of rodents (Nelson, 1987; Nelson et al., 1989). This contention is supported by a field study of winter nesting behavior of prairie voles (McShea, 1990). Most voles in the population studied were reproductively inactive during the winter and formed groups of huddling individuals. Two males, however, remained in breeding condition and were never observed to huddle with other animals. In pairwise tests of aggression, these two males were much more aggressive than reproductively quiescent individuals. In another study, reproductive status also influenced odor preferences of meadow voles maintained in simulated winter day lengths (Gorman et al., 1993). Males that retained reproductive capability in winter day lengths preferred the odors of females that also failed to inhibit reproduction during short days. This preference may facilitate the sporadic occurrences of winter breeding frequently reported for this species (reviewed in Nelson, 1987).

A decrease in circulating androgens associated with the cessation of reproduction may mediate the increase in male affiliative interactions during winter; males that maintain summer reproductive status may thereby also maintain summer patterns of aggression. This hypothesis is supported by the observation that castration results in decreased aggressiveness. Although the relation between castration and reduced male aggression is well established, anecdotal observations of male prairie voles suggest that low circulating testosterone concentrations are not sufficient to reduce aggressive behavior.

Castration did not reduce the frequency of male aggression in tests that involved resident–intruder, grouped aggression, and aggression against a lactating female interactions (Demas et al., 1999). Similarly, postpubertal castration of male dusky-footed wood rats also did not eliminate the marked vernal increase in aggression in laboratory encounters with castrated or gonadally intact opponents (Caldwell et al., 1984). Aggressive behavior may be independent of gonadal steroid hormones in some adult male rodents; further studies are needed to establish the generality of the notion that aggression is maintained by testicular androgens.

E. Brain Development

Seasonal changes in brain weight have been documented in rodents and shrews (e.g., *Clethrionomys glareolus, C. rutilus, M. oeconomus, M. gregalis, Sorex auraneus,* and *S. minutus*; Bielak and Pucek, 1960; Pucek, 1965; Yaskin, 1984). Brain weights tend to be higher in summer than winter (Yaskin, 1984). Seasonal variations in brain weight may decrease energy expenditure (Jacobs, 1996). Although the brain constitutes only 2–3% of the total body mass in rodents, it consumes a somewhat higher percentage of total energy expenditure (Mink et al., 1981). It has been suggested that minor reductions in brain mass could result in substantial energetic savings (Jacobs, 1996).

A significant part of the seasonal change in brain weight may be attributable to differences in water content; however, the neocortex and the basal portion of the brains (i.e., the corpus striatum) of rodents and shrews show seasonal cytoarchitectural changes. The relative weight of the forebrain declines during the winter, the relative weight of the hippocampus increases from winter to summer, and the relative weight of the olfactory bulbs, myelencephalon, and cerebellum increases during the winter (Yaskin, 1984). A sex difference in brain weight is observed among bank voles (*C. glareolus*) only during the winter months; male brains are heavier than female brains at this time. The absolute and relative weight of the hippocampus is significantly higher in males than in females throughout the year, but the difference is most pronounced during the winter (Yaskin, 1984). Meadow voles also show seasonal changes in brain weight. Photoperiod appears to organize the seasonal fluctuation in brain weight in meadow voles (Dark et al., 1987); males kept in short-day conditions have lighter brains than long-day animals. Meadow voles born into long day lengths have greater brain growth (i.e., more cells) than cohorts born in short day lengths (Dark et al., 1990). Furthermore, long days enhance myelination of both the midbrain and hindbrain regions of developing male meadow voles (Spears et al., 1990).

Photoperiodic effects on cell division in the dentate gyrus and subependymal zone of adult mammals were reported (Huang et al., 1998). Long-term exposure to short days in Syrian hamsters doubled the number of new neurons produced in these brain regions, as well as in the hypothalamus and cingulate-retrosplenial cortex (Huang et al., 1998). There were no appreciable photoperiodic differences in the brain volume of either the granule cell layer of the hippocampus or the dentate gyrus. A potential functional role for these photoperiodic effects is described later.

Sex differences in hippocampal size were evident in male polygamous meadow voles (M. pennsylvanicus), but not in monogamous pine voles (M. pinetorum; Jacobs et al., 1990). Similar sex differences, but not seasonal changes, were also reported for eastern gray squirrels (Sciurus carolinensis; Lavenex et al., 2000). In both cases, it was suggested that the larger hippocampal complex in males was related to their increased reliance on spatial memory in foraging and maintenance of territories (Jacobs, 1996). These results suggest that the developmental effects of steroids might mediate changes in hippocampal size. There was, however, no overall sex difference in hippocampal volume or dentate gyrus width in wild-captured male and female meadow voles (Galea et al., 1999). A sex difference in hippocampal volume emerged if only the males with relatively high circulating testosterone concentrations (top 50th percentile) were compared to females with relatively low circulating estradiol concentrations (bottom 50th percentile) (Galea et al., 1999).

Despite the evidence for seasonal changes in brain weight in rodents, there has been relatively little research investigating seasonal changes in learning among mammalian species (but see Jacobs, 1996). Voles trapped in winter make more errors and require longer to learn mazes than do summer-captured voles (Jacobs, 1996); the extent to which this seasonal change is mediated by day length remains uncertain.

Certainly, reproductive function diminishes in short days. The motoneurons of the spinal nucleus of the bulbocavernosus and their target muscles, the bulbocavernosus and levator ani are sexually dimorphic and control penile erection in rodents (Breedlove, 1992). Short days reduce the size and neuronal numbers in these regions in white-footed mice and Siberian hamsters (Forger and Breedlove, 1987; Hegstrom and Breedlove, 1999a).

The interaction of sex and seasonal differences is complex, but may be important in typical development. For example, the androgenic induction of sexual dimorphism in meadow voles proceeds under long, but not short, days (Kelly, 1993). The slight but significant increases in neurodevelopmental disorders associated with autumn conceptions may involve subtle interactions among sex steroid hormones, photoperiod, and brain development in humans (Liederman and Flannery, 1994).

F. Locomotor Activity

Long-term exposure to short days causes a marked reduction in daily locomotor activity in castrated male Syrian hamsters. Hormonal implants that increase blood testosterone concentrations restore wheel-running activity in hamsters maintained in long days, but are completely ineffective in short-day animals (Ellis and Turek, 1983). Short days render hamsters less responsive to the stimulatory effect of testosterone on locomotor activity. After 160–200 days in the short photoperiod, castrated hamsters whether treated with testosterone or not increased locomotor activity; this seasonal change coincides with the development of photorefractorinesss to melatonin and is a steroid-independent process (Ellis and Turek, 1983). Total amount of daily locomotor activity in hamsters is modulated by circulating testosterone concentrations in a manner that depends on ambient day length.

1. Daily Activity Patterns

Field observations of rodents (e.g., *Microtus agrestis, M. oeconomus, M. montanus, Clethrionomys gapperi,* and *C. glareolus*) have documented striking shifts in activity patterns (Fig. 19) (Erkinaro, 1961; Herman, 1977; Ostermann, 1956; Rowsemitt, 1986) with nocturnality predominating during the summer and diurnality

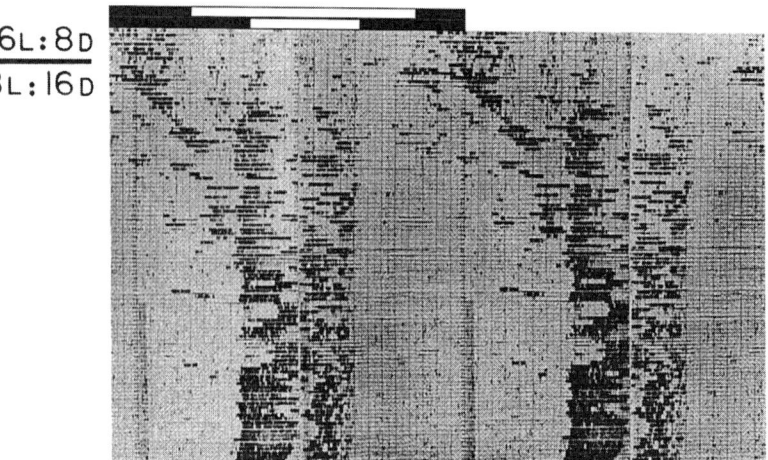

FIGURE 19 Double-plotted wheel-running activity record of an adult male montane vole prior to and after transfer from long (16L:8D) to short (8L:16D) day lengths. The animal's circadian locomotor activity rhythm was primarily nocturnal under long days, but free-ran ($\tau > 24$ hr) coinciding with the photoperiod switch (indicated by horizontal line) and established a new diurnal phase relationship approximately 1 month after transfer to short days. From Rowsemitt et al. (1982).

during the winter. By constraining the majority of its locomotor activity to the daylight hours during the winter, voles can avoid above-ground activity during the coldest part of the day; likewise, bouts of activity during summer nights allow the animal to minimize thermal stress or dehydration (Rowsemitt et al., 1982; Rowsemitt, 1986).

The seasonal shift in activity patterns in montane voles is mediated by testosterone. The castration of montane voles resulted in increased diurnal and decreased nocturnal wheel-running activity; this suggests that decreased testosterone secretion in short days induces the seasonal change in activity patterns. Castrates held in short days and treated with testosterone increased their nocturnal activity relative to untreated voles. Despite much individual variation in responses to hormone treatment, the results suggest that photoperiod is the primarily proximate cue that mediates the marked seasonal shift in activity patterns by decreasing androgen secretion (Rowsemitt, 1986). Environmental cues such as temperature, food quality, and food quantity may also affect activity patterns. Although many subtle influences of steroids on the timing of activity have been reported in other rodent species (Ellis and Turek, 1983; Morin and Cummings, 1981; Morin et al., 1977), their functional significance remains unknown.

G. Ultrasonic Vocalizations

Individuals of many species of rodents communicate with one another during sexual or parental interactions by emitting high-frequency vocalizations. In mice (Mus sp.), gonadal steroids are important for both eliciting and responding to ultrasonic vocalizations from conspecifics (Warburton et al., 1989). Exposure to short day lengths increased the rate of ultrasound vocalizations in Syrian hamsters (Matochik et al., 1986). Among gonadally intact male hamsters transferred to short days and presented with receptive females, the rates of ultrasonic vocalizations increased as blood concentrations of testosterone were decreasing (Matochik et al., 1986).

H. Odor Preferences

Individual rodents have characteristic chemical signatures or odors. Generally, individuals prefer familiar, conspecific, heterosexual odors (Fortier et al., 1996; Sawry and Dewsbury, 1994) over unfamiliar, heterospecific, same-sex odors. In some species, reliance on chemosensory information for reproductive decisions is pronounced (Carter et al., 1995). Odor preferences vary on a seasonal basis. Adult male meadow voles trapped in the field were more aggressive toward juvenile males during the first part of the breeding season (May through August) than during the later months; there were no seasonal differences in the males' responses to juvenile females (Ferkin, 1988). In contrast, adult female voles were more aggressive to juvenile males in later than in earlier parts of the breeding season. A seasonal shift in aggressiveness of adult voles toward juvenile males may facilitate the juveniles' dispersal, as well as the formation of overwintering aggregations, which typically include more females than males (Ferkin and Seamon, 1987).

Seasonal shifts in odor preference are affected by photoperiod and gonadal steroid hormones (Ferkin and Gorman, 1992; Ferkin et al., 1991, 1992). Long-day male meadow voles prefer female to male odors, whereas short-day males show no preference (Ferkin and Gorman, 1992). The preference of long-day male voles for female odors was eliminated by castration and restored by testosterone treatment; odor preference among short-day voles was unaffected by castration, but testosterone treatment induced a preference for female odors (Ferkin and Gorman, 1992). Short-day treatments do not abolish responsiveness to artificially elevated blood testosterone for this behavioral trait. Unlike the short-day-induced loss of responsiveness to testosterone in hamster reproductive neural circuitry, substrates that mediate odor preferences in male voles retain responsiveness to androgens out of season. Photoperiod also affects odor preferences in female voles. Unlike in males, steroid treatments reverse odor preferences in gonadectomized females housed in long day lengths, but are without effect on females housed in short days (Ferkin et al., 1991; Ferkin and Zucker, 1991). Prolactin and melatonin also influence the attractiveness of male odors to females (Ferkin and Kile, 1996; Ferkin et al., 1997; Leonard and Ferkin, 1999).

Photoperiod also affects odor perception. In contrast to commonly studied rodents, female prairie voles do not undergo spontaneous estrous cycles; rather, they are induced into estrus by exposure to chemosignals expressed in conspecific male urine (Carter et al., 1995). Seasonal breeding among female prairie voles in the field may reflect photoperiod-mediated changes in the responsiveness of the chemosensory system to male urine (Moffatt et al., 1995). Responsiveness was assessed by localizing the product of the *c-fos* immediate-early gene with an immunocytochemical procedure. Immunocytochemistry for Fos protein revealed an increased number of immunoreactive cells in the accessory olfactory system of female prairie voles, including the accessory olfactory bulbs, granule cell layer, and the medial and cortical divisions of the amygdala, 1 hr after exposure to a single drop of urine compared to individuals exposed to skim milk. The number of immunoreactive Fos cells induced in the accessory olfactory system of females by conspecific male urine was lower in short-day than long-day females (Moffatt et al., 1995).

I. Hibernation and Daily Torpor

Hibernation is an extreme form of seasonal thermoregulation displayed by mammalian species from several orders (Lyman et al., 1982). It presumably evolved in response to enduring seasonal food shortages and greatly reduces energy expenditure during winter. A typical rodent hibernator retires to an underground hibernaculum in the autumn and spends the winter months in a state of deep torpor. Torpor is not sustained continuously; animals arouse at species-specific intervals, which may be as short as 2 days or as long as 2 or more weeks, reestablish summer-like body temperatures for several hours, only to descend into torpor once again (Lyman et al., 1982). The intervals between successive arousals and the duration of individual torpor bouts vary as a function of stage during the hibernation season, tending to be longest during the mid-portion (Geiser et al., 1990). True hibernators reduce their body temperatures from euthermic values of 37°C to approximately 1–2°C above ambient temperature, sometimes, as in arctic ground squirrels, even slightly below 0°C (Barnes, 1989). The SCN remains disproportionately active compared to almost all other subcortical structures during deep hibernation (Kilduff et al., 1990) and is implicated in timing of the hibernation season (Ruby et al., 1996).

Other species display a shallow form of winter torpor during which body temperature is reduced from 37°C to approximately 15–20°C for 4–8 hours during the rest phase of the daily activity cycle (Hudson, 1978). The designation of this behavior as daily torpor refers to the duration of each torpor bout, not to the frequency of the behavior; most individuals display torpor two to three times per week during the winter months, and many do not undergo torpor at all in typical laboratory settings.

In Syrian hamsters and Siberian hamsters, seasonal rhythms of hibernation and torpor, respectively, are entrained by variations in day length and are displayed only after prolonged exposure to short day lengths. The combination of low temperatures and long day lengths does not elicit these behaviors. In Turkish hamsters (*Mesocricetus brandti*) and European hamsters (*Cricetus cricetus*), however, a decline in temperature is sufficient to induce hibernation, irrespective of the ambient day length, no doubt because the cold challenge triggers gonadal regression and decreased testosterone secretion (Goldman and Darrow, 1987; see below). Exposure to short day lengths and the associated long-duration nocturnal melatonin signals predispose several species of rodents to enter hibernation or to display daily torpor. Pinealectomized Turkish and Siberian hamsters neither hibernate nor display torpor when challenged with short day lengths and low temperatures (Goldman and Darrow, 1987).

Although melatonin is critical for induction of readiness to hibernate, it is not essential for the maintenance of ongoing hibernation or daily torpor. Thus, melatonin synthesis and secretion are suppressed during hibernation in hamsters and marmots (Florant *et al.*, 1984; Vanecek *et al.*, 1984; Darrow *et al.*, 1987), and Siberian hamsters that are manifesting torpor bouts continue to do so for several weeks after pinealectomy (Ruby *et al.*, 1989).

Hibernation is not dependent on the pineal gland in ground squirrels (Harlow *et al.*, 1980; Ralph *et al.*, 1982), even though some relatively subtle changes in the hibernation pattern are detectable after pinealectomy. The main role of pineal melatonin secretion in species with Type II rhythms is to transduce the variations in day length that entrain the hibernation rhythm to a period of 12 months (Hiebert *et al.*, 2000). Unlike species with Type I rhythms, melatonin is not an enabler of hibernation in ground squirrels.

Hibernation and reproduction have long been viewed as mutually incompatible processes (Wimsatt, 1969). Involution of the reproductive apparatus and a decline in androgen secretion appear to be preconditions for entry into hibernation by male mammals (Goldman and Darrow, 1987; Jansky, 1986). Males of several hamster species treated with testosterone forgo hibernation, as do hedgehogs (Saboureau, 1986) and ground squirrels (French, 1986; Lee *et al.*, 1990b).

Increased gonadal activity, specifically testosterone secretion in late winter, has been proposed as instrumental in terminating hibernation (Wimsatt, 1969; Goldman and Darrow, 1987; Darrow *et al.*, 1988). There were, however, no significant increases in blood testosterone concentrations in Turkish hamsters before the terminal arousal in the spring (Darrow *et al.*, 1987); nor were plasma testosterone concentrations elevated prior to the terminal arousal in edible dormice (*Glis glis*; Jallageas and Assenmacher, 1983), chipmunks (Scott *et al.*, 1981), and bats (Racey, 1974). Testosterone concentrations did increase in the blood of hedgehogs in the weeks preceding the end of hibernation (Saboureau, 1986). In golden-mantled ground squirrels, substantial testicular development begins shortly after the terminal arousal from hibernation; plasma concentrations of testosterone at the time of terminal arousal are no higher than values during the preceding month (Barnes *et al.*, 1988). Because substrate sensitivity to testosterone does not appear to change over the course of the hibernation season (Lee *et al.*, 1990b), the combined evidence does not indicate that testosterone is instrumental in provoking arousal from hibernation. The principal role of this hormone, at least in male golden-mantled ground squirrels, may be to determine whether the animal re-enters torpor at the end of an arousal bout. This conjecture was supported by the observation that male ground squirrels that had spontaneously terminated hibernation in the spring, reentered hibernation if gonadectomized 1–3 weeks after the terminal arousal (Dark *et al.*, 1996). A steroid-independent mechanism may control arousal from torpor at all phases of the hibernation season; increased androgen secretion during the terminal arousal, sustained for several weeks thereafter, may be the limiting factor on hibernation (Dark *et al.*, 1996).

Because estradiol was ineffective in terminating torpor in male ground squirrels (Lee *et al.*, 1990b), we infer that aromatization of testosterone is not implicated in hormonal control of hibernation; a direct action on androgen receptors in the nervous system seems more likely, at sites yet to be determined. Similar conclusions apply to Turkish hamsters (Goldman and Darrow, 1987).

The control of hibernation differs in male and female Belding's ground squirrels (*Spermophilus beldingi*).

Females do not obligatorily abandon hibernation in the spring at a fixed calendar date but instead monitor snow cover and food availability before terminating hibernation (French, 1988). In light of this observation, it is interesting that ovarian hormones have not been implicated in timing the end of the hibernation season (Hall and Goldman, 1982).

References

Ader, R., and Cohen, N. (1993). Psychoneuroimmunology: Conditioning and stress. *Annu. Rev. Psychol.* **44,** 53–85.

Almeida, O. F., and Lincoln, G. A. (1984). Reproductive photorefractoriness in rams and accompanying changes in the patterns of prolactin and melatonin secretion. *Biol. Reprod.* **30,** 143–158.

Aoyama, H., Mori, W., and Mori, N. (1986). Anti-glucocorticoid effects of melatonin in young rats. *Acta Pathol. Jpn.* **36,** 423–428.

Aoyama, H., Mori, W., and Mori, N. (1987). Anti-gluccocorticoid effects of melatonin in adult rats. *Acta Pathol. Jpn.* **37,** 1143–1148.

Arendt, J. (1995). "Melatonin and the Mammalian Pineal Gland." Chapman & Hall, London.

Arendt, J. (2000). Is melatonin a photoperiodic signal in humans? *In* "Melatonin After Four Decades" (J. Olcese, ed.). Kluwer Academic/Plenum Press, New York.

Badura, L. L., and Goldman, B. D. (1992). Central sites mediating reproductive responses to melatonin in juvenile male Siberian hamsters. *Brain Res.* **598,** 98–106.

Badura, L. L., and Nunez, A. A. (1989). Photoperiodic modulation of sexual and aggressive behavior in female Golden hamsters (*Mesocricetus auratus*): Role of the pineal gland. *Horm Behav.* **23,** 27–42.

Badura, L. L., Yant, W. R., and Nunez, A. A. (1987). Photoperiodic modulation of steroid-induced lordosis in Golden hamsters. *Physiol. Behav.* **40,** 551–554.

Bae, H. H., Mangels, R. A., Cho, B. S., Dark, J., Yellon, S. M., and Zucker, I. (1999). Ventromedial hypothalamic mediation of photoperiodic gonadal responses in male Syrian hamsters. *J. Biol. Rhythms* **14,** 391–401.

Barnes, B. M. (1989). Freeze avoidance in a mammal: Body temperatures below 0 degree C in an Arctic hibernator. *Science* **244,** 1593–1595.

Barnes, B. M., and York, A. D. (1990). Effect of winter high temperatures on reproduction and circannual rhythms in hibernating ground squirrels. *J. Biol. Rhythms* **5,** 119–130.

Barnes, B. M., Kretzmann, M., Zucker, I., and Licht, P. (1988). Plasma androgen and gonadotropin levels during hibernation and testicular maturation in golden-mantled ground squirrels. *Biol. Reprod.* **38,** 616–622.

Barrell, G. K., Thrun, L. A., Brown, M. E., Viguie, C., and Karsch, F. J. (2000). Importance of photoperiodic signal quality to entrainment of the circannual reproductive rhythm of the Ewe. *Biol. Reprod.* **63,** 769–774.

Bartholemew, G. A. (1987). Interspecific comparison as a tool for ecological physiologists. *In* "New Directions in Ecological Physiology" (M. E. Feder, A. E. Bennett, W. W. Burggren, and R. B. Huey, eds.), pp. 11–35. Cambridge University Press, Cambridge, UK.

Bartness, T. J., and Wade, G. N. (1984). Photoperiodic control of body weight and energy metabolism in Syrian hamsters (*Mesocricetus auratus*): Role of the pineal gland, melatonin, gonads, and diet. *Endocrinology (Baltimore)* **114,** 492–498.

Bartness, T. J., and Wade, G. N. (1985). Photoperiodic control of seasonal body weight cycles in hamsters. *Neurosci. Biobehav. Rev.* **9,** 599–612.

Bartness, T. J., Goldman, B. D., and Bittman, E. L. (1991). SCN lesions block responses to systemic melatonin infusions in Siberian hamsters. *Am. J. Physiol.* **260,** R102–R112.

Bartness, T. J., Powers, J. B., Hastings, M. H., Bittman, E. L., and Goldman, B. D. (1993). The timed infusion paradigm for melatonin delivery: What has it taught us about the melatonin signal, its reception, and the photoperiodic control of seasonal responses? *J. Pineal Res.* **15,** 161–190.

Baxter, J., and Forsham, P. (1972). The effects of gluccorticoids. *Am. J. Med.* **53,** 573–589.

Beck, W., and Wuttke, W. (1979). Annual rhythms of luteinizing hormone, follicle-stimulating hormone, prolactin and testosterone in the serum of male rhesus monkeys. *J. Endocrinol.* **82,** 131–139.

Bentley, G. R. (1999). Aping our ancestors: Comparative aspects of reproductive ecology. *Evol. Anthropol.* **7,** 175–185.

Bercovitch, F. B., and Harding, R. S. (1993). Annual birth patterns of savanna baboons (*Papio cynocephalus anubis*) over a ten-year period at Gilgil, Kenya. *Folia Primatol.* **61,** 115–122.

Berczi, I. (1986). The influence of the pituitary-adrenal axis on the immune system. *In* "Pituitary Function and Immunity" (I. Berczi, ed.), pp. 49–133. CRC Press, Boca Raton, FL.

Bernard, D. J., Losee-Olson, S., and Turek, F. W. (1997). Age-related changes in the photoperiodic response of Siberian hamsters. *Biol. Reprod.* **57,** 172–177.

Bernard, D. J., Abuav-Nussbaum, R., Horton, T. H., and Turek, F. W. (1999). Photoperiodic effects on gonadotropin-releasing hormone (GnRH) content and the GnRH-immunoreactive neuronal system of male Siberian hamsters. *Biol. Reprod.* **60,** 272–276.

Besedovsky, H. O., and del Rey, A. (1991). Feedback interactions between immunological cells and the hypothalamus-pituitary-adrenal axis. *Neth. J. Med.* **39,** 274–280.

Besedovsky, H. O., del Rey, A., Sorkin, E., and Dinarello, C. A. (1986). Immunoregulatory feedback between interleukin-1 and glucocorticoid hormones. *Science* **233**, 652–654.

Beutler, B., and Cerami, A. (1988). Cachectin, cachexia, and shock. *Annu. Rev. Med.* **39**, 75–83.

Bielak, T., and Pucek, Z. (1960). Seasonal changes in the brain weight of the common shrew (*Sorex araneus araneus* Linnaeus, 1758). *Acta Theriol.* **3**, 297–300.

Bittman, E. L., and Karsch, F. J. (1984). Nightly duration of pineal melatonin secretion determines the reproductive response to inhibitory day length in the ewe. *Biol. Reprod.* **30**, 585–593.

Bittman, E. L., and Lehman, M. N. (1987). Paraventricular neurons control hamster photoperiodism by a predominantly uncrossed descending pathway. *Brain Res. Bull.* **19**, 687–694.

Bittman, E. L., and Weaver, D. R. (1990). The distribution of melatonin binding sites in neuroendocrine tissues of the ewe. *Biol. Reprod.* **43**, 986–993.

Bittman, E. L., Goldman, B. D., and Zucker, I. (1979). Testicular responses to melatonin are altered by lesions of the suprachiasmatic nuclei in golden hamsters. *Biol. Reprod.* **21**, 647–656.

Bittman, E. L., Crandell, R. G., and Lehman, M. N. (1989). Influences of the paraventricular and suprachiasmatic nuclei and olfactory bulbs on melatonin responses in the Golden hamster. *Biol. Reprod.* **40**, 118–126.

Bittman, E. L., Hegarty, C. M., Layden, M. Q., and Jonassen, J. A. (1990). Influences of photoperiod on sexual behaviour, neuroendocrine steroid receptors and adenohypophysial hormone secretion and gene expression in female Golden hamsters. *J. Mol. Endocrinol.* **5**, 15–25.

Bittman, E. L., Bartness, T. J., Goldman, B. D., and De Vries G. J. (1991). Suprachiasmatic and paraventricular control of photoperiodism in Siberian hamsters. *Am. J. Physiol.* **260**, R90–R101.

Bittman, E. L., Thomas, E. M., and Zucker, I. (1994). Melatonin binding sites in sciurid and hystricomorph rodents: Studies on ground squirrels and guinea pigs. *Brain Res.* **648**, 73–79.

Bittman, E. L., Jetton, A. E., Villalba, C., and De Vries, G. J. (1996). Effects of photoperiod and androgen on pituitary function and neuropeptide staining in Siberian hamsters. *Am. J. Physiol.* **271**, R64–R72.

Black, P. H. (1994). Central nervous system-immune system interactions: Psychoneuroendocrinology of stress and its immune consequences. *Antimicrob. Agents Chemother.* **38**, 1–6.

Blank, J. L. (1992). Phenotypic variation in physiological response to seasonal environments. *In* "Mammalian Energetics: Interdisciplinary Views of Metabolism and Reproduction" (T. E. Tomasi and T. H. Horton, eds.), pp. 186–212. Cornell University Press, Ithaca, NY.

Blank, J. L., and Desjardins, C. (1986). Photic cues induce multiple neuroendocrine adjustments in testicular function. *Am. J. Physiol.* **250**, R199–R206.

Blank, J. L., and Freeman, D. A. (1991). Differential reproductive response to short photoperiod in deer mice: Role of melatonin. *J. Comp. Physiol. A* **169**, 501–506.

Blank, J. L., Nelson, R. J., Vaughan, M. K., and Reiter, R. J. (1988). Pineal melatonin content in photoperiodically responsive and non-responsive phenotypes of deer mice. *Comp. Biochem. Physiol. A* **91**, 535–537.

Bocquier, F., Bonnet, M., Faulconnier, Y., Guerre-Millo, M., Martin, P., and Chilliard, Y. (1998). Effects of photoperiod and feeding level on perirenal adipose tissue metabolic activity and leptin synthesis in the ovariectomized ewe. *Reprod. Nutr. Dev.* **38**, 489–498.

Bolinger, M., Olson, S. L, Delagrange, P., and Turek, F. W. (1996). Melatonin agonist attenuates a stress response and permits growth hormone release in male Golden hamsters. *5th Meet. Soc. Res. Biol. Rhythms,* Amelia Island, FL.

Boulos, Z., Terman, J. S., and Terman, M. (1996). Circadian phase-response curves for simulated dawn and dusk twilights in hamsters. *Physiol. Behav.* **60**, 1269–1275.

Bowers, C. W., Baldwin, C., and Zigmond, R. E. (1984). Sympathetic reinnervation of the pineal gland after postganglionic nerve lesion does not restore normal pineal function. *J. Neurosci.* **4**, 2010–2015.

Bradley, A. J., McDonald, I. R., and Lee, A. K. (1980). Stress and mortality in a small marsupial (*Antechinus stuarti* Macleay). *Gen. Comp. Endocrinol.* **40**, 188–200.

Brakefield, P. M. (1996). Seasonal polyphenism in butterflies and natural selection. *Trends Ecol. Evol.* **11**, 275–277.

Breedlove, S. M. (1992). Sexual dimorphism in the vertebrate nervous system. *J. Neurosci.* **12**, 4133–4142.

Breuner, C. W., Wingfield, J. C., and Romero, L. M. (1999). Diel rhythms of basal and stress-induced corticosterone in a wild, seasonal vertebrate, Gambel's white-crowned sparrow. *J. Exp. Zool.* **284**, 334–342.

Brewis, A., Laycock, J., and Huntsman, J. (1996). Birth non-seasonality on the Pacific equator. *Curr. Anthropol.* **37**, 842–851.

Bronson, F. H. (1985). Mammalian reproduction, an ecological perspective. *Biol. Reprod.* **32**, 1–26.

Bronson, F. H. (1989). "Mammalian Reproductive Biology." University of Chicago Press, Chicago.

Bronson, F. H. (1995). Seasonal variation in human reproduction: Environmental factors. *Q. Rev. Biol.* **70**, 141–164.

Bronson, F. H. (2000). Puberty and energy reserves: A walk on the wild side. *In* "Reproduction in Context" (K. Wallen and J. E. Schneider, eds.), pp. 15–33. MIT Press, Cambridge, UK.

Bronson, F. H., and Heideman, P. D. (1994). Seasonal regulation of reproduction in mammals. *In* "Physiology of Reproduction"

(E. Knobil and J. D. Neill, eds.), pp. 541–583. Raven Press, New York.

Caldwell, G. S., Glickman, S. E., and Smith, E. R. (1984). Seasonal aggression independent of seasonal testosterone in wood rats. *Proc. Natl. Acad. Sci. U.S.A.* **81**, 5255–5257.

Callard, G. V., Mak, P., and Solomon, D. J. (1986). Effects of short days on aromatization and accumulation of nuclear estrogen receptors in the hamster brain. *Biol. Reprod.* **35**, 282–291.

Campbell, C. S., Finkelstein, J. S., and Turek, F. W. (1978). The interaction of photoperiod and testosterone on the development of copulatory behavior in castrated male hamsters. *Physiol. Behav.* **21**, 409–415.

Campfield, L. A., Smith, F. J., Guisez, Y., Devos, R., and Burn, P. (1995). Recombinant mouse OB protein: Evidence for a peripheral signal linking adiposity and central neural networks. *Science* **269**, 546–549.

Cardinali, D. P., Brusco, L. I., Cutrera, R. A., Castrillon, P., and Esquifino, A. I. (1999). Melatonin as a time-meaningful signal in circadian organization of immune response. *Biol. Signals Recept.* **8**, 41–48.

Carlson, L. L., Zimmermann, A., and Lynch, G. R. (1989). Geographic differences for delay of sexual maturation in *Peromyscus leucopus*: Effects of photoperiod, pinealectomy, and melatonin. *Biol. Reprod.* **41**, 1004–1013.

Carlson, L. L., Weaver, D. R., and Reppert, S. M. (1991). Melatonin receptors and signal transduction during development in Siberian hamsters (*Phodopus sungorus*). *Dev. Brain Res.* **59**, 83–88.

Caroleo, M. C., Frasca, A. D., Nistico, G., and Doria, D. (1992). Melatonin as immunomodulator in immunodeficient mice. *Immunopharmacology* **23**, 81–89.

Carter, C. S, DeVries, A. C., and Getz, L. L. (1995). Physiological substrates of mammalian monogamy: The prairie vole model. *Neurosci. Biobehav. Rev.* **19**, 303–314.

Carter, D. S., and Goldman, B. D. (1983a). Antigonadal effects of timed melatonin infusion in pinealectomized male Djungarian hamsters (*Phodopus sungorus sungorus*): Duration is the critical parameter. *Endocrinology (Baltimore)* **113**, 1261–1267.

Carter, D. S., and Goldman, B. D. (1983b). Progonadal role of the pineal in the Djungarian hamster (*Phodopus sungorus sungorus*): Mediation by melatonin. *Endocrinology (Baltimore)* **113**, 1268–1273.

Christian, J. J. (1980). Regulation of annual rhythms of reproduction in temperate small rodents. *In* "Testicular Development, Structure and Function" (A. Steinberger and E. Steinberger, eds.), pp. 367–380. Raven Press, New York.

Chrousos, G. P. (1998). Ultradian, circadian, and stress-related hypothalamic-pituitary-adrenal axis activity—a dynamic digital-to-analog modulation. *Endocrinology (Baltimore)* **139**, 437–440.

Claman, H. N. (1972). Corticosteroids and lymphoid cells. *N. Engl. J. Med.* **287**, 388–397.

Clewe, T. H. (1969). Observations on reproduction of squirrel monkeys in captivity. *J. Reprod. Fertil.* **S6**, 151–156.

Clutton-Brock, T. (1991). "The Evolution of Parental Care." Cambridge University Press, Cambridge, UK.

Creel, S., and Creel, N. M. (1996). Limitation of African wild dogs by competition with larger carnivores. *Constr. Biol.* **10**, 526–538.

Czyba, J. C., Girod, C., and Durland, N. (1964). *C. R. Soc. Biol. Seances Ses. Fil.* **158**, 742.

Dallman, M. F., Strack, A. M., Akana, S. F., Bradbury, M. J., Hanson, E. S., Scribner, K. A., and Smith, M. (1993). Feast and famine: Critical role of glucocorticoids with insulin in daily energy flow. *Front. Neuroendocrinol.* **14**, 303–347.

Dark, J., and Zucker, I. (1983). Short photoperiods reduce winter energy requirements of the meadow vole, *Microtus pennsylvanicus*. *Physiol. Behav.* **31**, 699–702.

Dark, J., and Zucker, I. (1984a). Gonadal and photoperiodic control of seasonal body weight changes in male voles. *Am. J. Physiol.* **247**, R84–R88.

Dark, J., and Zucker, I. (1985). Seasonal cycles in energy balance: Regulation by light. *Ann. N.Y. Acad. Sci.* **453**, 170–181.

Dark, J., and Zucker, I. (1986a). Circannual rhythms of ground squirrels: Role of the hypothalamic paraventricular nucleus. *J. Biol. Rhythms* **1**, 17–23.

Dark, J., and Zucker, I. (1986b). Photoperiodic regulation of body mass and fat reserves in the meadow vole. *Physiol. Behav.* **38**, 851–854.

Dark, J., Johnston, P. G., Healy, M., and Zucker, I. (1983a). Latitude of origin influences photoperiodic control of reproduction of deer mice (*Peromyscus maniculatus*). *Biol. Reprod.* **28**, 213–220.

Dark, J., Zucker, I., and Wade, G. N. (1983b). Photoperiodic regulation of body mass, food intake, and reproduction in meadow voles. *Am. J. Physiol.* **245**, R334–R338.

Dark, J., Whaling, C. S., and Zucker, I. (1987). Androgens exert opposite effects on body mass of heavy and light meadow voles. *Horm. Behav.* **21**, 471–477.

Dark, J., Spears, N., Whaling, C. S., Wade, G. N., Meyer, J. S., and Zucker, I. (1990). Long day lengths promote brain growth in meadow voles. *Dev. Brain. Res.* **53**, 264–269.

Dark, J., Ruby, N. F., Wade, G. N., Licht, P., and Zucker, I. (1992). Accelerated reproductive development in juvenile male ground squirrels fed a high-fat diet. *Am. J. Physiol.* **262**, R644–R650.

Dark, J., Miller, D. R., and Zucker, I. (1994). Reduced glucose availability induces torpor in Siberian hamsters. *Am. J. Physiol.* **267**, R496–R501.

Dark, J., Miller, D. R., Licht, P., and Zucker, I. (1996). Glucoprivation counteracts effects of testosterone on daily torpor in Siberian hamsters. *Am. J. Physiol.* **270**, R398–R403.

Darrow, J. M., and Goldman, B. D. (1985). Circadian regulation of pineal melatonin and reproduction in the Djungarian hamster. *J. Biol. Rhythms* **1**, 39–54.

Darrow, J. M., Yogev, L., and Goldman, B. D. (1987). Patterns of reproductive hormone secretion in hibernating Turkish hamsters. *Am. J. Physiol.* **253**, R329–R336.

Darrow, J. M., Duncan, M. J., Bartke, A., Bona-Gallo, A., and Goldman, B. D. (1988). Influence of photoperiod and gonadal steroids on hibernation in the European hamster. *J. Comp. Physiol. A* **163**, 339–348.

Davis, D. E. (1976). Hibernation and circannual rhythms of food consumption in marmots and ground squirrels. *Q. Rev. Biol.* **51**, 477–514.

del Rey, A., Besedovsky, H., and Sorkin, E. (1984). Endogenous blood levels of corticosterone control the immunologic cell mass and B-cell activity in mice. *J. Immunol.* **133**, 572–575.

Demas, G. E., and Nelson, R. J. (1996). The effects of photoperiod and temperature on immune function of adult male deer mice (*Peromyscus maniculatus*). *J. Biol. Rhythms* **11**, 94–102.

Demas, G. E., and Nelson, R. J. (1998). Photoperiod, ambient temperature, and food availability interact to affect reproductive and immune function in adult male deer mice (*Peromyscus maniculatus*). *J. Biol. Rhythms* **13**, 253–262.

Demas, G. E., DeVries, A. C., and Nelson, R. J. (1997a). Effects of photoperiod and 2-deoxy-D-glucose-induced metabolic stress on immune function in female deer mice. *Am. J. Physiol.* **272**, R1762–R1767.

Demas, G. E., Chefer, V., Talan, M. C., and Nelson, R. J. (1997b). Metabolic costs of an antigen-stimulated immune response in adult and aged C57BL/6J mice. *Am. J. Physiol.* **273**, R1631–R1637.

Demas, G. E., Moffatt, C. A., Drazen, D. L., and Nelson, R. J. (1999). Castration does not inhibit aggressive behavior in adult male prairie voles (*Microtus ochrogaster*). *Physiol. Behav.* **66**, 59–62.

Desjardins, C., and Lopez, M. J. (1980). Sensory and nonsensory modulation of testis function. *In* "Testicular Development, Structure and Function" (A. Steinberger and E. Steinberger, eds.), pp. 381–388. Raven Press, New York.

Desjardins, C., and Lopez, M. J. (1983). Environmental cues evoke differential responses in pituitary-testicular function in deer mice. *Endocrinology (Baltimore)* **112**, 1398–1406.

Desjardins, C., Bronson, F. H., and Blank, J. L. (1986). Genetic selection for reproductive photoresponsiveness in deer mice. *Nature (London)* **322**, 172–173.

De Souza, C. J., and Meier, A. H. (1987). Circadian and seasonal variations of plasma insulin and cortisol concentrations in the Syrian hamster *Mesocricetus auratus*. *Chronobiol. Int.* **42**, 141–151.

Di Bitetti, M. S., and Janson, C. H. (2000). When will the stork arrive? Patterns of birth seasonality in neotropical primates. *Am. J. Primatol.* **50**, 109–130.

Dickert-Conlin, S., and Chandra, A. (1999). Taxes and the timing of births. *J. Political Econ.* **107**, 161–177.

Drazen, D. L., Kriegsfeld, L. J., Schneider, J. E., and Nelson, R. J. (2000). Leptin, but not immune function, is linked to reproductive responsiveness to photoperiod. *Am. J. Physiol.* **278**, R1401–R1407.

Donham, R. S., Palacio, E., and Stetson, M. H. (1994). Dissociation of the reproductive and prolactin photoperiodic responses in male golden hamsters. *Biol. Reprod.* **51**, 366–372.

Duncan, M. J., and Goldman, B. D. (1984). Hormonal regulation of the annual pelage color cycle in the Djungarian hamster, *Phodopus sungorus*. I. Role of the gonads and pituitary. *J. Exp. Zool.* **230**, 89–95.

Duncan, M. J., Goldman, B. D., DiPinto, M. N., and Stetson, M. H. (1985). Testicular function and pelage color have different critical daylengths in the Djungarian hamster, *Phodopus sungorus sungorus*. *Endocrinology (Baltimore)* **116**, 424–430.

Duncan, M. J., Takahashi, J. S., and Dubocovich, M. L. (1989). Characteristics and autoradiographic localization of 2-[^{125}I]iodomelatonin binding sites in Djungarian hamster brain. *Endocrinology (Baltimore)* **125**, 1011–1018.

Dunn, A. (1989). Psychoneuroimmunology for the psychoneuroendocrinologist: A review of animal studies of nervous system-immune system interactions. *Psychoneuroendocrinology* **14**, 251–274.

Elliott, A. S., and Nunez, A. A. (1992). Photoperiod modulates the effects of steroids on sociosexual behaviors of hamsters. *Physiol. Behav.* **51**, 1189–1193.

Elliott, J. A. (1974). Photoperiodic regulation of testis function in the Golden hamster: Relation to the circadian system. Unpublished Doctoral Dissertation, University of Texas at Austin.

Elliott, J. A. (1976). Circadian rhythms and photoperiodic time measurement in mammals. *Fed. Proc., Fed. Am. Soc. Exp. Biol.* **35**, 2239–2246.

Elliott, J. A., and Goldman, B. D. (1981). Seasonal reproduction:photoperiodism and biological clocks. *In* "Neuroendocrinology of Reproduction: Physiology and Behavior" (N. T. Adler, ed.), pp. 377–423. Plenum Press, New York.

Elliott, J. A., and Tamarkin, L. (1994). Complex circadian regulation of pineal melatonin and wheel-running in Syrian hamsters. *J. Comp. Physiol. A* **174**, 469–484.

Elliott, J. A., Stetson, M. H., and Menaker, M. (1972). Regulation of testis function in Golden hamsters: A circadian clock measures photoperiodic time. *Science* **178**, 771–773.

Elliott, J. A., Bartness, T. J., and Goldman, B. D. (1987). Role of short photoperiod and cold exposure in regulating daily torpor in Djungarian hamsters. *J. Comp. Physiol. A* **161**, 245–253.

Elliott, J. A., Bartness, T. J., and Goldman, B. D. (1989). Effect of melatonin infusion duration and frequency on gonad, lipid, and body mass in pinealectomized male Siberian hamsters. *J. Biol. Rhythms* **4**, 439–455.

Ellis, G. B., and Turek, F. W. (1980). Photoperiod-induced change in responsiveness of the hypothalamic-pituitary axis to exogenous 5-alpha-dihydrotestosterone and 17β-estradiol in castrated male hamsters. *Neuroendocrinology* **31**, 205–209.

Ellis, G. B., and Turek, F. W. (1983). Testosterone and photoperiod interact to regulate locomotor activity in male hamsters. *Horm. Behav.* **17**, 66–75.

Erkinaro, E. (1961). The seasonal change of the activity of *Microtus agrestis*. *Oikos* **12**, 157–163.

Eskes, G. A. (1983). Gonadal responses to food restriction in intact and pinealectomized male Golden hamsters. *J. Reprod. Fertil.* **68**, 85–90.

Eskes, G. A., Wilkinson, M., Moger, W. H., and Rusak, B. (1984). Periventricular and suprachiasmatic lesion effects on photoperiodic responses of the hamster hypophyseal-gonadal axis. *Biol. Reprod.* **30**, 1073–1081.

Farner, D. S. (1985). Annual rhythms. *Annu. Rev. Physiol.* **47**, 65–82.

Farrell, G., and Pease, K. (1994). Crime seasonality. *Br. J. Criminol.* **34**, 487–498.

Ferkin, M. H. (1988). The effect of familiarity on social interactions in meadow voles, *Microtus pennsylvanicus*: A laboratory and field study. *Anim. Behav.* **36**, 1816–1822.

Ferkin, M. H., and Gorman, M. R. (1992). Photoperiod and gonadal hormones influence odor preferences of the male meadow voles, *Microtus pennsylvanicus*. *Physiol. Behav.* **51**, 1087–1091.

Ferkin, M. H., and Kile, J. R. (1996). Melatonin treatment affects the attractiveness of the anogenital area scent in meadow voles (*Microtus pennsylvanicus*). *Horm. Behav.* **30**, 227–235.

Ferkin, M. H., and Seamon, J. O. (1987). Odor preference and social behavior in meadow voles, *Microtus pennsylvanicus*; seasonal differences. *Can. J. Zool.* **65**, 2931–2937.

Ferkin, M. H., and Zucker, I. (1991). Seasonal control of odour preferences of meadow voles (*Microtus pennsylvanicus*) by photoperiod and ovarian hormones. *J. Reprod. Fertil.* **92**, 433–441.

Ferkin, M. H., Gorman, M. R., and Zucker, I. (1991). Ovarian hormones influence odor cues emitted by female meadow voles, *Microtus pennsylvanicus*. *Horm. Behav.* **25**, 572–581.

Ferkin, M. H., Gorman, M. R., and Zucker, I. (1992). Influence of gonadal hormones on odours emitted by male meadow voles (*Mircrotus pennsylvanicus*). *J. Reprod. Fertil.* **95**, 729–736.

Ferkin, M. H., Sorokin, E. S., Renfroe, M. W., and Johnston, R. E. (1994). Attractiveness of male odors to females varies directly with plasma testosterone concentration in meadow voles. *Physiol. Behav.* **55**, 347–353.

Ferkin, M. H., Sorokin, E. S., and Johnston, R. E. (1997). Effect of prolactin on the attractiveness of male odors to females in meadow voles: Independent and additive effects with testosterone. *Horm. Behav.* **31**, 55–63.

Finck, B. N., Kelley, K. W., Dantzer, R., and Johnson, R. W. (1998). *In vivo* and *in vitro* evidence for the involvement of tumor necrosis factor-alpha in the induction of leptin by lipopolysaccharide. *Endocrinology (Baltimore)* **139**, 2278–2283.

Fine, J. B., and Bartness, T. J. (1996). Daylength and body mass affect diet self-selection by Siberian hamsters. *Physiol. Behav.* **59**, 1039–1050.

Fischette, C. T., Komisaruk, B. K., Edinger, H. M., Feder, H. H., and Siegel, A. (1980). Differential fornix ablations and the circadian rhythmicity of adrenal corticosteroid secretions. *Brain Res.* **195**, 373–387.

Fitzgerald, B. P., and McManus, C. J. (2000). Photoperiodic versus metabolic signals as determinants of seasonal anestrus in the mare. *Biol. Reprod.* **63**, 335–340.

Fleming, A. S., Cheung, U., Myhal, N., and Kessler, Z. (1989). Effects of maternal hormones on 'timidity' and attraction to pup-related odors in female rats. *Physiol. Behav.* **46**, 449–453.

Florant, G. L., Rivera, M. L., Lawrence, A. K., and Tamarkin, L. (1984). Plasma melatonin concentrations in hibernating marmots: Absence of a plasma melatonin rhythm. *Am. J. Physiol.* **247**, R1062–R1066.

Flores, J. A., Veliz, F. G., Perez-Villanueva, J. A., Martinez De La Escalera, G., Chemineau, P., Poindron, P., Malpaux, B., and Delgadillo, J. A. (2000). Male reproductive condition is the limiting factor of efficiency in the male effect during seasonal anestrus in female goats. *Biol. Reprod.* **62**, 1409–1414.

Flynn, A. K., Freeman, D. A., Zucker, I., and Prendergast, B. J. (2000). Testicular development in Siberian hamsters depends on frequency and pattern of melatonin signals. *Am. J. Physiol.* **279**, R1182–R1189.

Foley, R. A. (1993). The influence of seasonality on hominid evolution. *In* "Seasonality and Human Ecology" (S. J. Ulijaszek and S. S. Strickland, eds.), pp. 17–37. Cambridge University Press, Cambridge, UK.

Follett, B. K., Nicholls, T. J., Simpson, S. M., and Ellis, D. H. (1981). Photoperiodic clocks in birds and mammals Whither Bunning's hypothesis? *In* "Photoperiodism and Reproduction in Vertebrates" (R. Ortavant, J. Pelletier, and J.-P. Ravault, eds.), pp. 1–18. INRA, Paris.

Forger, N. G., and Breedlove, S. M. (1987). Seasonal variation in mammalian striated muscle mass and motoneuron morphology. *J. Neurobiol.* **18,** 155–165.

Fortier, G. M., Erskine, M. S., and Tamarkin, R. H. (1996). Female familiarity influences odor preferences and plasma estradiol levels in the meadow vole, *Microtus pennsylvanicus. Physiol. Behav.* **59,** 205–208.

Fowler, P. A., Townsend, C., Messinis, I. E., Cunningham, P., and Templeton, A. (1992). Gonadotropin surge-attenuating factor attenuates in-vitro LH secretion induced by gonadotropin-releasing hormone from cultured ovine pituitary cells only during the breeding season. *J. Endocrinol.* **135,** 221–227.

Freeman, D. A., and Goldman, B. D. (1997a). Evidence that the circadian system mediates photoperiodic nonresponsiveness in Siberian hamsters: The effect of running wheel access on photoperiodic responsiveness. *J. Biol. Rhythms* **12,** 100–109.

Freeman, D. A., and Goldman, B. D. (1997b). Photoperiod nonresponsive Siberian hamsters: Effect of age on the probability of nonresponsiveness. *J. Biol. Rhythms* **12,** 110–121.

Freeman, D. A., and Zucker, I. (2000). Temperature-independence of circannual variations in circadian rhythms of golden-mantled ground squirrels. *J. Biol. Rhythms* **15,** 336–343.

French, A. R. (1986). The interrelationship between testosterone production and the termination of hibernation in Belding's ground squirrels. *Proc. 66th Meet. Am. Soc. Mammal.,* Abstr., p. 4.

French, A. R. (1988). The patterns of mammalian hibernation. *Am. Sci.* **76,** 569–575.

Galea, L. A. M., Perrot-Sinal, T. S., Kavaliers, M., and Ossenkopp, K. P. (1999). Relations of hippocampal volume and dentate gyrus width to gonadal hormone levels in male and female meadow voles. *Brain Res.* **821,** 383–391.

Garcia, I. M., and Whitsett, J. M. (1983). Influence of photoperiod and social environment on sexual maturation in female deer mice (*Peromyscus maniculatus bairdii*). *J. Comp. Psychol.* **97,** 127–134.

Geiser, F., Hiebert, S., and Kenagy, G. J. (1990). Torpor bout duration during the hibernation season of 2 sciurid rodents—interrelations with temperature and metabolism. *Physiol. Zool.* **63,** 489–503.

Giordano, M., Vermeulen, M., and Palermo, M. S. (1993). Seasonal variations in antibody cellular cytotoxicity regulation by melatonin. *FASEB J.* **7,** 1052–1054.

Glass, J. D. (1986). Short photoperiod-induced gonadal regression: Effects on the gonadotropin-releasing hormone (GnRH) neuronal system of the white-footed mouse, *Peromyscus leucopus. Biol. Reprod.* **35,** 733–743.

Glass, J. D., and Dolan, P. L. (1988). Melatonin acts in the brain to mediate seasonal steroid inhibition of luteinizing hormone secretion in the white-footed mouse (*Peromyscus leucopus*). *Proc. Soc. Exp. Biol. Med.* **188,** 375–380.

Goldman, B. D. (1991). Parameters of the circadian rhythm of pineal melatonin secretion affecting reproductive responses in Siberian hamsters. *Steroids.* **56,** 218–225.

Goldman, B. D. (1999). The Siberian hamster as a model for study of the mammalian photoperiodic mechanism. *Adv. Exp. Med. Biol.* **460,** 155–164.

Goldman, B. D., and Darrow, J. M. (1987). Effects of photoperiod on hibernation in castrated Turkish hamsters. *Am. J. Physiol.* **253,** R337–R343.

Goldman, B. D., and Nelson, R. J. (1993). Melatonin and seasonality in mammals. *In* "Melatonin: Biosynthesis, Physiological Effects, and Clinical Applications" (H. S. Yu and R. J. Reiter, eds.), pp. 225–252. CRC Press, Boca Raton, FL.

Goldman, B. D., Darrow, J. M., and Yogev, L. (1984). Effects of timed melatonin infusions on reproductive development in the Djungarian hamster (*Phodopus sungorus*). *Endocrinology (Baltimore)* **114,** 2074–2083.

Goodman, R. L., Legan, S. J., Ryan, K. D., Foster, D. L., and Karsch, F. J. (1981). Importance of variations in behavioural and feedback actions of oestradiol to the control of seasonal breeding in the ewe. *J. Endocrinol.* **89,** 229–240.

Gorman, M. R., and Zucker, I. (1995). Seasonal adaptations of Siberian hamsters. II. Pattern of change in day length controls annual testicular and body weight rhythms. *Biol. Reprod.* **53,** 116–125.

Gorman, M. R., and Zucker, I. (1997). Environmental induction of photononresponsiveness in the Siberian hamster (*Phodopus sungorus*). *Am. J. Physiol.* **272,** R887–R895.

Gorman, M. R., and Zucker, I. (1998). Mammalian seasonal rhythms: New perspectives gained from the use of simulated natural photoperiods. *In* "Biological Clocks: Mechanisms and Applications" (Y. Touitou, ed.), pp. 195–204. Elsevier, Amsterdam.

Gorman, M. R., Ferkin, M. H., Nelson, R. J., and Zucker, I. (1993). Reproductive status influences odor preferences of the meadow vole, *Microtus pennsylvanicus,* in winter day lengths. *Can. J. Zool.* **71,** 1748–1754.

Goss, R. J. (1984). Photoperiodic control of antler cycles in deer. VI. Circannual rhythms on altered day lengths. *J. Exp. Zool.* **230,** 265–271.

Gower, B. A., Nagy, T. R., and Stetson, M. H. (1994). Effect of photoperiod, testosterone, and estradiol on body mass, bifid claw size, and pelage color in collared lemmings (*Dicrostonyx groenlandicus*). *Gen. Comp. Endocrinol.* **93,** 459–470.

Gram, W. D., Heath, H. W., Wichman, H. A., and Lynch, G. R. (1982). Geographic variation in *Peromyscus leucopus:* Short-day induced reproductive regression and spontaneous recrudescence. *Biol. Reprod.* **27,** 369–373.

Grimble, R. F. (1994). Malnutrition and the immune response. 2. Impact of nutrients on cytokine biology in infection. *Trans. Roy. Soc., Trop. Med. Hygiene* **88**, 615–619.

Gupta, D. (1990). The pineal gland: Its immunomodulatory role. *Adv. Pineal Res.* **4**, 265–285.

Gwinner, E. (1986). "Circannual Rhythms." Springer-Verlag, Berlin.

Gwinner, E., Ball, G. F., Goldman, B. D., Karsch, F. J., Saunders, D. S., and Zucker, I. (2001). Circannual rhythms and photoperiodism. *Proc. APS Conf.*

Hall, V. D., and Goldman, B. D. (1982). Hibernation in the female Turkish hamster (*Mesocricetus brandti*): An investigation of the role of the ovaries and of photoperiod. *Biol. Reprod.* **27**, 811–815.

Harlow, H. J., Phillips, J. A., and Ralph, C. L. (1980). The effect of pinealectomy on hibernation in two species of seasonal hibernators, *Citellus lateralis* and *C. richardsonii*. *J. Exp. Zool.* **213**, 301–303.

Hastings, M. (1996). Melatonin and seasonality: Filling the gap. *J. Neuroendocrinol.* **8**, 482–483.

Heath, W. H., and Lynch, G. R. (1982). Intraspecific differences for melatonin-induced reproductive regression and the seasonal molt in *Peromyscus leucopus*. *Gen. Comp. Endocrinol.* **48**, 289–295.

Hegstrom, C. D., and Breedlove, S. M. (1999a). Seasonal plasticity of neuromuscular junctions in adult male Siberian hamsters (*Phodopus sugorus*). *Brain Res.* **819**, 83–88.

Hegstrom, C. D., and Breedlove, S. M. (1999b). Social cues attenuate photoresponsiveness of the male reproductive system in Siberian hamsters (*Phodopus sungorus*). *J. Biol. Rhythms* **14**, 54–61.

Heideman, P. D., and Bronson, F. H. (1992). A pseudoseasonal reproductive strategy in a tropical rodent, *Peromyscus nudipes*. *J. Reprod. Fertil.* **95**, 57–67.

Heideman, P. D., and Bronson, F. H. (1993). Sensitivity of Syrian hamsters (*Mesocricetus auratus*) to amplitudes and rates of photoperiodic change typical of the tropics. *J. Biol. Rhythms.* **8**, 325–337.

Heideman, P. D., Deoraj, P., and Bronson, F. H. (1992). Seasonal reproduction of a tropical bat, *Anoura geoffroyi*, in relation to photoperiod. *J. Reprod. Fertil.* **96**, 765–773.

Heller, H. C., and Poulson, T. L. (1970). Circanian rhythms. II. Endogenous and exogenous factors controlling reproduction and hibernation in chipmunks (*Eutamias*) and ground squirrels (*Spermophilus*). *Comp. Biochem. Physiol.* **33**, 357–383.

Henken, A. M., and Brandsma, H. A. (1982). The effect of environmental temperature on immune response and metabolism of the young chicken. 2. Effect of the immune response to sheep red blood cells on energy metabolism. *Poult. Sci.* **61**, 1667–1677.

Herbert, J., and Klinowska, M. (1978). Day length and the annual reproductive cycle in the ferret (*Mustela furo*): The role of the pineal body. In "Environmental Endocrinology," (I. Assenmacher and D. S. Farner, eds.), pp. 87–93. Springer-Verlag, Berlin.

Herman, J. P., Watson, S. J., Chao, S. M., Corini, H., and McEwen, B. S. (1993). Diurnal regulation of glucocorticoid receptor and mineralocorticoid receptor mRNAs in rat hippocampus. *Mol. Cell. Neurosci.* **4**, 181–190.

Herman, T. B. (1977). Activity patterns and movements of subarctic voles. *Oikos* **29**, 434–444.

Herndon, J. G., Bein, M. L., Nordmeyer, D. L., and Turner, J. J. (1996). Seasonal testicular function in male rhesus monkeys. *Horm. Behav.* **30**, 266–271.

Hiebert, S. M., Lee, T. M., Licht, P., and Zucker, I. (1998). Estradiol phase shifts circannual body mass rhythms of male ground squirrels. *Am. J. Physiol.* **274**, R754–R759.

Hiebert, S. M., Thomas, E. M., Lee, T. M., Pelz, K. M., Yellon, S. M., and Zucker, I. (2000). Photic entrainment of circannual rhythms in golden-mantled ground squirrels: Role of the pineal gland. *J. Biol. Rhythms* **15**, 126–134.

Hileman, S. M., Kuehl, D. E., and Jackson, G. L. (1994). Effect of anterior hypothalamic area lesions on photoperiod-induced shifts in reproductive activity of the ewe. *Endocrinology (Baltimore)* **135**, 1816–1823.

Hill, K., and Hurtado, A. M. (1996). "Ache Life History." Aldine/de Gruyter, New York.

Hoffman, R. A., and Reiter, R. J. (1965). Pineal gland: Influence on gonads of male hamsters. *Science* **148**, 1609–1611.

Hoffmann, K. (1979). Photoperiod, pineal, melatonin and reproduction in hamsters. *Prog. Brain Res.* **52**, 397–415.

Hoffmann, K. (1982). The critical photoperiod in the Djungarian hamster *Phodopus sungorus*. In "Vertebrate Circadian Systems" (J. Aschoff, S. Daan, and G. Gross, eds.), pp. 297–304. Springer Verlag, Berlin.

Hoffmann, K., and Illnerova, H. (1986). Photoperiodic effects in the Djungarian hamster. Rate of testicular regression and extension of pineal melatonin pattern depend on the way of change from long to short photoperiods. *Neuroendocrinology* **43**, 317–321.

Hoffmann, K., Illnerova, H., and Vanecek, J. (1986). Change in duration of the nighttime melatonin peak may be a signal driving photoperiodic responses in the Djungarian hamster (*Phodopus sungorus*). *Neurosci. Lett.* **67**, 68–72.

Honrado, G. I., and Fleming, A. S. (1996). Chemical and behavioral stimulation from females accelerates recrudescence in male Syrian hamsters exposed to short days. *J. Biol. Rhythms* **11**, 103–112.

Honrado, G. I., Bird, M., and Fleming, A. S. (1991). The effects of short day exposure on seasonal and circadian reproductive rhythms in male Golden hamsters. *Physiol. Behav.* **49**, 277–287.

Horton, T. H. (1984). Growth and reproductive development of male *Microtus montanus* is affected by the prenatal photoperiod. *Biol. Reprod.* **31**, 499–504.

Horton, T. H. (1985). Cross-fostering of voles demonstrates in utero effect of photoperiod. *Biol. Reprod.* **33**, 934–939.

Horton, T. H., Ray, S. L., and Stetson, M. H. (1989). Maternal transfer of photoperiodic information in Siberian hamsters. III. Melatonin injections program postnatal reproductive development expressed in constant light. *Biol. Reprod.* **41**, 34–39.

Horton, T. H., Stachecki, S. A., and Stetson, M. H. (1990). Maternal transfer of photoperiodic information in Siberian hamsters. IV. Peripubertal reproductive development in the absence of maternal photoperiodic signals during gestation. *Biol. Reprod.* **42**, 441–449.

Huang, L. Y., De Vries, G. J., and Bittman, E. L. (1998). Photoperiod reglates neuronal bromodeoxyuridine labeling in the brain of a seasonally breeding mammal. *J. Neurobiol.* **36**, 410–420.

Hudson, J. W. (1978). Shallow daily torpor: A thermoregulatory adaptation. *In* "Strategies in the Cold" (J. W. Hudson and L. C. H. Wang, eds.), pp. 67–108. Academic Press, New York.

Huey, R. B., and Berrigan, D. (1996). Testing evolutionary hypotheses of acclimation. *Semin. Ser.—Soc. Exp. Biol.* **59**, 205–237.

Hutchison, R. E., Hutchison, J. B., Steimer, T., Steel, E., Powers, J. B., Walker, A. P., Herbert, J., and Hastings, M. H. (1991). Brain aromatization of testosterone in the male Syrian hamster: Effects of androgen and photoperiod. *Neuroendocrinology* **53**, 194–203.

Illnerova, H. (1991). The suprachiasmatic nucleus and rhythmic pineal melatonin production. *In* "Suprachiasmatic Nucleus: The Mind's Clock" (D. C. Klein, R. Y. Moore, and S. M. Reppert, eds.), pp. 197–216. Oxford University Press, New York.

Illnerova, H., Hoffmann, K., and Vanecek, J. (1984). Adjustment of pineal melatonin and N-acetyltransferase rhythms to change from long to short photoperiod in the Djungarian hamster *Phodopus sungorus*. *Neuroendocrinology* **38**, 226–231.

Iverson, S. L., and Turner, B. N. (1974). Winter weight dynamics in *Microtus pennsylvanicus*. *Ecology* **55**, 1030–1041.

Jablonski, N. G., Whitfort, M. J., Roberts-Smith, N., and Qinqi, X. (2000). The influence of life history and diet on the distribution of catarrhine primates during the Pleistocene in eastern Asia. *J. Hum. Evol.* **39**, 131–157.

Jacobs, L. F. (1996). The economy of winter: Phenotypic plasticity in behavior and brain structure. *Biol. Bull. (Woods Hole Mass.)* **191**, 92–100.

Jacobs, L. F., Gaulin, S. J., Sherry, D. F., and Hoffman, G. E. (1990). Evolution of spatial cognition: Sex-specific patterns of spatial behavior predict hippocampal size. *Proc. Natl. Acad. Sci. U.S.A.* **87**, 6349–6352.

Jallageas, M., and Assenmacher, I. (1983). Annual plasma testosterone and thyroxine cycles in relation to hibernation in the edible dormouse *Glis glis*. *Gen. Comp. Endocrinol.* **50**, 452–462.

Jannett, F. J. (1984). Reproduction of the montane vole, *Microtus montanus*, in subnivean populations. *Carnegie Mus. Nat. Hist., Spec. Publ.* **10**, 215–224.

Jansky, L. (1986). Pineal, gonads and hibernation. *Pineal Res. Rev.* **4**, 141–181

Jetton, A. E., Turek, F. W., and Schwartz, N. B. (1994). Effects of melatonin and time of day on *in vitro* pituitary gonadotropin basal secretion and GnRH responsiveness in the male Golden hamster. *Neuroendocrinology* **60**, 527–534.

Johnson, R. W. (1997). Inhibition of growth by pro-inflammatory cytokines: An integrative view. *J. Animal Sci.* **75**, 1244–1255.

Johnston, F. E. (1993). Seasonality and human biology. *In* "Seasonality and Human Ecology" (S. J. Ulijaszek and S. S. Strickland, eds.), pp. 5–16. Cambridge University Press, Cambridge, UK.

Johnston, P. G., and Zucker, I. (1980). Photoperiodic regulation of reproductive development in white-footed mice (*Peromyscus leucopus*). *Biol. Reprod.* **22**, 983–989.

Kaplan, J. N. (1977). Breeding and rearing squirrel monkeys (*Saimiri sciureus*) in captivity. *Lab. Anim. Sci.* **27**, 557–567.

Karp, J. D., and Powers, J. B. (1993). Photoperiodic and pineal influences on estrogen-stimulated behaviors in female Syrian hamsters. *Physiol. Behav.* **54**, 19–28.

Karsch, F. J., Robinson, J. E., Woodfill, C. J., and Brown, M. B. (1989). Circannual cycles of luteinizing hormone and prolactin secretion in ewes during prolonged exposure to a fixed photoperiod: Evidence for an endogenous reproductive rhythm. *Biol. Reprod.* **41**, 1034–1046.

Karsch, F. J., Dahl, G. E., Hachigian, T. M., and Thrun, L. A. (1995). Involvement of thyroid hormones in seasonal reproduction. *J. Reprod. Fertil.* **49**, 409–422.

Kaufman, C. M., and Menaker, M. (1991). Ontogeny of the pineal response to norepinephrine. *J. Pineal Res.* **11**, 173–178.

Kelley, K. W. (1985). Immunological consequences of changing environmental stimuli. *In* "Animal Stress" (G. P. Moberg, ed.), pp. 193–223. American Physiology Society, Bethesda, MD.

Kelley, K. W., and Dantzer, R. (1990). Neuroendocrine-immune interactions. *Adv. Veterinary Sci. Comp. Med.* **35**, 283–305.

Kelly, K. K. (1993). Androgenic induction of brain sexual dimorphism depends on photoperiod in meadow voles. *Physiol. Behav.* **53**, 245–249.

Kerbeshian, M. C., and Bronson, F. H. (1996). Running-induced testicular recrudescence in the meadow vole: Role of the circadian system. *Physiol. Behav.* **60**, 165–170.

Kerbeshian, M. C., LePhuoc, H., and Bronson, F. H. (1994). The effects of running activity on the reproductive axes of rodents. *J. Comp. Physiol. A* **174**, 741–746.

Kilduff, T. S., Miller, J. D., Radeke, C. M., Sharp, F. R., and Heller, H. C. (1990). 14C-2-deoxyglucose uptake in the ground squirrel brain during entrance to and arousal from hibernation. *J. Neurosci.* **10**, 2463–2475.

Kiltie, R. (1988). Gestation as a constraint on the evolution of seasonal breeding in mammals. *In* "Evolution of Life Histories of Mammals" (M. S. Boyce, ed.), pp. 257–289. Yale University Press, New Haven, CT.

Klein, D. C., Smoot, R., Weller, J. L., Higa, S., Markey, S. P., Creed, G. J., and Jacobowitz, D. M. (1983). Lesions of the paraventricular nucleus area of the hypothalamus disrupt the suprachiasmatic → spinal cord circuit in the melatonin rhythm generating system. *Brain Res. Bull.* **10**, 647–652.

Kliman, R. M., and Lynch, G. R. (1992). Evidence for genetic variation in the occurrence of the photoresponse of the Djungarian hamster, *Phodopus sungorus*. *J. Biol. Rhythms* **7**, 161–173.

Klingenspor, M., Dickopp, A., Heldmaier, G., and Klaus, S. (1996). Short photoperiod reduces leptin gene expression in white and brown adipose tissue of Djungarian hamsters. *FEBS Lett.* **399**, 290–294.

Klingenspor, M., Niggemann, H., and Heldmaier, G. (2000). Modulation of leptin sensitivity by short photoperiod acclimation in the Djungarian hamster, *Phodopus sungorus*. *J. Comp. Physiol. B* **170**, 37–43.

Kloner, R. A., Poole, W. K., and Perritt, R. L. (1999). When throughout the year is coronary death most likely to occur? A 12-year population-based analysis of more than 220,000 cases. *Circulation* **100**, 1630–1634.

Korytko, A. I., Marcelino, J., and Blank, J. L. (1995). Differential testicular responses to short daylength in deer mice are reflected by regional and morphological differences in the GnRH neuronal system. *Brain Res.* **685**, 135–142.

Korytko, A. I., Dluzen, D. E., and Blank, J. L. (1997). Photoperiod and steroid-dependent adjustments in hypothalamic gonadotropic hormone-releasing hormone, dopamine and norepinephrine content in male deer mice. *Biol. Reprod.* **56**, 617–624.

Korytko, A. I., Vessey, S. H., and Blank, J. L. (1998). Phenotypic differences in the GnRH neuronal system of deer mice *Peromyscus maniculatus* under a natural short photoperiod. *J. Reprod. Fertil.* **114**, 231–235.

Kriegsfeld, L. J., and Nelson, R. J. (1996). Gonadal and photoperiodic influences on body mass regulation in adult male and female prairie voles. *Am. J. Physiol.* **39**, R1013–R1018.

Kriegsfeld, L. J., Ranalli, N. J., Bober, M. A., and Nelson, R. J. (2000). Photoperiod and temperature interact to affect the gonadotropin-releasing hormone (GnRH) neuronal system of male prairie voles (*Microtus ochrogaster*). *J. Biol. Rhythms.* **15**(4), 306–316.

Kutzback, J. E., and Webb, T. (1993). Conceptual basis for understanding late quaternary climates. *In* "Global Climates Since the Last Glacial Maximum" (H. E. Wright, Jr., ed.), pp. 5–11. University of Minnesota Press, Minneapolis.

Lance, S. J., Miller, S. C., Holtsclaw, L. I., and Turner, B. B. (1998). Photoperiod regulation of mineralocorticoid receptor mRNA expression in hamster hippocampus. *Brain Res.* **780**, 342–347.

Larkin, J. E., Freeman, D. A., and Zucker, I. (2001). Low ambient temperatures accelerate short-day responses in Siberian hamsters by altering responsiveness to melatonin. *J. Biol. Rhythms* **16**, 76–86.

Lavenex, P., Steele, M. A., and Jacobs, L. F. (2000). Sex differences, but no seasonal variations in the hippocampus of food-caching squirrels: A stereological study. *J. Comp. Neurol.* **425**, 152–166.

Lee, T. M. (1993). Development of meadow voles is influenced postnatally by maternal photoperiodic history. *Am. J. Physiol.* **265**, R749–R755.

Lee, T. M., and Gorman, M. R. (2000). Timing of Reproduction by the Integration of Photoperiod and Other Seasonal Signals. *In* "Reproduction in Context" (K. Wallen and J. S. Schneider, eds.), pp. 191–218. MIT Press, Cambridge, MA.

Lee, T. M., and Zucker, I. (1988). Vole infant development is influenced perinatally by maternal photoperiodic history. *Am. J. Physiol.* **255**, R831–R838.

Lee, T. M., and Zucker, I. (1991). Suprachiasmatic nucleus and photic entrainment of circannual rhythms in ground squirrels. *J. Biol. Rhythms* **6**, 315–330.

Lee, T. M., and Zucker, I. (1992). Estradiol phase-shifts circannual rhythms of golden-mantled ground squirrels. *Am. J. Physiol.* **262**, R1096–R1099.

Lee, T. M., and Zucker, I. (1995). Seasonal variations in circadian rhythms persist in gonadectomized golden-mantled ground squirrels. *J. Biol. Rhythms.* **10**, 188–195.

Lee, T. M., Carmichael, M. S., and Zucker, I. (1986). Circannual variations in circadian rhythms of ground squirrels. *Am. J. Physiol.* **250**, R831–R836.

Lee, T. M., Smale, L., Zucker, I., and Dark, J. (1987). Influence of daylength experienced by dams on post-natal development of young meadow voles (*Microtus pennsylvanicus*). *J. Reprod. Fertil.* **81**, 337–342.

Lee, T. M., Spears, N., Tuthill, C. R., and Zucker, I. (1989). Maternal melatonin treatment influences rates of neonatal development of meadow vole pups. *Biol. Reprod.* **40**, 495–502.

Lee, T. M., Holmes, W. G., and Zucker, I. (1990a). Temperature dependence of circadian rhythms in golden-mantled ground squirrels. *J. Biol. Rhythms.* **5**, 25–34.

Lee, T. M., Pelz, K., Licht, P., and Zucker, I. (1990b). Testosterone influences hibernation in golden-mantled ground squirrels. *Am. J. Physiol.* **259**, R760–R767.

Lehman, M. N., Bittman, E. L., and Newman, S. W. (1984). Role of the hypothalamic paraventricular nucleus in neuroendocrine responses to daylength in the Golden hamster. *Brain Res.* **308**, 25–32.

Leonard, S. T., and Ferkin, M. H. (1999). Prolactin and testosterone affect seasonal differences in male meadow vole, *Microtus pennsylvanicus*, odor preferences for female conspecifics. *Physiol. Behav.* **68**, 139–143.

Lerner, A. B., Case, J. D., Lee, T. H., Takahashi, Y., and Mori, W. (1958). Isolation of melatonin, the pineal factor that lightens melanocytes. *J. Am. Chem. Soc.* **80**, 2587–2594.

Li, K., Reiter, R. J., Vaughan, M. K., Oaknin, S., and Troiani, M. E. (1987). Elevated ambient temperature retards the atrophic response of the neuroendocrine-reproductive axis of male Syrian hamsters to either daily afternoon melatonin injections or to short photoperiod exposure. *Neuroendocrinology* **45**, 356–362.

Licht, P., McCreery, B. R., Barnes, B. R., and Pang, R. (1983). Seasonal and stress related changes in plasma gonadotropins, sex steroids and corticosterone in the bullfrog, *Rana catesbeiana*. *Gen. Comp. Endocrinol.* **50**, 124–145.

Liederman, J., and Flannery, K. A. (1994). Fall conception increases the risk of neurodevelopmental disorder in offspring. *J. Clin. Exp. Neurospychol.* **16**, 754–768.

Lincoln, G. A. (1990). Correlation with changes in horns and pelage, but not reproduction, of seasonal cycles in the secretion of prolactin in rams of wild, feral and domesticated breeds of sheep. *J. Reprod. Fertil.* **90**, 285–296.

Lincoln, G. A. (1999). Melatonin modulation of prolactin and gonadotrophin secretion. Systems ancient and modern. *Adv. Exp. Med. Biol.* **460**, 137–153.

Lincoln, G. A., and Clarke, I. J. (1997). Refractoriness to a static melatonin signal develops in the pituitary gland for the control of prolactin secretion in the ram. *Biol. Reprod.* **57**, 460–467.

Lincoln, G. A., and MacKinnon, C. B. (1976). A study of seasonally delayed puberty in the male hare, *Lepus Europaeus*. *J. Reprod. Fertil.* **46**, 123–128.

Lincoln, G. A., and Short, R. V. (1980). Seasonal breeding: Nature's contraceptive. *Recent Prog. Horm. Res.* **36**, 1–52.

Lindburg, D. G. (1987). Seasonality of reproduction in primates. *In* "Comparative Primate Biology" (G. Mitchell and J. Erwin, eds.), Vol. 2, Part B, pp. 167–218. Liss, New York.

Lochmiller, R. L., and Deerenberg, C. (2000). Trade-offs in evolutionary immunology: Just what is the cost of immunity? *Oikos* **88**, 87–98.

Lochmiller, R. L., Vestey, M. R., and McMurry, S. T. (1994). Temporal variation in humoral and cell-mediated immune response in a *Sigmodon hispidus* population. *Ecology* **75**, 236–245.

Loudon, A. S. (1994). Photoperiod and the regulation of annual and circannual cycles of food intake. *Proc. Nutr. Soc.* **53**, 495–507.

Loudon, A. S. (1996). The photoperiodic response in Syrian hamster depends upon a melatonin-driven circadian rhythm of sensitivity to melatonin. *J. Neuroendocrinol.* **8**, 481–482.

Lummaa, V., Lemmetyinen, R., Haukioja, E., and Pikkola, M. (1998). Seasonality of births in *Homo sapiens* in pre-industrial Finland: Maximisation of offspring survivorship? *J. Evol. Biol.* **11**, 147–157.

Lyman, C. P., Willis, J. S., Malan, A., and Wang, L. C. H. (1982). "Hibernation and Torpor in Mammals and Birds." Academic Press, New York.

Lynch, G. R., Lynch, C. B., and Kliman, R. M. (1989). Genetic analyses of photoresponsiveness in the Djungarian hamster, *Phodopus sungorus*. *J. Comp. Physiol. A* **164**, 475–482.

MacMurray, J. P., Barker, J. P., Armstrong, J. D., Bozzetti, L. P., and Kuhn, I. N. (1983). Circannual changes in immune function. *Life Sci.* **32**, 2363–2370.

Madison, D. M., FitzGerald, R. W., and McShea, W. J. (1984). Dynamics of social nesting in overwintering meadow voles (*Microtus pennsylvanicus*): Possible consequences for population cycling. *Behav. Ecol. Sociobiol.* **15**, 9–17.

Maestroni, G. J. (1993). The immunoneuroendocrine role of melatonin. *J. Pineal Res.* **14**, 1–10.

Maestroni, G. J. (1995). T-helper-2 lymphocytes as a peripheral target of melatonin. *J. Pineal Res.* **18**, 84–89.

Maestroni, G. J., and Conti, A. (1990). The pineal neurohormone melatonin stimulates activated CD4+ Thy-1+ cells to release opioid agonists with immunoenhancing and anti-stress properties. *J. Neuroimmunol.* **28**, 167–176.

Mahmoud, I. Y., and Licht, P. (1997). Seasonal changes in gonadal activity and the effects of stress on reproductive hormones in the common snapping turtle, *Chelydra serpentina*. *Gen. Comp. Endocrinol.* **107**, 359–372.

Maier, S. F., and Watkins, L. R. (1999). Bi-directional communication between the brain and the immune system: Implications for behavior. *Anim. Behav.* **57**, 741–760.

Maier, S. F., Watkins, L. R., and Fleshner, M. (1994). Psychoneuroimmunology: The interface between behavior, brain, and immunity. *Am. Psychol.* **49**, 1004–1017.

Mangels, R. A., Powers, J. B., and Blaustein, J. D. (1998). Effect of photoperiod on neural estrogen and progestin receptor immunoreactivity in female Syrian hamsters. *Brain Res.* **796**, 63–74.

Mann, D. R., Akinbami, M. A., Gould, K. G., and Castracane, V. D. (2000). A longitudinal study of leptin during development in the male rhesus monkey: The effect of body composition and season on circulating leptin levels. *Biol. Reprod.* **62**, 285–291.

Margraf, R. R., Zlomanczuk, P., Liskin, L. A., and Lynch, G. R. (1991). Circadian differences in neuronal activity of the suprachiasmatic nucleus in brain slices prepared from photoresponsive and photo-non-responsive Djungarian hamsters. *Brain Res.* **544**, 42–48.

Martin, J. E., Engel, J. N., and Klein, D. C. (1977). Inhibition of the in vitro pituitary response to luteinizing hormone-releasing hormone by melatonin, serotonin, and 5-methoxytryptamine. *Endocrinology (Baltimore)* **100**, 675–680.

Martinet, L., and Spitz, F. (1971). Variations saisonnières de la croissance et de la mortalité du campagnol des champs, *Microtus arvalis*. Role du photopériodisme et de la végétation sur ces variations. *Mammalia* **35**, 38–84.

Mason, J. W. (1975). A historical view of the stress field. *J. Hum. Stress* **1**, 6–12.

Mather, J. G. (1981). Wheel running activity: A new interpretation. *Mammal. Rev.* **11**, 41–51.

Matochik, J. A., Miernicki, M., Powers, J. B., and Bergondy, M. L. (1986). Short photoperiods increase ultrasonic vocalization rates among male Syrian hamsters. *Physiol. Behav.* **38**, 453–458.

Maywood, E. S., and Hastings, M. H. (1995). Lesions of the iodomelatonin-binding sites of the mediobasal hypothalamus spare the lactotropic, but block the gonadotropic response of male Syrian hamsters to short photoperiod and to melatonin. *Endocrinology (Baltimore)* **136**, 144–153.

Maywood, E. S., Bittman, E. L., and Hastings, M. H. (1996). Lesions of the melatonin- and androgen-responsive tissue of the dorsomedial nucleus of the hypothalamus block the gonadal responses of male Syrian hamsters to programmed infusions of melatonin. *Biol. Reprod.* **54**, 470–477.

McShea, W. J. (1990). Social tolerance and proximate mechanisms of dispersal among winter groups of meadow voles, *Microtus pennsylvanicus*. *Anim. Behav.* **39**, 346–351.

Meek, L. R., and Lee, T. M. (1993a). Female meadow voles have a preferred mating pattern predicted by photoperiod, which influences fertility. *Physiol. Behav.* **54**, 1201–1210.

Meek, L. R., and Lee, T. M. (1993b). Prediction of fertility by mating latency and photoperiod in nulliparous and primiparous meadow voles (*Microtus pennsylvanicus*). *J. Reprod. Fertil.* **97**, 353–357.

Mehdi, A. Z., and Sandor, T. (1976). The effect of melatonin on the biosynthesis of corticosteroids in beef adrenal preparations *in vitro*. *J. Steroid Biochem.* **8**, 822–825.

Menaker, M., and Refinetti, R. (1993). The tau mutation in Golden hamsters. *In* "Molecular Genetics of Biological Rhythms" (M. W. Young, ed.), pp. 255–269. Dekker, New York.

Mendonca, M. T., and Licht, P. (1986). Seasonal cycles in gonadal activity and plasma gonadotropin in the musk turtle, *Sternotherus odoratus*. *Gen. Comp. Endocrinol.* **62**, 459–469.

Mercer, J. G. (1998). Regulation of appetite and body weight in seasonal mammals. *Comp. Biochem. Physiol. C* **119**, 295–303.

Mercer, J. G., Duncan, J. S., Lawrence, B., and Trayhurn, P. (1994). Effect of photoperiod on mitochondrial GDP binding and adenylate cyclase activity in brown adipose tissue of Djungarian hamsters. *Physiol. Behav.* **56**, 737–740.

Messager, S., Ross, A. W., Barrett, P., and Morgan, P. J. (1999). Decoding photoperiodic time through Per1 and ICER gene amplitude. *Proc. Natl. Acad. Sci. U.S.A.* **96**, 9938–9943.

Michael, R. P., and Bonsall, R. W. (1977). A 3-year study of an annual rhythm in plasma androgen levels in male rhesus monkeys (*Macaca mulatta*) in a constant laboratory environment. *J. Reprod. Fertil.* **49**, 129–131.

Miernicki, M., Karp, J. D., and Powers, J. B. (1990). Pinealectomy prevents short photoperiod inhibition of male hamster sexual behavior. *Physiol. Behav.* **47**, 293–299.

Milette, J. J., and Turek, F. W. (1986). Circadian and photoperiodic effects of brief light pulses in male Djungarian hamsters. *Biol. Reprod.* **35**, 327–335.

Millar, J., and Gyug, L. (1981). Initiation of breeding by northern *Peromyscus* in relation to temperature. *Can. J. Zool.* **59**, 1094–1098.

Millar, J. S., Wille, F. B., and Iverson, S. L. (1979). Breeding by *Peromyscus* in seasonal environments. *Can. J. Zool.* **57**, 719–727.

Miller, E. S., Klinger, J. C., Akin, C., Koebel, D. A., and Sonnenfeld, G. (1994). Inhibition of murine splenic T lymphocyte proliferation by 2-deoxy-D-glucose-induced metabolic stress. *J. Neuroimmunol.* **52**, 165–173.

Mink, J. W., Blumenschine, R. J., and Adams, D. B. (1981). Ratio of central nervous system to body metabolism in vertebrates: its constancy and functional basis. *Am. J. Physiol.* **241**, R203–R212.

Moffatt, C. A., and Nelson, R. J. (1994). Day length influences proceptive behavior of female prairie voles (*Microtus ochrogaster*). *Physiol. Behav.* **55**, 1163–1165.

Moffatt, C. A., DeVries, A. C., and Nelson, R. J. (1993). Winter adaptations of male deer mice (*Peromyscus maniculatus*) and prairie voles (*Microtus ochrogaster*) that vary in reproductive responsiveness to photoperiod. *J. Biol. Rhythms* **8**, 221–232.

Moffatt, C. A., Ball, G. F., and Nelson, R. J. (1995). The effects of photoperiod on olfactory c-fos expression in prairie voles, *Microtus ochrogaster*. *Brain Res.* **677**, 82–88.

Monjan, A. A. (1981). Stress and immunologic competence: Studies in animals. *In* "Psychoneuroimmunology" (R. Ader, ed.), pp. 185–228. Academic Press, New York.

Moore, R. Y. (1996). Neural control of the pineal gland. *Behav. Brain Res.* **73**, 125–130.

Moore, R. Y., and Klein, D. C. (1974). Visual pathways and the central neural control of a circadian rhythm in pineal serotonin N-acetyltransferase activity. *Brain Res.* **71**, 17–33.

Morgan, P. J., and Williams, L. M. (1989). Central melatonin receptors: Implications for a mode of action. *Experientia* **45**, 955–965.

Morin, L. P., and Cummings, L. A. (1981). Effect of surgical or photoperiodic castration, testosterone replacement or pinealectomy on male hamster running rhythmicity. *Physiol. Behav.* **26**, 825–838.

Morin, L. P., and Zucker, I. (1978). Photoperiodic regulation of copulatory behaviour in the male hamster. *J. Endocrinol.* **77**, 249–258.

Morin, L. P., Fitzgerald, K. M., and Zucker, I. (1977). Estradiol shortens the period of hamster circadian rhythms. *Science* **196**, 305–307.

Motta, M., Fraschini, F., and Martini, L. (1967). Endocrine effects of pineal gland and melatonin, *Proc. Soc. Exp. Biol. Med.* **126**, 431–435.

Motta, M., Fraschini, F., and Martini, L. (1969). Short feedback mechanisms in the control of anterior pituitary function. *In* "Frontiers in Neuroendocrinology" (W. F. Ganong and L. Martini, eds.), p. 212. Oxford University Press, Oxford.

Mrosovsky, N. (1985). Cyclical obesity in hibernators: The search for the adjustable regulator. *Recent Adv. Obes. Res.* **4**, 45–56.

Mrosovsky, N., Boshes, M., Hallonquist, J. D., and Lang, K. (1976). Circannual cycle of circadian cycles in a golden-mantled ground squirrel. *Naturwissenschaften* **63**, 298–299.

Munck, A., and Guyre, P. M. (1991). Glucocorticoids and immune function. *In* "Psychoneuroimmunology" (R. Ader, D. L. Felten, and N. Cohen, eds.), pp. 447–474. Academic Press, San Diego, CA.

Nagy, T. R. (1993). Effects of photoperiod history, and temperature on male collard lemmings, *Dicrostonyx groenlandicus*. *J. Mammal.* **74**, 990–998.

Nakano, K., Suzuki, S., and Oh, C. (1987). Significance of increased secretion of glucocorticoids in mice and rats injected with bacterial endotoxin. *Brain Behav. Immunol.* **1**, 159–172.

Nelson, R. J. (1985). Photoperiod influences reproduction in the prairie vole (*Microtus ochrogaster*). *Biol. Reprod.* **33**, 596–602.

Nelson, R. J. (1987). Photoperiod-nonresponsive morphs a possible variable in microtine population-density fluctuations. *Am. Nat.* **130**, 350–369.

Nelson, R. J., and Demas, G. E. (1996). Seasonal changes in immune function. *Q. Rev. Biol.* **71**, 511–548.

Nelson, R. J., and Demas, G. E. (1997). Role of melatonin in mediating seasonal energetic and immunologic adaptations. *Brain Res. Bull.* **44**, 423–430.

Nelson, R. J., and Drazen, D. L. (1999). Melatonin mediates seasonal adjustments in immune function. *Reprod. Nutr. Dev.* **39**, 383–398.

Nelson, R. J., Dark, J., and Zucker, I. (1983). Influence of photoperiod, nutrition and water availability on reproduction of male California voles (*Microtus californicus*). *J. Reprod. Fertil.* **69**, 473–477.

Nelson, R. J., Frank, D., Smale, L., and Willoughby, S. B. (1989). Photoperiod and temperature affect reproductive and nonreproductive functions in male prairie voles (*Microtus ochrogaster*). *Biol. Reprod.* **40**, 481–485.

Nelson, R. J., Demas, G. E., Klein, S. L., and Kriegsfeld, L. J. (1995). The influence of season, photoperiod, and pineal melatonin on immune function. *J. Pineal Res.* **19**, 149–165.

Nelson, R. J., Demas, G. E., and Klein, S. L. (1998). Photoperiodic mediation of seasonal breeding and immune function in rodents: A multi-factorial approach. *Am. Zool.* **38**, 226–237.

Nelson, R. J., Demas, G. E., Klein, S. L., and Kriegsfeld, L. J. (2001). "Seasonal Cycles in Immune Function and Disease Processes." Cambridge University Press, New York.

Nicholls, T. J., Follett, B. K., Goldsmith, A. R., and Pearson, H. (1988). Possible homologies between photorefractoriness in sheep and birds: The effect of thyroidectomy on the length of the ewe's breeding season. *Reprod. Nutr. Dev.* **28**, 375–385.

Nieuwenhuijsen, K., de Neef, K. J., van der Werff ten Bosch, J. J., and Slob, A. K. (1987). Testosterone, testis size, seasonality, and behavior in group-living stumptail macaques (*Macaca arctoides*). *Horm. Behav.* **21**, 153–169.

Niklowitz, P., Lerchl, A., and Nieschlag, E. (1994). Photoperiodic responses in Djungarian hamsters (*Phodopus sungorus*): Importance of light history for pineal and serum melatonin profiles. *Biol. Reprod.* **51**, 714–724.

Nozaki, M., Mitsunaga, F., and Shimizu, K. (1995). Reproductive senescence in female Japanese monkeys (*Macaca fuscata*): Age- and season-related changes in hypothalamic-pituitary-ovarian functions and fecundity rates. *Biol. Reprod.* **52**, 1250–1257.

O'Leary, A. (1990). Stress, emotion, and human immune function. *Psychol. Bull.* **108**, 363–382.

Orchinik, M., Licht, P., and Crews, D. (1988). Plasma steroid concentrations change in response to sexual behavior in *Bufo marinus*. *Horm. Behav.* **22**, 338–350.

Ostermann, K. (1956). Zur Aktivität heimischer Muriden und Gliriden. *Zool. Jahrb. Abt. All. Zool. Physiol.* **66**, 355–375.

Ottenweiler, J. E., Tapp, W. E., Pitman, D. L., and Natelson, B. H. (1987). Adrenal, thyroid, and testicular hormone rhythms in male Golden hamsters on long and short days. *Am. J. Physiol.* **253**, R322.

Parkinson, T. J., and Follett, B. K. (1994). Effect of thyroidectomy upon seasonality in rams. *J. Reprod. Fertil.* **101**, 51–58.

Pengelley, E. T., and Asmundson, S. J. (1974). Circannual rhythmicity in hibernating mammals. *In* "Circannual Clocks" (E. T. Pengelley, ed.), pp. 95–160. Academic Press, New York.

Pengelley, E. T., Aloia, R. C., Barnes, B. M., and Whitson, D. (1979). Differential temporal behavior between males and females in the hibernating ground squirrel, *Citellus lateralis*. *Comp. Biochem. Physiol. A* **64A**, 593–596.

Perret, M. (1992). Environmental and social determinants of sexual function in the male lesser mouse lemur (*Microcebus murinus*). *Folia Primatol.* **59**, 1–25.

Perret, M. (1997). Change in photoperiodic cycle affects life span in a prosimian primate (*Microcebus murinus*). *J. Biol. Rhythms.* **12**, 136–145.

Perret, M., and Schilling, A. (1993). Response to short photoperiod and spontaneous sexual recrudescence in the lesser mouse lemur: Role of olfactory bulb removal. *J Endocrinol.* **137**, 511–518.

Persengiev, S., Marinova, C., and Patchev, V. (1991a). Steroid hormone receptors in the thymus: A site of immunomodulatory action of melatonin. *Int. J. Biochem.* **23**, 1483–1485.

Persengiev, S., Patchev, V., and Velev, B. (1991b). Melatonin effects on thymus steroid receptors in the course of primary antibody responses: Significance of circulating glucocorticoid levels. *Int. J. Biochem.* **23**, 1487–1489.

Petterborg, L. J. (1978). Effect of photoperiod on body weight in the vole, *Microtus montanus. Can. J. Zool.* **56**, 431–435.

Pevet, P., Vivien-Roels, B., and Masson-Pevet, M. (1989). Low temperature in the Golden hamster accelerates the gonadal atrophy induced by short photoperiod but does not affect the daily pattern of melatonin secretion. *J. Neural. Transm.* **76**, 119–128.

Pickard, G. E., and Turek, F. W. (1983). The hypothalamic paraventricular nucleus mediates the photoperiodic control of reproduction but not the effects of light on the circadian rhythm of activity. *Neurosci. Lett.* **43**, 67–72.

Pioli, C., Carleo, C., Nistico, G., and Doria, G. (1993). Melatonin increases antigen presentation and amplifies specific and non-specific signals for T-cell proliferation. *Int. J. Immunopharmacol.* **15**, 463–468.

Pistole, D. H., and Cranford, J. A. (1982). Photoperiodic effects on growth in *Microtus pennsylvanicus. J. Mammal.* **63**, 547–553.

Pitrosky, B., and Pevet, P. (1997). The photoperiodic response in Syrian hamsters depends upon a melatonin-driven rhythm of sensitivity to melatonin. *Biol. Signals* **6**, 264–271.

Pitrosky, B., Kirsch, R., Vivien-Roels, B., Georg-Bentz, I., Canguilhem, B., and Pevet, P. (1995). The photoperiodic response in Syrian hamster depends upon a melatonin-driven circadian rhythm of sensitivity to melatonin. *J. Neuroendocrinol.* **7**, 889–985.

Pittendrigh, C. S. (1974). Circadian oscillations in cells and the circadian organization of multicellular systems. *In* "The Neurosciences: Third Study Program" (F. O. Schmitt and F. O. Worden, eds.), pp. 437–458. MIT Press, Cambridge, MA.

Plant, T. M., Zumpe, D., Sauls, M., and Michael, R. P. (1974). An annual rhythm in the plasma testosterone of adult male rhesus monkeys maintained in the laboratory. *J. Endocrinol.* **62**, 403–404.

Pleim, E. T., Lisciotto, C. A., and DeBold, J. F. (1990). Facilitation of sexual receptivity in hamsters by simultaneous progesterone implants into the VMH and ventral mesencephalon. *Horm. Behav.* **24**, 139–151.

Poon, A. M., Liu, Z. M., Tang, F., and Pang, S. F. (1994). Cortisol decreases 2[^{125}I] iodomelatonin binding sites in the duck thymus. *Eur. J. Endocrinol.* **130**, 320–324.

Pope, N. S., Gordon, T. P., and Wilson, M. E. (1986). Age, social rank and lactational status influence ovulatory patterns in seasonally breeding rhesus monkeys. *Biol. Reprod.* **35**, 353–359.

Pope, N. S., Wilson, M. E., and Gordon, T. P. (1987). The effect of season on the induction of sexual behavior by estradiol in female rhesus monkeys. *Biol. Reprod.* **36**, 1047–1054.

Pospichal, M. W., Karp, J. D., and Powers, J. B. (1991). Influence of daylength on male hamster sexual behavior: Masking effects of testosterone. *Physiol. Behav.* **49**, 417–422.

Potts, R. (1998). Environmental hypotheses of hominin evolution. *Yearbk. Phys. Anthropol.* **41**, 93–136.

Powers, J. B., Steel, E. A., Hutchison, J. B., Hastings, M. H., Herbert, J., and Walker, A. P. (1989). Photoperiodic influences on sexual behavior in male Syrian hamsters. *J. Biol. Rhythms* **4**, 61–78

Powers, J. B., Jetton, A. E., Mangels, R. A., and Bittman, E. L. (1997). Effects of photoperiod duration and melatonin signal characteristics on the reproductive system of male Syrian hamsters. *J. Neuroendocrinol.* **9**, 451–466.

Prendergast, B. J., and Freeman, D. A. (1999). Pineal-independent regulation of photo-nonresponsiveness in the Siberian hamster (*Phodopus sungorus*). *J. Biol. Rhythms* **14**, 62–71.

Prendergast, B. J., and Hugenberger, J. L. (1999). Frequency coding of melatonin signals sufficient to induce testicular growth in photoregressed Siberian hamsters. *J. Neuroendocrinol.* **11**, 237–241.

Prendergast, B. J., Kelly, K. K., Zucker, I., and Gorman, M. R. (1996). Enhanced reproductive responses to melatonin in juvenile Siberian hamsters. *Am. J. Physiol.* **271**, R1041–R1046.

Prendergast, B. J., Zucker, I., Yellon, S. M., Ringold, D. A, and Gorman, M. R. (1998). Melatonin chimeras alter reproductive development and photorefractoriness in Siberian hamsters. *J. Biol. Rhythms* **13**, 518–531.

Prendergast, B. J., Flynn, A. K., and Zucker, I. (2000). Triggering of neuroendocrine refractoriness to short-day patterns of melatonin in Siberian hamsters. *J. Neuroendocrinol.* **12**, 303–310.

Prendergast, B. J., Kriegsfeld, L. J., and Nelson, R. J. (2001). Photoperiodic polyphenisms in rodents: Neuroendocrine mechanisms, costs and functions. *Q. Rev. Biol.* **76**, 293–325.

Pucek, Z. (1965). Water contents and seasonal changes of the brain weight in shrews. *Acta Theriol.* **10**, 353–367.

Puchalski, W., and Lynch, G. R. (1986). Evidence for differences in the circadian organization of hamsters exposed to short day photoperiod. *J. Comp. Physiol. A* **159**, 7–11.

Puchalski, W., and Lynch, G. R. (1988). Daily melatonin injections affect the expression of circadian rhythmicity in Djungarian hamsters kept under a long-day photoperiod. *Neuroendocrinology* **48**, 280–286.

Puchalski, W., and Lynch, G. R. (1994). Photoperiodic time measurement in Djungarian hamsters evaluated from T-cycle studies. *Am. J. Physiol.* **267**, R191–R201.

Puchalski, W., Kliman, R., and Lynch, G. R. (1988). Differential effects of short day pretreatment on melatonin-induced adjustments in Djungarian hamsters. *Life Sci.* **43**, 1005–1012.

Pulver, A. E., Stewart, W., Carpenter, W. T., and Childs, B. (1983). Risk factors in schizophrenia: Season birth in Maryland, USA. *Br. J. Psychiatry* **143**, 389–396.

Racey, P. (1974). The reproductive cycle in male noctule bats, *Nyctalus noctula*. *J. Reprod. Fertil.* **41**, 169–182.

Ralph, C. L., Harlow, H. J., and Phillips, J. A. (1982). Delayed effect of pinealectomy on hibernation of the golden-mantled ground squirrel. *Int. J. Biometeorol.* **26**, 311–328.

Reiter, R. J. (1974). Influence of pinealectomy on the breeding capability of hamsters maintained under natural photoperiodic and temperature conditions. *Neuroendocrinology* **13**, 366–370.

Reiter, R. J. (1980). Photoperiod: Its importance as an impeller of pineal and seasonal reproductive rhythms. *Int. J. Biometeorol.* **24**, 57–63.

Reiter, R. J. (1998). Melatonin and human reproduction. *Ann. Med.* **30**, 103–108.

Reiter, R. J., Vaughn, M. K., Blask, D. E., and Johnson, L. Y. (1974). Melatonin: Its inhibition of pineal antigonadotrophic activity in male hamsters. *Science* **185**, 1169–1171.

Reiter, R. J., Vaughan, M. K., and Waring, P. J. (1977). Prevention by melatonin of short day induced atrophy of the reproductive systems of male and female hamsters. *Acta Endocrinol. (Copenhagen)* **84**, 410–418.

Reiter, R. J., Rudeen, P. K., Banks, A. F., and Rollag, M. D. (1979). Acute effects of unilateral or bilateral superior cervical ganglionectomy on rat pineal N-acetyltransferase activity and melatonin content. *Experientia* **35**, 691–692.

Richard, A. F., Dewar, R. E., Schwartz, M., and Ratsirarson, J. (2000). Mass change, environmental variability and female fertility in wild *Propithecus verreauxi*. *J. Hum. Evol.* **39**, 381–391.

Riesen, J. W., Meyer, R. K., and Wolf, R. C. (1971). The effect of season on occurrence of ovulation in the rhesus monkey. *Biol. Reprod.* **5**, 111–114.

Rivkees, S. A., Hall, D. A., Weaver, D. R., and Reppert, S. M. (1988). Djungarian hamsters exhibit reproductive responses to changes in daylength at extreme photoperiods. *Endocrinology (Baltimore)* **122**, 2634–2638.

Robinson, J. E., Wayne, N. L., and Karsch, F. J. (1985). Refractoriness to inhibitory day lengths initiates the breeding season of the Suffolk ewe. *Biol. Reprod.* **32**, 1024–1030.

Rodgers, J. L., Harris, D. F., and Vickers, K. B. (1992). Seasonality of first coitus in the United States. *Soc. Biol.* **39**, 1–14.

Roenneberg, T., and Aschoff, J. (1990a). Annual rhythm of human reproduction: I. Biology, sociology, or both? *J. Biol. Rhythms* **5**, 195–216.

Roenneberg, T., and Aschoff, J. (1990b). Annual rhythm of human reproduction: II. Environmental correlations. *J. Biol. Rhythms* **5**, 217–239.

Ronchi, E., Krey, L. C., and Pfaff, D. W. (1992). Steady state analysis of hypothalamic GnRH mRNA levels in male Syrian hamsters: Influences of photoperiod and androgen. *Neuroendocrinology* **55**, 146–155.

Ronchi, E., Spencer, R. L., Krey, L. C., and McEwen, B. S. (1998). Effects of photoperiod on brain corticosteroid receptors and the stress response in the Golden hamster (*Mesocricetus auratus*). *Brain Res.* **780**, 348–351.

Rostal, D. C., Glick, B. B., Eaton, G. G., and Resko, J. A. (1986). Seasonality of adult male Japanese macaques (*Macaca fuscata*): Androgens and behavior in a confined troop. *Horm. Behav.* **20**, 452–462.

Rowsemitt, C. N. (1986). Seasonal variations in activity rhythms of male voles: Mediation by gonadal hormones. *Physiol. Behav.* **37**, 797–803.

Rowesmitt, C. N., Petterborg, L. J., Claypool, L. E., and Hoppenstedt, F. C. (1982). Photoperiodic induction of diurnal locomotor activity in *Microtus montanus*, the montane vole. *Can. J. Zool.* **60**, 2798–2803.

Ruby, N. F., Ibuka, N., Barnes, B. M., and Zucker, I. (1989). Suprachiasmatic nuclei influence torpor and circadian temperature rhythms in hamsters. *Am. J. Physiol.* **257**, R210–R215.

Ruby, N. F., Dark, J., Heller, H. C., and Zucker, I. (1996). Ablation of suprachiasmatic nucleus alters timing of hibernation in ground squirrels. *Proc. Natl. Acad. Sci. U.S.A.* **93**, 9864–9868.

Ruby, N. F., Dark, J., Heller, H. C., and Zucker, I. (1998). Suprachiasmatic nucleus: Role in circannual body mass and hibernation rhythms of ground squirrels. *Brain Res.* **782**, 63–72.

Ruf, T. (1993). Individual energetic strategies in winter-adapted Djungarian hamsters: The relation between daily torpor, locomotion, and food consumption. *In* "Life in the Cold: Ecological, Physiological, and Molecular Mechanisms" (C. Carey, G. L. Florant, B. A. Wunder, and B. Horwitz, eds.), pp. 99–107. Westview Press, Boulder, CO.

Ruf, T., and Heldmaier, G. (1992). Reduced locomotor activity following daily torpor in the Djungarian hamster: Recovery from hypothermia? *Naturwissenschaften* **79**, 574–575.

Ruf, T., Korytko, A. I., Stieglitz, A., Lavenburg, K. R., and Blank, J. L. (1997). Phenotypic variation in seasonal adjustments of testis size, body weight, and food intake in deer mice: Role of pineal function and ambient temperature. *J. Comp. Physiol. B* **167**, 185–192.

Rusak, B., and Morin, L. P. (1976). Testicular responses to photoperiod are blocked by lesions of the suprachiasmatic nuclei in Golden hamsters. *Biol. Reprod.* **15**, 366–374.

Saboureau, M. (1986). Hibernation in the hedgehog: Influence of of external and internal factors. *In* "Living in the Cold: Physiological and Biochemical Adaptations" (H. C. Heller, X. J. Musacchia, and L. C. H. Wang, eds.), pp. 253–263. Am. Elsevier, New York.

Sadleir, R. M. F. S. (1969). "The Ecology of Reproduction in Wild and Domestic Mammals." Methuen, London.

Sandweiss, D. H., Maasch, K. A., and Anderson, D. G. (1999). Climate and culture—Transitions in the mid-Holocene. *Science* **283**, 499–500.

Sapolsky, R. M. (1992). "Stress, the Aging Brain, and the Mechanisms of Neuron Death." MIT Press, Cambridge, MA.

Sapolsky, R. M. (1998). "Why Zebras Don't Get Ulcers: An Updated Guide to Stress, Stress-Related Diseases, and Coping." Freeman, San Francisco.

Sapolsky, R. M., Krey, L., and McEwen, B. S. (1984). Glucocorticoid-sensitive hippocampal neurons are involved in terminating the adrenocortical stress response. *Proc. Natl. Acad. Sci. U.S.A.* **81**, 6174–6177.

Sapolsky, R. M., Romero, L. M., and Munck, A. U. (2000). How do glucocorticoids influence stress responses? Integrating permissive, suppressive, stimulatory, and preparative actions. *Endocr. Rev.* **21**, 55–89.

Sato, T., Attanasio, A., Wake, K., and Gupta, D. (1989). Rhythm development in pineal and circulating serotonin, N-acetylserotonin, and melatonin in Syrian hamsters. *J. Pineal Res.* **7**, 45–54.

Sawry, D. K., and Dewsbury, D. A. (1994). Conspecific odor preferences in montane voles (*Microtus montanus*): Effects of sexual experience. *Physiol. Behav.* **56**, 339–344.

Schiml, P. A., Mendoza, S. P., Saltzman, W., Lyons, D. M., and Mason, W. A. (1996). Seasonality in squirrel monkeys (*Saimiri sciureus*): Social facilitation by females. *Physiol. Behav.* **60**, 1105–1113.

Schiml, P. A., Mendoza, S. P., Saltzman, W., Lyons, D. M., and Mason, W. A. (1999). Annual physiological changes in individually housed squirrel monkeys (*Saimiri sciureus*). *Am. J. Primatol.* **47**, 93–103.

Schlatt, S., Niklowitz, P., Hoffmann, K., and Nieschlag, E. (1993). Influence of short photoperiods on reproductive organs and estrous cycles of normal and pinealectomized female Djungarian hamsters, *Phodopus sungorus*. *Biol. Reprod.* **49**, 243–250.

Schneider, J. E., Friedenson, D. G., Hall, A. J., and Wade, G. N. (1993). Glucoprivation induces anestrus and lipoprivation may induce hibernation in Syrian hamsters. *Am. J. Physiol.* **264**, R573–R577.

Schneider, J. E., Blum, R. M., and Wade, G. N. (2000). Metabolic control of food intake and estrous cycles in Syrian hamsters. I. Plasma insulin and leptin. *Am. J. Physiol.* **278**, R476–R485.

Scott, I., D'Agostino, G., Cernova, T., Becker, L., and Giovinazzo, L. (1981). Seasonal testosterone in the eastern chipmunk, *Tamias striatus*. *Cryobiology* **18**, 89 (abstr.).

Seegal, R. F., and Goldman, B. D. (1975). Effects of photoperiod on cyclicity and serum gonadotropins in the Syrian hamster. *Biol. Reprod.* **12**, 223–231.

Sheldon, B. C., and Verhulst, S. (1996). Ecological immunology: Parasite defences and trade-offs in evolutionary ecology. *Trends Ecol. Evol.* **11**, 317–321.

Sherwin, C. M. (1998). Voluntary wheel running: A review and novel interpretation. *Anim. Behav.* **56**, 11–27.

Sicard, B., Fuminier, F., Maurel, D., and Boissin, J. (1993). Temperature and water conditions mediate the effects of day length on the breeding cycle of a Sahelian rodent, *Arvicanthis niloticus*. *Biol. Reprod.* **49**, 716–722.

Sinclair, J. A., and Lochmiller, R. L. (2000). The winter immunoenhancement hypothesis: Associations among immunity, density, and survival in prairie vole (*Microtus ochrogaster*) populations. *Can. J. Zool.* **78**, 254–264.

Sinervo, B., and Basolo, A. L. (1996). Testing adaptation using phenotypic manipulation. *In* "Adaptation" (M. R. Rose and G. V. Lauder, eds.), pp. 149–185. Academic Press, San Diego, CA.

Smale, L., Nelson, R. J., and Zucker, I. (1985). Neuroendocrine responsiveness to oestradiol and male urine in neonatally androgenized prairie voles (*Microtus ochrogaster*). *J. Reprod. Fertil.* **74**, 491–496.

Smith, G. P., and Epstein, A. N. (1969). Increased feeding in response to decreased glucose utilization in the rat and monkey. *Am. J. Physiol.* **217**, 1083–1087.

Spears, N., and Clarke, J. R. (1986). Effect of male presence and of photoperiod on the sexual maturation of the field vole (*Microtus agrestis*). *J. Reprod. Fertil.* **78**, 231–238.

Spears, N., Meyer, J. S., Whaling, C. S., Wade, G. N., Zucker, I., and Dark, J. (1990). Long day lengths enhance myelination of midbrain and hindbrain regions of developing meadow voles. *Dev. Brain Res.* **55**, 103–108.

Speth, J. D. (1987). Early hominid subsistence strategies in seasonal habitats. *J. Archaeol. Sci.* **14**, 13–30.

Spurlock, M. E. (1997). Regulation of metabolism and growth during immune challenge: An overview of cytokine function. *J. Anim. Sci.* **75**, 1773–1783.

Stebbins, L. L. (1977). Some aspects of overwintering in *Peromyscus maniculatus. Can. J. Zool.* **56**, 386–390.

Steinlechner, S., Stieglitz, A., Ruf, T., Heldmaier, G., and Reiter, R. J. (1991). Integration of environmental signals by the pineal gland and its significance for seasonality in small mammals. *In* "Role of Melatonin and Pineal Peptides in Neuroimmunoregulation" (F. Fraschini and R. J. Reiter, eds.), pp. 159–163. Plenum Press, New York.

Stetson, M. H., Elliott, J. A., and Goldman, B. D. (1986). Maternal transfer of photoperiodic information influences the photoperiodic response of prepubertal Djungarian hamsters (*Phodopus sungorus sungorus*). *Biol. Reprod.* **34**, 664–669.

Stetson, M. H., Ray, S. L., Creyaufmiller, N., and Horton, T. H. (1989). Maternal transfer of photoperiodic information in Siberian hamsters. II. The nature of the maternal signal, time of signal transfer, and the effect of the maternal signal on peripubertal reproductive development in the absence of photoperiodic inputs. *Biol. Reprod.* **40**, 458–465.

Stewart, K. M. (1994). Early hominid utilization of fish resources and implications for seasonality and behavior. *J. Hum. Evol.* **27**, 229–245.

Stieglitz, A., Gwinner, K., Spiegelhalter, F., Wicherek, M., and Heldmaier, G. (1994). Urinary 6-sulphatoxymelatonin as an index of pineal function in the Djungarian hamster: Influence of photoperiod and ambient temperature. *Adv. Pineal Res.* **8**, 285–291.

Stirland, J. A., Mohammad, Y. N., and Loudon, A. S. (1996). A mutation of the circadian timing system (tau gene) in the seasonally breeding Syrian hamster alters the reproductive response to photoperiod change. *Proc. R. Soc. London, Ser. B* **263**, 345–350.

Struhsaker, T. T. (1997). "Ecology of an African Rain Forest: Logging in Kibale and the Conflict Between Conservation and Exploitation." University Press of Florida, Gainesville.

Sumova, A., Travnickova, Z., Peters, R., Schwartz, W. J., and Illnerova, H. (1995). The rat suprachiasmatic nucleus is a clock for all seasons. *Proc. Natl. Acad. Sci. U.S.A.* **92**, 7754–7758.

Takahashi, N., Waelput, W., and Guisez, A. (1999). Leptin is an endogenous protective protein against the toxicity exerted by tumor necrosis factor. *J. Exp. Med.* **189**, 207–212.

Tamarkin, L., Lefebvre, N. G., Hollister, C. W., and Goldman, B. D. (1977). Effect of melatonin administered during the night on reproductive function in the Syrian hamster. *Endocrinology (Baltimore)* **101**, 631–634

Turek, F. W., and van Cauter, E. (1994). Rhythms in reproduction. *In* "The Physiology of Reproduction" (E. Knobil and J. D. Neill, eds.), 2nd ed., Vols. 1 and 2, pp. 487–540. Raven Press, New York.

Turner, B. N., Perrin, M. R., and Iverson, S. L. (1975). Winter coexistence of voles in spruce forest: Relevance of seasonal changes in aggression. *Can. J. Zool.* **53**, 1004–1011.

Urbanski, H. F., Doan, A., and Pierce, M. (1991). Immunocytochemical investigation of luteinizing hormone-releasing hormone neurons in Syrian hamsters maintained under long or short days. *Biol. Reprod.* **44**, 687–692.

Vanecek, J. (1988). Melatonin binding sites. *J. Neurochem.* **51**, 1436–1440.

Vanecek, J., Jansky, L., Illnerova, H., and Hoffmann, K. (1984). Pineal melatonin in hibernating and aroused Golden hamsters (*Mesocricetus auratus*). *Comp. Biochem. Physiol. A* **77**, 759–762.

van Schaik, C. P., Terborgh, J. W., and Wright, S. J. (1993). The phenology of tropical forests—adaptive significance and consequences for primary consumers. *Annu. Rev. Ecol. Syst.* **24**, 353–377.

Vondrasova, D., Hajek, I., and Illnerova, H. (1997). Exposure to long summer days affects the human melatonin and cortisol rhythms. *Brain Res.* **759**, 166–170.

von Mutius, E. (2000). The environmental predictors of allergic disease. *J. Allergy Clin. Immunol.* **105**, 9–19.

Waage, A., Halstensen, A., Shalaby, R., Brandtzaeg, P., Kierulf, P., and Espevik, T. (1989). Local production of tumor necrosis factor alpha, interleukin 1, and interleukin 6 in meningococcal meningitis. Relation to the inflammatory response. *J. Exp. Med.* **170**, 1859–1867.

Wade, G. N., Bartness, T. J., and Alexander, J. R. (1986). Photoperiod and body weight in female Syrian hamsters: Skeleton photoperiods, response magnitude, and development of photorefractoriness. *Physiol. Behav.* **37**, 863–868.

Walkden-Brown, S. W., Martin, G. B., and Restall, B. J. (1999). Role of male-female interaction in regulating reproduction in sheep and goats. *J. Reprod. Fertil., Suppl.* **154**, 243–257.

Wallis, J. (1997). A survey of reproductive parameters in the free-ranging chimpanzees of Gombe National Park. *J. Reprod. Fertil.* **109**, 297–307.

Warburton, V. L., Sales, G. D., and Milligan, S. R. (1989). The emission and elicitation of mouse ultrasonic vocalizations:

The effects of age, sex and gonadal status. *Physiol. Behav.* **45**, 41–47.

Watson-Whitmyre, K., and Stetson, M. H. (1988). Reproductive refractoriness in hamsters: Environmental and endocrine etiologies. *In* "Processing of Environmental Information in Vertebrates" (M. H. Stetson, ed.), pp. 203–218. Springer-Verlag, New York.

Watts, D. P. (1998). Seasonality in the ecology and life histories of mountain gorillas (*Gorilla gorilla beringei*). *Int. J. Primatol.* **19**, 929–948.

Weaver, D. R., and Reppert, S. M. (1986). Maternal melatonin communicates daylength to the fetus in Djungarian hamsters. *Endocrinology (Baltimore)* **119**, 2861–2863.

Weaver, D. R., and Reppert, S. M. (1990). Melatonin receptors are present in the ferret pars tuberalis and pars distalis, but not in brain. *Endocrinology (Baltimore)* **127**, 2607–2609.

Weaver, D. R., Keohan, J. T., and Reppert, S. M. (1987). Definition of a prenatal sensitive period for maternal-fetal communication of day length. *Am. J. Physiol.* **253**, E701–E704.

Weaver, D. R., Rivkees, S. A., and Reppert, S. M. (1989). Localization and characterization of melatonin receptors in rodent brain by in vitro autoradiography. *J. Neurosci.* **9**, 2581–2590.

Webb, T. (1993). Vegetation, lake levels, and climate in eastern North America for the past 18,000 years. *In* "Global Climates Since the Last Glacial Maximum" (H. E. Wright, J. E. Kutzbach, T. Webb, W. F. Ruddiman, F. A. Street-Perrott, and P. J. Bartlein, eds.), pp. 415–467. University of Minnesota Press, Minneapolis.

Wehr, T. A. (1997). Melatonin and seasonal rhythms. *J. Biol. Rhythms* **12**, 518–527.

Weidenfeld, J., Siegel, R. A., Corcos, A. P., Heled, V., Conforti, N., and Chowers, I. (1984). ACTH and corticosterone secretion following 2-deoxyglucose administration in intact and in hypothalamic deafferentated male rats. *Brain Res.* **305**, 109–113.

West, S. D., and Dublin, H. T. (1984). Behavioral strategies of small mammals under winter conditions solitary or social. *Carnegie Mus. Nat. Hist., Spec. Publ.* **10**, 293–300.

Wetterberg, L. (1999). Melatonin and clinical application. *Reprod. Nutr. Dev.* **39**, 367–382.

Whitsett, J. M., and Lawton, A. D. (1982). Social stimulation of reproductive development in male deer mice housed on a short-day photoperiod. *J. Comp. Physiol. Psychol.* **96**, 416–422.

Whitsett, J. M., and Miller, L. L. (1982). Photoperiod and reproduction in female deer mice. *Biol. Reprod.* **26**, 296–304.

Wick, A. N., Drury, D. R., Nakada, H. I., and Wolfe, J. B. (1957). Localization of the primary metabolic block produced by 2-deoxy-glucose. *J. Biol. Chem.* **224**, 963–969.

Wickings, E. J., and Nieschlag, E. (1980). Seasonality in endocrine and exocrine testicular function of the adult rhesus monkey (*Macaca mulatta*) maintained in a controlled laboratory environment. *Int. J. Androl.* **3**, 87–104.

Widmaier, E. P., Long, J., Cadigan, B., Gurgel, S., and Kunz, T. H. (1997). Leptin, corticotropin-releasing hormone (CRH), and neuropeptide Y (NPY) in free-ranging pregnant bats. *Endocrine* **7**, 145–150.

Wilson, M. E., Pope, N. S., and Gordon, T. P. (1987). Seasonal modulation of luteinizing-hormone secretion in female rhesus monkeys. *Biol. Reprod.* **36**, 975–984.

Wimsatt, W. A. (1969). Some interrelations of reproduction and hibernation in mammals. *Symp. Soc. Exp. Biol.* **23**, 511–549.

Wolff, J. O., and Lidicker, W. Z. (1980). Population ecology of the tiaga vole, *Microtus xanthognathus*, in interior Alaska. *Can. J. Zool.* **58**, 1800–1812.

Wood, R. I. (1996). Estradiol, but not dihydrotestosterone, in the medial amygdala facilitates male hamster sex behavior. *Physiol. Behav.* **59**, 833–841.

Woodfill, C. J., Robinson, J. E., Malpaux, B., and Karsch, F. J. (1991). Synchronization of the circannual reproductive rhythm of the ewe by discrete photoperiodic signals. *Biol. Reprod.* **45**, 110–121.

Woodfill, C. J., Wayne, N. L., Moenter, S. M., and Karsch, F. J. (1994). Photoperiodic synchronization of a circannual reproductive rhythm in sheep: Identification of season-specific time cues. *Biol. Reprod.* **50**, 965–976.

Worth, R. W., Charlton, H. M., and Mackinnon, P. C. (1973). Field and laboratory studies on the control of luteinizing hormone secretion and gonadal activity in the vole, *Microtus agrestis*. *J. Reprod. Fertil.* **19**, 89–99.

Wunder, B. A. (1984). Strategies for, and environmental cueing mechanisms of, seasonal changes in thermoregulatory parameters of small mammals. *Carnegie Mus. Nat. Hist., Spec. Publ.* **10**, 165–172.

Wunder, B. A., Dobkin, D., and Gettinger, R. (1977). Shifts of thermogenesis in the prairie vole (*Microtus ochrogaster*). *Oecologia* **29**, 11–26.

Xu, Z. Z., McDonald, M. F., McCutcheon, S. N., and Blair, H. T. (1992). Effects of season and testosterone treatment on gonadotrophin secretion and pituitary responsiveness to gonadotrophin-releasing hormone in castrated Romney and Poll Dorset rams. *J. Reprod. Fertil.* **95**, 183–190.

Yaskin, V. A. (1984). Seasonal changes in brain morphology in small mammals. *Carnegie Mus. Nat. Hist., Spec. Publ.* **10**, 183–192.

Yaskin, V. A. (1998). Hippocampus mass dynamics and spatial behavior feature in annual cycle of bank voles. *Dokl. Akad. Nauk* **360**, 141–144.

Yellon, S. M. (1994). Effects of photoperiod on reproduction and the gonadotropin-releasing hormone-immunoreactive neuron system in the postpubertal male Djungarian hamster. *Biol. Reprod.* **50**, 368–372.

Yellon, S. M., and Goldman, B. D. (1984). Photoperiod control of reproductive development in the male Djungarian hamster *(Phodopus sungorus)*. *Endocrinology (Baltimore)* **114**, 664–670.

Yellon, S. M., Fagoaga, O. R., and Nehlsen-Cannarella, S. L. (1999). Influence of photoperiod on immune cell functions in the male Siberian hamster. *Am. J. Physiol.* **276**, R97–R102.

Ziegler, T., Hodges, K., Winkler, P., and Heistermann, M. (2000). Hormonal correlates of reproductive seasonality in wild female Hanuman langurs *(Presbytis entellus)*. *Am. J. Primatol.* **51**, 119–134.

Zucker, I. (1985). Pineal gland influences period of circannual rhythms of ground squirrels. *Am. J. Physiol.* **249**, R111–R115.

Zucker, I. (1988). Seasonal affective disorders: Animal models *non fingo*. *J. Biol. Rhythms* **3**, 209–223.

Zucker, I. (2001). Circannual rhythms: Mammals. *In* "Handbook of Behavioral Neurobiology" Vol. 12 : Circadian Clocks (J. Takahashi, F. W. Turek, and R. Y. Moore, eds.), pp. 509–528. Kluwer Academic/Plenum Press, New York.

Zucker, I., Fitzgerald, K. M., and Morin, L. P. (1980a). Sex differentiation of the circadian system in the golden hamster. *Am. J. Physiol.* **238**, R97–R101

Zucker, I., Johnston, P. G., and Frost, D. (1980b). Comparative, physiological, and biochronometric analyses of rodent seasonal reproductive cycles. *Prog. Reprod. Biol.* **5**, 102–133.

Zucker, I., Boshes, M., and Dark, J. (1983). Suprachiasmatic nuclei influence circannual and circadian rhythms of ground squirrels. *Am. J. Physiol.* **244**, R472–R480.

Zucker, I., Lee, T. M., and Dark, J. (1991). The suprachiasmatic nucleus and annual rhythms of mammals. *In* "The Suprachiasmatic Nucleus: The Mind's Clock" (D. C. Klein, R. Y. Moore, and S. M. Reppert, eds.), pp. 246–259. Oxford University Press, New York.

20

Thyroid Hormones in Neural Tissue

Ronald M. Lechan
Tupper Research Institute, New England Medical Center and Department of Neuroscience, Tufts University School of Medicine Boston, Massachusetts 02111

Roberto Toni
Department of Human Anatomy University of Parma School of Medicine Parma, Italy

I. INTRODUCTION

A. Historical Overview

Knowledge that the brain has a critical role in the control of thyroid hormone secretion from the thyroid gland is based on nearly a century of research beginning with the observation by Smith in 1916 that ablation of the tadpole pituitary gland prevents growth of the thyroid gland. The subsequent discovery of neurosecretion by the Scharrers between 1928 and 1940 (Scharrer, 1928; Scharrer and Scharrer, 1940, 1954), elucidation of the portal vessel chemotransmitter hypothesis by Harris (1955), demonstration by Halasz et al. (1962) that grafts of the anterior pituitary to the base of the hypothalamus but not other regions outside of the central nervous system (CNS) support function of the thyroid gland, and Greer's identification of the "thyrotropic area" within the hypothalamus (Greer, 1957), are among the many findings that established the importance of the brain in thyroid hormone secretion. Detailed historical accounts have been given by Reichlin (1966, 1989).

B. Importance of Feedback Regulation by Thyroid Hormone

The maintenance of normal thyroid function (euthyroidism) is now recognized to be dependent on a complex interplay between the hypothalamus, anterior pituitary, and thyroid gland as well as other factors that influence the function of these organ systems. The major hormone responsible for the secretion of thyroid hormone from the thyroid is thyroid-stimulating hormone (TSH), also termed thyrotropin. TSH is secreted from anterior pituitary thyrotropes, which comprise approximately 10% of the anterior pituitary cells, and in turn is positively regulated by thyrotropin-releasing hormone (TRH), originating in the hypothalamus. The free fraction of thyroid hormone circulating in the bloodstream (<1% of total, protein-bound thyroid hormone) feeds back both on the anterior pituitary and hypothalamus to inhibit the secretion of TSH and TRH, respectively, thereby completing what is recognized as a classic example of a negative feedback loop system (Fig. 1).

Ultimately, the role of the negative feedback system to control thyroid function is to maintain a constant level of free thyroid hormone in the bloodstream. In addition to important effects on peripheral tissues by affecting protein synthesis and/or altering the metabolic activity of cells, thyroid hormone is essential for normal brain development during fetal growth and early infancy. Cretinism, characterized by mental deficiency, spastic or ataxic gait, impaired voluntary motor activity, and defects in hearing and speech, occurs if thyroid hormone is not available during fetal development (Dussault and Ruel, 1987). This syndrome arises as a result of a number of structural and functional abnormalities

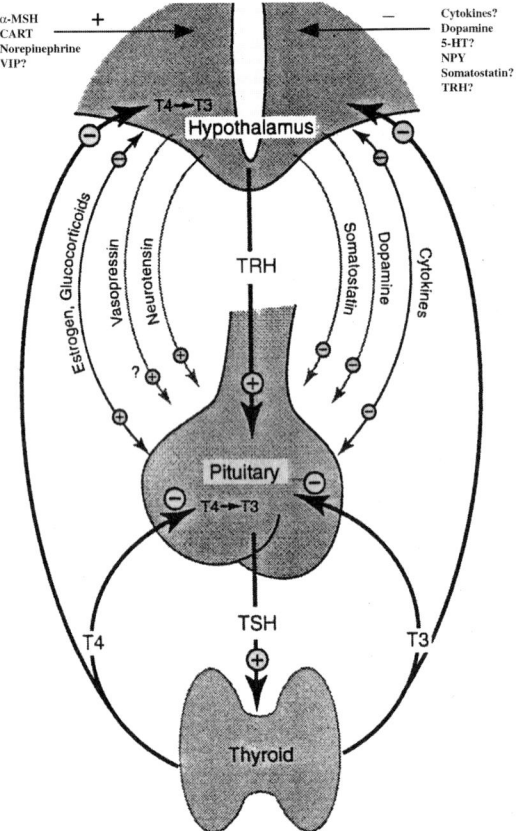

FIGURE 1 Schematic diagram of the neuroregulatory control systems involved in the secretion of thyroid hormone. Bold lines denote the negative feedback loop of thyroid hormone on TRH secretion from the hypothalamus and TSH secretion from the anterior pituitary. Both the hypothalamic TRH neurons and anterior pituitary thyrotropes are impinged on by numerous other potential regulatory influences that are activated under specific physiological or pathological conditions.

in the brain due to severe hypothyroidism, including poor neurite outgrowth and synapse formation, decreased myelination, reduction in the formation of microtubules, and delayed axoplasmic transport, diffusely throughout the brain but particularly in the cerebral cortex, cerebellum, and basal ganglia (see Chapter 74). Damage to the pyramidal and extrapyramidal system is usually permanent, whereas mental retardation can be prevented if thyroid hormone is replaced within a critical period following birth (approximately 1–3 months in man). Maintaining normal circulating levels of thyroid hormone is also important in the mature, adult brain, as thyroid hormone insufficiency or excess can result in a number of functional, neurological, and behavioral manifestations, as summarized in Table 1 and discussed in detail in Chapter 21.

Secretion of TSH by the pituitary is strongly influenced by the normal level of free thyroid hormone. If thyroid hormone levels fall below normal, there is an increase in TSH secretion to restore thyroid hormone levels back to normal; if thyroid hormone levels rise above normal, there is suppression of TSH secretion. The inverse relationship between thyroid hormone levels and TSH secretion is extremely precise such that slight increases or decreases in thyroid hormone levels circulating in the bloodstream, even within the normal range, can have inhibitory or stimulatory effects on the secretion of TSH (Snyder and Utiger, 1973; Saberi and Utiger, 1975). TRH also has an important influence on the set point for TSH secretion such that an increase or decrease in TRH secretion can alter the set point for feedback regulation of anterior pituitary TSH secretion by thyroid hormone. However, a number of factors, in addition to TRH, TSH, and thyroid hormone, can also be involved in the regulation of thyroid hormone secretion, including peptides, catecholamines, cytokines, steroid hormones, and nuclear regulatory factors, many originating in the brain.

II. MECHANISMS OF THYROID HORMONE ACTION IN THE CNS

A. Thyroid Hormone Transport in the Bloodstream

Thyroid hormone circulates primarily as L-thyroxine (T_4) and triiodothyronine (T_3), composed of two amino acids differing only in the number of iodine molecules on its tyrosine rings (Fig. 2). Because of their poor solubility in aqueous solutions, thyroid hormones are largely bound to plasma proteins that serve as reservoirs for their hormones. Only a small fraction of the total circulates as unbound (free) T_4 and free T_3, respectively. In man, the normal concentration of T_4 in the bloodstream ranges from 4.2 to 12.0 μg/dl of which 0.02% is free, and the normal concentration of T_3 ranges from 80 to 200 ng/dl, of which 0.3% is free. Nevertheless, the biological activity of thyroid hormone is exerted only by the fraction that is free in the plasma. This became apparent when Recant and Riggs (1952) and Robbins and Rall (1957) observed that conditions that increase or

TABLE 1
Clinical Manifestations of Thyroid Hormone Excess or Insufficiency on the Central and Peripheral Nervous Systems

Excess thyroid hormone	Insufficient thyroid hormone
Tremor	Cretinism (mental deficiency, defects in hearing and speech, spastic or ataxic gait, impaired voluntary motor activity, clonus)
Nervousness	
Tremulousness (hyperkinesis agitation, irritability)	
Insomnia	Sleep apnea
Vivid dreams and nightmares	Dysarthria
Decreased memory	Hypothermia
Impaired concentration	Hypoventilation
Seizures	Cerebellar ataxia
Chorea	Coma
Coma	Neuropsychiatric syndromes [myxedema madness (psychosis), dementia]
Neuropsychiatric syndromes (depression, anxiety, mania, dysphoria, emotional lability, attention deficit, weakness, delirium, paranoia)	Peripheral neuropathy (carpal tunnel syndrome, facial)

decrease the concentration thyroid hormone–binding proteins do not result hyper- or hypothyroidism, respectively, and that the concentration of free T_4 and T_3 in the plasma remain unaltered. The natural conclusion, therefore, is that feedback regulation of the hypothalamic-pituitary-thyroid axis occurs in response to the circulating levels of free but not total thyroid hormones.

On the basis of studies by Mendel *et al.* (1987), the importance of thyroid hormone–binding proteins is presumed to provide the uniform distribution of thyroid hormones to all cells of every tissue such that each cell sees the same concentration of circulating thyroid hormone. Thus, when rat liver was perfused through the portal vein with radiolabeled T_4 in the absence of thyroid hormone–binding proteins, T_4 was disproportionaly taken up by cells in the hepatic lobule—highly concentrated in the first cells it contacted, but unavailable to cells more distal to the portal vein. In contrast, when T_4 was perfused in the presence of thyroid hormone–binding proteins, T_4 was taken up uniformly by all cells. However, thyroid-binding proteins are not involved in the mechanism of cellular uptake of thyroid hormones. Therefore, the intracellular concentration of thyroid hormone can vary from tissue to tissue, depending partly on the rate of active transport of T_4 into the cell, but also the local conversion of T_4 to the more biologically active T_3 and the rate of intracellular elimination, either by transport and secretion or inactivation to reverse T_3 (rT_3) and T_2, as described more fully below. In this manner, thyroid hormone is utilized in a tissue-specific manner, presumably in a way that is necessary to preserve biological function. Thyroid hormone–binding proteins may also contribute to the conservation of iodine by preventing renal losses.

Thyroxine-binding globulin (TBG) is the major transport protein in man, binding approximately 70% of the circulating T_4 and 80% of circulating T_3. TBG is synthesized in the liver, has a molecular weight of approximately 44,000, and is a member of the serine antiprotease superfamily (Fink *et al.*, 1986). TBG levels are subject to change under certain conditions such as pregnancy and exogenous estrogen administration when the TBG concentration increases, but as stated above, the resulting increase in total T_4 and T_3 levels in the plasma are not associated with thyrotoxicosis because bound thyroid hormone is inactive, and free thyroid hormone levels remain unchanged.

Transthyretin (TTR), previously called thyroxine-binding prealbumin (TBPA), is similarly a major thyroid hormone–binding protein, carrying approximately 10% of the circulating total T_4 to which it binds with high affinity, and approximately 10% of circulating T_3 to which it binds with low affinity. TTR is synthesized in

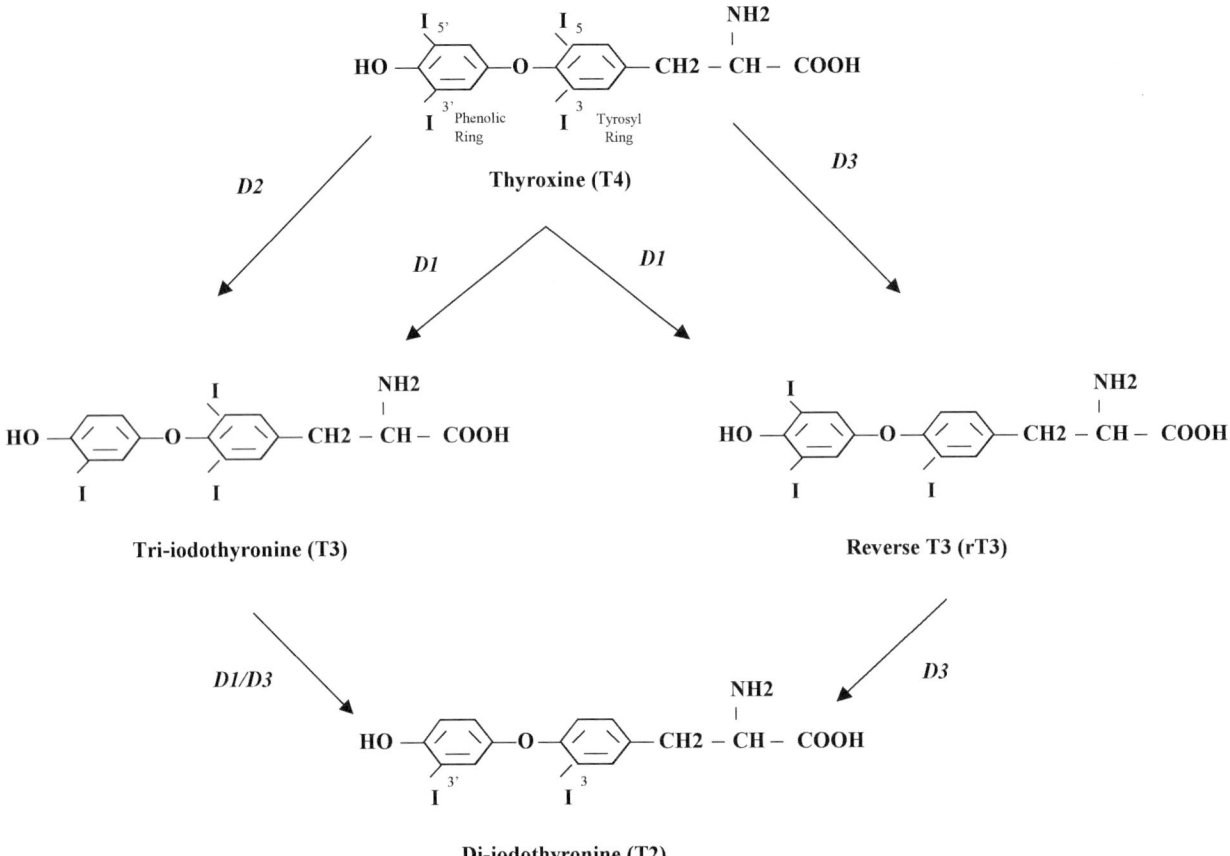

FIGURE 2 Chemical structures of L-thyroxine (T_4) and triiodothyronine (T_3) and their metabolites. The conversion of T_4 to T_3 and the inactivation of T_3 depend on membrane-bound enzymes called deiodinases. D_1, type 1 deiodinase; D_2, type 2 deiodinase; D_3, type 3 deiodinase. Reverse T_3 (rT_3) and diiodothyronine (T_2) are biologically inactive.

the liver and circulates as an approximately 55,000 MW protein composed for four, identical subunits with a central channel that contains two binding sites for thyroid hormone (Blake et al., 1974). Since binding to the first site reduces the affinity of thyroid hormone–binding to the second site, only a single binding site is occupied in a single tetramer of TTR. Dissociation of thyroid hormone from TTR is greater than from TBG (Hiller, 1971), but because so much more T_4 and T_3 are bound to TBG, the amounts of thyroid hormone released from both binding proteins are similar.

Albumin also binds thyroid hormone, although with a significantly weaker binding affinity for thyroid hormone than TBG or TTR. However, due to the high concentration of albumin in plasma, it accounts for the binding of approximately 20% of T_4 and 10% of T_3. The potential for changes in the concentration of free fatty acids to readily displace T_4 from albumin and increase the percentage of free T_4 (Mendel et al., 1987) makes albumin a rather poor transport protein for thyroid hormone in general. It is probably for this reason that genetic abnormalities characterized by the absence of both TBG and TTR have not been found in any animal species. Finally, a small percentage of the total circulating thyroid hormone is bound to apolipoprotein A1 and apolipoprotein B100 (Benvenga et al., 1989), as well as other blood components (Crispell and Coleman, 1956), but this is probably insignificant.

B. Thyroid Hormone Delivery across the Blood–Brain and Blood–CSF Barriers

Two mechanisms for transport of thyroid hormone from the peripheral circulation to the brain are known,

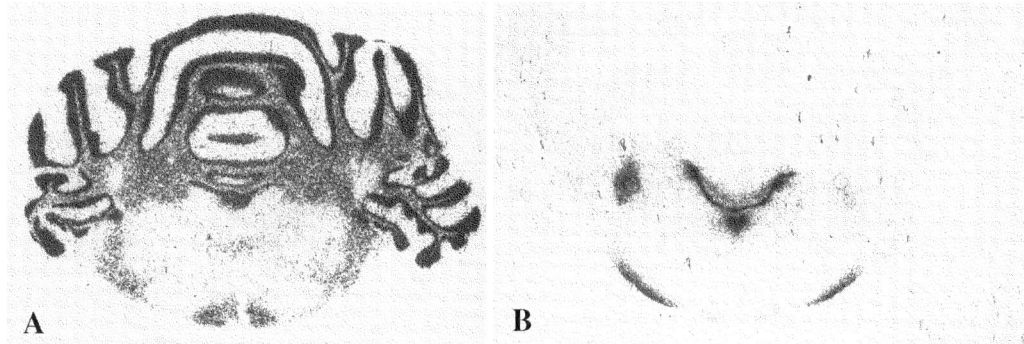

FIGURE 3 Distribution of ^{125}I-T$_3$ in the brain 48 hr after injection into the bloodstream (A) and the cerebrospinal fluid (B). Note the more uniform distribution of the radiolabeled material in the autoradiogram in (A). (From Dratman *et al.*, 1991, with permission.)

including movement through the blood-brain barrier across capillary endothelial cells, and through the blood–CSF barrier via the choroid plexus. On the basis that the surface area of the blood-brain barrier markedly exceeds the blood–cerebrospinal fluid (CSF) barrier, Pardridge (1979) proposed that the blood-brain barrier is the most important route for the transport of thyroid hormone to the brain. This concept would seem to be supported by the work of Dratman *et al.* (1976, 1982, 1987, 1991). Following the intravenous injection, radiolabeled T$_4$ and T$_3$ rapidly enter the brain in a diffuse pattern similar to the distribution of the cerebral blood flow. The concentration of thyroid hormone reaches a plateau within the first hour and is sustained within the brain for up to 48 hours, but in a distinct pattern, favoring the cerebral cortex, cerebellum, basal ganglia, and thalamus (Dratmen *et al.*, 1976, 1991) (Fig. 3A). Gordon *et al.* (1999) have proposed that following uptake into the brain, thyroid hormone can be further transported to distant destinations in the brain through anterograde transport in axons.

In contrast, injection of radiolabeled T$_4$ and T$_3$ into the CSF distributes only to regions immediately surrounding the ventricles and does not enter the deeper neuropil (Fig. 3B). Nevertheless, a considerable amount of attention has been focused on the choroid plexus as a point of entry of thyroid hormone into the brain. The choroid plexus is composed of epithelial cells that separate the peripheral vascular system from the CSF and has as one of its most important functions the synthesis of CSF. Following the intravenous administration of [^{125}I]T$_4$, the choroid plexus accumulates nearly 400 times more T$_4$ than any other region in the brain and even exceeds the concentration of radiolabeled T$_4$ in the liver (Fig. 4). This remarkable ability is primarily due to the synthesis of the thyroid hormone–binding protein TTR in choroid epithelial cells (Dickson *et al.*, 1985; Soprano *et al.*, 1985; Dickson and Schreiber, 1986; Herbert *et al.*, 1986). Thus, T$_4$ may bind TTR in choroid epithelial cells and then be extruded into the CSF together with TTR for transport within the ventricular system, or drawn across the choroid epithelial cells

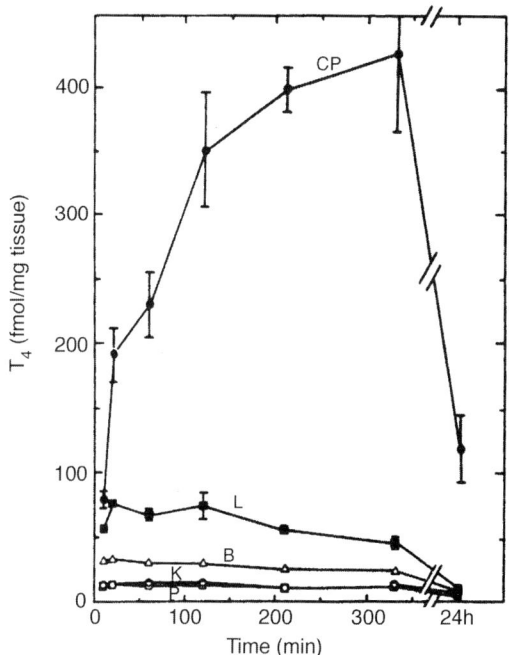

FIGURE 4 Kinetics of uptake of intraveneously injected ^{125}I-T$_4$ into the choroid plexus (CP), liver (L), kidney (K), and pituitary (P). (From Dickson *et al.*, 1986, with permission.)

to bind TTR secreted by the choroid into the CSF. In support of this hypothesis are the high concentration of TTR in the CSF, composing approximately 25% of the total CSF protein (Weisner and Roethig, 1983), the presence of bound and free thyroid hormones in the CSF (Hagen and Elliott, 1973; Thompson et al., 1982), and a reduction in CSF thyroid hormone levels when the binding of T_4 to TTR is competitively inhibited with the flavenoid EMD 21388 (Chanoine et al., 1992). Southwell et al. (1993) and Zheng et al. (1999) have similarly shown in two-chamber tissue culture system separated by a layer of choroid epithelial cells that competitive inhibition of T_4 binding to TTR by EMD 21388 or interference with TTR production by lead exposure prevents movement of T_4 across the choroid epithelial cells, establishing the importance of TTR in transcytosis of T_4 across the choroid plexus.

The possibility that the blood-CSF barrier may have an important role in the transport of thyroid hormone to the brain has been challenged by Palha et al. (1994, 2000), however, on the basis that deletion of the TTR gene in mice did not result in any phenotypic abnormalities and the free thyroid hormone levels were normal. The fact that TTR is preserved in the choroid plexus during vertebrate evolution from reptiles to man and appeared even before TTR expression in liver (Schreiber et al., 1995) however, suggests a fundamental importance for the presence of this thyroid hormone–binding protein in the brain that requires further elucidation.

C. Thyroid Hormone Transport into the CNS

It has been long postulated that thyroid hormone is actively transported across cell membranes by a saturable, energy-dependent mechanism and does not simply diffuse across cells (Krenning et al., 1978, 1981). Evidence that binding sites for T_3 could be identified on the surface of a variety of cell types (Cheng et al., 1980; Segal and Ingbar, 1982), that the uptake of T_4 and T_3 into hepatocytes could be inhibited by antibodies to a high molecular weight membrane-specific protein or by the Na,K-ATPase inhibitor ouabain (Hennemann et al., 1986), and that the intracellular concentration of T_3 is more than 100-fold greater than the plasma free levels (Oppenheimer and Schwartz, 1985) gave further credence to this hypothesis. It is now clear that a specific transport mechanism for the movement of thyroid hormone across cell membranes does indeed exist and is mediated by multispecific membrane transporter proteins that are also involved in the transport of bile salts, conjugated steroids, organic amines, and a number of drugs.

The superfamily of membrane transporter proteins is rapidly expanding, and a summary can be found in Table 2. These include the Oatp gene family of organic anion transporters, originally cloned from rat liver (Jacquemin et al., 1994) but subsequently found to be present in other tissues, including kidney and brain (Saito et al., 1996; Angeletti et al., 1997; Noe et al., 1997; Abe et al., 1998; Gao et al., 1999); the prostaglandin transporter PGT (Kanai et al., 1995); the rat liver–specific organic anion transporter rlst-1 (Kakyo et al., 1999); the sodium-dependent taurocholate transporting polypeptide ntcp (Hagenbuch et al., 1991); and the renal organic ion transporter 1, rROAT1, rOAT1, mROAT1, fROAT1, and hOAT1 (Cihlar et al., 1999). Characteristic of the Oatp proteins is their large size (approximately 75,000 MW) and location in cell surface membranes with 12 transmembrane spanning domains (Fig. 5). Rlst-1 contains eleven transmembrane spanning domains, resulting in termination of its C-terminal portion in the extracellular domain (Kakyo et al., 1999), ntcp contains seven transmembrane spanning domains (Hagenbuch et al., 1991), and similar to the Oatp family, ROAT1 and OAT1 proteins contain twelve transmembrane spanning domains (Cihlar et al., 1999). Polarization of membrane transporter proteins to only one side of the cell membrane is commonly observed. This is particularly the case for the Oatp proteins, where in some cells, such as choroid epithelial cells, Oatp1 is located on the apical, microvillus cell border in contact with the CSF, whereas Oatp2 is located on its basolateral cell surface in contact with the capillary bed (Angeletti et al., 1997; Gao et al., 1999). This organization suggests the possibility of coorporation between the different Oatp proteins in the transport of substances across the blood-CSF barrier. In contrast, Oatp2 is expressed both on the luminal and abluminal surface of brain endothelial cells, suggesting that only one Oatp isoform is involved in the movement of substances across the blood-brain barrier. Other membrane transporter

TABLE 2
Superfamily of Membrane Transporter Proteins

Type	Tissue expression
Organic Anion Transporting Polypeptides	
Oatp1	Liver, kidney, brain
Oatp2	Liver, brain, retina
Oatp3	Kidney
OATP	Liver, brain
OAT-K1	Kidney
Prostaglandin Transporters	
Rat matrin	Liver, kidney, brain, lung, stomach, small intestines,
Human PGT or matrin F/G	colon, testis, uterus, eye
Liver-Specific Organic Anion Transporters	
Rat lst-1	Liver
Human LST-1	Liver
Na^+-Dependent Taurochlate Transporting Polypeptides	
Rat Ntcp	Liver, kidney, ileum
Human NTCP	Liver
Rat ileal Na^+-dependent bile acid transporter	Ileum
Human Na^+-dependent bile acid transporter	Ileum, cecum, kidney
Renal Organic Anion Transporter Proteins	
Rat ROAT1	Kidney
Rat OAT1	Kidney
Mouse ROAT1 (mNKT)	Kidney, brain
Flounder ROAT1	Kidney
Human OAT1	Kidney, brain
Multidrug Resistance Efflux Proteins	
Rat mdr1a	Brain, adrenal gland, lung, heart, testis, skeletal muscle,
Rat mdr1b	livers, spleen, kidney, skin, intestine, pancreas
Rat mdr2 P-glycoprotein isoforms	
Human MDR1	
Human MDR3	
Rat Mrp1	Brain
Rat Mrp2	Liver
Human MRP1	Lung, brain
Human MRP2 (cMOAT)	Liver, brain, duodenum, kidney, peripheral nerve
Human MRP3	Liver, duodenum, colon, adrenal gland
Human MRP4	Cancer cells
Human MRP5	Brain, skeletal muscle, multiple tissues

proteins of the multidrug resistance family (Table 2) have also been identified in choroid epithelium and brain endothelium, including Mrp1 (multidrug resistance–associated protein), and P-glycoprotein or mdr1a/b (multidrug resistance) isoforms (Beaulieu *et al.*, 1997; Kusuhara *et al.*, 1998; Regina *et al.*, 1998;

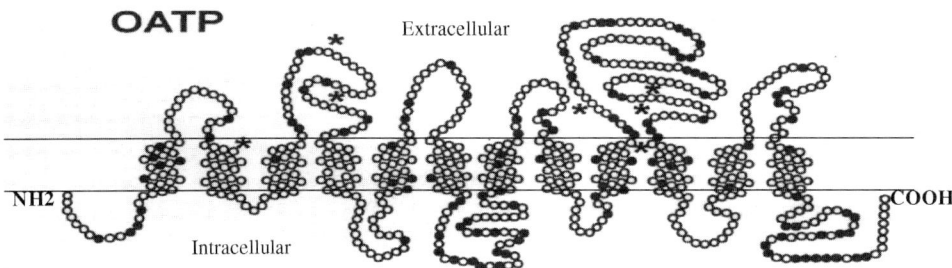

FIGURE 5 Predicted appearance of an organic anion transporter protein of the oatp gene family. The protein has 12 transmembrane-spanning domains and sites for phosphorylation and glycosylation (*). (Adapted from Abe, with permission.)

Nishino et al., 1999). However, these transporter proteins are thought to function primarily as efflux pumps, involved in the uptake and extrusion of toxic substances or drugs, and located only on the surface of these cells in contact with blood. Mrp1 and mdr1b have also been found in brain parenchyma exclusive of endothelial cells (Regina et al., 1998), suggesting the association with either glia or neurons. Finally, the mouse and human OAT1 have been identified in brain by reverse transcriptase–polymerase chain reaction (RT-PCR) (Lopez-Nieto et al., 1997; Cihlar et al., 1999), but its association with specific cell types is unknown.

While not known to be associated with the nuclear membrane, Oatp proteins contain zinc finger motifs (Noe et al., 1997), an unusual feature for surface membrane transporter proteins since zinc fingers are believed to be involved the binding of proteins to DNA (see Sec. I.E below). Therefore, the possibility that one or more of the known or yet to be discovered isoforms in the Oatp gene family are involved in transport to and from the nucleus must be considered. Other specializations of these proteins include glycosylation sites in the extracellular domain and multiple potential phosphorylation sites for cyclic adenosine monophosphate (cAMP)–dependent protein kinase and protein kinase C in the cytoplasmic domain (Noe et al., 1997; Abe et al., 1998).

When expressed in *Xenopus laevis* oocytes, T_4 and T_3 is transported in a dose-dependent, saturable manner by Oatp1, Oatp2, and Oatp3 (Friesema et al., 1998; Abe et al., 1998). The K_m values for transport are 6.53 ± 2.56 and 5.87 ± 1.06 μM, respectively for Oatp2, and 4.92 ± 1.79 and 7.33 ± 2.34 μM for Oatp3 (Abe et al., 1998). Thyroid hormone transport in oocytes has also been demonstrated for the sodium-dependent taurocholate-transporting polypeptide (ntcp) (Friesema et al., 1999), and by the human liver–specific transporter (LST-1) (Kakyo et al., 1999). As noted in Table 2, however, only Oatp1 and Oatp2 are expressed in the brain in association with the choroid plexus and brain capillary endothelial cells. Abe et al. (1998) have described Oatp2 mRNA in hippocampal pyramidal and dentate granule cell layers, cerebellar Purkinge and granule cell layers, olfactory nuclei, striatum, cerebral cortex, thalamus, and hypothalamus, but association of these transporter proteins with glial cells or neurons could not be confirmed by Gao et al. (1999). Nevertheless, evidence for a stereospecific, saturable transport mechanism for T_4 and T_3 in cultured glial cells and cerebrocortical neurons has been reported by Francon et al. (1989) and Chantoux et al. (1995), raising the possibility that other transporter proteins may ultimately be found in these cells.

D. Activation and Inactivation of Thyroid Hormone by Iodothyronine Deiodinases

Generation of the more biologically active metabolite of T_4, T_3, and the inactivation of T_4 and T_3, are mediated by a family of membrane-associated eukaryotic selenoproteins called iodothyronine deiodinases (Larsen, 1997; Kohrle, 1999) (Table 3). Three different deiodinases of similar molecular size ($\sim$28 to 32 kDa) have been identified, including type 1 (D_1), type 2 (D_2), and type 3 (D_3), and their cDNAs cloned (Berry et al., 1991; Mandel et al., 1992; St. Germain et al., 1994; Davey et al., 1995, 1999; Salvatore et al., 1995, Croteau et al., 1995, 1996). Characteristic of the mRNA encoding the deiodinases is the presence of a stem loop structure

TABLE 3
Characteristics of Iodothyronine Deiodinases

Parameters	D_1	D_2	D_3
Molecular weight (kDa)	29	30.5	31.5
Tissue distribution	Liver, kidney, CNS, pituitary, thyroid	CNS, pituitary, brown fat, placenta, thyroid, muscle	CNS, placenta, skin
Substrate preference	$rT_3 > T_4 > T_3$	$T_4 > rT_3$	T_3, T_4
Reaction kinetics	Ping-pong	Sequential	Sequential
Deiodination site	Phenolic/tyrosine rings	Phenolic ring	Tyrosine ring
Inhibitors	PTU, iopanoic acid	Iopanoic acid	Iopanoid acid
Hypothyroidism	Decrease	Increase	Decrease
Hyperthyroidism	Increase	Decrease	Decrease

Adapted from Larsen, 1997.

created by RNA-RNA interactions referred to as the selenocysteine insertion sequence (SECIS). SECIS is necessary to suppress an inframe UGA stop codon in the 3' untranslated region of deiodinase mRNA to permit encoding of the complete molecular structure of the deiodinases and to allow the insertion of the unique amino acid selenocysteine into the active center of the protein to permit maximal enzymatic activity. Although the amino acid sequences of D_1, D_2, and D_3 are generally dissimilar (Crouteau et al., 1996), there are some regions that show homology. These include the midregion of the molecule that contains the selenocysteine residue, necessary for catalysis of rat D_1, and a sequence of hydrophobic amino acids at the amino terminus of the molecule (Fig. 6). The latter region is believed to be the only membrane spanning domain of the deiodinases, associated with either the plasma membrane or the endoplasmic reticulum, allowing its catalytic domain to extend into the cytoplasmic compartment (Larsen, 1997).

Both D_1 and D_2 catalyze the removal of iodine from the outer (phenolic) ring (5'-position) of T_4, thus generating T_3 (Fig. 2). Therefore, these enzymes are activating enzymes since T_3 has 10- to 15-fold more affinity for binding to nuclear thyroid hormone receptors than T_4 (Larsen, 1997). D1 predominates in peripheral tissues but has a preference for rT_3 as a substrate and converts T_4 to T_3 with poor efficiency (Kaplan, 1984). D_2 has a preference for T_4, however, and is the major T_3-generating enzyme in the brain. In contrast, D_3 removes an iodine from the inner (tyrosyl) ring (5-position) of T_4 and T_3 to result in metabolites, rT_3 and T_2, that have a very low affinity for binding to nuclear thyroid hormone receptors. Consequently, D_3 is the major inactivating enzyme of thyroid hormone. D_1 can also remove iodine from the inner ring 5'-position, resulting in the inactivation of T_3 and T_4 and degradation of rT_3.

The distribution of the deiodinases is tissue specific and noted in Table 3. Within the CNS, D_1 and D_2 are present in the brain and pituitary whereas D_3 is expressed only in the brain. In the brain, D_2 is found in multiple regions but is highly expressed in the neocortex, basal ganglia, and hippocampus (Croteau et al., 1996). Croteau et al. (1996) have proposed that this distribution may suggest an important effect of

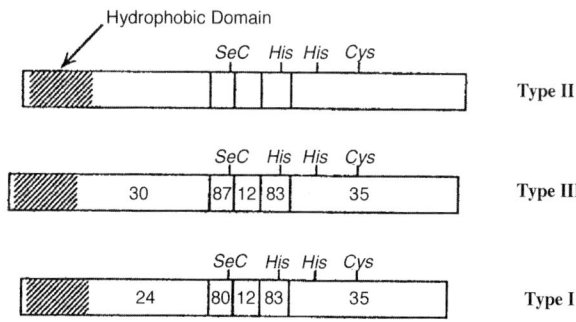

FIGURE 6 Schematic representation of type 1, type 2, and type 3 deiodinase showing regions of homology. Characteristic of these enzymes are an animo-terminal hydrophobic domain that is necessary for anchoring to membranes, and a selenocysteine residue (Sec) in the midportion of the protein. (From Davey et al., 1995, with permission.)

thyroid hormone on memory and learned patterns of movement. In these regions, D_2 is expressed primarily in the processes of glial cells (Guadano-Ferraz et al., 1997, 1999), suggesting that after transport of T_4 into the brain, T_4 is converted to T_3 by glial cells and then released locally to neurons via glial-neuronal interactions. Indeed, studies by Crantz and co-workers (1980, 1982) have demonstrated that most of the T_3 in the brain and pituitary is produced locally from the intracellular conversion of T_4 to T_3, whereas in the liver, kidneys, and skeletal muscle, T_3 is largely derived from the circulation. The hypothalamus also expresses high levels of D_2 activity (Riskind et al., 1987). Similar to other regions of the brain, D_2 mRNA is concentrated in glial cells (Tu et al., 1997; Guadano-Ferraz et al., 1997) but of a very specialized type that lines the floor and wall of the third ventricle, called *tanycytes*. These cells are in intimate contact with the CSF at their apical border through villus-like protrusions into the CSF, and with hypothalamic neurons and capillaries by way of long, basal cytoplasmic processes or tails that project into the adjacent neuropil (Fig. 7). Since tanycytes are phagocytic, they may be capable of extracting T_4 from the CSF by an absorptive process, conversion of T_4 to T_3, and then release of T_3 into the hypothalamus. Alternatively, because tanycytes also envelope blood vessels in the mediobasal hypothalamus and median eminence (ME), they may also be capable of extracting T_4 from the systemic circulation and releasing T_3 into the CSF. This may be an important mechanism for the accumulation of T_3 in the CSF as the choroid plexus does not contain D_2 mRNA (Tu et al., 1997).

D_3 is presumably also expressed in astrocytes in the brain on the basis that astroglial cells in culture have D_3 enzymatic activity (Cavalieri et al., 1986; Esfandiari et al., 1992). However, evidence for neuronal D_3 has also been given (Tu et al., 1999). D_3 mRNA is expressed widely in the brain but is particularly prominent in the cerebral cortex, hippocampus, and cerebellum (Tu et al., 1999; Bates et al., 1999). During development, D_3 is present primarily in the bed nucleus of the stria terminalis and the preoptic nucleus, suggesting a role in sexual development (Escamez et al., 1999).

All of the deiodinases are thyroid hormone responsive (Kaplan and Yaskoski, 1980; Leonard et al., 1981; Chopra et al., 1984; Escobar-Morreale et al., 1997; Croteau et al., 1996; Burmeister et al., 1997; Tu et al.,

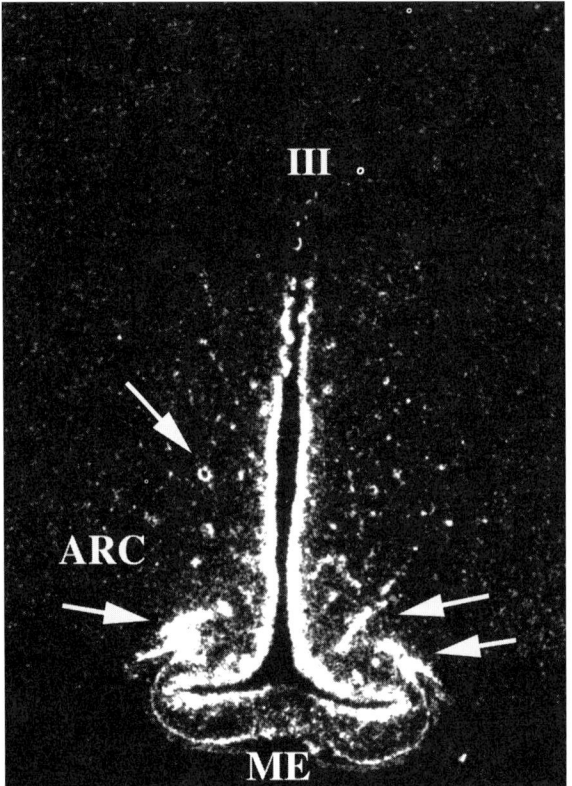

FIGURE 7 In situ hybridization autoradiogram of type 2 deiodinase (D_2) mRNA in a coronal section of the hypothalamus showing its association with tanycytes lining the walls and base of the third ventricle (III). Note D_2 mRNA in tanycyte cytoplasmic projections entering the adjacent arcuate nucleus (ARC) and surrounding blood vessels (arrows). ME = median eminence.

1997, 1999; Guadano-Ferraz et al., 1999). When thyroid hormone levels fall, D_2 mRNA and enzymatic activity markedly increase whereas D_1 and D_3 activity decreases. This control system helps to maintain normal intracerebral T_3 levels when circulating levels of thyroid hormone are low by shunting T_4 from the periphery to the brain, increasing intracerebral conversion of T_4 to T_3, and reducing the degradation of T_3 (Escobar-Morreale et al., 1997). Of interest, the signal for increased D_2 activity appears to be primarily the fall in T_4 since infusion of T_3 to hypothyroid animals does not normalize D_2 activity in the neocortex (Escobar-Morreale et al., 1997). Nevertheless, T_3 reduces D_2 mRNA in the cerebral cortex (Burmeister et al., 1997), indicating that the regulation of D_2 by thyroid hormone is complex. Increased D_2 activity is also observed in the anterior pituitary in hypothyroid states, but primarily in growth hormone– and prolactin-producing cells, and not thyroid-stimulating hormone (TSH)–producing cells (Koenig et al., 1984). Cell-specific expression of D_2 in the anterior pituitary is important to preserve the integrity of the negative feedback control system of the hypothalamic-pituitary-thyroid axis, since an increase in D_2 in thyrotropes during hypothyroidism would serve to inhibit TSH secretion. Conversely, when thyroid hormone levels are elevated, D_2 activity decreases whereas D_1 and D_3 activity increases (Kaplan and Yaskoski, 1980; Chopra et al., 1984), protecting the brain from the potentially harmful effects of excess thyroid hormone listed in Table 1.

E. Thyroid Hormone Receptors

Interaction of T_3 with proteins that bind DNA, thyroid hormone receptors (TRs), is the primary mechanism whereby thyroid hormone controls transcription of thyroid hormone–responsive genes. Two genes on separate chromosomes encode TRs. By alternative splicing, chromosome 17 gives rise to the α isoforms of the TRs, TRα1 and TRα2. While both isoforms bind DNA, only TRα1 binds T_3. Therefore, TRα2 is not considered to be a functional TR and, in fact, may act as a competitive antagonist of authentic TRs by binding to the same site in DNA. Chromosome 3 gives rise to the β TR isoforms, TRβ1 and TRβ2, which both bind T_3. All of the TR isoforms are found in hypophysiotropic TRH neurons in the hypothalamus, as well as in the anterior pituitary (Lechan et al., 1994). However, relative to the other TR isoforms, TRβ2 is highly expressed in the anterior pituitary (Bradley et al., 1992).

The TRs range in size from 47 to 57 kDa and are schematically illustrated in Fig. 8. Characteristic of these receptors are five discrete domains: an amino-terminal A/B domain that differs among the three active TRs; a highly homologous DNA binding or C domain; a hinge region or D domain; the ligand (T_3) binding or E domain; and the carboxyl-terminal AF-2 or F domain. The DNA binding domain consists of two cysteine-rich amino acid loops that chelate zinc, called zinc fingers, that are important for interaction with DNA. The T_3 binding and carboxy-terminal domains contain sequences not only for binding T_3 but also for dimerization with other TRs and nuclear proteins that allow transcriptional activation or repression.

The three-dimensional structure of rat TRα1 reveals that T_3 is deeply buried in the ligand binding domain as part of a hydrophobic core, and when T_3 binding occurs, a conformational change in the receptor results (Wagner et al., 1995).

TRs are members of a superfamily of ligand-regulated nuclear receptors listed in Table 4. However, as opposed to some of these receptors, such as the glucocorticoid receptor, which is found both in the cytoplasmic and nuclear compartments, TRs are found exclusively in the nucleus and can bind to 5' regulatory sequences in DNA, referred to as *thyroid hormone response elements* (TREs). TREs are mostly composed of two half-sites, represented by the nucleotide sequence TNAGGTCA (where N is any nucleotide) in a palandromic, directed or inverted repeat, separated by a gap of nucleotides, although single half-sites in certain thyroid hormone–regulated genes also occur (Katz and Koenig, 1993). Since T_3 disrupts the binding of TR homodimers to DNA (Yen et al., 1992), is not likely that homodimerization of TRs is important for thyroid hormone–regulated gene transcription. In contrast, heterodimerization of TRs with a separate family of nuclear proteins, the retinoid X receptors (RXRα, RXRβ, RXRγ), increases TR binding to TREs and augments thyroid hormone–mediated regulation of gene transcription (Chin, 1992). While 9-*cis*-retinoic acid is the natural ligand for RXR, no ligand binding of RXR occurs when TR/RXR heterodimers are formed (Forman et al., 1995).

Transcriptional activation of genes positively regulated by thyroid hormone occurs after T_3 binds to TR/RXR heterodimers bound to DNA as illustrated in Fig. 9. The unliganded TR tends to repress transcriptional activity, mediated by its interaction with corepressor proteins such as N-CoR (nuclear corepressor) and SMRT (silencing mediator of retinoid and thyroid receptors) (Koenig, 1998). These proteins bind to the D domain of the TRs (Chen and Evans, 1995) and lead to histone deacetylation by interacting with Sin3 (Alland et al., 1997). Histone deacetylation is believed to tighten DNA structure, making it difficult for other regulatory proteins to bind to DNA. The interaction of T_3 with the TR heterodimers alters the location of a critical sequence of nine amino acids called activator function 2 (AF-2) in the F domain, resulting in the dissociation of corepressors and allowing the binding of coactivators (Koenig, 1998). This sequence of events results in

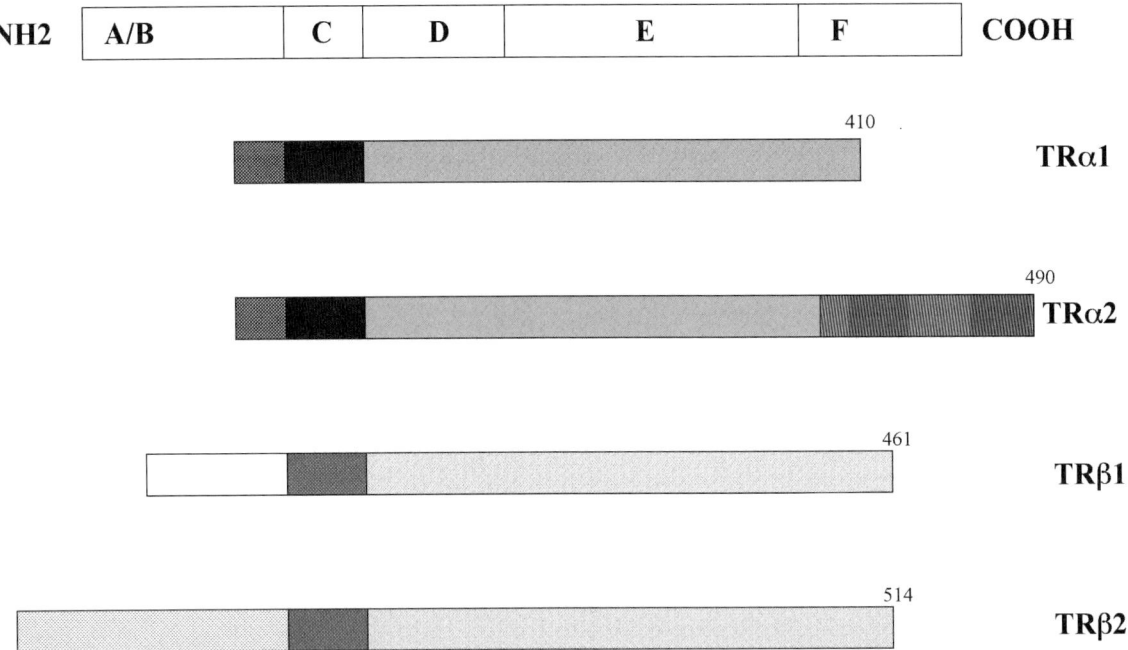

FIGURE 8 Schematic representation of the thyroid hormone receptors (TRs): TRα1, TRα2, TRβ1, and TRβ2. A/B, variable amino-terminal domain; C, DNA binding domain; D, hinge region; E, T_3 binding domain; F, cabroxyl-terminal AF-2 domain. (Adapted from Brent, G. A., 1994, with permission.)

transcriptional activation (Fig. 9A). Several coactivator proteins may be involved including SRC-1 (steroid receptor coactivator 1, also known as the nuclear coactivator, NcoA-1), a member of the p160 family, CREB (cAMP-responsive element binding protein), CBP (CREB-binding protein), p120, Trip 230 (thyroid hormone receptor and Rb interacting protein of 230 kDa), PGC-1 (PPAR-γ coactivator 1), PCAF, and the TATA-binding proteins, TAF$_{II}$110 and TAF$_{II}$60 (Onate et al., 1995; Kamei et al., 1996; Monden et al., 1997; Chang et al., 1997; Puigserver et al., 1998; Petty et al., 1996). Binding of T_3 to TR may allow SRC-1 to interact with the E domain (Takeshita et al., 1997), and by acetylating histones, SRC-1 may loosen chromatin structure and promote the recruitment of the other coactivators that allow transcriptional activation. The reason for the need for multiple coactivators to mediate the action of thyroid hormone is uncertain and may serve a redundant function or provide for a high degree of regulation of thyroid hormone activity depending on the availability of the coactivators in specific tissues (Lazar, 1997).

However, in the hypothalamic-pituitary-thyroid axis, the TRH and TSH (TSHα, TSHβ) genes are negatively regulated by T_3 (Feng et al., 1994; Hollenberg et al., 1995; Tagami et al., 1997). Thus, cotransfection of the human TRH promoter and unliganded TRα1, TRβ1, or TRβ2 into a neuroblastoma cell line activates basal promoter activity, while the addition of T_3 inhibits it (Feng et al., 1994). The mechanism by which thyroid hormone accomplishes negative regulation is not well understood. TRβ is required since natural mutations of the ligand binding domain of TRβ (which is identical in TRβ1 and TRβ2) in humans results in thyroid hormone resistance, i.e., elevation in serum TSH, T_4, and T_3 without signs or symptoms of thyrotoxicosis and poor response to inhibition to exogenous T_3 (Refetoff, 1994). TRβ2 may be more important than TRβ1 in negative regulation by thyroid hormone since TRβ2 achieves significantly greater T_3-independent activation of the TRH and TSHα genes in vitro (Langlois et al., 1997). In addition, mice with targeted disruption of TRβ2 but not the other TR isoforms show a similar degree of central resistance to thyroid hormone as mice with disruption of both TRβ1 and TRβ2 (Abel et al., 1999). The importance of the TRβ2 isoform in negative regulation by T_3 may be due to the A/B domain of TRβ2, since a chimeric TRβ isoform containing the TRβ2 amino terminus linked to the TRα1 DNA and

TABLE 4
Superfamily of Ligand-Regulated Nuclear Receptors

Aldosterone receptor
Androgen receptor
COUP-TF receptor
Ecdysone receptor
Estrogen receptor
   ERα
   ERβ
Glucocorticoid receptor
Mineralodorticoid receptor
Progesterone receptor
Retinoid acid receptor (RAR)
   RARα
   RARβ
   RARγ
Retinoid X receptor (RXR)
   RXRα
   RXRβ
   RXRγ
Thyroid hormone recetpor (TR)
   TRα1
   TRα2
   TRβ1
   TRβ2
Vitamin D receptor
Orphan receptors
   ARP-1
   COUP-TF
   ERR2
   PPAR
   TR4

ligand binding domains functions like the TRβ2 isoform (Langlois et al., 1997). Binding of coactivators to the A/B domain of the unliganded TRβ2 but not the other TR isoforms (Oberste-Berghaus et al., 2000) may explain these observations, and function by antagonizing the ability of corepressors to bind to the D domain. Thus far, no mutations of TRα1 are known to be associated with the syndrome of thyroid hormone resistance, although this does not absolutely exclude the importance of TRα1 in negative regulation by T_3.

Some of the same nuclear regulatory proteins involved in the regulation of T_3 positively regulated genes also appear to be involved in the regulation of negatively regulated genes. This is illustrated by the presence of thyroid hormone resistance in mice deficient in SRC-1 (Weiss et al., 1999). Because SRC-1 is a coactivator protein in T_3 positively regulated genes, however, the above observation would appear somewhat paradoxical as it suggests that SRC-1 is needed for transcriptional repression in T_3 negatively regulated genes. Similarly, Tagami et al. (1997) reported that SMRT and NCoR increase basal promoter activity (i.e., act as coactivators) in the TRH and TSH genes, contrary to their function in T_3 positively regulated genes where they function as corepressors. Indeed, severe resistance to thyroid hormone (extremely high circulating levels of T_4 and inappropriately elevated TSH levels) in man can be due to unusually strong interactions between NCoR and a mutation in the hinge region of TRβ, resulting in constitutive activation of the TSH genes and resistance to displacement of NCoR by T_3 (Tagami et al., 1998; Safer et al., 1998).

The possibility that negative regulation of genes by T_3 may not involve the binding of TRs to DNA but rather that TRs exist free in the nucleoplasm and function by sequestering nuclear regulatory factors, thereby allowing or disallowing these factors to interact with T_3-regulated genes, has also been suggested as a mechanism for T_3 negatively regulated genes. This hypothesis is supported by the observation that the TSHα gene does not contain a TRE; only a monomeric half-site can be found in the TSHβ gene (Hollenberg et al., 1995; Satoh et al., 1996), and deletion of two candidate half-sites for binding of TRs to DNA in the human TRH gene (between $-191/-184$ bp and $-166/-158$ bp) does not completely prevent T_3 inhibition of promoter activity (Feng et al., 1994). Such a mechanism has recently been proposed by Tagami et al. (1999) for the TSHα gene and is summarized in Fig. 9B. It is suggested that in the absence of T_3, TR in the nucleoplasm binds corepressors SMRT and NCoR, which then sequesters histone deacetylases from DNA, allowing for transcriptional activation of the TSHα gene under the stimulatory control of CREB and CBP. In the presence of T_3, the corepressors dissociate from the TR, allowing TR to bind coactivators such as CBP. As a result, CBP is competed away from CREB on the promoter of the

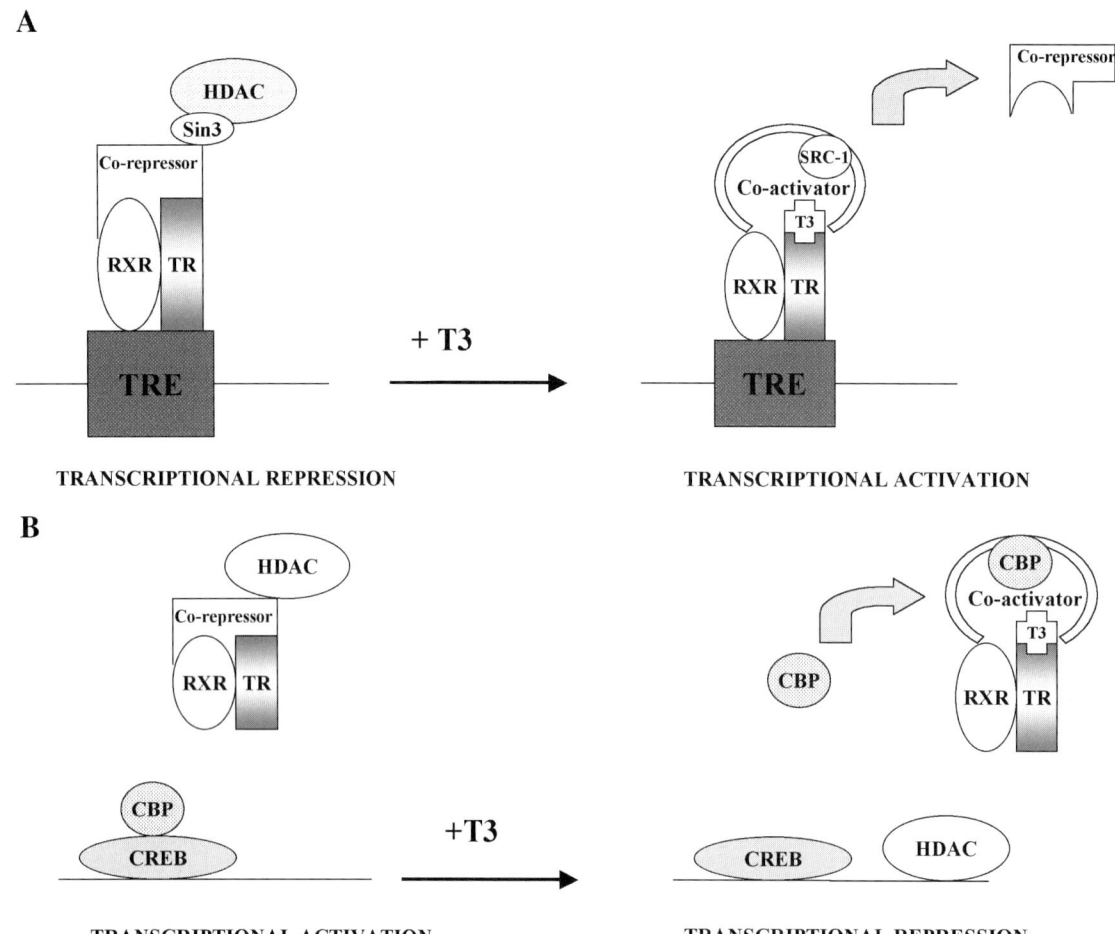

FIGURE 9 Models for genes positively (A) and negatively (B) regulated by T_3. (Adapted from Koenig et al., 1998, and Tagami et al., 1999, with permission.)

TSHα gene. Both events result in transcriptional repression by making histone deacetylase available to the promoter. Given that the 11-zinc-finger CCTC-binding factor, CTCF, has been recently shown to have an important role in negative transcriptional regulation by thyroid hormone in the c-Myc gene and genomic element 144, both of which have TREs (Awad et al., 1999; Perez-Juste et al., 2000), the mechanisms for the regulation of T_3-repressed genes is probably much more complex.

F. Nonnuclear Effects of Thyroid Hormone

In addition to nuclear effects of thyroid hormone, there is some evidence that T_3 can also have nonnuclear actions. T_3 has a very rapid effect on the stimulation of oxidative phosphorylation and mitochondrial O_2 consumption that is not dependent on protein synthesis, indicating that mitochondria could be an important target of T_3 (Wrutnaik et al., 1998). A truncated form of TRα1 has been identified in rat liver mitochondria that may mediate the effect of T_3 by binding to TREs present in the mitochondrial genome (Wrutnaik et al., 1998). Regulation of deiodinase (D_2) activity by thyroid hormone has also been proposed to occur via a nonnuclear mechanism, since its action is very rapid and independent of protein synthesis (Leonard et al., 1984). Disruption of this effect by cytochalasin B has suggested to Leonard et al. (1990) that the effect of thyroid hormone to regulate D_2 is due to T_4-mediated interactions between D_2 and the actin cytoskeleton.

III. HYPOTHALAMIC-PITUITARY-THYROID AXIS

A. Anatomy of the Hypophysiotrophic TRH Neuroregulatory System

1. TRH Tuberoinfundibular System

In the adult rat hypothalamus, immunoreactive (IR)-TRH axon terminals are found in increasing density from the lateral to the medial aspects of the external layer of the median eminence, in close apposition to capillaries of the hypophysial-portal system (Fig. 10A), establishing these fibers as part of the hypothalamic tuberoinfundibular system (Hökfelt et al., 1975; Choy and Walkins, 1977; Johansson and Hökfelt, 1980; Johansson et al., 1980; Lechan and Jackson, 1982). These axons originate from neuronal perikarya located in the paraventricular nucleus of the hypothalamus (PVN) (Fig. 10B), a region contained within the classic thyrotropic area (Aizawa and Greer, 1981), and whose destruction results in disappearance of more than 90% of TRH in the external layer of the median eminence (Brownstein et al., 1982) and depression of TSH secretion from the anterior pituitary gland (Aizawa and Greer, 1981). The axon trajectory of the PVN TRH neurons to the ME is primarily in a mediolateral direction. IR-TRH fibers arch above and around the fornix, extend toward the basal hypothalamus, and then course through the lateral retrochiasmatic area to terminate in the ME (Palkovits et al., 1982a). Few axons also descend along the wall of the third ventricle in the subependymal neuropil (Nishiyama et al., 1985), but contribute minimally to the total tuberoinfundibular IR-TRH fibers.

IR-TRH fibers also traverse the internal layer of the rat ME *en route* to a second destination, the posterior pituitary (Lechan and Jackson, 1982). The cells of origin of these axons are also the PVN, and destruction of the PVN leads to almost total depletion of TRH in the posterior lobe (Jackson and Reichlin, 1977). As opposed to the parvocellular TRH neurons in the PVN, whose axons terminate in the external zone of the ME, magnocellular TRH neurons in the PVN may project their neurites to the posterior pituitary (Meister et al., 1990). These magnocellular neurons may also contain oxytocin, vasopressin, vasoactive intestinal peptide (VIP), and

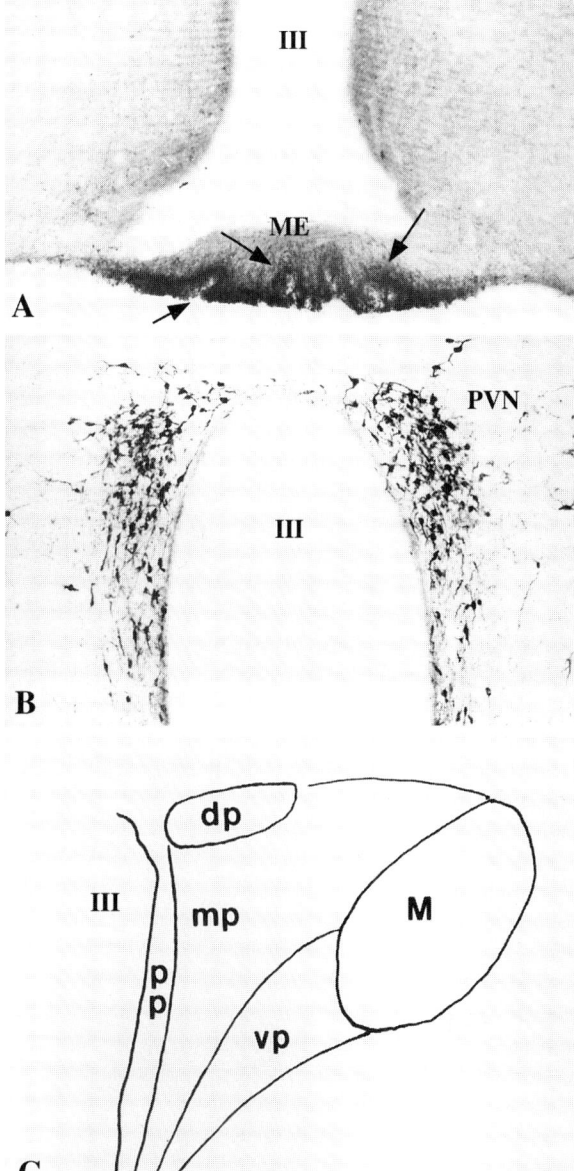

FIGURE 10 Immunocytochemical delineation of the TRH-tuberoinfundibular system. (A) Note dense concentration of TRH-containing axon terminals in the external zone of the median eminence (ME) in contact with capillaries of the portal system (arrows). (B) Their neurons originate in the parvocellular subdivision of the hypothalamic paraventricular nucleus (PVN). (C) Schematic representation of the PVN showing its major subdivisions. p, periventricular parvocellular subdivision; mp, medial parvocellular subdivision; dp, dorsal parvocellular subdivision; vp, ventral parvocellular subdivision; M, magnocellular division; III, third ventricle.

peptide histidine isoleucine (PHI) (Meister et al., 1990), suggesting that neurohypophysial TRH might act as coregulator for posterior pituitary function. Indeed, in the rat neurohypophysial system, both TRH and VIP stimulate vasopressin (VP) secretion (Weitzman et al., 1979; Ottensen et al., 1984; Bardrum et al., 1988) and are similarly affected by alterations in circulating thyroid hormone levels (Toni et al., 1992; Rondeel et al., 1995). Toni et al. (1994, 1995) have suggested that since hypothyroidism can be associated with disturbances in VP secretion leading to fluid and electrolyte imbalance (so-called syndrome of inappropriate secretion of antidiuretic hormone, SIADH) (Skowsky and Kikuchi, 1978), it is conceivable that colocalization of TRH and VIP may play a role to control by autocrine/paracrine action VP secretion from the neurohypophysial tract. Alternatively, TRH in the posterior pituitary might participate in the tuberoinfundibular TRH system to regulate anterior pituitary thyrotropes by secreting TRH into the short portal vessels that connect the posterior pituitary to the anterior pituitary (Lechan and Toni, 1992).

The PVN is a wing-shaped nucleus located at the dorsal margin of the third ventricle, which can be divided into two major portions based on the size of neuronal cell bodies: a magnocellular division of large neurons and a parvocellular division of small to medium-sized neurons (Fig. 10C). The parvocellular portion lies more medially, adjacent to the ependymal wall of the third ventricle (Swanson and Kuypers, 1980). Numerous TRH-synthesizing neurons have been found in the anterior, medial, and periventricular parvocellular subdivisions (Fig. 10B) and, to a lesser extent, in the dorsal and lateral subnuclei (Lechan and Jackson, 1982; Kawano et al., 1991), but neuroanatomical tracing methods have shown that only neurons in the medial and periventricular subnuclei densely project to the ME (Ishikawa et al., 1988; Kawano et al., 1991; Merchenthaler and Liposits, 1994).

Until recently, TRH tuberoinfundibular neurons were thought to co-contain very few peptides other than TRH itself and peptides derived from the cleavage of its precursor molecule (see Section III.B). Only rare TRH cells in the periventricular parvocellular subdivision were found to contain corticotropin-releasing factor, neurotensin (Ceccatelli et al., 1989), and pituitary adenylate cyclase–activating polypeptide (Legradi et al., 1997a).

However, Fekete et al. (2001) and Broberger (1999) have clearly demonstrated that the majority of hypophysiotropic TRH neurons contain CART (cocaine- and amphetamine-regulated transcript), raising the possibility of an important role for CART, independently or in concert with TRH, in the regulation of the thyroid axis.

In addition to the PVN, TRH is synthesized in neurons in many other regions of the hypothalamus, including the preoptic area; anterior hypothalamus; supraoptic, arcuate, dorsomedial, and premammillary nuclei; as well as basolateral and perifornical hypothalamus (Lechan and Jackson, 1982). However, these neurons do not contribute to TRH hypophysiotrophic axons in the tuberoinfundibular system (Ishikawa et al., 1988) and subserve other physiological functions in the brain (see Lechan and Toni, 1992 for review).

In the human brain, substantial amounts of IR-TRH have been detected by radioimmunoassay (RIA) in the PVN and stalk ME (Jackson and Reichlin, 1979; Borson-Chazot et al., 1986; Kopp et al., 1992). This has been confirmed by immunocytochemical and in situ hybridization histochemistochemical studies in adults (Fliers et al., 1994; Guldenaar et al., 1996; Mihaly et al., 2000), showing that TRH-synthesizing neurons, both of parvocellular and magnocellular type, are located in the PVN, and that a dense network of IR-TRH axons is present throughout the ME. These data indicate that the anatomical organization of the TRH tuberoinfundibular system is preserved across animal species. TRH has also been detected by RIA in the fetal hypothalamus as early as 9 to 10 weeks of gestation (Winters et al., 1974; Kaplan et al., 1976). Since the tuberoinfundibular tract is partially formed by the third month of intrauterine life (Hyyppa, 1972), functional, hypophysial-portal connections have been described at 12 weeks gestation (Thliveris and Currie, 1980), and since TSH is detectable in anterior pituitary thyrotrophs during the same period of time (Baker and Jaffe, 1974), it has been suggested that during early fetal development, hypophysiotropic TRH might be released from the human hypothalamus to initiate regulation of the pituitary-thyroid function (Pintar, 1996). Recent evidence in the mutant TRH null mice, however, shows that functional maturation of thyrotrophs in the mammalian pituitary is dependent on the presence of tuberoinfundibular TRH only at birth (Yamada et al.,

1997; Shibusawa et al., 2000). Alternatively, TRH and/or proTRH-derived peptides might contribute by paracrine/autocrine mechanisms to the maturation of the tuberal hypothalamus.

2. TRH Gene and Promoter Regulation

The TRH gene is located on chromosome 3 and contains three exons interrupted by two introns. The first exon encodes the 5′ untranslated sequence, the second encodes the signal peptide and the initial part of the prohormone, and the final exon encodes the bulk of the proTRH protein and the 3′ untranslated region (Lee, 1988; Yamada et al., 1990) (Fig. 11).

Analysis of the 5′ flanking sequence of the rat and human TRH gene has identified several regions that may be relevant to regulation of the TRH gene (Fig. 12). A single TATA consensus sequence is located within 29 nucleotides upstream from the transcriptional start site in both species. Two imperfect CREs that bind the CREB and may activate the TRH promoter (Stevenin and Lee, 1995; Wilber and Xu, 1998) are located within 100 bp of the transcriptional start site in both species. Of the two CREs, the site located closest to the transcriptional start site would appear to be multifunctional, as it also binds TRs. This site may contribute to negative regulation of the TRH gene by thyroid hormone if TRs compete with CREB at this site to result in inhibition of promoter activation (Wilber and Xu, 1998). Alternatively, as hypothesized by Tagami et al. (1999) for negative regulation of the TSHα gene by thyroid hormone, competition of the CBP away from CREB on the promoter of the TRH gene may lead to transcriptional repression.

Hollenberg et al. (1995) have identified several other potential half-sites for TRH binding between −150 and +55 bp in the human TRH gene (Fig. 12). Site-directed mutagenesis and deletional analysis of three of these sites between −60 and +55 have demonstrated their importance in negative regulation of the TRH gene by T_3. In addition to binding the TR monomer, the half-site between −53 and −60 may also be capable of binding the TR-RXR heterodimer (Hollenberg et al., 1995). Studies by Satoh et al. (1999) have further

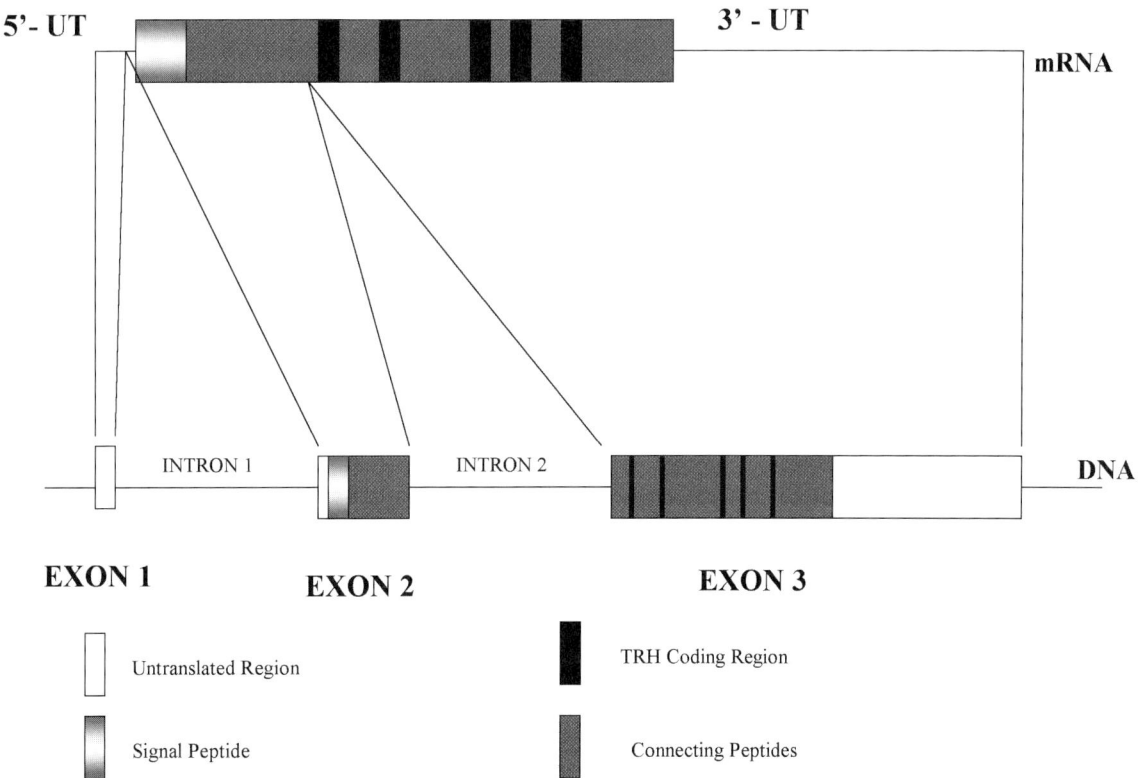

FIGURE 11 Structure of the rat preproTRH gene; genomic DNA is shown on the bottom and mRNA on the top. (From Stevenin and Lee, 1995, with permission.)

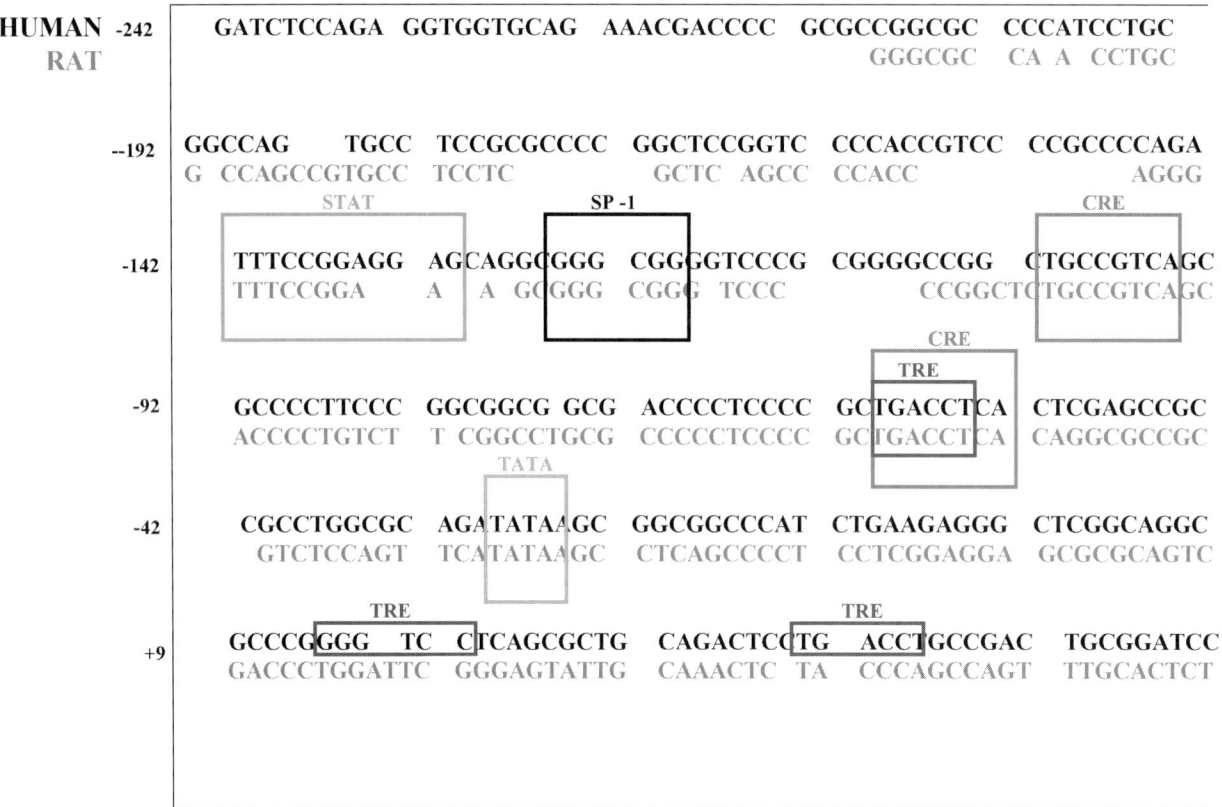

FIGURE 12 Promoter sequence of the human and rat TRH genes. Potential regions for regulation by thyroid hormone or CREB are enclosed in boxes. TRE, thyroid hormone response element; CRE, cAMP response element. (Adapted from Yamada et al., 1990, with permission.)

demonstrated activation of the TRH promoter by the retinoic acid receptor (RAR), but no specific binding site for RAR on the TRH gene has yet been identified.

A perfect glucocorticoid response element (GRE) approximately −200 bp from the transcriptional start site has been described by Lee (1988) in the rat TRH promoter, but a comparable site in the human TRH promoter has not been found. Harris et al. (2001) have also described a STAT binding site in the TRH promoter between −141 and −132 of the human gene, adjacent to an Sp-1 site. These sites may coorporate with each other to mediate the stimulatory effects of leptin on TRH gene expression (see below).

B. Biosynthesis and Processing of PreproTRH

TRH arises by an mRNA-directed ribosomal mechanism and posttranslational processing of a larger precursor prohormone. The complete sequences of the TRH precursors, deduced from its cDNA, have been elucidated for frog, rat, mouse, and man and are schematically illustrated in Fig. 13. Common to each prohormone are multiple copies of a progenitor sequence for TRH, Gln-His-Pro-Gly, flanked on either side by paired basic amino acids, Lys-Arg or Arg-Arg, that serve as processing signals (Fischer and Speiss, 1987) to result in the fully mature and biologically active TRH.

Rat preproTRH contains 255 amino acids and 5 copies of the TRH progenitor sequence (Lechan et al., 1986). It is approximately 88% homologous to the mouse preproTRH (Satoh et al., 1992), which contains 256 amino acids and also could give rise to five copies of TRH by proteolytic processing. The human preproTRH contains 242 amino acids but six copies of TRH of the progenitor sequence for TRH (Yamada et al., 1990). Frog brain has at least three different

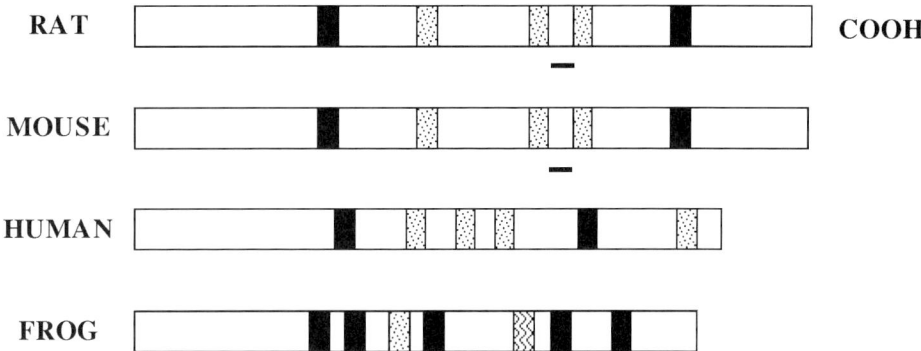

FIGURE 13 Schematic representation of rat, mouse, human, and frog preproTRH. Each contains multiple copies of a progenitor sequence to TRH (filled or textured boxes), flanked on either side by cleavage sites. ▬ denotes location of preproTRH 160–169.

TRH preprohormones ranging between 224 and 227 amino acids and contains seven copies of the TRH progenitor sequence (Kuchler et al., 1990; Bulant et al., 1992a). It is presumed that the presence of multiple copies of TRH in the precursor proteins is important to magnify the response to signals that trigger TRH secretion.

In addition to the sequences that give rise to TRH, the TRH precursor also contains several spacer peptides between the TRH progenitor sequences, and N- and C-terminal flanking peptides, but the biologic importance of these peptides is uncertain. Immunocytochemical studies using antisera directed against intact or partially processed proTRH (Lechan et al., 1986; Merchenthaler et al., 1989b) and the spacer or flanking peptides of the proTRH molecule (non-TRH peptides) (Lechan et al., 1987; Liao et al., 1988a,b; Toni et al., 1990a) have confirmed that these peptides are located in the same PVN parvocellular neurons as TRH. In addition, it has been possible to show that in neurons, proTRH immunolabeling is largely confined to the Golgi apparatus and to large, immature secretory granules in the neuronal perikaryon (Lechan et al., 1986; Nillni et al., 1993), whereas antisera directed against mature TRH and non-TRH peptides are associated with mature, dense core vesicles distributed throughout the perikaryon, processes, and axon terminals (Johansson et al., 1980; Hisano et al., 1986; Shioda et al., 1986; Liposits et al., 1987; Lechan et al., 1987; Liao et al., 1988a; Toni et al., 1990a). These observations indicate that proTRH-derived peptides are generated in the perikarya of PVN tuberoinfundibular and then transported to axon terminals in the ME.

The importance of transport of non-TRH peptides derived from proTRH in axons is unclear, but evidence suggests that some of these fragments may be biologically active. At least one peptide, preproTRH 160–169, a decapeptide containing the amino acid sequence Ser-Phe-Pro-Trp-Met-Glu-Ser-Asp-Val-Thr that follows the third TRH sequence in the rat prohormone (Fig. 13), is also present in the mouse preproTRH (Satoh et al., 1992) and has been isolated from bovine hypothalamus (Bulant et al., 1992b). By immunocytochemistry, this peptide is present in hypophysiotropic neurons in the PVN and transported to axon terminals in the ME (Valentijn et al., 1991) where it could be secreted into the portal capillary system. Bulant et al. (1988) and Roussel et al. (1991) have demonstrated that preproTRH 160–169 potentiates TRH-induced TSH release from perfused rat anterior pituitary fragments by a Ca^{2+}-dependent mechanism and increases prolactin synthesis and secretion independent of TRH. Biologic activity of preproTRH 160–169 has also been demonstrated by Yang and Taché (1994), showing that the decapeptide can potentiate gastric acid secretion stimulated by TRH after microinjection into the dorsal motor nucleus of the vagus. While the receptor for preproTRH 160–169 has not yet been characterized, specific binding sites for the decapeptide in pituitary tissue by radioceptor assay and autoradiography have been reported (Bulant et al., 1988; Ladram et al., 1994; Valentijn et al., 1998), establishing preproTRH 160–169 as an authentic neuropeptide. Interestingly, in the anterior pituitary, the preproTRH 160–169 receptor is present exclusively in folliculostellate cells (Valentijn *et al.*, 1998), a specialized glial cell, suggesting that the effect of this peptide on TSH and prolactin secretion is indirect. Paracrine interactions between the processes of folliculostellate cells and anterior pituitary thyrotropes and lactotropes probably mediate the potentiating actions of preproTRH 160–169 on TSH and prolactin secretion (Allaerts *et al.*, 1990).

PreproTRH 178–199, which separates the fourth and fifth progenitor TRH sequences, is also transported in axons to the ME and released by depolarizing agents (Liao *et al.*, 1988b; Valentijn *et al.*, 1991). Claims for biologic activity of this peptide have been based on the ability of preproTRH 178–199 to inhibit GH *in vitro* and act as a corticotropin-inhibiting factor by blocking adrenocorticotropin (ACTH) release and proopiomelanocortin (POMC) mRNA transcription (Redei *et al.*, 1995; McGivern *et al.*, 1997), but the latter has not been replicated by other laboratories (Nicholson and Orth, 1996). The fragments preproTRH 178–185 and 186–199, arising from the processing of preproTRH 178–199, have also been claimed to stimulate PRL secretion (Nillni *et al.*, 2001).

Bruhn *et al.* (1991) have shown that preproTRH 25–50, derived from the N-terminal portion of the TRH prohormone, is released from the ME in response to depolarizing stimuli. By immunocytochemistry, this peptide is present in hypophysiotropic neurons in the paraventricular nucleus and axon terminals in the external layer of the ME, where it could be secreted into the portal capillary system in response to hypothyroidism. The adjacent N-terminal peptide, preproTRH 53–74, is also highly expressed in the midbrain periaqueductal gray following opioid withdrawal (Legradi *et al.*, 1996). However, little more is known about the potential biologic activity of these peptides.

Processing of proTRH to its final products is region specific and dependent on the type of processing enzymes in the cell. In the hypothalamus, proTRH is fully processed to yield all five copies of TRH and each of the spacer peptides (Wu *et al.*, 1987; Wu and Jackson, 1988). In the olfactory lobes, C-terminal extended forms of TRH, preproTRH 154–169 and preproTRH 172–199, are the predominant end products, suggesting incomplete processing at Arg-Arg residues (Bulant *et al.*, 1990b). In addition, by immunocytochemistry, the mature form of TRH cannot be detected in the reticular nucleus of the thalamus, a sensory relay nucleus to the cerebral cortex, whereas the N-terminal peptide, preproTRH 25–250, and preproTRH mRNA are present in abundance in this region (Lechan *et al.*, 1987). These observations suggest that differential processing of the TRH precursor occurs in different regions of the brain.

Two enzymes that appear to be critical for the processing of proTRH are the proconvertase enzymes, PC1 and PC2. These enzymes cleave at the C-terminal end of single or paired basic amino acid residues (Rouille *et al.*, 1995), and the remaining basic amino acids are removed by carboxypeptidases. PC1 appears to be capable of processing the entire proTRH precursor to mature TRH, whereas PC2 processes only specific regions of the prohormone (Schaner *et al.*, 1997). Along these lines, it is of interest that both PC1 and PC2 are present in the majority of TRH neurons in paraventricular nucleus, whereas in the olfactory lobes, PC2 is primarily expressed (Pu *et al.*, 1996). Accordingly, differences in the expression of PC1 and PC2 in different regions of the brain may be responsible for the differential processing of proTRH observed in these regions.

A schema for the processing of proTRH has been proposed by Nillni *et al.* (1993, 1995) (Fig. 14) using cell lines that have been stably transfected with preproTRH cDNA that express PC1 and PC2 endogenously or in which preproTRH cDNA was cotransfected with PC1 or PC2 in cells that do not normally express these proteins (Friedman *et al.*, 1995; Nillni *et al.*, 1996; Schaner *et al.*, 1997). In this model, the 26-kDa prohormone is cleaved at one of two sites to generate either 15-kDa and 10-kDa fragments (preproTRH 25–151 and preproTRH 160–255) or 9.5-kDa and 16.5-kDa fragments (preproTRH 25–112 and preproTRH 115–255), respectively. This initial cleavage is believed to occur in the Golgi apparatus (Nillni *et al.*, 1993). Subsequently, the 15-kDa N-terminal fragment is processed to a 6-kDa intermediate (preproTRH 25–74) and a 3.8-kDa peptide (preproTRH 77–106), while the 10-kDa fragment produces a 5.6-kDa intermediate (preproTRH 160–199) and a 5.4-kDa intermediate corresponding to the C-terminal peptide, preproTRH 208–255. The 5.6-kDa

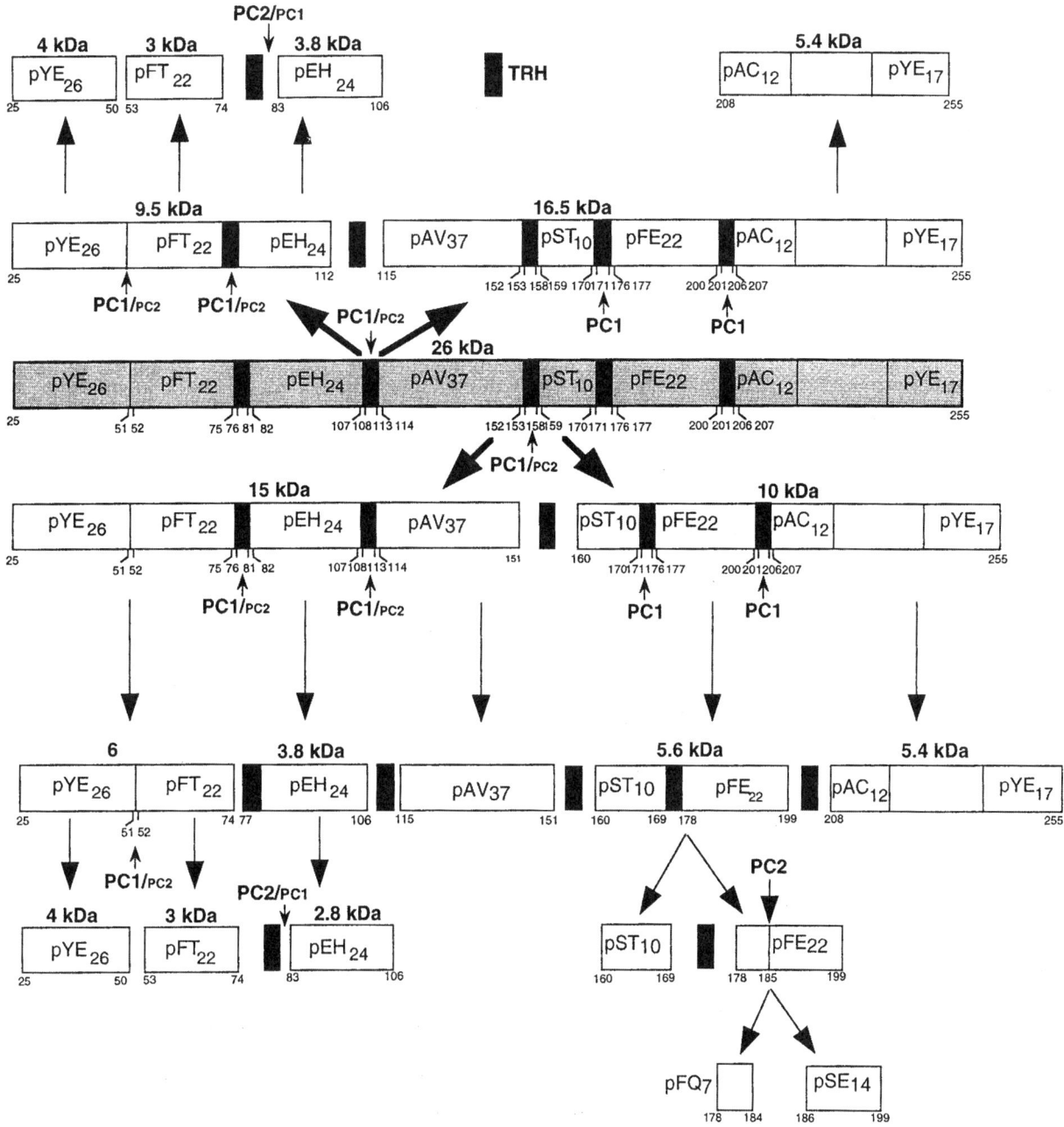

FIGURE 14 Proposed processing model of rat proTRH by proconvertase 1 (PC1) and proconvertase 2 (PC2). (From Nillni and Sevarino, 1999, with permission.)

fragment is then further processed to preproTRH 160–169 and preproTRH 178–199. PreproTRH 178–199 can then be further processed to the smaller peptides, preproTRH 178–184 and preproTRH 186–199, mediated by the action of PC2. Alternatively, processing of the 9.5-kDa N-terminal fragment is proposed to yield preproTRH 25–50, preproTRH 53–74, and preproTRH 83–106, and the 16.5-kDa C-terminal fragment to yield preproTRH 160–199 and preproTRH 208–255. Following cleavage at all paired basic residues, the mature TRH (pGlu-His-Pro-NH2) is generated by amidating the C-terminal end of the tripeptide using the glycine residue in the immediate precursor to TRH, TRH-Gly, as a substrate for the enzyme peptidylglyine α-amidating monooxygenase (PAM) (Bradbury et al., 1982), and cyclization of the N-terminal glutaminyl to pGlu by glytaminyl cyclase (Fisher and Spiess, 1987).

C. Feedback Regulation of Hypohysiotrophic TRH by Thyroid Hormone

The anatomical specificity of the neuronal populations giving rise to the rat TRH tuberoinfundibular system is also associated with a functional specificity of the constituent cells, as shown by the negative regulation by thyroid hormone in perikaryal size and content of proTRH-producing neurons (Nishiyama et al., 1985; Segerson et al., 1987; Liao et al., 1989) and proTRH mRNA (Koller et al. 1987; Zoeller et al., 1988; Dyess et al., 1988; Yamada and Wilber, 1990; Yamada et al. 1992a,b; Kakucska et al., 1992), only in parvocellular neurons of the medial and periventricular PVN subdivisions but not in other TRH-rich areas of the hypothalamus or forebrain (Fig. 15). The hypothyroidism-induced increase in IR-proTRH and proTRH mRNA levels in the medial and periventricular parvocellular neurons of the PVN is accompanied by a decline in the content of IR-TRH in both the PVN (Yamada et al., 1989; Yamada and Wilber, 1990; Yamada et al., 1992b) and the ME (Mori and Yamada, 1987; Yamada et al., 1992b), due to an increase in the secretion of TRH into the portal blood (Rondeel et al., 1992a; de Greef et al., 1992) for conveyance to the anterior pituitary. Dahl et al. (1994) have also reported markedly elevated levels of TRH in portal blood of hypothyroid sheep compared with euthyroid controls. Conversely, thyrotoxic levels of T_4 cause marked suppression of proTRH mRNA in the PVN compared with euthyroid controls (Segerson et al., 1987, 1989; Koller et al., 1987), and a reduction in the secretion of TRH into the portal plexus (de Greef et al., 1992), establishing an inverse relationship between thyroid hormone and the biosynthesis and secretion of hypophysiotropic TRH. In this manner, it is presumed that the concentration of TRH (and associated proTRH-derived peptides) in the portal capillary system can be regulated.

The increase or decrease in the amount of hypophysiotropic TRH secreted into the portal system

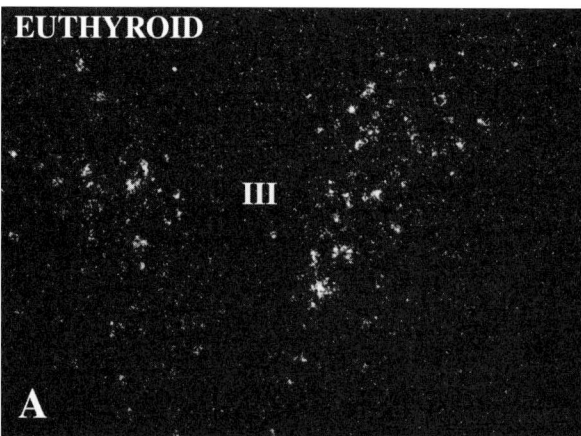

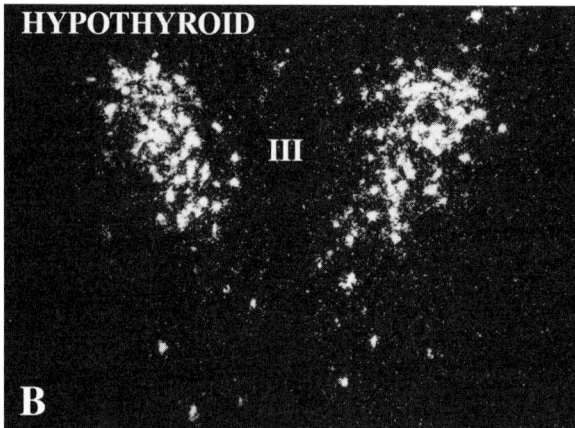

FIGURE 15 In situ hybridization autoradiogram of proTRH mRNA in a coronal section of the hypothalamus from (A) a euthyroid and (B) a hypothyroid animal. Note marked increase in silver grains selectively over TRH-synthesizing neurons in the hypothalamic paraventricular nucleus (PVN) in the hypothyroid animal. III = third ventricle.

for conveyance to the anterior pituitary, as dictated by variations in thyroid status, may be important to influence the set point for feedback regulation of thyroid hormone on anterior pituitary TSH secretion; when portal blood TRH concentrations are low, TSH can be suppressed by less T_4 (reduced set point), while high portal blood TRH concentrations raises the set point for feedback regulation of TSH. This concept was originally proposed by Reichlin and collaborators (Martin et al., 1970) on the basis that TSH in thyroidectomized animals with lesions of the hypothalamus that include the PVN can be suppressed by smaller doses of T_4 than animals with an intact hypothalamus, and by Kaplan et al. (1986) that

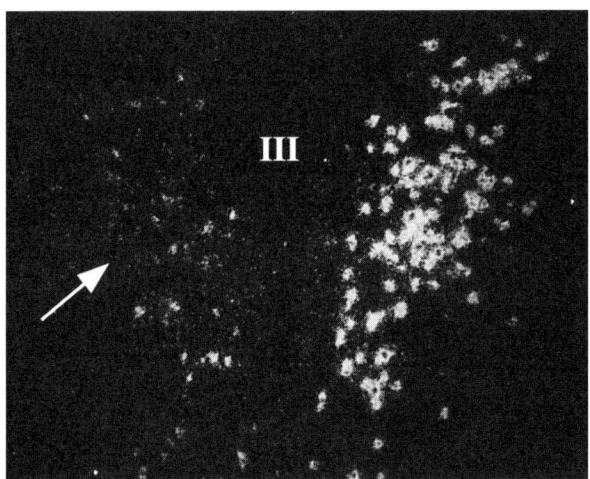

FIGURE 16 Effect of a unilateral microcrystalline implant of T_3 on one side of the hypothalamic paraventricular nucleus (PVN) in a hypothyroid animal. Marked inhibition of proTRH mRNA is seen on the side of the implant (arrow) in comparison with the opposite side. III = third ventricle.

chronic intrathecal infusion of TRH in man can elevate TSH and circulating free and total thyroid hormones. These observations have been confirmed by Greer et al. (1993).

The selectivity of TRH neurons in the medial and periventricular parvocellular subdivisions of the PVN to negative feedback regulation by thyroid hormone would appear to be an intrinsic property of these cells. Stereotactic implantation of microcrystals of T_3 adjacent to one side of the PVN in hypothyroid animals leads to marked inhibition of proTRH mRNA on that side (Fig. 16), confirming the early studies by Yamada and Greer (1959) that microinjection of T_4 into the thyrotropic area of rats reduces thyroid uptake of radioiodine, by Kniggee and Joseph (1971) that pellets of T_4 implanted in the preoptic area of cats prevent compensatory growth of hemithyroidectomized thyroid glands, and by Belchetz et al. (1978) that bilateral injection of T_3 into hypothyroid monkeys reduces plasma TSH concentrations. However, by using a more proximal end point for the response (proTRH mRNA content of PVN neurons), Dyess et al. (1988) avoided concerns expressed for the above studies that the implanted thyroid hormone had its effect on anterior pituitary TSH secretion by diffusing to the pituitary or stimulating somatostatin secretion into the portal capillary system. In addition, the presence of the thyroid hormone receptors TRα1 and TRβ2 in more than 80% of TRH-producing neurons in the PVN (Lechan et al., 1994) provides further support for a direct action of thyroid hormone on hypophysiotropic TRH neurons. In contrast, the relative paucity of TRα2 in hypophysiotropic TRH neurons may explain the unique responsiveness of these neurons to circulating thyroid hormone in contrast to TRH-producing neurons in other regions of the CNS that do not have a hypophysiotropic function.

The source of nuclear T_3 responsible for feedback regulation of TRH neurons in the PVN appears to differ from the source of T_3 in other regions of the CNS. The PVN contains little, if any, D_2 activity or D_2 mRNA (Riskind et al., 1987; Tu et al., 1997), indicating that cells in this region are not capable of intracellular conversion of T_4 to biologically active T_3. As opposed to the cerebral cortex and anterior pituitary where the majority of T_3 arises from intracellular conversion of T_4 to T_3 (Crantz et al., 1982; Silva and Leonard, 1985), hypophysiotropic TRH neurons in the PVN must receive T_3 from an exogenous source, either directly from the bloodstream, the CSF, or the adjacent glia, or by transneuronal transport (Dratman and Crutchfield, 1987; Dickson et al., 1990; Dratman et al., 1991). The possibility that feedback regulation by thyroid hormone on TRH neurons in the PVN is mediated exclusively by circulating levels of T_3 alone was dismissed after it was demonstrated that the systemic infusion of graded doses of T_3 to hypothyroid animals that restore plasma levels of T_3 to normal does not suppress proTRH mRNA levels in the PVN to euthyroid levels (Kakucska et al., 1992). Only after constant infusion with higher concentrations of T_3 that raise plasma T_3 to the supranormal range is there an apparent reduction in hybridization signal for proTRH mRNA to euthyroid levels. Thus, the calculated plasma level of T_3 required to suppress proTRH mRNA to normal is approximately 1.6 times euthyroid levels, highly reminiscent of the concentration of plasma T_3 required to reduce TSH to normal in the absence of T_4 (Connors and Hedge, 1980). Therefore, as in other regions of the brain, feedback regulation of thyroid hormone on TRH neurons in the PVN requires circulating T_4. Because the PVN lacks deiodinase, the monodeiodination of T_4 to T_3 must occur at another locus in the brain, such as in glial cells or other neuronal cells, and is then transported to the PVN.

D. Regulation of Hypophysiotropic TRH by Afferent Inputs

TRH-synthesizing neurons in the rat PVN are anatomically positioned to receive a large number of afferent, neuroendocrine inputs. Presumably, these inputs are important in establishing the set point at which thyroid hormone regulates the biosynthesis of TRH in the basal state, but more importantly, to alter this set point under certain physiological conditions elucidated below so as to increase or decrease circulating levels of thyroid hormone. Some of these inputs derive from the PVN itself, originating from peptidergic and aminergic neurons adjacent to TRH, hypophysiotropic cells. In fact, axon collaterals of parvocellular neurons ramify within the medial parvocellular PVN and establish numerous synaptic contacts with the perikarya and dendrites of other parvocellular as well as magnocellular neurons (Van den Pol, 1982). However, the majority of inputs to TRH neurons derive from other regions of the diencephalon, telencephalon, and brain stem. In the diencephalon, different nuclei in the periventricular, medial, and to a lesser extent lateral hypothalamic regions, the subthalamic zona incerta, the circumventricular subfornical organ, and the midline thalamic paraventricular nucleus, innervate the periventricular and medial parvocellular subdivisions of the PVN, largely through ipsilateral axons coursing in the periventricular fiber system and in the medial forebrain bundle (Sawchenko and Swanson, 1983) (Fig. 17). In the telencephalon, only the bed nucleus of the stria terminalis and the amygdaloid complex, primarily the medial and central nuclei, have direct projections to the periventricular and medial parvocellular PVN, through ispsilateral and partly contralateral pathways that course both in the stria terminalis and, more ventrally, in the substantia innominata and over the optic tract (Sawchenko and Swanson, 1983; Gray et al., 1989). In contrast, neurons in other limbic areas, including the lateral septum and the ventral subiculum of the hippocampus, project toward the PVN via the medial forebrain bundle and the medial corticohypothalamic tract of the postcommissural fornix, respectively, but their terminal fields remain outside the limits of the nucleus proper (Sawchenko and Swanson, 1983; Kohler, 1990). However, it is presumed that limbic imputs from the ventral subiculum of the hippocampus may establish a control over neurons in the medial parvocellular

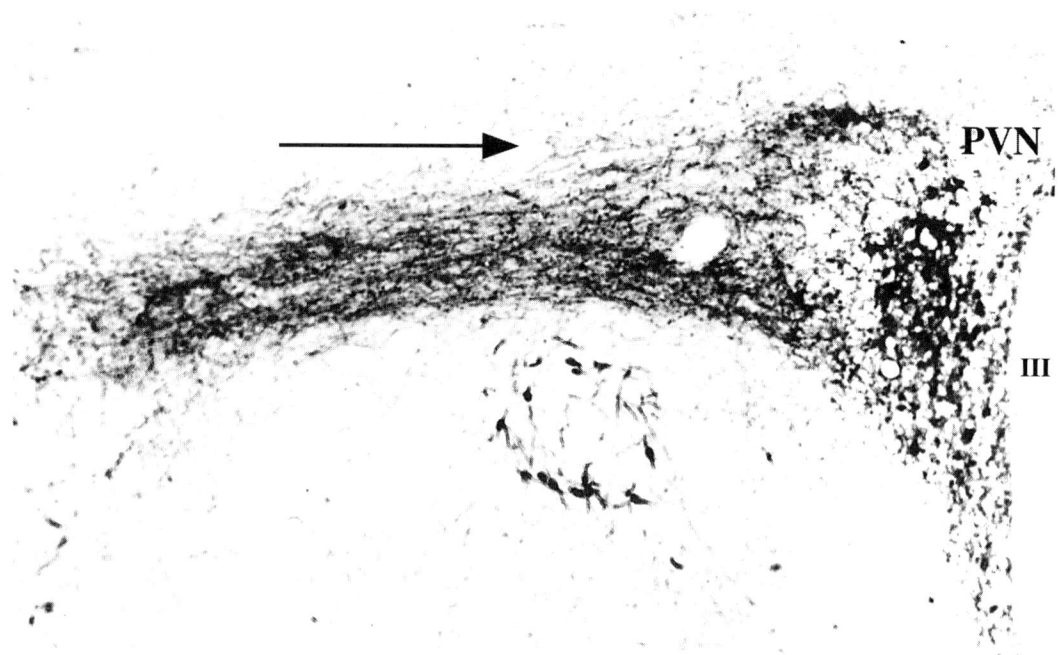

FIGURE 17 Immunocytochemical preparation showing afferent input to the paraventircular nucleus (PVN) via the median forebrain bundle (MFB). Arrow denotes the direction of projecting fibers to the PVN. III = third ventricle.

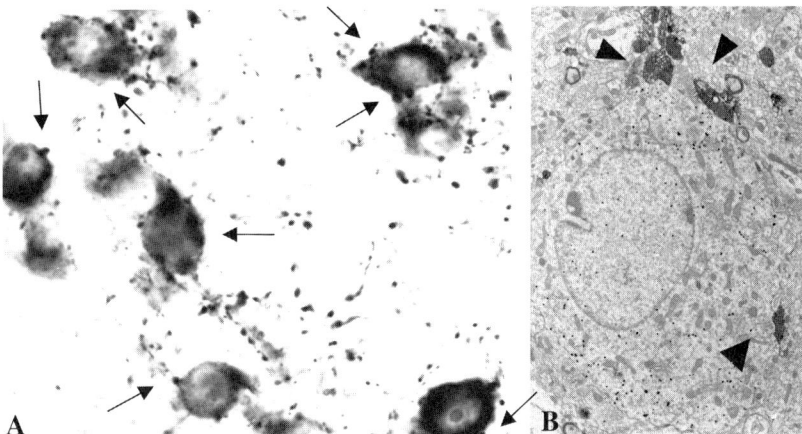

FIGURE 18 Dual immunolabeling for AGRP (fibers) and TRH (cell bodies) in the paraventricular nucleus (PVN). (A) At the light microscopic level, TRH neurons appear to receive numerous contacts from AGRP-containing axon terminals (arrows). (B) Electron micrograph reveals that axon terminals containing AGRP establish synaptic associations with TRH neurons (arrowheads) and that these contacts are primarily symmetric.

PVN through their monosynaptic connections with the bed nucleus of the stria terminalis (Cullinam et al., 1993). In the brain stem, different regions of the reticular formation, including the mesencephalic raphe nuclei, locus ceruleus, parabrachial nucleus, nucleus of the tractus solitarius, and specific ventral and dorsal neuronal groups in the medulla oblongata (described in detail below according to their neurotransmitter content), provide the greatest innervation to the periventricular and medial parvocellular subdivisions of the rat PVN by way of ventral and dorsal, primarily ipsilateral ascending pathways (Sawchenko and Swanson, 1982, 1983; Sawchenko et al., 1983, 1985).

Axon terminals within the medial and periventricular parvocellular PVN mainly establish axo-dendritic and, to a lesser extent, axo-somatic synapses (Fig. 18), giving off numerous axonal collaterals, some of which establish axo-axonic contacts, primarily with axons of magnocellular neurons (Van den Pol, 1982). As emphasized by Van den Pol (1982), the morphological organization of these contacts is relevant to their function: axo-somatic contacts are often invaginated in or surrounded by perikaryal plasmalemma, which may decrease neurotransmitter diffusion and thereby increase the efficacy of the postsynaptic response. In contrast, the axo-dendritic synapses mostly occur on thin, elongated dendritic appendages, which are less likely to generate high current flow and thereby decrease the efficacy of the postsynaptic response.

Morphologically distinct types of axon terminals preferentially establish synaptic contacts with either IR-TRH perikarya or dendrites. In particular, symmetric synapses established by axon terminals containing small and large electron-lucent vesicles predominate on TRH perikarya, whereas both symmetric and asymmetric contacts established by axonal boutons containing a mixed population of small, round, and oval clear vesicles are found on TRH dendrites (Kiss and Halasz, 1990; Toni and Lechan, 1993). As neurophysiological studies indicate that symmetric and asymmetric synapses may correlate with inhibitory and excitatory activity, respectively (Peters et al., 1970), regulation by different neurotransmitters on the activity of TRH hypophysiotropic neurons may occur at distinct loci, either on the cell body or dendrites.

In addition to the regulation of perikarya and dendrites within the PVN, regulation of TRH release may also occur in the external layer of the median eminence, where TRH axons terminate. The external layer of the rat ME is richly innervated by both aminergic and peptidergic axons primarily arising from nuclei in the periventricular and medial hypothalamus, including the PVN itself and to a lesser extent from neurons in the preoptic and septal regions (specifically the organum vasculosum of the lamina terminalis, diagonal band of Broca, and medial septum) and from a limited area in the reticular formation of the medulla oblongata, specifically the nucleus ambiguus region (Lechan et al., 1980, 1982; Weigand and Price, 1980) and from the mesencephalic raphe nuclei (Steinbush, 1984). Axons from these regions reach the ME by coursing through either the lateral retrochiasmatic area, periventricular fiber system (Palkovits, 1984), or the medial forebrain bundle (Conrad et al., 1974). In the human hypothalamus, primary sources of nerve fibers to the external layer of the ME are the arcuate (or infundibular) and periventricular nuclei, and there is indirect evidence that axons from these nuclei reach the ME through the lateral retrochiasmatic pathway (DeRooij and Hommes, 1974). Any of these axons are in a position to influence tuberoinfundibular TRH release by axo-axonal associations with TRH fibers, although true, axo-axonic synapses have been only rarely recognized in the mammalian ME (Knigge and Scott, 1970). The location of the nuclear groups contributing to the human tuberoinfundibular system is shown in Fig. 19.

The role of forebrain and brain stem inputs on the regulation of tuberoinfundibular TRH is only recently becoming better understood. It involves the regulation of circadian fluctuations in TSH levels, inhibition of TSH release during stress, and modulation of TSH secretion during adaptation to environmental temperature (Jackson and Reichlin, 1979; Reichlin, 1986a). The neuromediator substances thought to influence the thyroid axis by a central action include the biogenic amines, numerous neuropeptides and proteins, the neurotransmitter gamma aminobutyric acid (GABA), cytokines intrinsic and extrinsic to the CNS, and neurotrophic factors. Although the anatomical origin of each neurotransmitter-containing pathway that projects to hypophysiotropic TRH neurons is not precisely known, implications can be drawn from the anatomy of the innervation to the parvocellular PVN and ME. In particular, as the brain stem and, to a lesser extent, the diencephalon are the principal source of aminergic pathways to the hypothalamus, whereas the hypothalamus itself and the limbic system provide a major component of neuropeptidergic inputs to the diencephalon, it is reasonable to assume that aminergic inputs to the TRH tuberoinfundibular system primarily originate from the brain stem reticular formation and to a minor extent from specific regions of the diencephalon. In contrast, inputs containing neuropeptides, cytokines, and other factors arise largely in the periventricular hypothalamus and bed nucleus of the stria terminalis–amygdaloid complex (Toni and Lechan, 1993). As a consequence, it is presumed that aminergic pathways convey to the TRH hypophysiotropic neurons primarily autonomic sensory inputs of both somatic and visceral origin and/or act to modify their neuronal threshold to incoming stimuli of limbic origin (Nauta and Haymaker, 1969). Indeed, physiological evidence indicates that in the CNS the biogenic amines are more likely to facilitate and/or suppress other specific humoral and/or neurochemical information than to exert a direct inhibitory or stimulatory effect on target cells, depending on the type of pre- or postsynaptic receptor involved (Stricker and Zigmond, 1986). In contrast, peptidergic and other mediators containing afferents to the TRH tuberoinfundibular neurons are belived to convey selective information related to the initiation of specific homeostatic behaviors, like the sleep–wake cycle, thirst, hunger, thermoregulation, reproductive activity, aggressiveness, and affective sensations with compulsory component or motivation (Swanson, 1987), all involving a specific adaptation of the thyroid axis function (Toni and Lechan, 1993). It is therefore apparent why the importance of the anatomical origin and content of axons innervating TRH tuberoinfundibular neurons has been emphasized for many years (Joseph and Knigge, 1978; Reichlin, 1986a). The morphological organization as well as proposed physiological significance of these neuroendocrine inputs on the regulation of tuberoinfundibular TRH biosynthesis and/or secretion will be summarized below.

E. Biogenic Amines

1. Norepinephrine and Epinephrine

The periventricular and medial parvocellular subdivisions of the rat PVN are densely innervated by norepinephrine (NE)–containing axon terminals. These fibers originate from NE-containing A1 (lateral reticular nucleus), A2 (rostral to the nucleus of the tractus solitarius), A6 (rostral to the locus ceruleus), and epinephrine (E)–containing C1 (lateral paragigantocellular reticular nucleus), C2 (dorsal motor nucleus of the vagus nerve), and C3 (medial longitudinal fasciculus area) neuronal groups in the reticular formation of the ventrolateral (A1, C1) and dorsomedial (A2, C2,

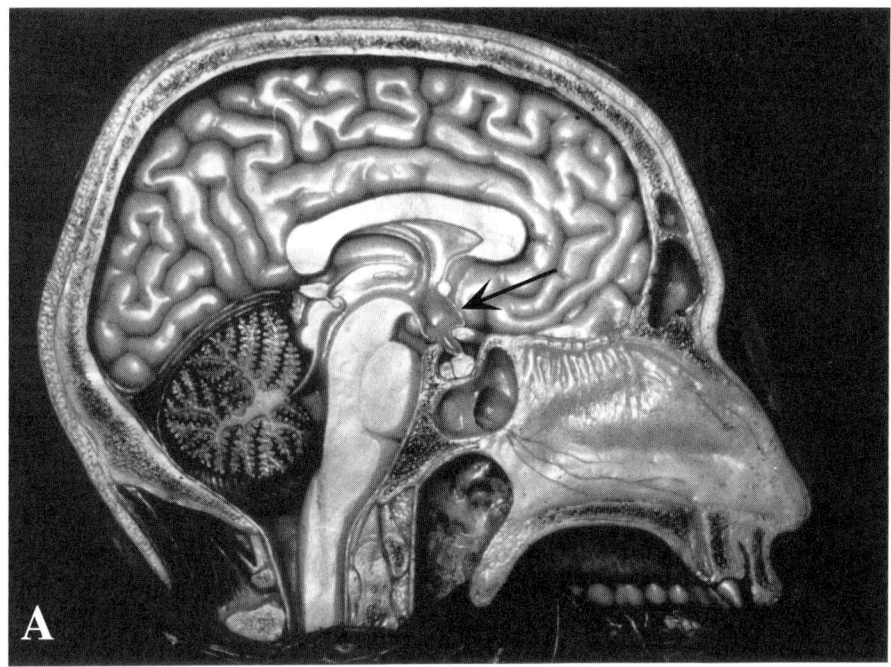

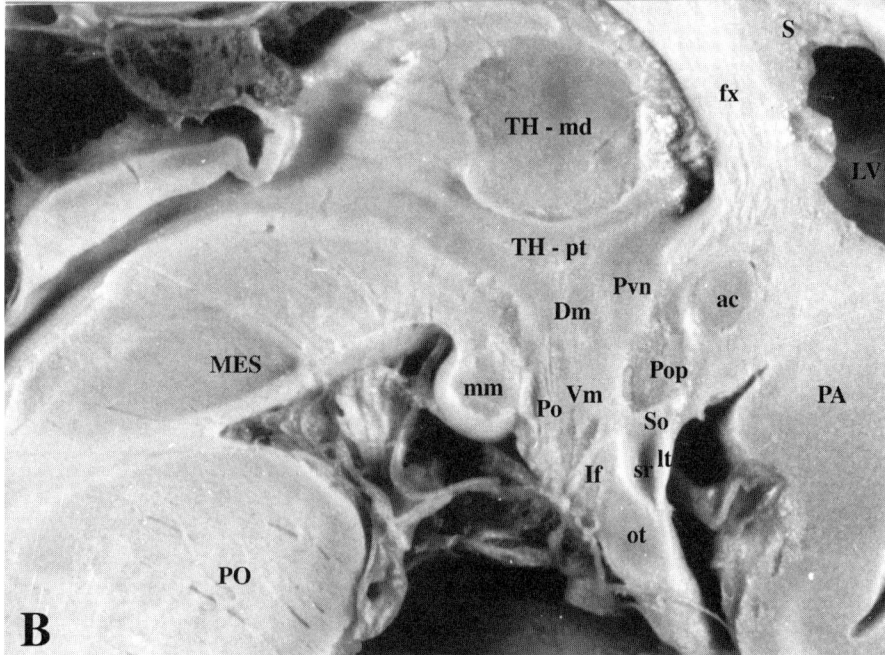

FIGURE 19 (A) Saggital section of a human skull showing the location of the hypothalamus (arrow) at the base of the brain. (From the anatomical wax collection at the University of Bologna, Italy.) In (B), the hypothalamus of a fixed, adult human brain is shown. It is bounded by the anterior commissure (ac) and lamina terminalis (lt) anteriorly, mammillary bodies with prominent medial mammillary nucleus (mm) and mesencephalon (MES) posteriorly, and the thalamus (TH) superiorly. The third ventricle makes up the core of the hypothalamus. Many of the major hypothalamic cell groups are located near the midline and contribute to the fiber pathways extending to the pituitary (or infundibular) stalk. These include the preoptic nucleus (Pop), paraventricular nucleus (Pvn), dorsomedial nucleus (Dm), ventromedial nucleus (Vm), arcuate (or infundibular) nucleus (If), supraoptic nucleus (So), and posterior hypothalamic nucleus (Po). Other abbreviations are as follows: fx, fornix; ot, optic tract; sr, supraoptic recess; LV, lateral ventricle; PA, paraolfactory area; PO, pons; S, septum; TH-md, thalamic mediodorsal nucleus; TH-pf, thalamic parafascicular nucleus.

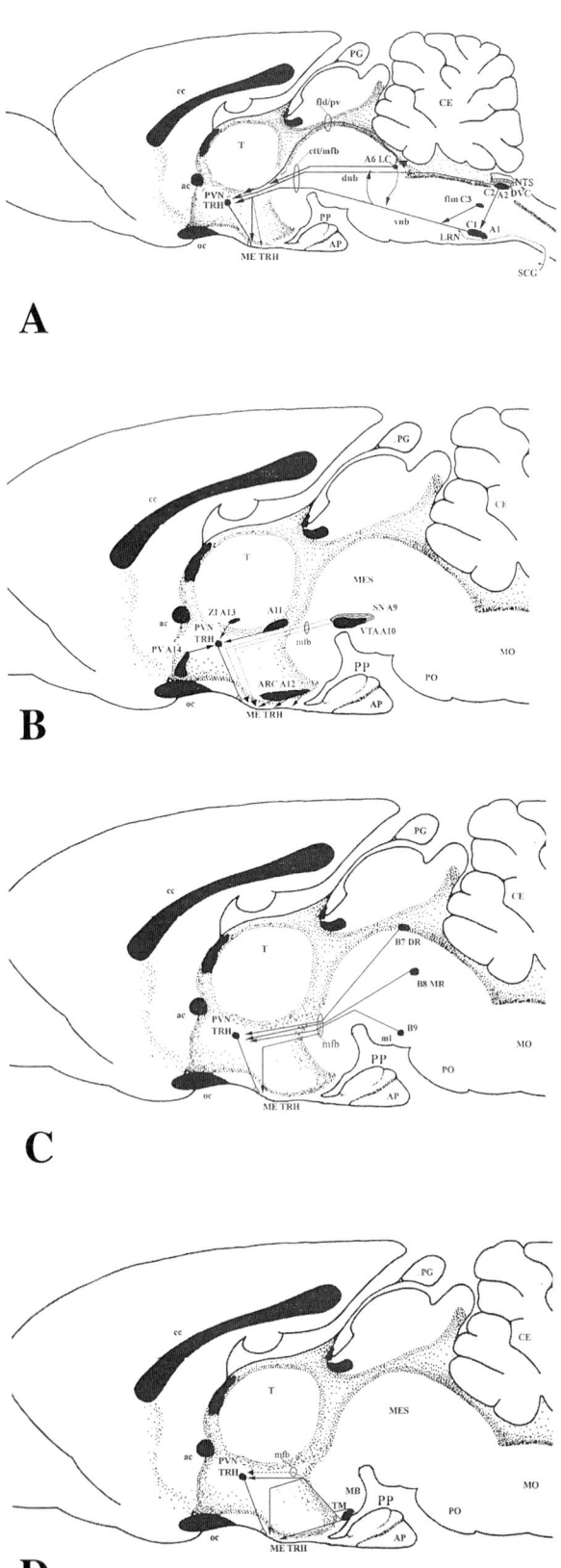

C3) medulla oblongata and pons (A6) (Sawchenko and Swanson, 1982; Sawchenko et al., 1983). As depicted in Fig. 20A, these axons course rostrally in the ventral (fibers from A1-C1 and A2-C2, C3) and dorsal (mainly fibers from A6) noradrenergic bundles as a part of the catecholaminergic central tegmental tract throughout the midbrain, and then enter the medial forebrain bundle to innervate the hypothalamus (Moore and Card, 1984; Nieuwenhuys, 1985; Bjorklund and Lindvall, 1986). Fibers from A6 and possibly A2 reach the PVN by traveling in the dorsal periventricular pathway, within the mesencephalic periaqueductal gray as a part of the dorsal longitudinal fasciculus (Nieuwenhuys, 1985; Bjorklund and Lindvall, 1986). Part of the fibers from A1-C1, A2, and, to a much lesser extent, C2 neuronal groups send collateral branches to the central nucleus of the amygdala, suggesting that brain stem catecholaminergic inputs to the periventicular and medial parvocellular PVN may coordinate endocrine with

---

FIGURE 20 Schematic representation of the origin of catecholamine-containing axon endings in the paraventricular nucleus (PVN). (A) norepinephrine; (B) dopamine; (C) serotonin; (D) histamine. Anatomical schema drawn on midline sagittal sections of the rat brain. Continuous lines illustrate pathways that are proven; dotted lines illustrate pathways that are hypothesized. Abbreviations are as follows: ac, anterior commissure; AMG, amygdala; AP, anterior pituitary; ARC, hypothalamic arcuate nucleus; BST, bed nucleus of the stria terminalis; cc, corpus callosum; cct/mflb, central tegmental tract/medial forebrain bundle; CE, cerebellum; DMN, hypothalamic dorsomedial nucleus; DVC, dorsal vagal complex; dnd, dorsal noradrenergic bundle; DR, dorsal raphe; fld/pv, fasciculus longitudinalis dorsalis/periventricular system; flm, fasciculus longitudinalis medialis; IGL, intergeniculate leaflet of the lateral geniculate body; LC, locus ceruleus, LHA, lateral hypothalamic area; LRN, lateral reticular nucleus; MB, mammillary body; ME, hypothalamic median eminence; MePO, hypothalamic median preoptic nucleus; MES, mesencephalon; mfb, medial forebrain bundle; MI, medial lemniscus; MO, medulla oblongata; MPA, hypothalamic medial preoptic area; MR, median raphe; NTS, nucleus of the tractus solitarius; oc, optic chiasm; PB, parabrachial nucleus; Pc, posterior commissure; PG, pineal gland; PO, pons; PP, posterior pituitary; PV, hypothalamic periventricular nucleus; PVN, hypothalamic paraventricular nucleus; SCG, superior cervical ganglion; SN, substantia nigra; vnd, ventral noradrenergic bundle; T, thalamus; TM, hypothalamic tuberomammillary nucleus; VTA, ventral tegmental tract; ZI, subthalamic zona incerta.

limbic responses to autonomic visceral stimuli (Petrov et al., 1993). A portion of the catecholaminergic fibers afferent to the PVN might also arise from epinephrine (E)-containing neurons intrinsic to the hypothalamus (Hokfelt et al., 1984). A similar distribution for neuroendocrine catecholamine afferents to the parvocellular PVN has also been found in primates (Ginsberg et al., 1993).

Evidence for direct innervation of TRH-synthesizing neurons in the PVN by catecholamine has been reported by Shioda et al. (1986) and Liposits et al. (1987). Using immunocytochemical techniques, these investigators provided morphological evidence for the presence of noradrenergic and adrenergic axons, respectively, in asymmetric synaptic contact with both the perikarya and dendrites of TRH tuberoinfundibular neurons. These data have been confirmed by Shioda and Nakay (1993) showing that ascending projections from the A1-C1 and A2 cell groups in the medulla oblongata establish synaptic contracts with IR-TRH perikarya and dendrites in the medial parvocellular PVN. Nakai et al. (1983) have found noradrenergic axon terminals in close apposition to TRH axons in the external layer of the rat median eminence, indicating that catecholaminergic inputs may influence TRH hypophysiotropic neurons not only through direct effects on their perikarya and dendrites but also on their axon terminals. These fibers originate from the A1 and A2 catecholaminergic centers in the medulla oblongata and possibly from the superior cervical ganglion (Moore and Card, 1984; Hokfelt et al., 1984; Gallardo et al., 1984).

The effect of NE and E on TRH release in the PVN is primarily stimulatory. Indirect evidence has shown that intracerebroventricular injections of either NE and E or α_2-adrenergic agonists stimulate basal TSH secretion, whereas blockade of the central noradrenergic tone by administration of inhibitors of either catecholaminergic biosynthesis or α_2-adrenergic transmission leads to a fall in basal TSH secretion (Annunziato et al., 1977; Vjivian et al., 1978; Montoya et al., 1979; Krulich, 1982; Terry, 1986). More direct evidence has been given by Grimm and Reichlin (1973) and Hirooka et al. (1978), showing that NE stimulates the release of TRH from mouse and rat hypothalamic preparations in vitro. Since the periventricular and medial parvocellular subdivisions of the PVN are rich in α_2-adrenoceptors (Young and Kuhar, 1980), it has been suggested that NE and E may exert a tonic, stimulatory regulation of TSH secretion at this level through an α_2-adrenoceptor (Muller and Nistico, 1989). Whether this stimulatory effect is due to a pre- or postsynaptic site of action remains to be clarified. In addition, NE may also stimulate TRH secretion from the ME; NE releases TRH from both isolated ME fragments in vitro and push–pull, cannulated ME in vivo (Tapia-Arancibia et al., 1985). This action occurs through a stimulatory postsynaptic α_1-adrenoceptor mechanism (Tapia-Arancibia et al., 1985) that may be mediated through α_1 binding sites in the external layer of the ME (Leibowitz et al., 1982).

The physiological correlate of the stimulatory action of NE and E on TRH secretion is seen in the response of the thyroid axis to cold exposure in experimental animals. Associated with an increase in thyroid hormone is a rapid rise in TSH, occurring within 30 min of the cold exposure (Krulich, 1982). The TSH rise is dependent on an intact, central noradrenergic innervation (Annunziato et al., 1979; Montoya et al., 1979; Schettini et al., 1979; Mannisto, 1983; Arancibia et al., 1989), particularly that coursing in the ventral noradrenergic bundle (Ishikawa et al., 1984). This view is supported by the observation that the TSH response to acute cold exposure does not occur during the first 10 days after birth in the rat (Ignar and Khun, 1988), when the hypothalamic, noradrenergic innervation is still immature (Fowlers and Kellogg, 1975), and that the TSH response to cold is blunted in aged rats (Reymond et al., 1989) in which there is a reduction in the neuronal density and immunoreactivity of medullary adrenergic C1 and C2 groups (Agnati et al., 1988). In addition, reduction of central catecholamines by α-methylparatyrosine, deafferentation of the medial basal hypothalamus, and intraventricular 6-hydroxydopamine each abolish the response (Annuziato et al., 1977; Schettini et al., 1979).

The rise in TSH is thought secondary to increased secretion of hypophysiotropic TRH on the basis that antiserum to TRH suppresses the response (Szabho and Frohman, 1977; Ishikawa et al., 1984), lesioning the PVN abolishes the response (Ishikawa et al., 1984), and push–pull perfusion studies show increased TRH in the ME (Arancibia et al., 1985). In addition, proTRH mRNA in PVN neurons increases within 60 min of cold exposure (Zoeller et al., 1990; Uribe et al., 1993), indicating that the response is mediated at the level of TRH gene transcription.

What is particularly intriguing about the acute cold-induced stimulation of the thyroid axis is that proTRH mRNA is increased at a time when circulating levels of thyroid hormone are high. This is contrary to the mechanism of inverse feedback regulation by thyroid hormone as discussed above, where inhibition of proTRH mRNA would be expected. Presumably, this can be interpreted to mean that cold exposure can override the feedback mechanism by altering the set point for inhibition by T_3 through the release of catecholamines. Catecholamines have also been proposed to have inhibitory effects on tuberoinfundibular TRH release, primarily acting in the ME (for review, see Toni and Lechan, 1993), but these data are mainly based on indirect evidence and require further confirmation. An extensive review on the mechanism of cold-induced activation of the thyroid axis has recently been given by Arancibia et al. (1996).

The release of catecholamines in contact with TRH neurons may be at least partly under the control of thyroid hormone. Andersson and Eneroth (1987) have reported increased NE levels and its utilization in the PVN of hypothyroid rats and reversal of this effect by thyroid hormone replacement. However, catecholamines, do not mediate negative feedback regulation exerted by thyroid hormone on TRH gene expression in the PVN. Depletion of catecholamine inputs to the rat PVN by either unilateral, stereotactoxic injections of the neurotoxin 6-hydroxydopamine, adjacent to the PVN or transection of the ascending catecholaminergic fibers to one side of the PVN at level of the rostral mesencephalon, does not alter the content of proTRH mRNA in hypothyroid animals (Dyess et al., 1988). Therefore, the effect of hypothyroidism-induced enhanced NE turnover in the PVN may be to facilitate the release of mature TRH and not to affect its biosynthesis. Other effects of catecholamines on TRH neurons in the PVN have been proposed by Yamashita et al. (1989), suggesting that NE inputs from A1 medullary neurons may stimulate PVN TRH neurons in response to a fall in arterial blood pressure and contribute to the increase in plasma TSH levels seen during hypovolemia and/or hypotension.

2. Dopamine

The PVN receives a conspicuous dopaminergic innervation from neuronal groups located in posterior and dorsal areas of the hypothalamus (group A11) as well as in the zona incerta of the subthalamic region (group A13); a minor projection field originates from the dopaminergic cell group in the anterior periventricular hypothalamus (group A14). Axons from these dopamine (DA)–containing neurons reach the PVN through the incerto-hypothalamic pathway and the periventricular system (Bjorklund and Lindvall, 1984, 1986; C. K. Wagner et al., 1995), but direct interactions with TRH neurons have not been established. Dopaminergic neurons in the arcuate nucleus and adjacent periarcuate area of the hypothalamus (group A12) provide a large terminal field of DA axons distributed in both medial and lateral aspects of the external layer in the rat ME (Bjorklund and Lindvall, 1984, 1986) where they could influence TRH secretion by contacts with TRH axons (Nakai et al., 1983). It has also been proposed that some fibers might originate from dopaminergic cell groups in the ventral midbrain (group A9: substantia nigra; group A10: reticular formation of the ventral tegmental area) and reach the ME through the nigrostriatal dopaminergic pathway within the medial forebrain bundle (for review, see Bjorklund and Lindvall, 1984). A similar distribution for neuroendocrine dopaminergic neurons has also been found in primates, human fetuses, and man (Muller and Nistico, 1989; Bjorklund and Lindvall, 1984, 1986). The origin of dopaminergic neurons that innervate the PVN and ME is schematically shown in Fig. 20B.

A number of studies suggest that DA exerts inhibitory regulation of TRH secretion in the rat, likely acting on TRH axons in the ME, but the evidence is indirect (Price et al., 1983). Enhancement of the central dopaminergic transmission by intracerebroventricular administration of high doses of DA (Vjivian et al., 1978; Mannisto et al., 1981) or peripheral administration of DA (Vjivian et al., 1978), DA receptor agonists (Krulich et al., 1977; Ranta et al., 1977; Mannisto and Ranta, 1978; Mannisto et al., 1979), and the DA precursor L-DOPA (Tuomisto et al., 1975; Krulich et al., 1977; Morley, 1981) has been found to inhibit basal and/or cold-stimulated TSH secretion. However, some studies, have failed to confirm these responses (Chen and Meites, 1975; Scapagnini et al., 1977; Annuziato et al., 1979). Conversely, administration of DA antagonists have resulted in stimulatory (Mueller et al., 1976; Krulich et al., 1977) or unmodified (Annuziato et al., 1979) basal and/or cold-stimulated TSH responses, while selective blockade of dopaminergic D_1 receptors has been shown to stimulate TSH secretion (Andersson, 1989). DA might also inhibit TSH release indirectly by stimulating somatostatin (somatotropin-release inhibiting factor, SRIF) secretion (Wakabayashi et al., 1977; Negro-Vilar et al., 1978; Chihara et al., 1979; Maeda and Frohman, 1980), which is inhibitory to TRH release (Hirooka et al., 1978). However, DA-induced SRIF release has not been confirmed by all authors (Terry et al., 1980).

As for NE and E, thyroid hormone may influence dopaminergic regulation of tuberoinfundibular TRH secretion by acting directly on TRH axons in the ME. This is supported by the decrease in DA concentration and utilization in the external layer of the ME in hypothyroid rats and its reversal by thyroid hormone replacement (Andersson and Eneroth, 1987). TSH might also be involved in the regulation of this response during hypothyroidism through a short feedback mechanism by increasing inhibitory dopaminergic influences on TRH release to counterbalance its own hypersecretion (Andersson et al., 1985), but these observations require confirmation.

In humans, DA exerts tonic regulation of TSH secretion, primarily acting at the level of the anterior pituitary (for review, see Krulich, 1982; Muller and Nistico, 1989). It may be important for the circadian variation of TSH (see later), but an effect on central TRH release is possible. Some studies have shown that a single dose of L-DOPA, which penetrates the blood-brain barrier, can lower basal TSH levels in hypothyroid patients without affecting the response of TSH to TRH (Rapoport et al., 1973; Feek et al., 1980), raising the possibility for an inhibitory action of DA on tuberoinfundibular TRH release. Furthermore, basal TSH secretion can be stimulated by DA antagonists that penetrate the blood-brain barrier, in both euthyroid (Healy and Burger, 1977; Massara et al., 1978; Scanlon et al., 1979) and hypothyroid (Massara et al., 1978; Scanlon et al., 1981) subjects, also suggesting a suprahypophysial site of action to regulate TSH secretion. Finally, DA might contribute to the pulsatile secretion of TSH by influencing TRH release (Brabant et al., 1991).

3. Serotonin

Only a few 5-hydroxytryptamine (5-HT, serotonin)–containing fibers innervate the PVN, primarily the periventricular and to a lesser extent the medial parvocellular subdivision of the rat PVN (Sawchenko et al., 1983). These fibers originate from neuronal groups in the raphe nuclei of the mesencephalic reticular formation (group B7: nucleus raphe dorsalis; group B8: nucleus raphe medianus or centralis superior of Bechterew; group B9: dorsal to the medial lemniscus) (Sawchenko et al., 1983) and reach the parvocellular PVN through the ventral ascending 5-HT pathway via the medial forebrain bundle (Nieuwenhuys, 1985; Jacobs and Azimita, 1992) (Fig. 20C). The rat hypothalamus also contains intrinsic 5-HT neurons (Steinbush, 1984), but their contribution to the innervation of the parvocellular PVN is not known. Some evidence for serotoninergic axon terminals in both asymmetric and symmetric synaptic contact as well as in close apposition without synaptic specializations with the perikarya and dendrites of TRH tuberoinfundibular neurons in the rat PVN has been provided by Shioda et al. (1986) and Kiss and Halasz (1990), suggesting that serotoninergic inputs might be involved in the neuroendocrine regulation of hypophysiotropic TRH release. Few 5-HT-containing fibers originating from the mesencephalic raphe nuclei described above are distributed to the external layer of the ME, mainly in its lateral part (Steinbush, 1984). Nakai et al. (1983) have observed close associations between ^{3}H-5-HT-containing axonal boutons and IR-TRH axons in the external layer of the ME, indicating that 5-HT inputs may influence TRH secretion through effects on perikarya, dendrites, and axon terminals of TRH tuberoinfundibular neurons. Mesencephalic 5-HT-containing neuronal groups analogous to those in the rat have also been recognized in primates (Nieuwenhuys, 1985; Jacobs and Azimita, 1992); therefore, it is conceivable that 5-HT innervation of tuberoinfundibular TRH neurons also occurs in higher mammals.

The role of 5-HT on hypophysiotropic TRH secretion and its involvement in the regulation of the TRH-TSH axis is far from clear. Inhibitory, excitatory, and no responses on TRH biosynthesis and/or release have been reported (Joseph-Bravo et al., 1979; Chen and Ramirez, 1981; Krulich, 1982; Coccaro et al., 1988; Muller and Nistico, 1989). One possibility that may account for these conflicting results is the complexity of the response to 5-HT release, dependent on the presence of the type of pre- and/or postsynaptic 5-HT receptors, including 5-HT$_1$ presynaptic, inhibitory autoreceptors located on 5-HT axon terminals and 5-HT$_2$ postsynatpic receptors located on target neurons (Jacobs and Azimita, 1992; Radja et al., 1991).

4. Histamine

A dense network of IR-histamine axons innervates the periventricular and medial parvocellular subdivisions of the rat and human PVN (Inagaki et al., 1988; Panula et al., 1989; Fekete et al., 1999). Steinbush (1984) has also observed a dense plexus of histamine-containing axons in the lateral part of the external layer of the rat ME. Histaminergic fibers largely emanate from neurons located in the ventral portion of the posterior hypothalamus, specifically in the tuberomammillary nuclei, and reach the PVN and possibly ME primarily by a periventricular route (Steinbush and Mulder, 1984; Schwartz et al., 1986; Inagaki et al., 1988; Panula et al., 1989; Fekete et al., 1999) (Fig. 20D). Lesion studies have suggested that some fibers may also be conveyed laterally by the medial forebrain bundle (Schwartz et al., 1986; Wada et al., 1991). Mast cells synthesizing histamine are also present in the rat ME and below the basal surface of the leptomeninges in close association with vascular elements, raising the possibility that histamine participates in the regulation of tuberoinfundibular blood flow to the anterior pituitary, or has direct effects on release of hypophysiotropic substances from axons terminating on the portal system (Steinbush and Mulder, 1984; Schwartz et al., 1986; Theoharides et al., 1995; Pang et al., 1996).

At present, there are no immunocytochemical data to establish an association between histamine-containing fibers and either IR-TRH perikarya and dendrites in the PVN or IR-TRH axon terminals in the median eminence. *In vitro* and *in vivo* studies indicate an involvement of histamine in the regulation of TRH release, although the data are contradictory. Some studies have shown that histamine induces the release of TRH from rat and sheep hypothalamic preparations *in vitro* (Charli et al., 1978; Joseph-Bravo et al., 1979; Bennett and Keeling, 1981), an effect that is blocked by H$_2$ receptor antagonists (Charli et al., 1978; Joseph-Bravo et al., 1979). In contrast, other studies have shown that the intracerebroventricular administration of histamine and H$_2$ receptor agonists decreases cold-induced TSH secretion (Mannisto, 1983; Tuominen et al., 1983, 1985), a response that requires the release of TRH (Szabo and Frohman 1977; Mori et al., 1978; Arancibia et al., 1983; Ishikawa et al., 1984). Stressful conditions, such as a low-calorie diet, hypoglycemia, and increased ambient temperature, stimulate the histaminergic transmission in the rat PVN (Sakata et al., 1997). Since these conditions also inhibit TRH biosynthesis and/or release (Blake et al., 1991; Yamaguchi et al., 1991; Arancibia et al., 1996), it is possibile that histamine inputs participate in stress-induced TSH inhibition though a central action on TRH neurons, as originally suggested by Knigge and Warberg (1991).

F. Neuropeptides, Proteins, and Amino Acids

1. Neuropeptide Y

The PVN receives a conspicuous innervation by neuropeptide Y (NPY)–containing fibers, most prominent in the periventricular and medial parvocellular subdivisions of the nucleus (Fig. 21A) where both classical synaptic contacts and close membrane associations without synaptic specializations (nonsynaptic varicosities) between IR-NPY axon terminals and PVN perikarya and dendrites have been recognized (Pelletier et al., 1984; Sawchenko and Pfeiffer, 1988). The origin of NPY neurons that innervate the PVN and ME is schematically shown in Fig. 21B. Some of these NPY axons originate from the A1, C1, C2, and C3 catecholaminergic neuronal groups in the medulla oblongata where NPY coexists with norepinephrine (in A1) and epinephrine (in C1, C2, C3), and reach the periventricular and medial parvocellular subdivisions of the PVN by traveling in the CA central tegmental tract, and then as a part of the medial forebrain bundle. Few IR-NPY nerve fibers originating from catecholamine centers in the medulla oblongata are also present in the external layer of the rat ME (Meister et al., 1989; Ciofi et al., 1991). Another major projection pathway arises from the hypothalamic arcuate nucleus (Bai et al., 1985; Kerkerian and Pelletier, 1986). Other NPY-containing axon terminals in the parvocellular PVN may derive from a number of other sources, including the dorsomedial nucleus (Kesterson et al., 1997), intergeniculate leaflet of the lateral geniculate body (Horvath, 1998), nuclei in the mesencephalic reticular formation, and

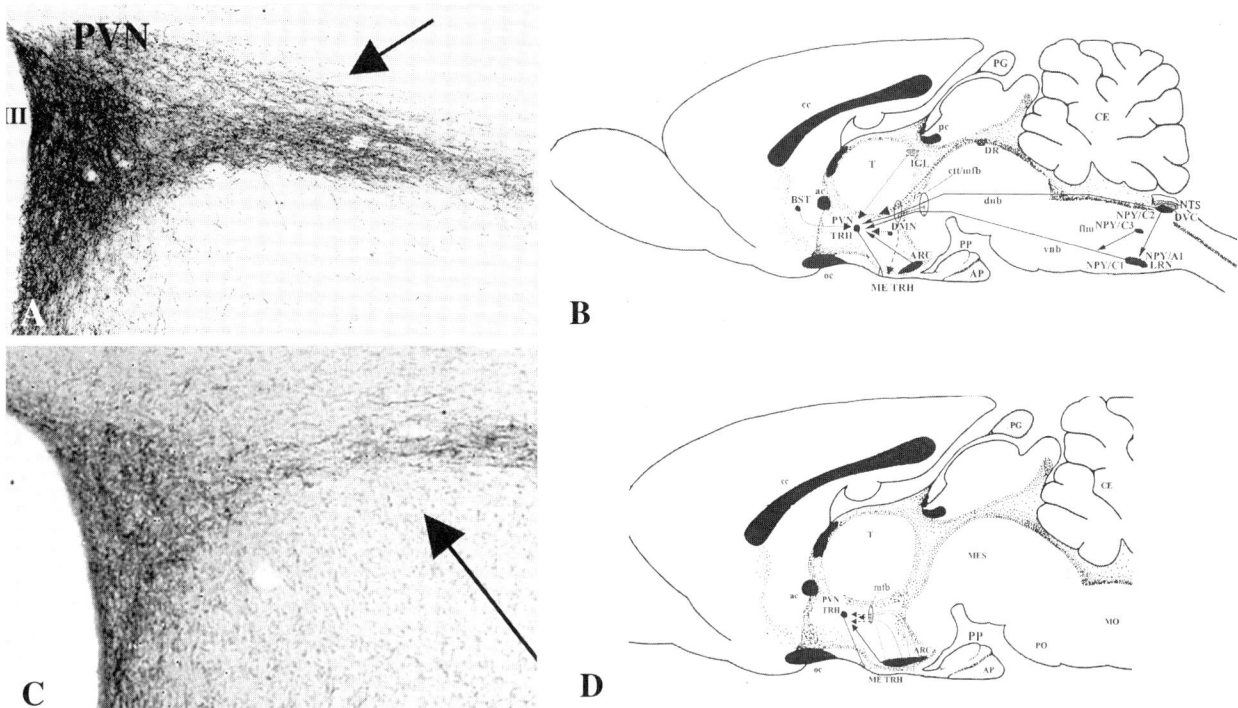

FIGURE 21 Immunolabeling of peptide-containing axon endings in the paraventricular nucleus (PVN) and schematic representation of the origin of their neuronal perikarya. (A,B) neuropeptide Y (NPY); (C,D) agouti-related peptide (AGRP). Arrow in (A) and (C) denotes pathway of fibers innervating the PVN. Abbreviations as in Fig. 20. III = third ventricle.

the bed nucleus of the stria terminalis (De Quidt and Emson, 1986), as all of these regions have known axonal projections to the parvocellular PVN (Swanson and Sawchenko, 1983). Similar innervation of IR-NPY in the PVN and ME has been found in monkeys (Smith et al., 1985) and man (Adrian et al., 1983; Mihaly et al., 2000).

IR-NPY axon terminals establish symmetric and sometimes asymmetric synaptic contacts with both IR-TRH perikarya and dendrites in the periventricular and medial parvocellular subdivisions of the rat PVN (Toni et al., 1990a; Legradi and Lechan, 1998). The arcuate-derived NPY inputs have a prominent association with cell bodies and proximal dendrites, whereas the brain stem–derived NPY/catecholamine afferents exhibit a selective location to the distal dentrites and spines of TRH neurons (Diano et al., 1998a). These findings have also provided a morphological basis for NPY-containing neuroendocrine pathways involved in the regulation of tuberoinfundibular TRH release and are consistent with the presence of NPY binding sites (NPY1 and NPY5 receptors) in the parvocellular PVN in both experimental animals and man (Harfstrand, 1987; Nichol et al., 1999). The predominance of symmetric synaptic contacts between NPY fibers and TRH neurons and their proximal location to the neuronal perikaryon is contrary to the catecholamine innervation of PVN TRH neurons, which establishes primarily asymmetric synaptic contacts (Liposits et al., 1987) on distal TRH dendritic appendages. Indeed, the major source for the NPY projection to TRH neurons in the PVN is the hypothalamic arcuate nucleus (Legradi and Lechan, 1998). Pharmacological obliteration of nearly all NPY neurons in the arcuate nucleus, but not NPY neurons in other regions of the brain, results in partial depletion of the NPY innervation of the PVN but an 82% reduction in the NPY innervation of TRH neurons in the PVN. In contrast, lesions in the brain stem that nearly deplete the catecholamine innervation of the PVN also result in a significant depletion of the NPY innervation to the PVN but do not result in a significant loss of the NPY innervation to hypophysiotropic TRH neurons in the PVN (Legradi and Lechan, 1998).

The functional significance of the target-specific innervation of TRH neurons by NPY fibers from the arcuate nucleus while other neurons in the PVN are innervated by NPY of brain stem or other origin may be seen in light of the potential role of NPY to reset the hypothalamic-pituitary-thyroid axis under certain physiological conditions. One of these conditions is fasting, in which substantial reductions in circulating thyroid hormone levels is accompanied by a paradoxical reduction in proTRH mRNA in hypophysiotropic neurons in the PVN and inappropriately normal or low circulating TSH levels (Blake et al., 1991; Rondeel et al., 1992b). These changes occur simultaneously with a marked increase in NPY gene expression in the arcuate nucleus and concomitant increase in NPY release in the PVN (Chua et al., 1991; Calza et al., 1989; Kalra et al., 1991). The up-regulation of NPY in the arcuato-paraventricular neuronal pathway has been implicated in the potent central stimulatory action of NPY on food intake (Kalra et al., 1991; Beck et al., 1990). Moreover, rats with streptozotocin-induced diabetes show alterations in the thyroid axis similar to those of starved rats (Gonzalez et al., 1980; Wilber et al., 1981) and also have an increased NPY content in the arcuate nucleus and the PVN (White et al., 1990; Abe et al., 1991). Conversely, studies by Legradi et al. (1997b) have demonstrated that the administration of leptin, a fat cell–derived hormone with anorectic activity that reduces the biosynthesis of NPY in the arcuate nucleus, prevents the fall in circulating thyroid hormone levels and the reduction of proTRH mRNA in the PVN. Since central administration of NPY reduces TSH secretion (Harfstrand, 1987), NPY may have direct inhibitory effects on hypophysiotropic TRH neurons. This has been demonstrated recently by Fekete et al. (2001), showing that intracerebroventricularly infused NPY substantially suppresses proTRH mRNA selectively in hypophysiotropic neurons in the PVN. Thus, NPY may modulate the set point for feedback regulation of hypophysiotropic TRH neurons during starvation by lowering the threshold of these neurons to feedback inhibition by circulating levels of thyroid hormone. NPY may also inhibit α-adrenergic neurotransmission at the postsynaptic level (Harfstrand, 1987), counteracting the stimulatory effects of norepinephrine. Finally, NPY may stimulate inhibitory regulators of TRH and TSH secretion by increasing the content of DA in the hypothalamus and external layer of the ME (Harfstrand, 1987; Heilig et al., 1990) and the release of somatostatin (Rettori et al., 1990).

2. Agouti-Related Protein

Agouti-related protein (AGRP) is a newly discovered protein (Shutter et al., 1997) and homolog of agouti, a well-characterized protein responsible for yellow coat pigmentation in mice. The observation that the agouti mouse is characterized not only by a light coat color but also by obesity and hyperphagia due to ectopic expression of agouti in the brain (Lu et al., 1994) led to the hypothesis that the brain may contain an endogenous substance closely related to agouti. The biologically active portion of AGRP is its C terminus, AGRP 83-132, which when administered intracerebroventricularly increases food intake (Rossi et al., 1998). Both agouti and AGRP exert its action on the melanocortin (MC) receptors. In the skin, agouti antagonizes the effect of α-melanocortin stimulating hormone (α-MSH) at the MC1 receptor to reduce pigmentation, and in the brain, AGRP antagonizes the anorectic effects of α-MSH by acting on the MC3 and MC4 receptors (Manne et al., 1995; Ollmann et al., 1997). The recognition that AGRP is synthesized only in the hypothalamic arcuate nucleus and colocalizes with NPY (Hahn et al., 1998; Broberger et al., 1998) raised the possibility that AGRP might also be contained in axon terminals that terminate on TRH neurons in the PVN.

Practically all detectable TRH neurons in the PVN are contacted by numerous nerve terminals containing AGRP, both on their cell bodies and on proximal dendrites (Legradi and Lechan, 1999) in a distribution similar to that described above for NPY. Axons appear to enter the PVN laterally from the median forebrain bundle just dorsal to the fornix. In contrast, TRH neurons in the adjacent perifornical group or lateral hypothalamus do not receive any contacts from AGRP-containing axon fibers. Pharmacological ablation of AGRP-synthesizing neurons in the arcuate nucleus results in the depletion of the ARGP innervation in the PVN (Broberger et al., 1998; Legradi and Lechan, 1998), establishing the arcuate nucleus as the sole origin of the AGRP innervation of TRH neurons (Fig. 21C, D).

Because AGRP gene expression increases with fasting and can be inhibited by leptin administration (Hahn et al. 1998; Mizuno and Mobbs, 1999), the possibility that AGRP might also contribute to the modulation of the thyroid axis during fasting as described above for NPY should be considered. This is further supported by the observation that mice with targeted deletion of the NPY gene retain the ability to suppress thyroid hormone levels with fasting (Erickson *et al.*, 1997), indicating that other mechanisms in addition to NPY may be operative. Thus, during fasting, the increased secretion of NPY, acting via NPY1 or NPY5 receptors, and AGRP, acting as an antagonist of the MC3/4 receptors, may work in concert on the surface of hypophysiotropic TRH neurons to increase the sensitivity of the TRH gene to circulating levels of thyroid hormone and reduce thyroid thermogenesis to preserve calories.

3. α-Melanocortin Stimulating Hormone

The presence of AGRP on the surface of hypophysiotropic TRH neurons strongly suggests that α-MSH is also involved in modulating hypophysiotropic TRH neurons, since AGRP has its primary action as an α-MSH receptor antagonist. Indeed, the PVN is heavily innervated by axons containing α-MSH. Whereas α-MSH is synthesized in two regions in the brain, the arcuate nucleus and the nucleus tractus solitarius (Dube *et al.*, 1978; Joseph *et al.*, 1983), the arcuate nucleus is probably the sole source for the α-MSH inervation of the PVN (Eskay *et al.*, 1979; Sawchenko *et al.*, 1982). Anatomical evidence to support a dual innervation of TRH neurons by α-MSH and AGRP has been demonstrated by Fekete *et al.* (2000a) in TRH neurons in the periventricular parvocellular subdivision of the PVN (Fig. 22). Since both peptides bind to the same receptors but have opposing actions, these data provide morphological evidence to suggest an interaction between melanocortin agonist and antagonistic effects directly on the surface of TRH neurons.

However, AGRP-containing axon terminals more heavily innervate TRH neurons in the PVN, however, and many examples of AGRP-innervated TRH neurons without α-MSH contacts are found in the medial parvocellular subdivision of the PVN (Fekete *et al.*, 2000a). Nevertheless, the intracerebroventricular infusion of

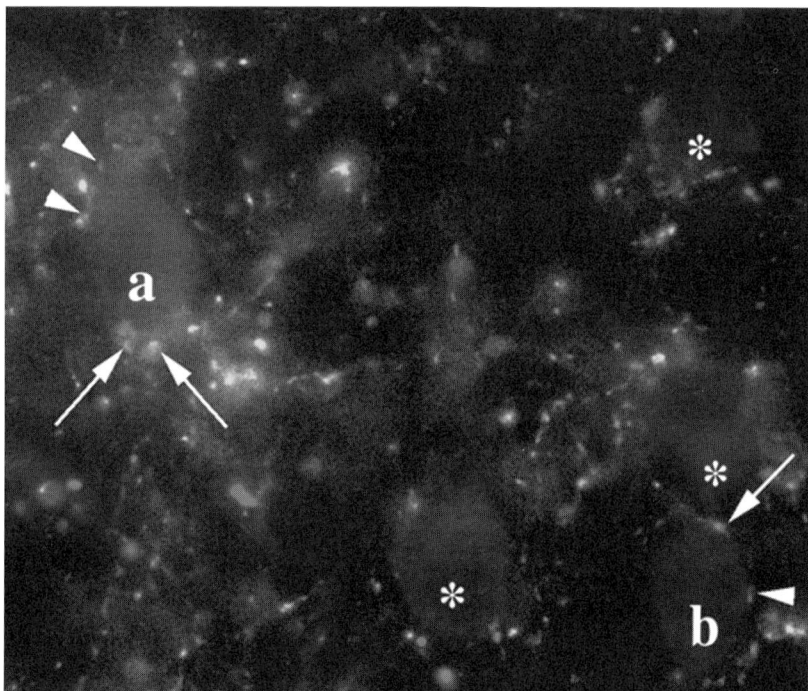

FIGURE 22 Dual innervation of a TRH neuron (a and b) in the paraventricular nucleus by axon terminals containing AGRP (arrows) and α-MSH (arrowheads). Neurons are innervated only by AGRP. (Courtesy of Dr. Csaba Fekete.) **See insert for a color version of this figure.**

α-MSH is capable of increasing the gene expression of TRH in fasting animals in all parvocellular subdivisions of the PVN, similar to that observed in fasting animals administered leptin (Legradi et al., 1997b). The anatomical selectivity of α-MSH-containing axon terminals for TRH neurons in the periventricular parvocellular subdivision of the PVN and the generalized effect of α-MSH to increase TRH gene expression in all hypophysiotropic neurons raises the possibility that α-MSH may exert both direct and indirect effect effects on parvocellular neurons in the PVN. Along these lines, the hypothalamic dorsomedial nucleus (DMN) has well-established projections to the parvocellular PVN (Ter Horst and Luiten, 1987; Thompson et al., 1996), and contains a subpopulation of neurons that are activated by the systemic administration of leptin (Elmquist et al., 1998). In addition, the DMN is one of the main targets for both α-MSH and AGRP-containing fibers (Jacobowitz and O'Donohue, 1978; Broberger et al., 1998), raising the possibility of a leptin-responsive, multisynaptic pathway, composed of α-MSH- and AGRP-producing neurons originating in the arcuate nucleus and influencing the activity of the PVN via direct afferents to the PVN and indirectly through afferents to the DMN.

While the intracerebroventricular infusion of α-MSH restores TRH mRNA levels in fasting animals to fed levels, its effect on peripheral thyroid hormone levels is only partial (Fekete et al., 2000a). Thyroid hormone levels rise to only approximately 50% of fed levels, in contrast to the administration of leptin to fasting animals, when circulating thyroid hormone levels fully return to normal fed levels (Legradi et al., 1997b). The ability of α-MSH to affect only part of the full regulatory effects of leptin on the thyroid axis, therefore, would suggest that other factors that respond to leptin administration and act in coordination with α-MSH downstream from the transcription of TRH are necessary to achieve the full regulatory response. Such factors may include NPY as discussed above, or other proteins that coexist with α-MSH in arcuate nucleus neurons as described below.

4. Cocaine- and Amphetamine-Regulated Transcript

Cocaine- and amphetamine-regulated transcript (CART), a 129- or 116-amino-acid prohormone deduced from its cDNA, is a newly discovered protein, named on the basis that its mRNA increases in the rat striatum after the acute administration of cocaine or amphetamine (Douglass et al., 1995). However, CART is present in many regions of the brain, including the hypothalamus (Koylu et al., 1998), and exerts a number of important central actions, including feeding behavior, sensory processing, reinforcement and reward, and stress (Kuhar and Vechia, 1999). It is presumed that the C-terminal portion of the prohormone gives rise to the biologically active CART as the peptide fragment, CART 55–102, is found in hypothalamic extracts and, when administered intraventricularly, inhibits food intake (Speiss et al., 1981; Kristensen et al., 1998).

The interst in CART as a potentially important peptide in the regulation of hypophysiotropic TRH neurons has arisen from its colocalization in POMC-producing neurons in the hypothalamic arcuate nucleus (Elias et al., 1998), and its presence in neurons in the hypothalamic PVN (Broberger, 1999) in a distribution highly reminiscent of the distribution of TRH neurons (Lechan and Jackson, 1982). Indeed, CART-containing axon terminals establish contacts with TRH-producing neurons in the PVN (Fekete et al., 2000). While many of these axon terminals co-contain α-MSH, suggesting a common origin from hypothalamic arcuate nucleus neurons, a separate, more delicate type of CART-containing axon terminal also innervates TRH neurons, presumably originating from a separate locus in the brain. These anatomical observations would suggest at least dual regulation of TRH neurons by CART. Since CART antagonizes the orexigenic effect of NPY (Lambert et al., 1998; Kristensen et al., 1998), and NPY may be inhibitory to TRH neurons (see above), we have hypothesized that CART may be stimulatory to hypophysiotropic TRH neurons and, in concert with α-MSH, contribute to the recovery of the hypothalamic-pituitary-thyroid axis in fasting animals that have been re-fed or treated with leptin (Fekete et al., 2000).

CART is also contained within TRH neurons in the PVN (Broberger, 1999; Fekete et al., 2000), but largely confined to TRH neurons in the medial and periventricular parvocellular subdivisions and their axon terminals in the ME (Fig. 23). To date, this is the only known peptide reported to colocalize with TRH in any substantial number of neurons in the PVN. The restriction to TRH neurons in the medial and periventricular

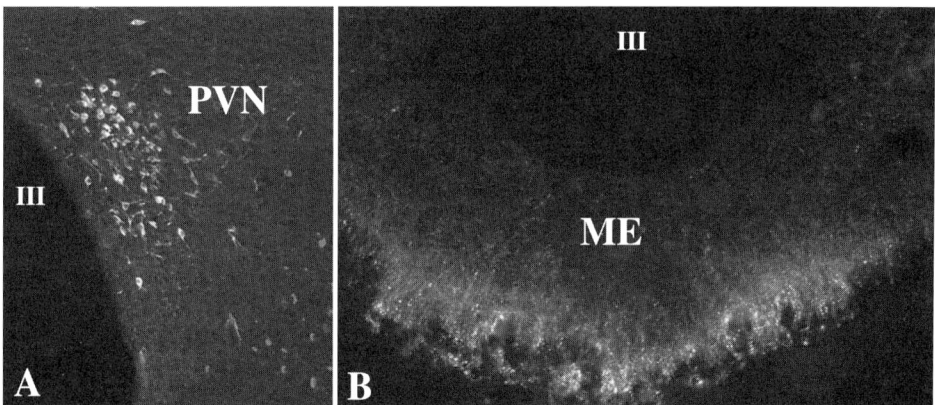

FIGURE 23 (A) Colocalization of CART with TRH in neuronal perikarya in the paraventricular nucleus (PVN) and (B) their axon terminals in the median eminence (ME). Neurons and axon terminals co-containing CART and TRH offer fellow. III = third ventricle. **See insert for a color version of this figure.**

parvocellular subdivisions would suggest a role for CART in hypophysiotropic regulation, since the anterior parvocellular subdivision TRH neurons do not project to the ME (Merchenthaler and Liposits, 1994). Thus, CART may be involved not only in the regulation of hypophysiotropic TRH neurons per se via secretion from axons in synaptic association with these neurons, but also the regulation of anterior pituitary TSH secretion after release from TRH-containing axon terminals in the ME, coordinating two components of the hypothalamic-pituitary-thyroid axis.

5. Thyrotropin-Releasing Hormone

The rat PVN is inundated by fine, beaded, IR-TRH fibers that are particularly dense in the periventricular and medial parvocellular subdivisions of the nucleus (Lechan and Jackson, 1982). Some of fibers innervate TRH hypophysiotropic neurons, primarily establishing symmetric synaptic contacts but also nonsynaptic interactions with their perikarya and dendrites (Toni et al., 1990b; Kiss and Halasz, 1990). The source of these inputs is not known, but could arise from recurrent axonal collaterals of tuberoinfundibular TRH neurons to mediate ultrashort feedback regulation of tuberoinfundibular TRH release (Renaud, 1978), or short projections from other TRH neurons within the PVN (Toni et al., 1990b). Van den Pol (1982) has described such short projections in the PVN. That TRH can regulate its own secretion by an autocrine mechanism as been reported by Bruhn et al. (1998) in anterior pituitary cultures.

TRH fibers might also originate from diencephalic and limbic regions. The hypothalamic medial preoptic area, dorsomedial nucleus, and bed nucleus of the stria terminalis each contain a dense collection of neuronal perikarya immunopositve for TRH prohormone–derived peptides (Lechan and Jackson, 1986; Lechan et al., 1987) and are known to innervate the parvocellular PVN (Swanson and Sawchenko, 1983). Of particular interest is the anatomical connection of the PVN with the DMN, in light of the effect of this region to regulate the set point for body energy stores (Bernardis and Bellinger, 1986; Choi et al., 1999; Choi and Dallman, 1999). As described above, the DMN is a target for a number of humoral and neuroendocrine inputs regulated by leptin (Elmquist et al., 1998) such as α-MSH and AGRP (Jacobowitz and O'Donohue, 1978; Broberger et al., 1998). Thus, if TRH-producing neurons in the DMN project to TRH neurons in the PVN, they would be in a position to contribute to a multisynaptic pathway regulated by leptin, to adjust thyroid function in relation to changes in nutrient intake.

A number of observations suggest that the effect of TRH on the secretion of tuberoinfundibular TRH is primarily inhibitory. This possibility was initially raised in the discussion of a paper from the laboratory of Luciano Martini where an unpublished observation reportedly showed that hypothalamic extracts containing TRH altered the content of TRH in the whole hypothalamus when injected systemically in hypophysectomized-thyroidectomized rats (Hyyppa et al., 1971). A direct inhibitory effect of TRH inputs is also suggested by the predominance of symmetric synapses between TRH axons and TRH neurons in the PVN (Toni et al., 1990b), similar to other peptide-producing tuberoinfundibular neurons, including SRIF, growth hormone–releasing hormone (GHRH), and luteinizing hormone–releasing hormone (LHRH), that make symmetric contacts and inhibit their own secretion (Jew et al., 1984; Witkin and Silverman, 1985; Leranth et al., 1985; Epelbaum et al., 1985, 1986; Richardson and Twente, 1986; DePaolo et al., 1987; Zanisi et al., 1987; Pelletier, 1987; Horvath and Palkovits, 1988).

6. Somatostatin

The periventricular and, to a lesser extent, medial parvocellular subdivisions of the rat PVN are innervated by IR-somatostatin fibers originating from both PVN neurons as well as more rostral neurons in the anteroventral portion of the periventricular nucleus (APv), whose axons reach the PVN by arching laterally and coursing caudally in the medial forebrain bundle (Krisch, 1979; Palkovits et al., 1982b). Minor projection fields arise from the arcuate (Finley et al., 1981; Moga and Saper, 1994; Shiosaka et al., 1981), lateral hypothalamus (Moga and Saper, 1994), and possibly parabrachial nucleus and nucleus of the tractus solitarius in the brain stem (Moga and Saper, 1994). In addition, one study has raised the possibility that somatostatin fibers from the amygdala and bed nucleus of the stria terminalis may innervate the parvocellular PVN by way of the stria terminalis (Sakanaka et al., 1981), but it is likely that the majority of these fibers remain outside the limits of the parvocellular PVN (Moga and Saper, 1994). A dense plexus of IR-somatostatin fibers is also present in the external layer of the rat ME, originating primarily from the APv nucleus (Ishikawa et al., 1987; Kawano and Daikoku, 1988; Merchenthaler et al., 1989a) and PVN (Krisch, 1979) and courses through both the retrochiasmatic area (Palkovits et al., 1980; Epelbaum et al., 1981; Makara et al., 1983) and periventricular pathway (Jew et al., 1984). IR-somatostatin fibers have also been observed in the human stalk ME and PVN and it has been suggested that they may originate from IR-SRIF perikarya in the arcuate nucleus (Desy and Pelletier, 1977).

Somatostatin-containing axon terminals innervate TRH-synthesizing neurons in the periventricular and, to a lesser extent, medial parvocellular subdivisions of the rat PVN (Toni and Lechan, 1990; Liao et al., 1992), establishing symmetric synaptic contacts with IR-TRH dendrites. In addition, Johansson and Hokfelt (1980) have found IR-somatostatin fibers in close proximity to TRH axons in the external layer of the rat ME. Collectively, these observations provide anatomical basis for a neuroendocrine regulation by somatostatin of TRH hypophysiotropic neurons.

The effect of somatostatin on TRH-producing neurons is likely inhibitory. This is supported by studies by Hirooka et al. (1978) who demonstrated that somatostatin inhibits TRH secretion from isolated rat hypothalamic fragments, and Arancibia et al. (1986) who reported that acute cold exposure induces a rapid decline in the levels of somatostatin followed by increased turnover of TRH in the rat ME. Somatostatin may also contribute to the inhibitory effects of cytokines on TRH gene expression since somatostatin mRNA is increased following the administration of interleukin (IL-1) to hypothalamic cell cultures (Scarborough et al., 1989).

7. Opioid Peptides

The rat parvocellular PVN is richly innervated by IR-enkephalin (ENK) fibers (including Leu- and Met-ENK peptides), primarily in its periventricular subdivision, that arise from the anterior hypothalamic and to lesser extent arcuate nucleus, and from the nucleus tractus solitarius in the brain stem (Kharchaturian et al., 1985; Moga and Saper, 1994). IR-dynorphin (DYN)–containing fibers have also been detected in the same location, possibly arising from the arcuate nucleus and/or the amygdaloid complex (Kharchaturian et al., 1985), the latter coursing in the stria terminalis and ventral amygdalofugal tract (Petruz et al., 1985). In addition, the external layer of the rat ME, particularly the lateral part, contains numerous IR-β-endorphin (END), IR-ENK, and IR-DYN axons, primarily arising from the arcuate nucleus, both in experimental animals and in humans (Meister et al., 1989; Petruz et al., 1985). Johansson and Hokfelt (1980) have described IR-ENK axons near TRH fibers in the external layer of the ME, and Liao et al. (1991) IR-ACTH/POMC fibers in strict association with IR-TRH perikarya in the PVN, raising the possibility of an interaction between EOPs and TRH at two different levels of the tuberoinfundibular system.

Several studies indicate that opiates may exert an inhibitory effect on tuberoinfundibular TRH release in the rat (Judd and Hedge, 1982, 1983). Both END and, to a lesser extent, ENK inhibit TRH release from the hypothalamus *in vitro* and can be inhibited by naloxone (Jordan *et al.*, 1986). In addition, *in vitro* and *in vivo* studies by Tapia-Arancibia and Astier (1983) and Arancibia *et al.* (1985), have shown that morphine and ENK inhibit TRH release from the ME. Jordan *et al.* (1986) have suggested that END is the major endogenous opioid peptide involved in the inhibition of TRH, based on the evidence that the inhibitory effect on hypothalamic TRH release is mediated primarily by μ receptors. In contrast, since ENK-containing fibers are densely distributed in the ME (Petruz *et al.*, 1985), ENK may inhibit TRH release at this level. Part of the effect of endogenous opioids on TRH release may be through effects on biogenic amines. Pretreatment of rats exposed to cold with the DA antagonist haloperidol eliminates the inhibitory effects of morphine on TSH secretion, a finding that led Sharp *et al.* (1981) to suggest that hypothalamic DA release mediates inhibition of TRH secretion in reponse to EOPs.

The physiological importance of an inhibitory opioidergic regulation of tuberoinfundibular TRH is unclear but may be involved in the control of the TSH response to environmental temperature and stress. Morphine injected into the third ventricle, ME, or peripheral circulation of rats exposed to cold decreases the cold-induced rise in TSH (Mannisto *et al.*, 1984; Sharp *et al.*, 1981) and increases the content of TRH in the whole hypothalamus, an effect prevented by the concurrent administration of naloxone (Sharp *et al.*, 1981). Morphine also prevents cold-induced increase of TRH turnover in the ME (Arancibia *et al.*, 1985).

8. Neurotensin

The periventricular and, to lesser extent, medial parvocellular subdivisions of the rat PVN are innervated by fibers containing neurotensin (NT), whose primary source is nuclei in the preoptic area of the hypothalamus, including the anteroventral portion of the periventricular nucleus (Moga and Saper, 1994) and the PVN itself (Ibata *et al.*, 1984). NT fibers are also present in the external layer of the ME arising from the arcuate nucleus and PVN (Emson *et al.*, 1985), but no data are available on potential axonal associations with TRH fibers in this site. In contrast, anatomical associations between NT fibers and TRH neurons in the PVN have been reported (Toni and Lechan, 1993), although little is known of their functional morphology; however, NT binding sites are present in these regions (Emson *et al.*, 1985; Meister *et al.*, 1989).

Data on the effect of NT on TRH release are limited but point to an inhibitory role. Studies by Maeda and Frohman (1978) have shown that intracerebroventricular NT inhibits basal TSH secretion. Part of the NT effect may be indirect and mediated by NT-induced DA (Myers and Lee, 1984) and somatostatin (Sheppard *et al.*, 1979; Maeda and Frohman, 1980; Abe *et al.*, 1981; Shimatsu *et al.*, 1982) release.

NT inputs to tuberoinfundibular TRH neurons could have a physiological role in modulating the response of TSH to environmental temperature. This possibility is supported by the inhibitory effect of NT on the cold-induced TSH rise (Nemeroff *et al.*, 1980). Sheppard *et al.* (1983; Sheppard and Sheennan, 1983) have also suggested that NT may participate in the inhibitory feedback regulation of thyroid hormone on tuberoinfundibular TRH release as thyroid hormone stimulates the secretion of NT from the hypothalamus and decreases hypothalamic NT content, whereas an insufficiency of thyroid hormone reduces the potassium-stimulated NT release and increases hypothalamic NT levels.

9. Corticotropin-Releasing Hormone

A dense cluster of small to medium-sized CRH-containing perikarya occupy the most dorsal and lateral portion of the medial parvocellular subdivision of the rat PVN, strictly adjacent to the bulk of TRH-synthezising cells, whereas few CRH-immunopositive neurons are present in the periventricular parvocellular subnucleus (for review, see Swanson *et al.*, 1986). These neurons send collateral axons throughout the medial parvocellular PVN (Liposits *et al.*, 1985) and massively project their axons outside the lateral margins of the nucleus, in a ventral direction toward the retrochiasmatic area, en route to the external layer of the ME where they extend thoughout its entire medial-lateral aspect (Aizawa and Greer, 1982; Antoni *et al.*, 1983; Merchenthaler *et al.*, 1984; Niimi *et al.*, 1988).

A moderate to light concentration of nerve fibers immunoreactive for CRH has also been observed in the medial and periventricular parvocellular subdivision of the rat PVN, primarily originating from the bed nucleus of the stria terminalis and, to a lesser extent, from the nucleus of the solitary tract and the hypothalamic preoptic nucleus (Moga and Saper, 1994).

Reciprocal synaptic associations between CRH- and TRH-synthesizing neurons have been observed primarily in the medial parvocellular PVN on both perikarya and dendrites (Hisano *et al.,* 1993). In addition, beaded CRH-containing fibers, possibly arising from other CRH-containing sources, have been found to surround TRH cell bodies in the same PVN location (Liao *et al.,* 1992). No data are available to show a direct association between CRH and TRH axons in the ME.

An inhibitory effect of CRH on hypothalamic TRH release *in vitro* has been reported by Mitsuma *et al.* (1987), and Hisano *et al.* (1993), suggesting that CRH inputs to TRH neurons might serve as a negative feedback circuitry to coordinate the activity of the thyroid with the adrenal axis.

10. Vasoactive Intestinal Peptide (VIP) and Pituitary Adenylate Cyclase Activating Polypeptide (PACAP)

VIP and the structurally and functionally related pituitary adenylate cyclase activating polypeptide (PACAP) have been found in fibers scattered thoughout the periventricular and medial parvocellular subdivisions of the PVN (Mezey and Kiss, 1985; Ceccatelli *et al.,* 1991; Koves *et al.,* 1991). Some of these fibers may originate from VIP or PACAP neurons in the PVN itself (Hokfelt *et al.,* 1987; Koves *et al.,* 1991); the ventral, retinal-recipient portion of the suprachiasmatic nucleus (SCN) (Watts and Swanson, 1987); and neurons outside the hypothalamus, primarily in the amygdaloid complex (Roberts *et al.,* 1980) or in the brain stem (Marley *et al.,* 1981; Legradi *et al.,* 1994). Few IR-VIP axons are present in the external layer of the ME in normal rats (Ceccatelli *et al.,* 1991), but after hypophysectomy, IR-PACAP fibers become evident in this location (Koves *et al.,* 1991). In humans, the ME contains high concentrations of VIP (Rostene, 1984), and its external layer contains numerous IR fibers for peptides that derive from the same precursor as VIP (Hokfelt *et al.,* 1987).

Rare reciprocal interactions of interneuronal types between VIP and TRH neurons in the medial parvocellular PVN have been seen in rats rendered hypothyroid by treatment with propylthiouracil (Toni and Lechan, 1993), and synaptic contacts between IR-PACAP axons and TRH-containing perikarya and dendrites have been shown in euthyroid animals in the same location (Legradi *et al.,* 1997a). These findings provide a morphological basis to suggest integration of responses between tuberoinfundibular VIP neurons, PACAP inputs, and TRH hypophysiotropic neurons under certain conditions.

Data on the effect of VIP on TRH release are limited but point to a stimulatory role. Observations by Mitsuma *et al.* (1984) have indicated that peripheral administration of VIP in high doses decreases TRH content in the whole hypothalamus while increasing plasma concentration of basal and cold-stimulated TSH. These data suggest that VIP may stimulate tuberoinfundibular TRH release. No data are available on the role exerted by PACAP on TRH or the thyroid axis at the hypothalamic level.

11. Gamma Aminobutyric Acid

The parvocellular subdivision in the rat PVN receives a dense innervation by axons containing the inhibitory amino acid gamma aminobutyric acid (GABA), primarily arising from GABA neurons in the PVN (Decavel and van den Pool, 1990; Roland and Sawchenco, 1993) and arcuate nucleus (Pu *et al.,* 1999). In addition, a large number of IR-GABA fibers are present in the external layer of the rat ME, originating in the hypothalamic arcuate nucleus (Meister *et al.,* 1989).

Although there are no immunocytochemical data demonstrating a GABAergic innervation of TRH tuberoinfundibular neurons in the PVN, indirect evidence suggests that GABA may primarily exert an inhibitory action on the TRH-TSH axis at the hypothalamic level (Vijayan and McCann, 1978; Mattila and Mannisto, 1980). This inhibitory action may be involved in the nocturnal restraint of tuberoinfundibular TRH release in the rat (Jordan *et al.,* 1983). Recent data by Pu *et al.* (1999) have also shown a role for GABA in the regulation of food intake in the PVN, where it may act as a comodulator of orexigenic NPY inputs from the arcuate nucleus, raising the possibility that

GABA may participate with NPY to inhibit the thyroid axis during fasting.

12. Cytokines

2 The CNS contains an endogenous cytokine system that includes IL-1, IL-2, IL-3, IL-6, tumor necrosis factor-α (TNFα), and interferon-γ (INFγ), synthesized and secreted by glial cells, endothelial cells, macrophages, and/or neurons (Reichlin, 1993). Of these, IL-1, IL-6, and TNFα have been the most extensively studied. IL-1β perikarya and fibers have been identified in the PVN and ME of both rat and man (Breder et al., 1988; Lechan et al., 1990), and IL-6 and IL-6 receptor mRNAs are present throughout the rostrocaudal extension of the rat periventricular hypothalamus (Schobitz et al., 1992).

Continuous infusion of IL-1 in rats suppresses TSH and thyroid hormone levels (Hermus et al., 1992), and studies by Kakucska et al. (1994) have demonstrated that intracerebroventricular administration of IL-1β inhibits TRH mRNA in the PVN. The effect of IL-1 on TRH could be direct via glial-neuronal or neuronal-neuronal interactions, or indirect and mediated through the inhibitory effects of somatostatin on TRH release. IL-1 stimulates somatostatin biosynthesis and release in fetal diencephalic cells *in vitro* (Scarborough et al., 1989); *in vivo*, immunoneutralization with antisomatostatin antiserum blocks the inhibitory effect of the bacterial endotoxin, lipopolysaccharide, on TSH secretion (Kasting and Martin, 1982).

Other cytokines, including IL-6 and TNFα, may influence tuberoinfundibular TRH release, but their effect is less clear. IL-6 depresses TSH secretion after intraventricular administration (McCann et al., 1990; Lyson and McCann, 1991; McCann, 1991), possibly by stimulating the release of somatostatin into the portal blood. TNFα administered into the cerebral ventricles reduces TSH secretion and may be due to direct effects on TRH neurons (Pang et al., 1989), although indirect effects through the release of IL-1 cannot be excluded. TNF-γ has also been proposed to act *in vivo* directly on the hypothalamus to inhibit TSH secretion, as it has no effect on TSH secretion from hemipituitaries *in vitro* (Gonzales et al., 1990).

The physiological significance of cytokine regulation of the TRH-TSH axis may relate to homeostatic mechanisms activated in the course of infection at the level of the CNS. During infection, release of endogenous cytokines in the hypothalamus as well as pituitary (Koenig et al., 1990) may act in concert with peripheral cytokines to reduce circulating thyroid hormone by inhibiting the secretion of TRH and TSH. This disorder, commonly referred to as "nonthyroidal illness syndrome" in patients with infection and chronic illnesses, may be important to retard the catabolic side effects of infectious illness, since restoration of normal thyroid hormone levels to rats with streptococcal pneumonia may increase the susceptibility to infection (Reichlin and Glaser, 1958).

13. Other Substances

A number of other neuromediators have been suggested to influence the thyroid axis at the hypothalamic level, but their site of action is unclear (for review, see Toni and Lechan, 1993). Included among them is the neuropeptide galanin. Galanin densely innervates parvocellular PVN in rats (Ching et al., 1985; Levin et al., 1987) and primates (Kordower et al., 1992). Since galanin induces NE release in the rat PVN (Kyrkouli et al., 1992), its content is reduced in the ME of hypothyroid rats (Hooi et al., 1990; Giardino et al., 1992), and it stimulates SRIF release from ME fragments *in vitro* (Aguila et al., 1992), galanin could exert a physiological effect in the regulation of the thyroid axis. However, no anatomical evidence is available to substantiate a neuroendocrine role for this neuromediator in the regulation of hypophysiotropic TRH.

G. Steroid Hormones

1. Glucocorticoids

Circulating levels of glucocorticoids (GCs) may both inhibit *in vivo* the biosynthesis of proTRH selectively in the rat PVN, but not in other TRH-rich areas of the dienchephalon (Kakucska et al., 1995), and reduce the release of TRH in the hypophysial portal blood (Van Haasteren et al., 1995). These effects are likely to occur primarily at the transcriptional level, since GC receptors are present in TRH tuberoinfundibular cells (Cintra et al., 1990, 1991) and a potential GC-responsive element, identical to the proposed consensus sequence for GC receptor binding, is located between 196 and 203 base pairs from the transcriptional initiation site of the TRH gene promoter (Jackson et al., 1990; Stevenin and Lee, 1995). The inhibitory effect of GC *in vivo* contrasts with its stimulation of TRH mRNA transcription *in vivo* in hypothalamic neurons (Luo *et al.*, 1993; Luo and Jackson, 1998; Pèrez-Martinez *et al.*, 1998); for this reason, it has been proposed that part of their effects in the PVN might be mediated by activation of inhibitory inputs to TRH neurons (Jackson, 1995). This possibility is consistent with the capacity of GCs to stimulate the biosynthesis of NPY (McKibbin *et al.*, 1992; White *et al.*, 1994; Mercer *et al.*, 1996; Zakrezewska *et al.*, 1999) that may inhibit TRH, or inhibit stimulators of TRH release such as catecholamines (Lechan *et al.*, 1992; Fuxe *et al.*, 1988). GC-induced inhibition of TRH release may contribute to the mechanism of suppression of the thyroid axis during fasting (van Haasteren *et al.*, 1995).

2. Gonadal Steroids

In the male rat, some data indicate that testosterone may exert a tonic stimulatory role on the thyroid axis (Rapp and Pyunn, 1974; Chen and Walfish, 1979; Christianson *et al.*, 1981). More direct evidence shows that castration inhibits the release of hypothalamic TRH *in vitro* (Pekary *et al.*, 1990) and increases its accumulation in the ME (Rondeel *et al.*, 1995), whereas testosterone reverses this effect (Pekary *et al.*, 1990), suggesting a tonic stimulatory role on tuberoinfundibular TRH release. Since changes in circulating levels of testosterone levels do not alter proTRH mRNA in the rat hypothalamus (Rondeel *et al.*, 1995), it is apparent that this regulation primarily occurs at a posttranscriptional level. This possibility is supported by evidence that testosterone administration reduces gonadectomy-induced accumulation of TRH in the posterior pituitary (Pekary *et al.*, 1990), indicating a stimulatory effect on intraneuronal TRH stores rather than on TRH biosynthesis. Part of the testosterone regulation might also be indirect through stimulation of substances that control the basal release of TRH from the PVN, such as catecholamines (Kalra and Kalra, 1984), or inhibition of substances that inhibit TRH secretion, such as somatostatin (Hirooka *et al.*, 1978). The basal release of somatostatin *in vitro* from hypothalamic explants has been shown to be inhibited by testosterone administration (Murray *et al.*, 1999).

Very limited data are available in the female rat. No effect of gonadectomy has been observed on the content of TRH in either the ME or the posterior pituitary (Rondeel *et al.*, 1995). However, *in vitro* data have shown that estradiol may stimulate hypothalamic TRH release (Franks *et al.*, 1984). Since this effect is observed *in vivo* when progesterone is simultaneously administered (Huang *et al.*, 1995), estradiol and progesterone may cooperate in regulating the thyroid axis at the hypothalamic level, possibly by acting on the neuroendocrine inputs that control TRH hypophysiotropic neurons (Toni and Lechan, 1993).

H. Hypothalamic Regulation of TSH

1. Molecular Structure and Glycosylation of TSH

TSH is a 28,000 MW heterodimer composed of two noncovalently linked glycosylated subunit polypeptides, α and β, derived from separate gene products. The α subunit is virtually identical to the α subunit in the other glycoprotein hormones, including luteinizing hormone (LH), follicle-stimulating hormone (FSH), and chorionic gonadotropin (CG), and is expressed in several different cell types. The β subunit is unique to TSH, expressed only in thyrotropes in the anterior pituitary, and confers biological and receptor binding specificity to the hormone. The α,β-heterodimer formation of the two subunits is essential for biological activity as the individual subunits are inactive.

In addition to heterodimerization of the subunits, glycosylation of asparagine residues (one in TSHβ and two in TSHα) are important for biologic activity (Magner, 1990; Grossmann *et al.*, 1997a). Newly synthesized α and β subunits are glycosylated in the endoplasmic reticulum with precursor oligosaccharides rich in mannose. This posttranslational modification facilitates combination of the two subunits into a heterodimer, retards aggregation of the individual subunits, and decreases intracellular proteolysis. High-mannose oligosaccharides on TSH then undergo multistep processing in the Golgi to more complex oligosaccharides in a hormonally dependent manner that requires an intact hypothalamus and is essential for the biopotency of mature TSH.

The three-dimensional structure of TSH is presumed similar to that of the other glycoprotein hormones CG, LH, and FSH. These molecules are members of the so-called cystine knot growth family, which also includes platelet-derived growth factor, nerve growth factor, vascular endothelial growth factor, and transforming

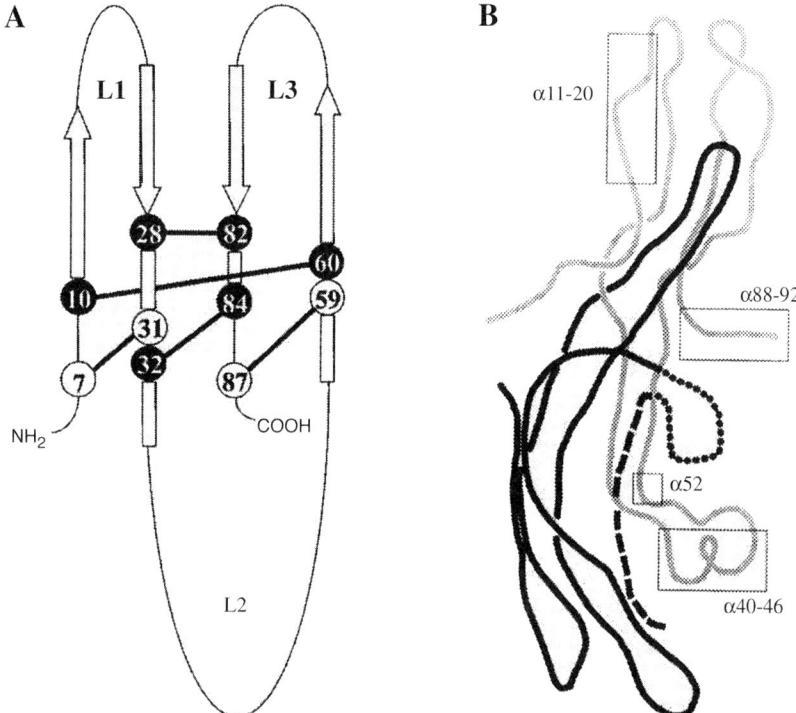

FIGURE 24 (A) Schematic diagram of the crystal structure of α subunit of glycoprotein hormones. The cysteine residues displayed as filled circles create disulfide bonds and form the "cystine knot." This creates three loops, designated L1, L2, and L3, respectively. (B) Schematic drawing of the presumed crystalline structure of hTSH showing the interaction between the α subunit (gray) and the β subunit (black). The seat belt region is shown by the interrupted line. [(A) From Darling *et al.*, 2000 and (B) from Grossmann *et al.*, 1997b, with permission.]

growth factor-β (Lapthorn *et al.*, 1994; Sun and Davis, 1995). The cystine knot is created by pairings of cysteine residues that are important for folding of the α and β chains of the glycoprotein hormones. This results in the subunits having two β-hairpin loops (L1 and L3) on one side of the cysteine knot, and a long loop of double-stranded β-sheet-like structure (L2) on the other side (Fig. 24A). The hairpin structure is stabilized by a hydrophobic core extending between the two loops (Lapthorn *et al.*, 1994). On the basis of studies on the crystalline structure of human chorionic gonadotropin (hCG), it is believed that heterodimer formation between the α and β subunits involves pairing of the segments near the cystine knot and aligns the long loop of the β subunit to the hairpin loops of the α subunit (Fig. 24B). The long loop of the β subunit can then surround the α subunit and covalently bind to itself through disulfide linkages, giving rise to what has been referred to as the "β-subunit seat belt loop." The seat belt region may be important for binding of TSH to the TSH receptor since creation of a TSHβ chimera containing the hCG seat belt sequence abolishes TSH receptor binding, whereas creation of an hCG chimera that contains the TSHβ seat belt sequence activates the TSH receptor (Grossmann *et al.*, 1997b). Genetic abnormalities that are associated with disruption of the cystine knot results in thyroid hormone deficiency (Hayashizaki *et al.*, 1989).

2. Feedback Regulation of TSH by Thyroid Hormone

The most important regulator of TSH is thyroid hormone. Thyroid hormone has a rapid effect on both the *TSHα* and *TSHβ* genes to result in a reduction in the steady-state levels of their mRNAs (Chin *et al.*, 1985) and the transcriptional rate of the *TSHβ* gene

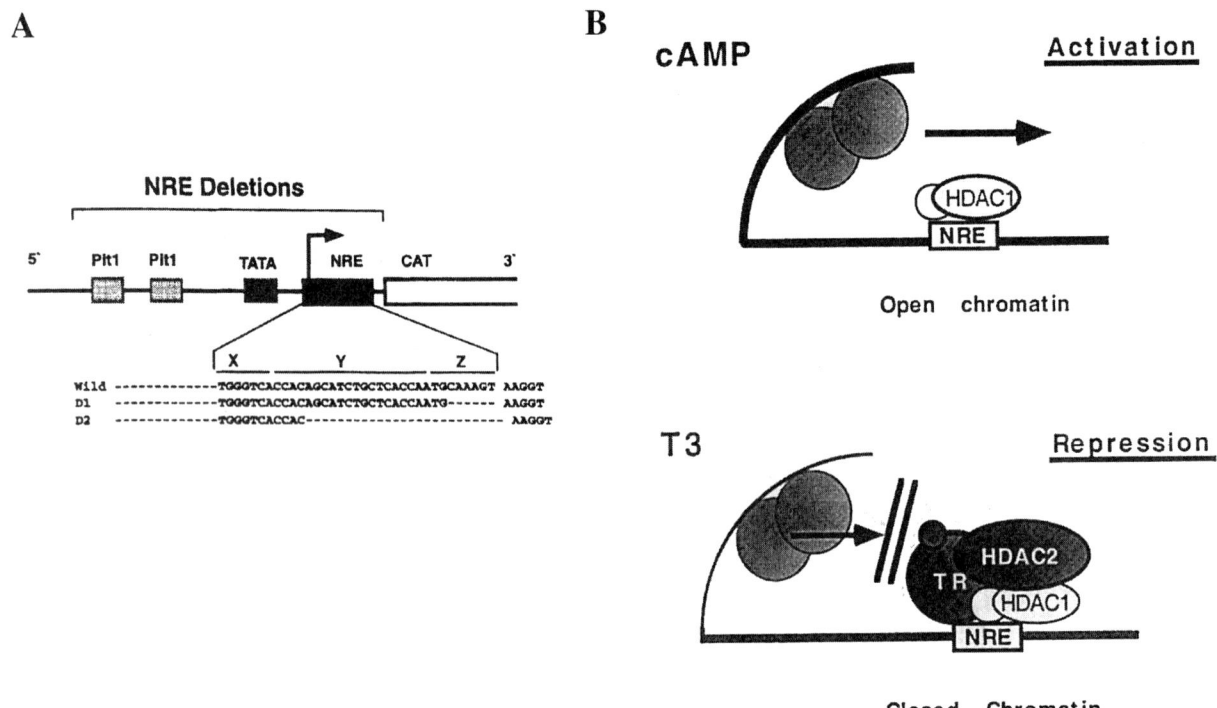

FIGURE 25 (A) Schematic structure of the TSHβ promoter showing the presence of the T_3 negative response element (NRE). (B) Model for T_3-mediated recruitment of histone deacetylase (HDAC) to the NRE in the TSHβ promoter. T_3 recruits the thyroid hormone receptor (TR) and HDAC2, resulting in closing of chromatin and transcriptional repression. (From Sasaki et al., 1999.)

(Shupnik et al., 1985). TSHα mRNA declines within 4 hr and TSHβ mRNA declines within 1 hr, and transcription rate within 1 hr and 30 min, respectively, of exposure to thyroid hormone. The effects of thyroid hormone are exerted directly on the TSHα and TSHβ genes as the inhibition of protein synthesis with cycloheximide does not prevent the inhibitory effects of thyroid hormone on the above responses (Shupnick et al., 1986).

The locus within the TSHβ gene that mediates the inhibitory effects of thyroid hormone (the negative thyroid hormone response element or NRE) is believed to reside downstream from the transcription start site of the TSHβ gene (Carr and Wong, 1994). This region contains a sequence, TGCAAAGT, that is conserved in the human, rat, and mouse TSHβ gene, as well as in the TSHα gene (Fig. 25A). When this region is deleted experimentally, it results in significantly less repression of the TSHβ gene by T_3 (Sasaki et al., 1999).

A mechanism whereby T_3 mediates repression of the TSHα gene has been proposed by Tagami et al. (1999) in which coactivators are competed away from the TSH promoter by T_3 bound to its receptor in the nucleoplasm, as discussed previously. However, an alternative mechanism by which T_3 could mediate repression of the TSHβ gene has been proposed by Sasaki et al. (1999). This model is depicted in Fig. 25B, in which T_3 induces recruitment of the histone deacetylase, HDAC2, and a TRβ monomer directly to the NRE of the TSHβ promoter. This results in repression of transcription by increasing the affinity of histones for DNA thereby reducing the accessibility of transcription factors to the promoter. Heterodimerization of TRβ to RXR is probably not necessary for T_3 repression of the TSHβ gene, as TRβ can bind to the NRE without RXR (Sasaki et al., 1999). Nevertheless, RXR may have an independent role in the regulation of TSHβ. RXR-selective retinoids have been shown to suppress TSHβ promoter activity through the −200 to −149 regions of the mouse and rat promoters (Haugen et al., 1997), a region distinct from the binding region for thyroid hormone receptors, and to suppress TSH secretion in human patients being treated with these agents for cutaneous T-cell lymphoma (Sherman et al., 1999). Since selective deficiency of RXRγ can replicate the central hyperthyroid state observed in vitamin A deficiency (Morley et al., 1978; Brown et al., 2000), and RXRγ is found exclusively in thyrotropes (Sugawra et al., 1995; Sanno et al., 1997), the RXRγ isoform may solely contribute to negative feedback regulation of RXR on the *TSHβ* gene.

Since both TRβ1 and TRβ2 are present in the anterior pituitary, until recently it was uncertain which of the isoforms (or both) contributes to the negative feedback effects of T_3 on TSH secretion. However, TRβ2 mRNA is more abundant than TRβ2 mRNA in the pituitary (Hodin, 1989), and mice with targeted disruption of the TRβ2 isoform have increased levels of TSHβ mRNA and only partial suppression of the *TSHβ* gene by thyroid hormone (Abel et al., 1999). Since TRβ1 is not affected in these TRβ2 knockout mice, these data would suggest a relatively unimportant role for TRβ1 in T_3 feedback regulation of the *TSHβ* gene and therefore that TRβ2 is the more potent negative regulator.

3. Regulation of TSH by TRH

While TSH secretion is regulated by feedback suppression of circulating thyroid hormone directly on anterior pituitary thyrotrophs, the hypothalamus serves an important function in determining the set point for thyroid hormone negative feedback on TSH secretion. The observations made in the 1930s by Houssay et al. (1935) and Cahane and Cahane (1936) that lesions in the hypothalamus can disrupt thyroid function were supported by a number of increasingly sophisticated studies over the next three decades showing that hypothalamic lesions reduce baseline levels of thyroid function and impair the TSH response to thyroid hormone deficiency (see Reichlin, 1966 for review). One of the most elegant demonstrations of this association was reported by Martin et al. in 1970 in which thyroidectomized rats with bilateral lesions in the PVN showed a considerably lower rise in TSH levels compared to intact animals, and a greater sensitivity in the suppression of plasma TSH to exogeneously administered thyroid hormone. It is now well recognized that TRH is the major hypothalamic peptide mediating control over the set point for anterior pituitary TSH secretion (see below), but it is also clear that other substances originating in the brain participate in the secretion of TSH either directly or by modulating the response of TSH to TRH.

4. TRH Receptor

TRH-induced secretion of TSH is primarily due to the activation of transcription of the *TSHβ* and *TSHα* genes after binding to a G-protein-coupled membrane receptor. Two TRH receptors have been cloned, TRH-R1 and TRH-R2, both members of the seven-transmembrane G-protein-coupled receptors (Straub et al., 1990; Matre et al., 1993; Itadani et al., 1998; Cao et al., 1998; Matre et al., 1999). Both receptors have similar binding affinities for TRH, which is thought to involve the third transmembrane helix (Perlman et al., 1994). However, in the pituitary, TRH-R1 is the predominant form (O'Dowd et al., 2000). Like the LHRH receptor, the TRH receptor is coupled to the pertussis toxin–insensitive G protein of the $G_{q/11}$ family (Hsieh and Martin, 1992). The binding of TRH to its receptors activates membrane-bound phospholipase C and hydrolysis of phosphatidylinositol 4,5-bisphosphate (PIP_2) to inositol 1,4,5-trisphosphate (IP_3) and diacylglycerol (DAG) (Gershengorn, 1989). These actions ultimately result in the phosphorylation or increased concentration of nuclear proteins that interact with the *TSHβ* and *TSHα* genes, and hence increase the transcription of these genes (Fig. 26). In addition, there is a biphasic increase in calcium, a transient increase due to the relase of Ca^{2+} from the endoplasmic reticulum, and a sustained Ca^{2+} elevation from increased influx through L-type calcium channels (Hinkle et al., 1996). The sex-related differences of TRH-induced TSH secretion in man (greater in females) may be due to stimulation of TRH receptor transcription by estrogen, thereby increasing binding sites for TRH (Kimura et al., 1994).

With continued stimulation of the TRH receptor by TRH, desensitization results, ultimately reducing the secretion of TSH. Desensitization is associated with the inability of TRH to stimulate IP_3 production (Yu and Hinkle, 1997) and depletion of intracellular Ca^{2+}, but the mechanism of TRH receptor uncoupling from the PIP_2 cascade is not known. Groarke et al. (1999) have proposed that TRH-induced TRH receptor down-regulation involves internalization of the TRH receptor from the cell membrane into clathrin-coated vessicles, mediated by β-arrestin. However, Yu and Hinkle (1998) have observed that desensitization can still occur without the TRH receptor undergoing endocytosis. Paradoxically, when thyroid hormone levels in the circulation fall and TRH increases in the portal capillary blood, there is an increase rather than a decrease in TRH receptors in the anterior pituitary (Yamada et al., 1992a), likely due to the overriding

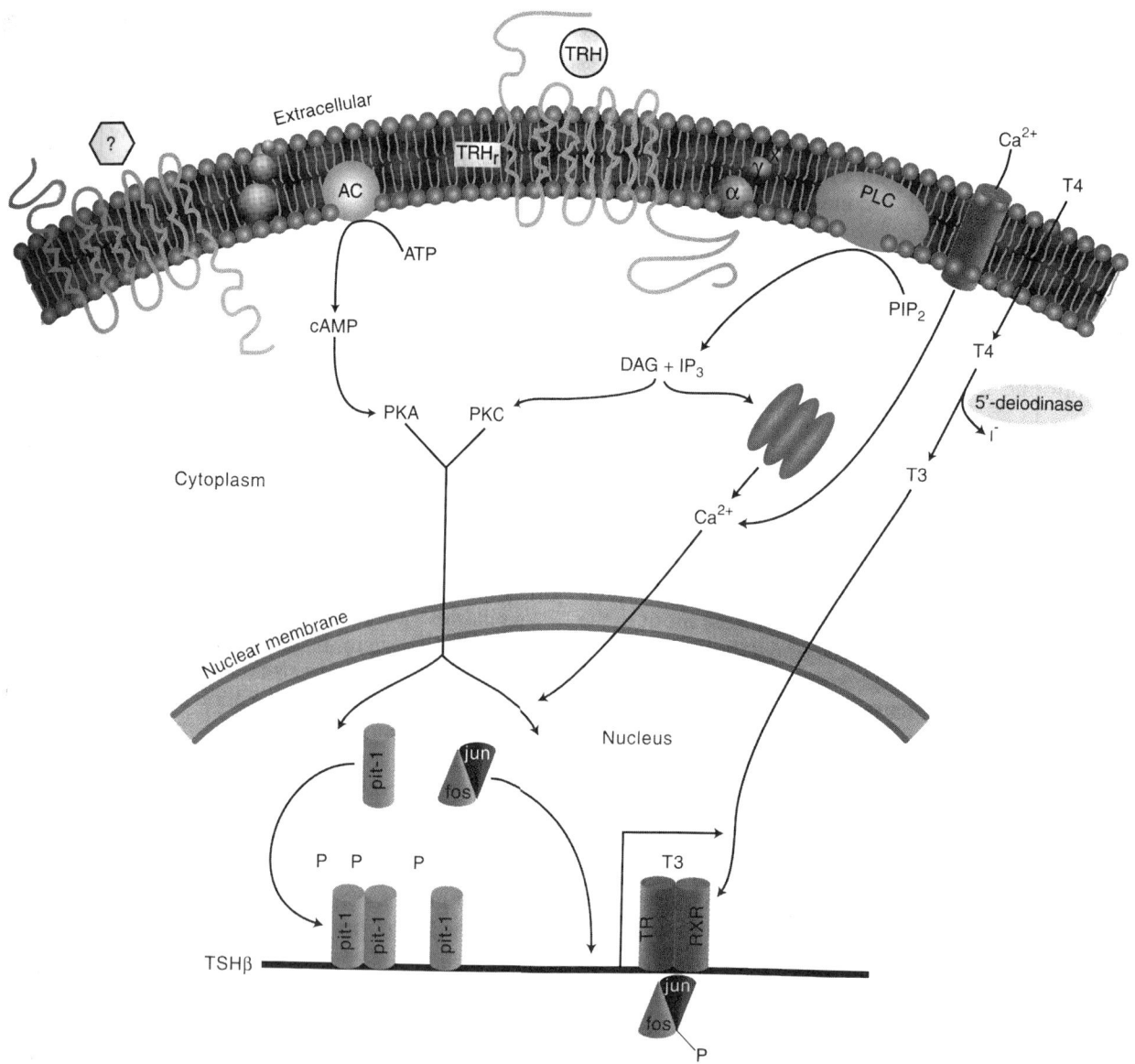

FIGURE 26 Simplified schema of the proposed regulation of TSHβ gene transcription by TRH and thyroid hormone. TRH activates PKC in the cytoplasm after binding to its receptor (TRHr) on the cell membrane. Protein kinase A (PKA) may also be activated by an unknown ligand. This results in phosphorylation of Pit-1 and AP-1 (fos-jun) in the nucleus, enhancing their binding to TRH-responsive regions in the TSHβ gene to activate the transcription of TSH. An increase in cytoplasmic free calcium (Ca^{2+}) also contributes to activation of the TSHβ gene but by unknown mechanism(s). Thyroid hormone is transported across the cell membrane, converted to T_3 in the cytoplasm by 5'-deiodinase, and then transported across the nuclear membrane. In the nucleus, T_3 binds to its receptor (TR). T_3 bound to its receptor may compete with AP-1 for binding to the same site in the TSHβ gene.

effects of T_3 deficiency on the stimulation of TRH receptor gene transcription. Conversely, excess T_3 reduces the concentration of TRH receptor mRNA in the anterior pituitary (Heuer et al., 1998), thereby contributing to the mechanism of T_3-induced suppression of TSH.

In the human TRH receptor gene, several response elements have been identified in its promoter region, including two GREs (one half site at −885 and one full site at −624), a CRE, and two sites for binding by the nuclear transcription factor Pit-1 (Matre et al., 1999). Gene expression of the TRH receptor after activation of the PIP$_2$ pathway is likely mediated *via* AP-1, a heterodimer of the protooncogene family jun and fos (Carr *et al.*, 1993; Kim *et al.*, 1993). Glucocorticoids have also been shown to increase TRH receptor expression as a result of increased transcription of the TRH receptor gene (Yang and Tashjian, 1993), with both GREs functioning in a cooperative manner (Hovring *et al.*, 1999).

5. Regulation of the TSHβ Subunit Gene by TRH

TRH and other substances that can activate the cAMP or PIP$_2$ signaling pathways, such as forskolin and phorbol esters, respectively, are important in stimulating the *TSHβ* gene (Shupnick *et al.*, 1990). One nuclear protein that appears to be critical in mediating this response is the pituitary-specific transcription factor Pit-1 (Steinfelder and Wondisford, 1997). Three Pit-1 binding sites have been identifed in the human *TSHβ* gene between −119 to −104, −104 to −89, and −73 to −58 from the transcriptional start site (Steinfelder *et al.*, 1991). By binding to the TSHβ promoter, Pit-1 can stimulate the transcription of TSH. This may involve phosphorylation of Pit-1 since the phosphorylated form of Pit-1 binds to the promoter of TSHβ better than the unphosphorylated form (Steinfelder *et al.*, 1992). Two of the Pit-1 binding sites, −119 to −104 and −73 to −58, may be particularly important as mutation of these sites results in 60 to 70% reduction in TSHβ expression by TRH and forskolin (Steinfelder *et al.*, 1992). Interaction of Pit-1 with thyrotrope-specific transcription factors, such as GATA-2, may be important in activating the *TSHβ* promoter (Gordon *et al.*, 1997).

In addition to the Pit-1 binding sites, a fourth TRH-responsive region located in the first exon of the human *TSHβ* gene (−1 to +6) overlaps with a DNA sequence that binds to the transcription factor AP-1 (Steinfelder *et al.*, 1991). Both protein kinase C and increased cytosolic calcium act in a coordinated fashion on AP-1 to mediate the effects of TRH by increasing the synthesis of c-jun and c-fos or increasing its affinity for binding to its target sequences. In addition, the action of AP-1 requires that Pit-1 be bound to its binding sites in the TSHβ promoter, suggesting coorporation between these two nuclear transcription factors to stimulate the TSHβ gene (Kim *et al.*, 1993). Of note is that the AP-1 binding site in the *TSH* gene overlaps with the region that binds thyroid hormone receptors (Fig. 24). The coincidence of these overlapping loci suggests a possible mechanism to explain feedback regulation of thyroid hormone on the secretion of TSH. Thus, TRH acting through AP-1 and T$_3$ acting through thyroid hormone receptors can compete for binding to a similar region in the *TSH* gene, thereby influencing the secretion of TSH (Wondisford *et al.*, 1993; Zhang *et al.*, 1991).

6. Regulation of TSHα Gene by TRH

The *TSHα* gene is coordinately regulated with the TSHβ gene but through different regulatory pathways. The *TSHα* gene contains consensus sequences for binding by the cAMP regulatory protein CREB, which mediates the stimulatory effects of cAMP (Deutsch *et al.*, 1987). TRH-responsive sites are also present in the *TSHα* gene but are separate from the CREB binding sites (Pennathur *et al.*, 1993). Therefore, how TRH induces α-gene transcription at these sites, is not yet understood.

7. Effect of TRH on Glycosylation of TSH

In addition to promoting the secretion of TSH, TRH also influences the final form of secreted TSH by altering the oligosaccharide content on both α and β subunits (Weintraub *et al.*, 1989; Grossmann *et al.*, 1997a). Primary hypothyroidism due to thyroidectomy, for example, is associated with the secretion of TSH that contains more complex oligosaccharides, partly due to the increased content of TRH in the portal system under these conditions (see above). This could result in conformational changes in TSH that enhance hormone action by a postreceptor mechanism. Thus, during hypothyroidism the glycosylation of TSH contributes to the mechanism of feedback regulation by thyroid hormone by providing a more potent biologically active TSH at the same time the secretion of TSH is increased. In contrast, hypothyroidism produced by a lesion in the hypothalamus that disrupts the TRH tuberoinfundibular pathway results in the secretion of TSH with more simplified carbohydrate structures and reduced bioactivity, but can be restored by the administration of TRH (Taylor and Weintraub, 1989).

8. TRH-Degrading Enzymes

The regulation of TSH secretion also depends on inactivation of TRH, mediated by a membrane-anchored peptidase, pyroglutamyl peptidase II, located on the surface of cells that has a high substrate specificity for TRH (Bauer, 1995). As a result of the latter property, this enzyme has also been termed TRH-degrading ectoenzyme. The rat TRH-degrading ectoenzyme is composed of 1025 amino acids and contains a 22-amino-acid transmembrane-spanning domain near the amino terminus and anchored intracellularly by an uncleaved signal sequence (Schauder et al., 1994). The large extracellular C-terminal domain contains 12 potential glycosylation sites and a consensus sequence, HEXXH, indicating that the enzyme is a zinc-dependent metallopeptidase. Comparison of the human TRH-degrading ectoenzyme to the rat reveals that it has been highly conserved, with 96% of the residues being identical (Schomburg et al., 1999).

TRH-degrading ectoenzyme is highly concentrated in the anterior pituitary and markedly increased by thyroid hormone (Bauer, 1987; Suen and Wilk, 1989; Heuer et al., 1998). Thus, increased TRH-degrading ectoenzyme works in concert with the TRH receptor, which is inversely regulated by thyroid hormone (see above), ultimately to reduce TSH secretion. Conversely, hypothyroidism is associated with a reduction in TRH-degrading ectoenzyme (Schomburg and Bauer, 1995), which may be partly due to low circulating thyroid hormone levels, but also due to increased secretion of TRH since the addition of TRH to anterior pituitary cultures reduces TRH-degrading ectoenzyme by nearly 50% of basal levels (Vargas et al., 1994).

9. Mechanism of Action of Other Hypothalamic Hormones on TSH Secretion

A number of hypothalamic substances released from axon terminals in the ME other than TRH could contribute to the regulation of TSH secretion (Morley, 1981). Of these, somatostatin and dopamine, both exerting inhibitory control over the secretion of TSH, have the most convincing effects of negative regulation of TSH secretion in man.

a) Somatostatin Somatostatin is a 14-amino-acid peptide that, like TRH, is carried to the anterior pituitary via the portal vascular system after being released from axon terminals in the external zone of the ME. The inhibitory effect of somatostatin on TSH secretion has been demonstrated experimentally both *in vitro* and *in vivo*, showing that somatostatin can inhibit TRH-induced TSH release and that antiserum to somatostatin can increase the secretion of TSH (Vale et al., 1975; Arimura and Schally, 1976). In man, the infusion of somatostatin into the bloodstream can reduce TRH-induced TSH secretion and abolish the nocturnal elevation in TSH (Legrand, 1979; Magner, 1990). In addition, growth hormone deficiency is associated with a greater than normal increase in TRH-induced TSH secretion, whereas the opposite effect is observed when there is growth hormone excess, likely due to the decreases and increases in somatostatin release, respectively. The mechanism of action of somatostatin on TSH secretion is presumably by reducing cAMP or free calcium accumulation in the cytoplasm, thereby interfering with the signal transduction pathways involved in stimulating the *TSHβ* and *TSHα* genes. However, whether there is a physiological role for endogenous somatostatin to regulate TSH secretion, is not known.

b) Dopamine In addition to local inhibitory actions of DA on TRH axon terminals in the median eminence, DA originating from a separate population of neurons in the arcuate nucleus (A12), just dorsal to the median eminence, is also conveyed to the anterior pituitary by the portal system where it inhibits TSH release. The action of DA is mediated by D_2 receptors on anterior pituitary thyrotropes as in man, a single dose of a selective D_2 antagonist, amisulpride, stimulates the release of TSH (Wetzel et al., 1994). Inhibitory effects of DA on TSH secretion, resulting from a reduction in cAMP in the cytoplasm, is even greater when thyroid hormone levels are low and TSH is elevated due to TSH-induced, increased numbers of D_2 receptors on anterior pituitary thyrotrophs (Foord et al., 1985).

c) Other Hypothalamic Substances Since the mechanism of action of TRH on TSH secretion is primarliy through the PIP_2 signaling pathway, it is not completely clear why the TSHβ promoter is so effectively stimulated by pharmacological substances that activate the cAMP signaling pathway, such as forskolin (Shupnick et al., 1990). This might suggest the presence of an endogenous mechanism other than TRH, originating in the hypothalamus, that can activate cAMP in thyrotrophs.

Potential candidates that increase TSH secretion and bind to G-protein-coupled receptors include vasopressin and neurotensin (Lumpkin *et al.*, 1983; Vijayan *et al.*, 1994). VIP and substance P also increase in the hypothyroid state but are probably involved in the regulation of prolactin and LH and not TSH secretion (Toni *et al.*, 1992; Toni and Lechan, 1993; Coiro *et al.*, 1995). Epinephrine and norepinephrine, while important in the regulation of TRH secretion in the hypothalamus, and with a TSH-stimulating action in rat and bovine anterior pituitary cultures (Scanlon *et al.*, 1980), probably do not have direct effects on anterior pituitary thyrotrophs in man (Al-Damluji and Francis, 1993).

An interesting possibility that deserves further study is that one or more processed forms of the TRH prohormone that are released simultaneously with TRH into the portal blood could activate the *TSHβ* gene through the cAMP signaling pathway. In the rat, prepro-TRH (160–169) potentiates the effect of TRH on TSH secretion, stimulates the *TSHβ* gene, and binds to a receptor presumed coupled to a pertussis toxin–sensitive G protein (Bulant *et al.*, 1990a; Carr *et al.*, 1993; Ladram *et al.*, 1994). The human preproTRH does not contain a homologous sequence to rat preproTRH (160–169) between the third and fourth progenitor sequences for TRH, but the potential biological activity of the spacer peptides in the human prohormone has not been investigated.

10. Paracrine/Autocrine Regulation of TSH

Regulation of anterior pituitary function via direct interactions between anterior pituitary cell types mediated by cell adhesion molecules and gap junctions and/or by secreted factors intrinsic to the pituitary is becoming increasingly apparent and has been recently reviewed by Denef (1994). In addition to the classic anterior pituitary hormones, the anterior pituitary also synthesizes a number of releasing hormones, neuropeptides, growth factors, cytokines, vasoactive peptides, and acetylcholine, which may contribute to the growth, differentiation, and secretion of the anterior pituitary. TRH, for example, is synthesized and secreted by somatotrophs (Bruhn *et al.*, 1994a) and gonadotrophs (Peters *et al.*, 1997), suggesting that TRH might contribute to the regulation of TSH secretion not only by release from the hypothalamus, but also by paracrine signaling after local release. This concept was demonstrated in experiments by Bruhn *et al.* (1998), in which the synthesis of TRH in anterior pituitary cultures was inhibited by the addition of the enzyme necessary for α-amidation of TRH (peptidyl-glycine α-amidating monooxygenase), resulting in the preferential release of the relatively biologically inactive TRH precursor, TRH-gly. As consequence, an approximately 40% reduction in basal TSH secretion from anterior pituitary cells in culture was observed, suggesting that TRH secreted by anterior pituitary cells exerts a tonic stimulatory effect on thyrotrophs. Conversely, the addition of dexamethasone to anterior pituitary cells in culture, which stimulates the release of intrinsic TRH (Bruhn *et al.*, 1994b), also increased TSH secretion (Bruhn *et al.*, 1998).

Equally as intriguing are data by Pazos-Moura *et al.* (1996) and Ortiga-Carvalho *et al.* (1995, 1996, 1997), showing that the bombesin-like peptide, neuromedin B, is synthesized exclusively in thyrotropes and inhibits the secretion of TSH. Neuromedin B is under the regulation of thyroid hormone such that during hypothyroidism the neuromedin B content in the anterior pituitary gland is reduced, and during hyperthyroidism it is increased (Ortiga-Carvalho *et al.*, 1996). Thus, neuromedin B may work in concert with thyroid hormones and be involved in the mechanism by which thyroid hormones regulate the secretion of TSH. Evidence for fasting-induced increase in neuromedin B concentration in the anterior pituitary has also been given (Ortiga-Carvalho *et al.*, 1997), raising the possibility that neuromedin B may contribute to the low circulating levels of TSH in fasting animals.

A molecular variant of prolactin produced by lactotrophs may also be a paracrine regulator or anterior pituitary thyrotropes. The cleaved form of prolactin (clPRL-1) between Tyr^{145} and Leu^{146} (Andries *et al.*, 1992) stimulates ^{3}H-thymidine incorporation into DNA of thyrotropes (Andries *et al.*, 1996) and therefore may act as a growth regulator for thyrotropes in the anterior pituitary. Finally, as noted previously, paracrine interaction between foliculostellate cells and thyrotropes may regulate TSH secretion and may be the mechanism by which preproTRH potentiates the action of TRH on TSH secretion (Allaerts *et al.*, 1990).

11. Pulsatility and Circadian Rhythm

TSH is secreted in a pulsatile manner with a frequency of one pulse every 90 to 180 min (or

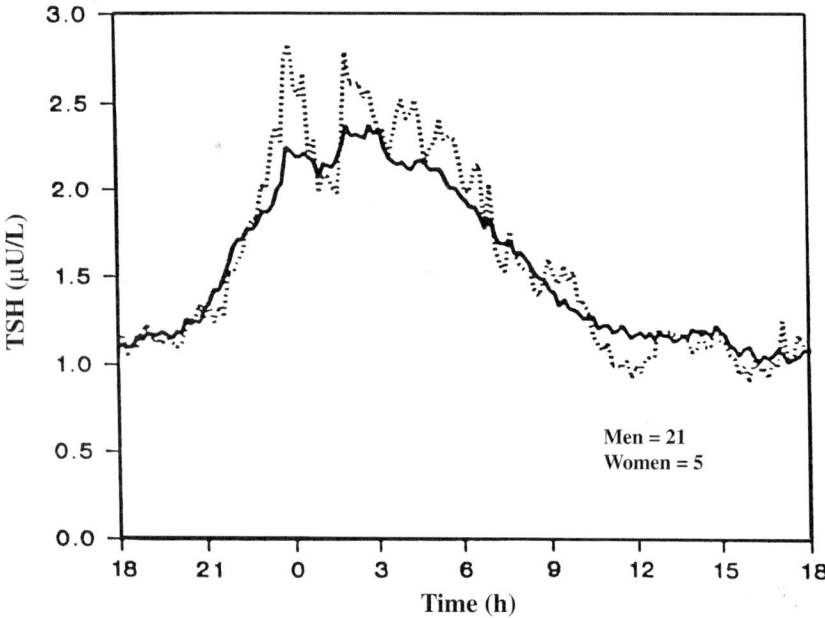

FIGURE 27 Mean TSH secretion in male (solid line) and female (broken line) subjects over 24 hr. (From Brabant et al., 1990.)

approximately 10 to 15 pulses/24 hr) in man (Brabant et al., 1990). The pulse frequency and amplitude tend to be greatest at night, but the pulse amplitude actually moves through three phases over a 24-hr period, including a rise during the evening until 4 AM, a decline until noon, and then a resting phase in the afternoon (Fig. 27). The evening rise in TSH is commonly referred to as the *nocturnal TSH surge*. Since the nocturnal surge begins 4 to 5 hr prior to sleep, sleep is not believed to be an important mechanism for induction of the TSH peak. In addition, sleep deprivation does not interefere with the circadian rhythmicity of TSH (Allan and Czeisler, 1994). In contrast, the endogenous rhythm of TSH can be phase shifted by exposure to bright light, indicating that as for other endogenous rhythmic functions controlled by the CNS, the suprachiasmatic nucleus, the major pacemaker in the hypothalamus, can influence the circadian timing of TSH secretion.

The mechanism responsible for the pulse frequency of TSH is probably the pulsatile secretion of hypothalamic TRH. Patients with large, destructive lesions of the hypothalamus have low TSH levels (central or tertiary hypothyroidism) without pulsations, which can be restored by the exogenous pulsatile administration of TRH (Brabant et al., 1990). The frequency of TRH pulsations from the hypothalamus are probably very rapid as a pulsatile TRH pattern can only be established in experimental animals if the release of TRH is sampled at 2-min intervals (Dahl et al., 1994). As noted for other neuroendocrine control systems, such as the hypothalamic-pituitary-gonadal axis, pulsatile secretion from the hypothalamus is essential for the biosynthesis and bioactivity of anterior pituitary hormones, and, in the case of TRH, its pulsatile secretion is necessary to stimulate the transcription of TSHβ subunit mRNA and influence the glycosylation of mature TSH (Haisenleder et al., 1992).

The mechanism for the nocturnal surge is less well understood. Clearly this also involves the hypothalamus since hypothalamic destruction abolishes the evening rise in TSH (Brabant et al., 1991). Intravenous infusion of somatostatin or DA can reduce the pulse amplitude (but not pulse frequency) of TSH in normal man (Brabant et al., 1991), raising the possibility that one or both of these hypothalamic substances are important in mediating the nocturnal rise. DA secretion from the hypothalamus, however, is greatest during the evening when TSH peaks (Scanlon et al., 1980), making it an unlikely candidate. The administration of naloxone, an opioid antagonist, also blunts the nocturnal surge (but not pulse frequency) in man, raising the possibility that endogenous opioids could influence the diurnal

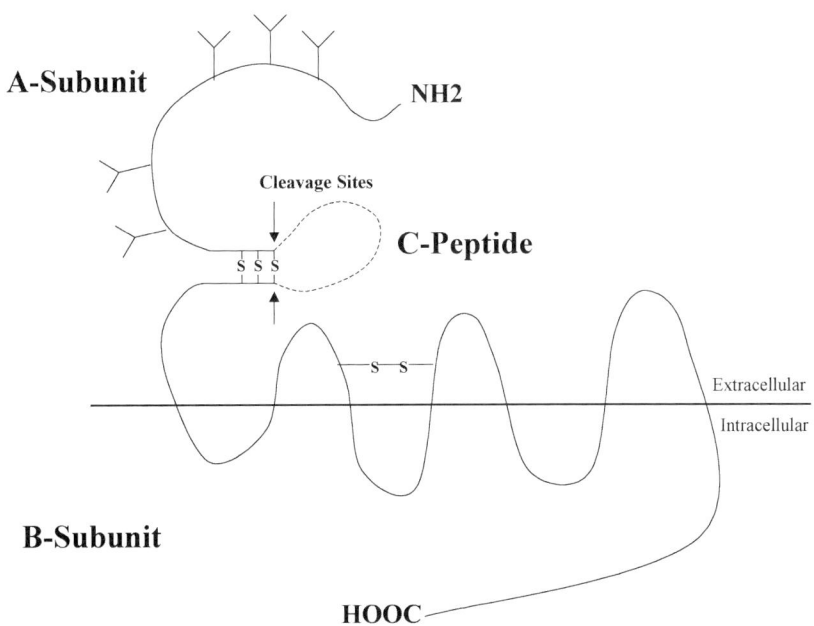

FIGURE 28 Schematic representation of the TSH receptor. (Adapted from Rapaport, 1998, with permission.)

variation of TSH (Samuels *et al.*, 1994). Finally, glucocorticoids can have a profound effect on the nocturnal surge of TSH by suppressing the pulse amplitude of TSH; this has been observed following the pharmacological administration of dexamethasone or in patients with Cushing's syndrome or depression in whom there is excessive secretion of cortisol from the adrenal glands (Bartalena *et al.*, 1991). Since glucocorticoids do not inhibit TSH β-subunit gene transcription, and in several studies the TSH response to exogeneously administered TRH is normal, the observed effects of glucocorticoids on TSH pulse amplitude may be due to direct hypothalamic effects. However, the parallel reduction in cortisol and TSH secretion during the morning between 8 AM and 12 noon, has raised doubt that cortisol is responsible for the circadian variation in TSH except under pharmacological or pathological circumstances (Adriaanse *et al.*, 1994).

I. Mechanism of Action of TSH on the Thyroid Gland

1. TSH Receptor

The TSH receptor is another member of the seven-transmembrane, G-protein-coupled receptors and closely related to other glycoprotein receptors, including the FSH, LH, and hCG receptors. Located on the long arm of chromosome 14, the TSH gene expands more than 60 kb and is composed of 10 exons. The first 9 exons encode the 398-amino-acid hyprophilic, amino-terminal extracellular domain that by posttranslational procesing can be glycosylated in six diffferent regions. The tenth exon encodes the entire carboxyl membrane-spanning segments and an intracellular tail (Nagayama and Rapoport, 1992; Vassart and Dumont, 1992).

The TSH receptor may exist in two forms, as a single-chain and/or as two subunits—subunit A and subunit B—linked by disulfide bonds (Fig. 28A). The subunits are formed by enzymatic cleavage at two separate sites of the extracellular domain and removal of a connecting peptide (C-peptide) (Chazenbalk *et al.*, 1997), analogous to the removal of the C-peptide from proinsulin to produce insulin. The importance of having two different forms of the TSH receptor that derive from the same mRNA is unclear, although evidence would suggest that both have a high affinity for TSH and are biologically active (Rapaport *et al.*, 1998).

The TSH binding sites are located in the enormous extracellular domain of the TSH receptor, although identification of the precise animo acid sequence(s) in contact with TSH has not been clearly identified. It was proposed by Rapaport *et al.* (1998) that the TSH binding site is highly conformational and that multiple discontinuous segments of the extracellular domain of the TSH receptor contribute to the TSH binding site. Observations that antibodies with thyroid-stimulating or thyroid-inhibiting activity in certain autoimmune diseases, such as Graves' disease (excess thyroid hormone secretion) and Hashimoto's thyroiditis (insufficient thyroid hormone secretion), respectively, bind to multiple regions of the extracellular domain of the TSH receptor (Nagayama *et al.*, 1991) would be consistent with the above proposal.

The transmembrane domain of the TSH receptor is important for regulation of G-protein interactions with the cAMP and PIP_2 signaling pathways. Mutations of the transmembrane domain of the TSH receptor in man have been associated with continuous activation of adenylate cyclase and thereby excessive secretion of thyroid hormone (Parma *et al.*, 1995). No one specific site in the transmembrane domain has been shown to induce constitutive activation of the TSH receptor, however, with more than 20 different mutations in practically all segments of the transmembrane being affected (Rapaport *et al.*, 1998). The C-terminal portion of the cytoplasmic tail can be removed without affecting receptor function (Vassart and Dumont, 1992). A two-state model of receptor activation has been proposed by Duprez *et al.* (1997) (Fig. 28B). In the unliganded state (TSH unbound to the receptor), the extracellular domain inhibits activation of the receptor. In the bound state, as a result of a conformational change in the extracellular domain of the receptor that may interfere with interactions between the intracellular and extracellular receptor domains, activation of the receptor takes place. The observations by Zhang *et al.* (2000) that truncation of the extracellular domain by 98% results in constitutive activation of the TSH receptor lends support to this hypothesis.

The 5' flanking region of the TSH receptor gene has been characterized by Ikuyama *et al.* (1992a). It contains cAMP- and cAMP-like response elements (CRE) and binding sites for several transcription factors (AP-1, AP-2, TTF-1, ETF), but does not have a TATA or CCAAT box. The CRE between -149 and -127 base pairs has been shown to act as a constitutive enhancer of TSH receptor promoter activity (Ikuyama *et al.*, 1992a). However, in cultures of the rat thyroid cell line FRTL5, TSH negatively regulates expression of its own receptor (Ikuyama *et al.*, 1992b), and this may be mediated by the second CRE upstream of the CRE (Ikuyama *et al.*, 1992a). Thyroid hormone also inhibits TSH receptor promoter activity, possibly via a TRE half-site contained between -139 and -130 (Saiardi *et al.*, 1994), thereby contributing to the overall regulation of thyroid hormone secretion during various states of thyroid function.

2. Regulation of Thyroid Follicular Cells by TSH

Binding of TSH to the TSH receptor activates two intracellular signaling pathways: the cAMP cascade and the PIP_2 cascade (Fig. 29). Practically all of the effects of TSH on thyroid follicular cells can be mediated through the cAMP cascade. However, in humans, the PIP2 cascade can also mediate several of the effects of TSH, although it requires concentrations of TSH 5 to 10 times higher than the cAMP cascade (Sho *et al.*, 1991). Included among the many actions of TSH after binding to the TSH receptor are active transport of iodide across the basolateral surface of the thyroid follicular cell via the sodium-iodine symporter, secretion of thyroglobulin into the lumen of thyroid follicles, oxidation of iodide at the apical surface of the follicular cell and its incorporation into tyrosyl residues mediated by thyroid peroxidase, endocytosis of formed thyroid hormones in the colloid, thyroid hormone secretion, and proliferation of follicular cells (Vassart and Dumont, 1992). Increased thyroglobulin induces pendrin mRNA (Royaux *et al.*, 2000), a second iodide transporter located in the apical membrane of follicular cells that allows translocation of iodide into the colloid. Activation of the PIP_2 pathway results in iodination of tyrosine residues and thus thyroid hormone synthesis, probably mediated through effects on H_2O_2 generation (Corvilain *et al.*, 1994).

3. Neural Regulation of the Thyroid Gland

It is well recognized that the peripheral nervous system, including autonomic motor and sensory branches, serves important physiological functions to modulate the secretory activity and blood supply of the thyroid gland. The thyroid gland, in fact, is richly innervated by both the sympathetic and parasympathetic, autonomic nervous system (Fig. 30). The sympathetic nerves derive from neuronal perikarya in the sympathetic

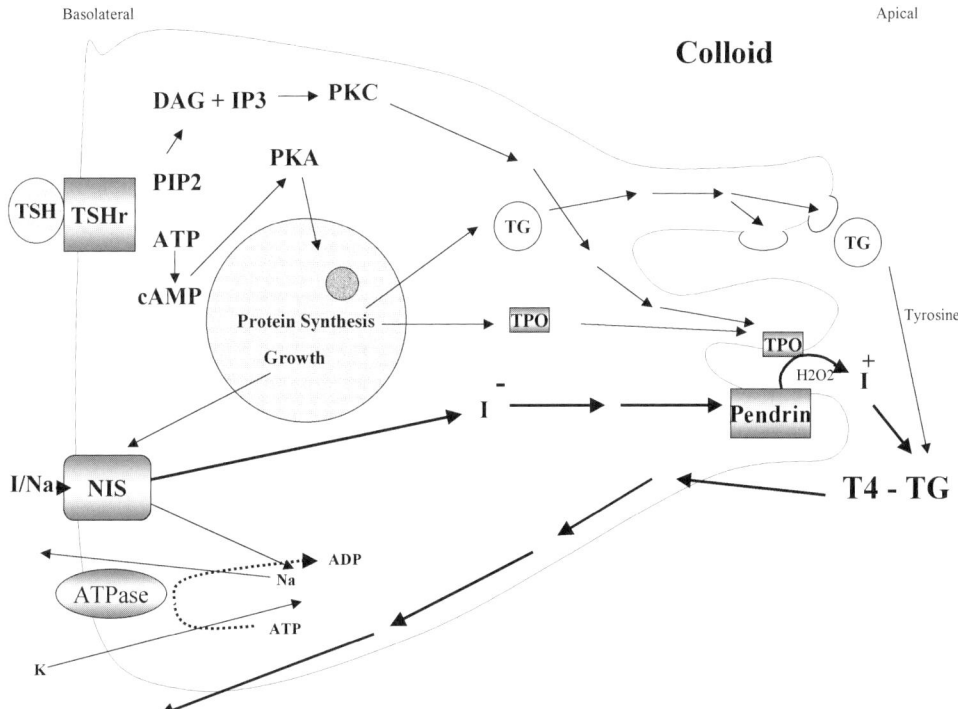

FIGURE 29 Schematic representation of a thyroid follicular cell showing the biosynthetic pathways involving iodine transport and thyroid hormone formation and secretion. H_2O_2, hydrogen peroxide; NIS, sodium-iodide symporter; TG, thyroglobulin; TPO, thyroperoxidase; TSH, thyroid-stimulating hormone; TSHr, thyroid stimulating hormone receptor. (Adopted from Spitzweg *et al.*, 2000, with permission.)

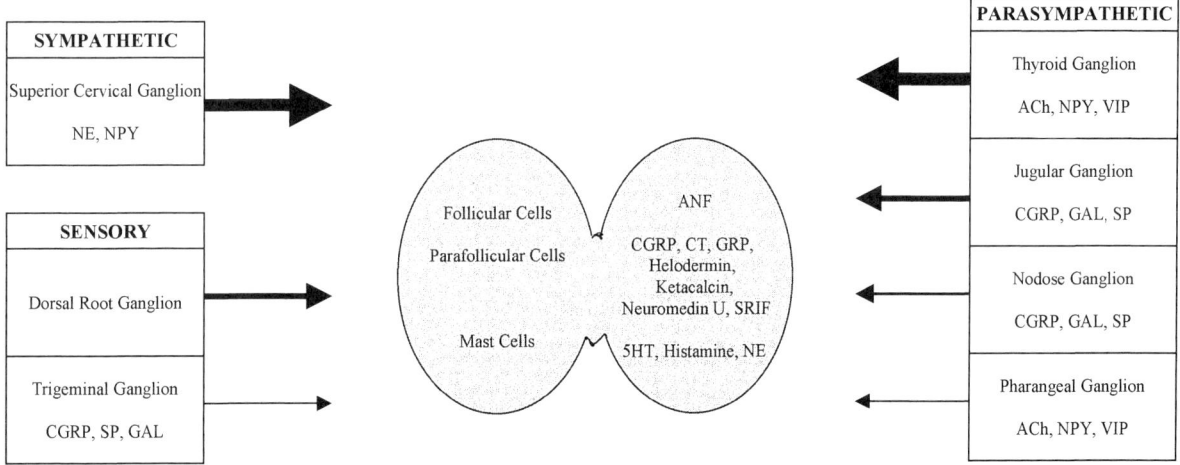

FIGURE 30 Schematic drawing summarizing the anatomical sources, principal neurotransmitters, and neuromediators intrinsic to the thyroid cells and contained in the thyroid nerves. Increasing thickness of arrows indicates increasing density of innervation. ACh, acetylcholine; ANF, atrial natriuretic factor; CGRP, calcitonin gene related peptide; CT, calcitonin; DA, dopamine; GAL, galanin; GRP, gastrin-releasing peptide; 5-HT, 5-hydroxytryptamine (serotonin); NE, norepinephrine; NPY, neuropeptide Y; SP, substance P; SRIF, somatostatin; VIP, vasoactive intestinal peptide. Arrow size reflects relative contribution of nerve fibers to the thyroid gland. (Adapted from Grunditz *et al.*, 1988.)

cervical ganglia, and reach the thyroid gland with the thyroid arteries and by joining the superior laryngeal nerve (Sodeberg, 1959). These fibers are vasomotor and secretomotor and contain noradrenaline and/or NPY (Grunditz et al., 1988). The parasympathetic nerve fibers emanate from neuronal perikarya located in ganglia juxtaposed and/or intrinsic to the thyroid gland (laryngeal and thyroid ganglia). These fibers are secretomotor and vasomotor and contain acetylcholine, VIP, and NPY (Grunditz et al., 1988). Separate contingent of sensory, parasympathetic fibers arise from neuronal perikarya in the jugular and nodose ganglia of the vagus nerve and reach the thyroid through the superior and inferior laryngeal nerves (Nonidetz, 1931; Harris and George, 1969). These fibers contain CGRP and/or susbstance P (SP) and/or galanin (Grunditz et al., 1988). Sensory fibers arise also from perikarya in the dorsal root ganglia of the cervical plexus (C2–C5) and in the trigeminal ganglion (Grunditz et al., 1988). They contain CGRP, SP, galanin (Grunditz et al., 1988), and Neurokinin A (Melander and Sundler, 1991). The autonomic fibers penetrate the thyroid parenchyma and terminate around follicular cells, separated only by the follicular basement membrane (Melander et al., 1975a), and in very close proximity to the walls of arterioles, capillaries, and, less frequently, venules (Melander and Sundler, 1991). This makes it likely that the released neurotransmitters may influence both thyroid hormone secretion and the thyroidal blood supply.

Autonomic fibers innervating the thyroid can be classified either vasomotor, secretomotor, or sensory. Vasomotor fibers of the sympathetic nervous system are involved in vasoconstriction of the thyroid arteries whereas parasympathetic nerves, primarily the laryngeal branches, elicit vasodilatation (Sodeberg, 1959; Harris and George, 1969). By altering thyroid blood flow and thus the presentation of TSH and iodine to thyroid follicular cells, the autonomic nervous system can modualte the secretion of thyroid hormone. The increase in the caliber of thyroid arteries and its blood flow during iodine deficiency (Michalkiewicz et al., 1989; Arntzenius et al., 1991) maximizes the delivery of iodine to the thyroid gland to allow synthesis of thyroid hormone and is believed to be mediated, at least in part, by the parasympathetic nervous system (Dey et al., 1993a). Secretomotor fibers of the sympathetic nervous system are involved in the accumulation of colloid droplets and presumably secretion of thyroid hormone from follicular cells since sympathectomy can reduce basal thyroid hormone secretion (Ahren, 1986). In contrast, vagotomy induces morphological changes that indicate increased secretory activity of the thyroid and are accompanied by increased levels of circulating T_3 (Ahren, 1986), suggesting an inhibitory effect on thyroid hormone secretion. However, some contradictory results indicate that stimulation of the parasympathetic nerves could also increase the release of ^{131}I-labeled hormones, a phenomenon presumably dependent on the presence of stimulators of thyroid hormone secretion in the parasympathetic fibers like VIP (Ahren, 1986). Whether this effect has physiological relevance and which conditions require such activation are not clear. The role of sensory fibers is presumed to be the mediation of sensory information from the thyroid parenchyma but virtually nothing is known about their physiological effects.

a) Adrenergic Regulation The presence of catecholamines in nerve terminals around follicular cells, arterioles, and capillaries was described more than 20 years ago by Melander et al. (1974) using fluorescence histochemistry, and it was found that these fibers are sympathetic (Melander et al., 1974, 1975b). A complex dual, opposite role has been proposed for noradrenaline on the thyroid. First, noradrenaline can stimulate basal thyroid hormone secretion by a cAMP-dependent mechanism after interacting with a β_2-adrenergic receptor (Ahren, 1986). However, noradrenaline may also inhibit TSH-induced thyroid hormone secretion via an α-adrenergic receptor (Ahren, 1986). Second, noradrenaline in high doses and injected systemically can have a direct effect on thyroid arteries and possibly thyroid veins by inducing vasoconstriction (Mawbray and Peart, 1960; Sodeberg, 1958). However, in low doses and injected locally into the thyroid arteries it may also induce vasodilatation (Mawbray and Peart, 1960). Other biogenic amines, including histamine, 5-HT, and DA, can also induce thyroid hormone secretion and vasodilatation of thyroid arterioles, but arise from mast cells and parafollicular C cells in the thyroid gland (Melander et al., 1975a) and may potentiate autonomic control by a paracrine mechanism (Melander and Sundler, 1991).

b) Cholinergic Regulation The follicular cells and thyroidal arterioles and capillaries are innervated by acetylcholinesterase-immunoreactive axon terminals (suggesting the presence of acetylcholine) originating from laryngeal branches of the vagus nerve (Grunditz *et al.*, 1988). Acetylcholine exerts an inhibitory effect on basal and TSH-dependent secretion of thyroid hormone (Ahren, 1986, 1991) through muscarinic receptors (Ahren, 1991) by increasing intracellular degradation of cAMP in thyroid follicular cells (Ahren, 1986). In addition, acetylcholine causes vasodilatation in the thyroid vessels (Sodeberg, 1959).

c) Peptidergic Regulation A number of peptides have been found in autonomic fibers innervating the thyroid gland, including NPY, VIP, PHI (which derives from the same precursor peptide as VIP), SP, CGRP, galanin, cholecistokinin, and neurokinin A (Melander and Sundler, 1991). Many other peptides are also present in the thyroid gland (e.g., atrial natriuretic factor, somatostain, ketacalcin, gastrin-releasing peptide, helodermin, neuromedin U, and a number of cytokines and growth factors) but arise from follicular cells, parafollicular C cells, resident monocytes, and other cells of mesenchymal origin (Ahren, 1991; Domin *et al.*, 1990).

4. Neuropeptide Y

NPY originates from noradrenaline-containing perikarya in the sympathetic cervical ganglia or from VIP-containing cell bodies in parasympathetic ganglia intrinsic to the thyroid (Grunditz *et al.*, 1988). NPY has a tonic, inhibitory role on thyroid blood flow by vasconstriction through a mechanism independent of noradrenaline (Michalkiewicz *et al.*, 1993; Dey *et al.*, 1993b). Whether this effect is mediated by NPY contained in sympathetic or parasympathetic fibers is not yet clear (Dey *et al.*, 1993c). As NPY can reverse the noradrenergic desensitization after prolonged sympathetic activity (Wahlestedt *et al.*, 1990), it has been suggested that this peptide might induce thyroidal vasoconstriction during stress (Dey *et al.*, 1993c). Similar to noradrenaline, a dual, opposite role has been proposed for NPY on thyroid function. NPY potentiates the noradrenaline-induced inhibition of TSH-stimulated release of thyroid hormone (Ahren, 1986, 1991), but it may also stimulate TSH-induced and VIP-induced release of thyroid hormone (Melander and Sundler, 1991; Grunditz *et al.*, 1984).

5. Vasoactive Intestinal Polypeptide/Peptide Histidine Isoleucine

VIP and PHI arise from perikarya in parasympathetic ganglia intrinsic to the thyroid gland and from sensory perikarya in the nodose ganglion (Grunditz *et al.*, 1988). VIP can induce the release of thyroid hormone from the thyroid gland, particularly under conditions of iodine deficiency (Pietrzyk *et al.*, 1992) through a cAMP-dependent mechanism (Ahren, 1986), and its action can be blocked by cholinergic antagonists (Ahren, 1986; Domin *et al.*, 1990), suggesting that VIP might be involved in the modulation of acetylcholine effects during parasympathetic neurotransmission. VIP is also a potent vasodilator in the thyroid (Huffman *et al.*, 1988a,b) and may increase thyroidal blood flow at doses that do not elicit any secretion of thyroid hormone (Huffman and Hedge, 1986). It has been suggested that this effect might favor thyroid hormone release in conditions of elevated thyroid activity, such as hyperthyroidism (Dey *et al.*, 1993a).

6. Other Peptides

CGRP, SP, and galanin are colocalized in unmyelinated fibers arising from sensory neurons of the C type in the jugular ganglion of the vagus nerve, the dorsal root ganglia of the cervical plexus (C2–C5), and the trigeminal ganglion (Grunditz *et al.*, 1988). Except for SP and CGRP, which have been shown to induce thyroid hormone secretion in the dog (Ahren, 1986) and enhance the secretory response to VIP (Melander and Sundler, 1991), there are no reported effects for the other peptides on thyroid hormone secretion and/or blood flow.

References

Abe, H., Chihara, K., Chiba, T., Shigeru, M., and Fujita, A. (1981). Effect of intraventricular injection of neurotensin and other various bioactive peptides on plasma immunoreactive somatostatin levels in rat hypophysial protal blood. *Endocrinology* **108**, 1939–1943.

Abe, M., Saito, M., Ikeda, H., and Shimazu, T. (1991). Increased neuropeptide Y content in the arcuato-paraventricular hypothalamic neuronal system in both insulin-dependent and non-insulin-dependent diabetic rats. *Brain Res.* **539**, 223–227.

Abe, T., Masayuki, K., Sakagami, H., Tokui, T., Nishio, T., Tanemoto, M., Nomura, H., Hebert, S. C., Matsuno, S., Kondo, H., and Yawo, H. (1998). Molecular characterization and tissue distrubition of a new organic anion transporter subtype (oatp3) that transports thyroid hormones and taurocholate and comparison with oatp2. *J. Biol. Chem.* **273**, 22395–22401.

Abel, E. D., Boers, M.-E., Pazos-Moura, C., Moura, E., Kaulbach, H., Zakaria, M., Lowell, B., Radovick, S., Liberman, M. C., and Wondisforn, F. (1999). Divergent roles for thyroid hormone receptor β isoforms in the endocrine axis and auditory system. *J. Clin. Invest.* **104**, 291–300.

Adriaanse, R., Brabant, G., Endert, E., and Wiersinga, W. M. (1994). Pulsatile thyrotropin secretion in patients with cushing's syndrome. *Metabolism* **43**, 782–786.

Adrian, T. E., Allen, J. M., Bloom, R. S., Ghatei, M. A., Rossor, M. N., Roberts, G. W., Crow, T. J., Tatemoto, K., and Polak, J. M. (1983). Neuropeptide Y distribution in human brain. *Nature* **306**, 584–586.

Agnati, L. F., Fuxe, K., Zoli, M., Zini, I., Harfstrand, A., Toffano, G., and Goldstein, M. (1988). Morphometrical and microdensitometrical studies on phenylethanolamine-N-methyltransferase- and neuropeptide Y-immunoreactive neurons in the rostral medulla oblongata of the adult and old male rat. *Neuroscience* **26**, 461–478.

Aguila, M. C., Marubayashi, U., and McCann, S. M. (1992). The effect of galanin and growth hormone-releasing factor and somatostatin release from median eminence fragments in vitro. *Neuroendocrinology* **56**, 889–894.

Ahren, B. (1986). Thyroid neuroendocrinology: Neural regulation of thyroid hormone secretion. *Endocr. Rev.* **7**, 149–155.

Ahren, B. (1991). Regulatory peptides in the thyroid gland—a review on their localization and funciton. *Acta Endocrinol.* **124**, 225–232.

Aizawa, T., and Greer, M. A. (1981). Delineation of the hypothalamic area controlling thyrotropin secretion in the rat. *Endocrinology* **109**, 1731–1738.

Aizawa, T., and Greer, M. A. (1982). The importance of the hypothalamic and retrochiasmatic area in the control of adrenocorticotropin and thyrotropin secretion. *Endocrinology* **110**, 1693–1699.

Al-Damluji, S., and Francis, D. (1993). Activation of central α1-adrenoceptors in humans stimulates secretion of prolactin and TSH, as well as ACTH. *Am. J. Physiol.* **264**, E208–E214.

Allaerts, W., Carmeliet, P., and Denef, C. (1990). New perspectives on the function of pituitary folliculo-stellate cells. *Mol. Cell. Endocrinol.* **71**, 73–81.

Allan, J. S., and Czeisler, C. A. (1994). Persistence of the circadian thyrotropin rhythm under constant conditions and after light-induced shifts of circadian phase. *J. Clin. Endocrinol. Metab.* **79**, 508–512.

Alland, L., Muhle, R., Hou, H. J., Potes, J., Chin, L., Schreiber-Agus, N., and DePinho, R. A. (1997). Role for N-CoR and histone deacetylase in sin3-mediated transcriptional repression. *Nature* **387**, 43–48.

Andersson, K. (1989). Involvement of D1 dopamine receptors in the control of TSH secretion in the male rat. *Acta Physiol. Scand.* **135**, 449–457.

Andersson, K., Eneroth, P., and Ross, P. (1985). Effects of TRH and a rat TSH preparation on discrete hypothalamic and forebrain catecholamine nerve terminal networks in the hypophysectomized male rat. *Eur. J. Pharmacol.* **111**, 295–307.

Andersson, K., and Eneroth, P. (1987). Thyroidectomy and central catecholamine neurons in the male rat. Evidence for the existence of an inhibitory dopaminergic mechanism in the external layer of the median eeminence and for a facilitatory noradrenergic mechanism in the paraventricular hypothalamic nucleus regulating TSH secretion. *Neuroendocrinology* **45**, 14–27.

Andries, M., Tilemans, D., and Denef, C. (1992). Isolation of cleaved prolactin variants that stimulate DNA synthesis in specific cell types in rat pituitary cell aggregates in culture. *Biochem. J.* **281**, 393–400.

Andries, M., Jacobs, G. F., Tilemans, D., and Denef, C. (1996). In vitro immunoneutralization of a cleaved prolactin variant: Evidence for a local paracrine action of cleaved prolactin in the development of gonadotrophs and thyrotrophs in rat pituitary. *J. Neuroendocrinol.* **8**, 123–127.

Angeletti, R. H., Novikoff, P. M., Juvvadi, S. R., Fritschy, J.-M., Meier, P. J., and Wolkoff, A. W. (1997). The choroid plexus epithelium is the site of the organic anion transport protein in the brain. *Proc. Natl. Acad. Sci. U.S.A.* **94**, 283–286.

Annunziato, L., DiRenzo, G., Lombardi, G., Scopacasa, F., Schettini, G., Preziosi, P., and Scapagnini, U. (1977). The role of central noradrenergic neurons in the control of thyrotropin secretion in the rat. *Endocrinology* **100**, 738–744.

Annunziato, L., DiRenzo, G. F., Schettini, G., Lombardi, G., Scopacasa, F., Scapagini, U., and Preziosi, P. (1979). Lack of evidence for an inhibitory role played by tuberoinfundibular dopaminergic neurons on TSH secretionin the rat. *Neuroendocrinolgy* **28**, 435–441.

Antoni, F. A., Palkovitz, M., Makara, G. B., Linton, E. A., Lowry, P. J., and Kiss J. Z. (1983). Immunoreactive corticotropin-releasing hormone in the hypothalamoinfundibular tract. *Neuroendocrinology* **36**, 415–423.

Arancibia, S., Tapic-Arancibia, L., Assenmacher, I., and Astier, H. (1983). Direct evidence of short-term cold-induced TRH release in the median eminence of unanesthetized rats. *Neuroendocrinology* **37**, 225–228.

Arancibia, S., Tapia-Arancibia, L., Roussel, J. P., Assenmacher, I., and Astier, H. (1986). Effect of morphine on cold-induced TRH release from the median eminence of anaesthetized rats. *Life Sci.* **38**, 59–66.

Arancibia, S., Tapia-Arancibia, L., Astier, H., and Assenmacher, I. (1989). Physiological evidence for alpha1-adrenergic facilitatory control of the cold-induced TRH release in the rat, obtained by push–pull cannulation of the median eminence. *Neurosci. Lett.* **100**, 169–174.

Arancibia, S., Rage, F., Astier, H., and Tapia-Arancibia, L. (1996). Neuroendocrine and autonomous mechanisms underlying thermoregulation in cold environment. *Neuroendocrinology* **64**, 257–267.

Arimura, A., and Schally, A. V. (1976). Increase in basal and thyrotropin-releasing hormone (TRH)-stimulated secretion of thyrotropin (TSH) by passive immunization with antiserum to somatostatin in rats. *Endocrinology* **98**, 1069–1072.

Arntzenius, A. B., Smit, L. J., Schipper, J., Heide, D., and van der, Meinders, A. E. (1991). Inverse relation between iodine intake and thyroid blood flow: Color doppler flow imaging in euthyroid humans. *J. Clin. Endocrinol. Metab.* **73**, 1051–1055.

Awad, T. A., Bigler, J., Ulmer, J. E., Hu, Y. J., Moore, J. M., Lutz, M., Neiman, P. E., Collins, S. J., Renkawitz, R., Lobanenkov, V. V., and Filippova, G. N. (1999). Negative transcriptional regulation mediated by thyroid hormone response element 144 requires binding of the multivalent factor CTCF to a novel target DNA sequence. *J. Biol. Chem.* **274**, 27092–27098.

Bai, F. L., Yamano, M., Shiotani, Y., Emson, P. C., Smith, A. D., Powell, J. F., and Tohyama, M. (1985). An arcuato-paraventricular and dorsomedial hypothalamic neuropeptide Y-containing system which lacks noradrenaline in the rat. *Brain Res.* **331**, 172–175.

Baker, B. L., and Jaffe, R. B. (1974). The genesis of cell types in the adenohypophysis of the human fetus as observed with immunocytochemistry. *Am. J. Anat.* **143**, 137–161.

Bardrum, B., Ottensen, B., Fahrenkrug, J., and Fuchs, A.-R. (1988). Release of oxytocin and vasopressin by intracerebroventricular vasoactive intestinal polypeptide. *Enodcrinology* **123**, 2249–2254.

Bartalena, L., Martino, E., Petrini, L., Velluzzi, F., Loviselli, A., Grasso, L., Mammoli, C., and Pinchera, A. (1991). The nocturnal serum thyrotropin surge is abolished in patients with adrenocorticotropin (ACTH)-dependent or ACTH-independent Cushing's syndrome. *J. Clin. Endocrinol. Metab.* **72**, 1195–1199.

Bates, J. M., St. Germain, D. L., and Galton, V. A. (1999). Expression profiles of the three iodothyronine deiodinases, D_1, D_2, and D_3, in the developing brain. *Endocrinology* **140**, 844–851.

Bauer, K. (1987). Adenohypophyseal degradation of thyrotropin-releasing hormone regulated by thyroid hormones. *Nature* **330**, 375–377.

Bauer, K. (1995). Inactivation of thyrotropin-releasing hormone (TRH) by hormonally regulated TRH-degrading ectoenzyme. *Trends Endocrinol. Metab.* **6**, 101–105.

Beaulieu, E., Demeule, M., Ghitescu, L., and Beliveau, R. (1997). P-glycoprotein is strongly expressed in the luminal membranes of the endothelium of blood vessels in the brain. *Biochem. J.* **326**, 539–544.

Beck, B., Jhanwar-Uniyal, M., Burlet, A., Chapleur-Chateau, M., Leibowitz, S. F., and Burlet, C. (1990). Rapid and localized alterations of neuropeptide Y in discrete hypothalamic nuclei with feeding status. *Brain Res.* **528**, 245–249.

Belchetz, P. E., Gredley, G., Bird, D., and Himsworth, R. L. (1978). Regulation of thyrotrophin secretion by negative feedback of tri-iodothyronine on the hypothalamus. *J. Endocr.* **76**, 439–448.

Bennett, G. W., and Keeling, M. (1981). H2-mediated histamine-induced release of thyrotropin releasing hormone (TRH) from hypothalamic synaptosomes: A neuroendocrine role for histamine. *Br. J. Pharmacol.* **72**, 151P–152P.

Benvenga, S., Cahnmann, H. J., Gregg, R. E., and Robbins, J. (1989). Characterization of the binding of thyroxine to high-density lipoproteins and apolipoproteins A–I. *J. Clin. Endocrinol. Metab.* **68**, 1067–1072.

Bernardis, L. L., and Bellinger, L. L. (1987). The dorsomedial hypothalamic nucleus revisited: 1986 update. *Brain Res. Rev.* **12**, 321–381.

Berry, M. J., Banu, L., and Larsen, P. R. (1991). Type I iodothyronine is a selenocysteine-containing enzyme. *Nature* **349**, 438–440.

Bjorklund, A., and Lindvall, O. (1984). Dopamine-containing systems in the CNS. *In* "Handbook of Chemical Neuroanatomy. Classical Transmitters in the CNS" (A. Bjorklund and Hokfelt, eds.), Vol. 2, Part 1, pp. 55–122. Elsevier, Amsterdam.

Bjorklund, A., and Lindvall, O. (1986). Catecholaminergic brain stem regulatory systems. *In* "Handbook of Physiology, The Nervous System, Section I: Neurophysiology" (V. B. Mountcastle, F. E. Bloom, and S. R. Geiger, eds.), Vol. 4, pp. 155–235. American Physiological Society, Bethesda, Maryland.

Blake, C. C. F., Geisow, M. J., and Swan, I. D. A. (1974). Structure of human plasma prealbumin at 2.4 Å resolution. A preliminary report on the polypeptide chain conformation, quaternary structure and thyroxine binding. *J. Mol. Biol.* **88**, 1–12.

Blake, N. G., Eckland, D. J., Goster, O. J., and Lightman, S. L. (1991). Inhibition of hypothalamic thyrotropin-releasing hormone messenger ribonucleic acid during food deprivation. *Endocrinology* **129**, 2714–2718.

Borson-Chazot, F., Jordan, D., Fèvre-Montange, M., Kopp, N., Tourniaire, J., Rouzioux, J. M., Veisseire, M., and Mornex, R. (1986). TRH and LH-RH distribution in discrete nuclei of the human hypothalamus: Evidence for a left predominance of TRH. *Brain Res.* **382**, 433–436.

Brabant, G., Prank, K., Ranft, U., Schuermeyer, T. H., Wagner, T. O. F., Hauser, H., Kummer, B., Feistner, H., Hesch, R. D., and von zur, Muhlen, A. (1990). Physiological regulation of circadian and pulsatile thyrotropin secretion in normal man and woman. *J. Clin. Endocrinol. Metab.* **70**, 403–409.

Brabant, G., Prank, K., Hoang-Vu, C., Hesch, R. D., and von zur Muhlen, A. (1991). Hypothalamic regulation of pulsatile thyrotropin secretion. *J. Clin. Endocrinol. Metab.* **72**, 145–150.

Bradbury, A. F., Finnie, M. D. A., and Smythe, D. G. (1982). Mechanism of C-terminal amide formation by pituitary enzymes. *Nature* **298**, 686–688.

Bradley, D. J., Towle, H. C., and Young III, W. S. (1992). Spatial and temporal expression of α and β-thyroid hormone receptor mRNAs, inlcuding the β2-subtype, in the developing mammalian nervous system. *J. Neurosci.* **12**, 2288–2302.

Breder, C. D., Dinarello, C. A., and Saper, C. B. (1988). Interleukin-1 immunoreactive innervation of the human hypothalamus, *Science* **240**, 321–324.

Brent, G. A. (1994). The molecular basis of thyroid hormone action. *N. Engl. J. Med.* **331**, 847–853.

Broberger, C. (1999). Hypothalamic cocaine- and amephtamine-regulated transcript (CART) neurons: Histochemical relationship to thyrotropin-releasing hormone, melanin-concentrating hormone, orexin/hypocretin and neuropeptide Y. *Brain Res.* **848**, 101–113.

Broberger, C., Johansen, J., Johansson, C., Schalling, M., and Hokfelt, T. (1988). The neuropeptide Y/agouti gene-related protein (AGRP) brain circuitry in normal, anorectic, and monosodium glutamate-treated mice. *Proc. Natl. Acad. Sci. U.S.A.* **95**, 15043–15048.

Brown, N. S., Smart, A., Sharma, V., Brinkmeier, M. L., Greenlee, L., Camper, S. A., Jensen, D. R., Eckel, R. H., Krezel, W., Chambon, P., and Haugen, B. R. (2000). Thyroid hormone resistance and increased metabolic rate in the RXR-γ-deficient mouse. *J. Clin. Invest.* **106**, 73–79.

Brownstein, M. J., Eskay, R. L., and Palkovits, M. (1982). Thyrotropin releasing hormone in the median eminence is in processes of paraventricular nucleus neurons. *Neuropeptides* **2**, 197–201.

Bruhn, T. O., Talpin, J. H., and Jackson, I. M. D. (1991). Hypothyroidism reduces content and increases in vitro release of pro-thyrotropin-releasing hormone peptides from the median eminence. *Neuroendocrinology* **53**, 511–515.

Bruhn, T. O., Bolduc, T. G., Rondeel, J. M. M., and Jackson, I. M. M. (1994a). Thyrotropin-releasing hormone (TRH) gene expression in the anterior pituitary. I. Presence of pro-TRH messenger ribonucleic acid and Pro-TRH-derived peptides in a subpopulation of somatortophs. *Endocrinology* **134**, 815–820.

Bruhn, T. O., Bolduc, T. G., Rondeel, J. M. M., and Jackson, I. M. D. (1994b). TRH gene expression in the anterior pituitary. II. Stimulation by glucocorticoids. *Endocrinology* **134**, 821–825.

Bruhn, T. O., Rondeel, J. M., and Jackson, I. M. (1998). Thyrotropin-releasing hormone gene expression in the anterior pituitary. IV. Evidence for paracrine and autocrine regulation. *Endocrinology* **139**, 3416–3412.

Bulant, M., Delfour, A., Vaudry, H., and Nicholas, P. (1988). Processing of thyrotropin-releasing hormone prohormone (pro-TRH) generates pro-TRH-connecting peptides. *J. Biol. Chem.* **263**, 17189–17196.

Bulant, M., Roussel, J.-P., Astier, H., Nicholas, P., and Vaudry, H. (1990a). Processing of thyrotropin-releasing hormone prohormone (pro-TRH) generates a biologically active peptide, prepro-TRH-(160-169), which regulates TRH-induced thyrotropin secretion. *Proc. Natl. Acad. Sci. U.S.A.* **87**, 4439–4443.

Bulant, M., Beauvillain, J. C., Delfourm, A., Vaudry, H., and Nicolas, P. (1990b). Processing of thyrotropin-releasing hormone (TRH) prohormone in the rat olfactory bulb generates novel TRH-related peptides. *Endocrinology* **127**, 1978–1985.

Bulant, M., Richter, K., Kuchler, K., and Kreil, G. (1992a). A cDNA from brain of *Xenopus laevis* coding for a new precursor of thyrotropin-releasing hormone. *FEBS Lett.* **296**, 292–296.

Bulant, M., Ladram, A., Montagne, J. J., Delfour, A., and Nicholas, P. (1992b). Isolation and amino acid sequence of the TRH-potentiating peptide from bovine hypothalamus. *Biochem. Biophys. Res. Commun.* **189**, 1110–1118.

Burmeister, L. A., Pachucki, J., and St. Germain, D. L. (1997). Thyroid hormones inhibit type 2 iodothyronine deiodinase in the rat cerebral cortex by both pre- and posttranslational mechanisms. *Endocrinology* **138**, 5231–5237.

Cahane, M., and Cahane, T. (1936). Sur certaine modifications des glands endocrine apres une lesion diencephalique. *Revue Francaise Endocrinologie* **14**, 472–487.

Calza, L., Giardino, L., Battistini, N., Zanni, M., Galetti, S., Protopapa, F., and Velardo, A. (1989). Increase of neuropeptide Y-like immunoreactivity in the paraventricular nucleus of fasting rats. *Neurosci. Lett.* **104**, 99–104.

Cao, J., O'Donnell, D., Vu, H., Payza, K., Pou, C., Godbout, C., Jakob, A., Pelletier, M., Membo, P., Ahmad, S., and Walker, P. (1998). Cloning and characterization of a cDNA encoding a novel subtype of rat thyrotropin-releasing hormone receptor. *J. Biol. Chem.* **273**, 32281–32287.

Carr, F. E., and Wong, N. C. W. (1994). Characteristics of a negative thyroid hormone response element. *J. Biol. Chem.* **269**, 4175–4179.

Carr, F. E., Fisher, C. U., Fein, H. G., and Smallridge, R. C. (1993). Thyrotropin-releasing hormone stimulates c-jun and c-fos messenger ribonucleic acid levels: Implications for calcium mobilization and protein kinase-C activation. *Endocrinology* **133**, 1700–1707.

Cavalieri, R. P., Gavin, L. A., Cole, R., and DeVellis, J. (1986). Thyroid hormone deiodinases in purified primary glial cell cultures. *Brain Res.* **364**, 382–385.

Ceccatelli, S., Eriksson, M., and Hokfelt, T. (1989). Distribution and coexistence of corticotropin-releasing factor-, neurotensin-, enkephalin-, cholecystokinin-, galinin-, and vasoactive intestinal polypeptide histidine isoleucine-like peptides in the parvocellular part of the paraventricular nucleus. *Neuroendocrinology* **49**, 309–322.

Ceccatelli, S., Fahrenkrug, J., Villar, M. J., and Hokfelt, T. (1991). Vasoactive intestinal polypeptide/peptide histidine isoleucine immunoreactive neuron systems in the basal hypothalamus of the rat with special reference to the portal vasculature: An immunohistochemical and in situ hybridization study. *Neuroscience* **4**, 483–502.

Chang, K. H., Chen, Y. M., Chen, T. T., Chou, W. H., Chen, P. L., Ma, Y. Y., Yang-Feng, T. L., Leng, X. H., Tsai, M.-J., O'Malley, V. W., and Lee, W. H. (1997). A thyroid hormone receptor coactivator negatively regulated by the retinoblastoma protein. *Proc. Natl. Acad. Sci. U.S.A.* **94**, 9040–9045.

Chanoine, J.-P., Alex, S., Fang, S. L., Stone, S., Leonard, J. L., Korhle, J., and Braverman, L. E. (1992). Role of transthyretin in the transport of thyroxine from the blood to the choroid plexus, the cerebrospinal fluid, and the brain. *Endocrinology* **130**, 933–938.

Chantoux, F., Blondeau, J.-P., and Francon, J. (1995). Characterization of the thyroid hormone transport system of cerebrocortical rat neurons in primary culture. *J. Neurochem.* **65**, 2549–2554.

Charli, J.-L., Joseph-Bravo, P., Palacios, J. M., and Kordon, C. (1978). Histamine-induced release of thyrotropin releasing hormone from hypothalamic slices. *Eur. J. Pharmacol.* **52**, 401–403.

Chazenbalk, G. D., Tanaka, K., Nagayama, Y., Kakinuma, A., Jaume, J. C. X., McLachlan, S. M., and Rapaport, B. (1997). Evidence that the thyrotropin receptor ectodomain contains not one, but two, cleavage sites. *Endocrinology* **138**, 2893–2899.

Chen, H. J., and Meites, J. (1975). Effects of biogenic amines and TRH on release of prolactin and TSH in the rat. *Endocrinology* **96**, 10–14.

Chen, H. J., and Walfish, P. G. (1979). Effect of age and testicular function on the pituitary–thyroid axis in male rats. *J. Endocrinol.* **82**, 53–59.

Chen, J. D., and Evans, R. M. (1995). A transcriptional corepressor that interacts with nuclear hormone receptors. *Nature* **377**, 454–457.

Chen, Y. F., and Ramirez, V. D. (1981). Serotonin stimulates thyrotropin-releasing hormone release from superfused rat hypothalami. *Endocrinology* **108**, 2359–2366.

Cheng, S.-Y., Maxfield, F. R., Robbins, J., Willingham, M. C., and Pastan, I. H. (1980). Receptor-mediated uptake of 3,3',5-triiodo-L-thyroxine by cultured fibroblasts. *Proc. Natl. Acad. Sci. U.S.A.* **77**, 3425–3426.

Chihara, K., Arimura, A., and Shally, A. V. (1979). Effect of intraventricular injection of dopamine, norepinephrine, acetylcholine and 5-hydroxytryptamine on immunoreactive somatostatin release into rat hypophyseal portal blood. *Endocrinology* **104**, 1656–1662.

Chin, W. W. (1992). Current concepts of thyroid hormone action: Progress notes for the clinician. *Thyroid Today* **15**(No. 3), 1–9.

Chin, W. W., Shupnik, M. A., Ross, D. S., Habener, J. F., and Ridgway, E. C. (1985). Regulation of the α and thyrotropin β-subunit messenger ribonucleic acids by thyroid hormones. *Endocrinology* **116**, 873–878.

Ching, J. L., Christofides, N. D., Anaud, P., Gibson, S. J., Allen, Y. S., Su, H. C., Tatemoto, K., Morrison, J. F. B., Polak, J. M., and Bloom, S. R. (1985). Distribution of galanin immunoreactivity in the central nervous system and the responses of galanin-containing neuronal pathways to injury. *Neuroscience* **16**, 343–354.

Choi, S., and Dallman, M. F. (1999). Hypothalamic obesity: Multiple routs mediate by loss of function of medial cell groups. *Endocrinology* **140**, 4081–4088.

Choi, S., Sparks, R., Caly, M., and Dallman, M. F. (1999). Rats with hypothalamic obesity are insensitive to central leptin injections. *Endocrinology* **140**, 4426–4433.

Chopra, I. J., Huang, T. S., Hurd, R. E., and Solomon, D. H. (1984). Effects of 3,5,3'-triiodothyronine-induced hyperthyroidism on iodothyronine metabolism in the rat: Evidence for tissue differences in metabolic responses. *Endocrinology* **114**, 1454–1459.

Choy, V. J., and Watkins, W. B. (1977). Immunohistochemical localization of thyrotropin-releasing factor in the rat median emenence. *Cell Tissue Res.* **177**, 371–374.

Christianson, D., Roti, E., Vagenakis, A. G., and Braverman, L. E. (1981). The sex-related difference in serum thyrotropin concentration is androgen mediated. *Endocrinology* **198**, 529–535.

Chua, S. C., Jr., Leibel, R. L., and Hirsch, J. (1991). Food deprivation and age modulate neuropeptide gene expression in the murine hypothalamus and adrenal gland. *Brain Res. Mol. Brain Res.* **9**, 95–101.

Cihlar, T., Lin, D. C., Pritchard, J. B., Ruller, M. D., Mendel, D. B., and Sweet, D. H. (1999). The antiviral nucleotide analogs cidofovir and adefovir are novel substrates for human and rat renal organic anion transporter 1. *Mol. Pharmacol.* **56**, 570–580.

Cintra, A., Fuxe, K., Wikstrom, A. C., Visser, T., and Gustafsson, J. A. (1990). Evidence for thyrotropin-releasing hormone and glucocorticoid receptor-immunoreactive neurons in various preoptic and hypothalamic nuclei of the male rat. *Brain Res.* **506**, 139–144.

Cintra, A., Fuxe, K., Solfrini, V., Agnati, L. F., Tinner, B., Wikstrom, A. C., Staines, W., Okret, S., and Gustafsson, J. A. (1991). Central peptidergic neurons as targets for glucocorticoid action. Evidence for the presence of glucocorticoid receptor immunoreactivity in various types of classes of peptidergic neurons. *J. Steroid Biochem. Mol. Biol.* **40**, 93–103.

Cioti, P., Fallon, J. H., Croix, D., Polak, J. M., and Tramu, G. (1991). Expression of neuropeptide Y precursor-immunoreactivity in the hypothalmic dopaminergic tuberoinfundibular system during lactation in rodents. *Endocrinology* **128**, 823–834.

Coccaro, E. F., Siever, L. J., Kaurides, I. A., Adam, F., Campel, G., and Davis, K. L. (1988). Central serotoninergic stimulation by fenfluramine challenge does not affect plasma thyrotropin-stimulating hormone levels in man. *Neuroendocrinology* **47**, 273–276.

Coiro, V., Volpi, R., Capretti, L., Gramellini, D., Cigarini, C., Papadia, C., Caiazza, A., Caffarri, G., Caffarra, P., and Chiodera, P. (1995). Effect of substance P on basal and thyrotropin-releasing hormone-stimulated thyrotropin release in humans. *Metab. Clin. Exp.* **44**, 474–477.

Connors, J. M., and Hedge, G. A. (1980). Feedback effectiveness of periodic versus constant triiodothyronine replacement. *Endocrinology* **106**, 911–917.

Conrad, L. C. A., Leonard, C. M., and Pfaff, D. W. (1974). Connetions of the median and dorsal raphe nuclei in the rat: An autoradiographic and degeneration study. *J. Comp. Neurol.* **156**, 179–206.

Corvilain, B., Laurent, E., Lecomte, M., Vansande, J., and Dumont, J. F. (1994). Role of the cyclic adenosine 3′,5′-monophosphate and the phosphatidylinositol-Ca^{2+} cascades in mediating the effects of thyrotropin and iodide on hormone synthesis and secretionin human thyroid slices. *J. Clin. Endocrinol. Metab.* **79**, 152–159.

Crantz, F. R., and Larsen, P. R. (1980). Rapid thyroxine to 3,5,3′-triiodothyronine conversion and nuclear 3,5,3′-triiodothyronine binding in rat cerebral cortex and cerebellum. *J. Clin. Invest.* **65**, 935–938.

Crantz, F. R., Silva, J. E., and Larsen, P. R. (1982). Analysis of the sources and quanitiy of 3,5,3′-triiodothyronine specifically bound to nuclear receptors in rat cerebral cortex and cerebellum. *Endocrinology* **110**, 367–375.

Crispell, K. R., and Coleman, J. (1956). A study of the relative binding capacity of plasma proteins, intact human red cells, and human red cell stroma for radioactive I-131 labeled L-thyroxine. *J. Clin. Invest.* **65**, 1032–1040.

Croteau, W., Whittemore, S. L., Schneider, M. J., and St. Germain, D. L. (1995). Cloning and expression of a cDNA for a mammalian type III iodothyronine deiodinase. *J. Biol. Chem.* **270**, 16569–16575.

Croteau, W., Davey, J. C., Galton, V. A., and St. Germain, D. L. (1996). Cloning of the mammalian type II iodothyronine deiodinase. *J. Clin. Invest.* **98**, 405–417.

Cullinam, W. E., Herman, J. P., and Watson, S. J. (1993). Ventral subicular interaction with the hypothalamic paraventricular nucleus: Evidence for a relay in the bed nucleus of the stria terminalis. *J. Comp. Neurol.* **332**, 1–20.

Dahl, G. E., Evans, N. P., Thrun, L. A., and Karsch, F. J. (1994). A central negative feedback action of thyroid hormones on thyrotropin-releasing hormone secretion. *Endocrinology* **135**, 2392–2397.

Darling, R. J., Ruddon, R. W., Perini, F., and Bedows, E. (2000). Cystine knot mutations affect the folding of the glycoprotein hormone alpha-subunit. Differential secretion and assembly of partially folded intermediates. *J. Biol. Chem.* **275**, 15413–15421.

Davey, J. C., Becker, K. B., Schneider, M. J., St. Germain, D. L., and Galton, V. A. (1995). Cloning of a cDNA for the type II iodothyronine deiodinase. *J. Biol. Chem.* **270**, 26786–26789.

Davey, J. C., Schneider, M. J., Becker, K. B., and Galton, V. A. (1999). Cloning of a 5.8 kb cDNA for mouse type 2 deiodinase. *Endocrinology* **140**, 1022–1025.

Decavel, C., and van den Pool, A. N. (1990). GABA: A dominant transmitter in the hypothalamus. *J. Comp. Neurol.* **302**, 1019–1037.

de Greef, W. J., Rondeel, J. M., van Haasteren, G. A., Klootwijk, W., and Visser, T. J. (1992). Regulation of hypothalamic TRH production and release in the rat. *Acta. Med. Austriaca.* **19**, 77–79.

Denef, C. (1994). Paracrine mechanisms in the pituitary. In "The Pituitary Gland" (H. Imura, ed.), pp. 351–378. Raven, New York.

DePaolo, L. V., King, R., and Carrillo, A. J. (1987). In vivo and in vitro examination of an autoregulatory mechanism for luteinizing hormone-releasing hormone. *Endocrinology* **120**, 272–279.

de Quidt, M. E., and Emson, P. C. (1986). Distribution of neuropeptide Y-like immunoreactivity in the rat central nervous system II. Immunohistochemical analysis. *Neuroscience* **18**, 545–618.

DeRooij, J. A. M., and Hommes, O. R. (1974). The tuberoinfundibular region in man. *In* Integrative hypothalamic activity. *Prog. Brain. Res.* **41**, 79.

Desy, L., and Pelletier, G. (1977). Immunohistochemical localization of somatostatin in the human hypothalamus. *Cell Tissue Res.* **184**, 491–497.

Deutsch, P. J., Jameson, J. L., and Habener, J. F. (1987). Cyclic AMP responsiveness of human gonadotropin-alpha gene transcription is directed by a repeated 18-base pair enhancer. alpha-promoter receptivity to the enhancer confers cell-preferential expression. *J. Biol. Chem.* **262**, 12169–12174.

Dey, M., Michalkiewicz, M., Huffman, L. J., and Hedge, G. A. (1993a). Thyroidal vascular responsiveness to parasympathetic stimulation is increased in hyperthyroidism. *Am. J. Physiol.* **264** (*Endocrinol. Metab.* 27), E398–E402.

Dey, M., Michalkiewicz, M., Huffman, L. J., and Hedge, G. A. (1993b). Sympathetic thyroidal vasoconstriction is not blocked by a neuropeptide Y antagonist or antiserum. *Peptides* **14**, 1179–1186.

Dey, M., Michalkiewicz, M., Huffman, L. J., and Hedge, G. A. (1993c). NPY is not a primary mediator of the acute thyroid blood flow response to sympathetic nerve stimulation. *Am J. Physiol.* **265** (*Endocrinol. Metab.* 28), E24–E30.

Diano, S., Naftolin, F., Goglia, F., and Horvath, T. L. (1998a). Segregation of the intra- and extrahypothalamic neuropeptide Y and catecholaminergic inputs on paraventricular neurons including those producing thyrotropin-releasing hormone. *Regul. Pept.* **75–76**, 117–126.

Diano, S., Naftolin, F., Goglia, F., and Horvath, T. L. (1998b). Fasting-induced increae in type II iodothyronine activity and messenger ribonucleic acid levels is not reversed by thyroxine in the rat hypothalamus. *Endocrinology* **139**, 2879–2884.

Dickson, P. W., and Schreiber, G. (1986). High levels of messenger RNA for transthyretin (prealbumin) in human choroid plexus. *Neurosci. Lett.* **66**, 311–315.

Dickson, P. W., Howlett, G. J., and Schreiber, G. (1985). Rat transthyretin (prealbumin). Molecular cloning, nucleotide sequence, and gene expression in liver and brain. *J. Biol. Chem.* **260**, 8214–8219.

Dickson, P. W., Aldred, A. R., Menting, J. G. T., Marley, P. D., Sawyer, W. H., and Schreiber, G. (1987). Thyroxine transport in choroid plexus. *J. Biol. Chem.* **262**, 13907–13915.

Dickson, P. W., Aldred, A. R., Menting, J. E., Marley, P. D., Sawyer, W. H., and Shreiber, G. (1990). Thyroxine transport from blood to brain via transthyretin synthesis in choroid plexus. *Am. J. Physiol.* **258**, R338–R345.

Docherty, K., and Steiner, D. F. (1982). Post-translational proteolysis in polypeptide hormone biosynthesis. *Annu. Rev. Physiol.* **44**, 625–638.

Domin, J., Al-Madani, A. M., Desperbasques, M., Bishop, A. E., Polak, J. M., and Bloom, S. R. (1990). Neuromedin U-like immunoreactivity in the thyroid gland of the rat. *Cell Tissue Res.* **260**, 131–135.

Douglass, J., McKinzie, A. A., and Couceyro, P. (1995). PCR differential display identified a rat brain mRNA that is transcriptionally regulated by cocaine and amphetamine. *J. Neurosci.* **15**, 2471–2481.

Dratman, M. B., and Crutchfield, F. L. (1987). Synaptosomal [^{123}I] triiodothyronine after intravenous [^{125}I] thyroxine. *Am. J. Physiol.* **235**, E638–E647.

Dratman, M. B., Crutchfield, F. L., Axelrod, J., Colburn, R. W., and Thoa, N. (1976). Localization of triiodothyronne in nerve ending fractions of rat brain. *Proc. Natl. Acad. Sci. U.S.A.* **73**, 941–944.

Dratman, M. B., Futaesaku, Y., Crutchfield, F. L., Berman, N., Payne, B., Sar, M., and Stumpf, W. E. (1982). Iodine-125-labeled triiodothyronine in rat brain: Evidence for localization in discrete neural systems. *Science* **215**, 309–312.

Dratman, M. B., Crutchfield, F. L., Futaesaku, Y., Goldberger, M. E., and Murray, M. (1987). [^{125}I] triiodothyronine in the rat brain: Evidence for neural localization and axonal transport derived from thaw-mount film autoradiography. *J. Comp. Neurol.* **260**, 392–408.

Dratman, M. B., Crutchfield, F. L., and Schoenhoff, M. B. (1991). Transport of iodothyronines from bloodstream to brain: Contributions by blood:brain and choroid plexus:cerebrospinal fluid barriers. *Brain Res.* **554**, 229–236.

Dube, D., Lissitzky, J. C., Leclerc, R., and Pelletier, G. (1978). Localization of alpha-melanocyte-stimulating hormone in rat brain and pituitary. *Endocrinology* **102**, 1283–1291.

Duprez, L., Parma, J., Costagliola, S., Hermans, J., Van Sande, J., Dumont, J. E., and Vassart, G. (1997). Constitutive activation of the TSH receptor by spontaneous mutations affecting the N-terminal extracellular domain. *FEBS Lett.* **409**, 469–474.

Dussault, J. H., and Ruel, J. (1987). Thyroid hormones and brain development. *Annu. Rev. Physiol.* **49**, 321–334.

Dyess, E. M., Segerson, T. P., Liposits, Z., Paull, W. K., Kaplan, M. M., Wu, P., Jackson, I. M. D., and Lechan, R. M. (1988). Triiodothyronine exerts direct cell-specific regulation of thyrotropin-releasing hormone gene expression in the hypothalamic paraventricular nucleus. *Endocrinology* **123**, 2291–2297.

Elias, C. F., Lee, C., Kelly, J., Aschkenasi, C., Ahima, R. S., Couceyro, P. R., Kuhar, M. J., Saper, C. B., and Elmquist, J. K. (1998). Leptin activates hypothalamic CART neurons projecting to the spinal cord. *Neuron* **21**, 1375–1385.

Elmquist, J. K., Ahima, R. S., Elias, C. F., Flier, J. S., and Saper, C. B. (1998). Leptin activtes distinct projections from the dorsomedial and ventromedial hypothalamic nuclei. *Proc. Natl. Acad. Sci. U.S.A.* **95**, 741–746.

Emson, P. C., Goedert, M., and Mantyh, P. W. (1985). Neurotensin-containing neurons. *In* "Handbook of Chemical Neuroanatomy. GABA and Neuropeptides" (A. Bjorklund and T. Hokfelt, eds.), Vol. 4, pp. 355–405. Elsevier, Amsterdam.

Epelbaum, J., Arancibia, L. T., Herman, J. P., Kordon, C., and Palkovits, M. (1981). Topography of median eminence somatostatinergic innervation. *Brain Res.* **230**, 412–416.

Epelbaum, J., Tapia-Arancibia, L., Alonso, G., and Assenmacher, I. (1985). Electron microscopic immunocytochemical study of somatostatin neurons in the periventricular nucleus of the rat hypothalamus with spcial reference to their relationship with homologous neuronal processes. *Neuroscience* **16**, 297–306.

Epelbaum, J., Tapia-Arancibia, L., Alonso, G., Astier, H., and Kordon, C. (1986). The anterior periventricular hypothalamus is the site of somatostatin inhibition on its own release: An in virto and immunocytochemical study. *Neuroendocrinology* **44**, 225–259.

Erickson, J. C., Ahima, R. S., Hollopeter, G., Flier, J. S., and Palmiter, R. D. (1997). Endocrine fucntion of neuropeptide Y knockout mice. *Regul. Pept.* **70**, 199–202.

Escamez, M. J., Guadano-Ferraz, A., Cuadrado, A., and Bernal, J. (1999). Type 3 iodothyronine deiodinase is selectively expressed in areas related to sexual differentiation in the newborn rat brain. *Endocrinology* **140**, 5443–5446.

Escobar-Morreale, H. F., Obregon, M. J., Hernandez, A., Del Rey, E., and De Escobar, G. M. (1997). Regulation of iodothyronine deiodinase activity as studied in thyroidectomized rats infused with thyroxine or triiodothyronine. *Endocrinology* **138**, 2559–2568.

Esfandiari, A., Courtein, F., Lennon, A.-M., Gavaret, J.-M., and Pierre, M. (1992). Induction of type III deiodinase activity in astroglial cells by thyroid hormones. *Endocrinology* **131**, 1682–1688.

Eskay, R. L., Giraud, P., Oliver, C., and Brown-Stein, M. J. (1979). Distribution of alpha-melanocyte-stimulating hormone in the rat brain: Evidence that alpha-MSH-containing cells in the arcuate region send projections to extrahypothalamic areas. *Brain Res.* **178**, 55–67.

Feek, C. M., Sawers, J. S. A., Brown, N. S., Seth, J., Irvine, W. J., and Toft, A. D. (1980). Influence of thyroid status on dopaminergic inhibition of thyrotropin and prolactin secretion: Evidence for an additional feedback mechanism in the control of thyroid hormone secretion. *J. Clin. Endocrinol. Metab.* **51**, 585–589.

Fekete, C. S., Stutton, P. H., Caganpang, F. R., Hrabosvsky, E., Kallo, I., Shughrue, P. J., Dobo, E., Mihaly, E., Barany, L., Okada, H., Panula, P., Merchenthaler, I., Coen, C. W., and Liposits, Z. S. (1999). Estrogen receptor immunoreactivity is present in the majority of central histaminergic neurons: Evidence for a new neuroendocrine pathway associated with luteinizing hormone-releasing hormone-synthesizing neurons in rats and humans. *Endocrinology* **140**, 4335–4341.

Fekete, C. S., Legradi, G., Mihaly, E., Huang, Q.-H., Tatro, J. B., Rand, W. M., Emerson, C. H., and Lechan, R. M. (2000a). α-Melanocyte-stimulating hormone is contained in nerve terminals innervating thyrotropin-releasing hormone-synthesizing neurons in the hypothalamic paraventricular nucleus and prevents fasting-induced supression of prothyrotropin-releasing hormone gene expression. *J. Neurosci.* **20**, 1550–1558.

Fekete, C. S., Mihaly, E., Luo, L.-G., Kelly, J., Clausen, J. T., Mao, Q., Rand, W. M., Moss, L. G., Kuhar, M., Emerson C. H., Jackson, I. M. D., and Lechan, R. M. (2000b). Association of CART-immunoreactive elements with thyrotropin-releasing hormone-synthesizing neurons in the hypothalamic paraventricular nucleus and its role in the regulation of the hypothalamic–pituitary–thyroid axis during fasting. *J. Neurosci.* **20**, 9224–9234.

Fekete, C., Kelly, J., Mihály, E., Sarkar, S., Rand, W. M., Légrádi, G., Emerson, C. H., and Lechan, R. M. (2001). Neuropeptide Y has a central inhibitory action on the hypothalamic-pituitary-thyroid axis. *Endocrinology* **142**, 2606–2613.

Feng, P., Li, Q. L., Satch, T., and Wilbur, J. F. (1994). Ligand (T3) dependent and independent effects of thyroid hormone receptors upon human TRH gene conscription in neuroblastoma cells. *Biochem. Biophys. Res. Commun.* **200**, 171–177.

Fink, I. L., Bailey, T. J., Gustafson, T. A., Markham, B. E., and Morkin, E. (1986). Complete amino acid sequence of human thyroxine-binding globulin deduced from cloned DNA: Close homology to the serine antiproteases. *Proc. Natl. Acad. Sci. U.S.A.* **83**, 7708–7712.

Finley, J. C. W., Maderdrut, J. L., Roger, L. J., and Petruz, P. (1981). The immunocytochemical localization of somatostatin-containing neurons in the rat central nervous system. *Neuroscience* **6**, 2173–2192.

Fisher, W. H., and Speiss, J. (1987). Identification of a mammalian glutaminyl cyclase converting glutaminyl into pyroglytamyl peptides. *Proc. Natl. Acad. Sci. U.S.A.* **84**, 3628–3632.

Fliers, E., Noppen, N. W. A. M., Wiersinga, W. M., Visser, T. J., and Swaab, D. F. (1994). Distribution of thyrotropin-releasing hormone (TRH)-containing cells and fibers in the human hypothalamus. *J. Comp. Neurol.* **350**, 311–323.

Foord, S. M., Peters, J. R., Dieguez, C., Shewring, A. G., Hall, R., and Scanlon, M. F. (1985). TSH regulates thyrotroph responsiveness to dopamine in vitro. *Endocrinology* **118**, 1319–1326.

Forman, B. M., Umesono, K., Chen, J., and Evans, R. M. (1995). Unique response pathways are established by allosteric interactions among nuclear hormone receptors. *Cell* **81**, 541–550.

Fowlers, S., and Kellogg, C. (1975). Ontogeny of thermoregulatory mechanisms in the rat. *J. Comp. Physiol. Psychol.* **7**, 738–746.

Francon, J., Chantoux, F., and Blondeau, J.-P. (1989). Carrier-mediated transport of thyroid hormones into rat glial cells in primary culture. *J. Neurochem.* **53**, 1456–1463.

Franks, S., Mason, H. D., Shennan, K. I., and Sheppard, M. C. (1984). Stimulation of prolactin secretion by oestradiol in the rat is associated with increased hypothalamic release of thyrotrophin-releasing hormone. *J. Endocrinol.* **103**(2), 257–261.

Friedman, T. C., Loh, Y. P., Cawley, N. X., Birch, N. P., Huang, S. S., Jackson I. M. D., and Nillni, E. A. (1995). Processing of pro-thyrotropin-releasing hormone (pro0TRH) by bovine intermediate lobe secretory vesicle membrane PC1 and PC2 enzymes. *Endocrinology* **136**, 4462–4472.

Friesma, E. C. H., Docter, R., Krenning, E. P., Everts, M. E., Hennemann, G., and Visser, T. J. (1998). Rapid sulfation of 3,3′,5′-triiodothyronine in native *Xenopus laevis* oocytes. *Endocrinology* **139**, 596–600.

Friesma, E. C. H., Docter, R., Moerings, E. P. C. M., Stieger, B., Hagenbuch, B., Meier, P. J., Krenning, E. P., Hennemann, G., and Visser, T. J. (1999). Identification of thyroid hormone transporters. *Biochem. Biophys. Res. Commun.* **254**, 497–501.

Fuxe, K., Agnati, L. F., Harfstrand, A., Cintra, A., Aronsson, M., Zoli, M., and Gustafsson, J. A. (1988). Principles for the hormone regulation of wiring transimission and volume transimission in the central nervous system. In "Neuroendocrinology of Mood. Current Topics in Neuroendocrinology" (D. Ganten and D. Pfaff, eds.), pp. 1–53. Springer-Verlag, Berlin and Heildelberg.

Gallardo, E., Chiocchio, S. R., and Tramezzani, J. H. (1984). Sympathetic innervation of the median eminence. *Brain Res.* **290**, 333–335.

Gao, B., Stieger, B., Noe, B., Fritschy, J.-M., and Meier, P. J. (1999). Localization of the organic anion transporting polypeptide 2 (Oatp2) in capillary endothelium and choroid plexus epithelium of rat brain. *J. Histochem. Cytochem.* **47**, 1255–1263.

Gershengorn, M. C. (1989). Mechanism of signal transduction by TRH. *Ann. N.Y. Acad. Sci.* **553**, 191–204.

Giardino, L., Velardo, A., Gallinelli, A., and Calzà, L. (1992). Deficit of galanin-like immunostaining in the median eminence of adult hypothyroid rats. *Neuroendocrinology* **55**, 237–247.

Ginsberg, S. D., Hof, P. R., Young, W. G., and Morrison, J. H. (1993). Noradrenergic innervation of the hypothalamus of Rhesus Monkeys: Distribution of dopamine-β-hydroxylase immunoreactive fibers and quantitative analysis of varicosities in the paraventricular nucleus. *J. Comp. Neurol.* **327**, 597–611.

Gonzales, M. C., Riedel, M., Rettori, V., Yu, W. H., and McCann, S. M. (1990). Effect of recombinant human gamma-interferon on the release of anterior pituitary hormones. *PNEI* **3**, 49–54.

Gonzalez, C., Montoya, E., and Jolin, T. (1980). Effect of streptozotocin diatetes on the hypothalamic–pituitary–thyroid axis in the rat. *Endocrinology* **107**, 2099–2103.

Gordon, D. F., Lewis, S. R., Haugen, B. R., James, R. A., McDermott, M. T., Wood, W. M., and Ridgway, E. C. (1997). Pit-1 and GATA-2 interact and functionally cooperate to activate the thyrotropin β-subunit promoter. *J. Biol. Chem.* **272**, 24339–24347.

Gordon, J. T., Kaminski, D. M., Rozanov, C. B., and Dratman, M. D. (1999). Evidence that 3,3′,5-triiodothyronine is concentrated in and delivered from the locus coeruleus to its noradrenergic targets via anterograde axonal transport. *Neuroscience* **93**, 943–954.

Gray, T. S., Carney, M. E., and Magnuson, D. J. (1989). Direct projection from the central amygdaloid neucleus to the hypothalamic paraventricular nucleus. Possible role in stress-induced adrenocorticotropin release. *Neuroendocrinology* **50**, 433–444.

Greer, M. A. (1957). Studies on the influence of the central nervous system on anterior pituitary function. *Recent Prog. Horm. Res.* **13**, 67–104.

Greer, M. A., Sato, N., Wang, X., Greer, S. E., and McAdams, S. (1993). Evidence that the major physiological role of TRH in the hypothalamic paraventricular nuclei may be to regulate the set-point for thyroid hormone negative feedback on the pituitary thyrotroph. *Neuroendocrinology* **57**, 569–575.

Grimm, Y., and Reichlin, S. (1973). Thyrotropin-releasing hormone (TRH): Neurotransmitter regulation of secretion by mouse hypothalamic tissue in vitro. *Endocrinology* **93**, 626–631.

Groarke, D. A., Wilson, S., Krasel, C., and Milligan, G. (1999). Visualization of agonist-induced association and trafficking of green fluorescent protein-tagged forms of both β-arrestin-1 and the thyrotropin-releasing hormone receptor-1. *J. Biol. Chem.* **274**, 23263–23269.

Grossmann, M., Weintraub, B. D., and Szkudlinski, M. W. (1997a). Novel insights into the molecular mechanisms of human thyrotropin action: Structural, physiological, and therapeutic implications for the glycoprotein hormone family. *Endocr. Rev.* **18**, 476–500.

Grossmann, M., Szudlinski, W., Wong, R., Dias, J. A., Ji, T. H., and Weintraub, B. D. (1997b). Substitution of the seat-belt region of the thyroid-stimulating hormone (TSH) β-subunit with the corresponding regions of choriogonadotropin or follitropin confers leuteotropic but not follitropic activity to chimeric TSH. *J. Biol. Chem.* **272**, 15532–15540.

Grunditz, T., Hakanson, R., Rerup, C., Sundler, F., and Uddman, R. (1984). Neuropeptide Y in the thyroid gland: Neuronal localization and enhancement of stimulated thyroid hormone secretion. *Endocrinology* **115**, 1537–1542.

Grunditz, T., Hakanson, R., Sundler, F., and Uddman, R. (1988). Neuronal pathways to the rat thyroid revealed by retrograde tracing and immunocytochemistry. *Neuroscience* **24**, 321–335.

Guadano-Ferraz, A., Obregon, M. J., St. Germain, D. L., and Bernal, J. (1997). The type 2 iodothyronine deiodinase is expressed primarily in glial cells in the neonatal rat brain. *Proc. Natl. Acad. Sci. U.S.A.* **94**, 10391–10396.

Guadano-Ferraz, A., Escamez, M. J., Rausell, E., and Bernal, J. (1999). Expression of type 2 iodothyronine deiodinase in hypothyroid rat brain indicates an important role of thyroid hormone in the development of specific primary sensory systems. *J. Neurosci.* **19**, 3430–3439.

Guldenaar, S. E. F., Veldkamp, B., Bakker, O., Wiersinga, W. M., Swaab, D. F., and Fliers, E. (1996). Thyrotropin-releasing hormone gene expression in the human hypothalamus. *Brian Res.* **743**, 93–101.

Hagen, G. A., and Elliott, W. J. (1973). Transport of thyroid hormones in serum and cerebrospinal fluid. *J. Clin. Endocrinol. Metab.* **37**, 415–422.

Hagenbuch, B., Stieger, B., Foguet, M., Lubbert, H., and Meier, P. J. (1991). Functional expression cloning and characterization of the hepatocyte Na^+/bile acid cotransport system. *Proc. Natl. Acad. Sci. U.S.A.* **88**, 10629–10633.

Hahn, T. M., Breininger, J. F., Baskin, D. G., and Schwartz, M. W. (1998). Coexpression of Agrp and NPY in fasting-activated hypothalamic neurons. *Nat. Neurosci.* **1**, 271–272.

Haisenleder, D. J., Ortolano, G. A., Dalkin, A. C., Yasin, M., and Marshall, J. C. (1992). Differential actions of thyrotropin (TSH)-releasing hormone pulses in the expression of prolactin and TSH subunit messenger ribonucleic acid in rat pituitary cells *in vitro*. *Endocrinology* **130**, 2917–2923.

Halasz, B., Pupp, L., and Uhlarik, S. (1962). Hypophysiotrophic area in the hypothalamus. *J. Endocrinol.* **25**, 147–154.

Harfstrand, A. (1987). Brain neuropeptide Y mechanisms: Basic aspects and involvement in cardiovascular and neuroendocrine regulation. *Acta. Physiol. Scand.* **131** (Suppl. 565), 1–83.

Harris, G. W. (1955). "Neural Control of the Pituitary Gland" Arnold, London.

Harris, G. W., and George, R. (1969). Neurohumoral control of the adenohypophysis and the regulation of the secretion of TSH, ACTH and growth hormone. In "The Hypothalamus" (W. Haymaker, E. Anderson, and W. J. H. Nauta, eds.), pp. 326–388. Thomas, Springfield.

Harris, M., Aschkenasi, C., Elias, C., Chandrankunnel, A., Nillni, E. A., Bjoerbaek, C., Elmquist, J. K., Flier, J. S., and Hollenberg, A. N. (2001). Transcriptional regulation of the thyrotropin-releasing hormone gene by leptin and melanocortin signaling. *J. Clin. Invest.* **107**, 111–120.

Haugen, B. R., Brown, N. S., Wood, W. M., Gordon, D. F., and Rudgway, E. C. (1997). The thyrotrope-restricted isoform of the retinoid X receptor (gamma 1) mediates 9-*cis* retinoic acid suppression of thyrotropin beta promoter activity. *Mol. Endocrinol.* **11**, 481–489.

Hayashizaki, Y., Hiraoka, Y., Miyai, K., and Matsubara, K. (1989). Thyroid-stimulating hormone (TSH) deficiency caused by a single base substitution in the CAGYC region of the beta-subunit. *EMBO J.* **8**(8), 2291–2296.

Healy, D. L., and Burger, H. G. (1977). Increased prolactin and thyrotropin secretion following oral metoclopramide: Dose response relationship. *Clin. Endocrinol.* **7**, 195–201.

Herbert, J., Wilcox, J. N., Pham, K.-T. C., Fremeau, R. T., Jr., Zeviani, M., Dwork, A., Soprano, D. R., Makover, A., Goodman, D. S., Zimmerman, E. A., Roberts, J. L., and Schon, E. A. (1986). Transthyretin: A choroid plexus-specific transport protein in human brain. *Neurology* **36**, 900–911.

Heilig, M., Vecsei, L., Wahlestedt, C., Alling, C., and Widerlov, E. (1990). Effects of centrally administered neuropeptide Y (NPY) and NPY 13-36 on the brain monoaminergic system of the rat. *J. Neural. Transm.* **79**, 193–208.

Hennemann, G., Krenning, E. P., Polhuts, M., Mol, J. A., Bernard, B. F., Visser, T. J., and Docter, R. (1986). Carrier-mediated transport of thyroid hormone into rat hepatocytes is rate-limiting in total cellular uptake and metabolism. *Endocrinology* **119**, 1870–1872.

Hermus, A. R. M. M., Sweep, C. G. J., van der Meer, M. J. M., Ross, H. A., Smals, A. G., Benraad, T. J., and Kloppenborg, P. W. (1992). Continuous injusion of interleukin-1β induces a nonthyroidal illness syndrome in the rat. *Endocrinology* **131**, 2139–2146.

Heuer, H., Ehrchen, J., Bauer K., and Schafer, M. K. H. (1998). Region-specific expression of thyrotrophin-releasing hormone-degrading ectoenzyme in the rat central nervous system and pituitary gland. *Eur. J. Neurosci.* **10**, 1465–1478.

Hiller, A. P. (1971). Human thyroxine-binding globulin and thyroxine-binding pre-albumin dissociation rates. *J. Physiol.* **217**, 625–634.

Hinkle, P. M., Nelson, E. J., and Ashworth, R. (1996). Characterization of the calcium response to thyrotropin-releasing hormone in lactotrophs and GH cells. *Trends Endocrinol. Metab.* **7**, 370–374.

Hirooka, Y., Hollander, C. S., Suzuki, S., Ferdinand, P., and Juan, S.-I. (1978). Somatostatin inhibits release of thyrotropin releasing factor from organ cultures of rat hypothalamus. *Proc. Natl. Acad. Sci. U.S.A.* **75**, 4509–4013.

Hisano, S., Ishizuka, H., Nishiyama, T., Tsuro, Y., Katoh, S., and Daikoku, S. (1986). Immunoelectron microscopic observations of hypothalamic TRH-containing neurons in rats. *Exp. Brain Res.* **63**, P495–P504.

Hisano, S., Yoshihiro, F., Chikamori-Aoyama, M., Aizawa, T., and Shibasaki, T. (1993). Reciprocal synaptic relations between CRF-immunoreactive and TRH-immunoreactive neurons in the paraventricular nucleus of the rat hypothalamus. *Brain Res.* **620**, 343–346.

Hodin, R. A., Lazar, M. A., Wintman, B. L., Darling, D. S., Koenig, R. J., Larson, P. R., Moore, D. D., and Chin, W. W. (1989). Identification of a thyroid hormone receptor that is pituitary-specific. *Science* **244**, 76–79.

Hökfelt, T., Fuxe, K., Johansson, O., Jeffcoate, S., and White, N. (1975). Distribution of thyrotropin-releasing hormone (TRH) in the central nervous system as revealed with immunocytochemistry. *Eur. J. Pharmacol.* **34**, 389–392.

Hökfelt, T., Johansson, O., and Goldstein, M. (1984). Central catecholamine neurons as revealed by immunocytochemistry with special reference to adrenaline neurons. *In* "Handbook of Chemical Neuroanatomy, Classical Transmitters in the CNS" (A. Bjorklund and T. Hokfelt, eds.), Vol. 2, Part 1, pp. 157–276. Elsevier, Amsterdam.

Hökfelt, T., Fahrenkrug, J., Ju, G., Ceccatelli, S., Tsuruo, Y., Meister, B., Mutt, V., Rundgren, M., Brodin, E., Terenius, L., Hulting, A.-L., Werner, S., Bjorklund, A., and Vale, W. (1987). Analysis of peptide histidine-isoleucine/vasoactive intestinal polypeptide-immunoreactive neurons in the central nervous system with special reference to their relation to corticotropin releasing factor- and enkephalin-like immunoreactivities in the praeventricular hypothalamic nucleus. *Neuroscience* **23**, 827–857.

Hollenberg, A. N., Monden, T., Flynn, T. R., Boers, M.-E, Cohen, O., and Wondisford, F. E. (1995). The human thyrotropin-releasing hormone gene is regulated by thyroid hormone through two distinct classes of negative thyroid hormone response elements. *Mol. Endocrinol.* **9**, 540–550.

Hooi, S. C., Koenig, J. I., Gabriel, S. M., Maiter, D., and Martin, J. B. (1990). Influence of thyroid hormone on the concentration of galanin in the rat brain and pituitary. *Neuroendocrinology* **51**(3), 351–356.

Horvath, S., and Palkovits, M. (1988). Synaptic interconnections among growth hormone-releasing hormone (GHRH)-containing neurons in the arcuate nucleus of the rat hypothalamus. *Neuroendocrinolgy* **48**, 471–476.

Horvath, T. L. (1998). An alternate pathway for visual signal integration into the hypothalamo–pituitary axis: Retinorecipient intergeniculate neurons project to various regions of the hypothalamus and innervate neuroendocrine cells including those producing dopamine. *J. Neurosci.* **18**, 1546–1558.

Houssay, B.-A., Biasotti, A., and Sammartino, R. (1935). Modifications functionnelles de l'hypophyse apres les lesions infundibulotuberiennes chez le crapaud. *C. R. Soc. Biol.* **110**, 834–836.

Hovring, P. I., Matre, V., Fjeldheim, A. K., Loseth, O. P., and Gautvik, K. M. (1999). Transcription of the human thyrotropin-releasing hormone receptor gene—analysis of basal promoter elements and glucocorticoid response elements. *Biochem. Biophys. Res. Commun.* **257**, 829–834.

Hsieh, K.-P, and Martin, T. F. J. (1992). Thyrotropin-releasing hormone and gonadotropin-releasing hormone receptors activate phospholipase C by complexing to the guanosine triphosphate-binding proteins Gq and G11. *Mol. Endocrinol.* **6**, 1773–1681.

Huang, S. W., Tsai, S. C., Tung, Y. F., and Wang, P. S. (1995). Role of progesterone in regulating the effect of estradiol on the secretion of thyrotropin-releasing hormone and dopamine in the hypophysial portal blood in ovariectomized rats. *Neuroendocrinology* **61**, 536–541.

Huffman, L. J., and Hedge, G. A. (1986). Effects of vasoactive intestinal peptide on thyroid blood flow and circulating thyroid hormone levels in the rat. *Endocrinology* **118**, 550–557.

Huffman, L. J., Conners, J. M., and Hedge, G. A. (1988a). VIP and its homologues increase vascular conductance in certain endorine and exocrine glands. *Am. J. Physiol.* **254**, (*Endocrinol. Metab.* **17**), E435–E442.

Huffman, L. J., Conners, J. M., White B. H., and Hedge G. A. (1988b). Vasoactive intestinal peptide treatment that increases thyroid blood flow fails to alter plasma T3 or T4 levels in the rat. *Neuroendocrinology* **47**, 567–574.

Hyyppa, M. (1972). Hypothalamic monoamines in human fetuses. *Neuroendocrinology* **9**, 257–266.

Hyyppa, M., Motta, M., and Martini, L. (1971). Ultrashort feedback control of follicle-stimulating hormone-releasing factor secretion. *Neuroendocrinology* **7**, 227–235.

Ibata, Y., Kawakami, F., Fukui, K., Obata-Tsuto, H. L., Tanaka, M., Kuba, T., Okamura, H., Morimoto, N., Yanaihara, C., and Yanaihara, N. (1984). Light and electron microscopic immunocytochemistry of neurotensin-like immunoreactive neurons in the rat hypothalamus. *Brain Res.* **302**, 221–230.

Ignar, D. M., and Khun, C. M. (1988). Relative ontogeny of opioid and catecholaminergic regulation of thyrotropin secretion in the rat. *Endocrinology* **123**, 567–571.

Ikuyama, S., Niller, H. H., Shimura, H., Akamizu, T., and Kohn, L. D. (1992a). Characterization of the 5′-flanking region of the rat thyrotropin receptor gene. *Mol. Endocrinol.* **6**, 793–804.

Ikuyama, S., Shimura, H., Hoeffler, J. P., and Kohn, L. D. (1992). Role of the cyclic adenosine 3′,5′-monophosphate response element in efficient expresion of the rat thyrotropin receptor promoter. *Mol. Endocrinol.* **6**(10), 1701–1715.

Inagaki, N., Yamatodani, A., Ando-Yamamoto, M., Tohyama, M., Watanabe, T., and Wada, H. (1988). Organization of histaminergic fibers in the rat brain. *J. Comp. Neurol.* **273**, 283–300.

Ishikawa, K., Kakegawa, T., and Suzuki, M. (1984). Role of the hypothalamic paraventricular nucleus in the secretion of thyrotorpin under adrenergic and cold-stimulated conditions in the rat. *Endocrinology* **114**, 352–358.

Ishikawa, K., Taniguchi, Y., Kurosumi, K., Suzuki, M., and Shioda, M. (1987). Immunohistochemical identification of somatostatin-containing neurons projecting to the median eminence of the rat. *Endocrinology* **121**, 94–97.

Ishikawa, K., Taniguchi, Y., Inoue, K., Kurosumi, K., and Suzuki, M. (1988). Immunocytochemical delineation of thyrotropic area: Oregin of thyrotropin-releasing hormone in the median eminence. *Neuroendocrinology* **47**, 384–388.

Itadani, H., Nakamura, T., Itoh, J., Iwaasa, H., Kanatani, A., Borkowski, J., Ihara, M., and Ohta, M. (1998). Cloning and characterization of a new subtype of thyrotropin-releasing hormone receptors. *Biochem. Biophys. Res. Commun.* **250**, 68–71.

Jackson, I. M. D. (1995). TRH and CRH. What's the message? *Endocrinology* **136**, 2793–2794.

Jackson, I. M., and Reichlin, S. (1977). Brain thyrotropin-releasing hormone is independent of the hypothalamus. *Nature* **267**, 853–854.

Jackson, I. M. D., and Reichlin, S. (1979). Distribution and biosynthesis of TRH in the nervous system. *In* "Central Nervous System Effects of Hypothalamic Hormones and Other Peptides" (R. Collu, A. Barbeau, S. R Duchaine, and J. G Rochefort, eds.), pp. 3–56. Raven, New York.

Jackson, I. M. D., Lechan, R. M., and Lee, S. L. (1990). TRH prohormone: Biosynthesis, anatomic distribution and processing. *Front. Neuroendocrinol.* **11**, 267–312.

Jacobowitz, D. M., and O'Donohue, T. L. (1978). Alpha-melanocyte stimulating hormone: Immunohistochemical identification and mapping in neurons of rat brain. *Proc. Natl. Acad. Sci. U.S.A.* **75**, 6300–6304.

Jacquemin, E., Hagenbuch, B., Stieger, B., Wolkoff, A. W., and Meier, P. J. (1994). Expression cloning of a rat liver Na (+)-independent organic anion transporter. *Proc. Natl. Acad. Sci. U.S.A.* **91**, 133–137.

Jacobs, B. L., and Azimita, E. C. (1992). Structure and function of the brain serotonin system. *Physiol. Rev.* **72**, 165–229.

Jew, J., Leranth, C. S., Arimura, A., and Palkovits, M. (1984). Preoptic LHRH and somatostatin in the rat median eminence. An experimental light and electron microscopic immunohistochemical study. *Neuroendocrinology* **38**, 169–175.

Johansson, O., and Hokfelt, T. (1980). Thyrotropin releasing hormone, somatostatin, and enkephalin: Distribution studies using immunohistochemical techniques. *J. Histochem. Cytochem.* **28**, 364–366.

Johansson, O., Hokfelt, T., Jefcoate, S. L., White N., and Sternberger, L. A. (1980). Ultrastructural localization of TRH-like immunoreactivity. *Exp. Brain Res.* **38**, 1–10.

Jordan, D., Poncet, C., Veisseire, M., and Mornex, R. (1983). Role of GABA in the control of thyrotropin secretion in the rat. *Brain Res.* **268**, 105–110.

Jordan, D., Veisseire, M., Borson-Charzot, F., and Mornex, R. (1986). In vitro effects of endogenous opiate peptides on thyrotropin function: Inhibition of thyrotropin-releasing hormone release and absence of effect on thyrotropin release. *Neurosci. Lett.* **67**, 289–294.

Joseph, S. A., and Knigge, K. M. (1978). The endocrine hypothalamus: Recent anatomical studies. *In* "The Hypothalamus" (S. Reichlin, R. J. Baldessarini, and J. B. Martin, eds.), pp. 15–47. Raven, New York.

Joseph, S. A., Pilcher, W. H., and Bennett-Clarke, C. (1983). Immunocytochemical localization of ACTH perikarya in nucleus tractus solitarius: Evidence for a second opiocortin neuronal system. *Neurosci. Lett.* **38**, 221–225.

Joseph-Bravo, P., Charli, J. L., Palacios, J. M., and Kordon, C. (1979). Effect of neurotransmitters on the in vitro release of immunoreactive thyrotropin-releasing hormone from rat mediobasal hypothalamus. *Endocrinology* **104**, 801–806.

Judd, A. M., and Hedge, G. A. (1982). The roles of the opiod peptides in controlling thyroid stimulating hormone release. *Life Sci.* **31**, 2529–2536.

Judd, A. M., and Hedge, G. A. (1983). Direct pituitary stimulation of thyrotropin secretion by opioid peptides. *Endocrinology* **113**(2), 706–710.

Kakucska, I., Rand, W., and Lechan, R. M. (1992). Thyrotropin-releasing hormone gene expression in the hypothalamic paraventricular nucleus is dependent upon feedback regulation by both triiodothyronine and thyroxine. *Endocrinology* **130**, 2845–2850.

Kakucska, I., Romero, L. I., Clark, B. D., Rondeel, J. M. M., Qi, Y., Alex, S., Emerson, C. H., and Lechan, R. M. (1994).

Suppression of thyrotropin-releasing hormone gene expression by interleukin-1-β in the rat: Implications for nonthyroidal illness. *Neuroendocrinology* **59**, 129–137.

Kakucska, I., Qi, Y., and Lechan, T. M. (1995). Changes in adrenal status affect hypothalamic thyrotropin-releasing hormone gene expression in parallel with corticotropin-releasing hormone. *Endocrinology* **136**, 2795–2802.

Kakyo, M., Unno, M., Tokui, T., Nakagomi, R., Nisho, T., Iwasashi, H., Nakai, D., Seki, M., Suzuki, M., Naitoh, T., Matsuno, S., Yawo, H., and Abe, T. (1999). Molecular characterization and functional regulation of a novel rat liver-specific organic anion transporter rlst-1. *Gastroenterology* **117**, 770–775.

Kalra, S. P., and Kalra, P. S. (1984). Opioid-adrenergic-steroid connection in the regulation of luteinizing hormone secretion in the rat. *Neuroendocrinology* **38**, 418–426.

Kalra, S. P., Dube, M. G., Sahu, A., Phelps, C. P., and Kalra, P. S. (1991). Neuropeptide Y secretion increases in the paraventricular nucleus in association with increased appetite for food. *Proc. Natl. Acad. Sci. U.S.A.* **88**, 10931–10935.

Kamei, Y., Xu, L., Heinzel, T., Torchia, J., Jurokawa, R., Gloss, B., Lin, S.-C., Heyman, R. A., Rose, D. W., Glass, C. K., and Rosenfeld, M. G. (1996). A CBP integrator complex mediates transcriptional activation and AP-1 inhibition by nuclear receptors. *Cell* **85**, 403–414.

Kanai, N., Lu, R., Satriano, J. A., Bao, Y., Wolkoff, A. W., and Schuster, V. L. (1995). Identification and characterization of a prostaglandin transporter. *Science* **268**, 866–869.

Kaplan, M. M. (1984). The role of thyroid hormone deiodination in the regulation of hypothalamo–pituitary function. *Neuroendocrinology* **38**, 254–260.

Kaplan, M. M., and Yaskoski, K. A. (1980). Phenolic and tyrosyl ring deiodination of iodothyronines in rat brain homogenates. *J. Clin. Invest.* **66**, 551–562.

Kaplan, M. M., Taft, J. A., Reichlin, S., and Munsat, T. (1986). Sustained rises in serum thyrotropin, thyroxine, and triiodothyronine during long-term, continuous thyrotropin-releasing hormone treatment in patients with amyotrophic lateral scloersis. *J. Clin. Endocrinol. Metab.* **63**, 808–814.

Kaplan, S. L., Grumbach, M. M., and Aubert, M. L. (1976). The ontogenesis of pituitary hormones and hypothalamic factors in the human fetus: Maturation of the central nervous system regulation of anterior pituitary function. *Recent Prog. Horm. Res.* **32**, 161–243.

Kasting, N. W., and Martin, J. B. (1982). Altered release of growth hormone and thyrotropin induced by endotoxin in the rat. *Am. J. Physiol.* **243**, E332–E337.

Katz, R. W., and Koenig, R. J. (1993). Nonbiased identification of DNA sequences that bind thyroid hormone receptor alpha 1 with high affinity. *J. Biol. Chem.* **268**, 19392–19297.

Kawano, H., and Daikoku, S. (1988). Somatostatin-containing neurons systems in the rat hypothalamus: Retrograde tracing and immunohistochemical studies. *J. Comp. Neurol.* **272**, 293–299.

Kawano, H., Tsuruo, Y., Bando, H., and Daikoku, S. (1991). Hypophysiotrophic TRH-producing neurons identified by combining immunohistochemistry for proTRH and retrograde tracing. *J. Comp. Neurol.* **307**, 531–538.

Kerkerian, L., and Pelletier, G. (1986). Effect of monosodium L-glutamate administration on neuropeptide Y-containing neurons in the rat hypothalamus. *Brain Res.* **369**, 388–390.

Kesterson, R. A., Huzar, D., Lynch, C. A., Simerly, R. B., and Cone, R. D. (1997). Induction of neuropeptide Y gene expression in the dorsal medial hypothalamic nucleus in two models of the agouti obesity syndrome. *Mol. Endocrinol.* **11**, 630–637.

Kharchaturian, H., Lewis, M. E., Tsou, K., and Watson, S. J. (1985). Beta-endorphin, alpha-MSH, ACTH, and related peptides. In "Handbook of Chemical Neuroanatomy, GABA and Neuropeptides" (A. Bjorklund and T. Hokfelt, eds.), Vol. 4, pp. 216–272. Elsevier, Amsterdam.

Kim, M. K., McClaskey, J. H., Bodenner, D. L., and Weintraub, B. D. (1993). An AP-like factor and the pituitary-specific factor Pit-1 are both necessary to mediate hormonal induction of human thyrotropin β gene expression. *J. Biol. Chem.* **268**, 23366–23375.

Kimura, N., Arai, K., Sahara, Y., Suzuki, H., and Kimura, N. (1994). Estradiol transcriptionally and posttranscriptionally up-regulates thyrotropin-releasing hormone receptor messenger ribonucleic acid in rat pituitary cells. *Endocrinology* **134**, 432–440.

Kiss, J., and Halasz, B. (1990). Ultrastructural analysis of the innervation of TRH-immunoreactive neuronal elements located in the periventricular subdivision of the paraventricular nucelus of the rat hypothalamus. *Brain Res.* **532**(1–2), 107–114.

Knigge, K. M., and Joseph, A. S. (1971). Neural regulation of TSH secretion: Sites of thyroxine feedback. *Neuroendocrinology* **8**, 273–288.

Kniggee, K. M., and Scott, D. E. (1970). Structure and function of the median eminence. *Am. J. Anat.* **129**, 223–243.

Knigge, U., and Warberg, J. (1991). The role of histamine in the neuroendocrine regulation of pituitary hormone secretion. *Acta Endocrinol.* **124**, 609–619.

Koenig, J. I., Snow, K., Clark, B. D., Toni, R., Cannon, J. G., Shaw, A. R., Dinarello, C. A., Reichlin, S., Lee, S. I., and Lechan, R. M. (1990). Intrinsic pituitary interleukin-1 beta is induced by bacterial lipopolysaccharide. *Endocrinology*, **126**(6), 3053–3058.

Koenig, R. J., Leonard, J. L., Denator, D., Raparpot, N., Watson, A. Y., and Larsen, P. R. (1984). Regulation of thyroxine 5′-deiodinase activity by 3,5,3′-triiodothyronine in cultured rat anterior pituitary cells. *Endocrinology* **115**, 324–329.

Koenig, R. J. (1998). Thyroid hormone receptor coactivators and corepressors. *Thyroid* **8**, 703–713.

Kohler, C. (1990). Subicular projections to the hypothalamus and brain stem: Some novel aspects revealed by the anterograde *Phaseolus vulgaris* leukoagglutinin (PHA-L) tracing method. *Prog. Brain Res.* **83**, 59–69.

Kohrle, J. (1999). Local activation and inactivation of thyroid hormones: The deiodinase family. *Mol. Cell. Endocrinol.* **25**, 103–119.

Koller, K. J., Wolff, R. S., Warden, M. K. L., and Koller, R. T. (1987). Thyroid hormones regulate levels of thyrotropin-releasing hormone mRAN in the paraventricular nucleus. *Proc. Natl. Acad. Sci. U.S.A.* **84**, 7329–7333.

Kopp, N., Najimi, M., Campier, J., Chigr, F., Charnay, Y., Epelbaum, J., and Jordan, D. (1992). Ontogeny of peptides in human hypothalamus in relation to sudden infant death syndrome (SIDS). *Prog. Brain Res.* **93**, 167–188.

Kordower, J. H., Le, H. K., and Mufson, E. J. (1992). Galanin immunoreactivity in the primate central nervous system. *J. Comp. Neurol.* **319**, 479–500.

Koves, K., Arimura, A., Gorcs, T. J., and Somogy-Vigh, A. (1991). Comparative distribution of pituitary adenylate cyclase activating polypeptide (PACAP) and vasoactive intestinal polypeptide (VIP) in rat forebrain. *Neuroendocrinology* **54**, 159–169.

Koylu, E. O., Couceyro, P. R., Lambert, P. D., and Kuhar, M. J. (1998). Cocaine- and amphetamine-regulated transcript peptide immunohistochemical localization in the rat brain. *J. Comp. Neurol.* **391**, 115–132.

Krenning, E. P., Docter, R., Bernard, H. F., Visser, T. J., and Hennemann, G. (1978). Active transport of triiodothyronine (T3) into isolated rat liver cells. *FEBS Lett.* **91**, 113–116.

Krenning, E., Docter, R., Bernard, B., Visser, T., and Hennemann, G. (1981). Characteristics of active transport of thyroid hormone into rat hepatocytes. *Biochim. Biophys. Acta.* **676**, 314–320.

Krisch, B. (1979). Immunohistochemical results on the distribution of somatostatin in the hypothalamus and in limbic structures of the rat. *J. Histochem. Cytochem.* **27**, 1389–1390.

Kristensen, P., Judge, M. E., Thim, L., Ribel, U., Christjansen, K. N., Wulff, B. S., Clausen, J. T., Jensen, P. B., Madsen, O. D., Vrang, N., Larsen, P. J., and Hastrup, S. (1998). Hypothalamic CART is a new anorectic peptide regulated by leptin. *Nature* **393**, 72–76.

Krulich, L. (1982). Neurotransmitter control of thyrotropin secretion. *Neuroendocrinology* **35**, 139–147.

Krulich, L., Giachetti, A., Marchlewska-Koj, A., Hefco, B., and Jameson, H. E. (1977). On the role of central noradrenergic and dopaminergic system in the regulation of TSH secretion in the rat. *Endocrinology* **100**, 496–505.

Kuchler, K., Richter, K., Trnovsky, J., Egger, R., and Kreil, G. (1990). Two precursors of thyrotropin-releasing hormone from skin of *Xenopus laevis*. *J. Biol. Chem.* **265**, 11731–11733.

Kuhar, M. J., and Vechia, S. E. D. (1999). CART peptides: Novel addiction- and feeding-related neuropeptides. *Trends Neurosci.* **22**, 316–320.

Kusuhara, H., Suzuki, H., Naito, M., Tsuruo, T., and Sugiyama, Y. (1998). Characterization of efflux transport of organic anions in a mouse brain capillary endothelial cell line. *Pharmacology* **285**, 1260–1265.

Krykouli, S. E., Stanley, B. G., and Leibowitz, S. F. (1992). Differential effects of galanin and neuropeptide Y on extracellular norepinephrine levels in the paraventricular hypothalamic nucleus of the rat: A microdialysis study. *Life Sci.* **51**(3), 203–210.

Lachuer, J., Buda, M., and Tappaz, M. (1992). Diffrential time course activation of the brain stem catecholaminergic groups following adrenalectomy. *Neuroendocrinology* **56**, 125–132.

Ladram, A., Bulant, M., Montagne, J. J., and Nicolas, P. (1994). Distribution of TRH potentiating peptide (PS4) and its receptors in rat brain and peripheral tissues. *Biochem. Biophys. Res. Commun.* **200**, 958–965.

Lambert, P. D., Couceyro, P. R., McGirr, K. M., Vechia, S. E. D., Smith, Y., and Kuhar, M. J. (1998). CART peptides in the central control of feeding and interactions with neuropeptide Y. *Synapse* **29**, 293–298.

Langlois, M.-F., Zanger, K., Monden, T., Safer, J. D., Hollenberg, A. N., and Wondisford, F. E. (1997). A unique role of the β-2 thyroid hormone receptor isoform in negative regulation by thyroid hormone. *J. Biol. Chem.* **272**, 24927–24933.

Lapthorn, A. J., Harris, D. C., Littlejohn, A., Lustbader, J. W., Canfield, R. E., Machin, K. J., Morgan, F. J., and Isaacs, N. W. (1994). Crystal structure of human chorionic gonadotropin. *Nature* **369**, 455–461.

Larsen, P. R. (1997). Update on the human iodothyronine selenodeiodinases, the enzymes regulating the activation and inactivation of thyroid hormone. *Biochem. Soc. Trans.* **25**, 588–592.

Lazar, M. A. (1997). Recent progress in understanding thyroid hormone action. *Thyroid Today* **20**(4), 1–9.

Lelbowitz, S. F., Jhanwar-Uniyal, M., Dvorkin, B., and Makman, M. H. (1982). Distribution of alpha-adrenergic, beta adrenergic and dopaminergic receptors in discrete hypothalamic areas of the rat. *Brain Res.* **233**, 97–114.

Lechan, R. M., and Jackson, I. M. D. (1982). Immunohistochemical localization of thyrotropin-releasing hormone in the rat hypothalamus and pituitary. *Endocrinology* **111**, 55–65.

Lechan, R. M., Wu, P., and Jackson, I. M. D. (1986). Immunolocalization of the thyrotropin-releasing hormone prohormone in the rat central nervous system. *Endocrinology* **119**, 1210–1216.

Lechan, R. M., Wu, P., and Jackson, I. M. D. (1987). Immunocytochemical distribution in rat brain of putative peptides derived from thyrotropin-releasing hormone prohormone. *Endocrinology* **121**, 1879–1891.

Lechan, R. M., and Toni, R. (1992). Thyrotropin-releasing hormone neuronal systems in the central nervous system. In "Neuroendocrinology" (C. B. Nemeroff, ed.), pp. 279–330. CRC Press, Boca Raton, Florida.

Lechan, R. M., Nestler, J. L., Jacobson, S., and Reichlin, S. (1980). The hypothalamic tuberoinfundibular system of the rat as demonstrated by horseradish peroxidase (HRP) microiontophoresis. *Brain Res.* **195**, 13–27.

Lechan, R. M., Nestler, J. L., and Jacobson, S. (1982). The tuberoinfundibular system of the rat as demonstrated by immunohistochemical localization of retrogradely transported wheat germ agglutinin (WGA) from the median eminence. *Brain Res.* **243**, 1–15.

Lechan, R. M., Toni, R., Clarke, D. B., Cannon, J. G., Shaw, A. R., Dinarello, C. A., and Reichlin, S. (1990). Immunoreactive interleukin 1-beta localization in the rat forebrain. *Brain Res.* **514**, 135–140.

Lechan, R. M., Qi, Y., Jackson, I. M. D., and Mahdavi, V. (1994). Identification of thyroid hormone receptor isoforms in thyrotropin-releasing hormone neurons of the hypothalamic paraventricular nucleus. *Endocrinology* **135**, 92–100.

Lee, S. L. (1988). Structure of the gene encoding rat thyrotropin releasing hormone. *J. Biol. Chem.* **263**, 16604–16609.

Legradi, G., and Lechan, R. M. (1999). Agouti-related protein containing nerve terminals innervate thyrotropin-releasing hormone neurons in the hypothalamic paraventricular nucleus. *Endocrinology* **140**(8), 3643–3652.

Legradi, G., Shioda, S., and Arimura, A. (1994). Pituitary adenylate cyclase-activating polypeptide-like immunoreactivity in autonomic regulatory areas of the rat medulla oblongata. *Neurosci. Lett.* **176**(2), 193–196.

Legradi, G., and Lechan, R. M. (1998). The arcuate nucleus is the major source of neuropeptide Y-innervation of thyrotropin-releasing hormone neurons in the hypothalamic paraventricular nucleus. *Endocrinology* **139**, 3262–3270.

Legradi, G., Rand, W. M., Hitz, S., Nillni, E. A., Jackson, I. M. D., and Lechan, R. M. (1996). Opiate withdrawal increases proTRH gene expression in the ventrolateral column of the midbrain periaqueductal gray. *Brain Res.* **729**, 10–19.

Legradi, G., Hannibal, J., and Lechan, R. M. (1997a). Association between pituitary adenylate-cyclase-activating polypeptide and thyrotropin-releasing hormone in the rat hypothalamus. *J. Chem. Neuroanat.* **13**, 265–269.

Legradi, G., Emerson, C. H., Ahima, R. S., Flier, J. S., and Lechan, R. M. (1997b). Leptin prevents fasting-induced suppression of prothyrotropin-releasing hormone messenger ribonucleic acid in neurons of the hypothalamic paraventricular nucleus. *Endocrinology* **138**, 2569–2576.

Legrand, J. (1979). Morphogenetic action of thyroid hormones. *Trends Neurosci.* **2**, 234–236.

Leonard, J. L., Kaplan, M. M., Visser, T. J., Silva, J. E., and Larsen, P. R. (1981). Cerebral cortex responds rapidly to thyroid hormones. *Science* **214**, 571–573.

Leonard, J. L., Silva, J. E., Kaplan, M. M., Mellen, S. A., Visser, T. J., and Larsen, P. R. (1984). Acute posttranscriptional regulation of cerebrocortical and pituitaryiodothyronine 5'-deiodinases by thyroid hormone. *Endocrinology* **114**, 998–1004.

Leonard, J. L., Siegrist-Kaiser, C. A., and Zuckerman, C. J. (1990). Regulation of type II iodothyronine 5'-deiodinase by thyroid hormone. *J. Biol. Chem.* **265**, 940–946.

Leranth, C. S., Segura, L. M. G., Palkovits, M., MacLusky, N. J., Shanabrough, M., and Naftolin, F. (1985). The LH-RH-containing neuronal network in the preoptic area of the rat: Demonstration of LH-RH-containing nerve terminals in synaptic contact with LH-RH neurons. *Brain Res.* **345**, 332–336.

Levin, M. C., Sawchenko, P. E., Howe, P. R., Bloom, S. R., and Polak, J. M. (1987). Organization of galanin-immunoreactive inputs to the paraventricular nucleus with special reference to their relationship to catecholaminergic afferents. *J. Comp. Neurol.* **261**(4), 562–582.

Liao, N., Bulant, M., Nicholas, P., Vaudry, H., and Pelletier, F. (1988a). Electron microscope immunocytochemical localization of thyrotropin-releasing hormone (TRH) prohormone in the rat hypothalamus. *Neuropeptides* **11**, 107–110.

Liao, N., Bulant, M., Nicolas, P., Vaudry, H., and Pelletier, G. (1988b). Immunocytochemical distribution of neurons containing a peptide derived from thyrotropin-releasing hormone precursor in the rat brain. *Neurosci. Lett.* **85**, 24–28.

Liao, N., Bulant, M., Nicolas, P., Vaudry, H., and Pelletier, G. (1989). Thyroid hormone regulation of neurons staining for a pro-TRH-derived cryptic peptide sequence in the rat hypothalmic paraventricular nucleus. *Neuroendocrinology* **50**, 217–221.

Liao, N., Bulant, M., Nicolas, P., Vaudry, H., and Pelletier, G. (1991). Anatomical interactions of proopiomelanocortin (POMC)-related peptides, neuropeptide Y(NPY) and dopamine beta-hydroxylase (D beta H) fibers and thyrotropin-releasing hormone (TRH) neurons in the paraventricular nucleus of the rat hypothalamus. *Neuropeptides* **18**, 63–67.

Liao, N., Vaudry, H., and Pelletier, G. (1992). Neuroanatomical connections between corticotropin-releasing factor (CRF) and somatostatin (SRIF) nerve endings and thyrotropin-releasing hormone (TRH) neurons in the paraventricular nucleus of the rat hypothalamus. *Peptides* **13**, 677–680.

Liposits, Z. S., Paull, W. K., Setalo, G., and Vigh, S. (1985). Evidence for local corticotropin releasing factor (CRF)-immunoreactive neuronal circuitries in the paraventricular nucleus of the rat hypothalamus. An electron microscopic immunohistochemical analysis. *Histochemistry* **83**, 5–16.

Liposits, Z. S., Paull, W. K., Wu, P., Jackson, I. M. D., and Lechan, R. M. (1987). Hypophysiotropic thyrotropin releasing hormone (TRH) synthesizing neurons. Ultrastructure, adrenergic innervation and putative transmitter action. *Histochemistry* **88**, 1–10.

Lopez-Nieto, C. E., You, G., Bush, K. T., Barros, E. J., Beier, D. R., and Nigam, S. K. (1997). Molecular cloning and characterization of NKT, a gene product related to the organic cation transporter family that is almost exclusively expressed in the kidney. *J. Biol. Chem.* **272**, 6471–6478.

Lu, D., Willard, D., Patel, I. R., Kadwell, S., Overton, L., Kost, T., Luther, M., Chen, W., Woychik, R. P., Wilkison, W. O., and Cone, R. D. (1994). Agouti protein is an antagonist of the melanocyte-stimulating-hormone receptor. *Nature* **371**, 799–802.

Lumpkin, M. D., Samson, W. K., and McCann, S. M. (1983). Arginine vasopressin releases thyroid stimulating hormone in vitro and in vivo. *Fed. Proc.* **42**, 973 (Abstract).

Luo, L. G., and Jackson, I. M. D. (1998). Glucocorticoids stimulates TRH and c-fos/c-jun co-expression in cultured hypothalamic neurons. *Brain Res.* **791**, 56–62.

Luo, L. G., Bruhn, T. P., and Jackson, I. M. D. (1993). Glucocorticoids stimulates thyrotropin-releasing hormone gene expression in cultured hypothalamic neurons. *Endocrinology* **36**, 4945–4950.

Lyson, K., and McCann, S. M. (1991). The effect of interlukin-6 on pituitary hormone release in vivo and in vitro. *Neuroendocrinology* **54**(3), 262–266.

McCann, S. M. (1991). The effect of interleukin-6 on pituitary hormone release in vivo and in vitro. *Neuroendocrinology* **54**, 262–266.

McCann, S. M., Rettori, V., Milenkovic, L., Jurcovica, J., and Gonzales, M. C. (1990). Role of monokines in control of anterior pituitary hormone release. In "Circulating Regulatory Factors and Neuroendocrine Function" (J. C. Porter and D. Jezova, eds.), pp. 315–329. Plenum, New York.

McGivern, R. F., Rittenhouse, P., Aird, F., Van de Kar, L. D., and Redei, E. (1997). Inhibition of stress-induced neuroendocrine and behavioral responses in the rat by prepro-thyrotropin-releasing hormone 178-199. *J. Neurosci.* **17**, 4886–4894.

McKibbin, P. E., Cotton, S. J., McCarthy, H. D., and Williams, G. (1992). The effect of dexamethasone on neurpeptide Y concentrations in specific hypothalamic regions. *Life Sci.* **51**, 1301–1307.

Maeda, K., and Frohman, L. A. (1978). Dissociation of systemic and central effects of neurotensin on the secretion of growth hormone, prolactin, and thyrotropin. *Endocrinology* **103**, 1903–1909.

Maeda, K., and Frohman, L. A. (1980). Release of somatostatin and thyrotropin-releasing hormone from rat hypothalamic fragments in vitro. *Endocrinology* **106**, 1837–1842.

Magner, J. A. (1990). Thyroid-stimulating hormone: Biosynthesis, cell biology, and bioactivity. *Endocr. Rev.* **11**, 354–385.

Makara, G. B, Palkovits, M., Antoni, F. A., and Kiss, J. Z. (1983). Topography of the somatostatin-immunoreactive fibers to the stalk-median eminence of the rat. *Neuroendocrinology* **37**, 1–8.

Mandel, S. J., Berry, M. J., Kieffer, J. D., Harney, J. W., Warne, R. L., and Larsen, P. R. (1992). Cloning and in vitro expression of the human selenoprotein, type I iodothyronine deiodinase. *J. Clin. Endocrinol. Metab.* **75**, 1133–1139.

Manne, J., Argeson, A. C., and Siracusa, L. D. (1995). Mechanisms for the pleiotropic effects of the agouti gene. *Proc. Natl. Acad. Sci. U.S.A.* **92**, 4721–4724.

Mannisto, P. T. (1983). Central regulation of thyrotropin secretion in rats: Methodological aspects, problems and some progress. *Med. Biol.* **6**, 92–100.

Mannisto, P., and Ranta, T. (1978). Neurotransmitter control of thyrotropin secretion in hypothyroid rats. *Acta. Endocrinol.* **89**, 100–107.

Mannisto, P., Ranta, T., and Tuomisto, J. (1979). Dual action of adrenergic system on the regulation of thyrotropin secretion in the male rat. *Acta. Endocrinol.* **90**, 249–258.

Mannisto, P., Mattia, J., and Kaakkola, S. (1981). Possible involvement of nigrostriatal dopamine system in the inhibition of thyrotrophin secretion in the rat. *Eur. J. Pharmacol.* **76**, 403–409.

Mannisto, P. T., Rauhala, P., Tuominen, R., Tuomisto, R., and Mattial, J. (1984). Dual action of morphine on cold-stimulated thyrotropin secretion in male rats. *Life Sci.* **35**, 1101–1107.

Marley, P. D., Emson, P. C., Hunt, S. P., and Fahrenkrug, J. (1981). A long ascending projection in the rat brain containing vasoactive intestinal polypeptide. *Neurosci. Lett.* **27**, 261–266.

Martin, J. B., Boshans, R., and Reichlin, (1970). Feedback regulation of TSH secretion in rats with hypothalamic lesions. *Endocrinology* **87**, 1032–1040.

Massara, F., Camanni, F., Belforte, L., Vergano, V., and Molinatti, G. M. (1978). Increased thyrotropin secretion induced by sulpiride in man. *Clin. Endocrinol.* **97**, 419–428.

Matre, V., Karlsen, H. E., Wright, M. S., Lundell, I., Fjeldheim, A. K., Gabrielson, O. S., Larhammar, D., and Gautvik, K. M. (1993). Molecular cloning of a functional human thyrotropin-releasing hormone receptor. *Biochem. Biophys. Res. Commun.* **195**, 179–185.

Matre, V., Hovring, P. I., Orstavik, S., Frengen, E., Rian, E., Velickovic, Z., Murray-McIntosh, R. P., and Gautvik, K. M. (1999). Structural and functional organization of the gene encoding the human thyrotropin-releasing hormone receptor. *J. Neurochem.* **72**(1), 40–50.

Mattila, J., and Mannisto, P. (1980). Modification of GABAergic activity and TSH secretion. *Acta. Pharmacol. Toxicol.* **47**, 241–248.

Meister, B., Ceccatelli, S., Hökfelt, T., Anden, N.-E., Anded, M., and Theodorsson, E. (1989). Neurotransmitters, neuropeptides and binding sites in the rat mediobasal hypothalamus; effects of monosodium glutamate (MSG) lesions. *Exp. Brain Res.* **76**, 343–368.

Meister, B., Villar, M. J., Ceccatelli, S., and Hökfelt, T. (1990). Localization of chemical messengers in magnocellular neurons of the hypothalamic supraoptic and paraventricular nuclei: An immunohistochemical study using experimental manipulations. *Neuroscience* **37**, 603–633.

Melander, A., and Sundler, F. (1991). Autonomic nervous control: Adrenergic, cholinergic,and peptidergic regulation. *In* "Werner's and Ingbar's The Thyroid. A Fundamental and Clinical Text" (L. E. Braverman and R. D. Utiger, eds.), 6th Ed., pp. 313–321. Lippincott, Philadelphia.

Melander, A., Ericson, L. E., Liunggren, J.-G., Norberg, K.-A., Persson, B., Sundler, F., Tibblin, S., and Westgren, U. (1974). Sympathetic innervation of the normal human thyroid. *J. Clin. Endocrinol. Metab.* **39**, 713–718.

Melander, A., Ericson, L. E., Sundler, F., and Westgren, U. (1975a). Intrathyroidal amines in the regulation of thyroid activity. *Rev. Physiol. Biochem. Pharmacol.* **73**, 39–71.

Melander, A., Sundler, F., and Westgren, U. (1975b). Sympathetic innervation of the thyroid: Variations with species and age. *Endocrinology* **96**, 102–106.

Mendel, C. M., Weisiger, R. A., Jones, A. L., and Cavalieri, R. R. (1987). Thyroid hormone-binding proteins in plasma facilitate uniform distribution of thyroxine within tissues: A perfused rat liver study. *Endocrinology* **120**, 1742–1749.

Mercer, J. G., Lawrence, C. B., and Atkinson, T. (1996). Hypothalamic NPY and CRF gene expression in the food-deprived Syrian hamster. *Physiol. Behav.* **60**, 121–127.

Merchenthaler, J., Hynes, M. A., Vigh, S., Schally, A. V., and Petrusz, P. (1984). Corticotropin releasing factor (CRF): Origin and course of afferent pathways to the median eminence (ME) of the rat hypothalamus. *Neuroendocrinology* **39**, 296–306.

Merchenthaler, I., and Liposits, Z. S. (1994). Mapping of thyrotropin-releasing hormone (TRH) neuronal systems of rat forerain projecting to the median eminence and the OVLT. Immunocytochemistry combined with retrograde labeling at the light and electron microscopic levels. *Acta. Biol. Hung.* **45**, 361–374.

Merchenthaler, I., Setalo, G., Csontos, C., Petruz, P., Flerko, B., and Negro-Vilar, A. (1989a). Combined retrograde tracing and immunocytochemical identification of luteinizing hormone-releasing hormone- and somatostatin-containing neurons projecting to the median eminence of the rat. *Endocrinology* **125**, 2812–2821.

Merchenthaler, I., Meeker, M., Petrusz, P., and Kizer, J. S. (1989b). Identification and immunocytochemical localization of a new thyrotropin-releasing hormone precursor in rat brain. *Endocrinology* **124**, 1888–1897.

Mezey, E., and Kiss, J. Z. (1985). Vasoactive intestinal peptide-containing neurons in the paraventricular nucleus may participate in regulating prolactin secretion. *Proc. Natl. Acad. Sci. U.S.A.* **82**, 245–247.

Michalkiewicz, M., Huffman, L. J., Coonnor, J. M., and Hedge, G. A. (1989). Alteration in thyroid blood flow induced by varying levels of iodine intake in the rat. *Endocrinology* **125**, 54–60.

Michalkiewicz, M., Huffman, L. J., Dey, M., and Hedge, G. A. (1993). Endogenous neuropeptide Y regulates thyroid blood flow. *Am J. Phsysiol.* **264** (*Endocrinol. Metab.* **27**), E699–E705.

Mihaly, E., Fekete, C. S., Tatro, J. B., Liposits, Z. S., Stopa, E. G., and Lechan, R. M. (2000). Hypophysiotropic thyrotropin-releasing hormone-synthesizing neurons in the human hypothalamus are innervated by neuropeptide Y, agouti-related protein, and alpha-melanocyte-stimulating hormone. *J. Clin. Endocrinol. Metab.* **85**, 2596–2603.

Mitsuma, T., Nogimori, T., and Chaya, M. (1984). Effects of vasoactive intestinal polypeptide on hypothalamic–pituitary–thyroid axis in rats. *Endocr. Exp.* **18**, 93–100.

Mitsuma, T., Nogimori, T., and Hirooka, Y. (1987). Effects of growth hormone-releasing hormone and corticotropin-releasing hormone on the release of thyrotropin-releasing hormone from the rat hypothalamus in vitro. *Exp. Clin. Endocrinol.* **90**, 365–368.

Mizuno, T. M., and Mobbs, C. V. (1999). Hypothalamic agouit-related protein messenger ribonucleic acid is inhibited by leptin and stimulated by fasting. *Endocrinology* **140**, 814–817.

Mizuno, T. M., Kleopoulos, S. P., Bergen, H. T., Roberts, J. L., Priest, C. A., and Mobbs, C. V. (1998). Hypothalamic pro-opiomelanocortin mRNA is reduced by fasting and in ob/ob and db/db mice, but is stimulated by leptin. *Diabetes* **47,** 294–297.

Moga, M. M., and Saper, C. B. (1994). Neuropeptide-immunoreactive neurons projecting to the praventricular hypothalamic nucleus of the rat. *J. Comp. Neurol.* **346,** 137–150.

Monden, T., Wondisford, E. E., and Hollenberg, A. N. (1997). Isolation and characterization of a novel ligand-dependent thyroid hormone receptor-coactivating protein. *J. Biol. Chem.* **272,** 29834–29841.

Montoya, E., Wilber, J. F., and Lorinez. M. (1979). Catecholominergic control of thyrotropin secretion. *J. Lab. Med.* **93,** 887–894.

Moore, R. Y., and Card, J. P. (1984). Noradrenaline-containing neuron systems. *In* "Handbook of Chemical Neuroanatomy" (A. Bjorklund and T. Hokfelt, eds.), Vol. 2, Part 1, pp. 125–156. Elsevier, Amsterdam.

Mori, M., and Yamada, M. (1987). Thyroid hormone regulates the amount of thyrotrophin-releasing hormone in the hypothalamic median eminence. *J. Endocrinol.* **114,** 443–448.

Mori, M., Kobayashi, I., and Wakabayashi, K. (1978). Suppression of serum thyrotropin concentrations following thyroidectomy and cold exposure by passive immunization with antiserum to thyrotropin-releasing hormone in rats. *Metabolism* **27,** 1485–1490.

Morley, J. E. (1981). Neuroendocrine control of thyrotropin secretion. *Endocr. Rev.* **2,** 396–436.

Morley, J. E., Damassa, D. A., Gordon, J., Pekary, A. E., and Hershman, J. M. (1978). Thyroid function and vitamin A deficiency. *Life Sci* **22,** 1901–1906.

Mowbray, J. F., and Peart, W. S. (1960). Effects of noradrenaline and adrenaline on the thyroid. *J. Physiol.* **151,** 261–271.

Mueller, G. P., Simpkins, J., Meites, J., and Moore, K. E. (1976). Differential effects of dopamine agonists and haloperidol on release of prolactin, thyroid stimulating hormone, growth hormone and luteinizing hormone in rats. *Neuroendocrinology* **20,** 121–135.

Muller, E. E., and Nistico, G. (1989). "Brain Messengers and the Pituitary." Academic Press, San Diego.

Murray, H. E., Simonian, S. X., Herbison, A. E., and Gillies, G. E. (1999). Correlation of hypothalamic somatostatin mRNA expression and peptide content with secretion: Sexual dimorphism and differential regulation by gonadal steroids. *J. Neuroendocrinol.* **11,** 27–33.

Myers, R. D., and Lee, T. F. (1984). Neurotensin perfusion of rat hypothalamus: Dissociation of dopamine release from body temperature change. *Neuroscience* **12,** 241–253.

Nagayama, Y., and Rapoport, B. (1992). The thyrotropin receptor 25 years after its discovery: New insight after its molecular cloning. *Mol. Endcrinol.* **6,** 145–156.

Nagayama, Y., Wadsworth, H. L., Russo, D., Chazenbalk, G. D., and Rapoport, B. (1991). Binding domains of stimulatory and inhibitory thyrotropin (TSH) receptor autoantibodies determined with chimeric TSH-lutropin/chorionic gonadotropin receptors. *J. Clin. Invest.* **88,** 336–340.

Nakai, Y., Shioda, S., Ochai, H., Kudo, J., and Hashimoto, A. (1983). Ultrastructural relationship between monoamine- and TRH-containing axons in the rat median eminence as revealed by combined autoradiography and immunocytochemistry in the same tissue section. *Cell Tissue Res.* **230,** 1–14.

Nauta, W. J. H., and Haymaker, W. (1969). Hypothalamic nuclei and fiber connections. *In* "The Hypothalamus" (W. Haymaker, E. Anderson, and W. J. H. Nauta, eds.), pp. 136–209. Thomas, Springfield,

Negro-Vilar, A., Ojeda, S. R., Arimura, A., and McCann, S. M. (1978). Dopamine and norepinephrine stimulate somatostatin release by median eminence fragments in vitro. *Life Sci.* **23,** 1493–1497.

Nemeroff, C. B., Bissette, G., Manberg, P. J., Osbahr III, A. J., Breese, G. R., and Prange, A. J. Jr. (1980). Neurotensin-induced hypothermia: Evidence for an interaction with dopamnergic systems and the hypothalamic–pituitary–thyroid axis. *Brain Res.* **195,** 69–84.

Nichol, K. A., Morey, A., Couzens, M. H., Shine, J., Herzog, H., and Cunningham, A. M. (1999). Conservation of expression of neuropeptide Y5 receptor between human and rat hypothalamus and limbic regions suggest an integral role in central neuroendocrine control. *J. Neurosci.* **19,** 10295–10304.

Nicholson, W. E., and Orth, D. N. (1996). Preprothyrotropin-releasing hormone-(178-199) does not inhibit corticotropin release. *Endocrinology* **137,** 2171–2174.

Nieuwenhuys, R. (1985). "Chemoarchitecture of the Brain." Springer-Verlag, Berlin and Heidelberg.

Niimi, M., Takahara, J., Hashimoto, K., and Kawanishi, K. (1988). Immunohistochemical indentification of corticotropin releasing factor-containing neurons projecting to the stalk-median eminence of the rat. *Peptides* **9,** 589–593.

Nillni, E. A., and Sevarino, K. A. (1999). The biology of pro-thyrotropin-releasing hormone-derived peptides. *Endocr. Rev.* **20,** 599–648.

Nillni, E. A., Sevarino, K. A., and Jackson, I. M. D. (1993). Identification of the thyrotropin-releasing hormone prohormone and its post-translational processing in a transfected AtT20 tumoral cell line. *Endocrinology* **132,** 1260–1270.

Nillni, E. A., Friedman, T. C., Todd, R. B., Birch, N. P., Loh, Y. P., and Jackson, I. M. D. (1995). Pro-thyrotropin-releasing hormone processing by recombinant PC1. *J. Neurochem.* **65**, 2462–2472.

Nillni, E. A., Luo, L. G., Jackson, I. M. D., and McMillan, P. (1996). Identification of the thyrotropin-releasing hormone precursor, its processing products and its coexpression with convertase 1 in primary cultures of hypothalamic neurons. Anatomic distribution of PC1 and PC2. *Endocrinology* **137**, 5651–5661.

Nillni, E. A., Aird, F., Seidah, N. G., Todd, R. B., and Koenig, J. L. (2001). PreproTRH(178–199) and two novel peptides (pFQ7 and pSE14) derived from its processing, which are produced in the paraventricular nucleus of the rat hypothalamus, are regulated during suckling. *Endocrinology* **142**(2), 896–906.

Nishino, J.-I., Suzuki, H., Sugiyama, D., Kitazawa, T., Ito, K., Hannano, M., and Sugiyama, Y. (1999). Transepithelial transport of organic anions across the choroid plexus: Possible involvement of organic anion transporter and multidrug resistance-associated protein. *J. Pharmacol. Exp. Ther.* **290**, 289–294.

Nishiyama, T., Kawano, H., Tsuruo, Y., Maegawa, M., Hisano, S., Adachi, T., Daikoku, S., and Suzuki, M. (1985). Hypothalamic thyrotropin-releasing hormone (TRH)-containing neurons involved in the hypothalamic–hypophysial–thyroid axis. Light microscopic immunocytochemistry. *Brain Res.* **345**, 205–218.

Noe, B., Hagenbuch, B., Stieger, B., and Meier, P. J. (1997). Isolation of a multispecific organic anion and cardiac glycoside transporter from rat brain. *Proc. Natl. Acad. Sci. U.S.A.* **94**, 10346–10350.

Nonidetz, G. F. (1931). Innervation of the thyroid gland. II Origin and course of the thyroid nerves in the dog. *Am. J. Anat.* **48**, 299–329.

Oberste-Berghaus, C., Zanger, K., Hashimoto, K., Cohen, R. N., Hollenberg, A. N., and Wondisford, F. E. (2000). Thyroid hormone-independent interaction between the thyroid hormone receptor β2 amino terminus and coactivators. *J. Biol. Chem.* **275**, 1787–1792.

O'Dowd, B. F., Lee, D. K., Huang, W., Nguyen, T., Cheng, R., Liu, Y., Wang, B., Gershengorn, M. C., and George, S. R. (2000). TRH-R2 exhibits similar binding and acute signaling but distinct regulation and anatomic distribution compared with TRH-R1. *Mol. Endocrinol.* **14**, 183–193.

Ollmann, M. M., Wilson, B. D., Yang, Y. K., Kerns, J. A., Chen, Y., Gantz, I., and Barsh, G. S. (1997). Antagonism of central melanocortin receptors *in vitro* and *in vivo* by agouti-related protein. *Science* **278**, 135–138.

Onate, S. A., Tsai, S. Y., Tsai, M.-J., and O'Malley, B. W. (1995). Sequence and characterization of a coactivator for the steroid hormone receptor superfamily. *Science* **270**, 1354–1357.

Oppenheimer, J. H., and Schwartz, H. L. (1985). Stereospecific transport of triiodothyronine from plasma to cytosol and from cytosol to nucleus in rat liver, kidney, brain and heart. *J. Clin. Invest.* **75**, 147–154.

Ortiga-Carvalho, T. M., Curty, F. H., and Pazos-Moura, C. C. (1995). Acute effect of thyroxine on pituitary neuromedin B content of hypothyroid rats and its correlation with TSH secretion. *Braz. J. Med. Biol. Res.* **28**, 715–719.

Ortiga-Carvalho, T. M., Polak, J., McCann, S., and Pazos-Moura, C. C. (1996). Effect of thyroid hormones on pituitary neuromedin B and possible interaction between thyroid hormones and neuromedin B on thyrotropin secretion. *Regul. Pept.* **14**, 47–53.

Ortiga-Carvalho, T. M., Curty, F. H., Nascimento-Saba, C. C., Moura, E. F., Polak, J., and Pazos-Moura, C. C. (1997). Pituitary neuromedin B content in experimental fasting and diabetes mellitus and correlation with thyrotropin secretion. *Metabolism* **46**, 149–153.

Ottensen, B., Hansen, B., Fahrenkrug, J., and Fuchs, A.-R. (1984). Vasoactive intestinal polypeptide stimulates oxytocine and vasopressin release from the neurohypophysis. *Endocrinology* **115**, 1648–1650.

Palha, J. A., Episkopou, V., Maeda, S., Shimada, K., Gottesman, M. E., and Saraiva, M. J. M. (1994). Thyroid hormone metabolism in a transthyretin-null mouse strain. *J. Biol. Chem.* **269**, 33135–33139.

Palha, J. A., Fernandes, R., deEscobar, G. M., Epistrore, V., Gottesman, M., and Saraiva, M. J. (2000). Transthyretin regulates thyroid hormone levels in the choroid plexus, but not in the brain parenchyma: Study in a transthyretin-null mouse model. *Endocrinology*, **141**, 3267–3272.

Palkovits, M. (1984). Neuropeptides in the hypothalamo–hypophyseal system: Lateral retrochiasmatic area as a common gate for neuronal fibers towards the median eminence. *Peptides* **5**(Suppl.), 35–39.

Palkovits, M., Kobayashi, R. M., Brown, M., and Vale, W. (1980). Changes in hypothalamic, limbic and extrapyramidal somatostatin levels following various hypothalamic transections in rat. *Brain Res.* **195**, 499–505.

Palkovits, M., Eskay, R. L., and Brownstein, M. J. (1982a). Course of thyrotropin-releasing hormone fibers in the median eminence in rats. *Endocrinology* **110**, 1526–1528.

Palkovits, M., Tapia-Arancibia, L., Kordon, C., and Epelbaum, J. (1982b). Somatostatin connections between the hypothalamus and the limbic system in the rat brain. *Brain Res.* **250**, 223–228.

Pang, X.-P., Hershman, J. M., Mirell, C. J., and Pekary, A. E. (1989). Impairment of hypothalamic–pituitary–thyroid function in rats treated with human recombinant tumor necrosis factor-alpha (Cachectin). *Endocrinology* **125**, 76–84.

Pang, X., Letourneau, R., Rozniecki, J. J., Wang, L., and Theoharides, T. C. (1996). Definitive characterization of rat hypothalamic mast cells. *Neuroscience* **73**, 889–902.

Panula, P., Pirvola, U., Auvinen, S., and Airaksinen, M. S. (1989). Histamine-immunoreactive nerve fibers in the rat brain. *Neuroscience* **28**, 585–610.

Pardridge, W. M. (1979). Carrier-mediated transport of thyroid hormones through the rat blood–brain barrier: Primary role of albumin-bound hormone. *Endocrinology* **105**, 605–612.

Parma, J., van Sande, J., Swillens, S., Tonacchera, M., Dumont, J., and Vassart, G. (1995). Somatic mutations causing constitutive activity of the thyrotropin receptor are the major cause of hyperfunctioning thyroid adenomas: Identification of additional mutations activating both the cyclic adenosine $3',5'$-monophosphate and inositol phosphate-Ca^{2+} cascades. *Mol. Endocrinol.* **9**, 725–733.

Pazos-Moura, C. C., Moura, E. G., Rettori, V., Polak, J., and McCann, S. M. (1996). Role of neuromedin B in the in vitro thyrotropin release in response to thyrotropin-releasing hormone from anterior pituitaries of eu-, hypo-, and hyperthyroid rats. *Proc. Soc. Exp. Biol.* **211**, 353–358.

Pekary, A. E., Knoble, M., Garcia, N. H., Bhasin, S., and Hershman, J. M. (1990). Testosterone regulates the secretion of thyrotropin-releasing hormone (TRH) and TRH precursor in rat hypothalamic–pituitary axis. *J. Endocrinol.* **125**, 263–270.

Pelletier, G. (1987). Demonstration of contacts between neurons staining for LHRH in the preoptic area of the rat brain. *Neuroendocrinology* **46**, 457–459.

Pelletier, G., Guy, J., Allen, Y. S., and Polak, J. M. (1984). Electron microscopic immunocytochemical localization of neuropeptide Y (NPY) in the rat brain. *Neuropeptides* **4**, 319–324.

Pennathur, S., Madison, L. D., Kay, T. W., and Jameson, J. L. (1993). Localization of promoter sequences required for thyrotropin-releasing hormone and thyroid hormone responsiveness of the glycoprotein hormone alpha-gene in primary cultures of rat pituitary cells. *Mol. Endocrinol.* **7**, 797–805.

Perez-Juste, G., Garcia-Silva, S., and Aranda, A. (2000). An element in the region responsible for premature termination of transcription mediates repression of c-myc gene expression by thyroid hormone in neuroblastoma cells. *J. Biol. Chem.* **275**, 1307–1314.

Pèrez-Martinez, L., Carrèon-Rodriguez, A., Gonzalez-Alzati, M. E., Morale, C., Chali, J. L., and Joseph-Bravo, P. (1998). Dexamethasone rapidly regulates TRH mRNA levels in hypothalamic cell cultures: Interactions with cAMP pathway. *Neuroendocrinology* **68**, 345–354.

Perlman, J. H., Laakkonen, L., Osman, R., and Gershengorn, M. C. (1994). A model of the thyrotropin-releasing hormone (TRH) receptor binding pocket. *J. Biol. Chem.* **269**, 23383–23386.

Peters, A. Palay, S. L., and Webster H de F. (1970)."The Fine Structure of the Nervous System, The Cells and Their Processes" p. 132. Harper & Row, New York.

Peters, A., Heuer, H., Schomburg, L., De Greef, W. J., Visser, T. J., and Bauer, K. (1997). Thyrotropin-releasing hormone gene expression by anterior pituitary cells in long-term cultures is influenced by the culture conditions and cell-to-cell interactions. *Endocrinology* **138**, 2807–2812.

Petrov, T., Krukoff, T. L., and Jhamandas, J. H. (1993). Branching projections of catecholaminergic brain stem neurons to the paraventricular hypothalamic nucleus and the central nucleus of the amygdala in the rat. *Brain Res.* **609**, 81–92.

Petruz, P., Merchenthaler, I., and Maderdrut, J. L. (1985). Distribution of enkephalin-containing neurons in the central nervous system. *In* "Handbook of Chemical Neuroanatomy, GABA and Neuropeptides" (A. Bjorklund and T. Hokfelt, eds.), Vol. 4, Part 1, pp. 273–334. Elsevier, Amsterdam.

Petty, K. J., Krimkevich, Y. I., and Thomas, D. (1996). A TATA binding protein-associated factor functions as a coactivator for thyroid hormone receptors. *Mol. Endocrinol.* **10**, 1632–1645.

Pietrzyk, Z., Michalkiewicz, M., Huffman, L. J., and Hedge, G. A. (1992). Vasoactive intestinal peptide enhances thyroidal iodide uptake during dietary iodine deficiency. *Endocr. Res.* **18**, 213–228.

Pintar, J. E. (1996). Normal development of the hypothalamic–pituitary–thyroid axis. *In* "Werner and Ingbar's The Thyroid, A Fundamental and Clinical Text" (L. E. Braverman and R. D. Utiger, eds.), 7th Ed., pp. 6–18. Lippincott-Raven, Philadelphia and New York.

Price, J., Grossman, A., Besser, G. M., and Rees, L. H. (1983). Dopaminergic control of the rat thyrotroph. *Neuroendocrinology* **36**, 125–129.

Pu, L. P., Ma, W., Barker, J. L., and Loh, Y. P. (1996). Differential coexpression of genes encoding prothyrotropin-releasing hormone (proTRH) and prohormone convertases (PC1 and PC2) in rat brain neurons: Implications for differential processing of pro-TRH. *Endocrinology* **137**, 1233–1241.

Pu, S., Jain, M. R., Horvath, T. L., Diano, S., Kalra, P. S., and Kalra, S. P. (1999). Interactions between neuropeptide Y and gamma-aminobutyric acid in stimulation of feeding: A morphological and pharmacological analysis. *Endocrinology* **140**, 933–940.

Puigserver, P., Wu, Z., Park, C. W., Graves, R., Wright, M., and Spiegelman, B. M. (1998). A cold-inducible coactivator of nuclear receptors linked to adaptive thermogenesis. *Cell* **92**, 829–839.

Radja, F., Laporte, A.-M., Daval, G., Verge, D., Gozlan, H., and Hamon, M. (1991). Autoradiography of serotonin receptor subtypes in the central nervous system. *Neurochem. Int.* **18**, 1–15.

Ranta, T., Mannisto, P., and Tuomisto, A. J. (1977). Evidence for dopaminergic control of thyrotropin secretion in the rat. *J. Endocrinol.* **72**, 329–335.

Rapaport, B., Refetoff, S., Fang, V. S., and Frisen, H. G. (1973). Suppression of serum thyrotropin (TSH) by L-dopa in chronic hypothyroidism: Interrelationships in the regulation of TSH and prolactin secretion. *J. Clin. Endocrinol. Metab.* **36**, 256–262.

Rapaport, B., Chazenbalk, G. D., Jaume, J. C., and McLachlan, S. M. (1998). The thyrotropin (TSH)-releasing hormone receptor: Interaction with TSH and autoantibodies. *Endocr. Rev.* **19**, 673–716.

Rapp, J. P., and Pyunn, L. L. (1974). A sex difference in plamsa thyroxine and thyroid stimulating hormone in rats. *Proc. Soc. Exp. Biol. Med.* **146**, 1021–1023.

Recant, L., and Riggs, D. S. (1952). Thyroid function in nephrosis. *J. Clin. Invest.* **31**, 789–797.

Redei, E., Hilderbrand, H., and Aird, F. (1995). Corticotropin release inhibiting factor is encoded within preproTRH. *Endocrinology* **136**, 1813–1816.

Refetoff, S. (1994). Resistance to thyroid hormone: An historical overview. *Thyroid* **4**, 345–349.

Regina, A., Koman, A., Piciotti, M., Hafny, B. E., Center, M. S., Berrgmann, R., Couraud, P.-O., and Roux, F. (1998). Mrp1 multidrug resistance-associated protein and P-glycoprotein expression in rat brain microvessel endothelial cells. *J. Neurochem.* **71**, 705–715.

Reichlin, S. (1966). Control of thyrotropic hormone secretion. *In* "Neuroendocrinology" (L. Martini and W. F. Ganong, eds.), pp. 445–536. Academic Press, New York.

Reichlin, S. (1986a). Neural functions of TRH. *Acta Endocrinol.* **112**(Suppl. 276), 21–33.

Reichlin, S. (1986b). Neuroendocrine control of thyrotropin secretion. *In* "Werner's, The Thyroid" (S. H. Ingbar and L. E. Braveman, eds.), 5th Ed., p. 241. Lippincott, Philadephia.

Reichlin, S. (1989). TRH: Historical aspects. *Ann. N.Y. Acad. Sci.* **553**, 1–6.

Reichlin, S. (1993). Neuroendocrine–immune interactions. *N. Engl. J. Med.* **329**, 1246–1253.

Reichlin, S., and Glaser, R. J. (1958). Thyroid function in experimental streptococcal pneumonia in the rat. *J. Exp. Med.* **107**, 219–235.

Renaud, L. P. (1978). Neurophysiological organization of the endocrine hypothalamus. *In* "The Hypothalamus" (S. Reichlin, R. J. Baldessarini, and J. B. Martin, eds.), pp. 269–301. Raven, New York.

Rettori, V., Milenkovic, L., Aguila, M. C., and McCann, S. M. (1990). Physiologically significant effect of neuropeptide Y to suppress growth hormone release by stimulating somatostatin discharge. *Endocrinology* **126**, 2296–2301.

Reymond, M. J., Donda, A., and Lemarchand-Beraud, T. (1989). Neuroendocrine aspects of aging: Experimental data. *Horm. Res.* **31**, 32–38.

Richardson, S. B., and Twente, S. (1986). Inhibition of rat hypothalamic somatostatin released by somatostatin. Evidence for somatostatin ultrashort loop feedback. *Endocrinology* **118**, 2076–2082.

Riskind, P. N., Kolodny, J. M., and Larsen, P. R. (1987). The regional hypothalamic distribution of type II 5'-monodeiodinase in euthyroid and hypothyroid rats. *Brain Res.* **420**, 194–198.

Robbins, J., and Rall, J. E. (1957). The interaction of thyroid hormones and protein in biological fluids. *Recent Prog. Horm. Res.* **13**, 161–208.

Roberts, G. W., Woodhams, P. L., Bryant, M. G., Crow, T. J., Bloom, S. R., and Polak, J. M. (1980). VIP in the rat brain: Evidence for a major pathway linking the amygdala and hypothalamus via the stria terminalis. *Histochemistry* **65**, 103–119.

Roland, B. L., and Sawchenko, P. E. (1993). Local distribution and origins of some GABAergic projections to the paraventricular and supraoptic nuclei in the hypothalamus of the rat. *J. Comp. Neurol.* **332**, 123–143.

Rondeel, J. M., de Greef, W. J., Klootwijk, W., and Visser, T. J. (1992a). Effects of hypothyroidism on hypothalamic release of thyrotropin-releasing hormone in rats. *Endocrinology* **130**, 651–665.

Rondeel, J. M., Heide, R., de Greef, W. J., van Toor, H., van Haasteren, G. A., Klootwijk, W., and Visser, T. J. (1992b). Effect of starvation and subsequent refeeding on thyroid function and release of hypothalamic thyrotropin-releasing hormone. *Neuroendocrinology* **56**, 348–353.

Rondeel, J. M. M., Klootwijk, W., Linkels, E., van Haasteren, G. A. C., de Greef, W. J., and Visser, T. J., (1995). Regulation of thyrotropin-releasing hormone in the posterior pituitary. *Neuroendocrinology* **61**, 421–429.

Rossi, M., Kim, M. S., Small, M. C. J., Edwards, C. M. B., Sunter, D., Abusnana, S., Goldstone, A. P., Russell, S. H., Stanley, S. A., Smith, D. M., Yagaloff, K., Ghatei, M. A., and Bloom, S. R. (1998). A C-terminal fragment of Agouti-related protein increases feeding and antagonizes the effect of alpha-melanocyte stimulating hormone *in vivo. Endocrinology* **139**, 4428–4431.

Rostene, W. H. (1984). Neurobiological and neuroendocrine functions of the vasoactive intestinal peptide (VIP). *Prog. Neurobiol.* **22**, 103–129.

Rouille, Y., Duguay, S. J., Lund, K., Furuta, M., Gong, Q., Lipkind, G., Oliva, A. A., Jr., Chan, S. J., and Steiner, D. F. (1995). Proteolytic processing mechanisms in the biosynthesis of neuroendocrine peptides: The subtilisin-like proprotein convertases. *Front. Neuroendocrinol.* **16**, 332–361.

Roussel, J. P., Hollande, F., Bulant, M., and Astier, H. (1991). A prepro-TRH connecting peptide (prepro-TRH 160–169) potentiates TRH-induced TSH release from rat perifused pituitaries by stimulating dihydropyridine-and omega-conotoxin-sensitive Ca^{2+} channels. *Neuroendocrinology* **54**, 559–565.

Royaux, I. E., Suzuki, K., Mori, A., Katoh, R., Everett, L. A., Kohn, L. D., and Green, E. D. (2000). Pendrin, the protein encoded by the Pendred syndrome gene (PDS), is an apical porter of iodide in the thyroid and is regulated by thyroglobulin in FRTL-5 cells. *Endocrinology* **141**(2), 839–845.

Saberi, M., and Utiger, R. D. (1975). Augmentation of thyrotropin responses to thyrotropin-releasing hormone following small decreases in serum thyroid hormone concentrations. *J. Clin. Endocrinol. Metab.* **40**, 432–441.

Safer, J. D., Cohen, R. N., Hollenberg, A. N., and Wondisford, F. E. (1998). Defective release of corepressor by hinge mutants of the thyroid hormone receptor found in patients with resistance to thyroid hormone. *J. Biol. Chem.* **273**, 30175–30182.

Saiardi, A., Falasca, P., and Civitareate, D. (1994). The thyroid hormone inhibits the thyrotropin receptor promoter activity: Evidence for a short loop regulation. *Biochem. Biophys. Res. Commun.* **205**, 230–237.

Saito, H., Masuda, S., and Inui, K. (1996). Cloning and functional characterization of a novel rat organic anion transporter mediating basolateral uptake of methotrexate in the kidney. *J. Biol. Chem.* **271**, 20710–20725.

Sakanaka, M., Shiosaka, S., Takatsuki, K., Inagaki, S., Takagi, H., Senba, E., Kawai, Y., Matsuzaki, T., and Tohyama, M. (1981). Experimental immunohistochemical studies on the amygdalofugal peptidergic (substance P and somatostatin) fibers in the stria terminalis of the rat. *Brain Res.* **221**(2), 231–242.

Sakata, T., Yoshimatsu, H., and Kurokawa, M. (1997). Hypothalamic neuronal histamine: Implications of its homeostatic control of energy metabolism. *Nutrition* **13**, 403–411.

Salvatore, D., Low, S. C., Berry, M., Maria, A. L., Harney, J. W., Croteau, W., St. Germain, D. L., and Larsen, P. R. (1995). Type 3 iodothyronine deiodinase: Cloning, in vitro expression, and functional analysis of the placental selenoenzyme. *J. Clin. Invest.* **96**, 2421–2430.

Samuels, M. H., Kramer, P., Wilson, D., and Sexton, G. (1994). Effects of naloxone infusions on pulsatile thyrotropin secretion. *J. Clin. Endocrinol. Metab.* **78**, 1249–1252.

Sanno, N., *et al.* (1997). Immunohistochemical expression of retinoid X receptor isoforms in human pituitaries and pituitary adenomas. *Neuroendocrinology* **65**, 73–79.

Sasaki, S., Lesoon-Wood, L., Dey, A., Kuwata, T., Weintraub, B. D., Humphrey, G., Yang, W.-M., Seto, E., Yen, P. M., Howard, B. H., and Ozato, K. (1999). Ligand-induced recruitment of a histone deacetylase in the negative-feedback regulation of the thyrotorpin β gene. *EMBO J.* **18**, 5389–5398.

Satoh, T., Yamada, M., Monden, T., Iizuka, M., and Mori, M. (1992). Cloning of the mouse hypothalamic preprothyrotropin-releasing hormone (TRH) cDNA and tissue distribution of its mRNA. *Mol. Brain Res.* **14**, 131–135.

Satoh, T., Yamada, M., Iwasaki, T., and Mori, M. (1996). Negative regulation of the gene for preprothyrotropin-releasing hormone from the mouse by thyroid hormone requires additional factors in conjunction with thyroid receptors. *J. Biol. Chem.* **271**, 27919–27926.

Satoh, T., Ishizuka, T., Monden, T., Shibusawa, N., Hashida, T., Kishi, M., Yamada, M., and Mori, M. (1999). Regulation of the mouse preprothyrotropin-releasing hormone gene by retinoic acid receptor. *Endocrinology* **140**, 5004–5013.

Sawchenko, P. E., and Pfeiffer, S. W. (1988). Ultrastructural localization of neuropeptide Y and galanin immunoreactivity in the paraventricular nucleus of the hypothalamus in the rat. *Brain Res.* **474**, 231–245.

Sawchenko, P. E., and Swanson, L. W. (1983). The organization of forebrain afferents to the paraventricular and supraoptic nuclei of the rat. *J. Comp. Neurol.* **218**, 121–144.

Sawchenko, P. E., and Swanson, L. W. (1982). The organization of noradrenergic pathways from the brain stem to the paraventricular and supraoptic nuclei in the rat. *Brain Res. Rev.* **4**, 275–325.

Sawchenko, P. E., Swanson, L. W., and Joseph, S. A. (1982). The distribution and cells of origin of ACTH (1-39)-stained varicosities in the paraventricular and supraoptic nuclei. *Brain Res.* **232**, 365–374.

Sawchenko, P. E., Swanson, L. W., Steinbush, H. W. M., and Verhofstad, A. A. J. (1983). The distribution and cells of origin of serotoninergic inputs to the paraventricular and supraoptic nuclei of the rat. *Brain Res.* **277**, 355–3360.

Sawchenko, P. E., Swanson, L. W., Grzanna, R., Howe, P. R. C., Bloom, S. R., and Polak, J. M. (1985). Colocalization of neuropeptide Y immunoreactivity in brain stem catecholaminergic neurons that project to the paraventricular nucleus of the hypothalamus. *J. Comp. Neurol.* **241**, 138–153.

Scanlon, M. F., Weightman, D. R., Shale, D. J., Mora, B., Heath, M., Snow, M. H., Alewis, M., and Hall, R. (1979). Dopamine is a physiological regulator of thyrotropin (TSH) secretion in normal men. *Clin. Endocrinol.* **10**, 7–15.

Scanlon, M. F., Weetman, A. P., and Lewis, M., et al. (1980). Dopaminergic modulation of circadian thyrotropin rhythms and thyroid hormone levels in euthyroid subjects. *J. Clin. Endocrinol.Metab.* **51**, 1251–1256.

Scanlon, M. F., Chan, V., Health, M., Pourmand, M., Rodriguez-Anao, M. D., Weightman, D. R., Lewis, M., and Hall, R. (1981). Dopaminergic control of thyrotropin, alpha-subunit, thyrotropin beta-subunit, and prolactin in euthyroidism and hypothyroidism. Dissociated responses to dopamine receptor blockade with metoclopramide in hypothyroid subjects. *J. Clin. Endocrinol. Metab.* **53**, 360–365.

Scapagnini, U., Annunziato, L., Di Renzo, G. F., Schettini, G., and Preziosi, P. (1977). Role of tuberoinfundibular dopaminergic neurons in TRH-TSH secretion. *Adv. Biochem. Psychopharmacol.* **16**, 369–375.

Scarborough, D. E., Lee, S. L., Dinarello, C. A., and Reichlin, S. (1989). Interleukin-1 beta stimulates somatostatin biosynthesis in primary culture of fetal rat brain. *Endocrinology* **124**, 549–551.

Schaner, P., Todd, R. B., Seidah, N. G., and Nillni, E. A. (1997). Processing of prothyrotropin releasing hormone by the family of prohormone convertases. *J. Biol. Chem.* **272**, 19958–19968.

Scharrer, E. (1928). Die Lichtempfindlichkeit blinder Elritzen (Untersuchungen uber das Zweischenhirn der r. I). *Z. Vgl. Physiol.* **7**, 1–38.

Scharrer, E., and Scharrer, B. (1940). Secretory cells within the hypothalamus. *Res. Publ. Assoc. Res. Nerv. Ment. Dis.* **20**, 170–194.

Scharrer, E., and Scharrer, B. (1954). Hormones produced by neurosecretory cells. *Recent Prog. Horm. Res.* **10**, 183–232.

Schauder, B., Schomburg, L., Kohrle, J., and Bauer, K. (1994). Cloning of a cDNA encoding an ectoenzyme that degrades thyrotropin-releasing hormone. *Proc. Natl. Acad. Sci. U.S.A.* **91**, 9534–9538.

Schettini, G., Quattrone, A., DiRenzo, G., Lombardi, G., and Preziosi, P. (1979). Effect of 6-hydroxydopamine treatment on TSH secretion in basal and cold-stimulated conditions in the rat. *Eur. J. Pharmacol.* **56**, 153–157.

Schobitz, B., Voorhuis, A. M., and DeKloet, E. R. (1992). Localization of interleukin 6 mRNA and interleukin 6 receptor mRNA in rat brain. *Neurosci. Lett.* **136**, 189–192.

Schomburg, L., and Bauer, K. (1995). Thyroid hormones rapidly and stringently regulate the messenger RNA levels of the thyrotropin-releasing hormone (TRH) receptor and the TRH-degrading ectoenzyme. *Endocrinology* **136**, 3480–3485.

Schomburg, L., Turwitt, S., Prescher, G., Lohmann, D., Horsthemke, B., and Bauer, K. (1999). Human TRH-degrading ectoenzyme cDNA cloning, functional expression, genomic structure and chromosomal assignment. *Eur. J. Biochem.* **265**, 415–422.

Schreiber, G., Southwell, B. R., and Richardson, S. J. (1995). Hormone delivery systems to the brain—transthyretin. *Exp. Clin. Endocrinol.* **103**, 75–80.

Schwartz, J. C., Garbar, M., and Pollard, H. (1986). Histaminertic transmission in the brain. *In* "Handbook of Physiology, The Nervous System, Section I: Neurophysiology" (V. B. Mountcastle, F. E. Bloom, and S. R. Geiger, eds.), Vol. 4, pp. 257–316. American Physiological Society, Bethesda, Maryland.

Segal, J., and Ingbar, S. H. (1982). Specific binding sites for triiodothyronine in the plasma membrane of rat thymocytes: Correlation biochemical responses. *J. Clin. Invest.* **70**, 919–926.

Segerson, T. P., Kauer, J., Wolfe, H. C., Mobtaker, H., Wu, P., Jackson, I. M. D., and Lechan, R. M., (1987). Thyroid hormone regulates TRH biosynthesis in the paraventricular nucleus of the rat hypothalamus. *Science* **238**, 78–80.

Sharp, B., Morley, J. E., Carlson, H. E., Gordon, J., Briggs, J., Melmed, S., and Hershman, M. (1981). The role of opiates and endogenous opiod peptides in the regulation of rat TSH secretion. *Brain Res.* **219**, 335–334.

Sheppard, M. C., and Sheennan, K. I. (1983). The effect of thyroid hormones *in vitro* and *in vivo* on hypothalamic neurotensin release and content. *Endocrinology* **112**, 1996–1998.

Sheppard, M. C., Kronheim, S., and Pimstone, B. L. (1979). Effect of substance P, neurotensin and the enkephalins on somatostatin release from the rat hypothalamus *in vitro*. *J. Neurochem.* **32**, 647–649.

Sheppard, M. C., Askew, R. D., Shennan, K. I. J., Franks, S., and Ramsden, D. B. (1983). Neurotensin regulation of TSH secretion in the rat. *Biochem. Biophys. Res. Commun.* **113**, 248–254.

Sherman, S. I., Gopal, J., Haugen, B. R., Chiu, A. C., Whaley, K., Nowlakha, P., and Duvic, M. (1999). Central hypothyroidism associated with retinoid X receptor-selective ligands. *N. Engl. J. Med.* **340**, 1075–1079.

Shibusawa, N., Yamada, M., Hirato, J., Monden, T., Satoh, T., and Mori, M. (2000). Requirement of thyrotropin-releasing hormone for the postnatal functions of pituitary thyrotrophs: Ontogeny study of congenital tertiary hypothyroidism in mice. *Mol. Endocrinol.* **14**, 137–146.

Shimatsu, A., Kato, Y., Matsushita, N., Katakami, H., Yanaihara, H., and Imura, H. (1982). Effect of glucagon, neurotensin, and vasoactive intestinal polypeptide on somatostatin release from perfused rat hypothalamus. *Endocrinology* **110**, 2113–2117.

Shioda, S., and Naki, Y. (1993). Medullary synaptic inputs to hytrotropin-releasing hormone (TRH)-containing neurons in the hypothalamus: An ultrastructural study combining WGA-HRP anterograde tracing with TRH immunocytochemistry. *Brain Res.* **625**, 9–15.

Shioda, S., Nakai, Y., Sato, A., Sunayama, S., and Shimoda, Y. (1986). Electron-microscopic cytochemistry of the catecholaminergic innervation of TRH neurons in the rat hypothalamus. *Cell Tissue Res.* **245**, 247–252.

Shiosaka, S., Takatsuki, K., Sakanaka, M., Inagaki, S., Takagi, H., Senba, E., Kawai, Y., Iida, H., Minigawa, H., Hara, Y., Matsuzaki, T., and Toyama, M. (1981). Ontogeny of somatostatin-containing neuron systems of the rat: Immunocytochemical analysis. II. Forebrain and diencephalon. *J. Comp. Neurol.* **204**, 211–224.

Sho, K., Okajiima, F., Majid, M. A., and Kondo, Y. (1991). Riciprocal modulation of thyrotropin actions by P1-purinergic agonists in FRTL-5 thyroid cells. *J. Biol. Chem.* **266**, 12180–12184.

Shupnick, M. A., Chin, W. W., Habener, J. F., and Ridgway, E. C. (1985). Transcriptional regulation of the thyrotropin subunit genes by thyroid hormone. *J. Biol. Chem.* **260**, 2900–2903.

Shupnick, M. A., Ardisson, L. J., Meskell, M. J., Bornstein, J., and Ridgway, E. C. (1986). Triiodothyronine (T3) regulation of thyrotropin subunit gene transcription is proportional to T3 nuclear receptor occupancy. *Endocrinology* **118**(1), 367–371.

Shupnick, M. A., Rosenzweig, B. A., and Showers, M. O. (1990). Interactions of thyrotropin-releasing hormone, phorbol ester, and forskolin-sensitive regions of the rat thyrotropin β gene. *Mol. Endocrinol.* **4**, 829–836.

Shutter, J. R., Graham, M., Kinsey, A. C., Scully, S., Luthy, R., and Stark, K. L. (1997). Hypothalamic expression of ART, a novel gene related to agouti, is up-regulated in obese and diabetic mutant mice. *Genes Dev.* **11**, 593–602.

Silva, J. E., and Leonard, J. L. (1985). Regulation of rat cerebrocortical and adenohypophyseal type II 5′-deiodinase by thyroxine, triiodothyronine, and reverse triiodothyronine. *Endocrinology* **116**, 1627–1635.

Skowsky, W. R., and Kikuchi, T. A. (1978). The role of vasopressin the impaired water excretion of myxedema. *Am. J. Med.* **64**, 613–621.

Smith. Y., Parent, A., Kerkerian, L., and Pelletier, G. (1985). Distribution of neuropeptide Y immunoreactivity in the basal forebrain and upper brain stem of the Squirrel monkey (*Saimri sciureus*). *J. Comp. Neurol.* **236**, 71–89.

Snyder, P. J., and Utiger, R. D. (1973). Repetitive administration of thyrotropin-releasing hormone results in small elevations of serum thyroid hormones and in marked inhibition of thyrotropin response. *J. Clin. Invest.* **52**, 2305–2312.

Sodeberg, U. (1958). Short-term reaction in the thyroid gland revealed by continuous measurement of blood flow, rate of uptake of radioactive iodine and rate of release of labelled hormones. *Acta Physiol. Scand.* **42**(Suppl. 147), 1–112.

Sodeberg, U. (1959). Temporal characteristics of thyroid activity. *Physiol Rev.* **39**, 777–810.

Soprano, D. R., Herbert, J., Soprano, K. J., Schon, E. A., and Goodman, D. S. (1985). Demonstration of transthyretin mRNA in the brain and other extrahepatic tissues in the rat. *J. Biol. Chem.* **200**, 11793–11798.

Southwell, B. R., Duan, W., Alcorn, D., Brack, C., Richardson, S. J., Khorle, J., and Shreiber, G. (1993). Thyroxine transport to the brain: Role of protein synthesis by the choroid plexus. *Endocrinology* **133**, 2116–2126.

Spiess, J., Villarreal, J., and Vale, W. (1981). Isolation and sequence analysis of a smoatostatin-like polypeptide from ovine hypothalamus. *Biochemistry* **20**, 1982–1988.

Spitzweg, C., Heufelder, A. E., and Morris, J. C. (2000). Thyroid iodine transport. *Thyroid* **10**, 321–330.

Steinbush, H. W. M. (1984). Serotonin-immunoreactive neurons and their projections in the CNS. In "Handbook of Chemical Neuroanatomy. Classical Transmitters and Transmitter Receptors in the CNS" (A. Bjorklund, T. Hökfelt, and M. J. Kuhar, eds.), Vol. 3, Part 2, pp. 68–125. Elsevier, Amsterdam.

Steinbush, H. W. M., and Mulder, A. H. (1984). Immunohistochemical localization of histamine in neurons and mast cells in the rat brain. In "Handbook of Chemical Neuroanatomy. Classical Transmitters and Transmitter Receptors in the CNS" (A. Bjorklund, T. Hökfelt, and M. J. Kuhar, eds.), Vol. 3, Part 2, pp. 126–140. Elsevier, Amsterdam.

Steinfelder, H. J., and Wondisford, F. E. (1997). Thyrotropin (TSH)β-subunit gene expression—an example for the complex regulation of pituitary hormone genes. *Exp. Clin. Endocrinol. Diabetes* **105**, 196–203.

Steinfelder, H. J., Hauser, P., Nakayama, Y., Radovick, S., McClasky, J. H., Taylor, T., Weintraub, B. D., and Wondisford, F. E. (1991). Thyrotropin-releasing hormone regulation of human TSHβ expression: Role of a pituitary-specific transcription factor (Pit-1/GHF-1) and potential interaction with a thyroid hormone-inhibitory element. *Proc. Natl. Acad. Sci. U.S.A.* **88**, 3130–3134.

Steinfelder, H. J., Radovick, S., and Wondisford, F. E. (1992). Hormonal regulation of the thyrotropin β-subunit gene by phosphorylation of Pit-1. *Proc. Natl. Acad. Sci. U.S.A.* **89**, 5942–5945.

Stevenin, B., and Lee, S. L. (1995). Hormonal regulation of the thyrotropin releasing hormone (TRH) gene. *Endocrinologist* **5**, 286–296.

St. Germain, D. L., Schwartzman, R., Croteau, W., Kanamori, A., Wang, Z., Brown, D. D., and Galton, V. A. (1994). A thyroid hormone regulated gene in *Xenopus laevis* encodes a type II iodothyronine-5-deiodinase. *Proc. Natl. Acad. Sci. U.S.A.* **91**, 11282.

Straub, T. E., Frech, G. C., Joho, R. H., and Gershiengorn, M. C. (1990). Expression cloning of a cDNA encoding the mouse pituitary thyrotropin-releasing hormone receptor. *Proc. Natl. Acad. Sci. U.S.A.* **87**, 9514–9618.

Stricker, E. M., and Zigmond, M. J. (1986). Brain monoamines, homeostasis, and adaptive behavior. *In* "Handbook of Physiology, The Nervous System, Section I: Neurophysiology" (V. B. Mountcastle, F. E. Bloom, and S. R. Geiger, eds.), Vol 4, pp. 677–700. American Physiological Society, Bethesda, Maryland.

Suen, C.-S., and Wilk, S. (1989). Regulation of thyrotropin releasing hormone degrading enzymes in rat brain and pituitary by L-3,5,3′-triiodothyronine. *J. Neurochem.* **52**, 884–888.

Sugawra, A., Yen, P. M., Qi, Y., Lechan, R. M., and Chin, W. W. (1995). Isoform-specific retinoid-X receptor (RXR) antibodies detect differential expression of RXR proteins in the pituitary gland. *Endocrinology* **136**, 1766–1774.

Sun, P. D., and Davis, D. R. (1995). The cystine-knot growth factor superfamily. *Annu. Rev. Biophys. Biomol. Struct.* **24**, 269–291.

Swanson, L. W. (1987). *In* "The Hypothalamus" (A. Bjorklund, T. Hökfelt, and L. W. Swanson, eds.), Part 1, pp. 1–124. Handbook of Chemical Neuroanatomy, Volume 5, Integrated Systems in the CNS, Elseveir, Amsterdam.

Swanson, L. W., and Kuypers, H. G. J. M. (1980). The paraventricular nucleus of the hypotalamus cytoarchitectonic subdivisions and organization of projections to the pituitary, dorsal vagal complex, and spinal cord as demonstrated by retrograde fluorescence double-labeling methods. *J. Comp. Neurol.* **192**, 555–570.

Swanson, L. W., and Sawchenko, P. E. (1983). Hypothalamic integration: Organization of the paraventricular and supraoptic nuclei. *Annu. Rev. Neurosci.* **6**, 269–324.

Swanson, L. W., Sawchenko, P. E., and Lind, R. S. (1986). Regulation of multiple peptides in CRF parvocellular neurosecretory neurons: Implications for the stress response. *Prog. Brain Res.* **68**, 169–190.

Szabo, M., and Frohman, L. A. (1977). Suppression of cold-stimulated thyrotropin secretion by antiserum to thyrotropin-releasing hormone. *Endocrinology* **101**, 1023–1033.

Tagami, T., Madison, L. D., Nagaya, T., and Jameson, J. L. (1997). Nuclear receptor corepressors activate rather than suppress basal transcription of genes that are negatively regulated by thyroid hormone. *Mol. Cell. Biol.* **17**, 2642–2648.

Tagami, T., Gu, W.-X., Peairs, P. T., West, B. L., and Jameson, J. L. (1998). A novel natural mutation in the thyroid hormone receptor defines a dual functional domain that exchanges nuclear receptor corepressors and coactivators. *Mol. Endocrinol.* **12**, 1888–1902.

Tagami, T., Park, Y., and Jameson, J. L. (1999). Mechanisms that mediate negative regulation of the thyroid-stimulating hormone α gene by the thyroid hormone receptor. *J. Biol. Chem.* **274**, 22345–22353.

Takeshita, A., Cardona, G. R., Koibuchi, N., Suen, C. S., and Chin, W. W. (1997). TRAM-1, a novel 160 kDa thyroid hormone receptor activator molecule, exhibits distinct properties from steroid receptor coactivator-1. *J. Biol. Chem.* **272**, 27628–27634.

Tapia-Arancibia, L., and Astier, H. (1983). Opiate inhibition of K^+ induced TRH release from superfused mediobasal hypothalamus in rats. *Neuroendocrinology* **37**, 166–168.

Tapia-Arancibia, L., Arancibia, S., and Astier, H. (1985). Evidence for alpha 1-adrenergic stimulatory control of in vitro release of immunoreactive thyrotropin-releasing hormone from rat median eminence: In vivo corroboration. *Endocrinology* **116**, 2314–2319.

Taylor, T., and Weintraub, B. D. (1989). Altered thyrotropin (TSH) carbohydrate structures in hypothalamic hypothyroidism created by paraventricular nuclear lesions are corrected by *in vivo* TSH-releasing hormone administration. *Endocrinology* **125**, 2198–2203.

Ter Horst, G. J., and Luiten, P. G. (1987). *Phaseolus vulgaris* leuco-agglutinin tracing of intrahypothalamic connections of the lateral, ventromedial, dorsomedial and paraventricular hypothalamic nuclei in the rat. *Brain Res. Bull.* **18**, 191–203.

Terry, L. C. (1986). Regulation of thyrotropin secretion by central epinephrine system, *Neuroendocrinology* **42**, 102–108.

Terry, L. C., Rostad, O. P., and Martin, J. B. (1980). The release of biologically and immunologically reactive somatostatin from perifused hypothalamic fragments. *Endocrinology* **100**, 794–800.

Theoharides, T. C., Spanos, C., Pang, X., Alferes, L., Ligris, K., Letourneau, R., Rozniecki, J. J., Webster, E., and Chrousos, G. P. (1995). Stress-induced intracranial mast cell degranulation: A corticotropin-releasing hormone-mediated effect. *Endocrinology* **136**, 5745–5750.

Thliveris, J. A., and Currie, R. W. (1980). Observations on the hypothalamic–hypophysial portal vasculature in the developing human fetus. *Am. J. Anat.* **157**, 441–444.

Thompson, P., Jr., Burman, K. D., Wright, F. D., Potter, M. W., and Wartofsky, L. (1982). Iodothyronine levels in human cerebrospinal fluid. *J. Clin. Endocrinol. Metab.* **54**, 653–655.

Thompson, R. H., Canteras, N. S., and Swanson, L. W. (1996). Organization of projections from the dorsomedial nucleus of the hypothalamus: A PHA-L study in the rat. *J. Comp. Neurol.* **376**, 143–173.

Toni, R., and Lechan, R. M. (1990). 1-Naphthol pyronin B as a novel substrate for silver intensification: Application to light and electron microscopic immunocytochemistry of neuroendocrine systems. *J. Histochem. Cytochem.* **38**, 1209–1214.

Toni, R., and Lechan, R. M. (1993). Neuroendocrine regulation of thyrotropin-releasing hormone (TRH) in the tuberoinfundibular system. *J. Endocrinol. Invest.* **16**, 715–753.

Toni, R., Jackson, I. M. D., and Lechan, R. M. (1990a). Neuropeptide-Y-immunoreactive innervation of thyrotropin-releasing hormone-synthesizing neurons in the rat hypothalamic paraventricular nucleus. *Endocrinology* **26**, 2444–2453.

Toni, R., Jackson, I. M. D., and Lechan, R. M. (1990b). Thyrotropin-releasing hormone-immunoreactive innervation of thyrotropin-releasing hormone-tuberoinfundibular neurons in rat hypothalamus: Anatomical basis to suggest ultrashort feedback regulation. *Neuroendocrinology* **52**, 422–428.

Toni, R., Kakucska, I., Mosca, S., Marrama, P., and Lechan, R. M. (1992). Hypothyroidism increases vasoactive intestinal polypeptide (VIP) immunoreactivity and gene expression in the rat hypothalamic paraventricular nucleus. *Endocrinology* **131**, 976–978.

Toni, R., Mosca, S., Lechan, R. M. N., and Vezzadini, P. (1994). Role of forebrain VIP in the neuroendocrine pathophysiology of SIADH in hypothyroidism. *Front. Endocrinol.* **9**, 71–76.

Toni, R., Mosca, S., Ruggeri, F., Valmori, A., Orlandi, G., Toni, G., Lechan, R. M., and Vezzadini, P. (1995). Effect of hypothyroidism on vasoactive intestinal polypeptide-immunoreactive neurons in forebrain-neurohypophysial nuclei of the rat brain. *Brain Res.* **682**, 101–115.

Tu, H. M., Kim, S.-W., Salvatore, D., Bartha, T., Legradi, G., Larsen, P. R., and Lechan, R. M. (1997). Regional distribution of type 2 thyroxine deiodinase messenger ribonucleic acid in rat hypothalamus and pituitary and its regulation by thyroid hormone. *Endocrinolgy* **138**, 3359–3368.

Tu, H., Legradi, G., Bartha, T., Salvatore, D., Lechan, R. M., and Larsen, P. R. (1999). Regional expression of the type 3 iodothyronine deiodinase messenger ribonucleic acid in the rat central nervous system and its regulation by thyroid hormone. *Endocrinology* **140**, 784–790.

Tuominen, R. K., Mattila, J., and Mannisto, P. T. (1983). Inhibition of the TSH secretion by histamine in male rats. *Acta Endocrinol.* **103**, 88–94.

Tuominen, R. K., Mannisto, P. T., and Mattila, J. (1985). Studies on the site and mechanism of the inhibitory action of intracerebral histamine on the cold stimulated thyrotropin secretion in male rats. *Brain Res.* **343**, 329–335.

Tuomisto, J., Ranta, T., Mannisto, P., Saarinen, A., and Leppalioto, J. (1975). Neurotransmitter control of thyrotropin secretion in the rat. *Eur. J. Pharmacol.* **30**(2), 221–229.

Uribe, R. M., Redondo, J. L., Charli, J.-L., and Joseph-Bravo, P. (1993). Suckling and cold stress rapidly and transiently increase TRH mRNA in the paraventricular nucleus. *Neuroendocrinology* **58**, 140–145.

Vale, W., Brazeau, P., Rivier, C., Brown, M., Boss, B., Rivier, J., Burgus, R., Ling, N., and Guillemin, R. (1975). Somatostatin. *Recent Prog. Horm. Res.* **31**, 365–397.

Valentijn, K., Bunel, D. T., Liao, N., Pelletier, G., and Vaudry, H. (1991). Release of pro-thyrotropin-releasing hormone connecting peptides Ps4 and Ps5 from perifused rat hypothalamic slices. *Neuroscience* **44**, 223–233.

Valentijn, K., Vandenbulcke, F., Piek, E., Beauvillain, J. C., and Vaudry, H. (1998). Distribution, cellular localization, and ontogeny of preprothyrotropin-releasing hormone-(160-169) (Ps4)-binding sites in rat pituitary. *Endocrinology* **139**, 1306–1313.

Van den Pol, A. N. (1982). The magnocellular and parvocellular paraventricular nucleus of rat: Intrinsic organization. *J. Comp. Neurol.* **206**, 317–345.

Van Haasteren, G. A., Linkels, E., Klootwijk, W., van Toor, H., Rondeel, J. M., Themmen, A. P., de Jong, F. H., Valentijn, K., Vaudry, H., and Bauer, K. (1995). Stravation-induced changes in hypothalamic content of prothyrotropin-releasing hormone (proTRH) mRNA and the hypothalamic release of proTRH-derived peptides: Role of the adrenal gland. *J. Endocrinol.* **145**, 143–153.

Vargas, M. A., Joseph-Bravo, P., and Charli, J. L. (1994). Thyrotropin-releasing hormone downregulates pyroglutamyl peptidase II activity in adenohypophyseal cells. *Neuroendocrinology* **60**, 323–330.

Vassart, G., and Dumont, J. E. (1992). The thyrotropin receptor and the regulation of thyrocyte function and growth. *Endocr. Rev.* **13**, 596–611.

Vijayan, E., and McCann, S. M. (1978). Effects of intraventricular injection of gamma-aminobutyric acid (GABA) on plasma growth hormone and thyrotropin in conscious ovariectomized rats. *Endocrinology* **103**, 1888–1893.

Vijayan, E., Carraway, R., Leeman, S. E., and McCann, S. M. (1994). Physiological significance of neurotensin in pituitary glycoprotein hormone release as revealed by *in vivo* and *in vitro* studies with neurotensin antiserum. *Neuroendocrinology* **60**, 157–164.

Vjivian, E., Krulich, L., and McCann, S. M. (1978). Catecholaminergic regulation of TSH and growth hormone release in ovariectomized and ovariectomized, steroid-primed rats. *Neuroendocrinology* **26**, 174–185.

Wada, H., Inagaki, N., Yamatodani, A., and Watanabe, T. (1991). Is the histaminergic neurons system a regulatory center for whole-brain activity? *Trends Neurosci.* **14**, 415–418.

Wagner, C. K., Eaton, M. J., Moore, K. E., and Lookingland, K. J. (1995). Efferent projections from the region of the medial zona incerta containing A13 dopaminergic neurons: A PHA-L anterograde tract-tracing study in the rat. *Brain Res.* **677**, 229–237.

Wagner, R. L., Apriletti, J. W., McGrath, M. E., West, B. L., Baxter, J. D., and Fletterick, R. J. (1995). A structural role for hormone in the thyroid hormone receptor. *Nature* **378**, 690–697.

Wahlestedt, C., Hakanson, R., Vaz, C. A., and Zukowska-Grojec, Z. (1990). Norepinephrine and neuropeptide Y: Vasoconstrictor cooperation *in vivo* and *in vitro*. *Am. J. Physiol.* **258** (*Regulatory Integrative Comp. Physiol.*) **27**, R736–R742.

Wakabayashi, I., Miyazawa, Y., Kanda, M., Miki, N., Demura, H., and Shizume, K. (1997). Stimulation of immunoreactive somatostatin release from hypothalamic synaptosomes by high K^+ and dopamine. *Endocrinol. Jpn.* **25**, 601–604.

Watts, A. G., and Swanson, L. W. (1987). Efferent projections of the suprachiasmatic nucleus. II. Studies using retrograde transport of fluorescent dyes and simultaneous peptide immunohistochemistry in the rat. *J. Comp. Neurol.* **258**, 230–252.

Weigand, S. J., and Price, J. L. (1980). The cells of the afferent fibers to the median eminence in the rat. *J. Comp. Neurol.* **192**, 1–19.

Weintraub, B., Gesundheit, N., Taylor, T., and Gyves, P. W. (1989). Effect of TRH and TSH glycosylation and biological action. *Ann. N. Y. Acad. Sci.* **553**, 205–213.

Weisner, B., and Roethig, H.-J. (1983). The concentration of prealbumin in cerebrospinal fluid, indicator of CSF circulation disorders. *Eur. Neurol.* **22**, 96–105.

Weiss, R. E., Xu, J., Ning, G., Pohlenz, J., O'Malley, B. W., and Refetoff, S. (1999). Mice deficient in the steroid receptor co-activator 1 (SRC-1) are resistant to thyroid hormone. *EMBO J.* **18**, 1900–1904.

Weitzman, R. E., Firemark, H. M., Glatz, T. H., and Fisher, D. (1979). Thyrotropin-releasing hormone stimulates release of arginine vasopressin and oxytocin in vivo. *Endocrinology* **104**, 904–907.

Wetzel, H., Wiesner, J., Hiemke, C., and Benkert, O. (1994). Acute antagonism of dopamine D2-like receptors by amisulpride: Effects on hormone secretion in healthy volunteers. *J. Psychiatr. Res.* **28**, 461–473.

White, B. D., Dean, R. G., Edwards, G. L., and Martin, R. J. (1994). Type II corticosteroids receptor stimulation increases NPY gene expression in basomedial hypothalamus of rats. *Am. J. Physiol.* **266**, R1523–R1529.

White, J. D., Olchovsky, D., Kershaw, M., and Berelowitz, M. (1990). Increased hypothalamic content of preproneuropeptide-Y messenger ribonucleic acid in streptozotocin-diabetic rats. *Endocrinology* **126**, 223–227.

Wilber, J. F., Banerji, A., Prasad, C., and Mori, M. (1981). Alterations in hypothalamic–pituitary–thyroid regulation produced by diabetes mellitus. *Life Sci.* **28**, 1757–1763.

Wilber, J. F., and Xu, A. H. (1998). The thyrotropin-releasing hormone gene 1998: Cloning, characterization, and transcriptional regulation in the central nervous system, heart, and testis. *Thyroid* **10**, 897–901.

Winters, A. J., Eskay, R. L., and Porter, J. C. (1974). Concentration and distribution of TRH and LRH in the human fetal brain. *J. Clin. Endocrinol. Metab.* **39**, 960–963.

Witkin, J. S., and Silverman, A. J. (1985). Synaptology of luteinizing hormone-releasing hormone neurons in rat preoptic area. *Peptides* **6**, 263–271.

Wondisford, F. E., Steinfelder, H. J., Nations, M., and Radovick, S. (1993). AP-1 antagonizes thyroid hormone receptor action on the thyrotropin β-subunit gene. *J. Biol. Chem.* **268**, 2749–2754.

Wrutniak, C., Rochard, P., Casas, F., Fraysse, A., Charrier, J., and Cabello, G. (1998). Physiological importance of the T3 mitochondrial pathway. *Ann. N.Y. Acad. Sci.* **839**, 93–100.

Wu, P., and Jackson, I. M. D. (1988). Post-translational processing of thyrotropin-releasing hormone precursor in rat brain: Identification of 3 novel peptides derived from pro-TRH. *Brain Res.* **456**, 22–28.

Wu, P., Lechan, R. M., and Jackson, I. M. D. (1987). Identification and characterization of thyrotropin-releasing hormone precursor peptides in rat brain. *Endocrinology* **121**, 108–115.

Yamada, T., and Greer, M. A. (1959). Studies on the mechanism of hypothalamic control of thyrotropin secretion: Effect of thyroxine injection into the hypothalamus or the pituitary on thyroid hormone release. *Endocrinology* **64**, 559–566.

Yamada, M., and Wilber, J. F. (1990). Reciprocal regulation of preprothyrotropin-releasing hormone (TRH) mRNA in the rat anterior hypothalamus by thyroid hormone: Dissociation from TRH concentrations during hypothyroidism. *Neuropeptides* **15**, 49–53.

Yamada, M., Rogers, D., and Wilber, J. F. (1989). Exogenous triiodothyronine lowers thyrotropin-releasing hormone concentration in the specific hypothalamic nucleus (paraventricular) involved in thyrotropin regulation and also in posterior nucleus. *Neuroendocrinology* **50**, 560–563.

Yamada, M., Radovick, S., Wondisford, F. E., Nakayama, Y., Weintraub, B. D., and Wilber, J. F. (1990). Cloning and structure of human genomic DNA and hypothalamic cDNA encoding human preprothyrotropin-releasing hormone. *Mol. Endocrinol.* **4**, 551–556.

Yamada, M., Monden, T., Satoh, T., Izuka, M., Murakami, M., Iriuchijima, T., and Mori, M. (1992a). Differential regulation of thyrotropin-releasing hormone receptor mRNA levels by thyroid hormone in vivo and in vitro (GH3 cells). *Biochem. Biophys. Res. Commun.* **184**, 367–372.

Yamada, M., Satoh, T., Monden, T., Murakami, M., Iriuchijima, T., Wilber, J. F., and Mori, M. (1992b). Influence of hypothyroidism on TRH concentrations and preproTRH mRNA levels in rat hypothalamus: A simple and reliable method to detect preproTRH mRNA. *Neuroendocrinology* **55**, 317–320.

Yamada, M., Saga, Y., Shibusawa, N., Hirato, J., Murakami, M., Iwasaki, T., Hashimoto, K., Satoh, T., Wakabayashi, K., Taketo, M. M., and Mori, M. (1997). Tertiary hypothyroidism and hyperglycemia in mice with targeted disruption of the thyrotropin-releasing hormone gene. *Proc. Natl. Acad. Sci. U.S.A.* **94**, 10862–10867.

Yamaguchi, M., Iriuchijima, T., Michimata, T., and Mori, M. (1991). Glucose affects the release of thyrotropin-releasing hormone from the rat hypothalamus. *Neuroendocrinology* **53**, 423–427.

Yamashita, H., Kannan, H., and Ueta, Y. (1989). Involvement of caudal ventrolateral medulla neurons in mediating viscero-receptive information to the hypothalamic paraventricular nucleus. The central neural organization of cardiovascular control. *Prog. Brain Res.* **81**, 293–302.

Yang, H., and Tache, Y. (1994). Prepro-TRH-(160–169) potentiates gastric acid secretion stimulated by TRH microinjected into the dorsal motor nucleus of the vagus. *Neurosci. Lett.* **174**, 43–50.

Yang, J., and Tashjian, A. H., Jr. (1993). Transcriptional regulation by dexamethasone of endogenous thyrotropin-releasing hormone receptor messenger ribonucleic acid in rat pituitary GH4C1 cells. *Endocrinology* **133**, 487–490.

Yen, P. M., Darling, D. S., Carter, R. L., Forgione, M., Umeda, P. K., and Chin, W. W. (1992). Triiodothyronine (T3) decreases binding to DNA by T3-receptor homodimers but not receptor–auxiliary protein heterodimers. *J. Biol. Chem.* **267**, 3565–3568.

Young III, W. S., and Kuhar, M. J. (1980). Noradrenergic alpha-1 and alpha-2 receptors: Light microscopic autoradiographic localization. *Proc. Natl. Acad. Sci. U.S.A.* **77**, 1696–1700.

Yu, R., and Hinkle, P. M. (1997). Desensitization of thyrotorpin-releasing hormone receptor-mediated responses involves multiple steps. *J. Biol. Chem.* **272**, 28301–28307.

Yu, R., and Hinkle, P. M. (1998). Signal transduction, desensitization, and recovery of responses to thyrotropin-releasing hormone after inhibition of receptor internalization. *Mol. Endocrinol.* **12**, 737–749.

Zakrzewska, K. E., Cusin, I., Stricker-Krongrad, A., Boss, O., Ricquier, D., Jeanrenaud, B., and Rohner-Jeanrenaud, F. (1999). Induction of obesity and hyperleptinemia by central glucocorticoid infusion in the rat. *Diabetes* **48**, 365–370.

Zhang, M., Tong, K. P. T., Fremont, V., Chen, J., Marayan, P., Puett, D., Weintraub, B. D., and Szkudlinski, M. W. (2000). The extracellular domain suppresses constitutive activity of the transmembrane domain of the human TSH receptor: Implications for hormone–receptor interaction and antagonist design. *Endocrinology* **141**, 3514–3517.

Zhanisi, M., Messo, E., Mottta, M., and Martini, L. (1987). Ultrashort feedback control of luteinizing hormone-releasing hormone secretion in vitro. *Endocrinology* **121**, 2199–2204.

Zhang, X.-K., Wills, K. W., Husmann, M., Hermann, T., and Pfahl, M. (1991). Novel pathway for thyroid hormone receptor actions through interactions with Jun and Fos oncogene activation. *Mol. Cell. Biol.* **11**, 6016–6025.

Zheng, W., Blaner, W. S., and Zhao, Q. (1999). Inhibition by lead of production and secretion of transthyretin in the choroid plexus: Its relation to thyroxine transport at blood–CSF barrier. *Toxicol. Appl. Pharmacol.* **155**, 24–31.

Zoeller, R. T., Wolff, R. S., and Koller, K. J. (1988). Thyroid hormone regulation of messenger ribonucleic acid encoding thyrotropin (TSH)-releasing hormone is independent of the pituitary and TSH. *Mol. Endocrinol.* **2**, 248–252.

Zoeller, R. T., Kabeer, N., and Albers, E. (1990). Cold exposure elevates cellular levels of messenger ribonucleic acid encoding thyrotropin-releasing hormone in paraventricular nucleus despite elevated levels of thyroid hormones. *Endocrinology* **127**, 2955–2962.

21

Thyroid Hormone, Brain, and Behavior

Michael Bauer and Peter C. Whybrow

Neuropsychiatric Institute and Hospital
Department of Psychiatry and Biobehavioral Sciences
University of California at Los Angeles
Los Angeles, California 90024

I. INTRODUCTION TO THE THYROID SYSTEM AND BEHAVIOR

A. Historical Perspective

The association between thyroid function and behavior was first noticed early in the nineteenth century. Hyperfunction of the thyroid gland was first described by Parry in 1825, who attributed the observed symptoms to a prior frightening experience suffered by the patient. In 1835, Graves described the syndrome named after him and suggested a relation between the thyroid gland and the syndrome globus hystericus, but it was not until the end of the nineteenth century that a thyrotoxic syndrome of endocrine origin was clearly distinguished from the group of neurosis. In the 1880s, behavioral changes in hypothyroid patients had been noted, culminating in a report in 1888 from the Clinical Society of London describing a variety of mental disturbances. Over subsequent decades, systematic studies revealed that disorders of the thyroid gland are frequently associated with mental disturbances (Whybrow and Bauer, 2000a,b). The most common psychiatric symptoms associated with hypothyroidism are depression and cognitive dysfunction. In severe forms of hypothyroidism (myxedema), psychotic and delusional symptoms may occur and the syndrome may mimic melancholic depression and dementia (Treadway et al., 1967).

During the twentieth century, interest in the relation between thyroid function and mental disorders, in particular mood disorders, grew significantly. During this time, the understanding of brain function was expanding rapidly with the identification of the role of neurotransmitters in controlling behavior and increasing knowledge of neurotransmitter metabolism and the complexity of neuronal interactions. In addition, the release of drugs to alter neurotransmitter function was revolutionizing psychiatric treatment. Given the apparent clinical relationship between thyroid function and behavior, early attention focused on the role of thyroid hormones in the pathophysiology of psychiatric disorders.

A causative role of hypothyroidism in psychopathology was demonstrated in 1949 by Asher in a case series describing that thyroid hormone deficiency may lead to depression and psychosis (myxedematous madness) and be reversed by the administration of desiccated thyroid. Later, the therapeutic effects of synthetic thyroid hormones alone and in combination with traditional psychotropic drugs were studied repeatedly in the treatment of mood disorders. In the 1960s, thyroid enhancement of the effects of tricyclic antidepressants (TCA) was discovered (Prange et al., 1969). Continued studies of the function of the hypothalamic-pituitary-thyroid (HPT) system and neuronal interactions led to the hypothesis that thyroid hormones play an important role in modulating catecholamine neurotransmission

(Whybrow and Prange, 1981). This hypothesis has since been modified to extend the modulating influence of thyroid hormone to other neurotransmitters and to intracellular mechanisms.

In this chapter we review some of the clinically relevant associations among the thyroid axis, mental functions, and the neuronal systems that are putatively involved in the regulation and modulation of mood.

B. Organization and Regulation of the Hypothalamic-Pituitary-Thyroid System

Thefunctionally interrelated HPT system is a typical endocrine system with a hierarchic organization. Thyrotropin-releasing hormone (TRH) is a hypothalamic tripeptide synthesized in the paraventricular nucleus (PVN) and released from the median eminence into the primary plexus of the portal venous system to thus reach the secondary plexus adjacent to the anterior pituitary sinusoids (Grant et al., 1972; Reichlin, 1998). Its synthesis and release are regulated by afferent influences from the limbic forebrain, where TRH also functions as a neurohormone or modulator of neuronal functioning. TRH release is stimulated centrally by α-noradrenergic and dopaminergic pathways and inhibited by a negative feedback effect of circulating triiodothyronine (T_3) and thyroxine (T_4). Somatostatin-containing axons also contribute to the negative regulation of TRH synthesis (Morley, 1981; Mason et al., 1995; Thorner et al., 1998; Scanlon and Toft, 2000).

In the pituitary, TRH binds to membrane receptors and induces the production of thyroid-stimulating hormone (TSH). After release into the general circulation, TSH binds to a specific TSH receptor (TSH-R) on the thyroid cell membrane, activating both the G-protein adenylylcyclase-cyclic adenosine monophosphate (cAMP) and the phospholipase C signaling systems (Morley, 1981; Reichlin, 1998). The activity of the thyroid gland is predominantly regulated by the concentration of TSH. In the absence of pituitary function, hypothyroidism occurs. Thus, the regulation of thyroid function in healthy individuals is to a large extent determined by the factors that regulate the synthesis and secretion of TSH (Scanlon and Toft, 2000).

The thyroid gland is the largest endocrine organ in the human body. In healthy humans, the thyroid gland produces predominantly the pro-hormone T_4, together with a small amount of the bioactive hormone T_3. These two hormones have traditionally been referred to as thyroid hormones (Chopra and Sabatino, 2000). TSH stimulates and regulates the production of the thyroid hormones, synthesized from the incorporation of iodide into thyroglobulin. T_4, the major secretion product of the thyroid gland, is converted to its biologically active metabolite, T_3, by widely distributed enzymes called iodothyronine 5′-monodeiodinases (deiodinases). Thus, T_4 is the precursor for the more potent hormone, T_3. After their release into the general circulation, thyroid hormones are necessary for the regulation of various metabolic functions in all body tissues throughout the life span. In addition, T_3 and T_4 exert feedback on the thyroid economy at pituitary and hypothalamic levels (Larsen et al., 1998).

C. Developmental and Metabolic Effects of Thyroid Hormones

The effects of thyroid hormones can be ascribed to two categories of biological response: (1) effects on cellular differentiation and development, and (2) effects on metabolic pathways (Bernal and Nunez, 1995; Larsen et al., 1998). Thyroid hormones play a critical role in the regulation of metabolism and in various processes that underlie the maturation and differentiation of the human brain, affecting such diverse events as neuronal development and integration, glial cell proliferation, myelination, and the synthesis of key enzymes required for neurotransmitter synthesis (Porterfield and Hendrich, 1993; Bernal and Nunez, 1995). Some of the most prominent effects of thyroid hormone occur during fetal development and in early childhood. In humans, the developmental role of the thyroid hormones is underscored by the syndrome cretinism (Porterfield and Hendrich, 1993). Delayed growth curves are characteristic of hypothyroidism during childhood, however, growth is restored rapidly after the institution of treatment (Dussault and Ruel, 1987). In adults, the primary effects of thyroid hormones are manifested by alterations in metabolism. Depending on whether they are present at elevated or reduced levels, the thyroid hormones have a wide range of effects in humans that are evident at many different levels of organization; these effects range from behavioral changes, growth effects, changes in cardiac output, gastrointestinal function and tissue oxygen consumption. In addition, thyroid hormones also change the synthesis and degradation rates of a variety of other growth factors and hormones, such that many of its effects emerge as secondary influences on other endocrine pathways (Larsen et al., 1998; Smallridge, 2000). The clinical features of hypothyroidism and hyperthyroidism emphasize the pleiotropic effects of thyroid hormones on many different pathways and target organs, including the brain.

D. Molecular and Cellular Effects of Thyroid Hormones in the Brain

Despite an accepted body of knowledge on the essential role of thyroid hormones on the maturation and differentiation of the brain, and in disregard of the clinical and therapeutic observations in association with affective illness, the action of thyroid hormones in central nervous system (CNS) function in adults has not been widely acknowledged or a focus of study by endocrinologists. This lack of interest seems to have originated in the 1950s and 1960s, when early physiological studies suggested that oxygen consumption in the mature human brain did not change with changing thyroid status (Sokoloff et al., 1953; Sensenbach et al., 1954; O'Brien and Harris, 1968). Thus, in contrast to our understanding of the thyroid hormone's critically important role in the development of the CNS, little has been known about the function and actions of thyroid hormones in the mature mammalian brain until recently (Anderson et al., 2000). However, with improved methods in basic science, there are now several lines of evidence suggesting that thyroid hormones affect mature brain function (Henley and Koehnle, 1997) (Table 1).

1. Thyroid Economy of the Brain

From studies in animals, it is well established that the brain's thyroid economy is tightly regulated and largely independent of peripheral metabolic shifts in thyroid

TABLE 1
Molecular and Cellular Sites of Action of Thyroid Hormones in the Adult Mammalian Brain

Site of action	Effects of thyroid hormones
Nucleus/genome	⇒ Binding to nuclear thyroid hormone receptors (TR)
	⇒ T_3-TR complex binds to DNA hormone-response elements (thyroid hormone–response elements, TRE)
	⇒ Genetic loci responsive to thyroid hormone
	Growth hormone (GH)
	RC3/neurogranin
	Brain-derived neurotrophic factor (BDNF)
	Neurotrophin 3
	Corticotropin-releasing hormone (CRH)
	Thyrotropin-releasing hormone (TRH)
	Angiotensinogen (AOG)
	Vasoactive intestinal peptide (VIP)
	Cerebral glucose transporter one (GLUT-1)
Synapse	⇒ Selective uptake of T_3 into synaptosomes
	⇒ Inhibition of GABA uptake into synaptosomes
	⇒ Enhancement of depolarization-induced Ca^{2+} uptake into synapse
Receptors	Receptor up- and down-regulation with change in thyroid status
	Serotonin receptors (5-HT_{1A}, 5-HT_2)
	Catecholaminergic receptors (α_2- and β-adrenergic)
Postreceptor sites	⇒ Influence on intracellular signaling pathways
	G-protein (G_i, G_0) synthesis and activity
	Adenylate cyclase activity

function (Dratman *et al.*, 1983). In contrast to most peripheral tissues, which uptake T_3 directly from the blood, the brain appears to regulate its interstitial levels of T_3 by local deiodination of T_4 (Crantz *et al.*, 1982). Thus, the brain is essentially dependent on the uptake of T_4 from the circulation. Subsequent local enzymatic deiodination of T_4 is the major source of nuclear T_3 in the cerebral cortex (Leonard and Koehrle, 2000). Studies in rats have shown that more than 70% of the T_3 that is bound to intranuclear receptors in the brain is locally derived from T_4 by deiodination (Crantz *et al.*, 1982).

The process of deiodination by which T_4 is metabolized to potent iodothyronines has been demonstrated to be different in the adult brain than in peripheral tissues. Specifically, the type II (D2) and type III (D3) deiodinases catalyze these metabolic processes in spatially distinct patterns in the CNS and appear to be segregated into specific cell types (St. Germain and Galton, 1997). D2 is expressed primarily in the brain and anterior pituitary gland where it metabolizes T_4 to T_3. The activity of D2 in anatomically distinct regions of the brain varies widely, with the highest levels found in cortical areas and lesser amounts in the midbrain, pons, hypothalamus and brain stem (van Doorn *et al.*, 1985). In the rat brain, D2 is expressed in neurons, in particular in nerve terminals, although astrocytes may be stimulated to express D2 by intracellular cAMP levels (Leonard, 1988).

2. Genomic and Extranuclear Effects

One of the most important findings supporting the view that the adult brain is a site of action of thyroid hormones was the presence of nuclear receptors in the adult rat brain (Oppenheimer *et al.*, 1974). Nuclear receptors for T_3 (the thyroid hormone with the highest biological activity) are widely distributed in the adult rat brain, with higher densities of nuclear T_3 receptors in phylogenetically younger brain regions—the amygdala and hippocampus—and low densities in the brain stem and cerebellum (Schwartz and Oppenheimer, 1978; Ruel *et al.*, 1985). The nuclear thyroid hormone receptors (TRs) are members of a large superfamily that includes receptors for steroid hormones, vitamin D, and retinoic acid (Evans, 1988). The T_3-receptor complex interacts with specific sequences in DNA regulatory regions, known as thyroid hormone response elements, and modifies the expression of target genes (Brent, 1994; Anderson *et al.*, 2000).

Molecular studies have shown that the adult brain has various genetic loci that are responsive to thyroid hormones (Köhrle, 2000). Among the most extensively studied loci is RT3/neurogranin, a brain-specific gene encoding a protein kinase C substrate that binds calmodulin and is located in dendritic spines and forebrain neurons (Bernal *et al.*, 1992); in these studies, adult-onset hypothyroidism led to a decrease of RC3/neurogranin, an effect that was reversible with T_4 treatment (Iniguez *et al.*, 1991). Thyroid hormone also modulates glucose transport processes across the blood–brain barrier (BBB) (Mooradian, 1990) and in astrocytes (Roeder *et al.*, 1988) and may alter the expression of the glucose transporter one (GLUT-1) gene, the principal isoform responsible for glucose transport across the BBB (Pardrige *et al.*, 1990). Furthermore, the effects of thyroid hormones on CNS gene expression have been demonstrated for various other neuroactive peptides—TRH (Segerson *et al.*, 1987), corticotropin-releasing hormone (CRH) (Ceccatelli *et al.*, 1992), brain-derived neurotrophic factor, nerve growth factor and neurotrophin 3 (Giordano *et al.*, 1992; Alvarez-Dolado *et al.*, 1994), vasoactive intestinal peptide (VIP) (Giardino *et al.*, 1994), and angiotensinogen (Hong-Brown and Deschepper, 1992). However, although molecular studies clearly indicate that thyroid hormones actively regulate a broad spectrum of genes in the adult brain, its significance is unknown.

In addition to the T_3 effects that are mediated through nuclear receptors, there appears to be one action of T_4 in the brain that is independent of nuclear mechanisms, the regulation of D2. It has been proposed that T_4 acts to maintain actin polymerization, which is required for the enzyme activity of D2 (Oppenheimer and Schwartz, 1997).

In summary, evidence has accumulated in the past decade that the mammalian adult brain is also responsive to thyroid hormone after the critical period of brain development, which occurs in the rat before postnatal days 15–20, and that thyroid hormones may also have genomic and nongenomic mechanisms of action in the adult mammalian brain. However, the physiological importance of the effects of thyroid hormones in the adult brain is not well understood (Mason *et al.*,

1993; Dratman and Gordon, 1996; Martin et al., 1996; Henley and Koehnle, 1997).

II. NEUROPSYCHIATRIC AND BEHAVIORAL MANIFESTATIONS IN DISORDERS OF THE THYROID GLAND

As stated earlier, virtually all individuals with clinical evidence of thyroid dysfunction have mental disturbances that usually remit with the correction of thyroid status, confirming the critical involvement of the HPT system in modulating behavior (Whybrow, 1995). Thus, thyroid dysfunctions may be of particular relevance for the study of the pathophysiology of mental disorders and behavioral dysfunction. In the following chapters we review (1) the psychiatric and behavioral manifestations in subjects with hyperthyroidism (thyrotoxicosis) and hypothyroidism and (2) the behavioral effects of changes in thyroid status and thyroid axis hormones, including TRH in rodents.

A. Psychiatric and Behavioral Aspects of Thyrotoxicosis

Thyrotoxicosis is the clinical syndrome of hypermetabolism that results when the serum concentrations of free thyroxine (fT_4), free triiodothyronine (fT_3), or both are increased. Subsequently, the secretion of TSH is suppressed, resulting in decreased serum TSH concentrations. The term hyperthyroidism is used to mean sustained increases in thyroid hormone biosynthesis and secretion by the thyroid gland (Braverman and Utiger, 2000a). The clinical manifestations of an excess availability of thyroid hormones are numerous and found in all systems of the body. Symptoms include weight loss, tachycardia, heat intolerance, tremor, fatigue, muscle weakness and wasting, warm skin, and palpitations (Larsen et al., 1998). Graves' disease is the most frequent cause of hyperthyroidism and is associated with a diffuse toxic goiter and exopthalmos. Graves disease is an autoimmune thyroid disease (AITD) that occurs most frequently in women ages 20–40 years. Patients with AITD show immune reactivity, both antibodies and cell-mediated immunity, directed predominantly at three thyroid autoantigens, thyroglobulin (Tg), thyroid peroxidase (TPO) and the TSH receptor (Marcocci and Chiovato, 2000). Less frequent causes of hyperthyroidism are toxic multinodular goiter and excessive replenishment in hypothyroidism (Larsen et al., 1998).

1. Neuropsychiatric Signs and Symptoms in Hyperthyroidism

There are a variety of neuropsychiatric symptoms of thyrotoxicosis, although overt psychiatric illness is rare in those without a concurrent diagnosis or family history of psychiatric disorders (Whybrow and Bauer, 2000a). Common complaints include anxiety, dysphoria, emotional lability, restlessness, and impaired concentration. Patients feel irritable and jittery and have episodic anxiety; they also have insomnia with fatigue and often feel too weak and tired to carry through with their plans. Speech can be rapid and disjointed. An uncommon presentation of behavioral change with thyrotoxicosis mimics a depressive disorder and usually occurs in elderly patients. These patients feel apathy, lethargy, pseudodementia, and depressed mood and often lack the standard physical findings associated with hyperthyroidism in younger people (Taylor, 1975; Peake, 1981).

The systematic investigation of the neuropsychiatric status of thyrotoxic patients has confirmed the clinical impressions of mood, anxiety, and cognitive disturbances. In studies in patients with thyrotoxicosis using modern diagnostic criteria, the prevalence of anxiety disorders was approximately 60% and of depressive disorders between 31% and 69% (Kathol and Delahunt, 1986; Trzepacz et al., 1988). Studies using objective neuropsychiatric measurements have confirmed these clinical impressions. A study using the Clyde mood scale found an increased jittery score and reduced score for clear thinking (Robbins and Vinson, 1960). Studies have also shown increased anxiety (Greer et al., 1973) on a standardized questionnaire, increased depression in the Minnesota Multiphasic Personality Inventory (MMPI) scale (Artunkel and Togrol, 1964), and increased depression and anxiety on the MMPI in another study (MacCrimmon et al., 1979).

Changes in cognition, including impaired memory and decreased concentration, are also directly correlated with the thyrotoxic state. Using standardized measures to assess neurotic and cognitive traits, patients with thyrotoxicosis were found to resemble those with an organic brain syndrome (Robbins and Vinson, 1960). Patients with thyrotoxicosis were also shown to perform poorly on the Porteus maze and trail-making tests, indicating impairment of cognition (Whybrow et al., 1969). Performance on tasks requiring concentration and memory was shown to decline in direct proportion to the degree of increase in serum T_4 (MacCrimmon et al., 1979).

2. Overt Psychiatric Manifestations

Overt psychiatric illness due to thyrotoxicosis is uncommon, occurring only in about 10% of patients (Lidz and Whitehorn, 1949; Bursten, 1961). Psychosis, mania, and delirium have been reported and may accompany a thyrotoxic storm (a relatively rare but life-threatening syndrome characterized by exaggerated manifestations of thyrotoxicosis) (Greer and Parsons, 1968; Wartofsky, 2000). Typically, patients who develop a true manic episode while thyrotoxic have an underlying mood disorder or family history of mood disorder (Checkley, 1978; Hasan and Mooney, 1981; Reus et al., 1979). In the few patients who develop a psychotic illness, evidence of delirium is usually present (Whybrow et al., 1969; Beierwaltes and Ruff, 1958).

3. Treatment Outcome of Neuropsychiatric Symptoms

After successful treatment of thyrotoxicosis, the psychiatric symptoms usually remit. Eight of ten studies conducted between 1956 and 1993 found the substantial improvement in neuropsychiatric symptoms to parallel resolution of the thyrotoxicosis. After return to a normal thyroid status, patients had improvement in cognitive function (Robbins and Vinson, 1960; MacCrimmon et al., 1979), and all 20 patients had improved MMPI profiles in a study by Artunkel and Togrol (1964). Whybrow et al. (1969) found improvement in nervousness, anxiety, and motor tension. However, some studies have shown incomplete neuropsychiatric recovery after patients become euthyroid. One study found only 8 of 17 patients with various nonpsychotic and psychotic symptoms to be improved with the reestablishment of normal thyroid status (Kleinschmidt and Waxenberg, 1956). Of 51 patients who were hyperthyroid 10 years previously, 25% were found to have markedly impaired neuropsychological functioning (Bommer et al., 1990). Trzepacz et al. (1988) reported that patients had recovery from mood and anxiety symptoms, but some attention deficit remained. A study that investigated the epidemiology of somatic and somatopsychic complaints in patients with remitted hyperthyroidism confirmed the impression of residual symptomatology—one-third of patients had long-term mental sequelae and residual complaints, including lack of energy (Fahrenfort et al., 2000). The incomplete remission of neuropsychiatric symptoms in some patients after return to euthyroid status is indicative of irreversible CNS damage, although the underlying pathophysiological mechanisms are unknown. We may speculate that the autoimmune processes associated with thyrotoxicosis may play a significant role. In one study, a higher number of previous hyperthyroid episodes was associated with more residual neuropsychiatric symptoms, indicating a relationship between the severity of the disease and treatment outcome (Bommer et al., 1990).

In summary, in most studies, the scores on various mood, anxiety, and cognitive tests returned to normal after hormonal normalization. The reversible nature of most psychiatric symptoms after treatment of the thyroid disorder suggests that they are secondary to the hormonal abnormality. However, in some patients, neuropsychiatric sequelae may persist in spite of a return to euthyroid status, indicating irreversible CNS damage.

B. Psychiatric and Behavioral Aspects of Hypothyroidism

Hypothyroidism is defined as deficient thyroidal production of thyroid hormone. The fall in serum concentrations of thyroid hormone causes an increased secretion of TSH, resulting in elevated serum TSH levels. Hypothyroidism is the most common clinical disorder of thyroid function (Braverman and Utiger, 2000b). Iodine deficiency persists in many parts of the world and is the most common cause of hypothyroidism worldwide (Braverman and Utiger, 2000b). In the industrialized countries, where iodine supplementation is available, thyroid hormone deficiency is most frequently caused by inadequate production and secretion of thyroid hormones due to the destruction of the thyroid gland as a consequence of disease or therapies to control thyrotoxicosis (Larsen et al., 1998). In the United States, the most frequent cause of hypothyroidism is iatrogenic from postsurgical or postradiation ablation of the thyroid gland to treat Graves disease. Idiopathic hypothyroidism in adults is more common in females than males and usually occurs between ages 40 and 60. Up to 80% of these patients have antithyroid antibodies and many have additional autoimmune illnesses (Weetman, 2000). The elevated TSH found in Hashimoto's thyroiditis (thought to be immunologically mediated) might result in enlargement of the thyroid. Rarely, pituitary failure leads to secondary hypothyroidism from inadequate TSH release.

The onset of hypothyroidism is usually insidious in adults. Physical symptoms include enlarged thyroid, constipation, cold intolerance, weight increase with decreased appetite, fatigue, dry and rough skin, hair loss, puffiness of the face, lethargy, and slowed motor activity (Braverman and Utiger, 2000b). Hypothyroidism is a graded phenomenon, ranging from mild cases, in which the only indication of disorder is an abnormal laboratory value, to severe cases with widespread symptoms that can progress into life-threatening myxedema coma (Larsen et al., 1998). The clinical expression of thyroid hormone deficiency varies considerably among individuals, depending on the cause, duration, and severity of the hypothyroid state. Characteristically there is a slowing of physical and mental activity and of many organ functions.

1. Neuropsychiatric Signs and Symptoms in Hypothyroidism

Studies using magnetic resonance spectroscopy (MRS) and positron emission tomography (PET) technology have indicated that the adult human brain, particularly the frontal lobe, is responsive to thyroid hormone (Smith and Ain, 1995; Silverman et al., 2001) and provide a biological basis for the prevalent neurological and psychiatric signs found in hypothyroidism (Dugbartey, 1998). The wide variety of neuropsychiatric symptoms associated with hypothyroidism includes impaired cognition, mood changes, irritability, and psychosis (Fig. 1). Mild hypothyroidism may appear as vague symptoms or inattentiveness, slowing of thought, weakness, and poor memory. Depressive mood is the most common mood change, but may be accompanied by anxiety and insomnia. Gradually, the patient's ability to carry out daily activities or to interact with others deteriorates. Impaired perception with paranoia and visual hallucinations may develop (Whybrow et al., 1969; Whybrow and Bauer, 2000b). The few studies of behavioral changes that have been

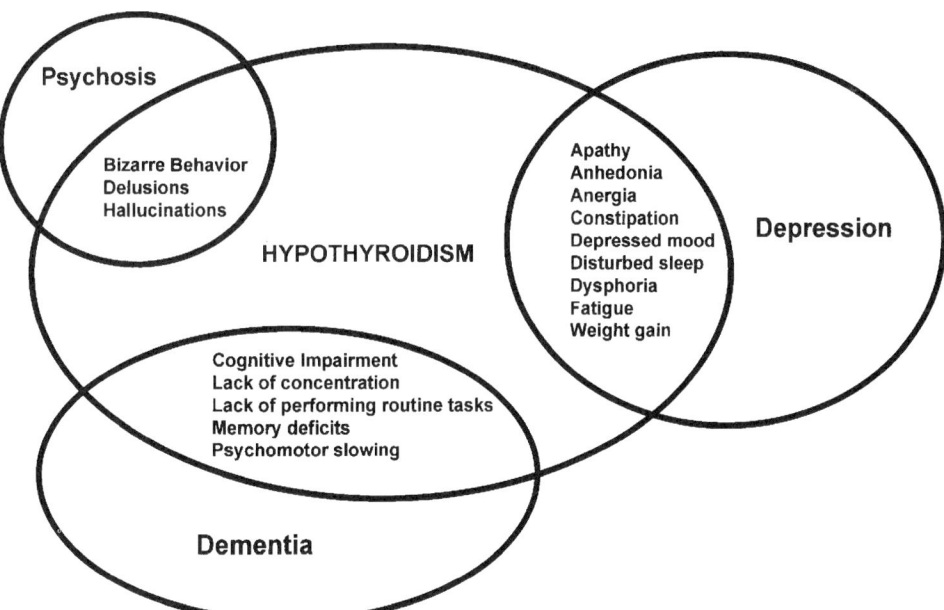

FIGURE 1 Most common psychiatric syndromes in hypothyroidism.

conducted have confirmed these clinical impressions. In one study, five of seven consecutive patients with hypothyroidism were depressed and one was anxious (Whybrow et al., 1969). Of 30 consecutive patients with hypothyroidism, 22 had some psychopathology, but the severity of the hypothyroidism and the psychiatric symptoms were unrelated (Jain, 1972). In this study, 43% had depression and 33% had anxiety. Of 31 patients at risk for hypothyroidism but with no manifestations of the disease, 16 were found to have subclinical hypothyroidism. These patients were significantly more likely to have a lifetime history of depression than a matched control group of 15 euthyroid women (Haggerty et al., 1993).

Hypothyroidism causes significant cognitive impairment, including short-term memory loss; disorientation; and impaired perception, attention, and problem solving (Dugbartey, 1998). The classic study of untreated myxedema by the Clinical Society of London (1888) found intellectual slowness in almost all cases. In a study in which the intellectual function of 15 patients with hypothyroidism was compared with age- and sex-matched controls diagnosed with brain damage or neurosis, "a generalized suppression of intellectual functions in myxedema which would become statistically significant if the groups were larger" [p. 444] was found (Reitan, 1953). In another objective study, disorientation was found in six of seven consecutive patients with hypothyroidism (Whybrow et al., 1969).

2. Overt Psychiatric Manifestations

Psychosis may occur in 5% of all patients with hypothyroidism. Gross mental changes may include disorientation, distractibility, hallucinations, and paranoia. Visual and auditory distortions may result in bizarre behavior and paranoid ideas (Whybrow and Bauer, 2000b). In the study of untreated myxedema in 1888, the Clinical Society of London found delusions and hallucinations in almost half of the 109 cases studied.

Thyroid function abnormalities are classified as grade I, decreased serum T_4 level; grade II, increased serum basal TSH with normal serum T_4 level; and grade III, presence of an isolated exaggeration of the TSH response to TRH stimulation, with normal basal TSH levels (Wenzel et al., 1974). Investigators have become increasingly aware of an association between grade II and III hypothyroidism and mood disorders. Grade II or III hypothyroidism was found in 20 of 250 consecutive persons with major depression admitted to an inpatient unit (Gold et al., 1981). Among women with postpartum depression, about 5% also have postpartum thyroiditis. A study of 145 women with high serum thyroid antibody concentrations (Tg and microsomal antibodies) 6 weeks postpartum, 47% had significant symptoms of depression compared with 32% of women with normal serum antibody concentrations (Harris et al., 1992).

3. Treatment Outcome of Neuropsychiatric Symptoms

In most cases, the behavioral changes associated with hypothyroidism remit after treatment with thyroid hormone and the return to euthyroid status. Residual symptoms sometimes remain, especially after severe and prolonged hypothyroidism (Whybrow et al., 1969). If the patient with hypothyroidism has an underlying depression, correction of the thyroid status may improve the cognition but not the depression (Treadway et al., 1967). If the patient has a family history of affective disorder, especially bipolar, initiation of treatment to correct hypothyroidism may precipitate mania. In such cases, the addition of a mood-stabilizing agent may be needed. A review article revealed 18 hypothyroid cases of significant psychiatric sequelae, predominantly mania, during hormone replacement for hypothyroidism (Josephson and Mackenzie, 1980). All but one of these cases had psychiatric symptoms prior to initiation of treatment. This suggests the need to proceed cautiously when correcting hypothyroid status in patients who experienced significant behavioral changes. Although subclinical hypothyroidism is associated with fewer mood syndromes, it is not established if correcting the thyroid deficit will reverse such symptoms (Haggerty et al., 1990).

In summary, the majority of patients who experience mood, cognitive, and psychotic changes due to hypothyroidism return to normal with treatment. However, the response is not uniform; differences may be due to other psychiatric illnesses or the duration or severity of the hypothyroidism (Whybrow and Bauer, 2000b).

C. Behavioral Effects of Thyrotropin-Releasing Hormone and Changes in Thyroid Status in Animals

In addition to its important physiological role as a hypothalamic-releasing hormone, TRH seems to function in the brain as a neurotransmitter or neuromodulator (Jackson, 1982; Mason et al., 1995). TRH and TRH receptors are widely distributed in the CNS, including the various limbic structures, midbrain, and the raphe nuclei of the medulla (Tsuruo et al., 1987). Thus, it was assumed that TRH exerts direct behavioral effects, prompting an examination of such effects in animal studies. The most consistent finding is the stimulant behavioral effects of TRH that were demonstrated in many different test situations in animal studies. TRH has been found to antagonize the sedation and motor impairment of various sedative drugs, including alcohol, benzodiazepines, barbiturates, and ketamine (Nemeroff et al., 1984). This antagonistic action of TRH is not blocked by the removal of the thyroid or the pituitary gland, indicating that the effect is independent of the TRH function that it exerts in the regulation of the HPT axis (Mason et al., 1995). TRH was also found to potentiate the arousing and locomotor-stimulating effects observed in the L-dihydroxyphenylalanine (L-DOPA) (a catecholamine precursor) and the 5-hydroxytryptophan (5-HTP; a serotonin precursor) potentiation tests. Based on the latter results, it has been suggested that the analeptic effects of TRH result, at least in part, from an interaction with central catecholaminergic and serotonergic systems (Nemeroff et al., 1984; Collu et al., 1992).

The influence of changes in thyroid hormone status on behavior has also been studied in various animal models. The learned helplessness paradigm in rats, an animal analog of the clinical syndrome depression, has been one focus of research. Pretreatment with T_3 for 4 days prevented escape and avoidance deficits produced by inescapable shock (Martin et al., 1985). Also, T_3 administration has been shown to significantly hasten antidepressant-induced reversal of learned helplessness (Brochet et al., 1987). Subsequently, it has been demonstrated that hypothyroid status can produce an escape deficit in rats, whereas sham-operated rats improved their performance on a simple escape task over 3 days of testing, thyroparathyroidectomized rats showed a pronounced decrease in their responses (Levine et al., 1990). Another line of evidence that alterations in thyroid status may change animal behavior stem from reports that applied catecholaminergic or serotonergic challenges. For example, an increase in hyperactivity to central serotonin- and dopamine-mediated behavioral responses has been observed with the administration of T_3 (Atterwill, 1981). In another study, the head twitch response to the administration of 5-HTP was potentiated by additional administration of T_3 (Brochet et al., 1985).

In summary, animal behavior models have provided some important mechanistic insights into thyroid hormone–dependent influences on affective state in humans.

III. HYPOTHALAMIC-PITUITARY-THYROID AXIS DYSFUNCTION IN AFFECTIVE ILLNESS

The early observation that symptoms of depression are commonplace in thyroid disorders has stimulated psychiatric research into possible links between thyroid hormone homeostasis and affective illness over many years. As noted earlier, disorders of the thyroid gland are frequently associated with disturbed mood, and primary mood disorders may present with abnormalities in the HPT system. Although most subjects presenting with depression do not have biochemical evidence of hypothyroidism, they do share many clinical factors with the endocrine disorder (Fig. 1). Many symptoms of depression, such as lowered mood, apathy, constipation, anhedonia, anergia, cognitive impairment, decreased libido, fatigue, decreased appetite, lethargy, lowered mood, and psychomotor retardation, resemble those of hypothyroidism. These clinical manifestations in common have been the impetus for investigating the HPT system in affective illness. As knowledge of the regulatory mechanisms underlying the normal HPT system increased and technology advanced, the study of the thyroid axis gained specificity and these more sophisticated studies have improved our understanding of the brain–thyroid interrelationship.

A. Peripheral Thyroid Hormone in Depression

Studies that investigated circulating (peripheral) concentrations of thyroid hormones in affective disorders have shown largely inconsistent results (Bauer and Whybrow, 1988; Baumgartner, 1993; Joffe and Sokolov, 1994). Despite the assumptions derived from studies of primary thyroid disorders that thyroid hypofunction predisposes to depression, the vast majority of patients with primary affective disorders have thyroid hormone blood levels within the normal (euthyroid) range (Baumgartner et al., 1988; Baumgartner, 2000). However, there is a large variability and often conflicting interpretations of the results. Joffe and Sokolov (1994) suggested methodological limitations (e.g., small sample sizes, variable diagnostic criteria of depression, lack of comparison groups, and different severity of depression) as responsible for the conflicting results in studies. Despite these inconsistencies across studies, some authors suggested that elevated serum concentrations of total and free T_4 (with normal T_3 levels), compared to healthy or psychiatric control groups, are the most common thyroid abnormalities in affective illness (Kirkegaard and Faber, 1998). In contrast, other studies have reported lower levels of T_4 in depressed patients compared to controls (reviewed in Bauer and Whybrow, 1988; Baumgartner et al., 1988).

The apparent paradox of increased serum T_4 parameters in some depressed patients and decreased levels in others cannot be resolved at present. It has been argued that it results from a nonspecific stress effect or environmental cicrcumstances (e.g., hospitalization) and does not play a particular pathogenetic role in affective disorders (Bauer and Whybrow, 1988).

B. The Thyrotropin-Releasing Hormone Test in Depression

The TSH response to TRH (TRH test) has been widely used as a standard endocrine procedure that involves measurement of TSH levels following the IV injection of a single TRH dose (Loosen, 1985). Studies have reported a blunted TSH response to TRH stimulation in approximately 25–30% of patients with depression (reviewed in Loosen, 1985). Two leading hypotheses used to interpret a blunted TSH response in depression are transient hyperthyroxinemia and hypersecretion of hypothalamic TRH (Mason et al., 1995). In contrast, in 10% of depressed patients, an exaggerated response in the TRH test occurs. This latter phenomenon supports the hypothesis of an association of depression with (subclinical) hypothyroidism (Mason et al., 1995).

Also of interest are studies by Duval et al., (1990) demonstrating that TRH stimulation in the evening (11 P.M.) produced greater Δ TSH differences between depressed patients and controls than did stimulation in the morning (8 A.M.). The abnormalities in the TRH test appear to be a state rather than a trait marker because clinical recovery is usually associated with the normalization of the TSH response. Another indication of altered TSH secretion in depression is the loss of the nocturnal TSH rise, which usually occurs between midnight and the early morning hours; this robust finding has been confirmed by different groups and is believed to be a more sensitive marker of a HPT system abnormality than the blunted TSH response in the TRH stimulation test (Sack et al., 1988; Bartalena et al., 1990). The lack of a nocturnal TSH surge and a blunted response in the TRH test may reflect elevations of thyroid hormones in these patients, with resulting alteration of pituitary or central regulatory mechanisms involved in the feedback control of TRH output including desensitization of TRH receptors in the pituitary (Mason et al., 1995). A decreased TSH secretion could be explained by a hypersecretion of hypothalamic TRH with the consequence of decreasing the number of pituitary TRH receptors (Holsboer, 1995). In accordance with the hypotheses of hypothalamic TRH hypersecretion are findings that TRH is elevated in cerebrospinal fluid (CSF) of patients with depression (Banki et al., 1988).

To summarize, only in a minority of patients with affective illness have abnormalities of the HPT system been described. The results are in some instances contradictory, and it remains unsolved whether the HPT system in affective illness is hyperactive or hypoactive. Whether the abnormalities of the HPT system in affective disorders are the result of a nonspecific stress effect or whether they reflect a specific pathogenic or compensatory process is yet to be determined.

C. Effects of Antidepressant Treatments on Peripheral Thyroid Hormone Levels

A broad range of treatments for affective disorders have been shown to decrease peripheral thyroid hormone levels, particularly those of total T_4 and free T_4 levels. This effect has been demonstrated for electroconvulsive therapy (ECT); various antidepressants such as imipramine, desipramine, clomipramine, and maprotiline; carbamazepine; cognitive psychotherapy; and bright and dim light therapy (Whybrow et al., 1972; Kirkegaard and Faber, 1981; Roy-Byrne et al., 1984; Baumgartner et al., 1988, 1996; Joffe and Singer, 1990a; Joffe et al., 1996). The few negative studies usually involved small study groups and, thus, reduced statistical power (Joffe and Sokolov, 1994).

In the majority of all studies published, the reductions in serum concentrations of T_4 during antidepressive treatment were significantly correlated to the degree of clinical response (Kirkegaard and Faber, 1981; Roy-Byrne et al., 1984; Baumgartner et al., 1988, 1996; Joffe and Singer, 1990a; Joffe et al., 1996). Specifically, a reduction of serum T_4 levels has been correlated with improvement in depression during antidepressant treatment. Studies have shown that high serum concentrations of T_4 predict a favorable response to various antidepressant therapies, such as antidepressant drugs (Whybrow et al., 1972; Baumgartner et al., 1988), total and partial sleep deprivation (Baumgartner et al., 1990; Szuba et al., 1992), and augmentation with T_3 (Sokolov et al., 1997). In these studies, there was no substantial clinical effect on TSH levels, despite reductions in mean T_4 and f T_4 levels of up to 30% (Joffe and Sokolov, 1994).

A series of animal experiments has shown that the declines in serum concentrations of T_4 seen during antidepressant treatment are probably due to enhanced degradation of T_4 to T_3, that is, enhanced activity of the D2 isoenzyme in the CNS (Campos-Barros and Baumgartner, 1994; Baumgartner et al., 1994b; Eravci et al., 2000). As a result, the concentrations of T_3 rise in various regions of the rat CNS following subchronic administration of various antidepressant drugs, such as desipramine and fluoxetine, as well as after sleep deprivation (Campos-Barros et al., 1993, 1995; Baumgartner et al., 1994b; Campos-Barros and Baumgartner, 1994). An increase in the activity of D2 and an inhibition of the activity of the D3 isoenzyme have now also been reported after the administration of lithium and carbamazepine for 14 days (Baumgartner et al., 1997).

In summary, a broad range of antidepressant and prophylactic treatments seem to affect thyroid hormone metabolism in the CNS, probably by enhancing the degradation of T_4 and increasing tissue concentrations of T_3. Thus, some antidepressants, and also lithium and carbamazepine, may need T_4 to unfold their specific actions in patients with depression. If so, the more T_4 that is available to the brain, the more effective antidepressant therapies may be. This hypothesis also explains why suprapahysiological T_4 treatment is effective only when given together with a conventional antidepressant or prophylactic drug, although this has not been studied systematically (see below). However, Baumgartner and colleagues have suggested that the same described effects of antidepressants and mood stabilizers on brain deiodinase activities in the rat brain may also be induced by stress and by novel neuroleptic drugs (Baumgartner, 2000).

D. Thyroid Dysfunction in Bipolar Affective Disorder

Abnormalities in thyroid function are of particular importance in the clinical course of bipolar affective disorder, especially rapid cycling disorder, a malignant form of the illness. Patients with a rapid cycling course of the disease, 70–90% of whom are women, by definition suffer four or more episodes of illness per year (Bauer and Whybrow, 1991). They have a much higher incidence (~25%) of grade II hypothyroidism than depressed patients in general (2–5%) or those taking lithium carbonate (9%) (Cowdry et al., 1983; Bauer and Whybrow, 1991). Challenge with therapeutic doses of lithium, an established drug for the prophylaxis of bipolar disorder with antithyroid properties (Lazarus, 1998), resulted in significantly higher changes in TSH after TRH stimulation in unmedicated rapid cycling bipolar patients than in healthy controls (Gyulai et al., 1999). This suggests that the thyroid axis plays a key role in the development of a rapid cycling pattern in bipolar disorder.

The neurobiological mechanisms that might underlie the exaggerated TSH response to TRH in rapid cycling patients after lithium challenge are unknown. Lithium is concentrated in the pituitary gland as well as in the hypothalamus and may interfere with cellular metabolism in these tissues as a result (Lazarus, 1986). One of the consequences of this interference is evidenced in reports of cross-sectional studies describing an exaggerated TSH response to TRH stimulation in 50–100% of lithium-treated patients (reviewed in

Lazarus, 1998). St. Germain (1987) was among the first to study the neuropharmacological effects of lithium on brain-thyroid metabolism in murine neural and anterior pituitary tissue. His research demonstrated that lithium inhibits the activity of D2 in mouse neuroblastoma and rat GH3 pituitary cell lines *in vitro*. As noted earlier, this is the predominate enzyme in the brain that catalyzes the deiodination of T_4 and thus provides neural tissue with the biologically active thyroid hormone T_3. Later, Baumgartner *et al.* (1997) showed that the administration of lithium for 14 days in dosages employed in the prophylaxis of affective disorders significantly inhibited the D2 activity in various regions in the rat brain (e.g., the parieto-occipital cortex, septum, and hypothalamus). Lithium also modulates the gene expression of thyroid hormone receptors in the rat brain *in vivo* (Hahn *et al.*, 1999a), and in rat pituitary GH3 and neuroblastoma B103 cell lines (Hahn *et al.*, 1999b). Hence, when used in patients with bipolar disorder, lithium may burden the thyroid economy of the brain, potentially creating a relative neuronal thyroid hormone deficiency in predisposed (vulnerable) individuals, thus stimulating an increase in pituitary TSH and possible up-regulation of pituitary TRH receptors. A greater sensitization to lithium at the level of the pituitary or a disturbance of central neurobiological mechanisms that regulate the HPT system may also account for the exaggerated TSH response to TRH stimulation in rapid cycling patients (Gyulai *et al.*, 1999).

A latent hypofunction of the thyroid axis in rapid cycling bipolar disorder may also explain why high doses of T_4 added to the established treatment with lithium and other psychotropic drugs can reverse the rapid cycling pattern (Bauer and Whybrow, 1990) and reduce the number of episodes in otherwise refractory bipolar disorder (Baumgartner *et al.*, 1994a; Bauer *et al.*, 2002).

IV. THYROID HORMONE AND MOOD MODULATION

A. Hormones of the Hypothalamic-Pituitary-Thyroid System in the Treatment of Mood Disorders

1. Historical Perspective

The use of thyroid hormones as a treatment in modern psychiatry has existed since the early twentieth century. In the 1930s to 1940s, Norwegian physicians were the first to use hypermetabolic doses of desiccated sheep thyroid gland to successfully treat patients with cyclic mood disorders and periodic catatonia (Gjessing, 1938; Gjessing and Jenner, 1976). The fact that thyroid hormone deficiency may lead to depression and psychosis (myxedematous madness) and be reversed by desiccated thyroid administration was demonstrated in a case series by Asher in 1949. Subsequently, with the identification of T_3 and T_4 as the natural thyroid hormones in the 1950s and their subsequent availability as pharmaceutical drugs, as well as the discovery of TRH and TSH, the effects of synthetic hormones of the HPT system (T_3, T_4, TRH, and TSH) alone and in combination with traditional psychotropic drugs have been studied repeatedly in the treatment of affective disorders.

2. Treatment with Thyrotropin-Releasing Hormone and Thyroid-Stimulating Hormone

Soon after the identification and purification of TRH from sheep hypothalami in the late 1960s, two initial reports suggested that 500 μg of TRH administered intravenously produced rapid (within hours) antidepressant effects that persisted up to 3 days (Kastin *et al.*, 1972; Prange *et al.*, 1972). However, several attempts to replicate this finding, including controlled double-blind studies and doses up to 1000 μg of TRH intravenously, showed inconsistent results (Stein and Avni, 1988). Various routes of TRH administration (oral, intravenous, subcutaneous, and intrathecal) have been applied in depression (Lasser and Baldessarini, 1997). Studies have shown promising antidepressant effects for TRH by intrathecal infusion (Marangell *et al.*, 1997a) and longer-term intravenous or subcutaneous injection (Callahan *et al.*, 1997). Despite contradictory results, some interesting observations have emerged from these studies, suggestive of an increased likelihood of response to TRH infusion in women and in patients with bipolar disorder (Frye *et al.*, 1999).

There is one randomized placebo-controlled study in the literature that showed a beneficial acceleration effect of TSH administered intramuscularly when given in addition to a tricyclic antidepressant in 30 subjects (Prange *et al.*, 1970). A high proportion (89%) of subjects responded in the group that had received imipramine and TSH, compared to only 44% in the group given imipramine plus the placebo. The authors concluded that the thyroid stimulation caused by TSH was most likely the reason for the therapeutic effects; however they did not rule out that TSH might exert a direct behavioral effect as well. These findings have not been replicated or pursued by other authors, perhaps because of the more complicated route of administration.

3. Treatment with Thyroid Hormones Alone

Thyroid hormones alone, without the concomitant use of psychoactive drugs, have only rarely been studied in affective disorders. Although it is well established that symptoms of depression that occur in hypothyroid conditions usually resolve after the euthyroid status has been restored, this area of research has not been systematically examined. The first two reports were case series, and the results were inconclusive (Flach et al., 1958; Feldmesser-Reiss, 1958). Later, Wilson et al. (1974) compared up to 62.5 µg/day T_3 alone with imipramine in depressed patients in a double-blind study. At a dose of 50 µg/day, T_3 alone was as effective as imipramine. However, later in the study, when T_3 doses reached 62.5 µg/day, patients showed mild thyrotoxicity, and the study was terminated. Therefore, the study left unanswered the question of whether T_3 alone in doses of 50 µg or less might prove a sufficient treatment for depression (Prange et al., 1976). Okuno and Nakayasu (1988) administered 50–100 µg/day T_4 alone for 2 weeks to patients with primary major depressive disorder without apparent thyroid dysfunction; the average effects were modest, although some patients improved markedly.

4. Thyroid Hormone Supplementation in Mood Disorders

The use of synthetic thyroid hormones, T_3 and T_4, as supplement agents in affective illness has a long history, with the first reports published in the late 1960s (Prange et al., 1969). Three main groups of studies on the technique of thyroid supplementation (potentiation) of antidepressant or mood-stabilizing drugs must be distinguished. The first group, the acceleration studies, involves the use of supplementation with thyroid hormone at the initiation of an antidepressant trial to speed up time to response. The second group, the augmentation studies, involves the supplementation with thyroid hormone after 4–6 weeks of an antidepressant trial and has resulted in no response or in a partial antidepressant response. The third group, the prophylactic studies, uses supplementation with thyroid hormone to prevent future episodes in recurrent mood disorders. These are summarized in Table 2.

TABLE 2
Hormones of the Hypothalamic-Pituitary-Thyroid Axis in the Treatment of Thyroid and Mood Disorders

Disease group	Type of hormone[a]	Clinical syndrome	Specific indication	Efficacy[b]
Primary thyroid disorders	T_4 (RD)	Hypothyroidism with depression and/or cognitive dysfunction	Treatment of thyroid hormone deficiency[c]	up to 90%
Mood disorders	T_3	Major depression	Acceleration of antidepressants[d]	40–80%
	T_3	Refractory depression	Augmentation of antidepressants[d]	40–60%
	T_4 (RD)	Refractory depression	Augmentation of antidepressants[d]	20%
	T_4 (SD)	Refractory depression	Augmentation of antidepressants[e]	50–60%
	T_4 (SD)	Prophylaxis-resistant recurrent mood disorders	Augmentation of mood stabilizers[e]	60%
	T_4 (SD)	Rapid Cycling Bipolar Disorder	Augmentation of mood stabilizers[e]	50–60%
	TRH	Major depression	Antidepressant response[c]	60%

[a]RD, replacement (low) dose; SD, supraphysiological (high) dose; T_4, thyroxine; T_3, triiodothyronine; TRH, thyrotropin-releasing hormone.
[b]Approximate response rates.
[c]Double-blind controlled studies.
[d]Double-blind placebo-controlled studies.
[e]Open studies.

a) Triiodothyronine Acceleration Studies The immediate addition of thyroid hormone to speed antidepressant treatment response was first reported in a controlled design in the classic study by Prange and associates in the late 1960s (Prange *et al.*, 1969). Despite several controlled studies with positive outcomes in the early 1970s following the initial report by Prange, the thyroid hormone acceleration paradigm has received little attention in the past two decades. We conducted a meta-analysis with the goal of determining whether evidence exists to support the clinical efficacy of thyroid hormone acceleration in depression (Altshuler *et al.*, 2001). Five of six double-blind placebo-controlled studies (comprising 125 patients) found that the addition of T_3 had a statistically significant effect on the time to response compared with the effects of placebo (Prange *et al.*, 1969; Wilson *et al.*, 1970, 1974; Wheatley, 1972; Coppen *et al.*, 1972; Feighner *et al.*, 1972). The results of this meta-analysis support an acceleration of antidepressant response when adjunctive T_3 is included early in antidepressant treatment; it also revealed that women may be more likely than men to benefit from the addition of T_3 (Altshuler *et al.*, 2001). It must be emphasized, that the studies included in this meta-analysis were performed in the 1970s and thus have methodological limitations. However, they were homogeneous with respect to the type of antidepressant (all TCAs: five of six studies used the tricyclic antidepressant imipramine; one used amitriptyline), the dose of T_3 (20–25 μg/day) and rating scale to measure the clinical outcome (Hamilton Rating Scale for Depression). These results point to the need for further studies to assess the efficacy of T_3 acceleration with the newer, more selective antidepressant agents and to evaluate specifically the use of T_3 as an acceleration agent in women.

b) Triiodothyronine Augmentation Studies Studies assessing the effects of thyroid hormones in treatment-resistant depression have largely focused on T_3 as the augmenting thyroid hormone. Numerous case series and at least 13 prospective trials (nine open and four controlled double-blind studies) have evaluated the use of T_3 (most studies have used 25–50 μg/day) to potentiate the response to tricyclic antidepressants in nonresponders to treatment. The open studies consistently showed that approximately 50% of TCA nonresponders are converted to responders within 2 to 3 weeks after the addition of T_3. The largest placebo-controlled study in 33 unipolar depressed outpatients (11 women, 22 men), showed significant improvement with T_3 compared to placebo after 2 weeks of treatment (Joffe *et al.*, 1993b). However, not all controlled double-blind studies showed significant results in favor of T_3; thus, the data are only partially supportive of the results given in the open studies (Steiner *et al.*, 1978; Gitlin *et al.*, 1987). For example, in a randomized crossover study of 16 unipolar depressed outpatients (7 women, 9 men), there was no significant effect of T_3 compared to the placebo (Gitlin *et al.*, 1987). As a result of these data, the efficacy of T_3 augmentation has been met with criticism in the literature, specifying methodological deficiencies in studies, for example, lack of power in the randomized controlled trials due to small sample sizes (Stein and Avni, 1988; Baumgartner, 1993; Patten *et al.*, 1992). Subsequently, a meta-analysis did not show consistent results in favor of T_3 augmentation (Aronson *et al.*, 1996). In this meta-analysis, improvements in depression scores were moderately large; however, study quality was uneven, and among the four randomized double-blind studies (Steiner *et al.*, 1978; Gitlin *et al.*, 1987; Joffe and Singer, 1990b; Joffe *et al.*, 1993b) the pooled effects were not significant. Aggregating eight prospective studies (unblinded and double-blinded studies) with a total of 292 patients gives the result that patients treated with T_3 augmentation were twice as likely to respond as controls. As a result of their meta-analysis, Aronson *et al.* (1996) concluded that "T_3 augmentation may be an effective empirical method of increasing response rates and decreasing depression severity scores in a subgroup of patients with depression refractory to tricyclic antidepressant therapy, but the total number of patients randomized was small, and additional placebo-controlled data are required for a definite verdict" [p. 842]. In all the studies to date, antidepressant response to T_3 was not affected by gender, bipolar/unipolar diagnosis, type of antidepressant used, or the pre-augmentation thyroid status of the patients (Joffe *et al.*, 1993a; Joffe and Sokolov, 1994). Furthermore, the efficacy of T_3 augmentation with today's widely used non-tricyclic antidepressants, e.g., SSRIs has only been studied in case series (Joffe, 1992).

c) Thyroxine Augmentation Studies Compared to the large number of trials on T_3 supplementation, adjunctive treatment with T_4 has been studied less frequently in the acute treatment of depressive disorders. Joffe and Singer (1990b) directly compared the augmenting effects of T_3 (37.5 μg/day) versus T_4 (replacement dose, 150 μg/day) in depressed patients. In this 3-week randomized double-blind study, 9 of 17 patients (response rate, 53%) responded to T_3, which was a significantly higher rate than the response to T_4 (4 of 21 patients; 19%). However, it must be emphasized that due to the long half-life of T_4 (1 week, leading to a steady state of approximately 3–4 weeks after the last dose increase) the therapeutic effects of T_4 may not have been evident in a 3-week trial, as suggested by the authors in a later review (Joffe and Sokolov, 1994). In an 8-week randomized double-blind crossover study, Spoov and Lahdelma (1998) compared lithium augmentation, an established strategy for refractory depressed patients, with T_4 augmentation (T_4 dose, 200 μg/day) in a group of unipolar depressed patients. The percentage reduction in the Montgomery-Asberg Depression Rating Scale (MADRS) was significantly greater in patients who started on T_4. However, the lithium dose was relatively small in this study, making the comparison somewhat unfair for lithium (Spoov and Lahdelma, 1998). Data from two open trials suggested that augmentation with supraphysiological doses of T_4 may cause substantial improvement in patients with treatment-resistant and chronic depression (Bauer *et al.*, 1998; Rudas *et al.*, 1999). In an 8-week open study of 17 patients (16 women, 1 man) with acute treatment-resistant depressive disorders (bipolar and unipolar), significant improvement was achieved in approximately 50% of patients between weeks 4 and 8 of treatment with T_4 (mean dose, 377 μg/day) (Bauer *et al.*, 1998). Rudas *et al.* (1999) reported that an 8-week augmentation trial with high-dose T_4 (mean dose, 235 μg/day) showed antidepressant effects in six of seven patients with chronic depression and dysthymia. Placebo-controlled studies are warranted to objectively assess the augmenting effects of supraphysiological T_4 doses in acute depression.

d) Thyroxine Prophylaxis Studies In a series of open studies investigating the prophylactic effects of supraphysiological T_4 doses alone (Stancer and Persad, 1982) or in addition to conventional mood stabilizers, it has been suggested that T_4 may improve the course of patients with rapid cycling and nonrapid cycling bipolar disorder (Bauer and Whybrow, 1990; Baumgartner *et al.*, 1994a; Afflelou *et al.*, 1997; Bauer *et al.*, 2001b, 2002a).

In one study that used T_4 alone as a prophylactic medication, Stancer and Persad (1982) reported that rapid cycling ceased in five of eight women with bipolar disorder, but did not in two men, following treatment with supraphysiological doses with up to 500 μg/day T_4. In prospective open studies, our investigations showed that adjunctive supraphysiological doses of T_4 may be beneficial in patients with mood disorders resistant to established medications for these disorders. Initially, the effects of adjunctive supraphysiological doses of T_4 in 11 patients (10 women, 9 of them were premenopausal; 1 male) with refractory rapid cycling bipolar illness were studied (Bauer and Whybrow, 1990). Adjunctive treatment with T_4 reduced the manic and the depressive phases in both amplitude and frequency and even led to remittance in some patients. Four patients also underwent single- or double-blind placebo substitution: three patients relapsed into depression or cycling after switching to the placebo (Bauer and Whybrow, 1990). Later, in a 8-year long-term study, adjunctive treatment of seriously ill and previously prophylaxis-resistant unipolar and bipolar patients with supraphysiological doses of T_4 also proved successful in preventing affective episodes in approximately 70% of patients. There was a significant reduction of the number of affective recurrences and Morbidity Indexes during T_4 treatment, compared with the same time period before T_4 administration. Although results must be seen as preliminary, these studies indicate that in otherwise refractory patients with affective disorders, treatment with supraphysiological doses of T_4 is a viable augmentation strategy (Bauer *et al.*, 2001b, 2002a).

There have been concerns in the literature about the high doses of T_4 administered in these studies. With respect to bone demineralization, it was demonstrated that pre- and postmenopausal women with mood disorders who received supraphysiological T_4 treatment for 12 months or longer had no clinically significant loss of bone mineral density (Gyulai *et al.*, 1997, 2001). With respect to the cardiovascular system, monitored with electrocardiograms, measurements of blood pressure, and measurements of body weight, we did not see changes or adverse effects during long-term treatment with T_4 (Bauer et al., 2002a). The long-term effects of treatment with supraphysiological doses of T_4 on other cardiovascular functions (e.g., ventricular function, cardiac output, and systemic vascular resistance) remain to be objectively studied. However, there is no evidence from preliminary follow-up studies that the cardiovascular system is clinically impaired during supraphysiological T_4 treatment in patients with affective disorders. Therefore, we continue to recommend adjunctive supraphysiological doses of T_4 for patients with the most refractory affective disorders.

V. ADULT BRAIN—A SITE OF THYROID HORMONE ACTION

Since the 1980s, we have witnessed dramatic changes in the concepts of thyroid hormone action in the adult brain (Oppenheimer, 1999). As outlined earlier in this chapter, methodological and technical progress in basic science has provided the biological bases for a better understanding of thyroid hormone action in mature neurons. Some of the interactions of thyroid hormones with neuronal systems that may have importance for the understanding of the mood-modulating properties of thyroid hormones are discussed here.

A. Thyroid-Monoamine Systems Interaction

Are changes of the brain–thyroid economy important to the aberrant behavior of patients with thyroid dysfunction and psychiatric disease? Strong clinical evidence in support of such speculation exists: the role of subclinical hypothyroidism in depressive illness; the association of the rapid cycling variant of bipolar illness with hypothyroidism; the adjunctive therapeutic role of thyroid hormones in both depression and bipolar illness; and the profound mental disturbances that are found in both hypo- an hyperthyroidism.

The mood disturbances that occur in patients with hypothyroidism are of great interest because they suggest the possibility that a common pathophysiology contributes to the behavioral dysfunction seen in affective disorders and to thyroid disease. In this, the biogenic amines, putatively disturbed in both disorders, may form a linkage (Whybrow and Prange, 1981). Over the past three decades it has become apparent that the monoamines, specifically norepinephrine and serotonin, play a major modulatory role in mood and that these systems are intimately involved in the pathogenesis of depression (Coppen, 1967; Asberg et al., 1976; Blier and de Montigny, 1994; Maes and Meltzer, 1995). These long fiber systems, which have their origin in the brainstem and extend through the midbrain into the limbic system and cortex, modulate the activity of many of the brain regions related to emotion, mood and memory. The interdependence of these monoamine systems with thyroid hormone metabolism has become better understood as technology has improved over the past two decades.

1. Thyroid–Catecholamine Interaction

The catecholaminergic system was initially investigated because of the known physiological association between sympathetic nervous system activity and thyroid hormones (Harrison, 1964). Thyroid hormones appear to play an important role in regulating central noradrenergic (NA) function and it has been suggested that thyroid dysfunction may be linked with abnormalities in central NA neurotransmission (Whybrow and Prange, 1981). In the rat brain, the noradrenergic receptor systems are responsive to changes in HPT-axis function; studies demonstrated that thyroidectomy results in region- and receptor-specific pre- and postsynaptic NA system changes (Tejani-Butt et al., 2000). Thyroidectomy decreases ligand binding to β- and α_2-adrenergic receptors in the cortex and limbic regions in the rat brain, changes that can be reversed by the administration of T_4, suggesting a neuromodulatory link between thyroid hormones and central NA systems (Tejani-Butt and Yang, 1994). Further evidence for a thyroid–NA interaction derives from immunohistochemical mapping studies demonstrating that T_3 is concentrated in both nuclei and projection sites of central NA systems (Rozanov and Dratman, 1996). Evidence that T_3 is also delivered from the locus coeruleus to its NA targets via anterograde axonal transport indicates that T_3 may function as a cotransmitter with norepinephrine in the adrenergic nervous system (Gordon et al., 1999).

2. Thyroid–Serotonin Interaction

Studies in animals and humans have shown that thyroid hormones also influence the activity of serotonin (5-HT), as well as the functioning of its receptors (Tejani-Butt et al., 1993; Kulikov et al., 1999). From research in humans with thyroid dysfunction, there is some evidence from neuroendocrine challenge studies that the hypothyroid status is associated with a reduced 5-HT responsiveness and that this is reversible with thyroid replacement therapy (Cleare et al., 1995, 1996a,b). Results from studies in animals provide evidence that the thyroid status has a considerable impact in serotonergic neurotransmission in the adult brain (reviewed in Bauer et al., 2002b). Experimentally induced hypothyroid states result in an increase in 5-HT turnover in the brain stem (Henley and Koehnle, 1997). Thyroid hormone application may increase cortical serotonergic neurotransmission via two independent mechanisms. First, an *in vivo* microdialysis study by Gur et al. (1999) indicated a loss of autoinhibitory 5-HT$_{1A}$-receptor sensitivity mediated by T$_3$. In this study, the decrease in hippocampal and cortical serotonin release that should follow the application of a 5-HT$_{1A}$ agonist was significantly reduced by the administration of T$_3$ or combined T$_3$ and clomipramine in euthyroid rats (Gur et al., 1999). The results indicated that thyroid hormone application may desensitize autoinhibitory 5-HT$_{1A}$ receptors, and thus increase cortical and hippocampal serotonin release. Second, increasing cortical 5-HT$_2$-receptor sensitivity is potentially an independent way of increasing 5-HT transmission (Heal and Smith, 1988). Another reported interaction between the thyroid and 5-HT systems indicated synergistic effects of T$_3$ and 5-HT$_{1A}$ receptors on hippocampal brain-derived neurotrophic factor (BDNF) expression. Chronic T$_3$ administration prior to treatment with a 5-HT$_{1A}$ agonist caused a down-regulation of hippocampal BDNF mRNA expression in adult rats (Vaidya et al., 2001).

In conclusion, the interaction of thyroid hormone with brain noradrenergic and serotonergic systems may have relevance for the understanding of the mood modulating effects of thyroid hormones in the clinical setting and thus may enhance the understanding of the pathophysiology and treatment of mood disorders (Bauer et al., 2002b). However, the exact molecular actions underlying the efficacy of thyroid hormone treatment in patients with mood disorders and in patients with primary hypothyroidism who have comorbid depression remain to be elucidated.

B. Modulatory Effects of Thyroid Hormones on the γ-Aminobutyric Acid System

It has been suggested that thyroid hormones may also have effects via a more direct influence on neurotransmission at the level of the synapse (Mason et al., 1993; Dratman and Gordon, 1996). Evidence for this hypothesis derived initially from studies showing that thyroid hormones are selectively taken up and metabolized in the synaptosomal fraction of the rat brain (Dratman et al., 1976) and showing the existence of specific T$_3$-binding sites in synaptosomes in the rat cerebral cortex (Mashio et al., 1982). Mason and colleagues reported that T$_3$ specifically inhibits the neuronal uptake γ-aminobutyric acid (of GABA) into the synaptosomes (Mason et al., 1987), enhances depolarization-induced Ca^{2+}-uptake (Mason et al., 1990), and is also released from depolarized synaptosomes by a Ca^{2+}-dependent process (Mason et al., 1993). Later, thyroid hormones have been found to modulate the activity of the GABA$_A$ receptor in rat brain. It has been demonstrated that the binding of ligands to the benzodiazepine recognition site on the GABA$_A$ receptor is inhibited by micromolar concentrations of thyroid hormones (Narihara et al., 1994) and that thyroid hormones exert inhibitory action on GABA$_A$-stimulated Cl$^-$ flux into synaptosomes (Martin et al., 1996). Thus, some authors have postulated that T$_3$ may act as a central neurotransmitter (Mason et al., 1993).

C. Effects of Thyroid Hormones on Postreceptor Mechanisms and Signal Transduction

The review of the variety of effects that thyroid hormones exert on neurotransmission is completed by a series of studies indicating that signaling pathways downstream from receptors are influenced by changes in thyroid status. The influence of thyroid hormones on G-protein synthesis, receptor-G-coupling events, adenylate cyclase activity, and phosphorylation events involved in transcriptional activities in the adult CNS is well established (Henley and Koehnle, 1997).

A significant up-regulation of G-protein abundances in synaptosomal membranes from various brain regions was found in experimentally induced hypothyroidism in rats (Orford et al., 1991). In subsequent studies, the same authors later demonstrated that treatment with T_3 decreased the abundance of the α-subunits of G_i in synaptosomal membranes in the cerebral cortex of euthyroid rats (Orford et al., 1992). Impaired signal transduction via adenylate cyclase and inositol phosphatase has also been demonstrated in the brain of hypothyroid rats. The inhibition of adenylate cyclase in rat synaptosomal membranes by guanosine triphosphate (GTP) was significantly enhanced in hypothyroid rats (Mazurkiewicz and Saggerson, 1989). Also, hypothyroidism caused decreased formation of inositol phosphate in response to the muscarinic cholinergic agonist carbachol in the adult rat (Iriuchijima et al., 1991).

Thus, it appears that thyroid hormones exert an important influence on the activity and synthesis of G-proteins in the adult brain and that a lack of thyroid hormone leads to an impairment in adenylate cyclase and phosphoinositide-based signaling pathways.

D. Novel Approaches to Study the Thyroid System and Brain Activity *in Vivo*

Despite the evidence of a close relationship between thyroid status and behavioral disturbances, metabolic effects of thyroid hormones in the adult mammalian brain have rarely been investigated *in vivo*. No methods for direct *in vivo* measurements of brain thyroid metabolism exist. However, brain-imaging techniques, such as positron emission tomography (PET) and magnetic-resonance spectroscopy (MRS), to evaluate the relationship among the brain, thyroid hormones, and behavior have been initiated and may provide such assessment. A study by Smith and Ain (1995) indicated that hypothyroid patients exhibit decreased cerebral metabolism in the frontal lobes, as measured by 31^PMRS, that returned to normal after T_4 replacement therapy. Other indications that the adult brain is metabolically responsive to thyroid hormone status derive from studies in adult rats using ^{13}C nuclear magnetic resonance (NMR) spectroscopy. Such studies revealed that experimentally induced hypothyroidism markedly reduces the cerebral metabolism of acetate and increases the concentrations of glutamate and GABA (Chapa et al., 1995). Calza et al. (1997) found a significant decline in ^{14}C-2-deoxyglucose uptake in hypothyroid adult rats throughout the brain, except for the brain stem and pons, indicating a general decline in metabolic and functional activity during thyroid hormone deficiency.

In patients with major depression, Marangell et al. (1997b) investigated relationships between serum levels of hormones of the HPT system, cerebral blood flow (CBF), and cerebral glucose metabolism using PET. Serum TSH (putatively the best marker of thyroid status) was inversely related to both global and regional CBF and cerebral glucose metabolism. Left dorsolateral and mesial prefrontal cortices were the areas of maximal negative correlation between regional CBF and TSH (Marangell et al., 1997b). In another study, the effects of supraphysiological doses of T_4 on regional cerebral glucose metabolism in women with bipolar depression were determined using PET with [^{18}F]-fluorodeoxyglucose (Bauer et al., 2001a). The treatment with T_4 significantly improved mood and was accompanied by regional cerebral metabolic effects. Preliminary analyses indicated a relative increase in metabolism in the left middle frontal gyrus and a decrease in the left hippocampus; statistical parametric mapping (SPM99) analysis revealed that the T_4-induced reduction in hippocampal activity was part of a widespread deactivation of limbic and subcortical structures, including the amygdala. This deactivation was maximal in the parahippocampal gyri and the thalamus. The findings suggest that T_4 produces improvement in mood by actions on specific cortical, subcortical, and limbic circuits that have been implicated in the pathophysiology of mood disorders (Bauer et al., 2001a). Thus, using functional brain-imaging techniques to further elucidate the relationship among thyroid status, brain, and mood disorders may also provide new insights into the pathophysiology and treatment of these disorders.

VI. SUMMARY

An intimate association between disturbances of thyroid hormone homeostasis, mood, and behavior has been recognized since the earliest desciptions of thyroid disorders in the nineteenth century. Disorders of the thyroid gland are frequently associated with mental disturbances. Hyper- and hypothyroidism can induce disturbances of mood and intellectual function, and in severe states there may be a profound disturbance of behavior that can mimic melancholic depression and dementia. The mental changes accompanying thyroid gland dysfunction are usually reversed with return to euthyroid status. Reciprocally, disturbances of affect and mood such as major depression and bipolar affective disorder have associated with them disturbances of the peripheral thyroid hormone metabolism.

Thyroid hormones have a profound influence on behavior and appear to be capable of modulating the phenotypic expression of major affective illness. The value of thyroid hormone supplementation as an adjunct treatment in affective disorders has been studied since the 1970s and it is now widely accepted as an effective treatment option. Specifically, there is good evidence that T_3 may accelerate the antidepressant response to tricylic antidepressants, and some studies suggest that T_3 may augment the therapeutic response to antidepressants in refractory depressed patients. Studies have also shown that adjunctive supraphysiological doses of T_4 can ameliorate depressive symptomatology and improve the course of illness in bipolar and unipolar patients, especially women refractory to standard psychiatric medications.

The specific neurochemical basis and functional pathways for the observed therapeutic effects of thyroid hormones on mental functions are unknown. The influence of the thyroid system on neurotransmitters that putatively play a major role in the regulation of mood and behavior, particularly serotonin and norepinephrine, may contribute to the mechanisms of action.

Acknowledgment

This work was supported by a grant from Deutsche Forschungsgemeinschaft (Ba 1504/3-1) to M. Bauer.

References

Afflelou, S., Auriacombe, M., Cazenave, M., Chartres, J. P., and Tignol, J. (1997). Administration of high dose levothyroxine in treatment of rapid cycling bipolar disorders. Review of the literature and initial therapeutic application apropos of 6 cases (in French). *Encephale* **23**, 209–217.

Altshuler, L., Bauer, M., Frye, M., Gitlin, M., Mintz, J., Szuba, M., Leight, K., and Whybrow, P. C. (2001). Does thyroid supplementation accelerate antidepressant response? A review and meta-analysis of the literature. *Am. J. Psychiatry* **158**, 1617–1622.

Alvarez-Dolado, M., Iglesias, T., Rodriguez-Pena, A., Bernal, J., and Munoz, A. (1994). Expression of neurotrophins and the trk family of neurotrophin receptors in normal and hypothyroid rat brain. *Brain Res. Mol. Brain Res.* **27**, 249–257.

Anderson, G. W., Mariash, C. N., and Oppenheimer, J. H. (2000). Molecular actions of thyroid hormone. *In* "Werner & Ingbar's The Thyroid: A Fundamental and Clinical Text" (L. E. Braverman and R. D. Utiger, eds.), 8th ed., pp. 174–195. Lippincott Williams & Wilkins, Philadelphia.

Aronson, R., Offman, H. J., Joffe, R. T., and Naylor, D. (1996). Triiodothyronine augmentation in the treatment of refractory depression. A meta-analysis. *Arch. Gen. Psychiatry* **53**, 842–848.

Artunkel, S., and Togrol, S. (1964). "Psychological Studies in Hyperthyroidism in Brain Thyroid Relationships." Little, Brown, Boston.

Asberg, M., Thoren, P., Traskman, L., Bertilsson, L., and Ringberger, V. (1976). "Serotonin depression"—a biochemical subgroup within the affective disorders? *Science* **191**, 478–480.

Asher, R. (1949). Myxoedematous madness. *Br. Med. J.* **22**, 555–562.

Atterwill, C. K. (1981). Effect of acute and chronic triiodothyronine (T_3) administration to rats on central 5-HT and dopamine-mediated behavioral responses and related brain biochemistry. *Neuropharmacology* **20**, 131–144.

Banki, C. M., Bissette, G., Arato, M., and Nemeroff, C. B. (1988). Elevation of immunoreactive CSF TRH in depressed patients. *Am. J. Psychiatry* **145**, 1526–1531.

Bartalena, L., Placidi, G. F., Martino, E., Falcone, M., Pellegrini, L., Dell'Osso, L., Pacchiarotti, A., and Pinchera, A. (1990). Nocturnal serum thyrotropin (TSH) surge and the TSH response to TSH-releasing hormone: Dissociated behavior in untreated depressives. *J. Clin. Endocrinol. Metab.* **71**, 650–655.

Bauer, M. S., and Whybrow, P. C. (1988). Thyroid hormones and the central nervous system in affective illness: Interactions that may have clinical significance. *Integr. Psychiatry* **6**, 75–100.

Bauer, M. S., and Whybrow, P. C. (1990). Rapid cycling bipolar affective disorders. II. Treatment of refractory rapid cycling with high-dose levothyroxine: A preliminary study. *Arch. Gen. Psychiatry* **47**, 435–440.

Bauer, M. S., and Whybrow, P. C. (1991). Rapid cycling bipolar disorder: Clinical features, treatment, and etiology. *Adv. Neuropsychiatry Psychopharmacol.* **2**, 191–208.

Bauer, M., Hellweg, R., Gräf, K. J., and Baumgartner, A. (1998). Treatment of refractory depression with high-dose thyroxine. *Neuropsychopharmacology* **18**, 444–455.

Bauer, M., London, E. D., Rasgon, N., Berman, S., Mandelkern, M., Frye, M., Mazziotta, J. J., Altshuler, L., Shinn, A. K., Gitlin, M., and Whybrow, P. C. (2001a). Effects of supraphysiological levothyroxine (T₄) on cerebral glucose metabolism in bipolar depression: Findings from a positron emission tomographic study. *Bipolar Disord.* (abstr.) **3**, Suppl. 1, 25.

Bauer, M., Priebe, S., Berghöfer, A., Bschor, T., Kiesslinger, K., and Whybrow, P. C. (2001b) Subjective response to and tolerability of long-term supraphysiological doses of levothyroxine in refractory mood disorders. *J. Affect. Disord.* **64**, 35–42.

Bauer, M., Berghöfer, A., Bschor, T., Baumgartner, A., Kiesslinger, U., Hellweg, R., Adli, M., Baethge, C., and Müller-Oerlinghausen, B. (2002a). Suprahysiological doses of thyroxine in the maintenance treatment of prophylaxis-resistant bipolar, unipolar and schizoaffective disorders. *Neuropsychopharmacology* (in press).

Bauer, M., Heinz, A., and Whybrow, P. C. (2002b). Thyroid hormones, serotonin and mood: Of synergy and significance in the adult brain. *Mol. Psychiatry* **7**, 140–156.

Baumgartner, A. (1993). Thyroid hormones and depressive illness. I. Clinical aspects (in German). *Nervenarzt* **64**, 1–10.

Baumgartner, A. (2000). Thyroxine and the treatment of affective disorders: An overview of the results of basic and clinical research. *Int. J. Neuropsychopharmacol.* **3**, 149–165.

Baumgartner, A., Gräf, K. J., Kürten, I., and Meinhold, H. (1988). The hypothalamic-pituitary-thyroid axis in psychiatric patients and healthy subjects: Parts 1–4. *Psychiatry Res.* **24**, 271–332.

Baumgartner, A., Gräf, K. J., Kürten, I., Meinhold, H., and Scholz, P. (1990). Neuroendocrinological investigations during sleep deprivation in depression. *Biol. Psychiatry* **28**, 556–568.

Baumgartner, A., Bauer, M., and Hellweg, R. (1994a). Treatment of intractable non-rapid cycling bipolar affective disorder with high-dose thyroxine: An open clinical trial. *Neuropsychopharmacology* **10**, 183–189.

Baumgartner, A., Dubeyko, M., Campos-Barros, A., Eravci, M., and Meinhold, H. (1994b). Subchronic administration of fluoxetine to rats affects triiodothyronine production and deiodination in regions of the cortex and the limbic forebrain. *Brain Res.* **635**, 68–74.

Baumgartner, A., Volz, H. P., Campos-Barros, A., Stieglitz, R. D., Mansmann, U., and Mackert, A. (1996). Serum concentrations of thyroid hormones in patients with nonseasonal affective disorders during treatment with bright and dim light. *Biol. Psychiatry* **40**, 899–907.

Baumgartner, A., Pinna, G., Hiedra, L., Gaio, U., Hessenius, C., Campos-Barros, A., Eravci, M., Prengel, H., Thoma, R., and Meinhold, H. (1997). The effects of lithium and carbamazepine on thyroid hormone metabolism in rat brain. *Neuropsychopharmacology* **16**, 25–41.

Beierwaltes, W. H., and Ruff, G. E. (1958). Thyroxin and triiodothyronine in excessive dosage to euthyroid humans. *Arch. Intern. Med.* **101**, 569–576.

Bernal, J., and Nunez, J. (1995). Thyroid hormones and brain development. *Eur. J. Endocrinol.* **133**, 390–398.

Bernal, J., Rodriguez-Pena, A., Iniguez, M. A., Ibarrola, N., and Munoz, A. (1992). Influence of thyroid hormone on brain gene expression. *Acta Med. Austriaca* **19**(Suppl. 1), 32–35.

Blier, P., and de Montigny, C. (1994). Current advances and trends in the treatment of depression. *Trends Pharmacol. Sci.* **15**, 220–226.

Bommer, M., Eversmann, T., Pickardt, R., Leonhardt, A., and Naber, D. (1990). Psychopathological and neuropsychological symptoms in patients with subclinical and remitted hyperthyroidism. *Klin. Wochenschr.* **68**, 552–558.

Braverman, L. E., and Utiger, R. D. (2000a). Introduction to thyrotoxicosis. In "Werner & Ingbar's The Thyroid: A Fundamental and Clinical Text" (L. E. Braverman and R. D. Utiger, eds.), 8th ed., pp. 515–517. Lippincott Williams & Wilkins, Philadelphia.

Braverman, L. E., and Utiger, R. D. (2000b). Introduction to hypothyroidism. In "Werner & Ingbar's The Thyroid: A Fundamental and Clinical Text" (L. E. Braverman and R. D. Utiger, eds.), 8th ed., pp. 719–720. Lippincott Williams & Wilkins, Philadelphia.

Brent, G. A. (1994). The molecular basis of thyroid hormone action. *N. Engl. J. Med.* **29**, 847–853.

Brochet, D. M., Martin, P., Soubrie, P., and Simon, P. (1985). Effects of triiodothyronine on the 5-hydroxytryptophan-induced head twitch and its potentiation by antidepressants in mice. *Eur. J. Pharmacol.* **112**, 411–414.

Brochet, D. M., Martin, P., Soubrie, P., and Simon, P. (1987). Triiodothyronine potentiation of antidepressant-induced reversal of learned helplessness in rats. *Psychiatry Res.* **21**, 267–275.

Bursten, B. (1961). Psychoses associated with thyrotoxicosis. *Arch. Gen. Psychiatry* **6**, 267.

Callahan, A. M., Frye, M. A., Marangell, L. B., George, M. S., Ketter, T. A., L'Herrou, T., and Post, R. M. (1997). Comparative antidepressant effects of intravenous and intrathecal thyrotropin-releasing hormone: Confounding effects of tolerance and implications for therapeutics. *Biol. Psychiatry* **41**, 264–272.

Calza, L., Aloe, L., and Giardino, L. (1997). Thyroid hormone-induced plasticity in the adult rat brain. *Brain Res. Bull.* **44**, 549–557.

Campos-Barros, A., and Baumgartner, A. (1994). Effects of chronic desipramine treatment on thyroid hormone concentrations in rat brain: Dependency on drug dose and brain area. *Biol. Psychiatry* **35**, 214–216.

Campos-Barros, A., Köhler, R., Müller, F., Eravci, M., Meinhold, H., Wesemann, W., and Baumgartner, A. (1993). The influence of sleep deprivation on thyroid hormone metabolism in rat frontal cortex. *Neurosci. Lett.* **162**, 145–148.

Campos-Barros, A., Meinhold, H., Köhler, R., Müller, F., Eravci, M., and Baumgartner, A. (1995). The effects of desipramine on thyroid hormone concentrations in rat brain. *Naunyn-Schmiedeberg's Arch. Pharmacol.* **351**, 469–474.

Ceccatelli, S., Giardino, L., and Calza, L. (1992). Response of hypothalamic peptide mRNAs to thyroidectomy. *Neuroendocrinology* **56**, 694–703.

Chapa, F., Kunnecke, B., Calvo, R., Escobar del Rey, F., Morreale de Escobar, G., and Cerdan, S. (1995). Adult-onset hypothyroidism and the cerebral metabolism of (1,2–13C2). Acetate as detected by 13C nuclear magnetic resonance. *Endocrinology (Baltimore)* **136**, 296–305.

Checkley, S. A. (1978). Thyrotoxicosis and the course of manic depressive illness. *Br. J. Psychiatry* **133**, 219.

Chopra, I. J., and Sabatino, L. (2000). Nature and sources of circulating thyroid hormone. *In* "Werner & Ingbar's The Thyroid: A Fundamental and Clinical Text" (L. E. Braverman and R. D. Utiger, eds.), 8th ed., pp. 121–135. Lippincott Williams & Wilkins, Philadelphia.

Cleare, A. J., McGregor, A., and O'Keane, V. (1995). Neuroendocrine evidence for an association between hypothyroidism, reduced central 5-HT activity and depression. *Clin. Endocrinol. (Oxford)* **43**, 713–719.

Cleare, A. J., McGregor, A., Chambers, S. M., Dawling, S., and O'Keane, V. (1996a). Thyroxine replacement increases central 5-hydroxytryptamine activity and reduces depressive symptoms in hypothyroidism. *Neuroendocrinology* **64**, 65–69.

Cleare, A. J., Murray, R. M., and O'Keane, V. (1996b). Reduced prolactin and cortisol responses to d-fenfluramine in depressed compared to healthy matched control subjects. *Neuropsychopharmacology* **14**, 349–354.

Clinical Society of London (1888). Report on myxedema. *Trans. Clin. Soc. London,* Suppl. **21**, 18.

Collu, M., D'Aquila, P. S., Gessa, G. L., and Serra, G. (1992). TRH activates mesolimbic dopamine system: Behavioral evidence. *Behav. Pharmacol.* **3**, 639–641.

Coppen, A. (1967). The biochemistry of affective disorders. *Br. J. Psychiatry* **113**, 1237–1264.

Coppen, A., Whybrow, P., Noguera, R., Maggs, R., and Prange, A., Jr. (1972). The comparative antidepressant value of L-tryptophan and imipramine with and without attempted potentiation by liothyronine. *Arch. Gen. Psychiatry* **26**, 234–241.

Cowdry, R. W., Wehr, T. A., Zis, A. P., and Goodwin, F. K. (1983). Thyroid abnormalities associated with rapid-cycling bipolar illness. *Arch. Gen. Psychiatry* **40**, 414–420.

Crantz, F. R., Silva, J. E., and Larsen, P. R. (1982). Analysis of the sources and quantity of 3,5,3'-iodothyronine specifically bound to nuclear receptors in rat cerebral cortex and cerebellum. *Endocrinology (Baltimore)* **110**, 367–375.

Dratman, M. B., and Gordon, J. T. (1996). Thyroid hormones as neurotransmitters. *Thyroid* **6**, 639–647.

Dratman, M. B., Crutchfield, F. L., Axelrod, J., Colburn, R. W., and Thoa, N. (1976). Localization of triiodothyronine in nerve ending fractions of rat brain. *Proc. Natl. Acad. Sci. U.S.A.* **73**, 941–944.

Dratman, M. B., Crutchfield, F. L., Gordon, J. T., and Jennings, A. S. (1983). Iodothyronine homeostasis in rat brain during hypo- and hyperthyroidism. *Am. J. Physiol.* **245**, E185–E193.

Dugbartey, A. T. (1998). Neurocognitive aspects of hypothyroidism. *Arch. Intern. Med.* **158**, 1413–1418.

Dussault, J. H., and Ruel, J. (1987). Thyroid hormones and brain development. *Annu. Rev. Physiol.* **49**, 321–334.

Duval, F., Macher, J. P., and Mokrani, M. C. (1990). Difference between evening and morning thyrotropin responses to protirelin in major depressive episode. *Arch. Gen. Psychiatry* **47**, 443–448.

Eravci, M., Pinna, G., Meinhold, H., and Baumgartner, A. (2000). Effects of pharmacological and nonpharmacological treatments on thyroid hormone metabolism and concentrations in rat brain. *Endocrinology (Baltimore)* **141**, 1027–1040.

Evans, R. M. (1988). The steroid and the thyroid hormone receptor superfamily. *Science* **240**, 889–895.

Fahrenfort, J. J., Wilterdink, A. M., and van der Veen, E. A. (2000). Long-term residual complaints and psychosocial sequelae after remission of hyperthyroidism. *Psychoneuroendocrinology* **25**, 201–211.

Feighner, J. P., King, L. J., Schuckit, M. A., Croughan, J., and Briscoe, W. (1972). Hormonal potentiation of imipramine and ECT in primary depression. *Am. J. Psychiatry* **128**, 1230–1238.

Feldmesser-Reiss, E. E. (1958). The application of triiodothyronine in the treatment of mental disorders. *J. Nerv. Ment. Dis.* **127**, 540–546.

Flach, F. F., Celian, C. I., and Rawson, R. W. (1958). Treatment of psychiatric disorders with triiodothyronine. *Am. J. Psychiatry* **114**, 841–842.

Frye, M. A., Gary, K. A., Marangell, L. B., George, M. S., Callahan, A. M., Little, J. T., Huggins, T., Cora-Locatelli, G., Osuch,

E. A., Winokur, A., and Post, R. M. (1999). CSF thyrotropin-releasing hormone gender difference: Implications for neurobiology and treatment of depression. *J. Neuropsychiatry Clin. Neurosci.* **11**, 349–353.

Giardino, L., Ceccatelli, S., Zanni, M., Hokfelt, T., and Calza, L. (1994). Regulation of VIP mRNA expression by thyroid hormone in different brain areas of adult rat. *Mol. Brain Res.* **27**, 87–94.

Giordano, T., Pan, J. B., Casuto, D., Watanabe, S., and Arneric, S. P. (1992). Thyroid hormone regulation of NGF, NT-3 and BDNF RNA in the adult rat brain. *Mol. Brain Res.* **16**, 239–245.

Gitlin, M. J., Weiner, H., Fairbanks, L., Hershman, J. M., and Friedfeld, N. (1987). Failure of T_3 to potentiate tricyclic antidepressant response. *J. Affect. Disord.* **13**, 267–272.

Gjessing, R. (1938). Disturbances of somatic function in catatonia with a periodic course and their compensation. *J. Ment. Sci.* **84**, 608–621.

Gjessing, R., and Jenner, A. (1976). "Contributions to the Somatology of Periodic Catatonia." Pergamon Press, Oxford.

Gold, M. S., Pottash, A. L. C., Extein, I., and Sweeney, D. R. (1981). Hypothyroidism and depression: Evidence from complete thyroid function evaluation. *JAMA, J. Am. Med. Assoc.* **245**, 1919–1922.

Gordon, J. T., Kaminski, D. M., Rozanov, C. B., and Dratman, M. B. (1999). Evidence that 3,3′,5-triiodothyronine is concentrated in and delivered from the locus coeruleus to its noradrenergic targets via anterograde axonal transport. *Neuroscience* **93**, 943–954.

Grant, G., Vale, W., and Guillemin, R. (1972). Interactions of thyrotropin-releasing factor with membrane receptors of pituitary cells. *Biochem. Biophys. Res. Commun.* **46**, 28–34.

Graves, R. J. (1835). Newly observed affection of the thyroid gland in females. *London Med. Surg. J.* **7**, 516.

Greer, S., and Parsons, V. (1968). Schizophrenia-like psychosis in thyroid crisis. *Br. J. Psychiatry* **114**, 1357.

Greer, S., Ramsey, I., and Bagley, C. (1973). Neurotic and thyrotoxic anxiety: Clinical, psychological and physiological measurements. *Br. J. Psychiatry* **122**, 549.

Gur, E., Lerer, B., and Newman, M. E. (1999). Chronic clomipramine and triiodothyronine increase serotonin levels in rat frontal cortex in vivo: Relationship to serotonin autoreceptor activity. *J. Pharmacol. Exp. Ther.* **288**, 81–87.

Gyulai, L., Whybrow, P. C., Jaggi, J., Bauer, M. S., Younkin, S., Rubin, L., and Attie, M. (1997). Bone mineral density and L-thyroxine treatment in rapidly cycling bipolar disorder. *Biol. Psychiatry* **41**, 503–506.

Gyulai, L., Bauer, M., Bauer, M. S., Garcia-Espana, F., and Whybrow, P. C. (1999). Lithium challenge to the hypothalamic-pituitary-thyroid (HPT) system in rapid cycling bipolar affective disorder. *Bipolar Disord.* **1**(Suppl. 1), 33.

Gyulai, L., Bauer, M., Espana-Garcia, F., Hierholzer, J., Baumgartner, A., Berghöfer, A., and Whybrow, P. C. (2001). Bone mineral density in pre- and post-menopausal women with affective disorder treated with long-term L-thyroxine augmentation. *J. Affect. Disord.* **66**, 185–191.

Haggerty, J. J., Jr., Garbutt, J. C., Evans, D. L., Golden, R. N., Pedersen, C., Simon, J. S., and Nemeroff, C. B. (1990). Subclinical hypothyroidism: A review of neuropsychiatric aspects. *Int. J. Psychiatry Med.* **20**, 193–208.

Haggerty, J. J., Jr., Stern, R. A., Mason, G. A., Beckwith, J., and Morey, C. E. (1993). Subclinical hypothyroidism: A modifiable risk factor for depression? *Am. J. Psychiatry* **150**, 508–510.

Hahn, C. G., Pawlyk, A. C., Whybrow, P. C., Gyulai, L., and Tejani-Butt, S. M. (1999a). Lithium administration affects gene expression of thyroid hormone receptors in rat brain. *Life Sci.* **64**, 1793–1802.

Hahn, C. G., Pawlyk, A. C., Whybrow, P. C., and Tejani-Butt, S. M. (1999b). Differential expression of thyroid hormone receptor isoforms by thyroid hormone and lithium in rat GH3 and B103 cells. *Biol. Psychiatry* **45**, 1004–1012.

Harris, B., Othman, S., Davies, J. A., Weppner, G. J., Richards, C. J., Newcombe R. G., Lazarus, J. H., Parkes, A. B., Hall, R., and Phillips, D. I. (1992). Association between postpartum thyroid dysfunction and thyroid antibodies and depression. *Br. Med. J.* **305**, 152–156.

Harrison, T. S. (1964). Adrenal, medullary, and thyroid relationships. *Physiol. Rev.* **44**, 161–185.

Hasan, M. K., and Mooney, R. P. (1981). Mania and thyrotoxicosis. *J. Fam. Pract.* **13**, 113.

Heal, D. J., and Smith, S. L. (1988). The effects of acute and repeated administration of T3 to mice on 5-HT1 and 5-HT2 function in the brain and its influence on the actions of repeated electroconvulsive shock. *Neuropharmacology* **27**, 1239–1248.

Henley, W. N., and Koehnle, T. J. (1997). Thyroid hormones and the treatment of depression: An examination of basic hormonal actions in the mature mammalian brain. *Synapse* **27**, 36–44.

Holsboer, F. (1995). Neuroendocrinology of mood disorders. In "Psychopharmacology: The Fourth Generation of Progress" (F. E. Bloom and D. J. Kupfer, eds.), pp. 957–969. Raven Press, New York.

Hong-Brown, L. Q., and Deschepper, C. F. (1992). Effects of thyroid hormones on angiotensinogen gene expression in rat liver, brain, and cultured cells. *Endocrinology (Baltimore)* **130**, 1231–1237.

Iniguez, M. A., Rodriguez-Pena, A., Ibarrola, N., Morreale de Escobar, G., and Bernal, J. (1991). Adult rat brain is sensitive to thyroid hormone. Regulation of RC3/neurogranin mRNA. *J. Clin. Invest.* **90**, 554–558.

Iriuchijima, T., Michimata, T., Mizuma, H., Murakami, M., Yamada, M., and Mori, M. (1991). Hypothyroidism inhibits the formation of inositol phosphate in response to carbachol in the striatum of adult rat. *Res. Commun. Chem. Pathol. Pharmacol.* **73**, 173–180.

Jackson, I. M. D. (1982). Thyrotropin-releasing hormone. *N. Engl. J. Med.* **306**, 145–155.

Jain, V. (1972). A psychiatric study of hypothyroidism. *Psychiatr. Clin.* **5**, 121–130.

Joffe, R., Segal, Z., and Singer, W. (1996). Change in thyroid hormone levels following response to cognitive therapy for major depression. *Am. J. Psychiatry* **153**, 411–413.

Joffe, R. T. (1992). Triiodothyronine potentation of fluoxetine in depressed patients. *Can. J. Psychiatry* **37**, 48–50.

Joffe, R. T., and Singer, W. (1990a). The effect of tricyclic antidepressants on basal thyroid hormone levels in depressed patients. *Pharmacopsychiatry* **23**, 67–69.

Joffe, R. T., and Singer, W. (1990b). A comparison of triiodothyronine and thyroxine in the potentiation of tricyclic antidepressants. *Psychiatry Res.* **32**, 241–251.

Joffe, R. T., and Sokolov, S. T. H. (1994). Thyroid hormones, the brain, and affective disorders. *Crit. Rev. Neurobiol.* **8**, 45–63.

Joffe, R. T., Levitt, A. J., Bagby, R. M., MacDonald, C., and Singer, W. (1993a). Predictors of response to lithium and triiodothyronine augmentation of antidepressants in tricyclic non-responders. *Br. J. Psychiatry* **163**, 574–578.

Joffe R. T., Singer, W., Levitt, A. J., MacDonald, C. (1993b). A placebo-controlled comparison of lithium and triiodothyronine augmentation of tricyclic antidepressants in unipolar refractory depression. *Arch. Gen. Psychiatry* **50**, 387–393.

Josephson, A. M., and Mackenzie, T. B. (1980). Thyroid induced manias in hypothyroid patients. *Br. J. Psychiatry* **137**, 222–228.

Kastin, A. J., Ehrensing, R. H., Schalch, D. S., and Anderson, M. S. (1972). Improvement in mental depression with decreased thyrotropin response after administration of thyrotropin-releasing hormone. *Lancet* **2**, 740–742.

Kathol, R. G., and Delahunt, J. W. (1986). The relationship of anxiety and depression to symptoms of hyperthyroidism using operational criteria. *Gen. Hosp. Psychiatry* **8**, 23–28.

Kirkegaard, C., and Faber, J. (1981). Altered serum levels of thyroxine, triiodothyronines and diiodothyronines in endogenous depression. *Acta. Endocrinol. (Copenhagen)* **96**, 199–207.

Kirkegaard, C., and Faber, J. (1998). The role of thyroid hormones in depression. *Eur. J. Endocrinol.* **138**, 1–9.

Kleinschmidt, H., and Waxenberg, S. (1956). Psychophysiology and psychiatric management of thyrotoxicosis: A two year follow up study. *Mt. Sinai J. Med. (NY)*. **23**, 131–153.

Köhrle, J. (2000). Thyroid hormone metabolism and action in the brain and pituitary. *Acta Med. Austriaca* **27**, 1–7.

Kulikov, A., Moreau, X., and Jeanningros, R. (1999). Effects of experimental hypothyroidism on 5-HT1A, 5-HT2A receptors, 5-HT uptake sites and tryptophan hydroxylase activity in mature rat brain. *Neuroendocrinology* **69**, 453–459.

Larsen, P. R., Davies, T. F., and Hay, I. D. (1998). The thyroid gland. *In* "Williams Textbook of Endocrinology" (J. D. Wilson, D. W. Foster, H. M. Kronenberg, and P. R. Larsen, eds.), 9th ed., pp. 389–515. Saunders, Philadelphia.

Lasser, R. A., and Baldessarini, R. J. (1997). Thyroid hormones in depressive disorders: A reappraisal of clinical utility. *Harv. Rev. Psychiatry* **4**, 291–305.

Lazarus, J. H. (1986). Effect of lithium on the thyroid gland. *In* "Endocrine and Metabolic Effects of Lithium" (J. H. Lazarus and K. J. Collard, eds.), pp. 99–124. Plenum Medical Book Company, New York.

Lazarus, J. H. (1998). The effects of lithium therapy on thyroid and thyrotropin-releasing hormone. *Thyroid* **8**, 909–913.

Leonard, J. L. (1988). Dibutyryl cAMP induction of type II 5'deiodinase activity in rat brain astrocytes in culture. *Biochem. Biophys. Res. Commun.* **151**, 1164–1172.

Leonard, J. L., and Koehrle, J. (2000). Intracellular pathways of iodothyronine metabolism. *In* "Werner & Ingbar's The Thyroid. A Fundamental and Clinical Text" (L. E. Braverman and R. D. Utiger, eds.), 8th ed., pp. 136–171. Lippincott Williams & Wilkins, Philadelphia.

Levine, J. D., Strauss, L. R., Munez, L. R., Dratman, M. B., Stewart, K. T., and Adler, N. T. (1990). Thyroparathyroidectomy produces a progressive escape deficit in rats. *Physiol. Behav.* **48**, 165–167.

Lidz, T., and Whitehorn, J. C. (1949). Psychiatric problems in a thyroid clinic. *JAMA, J. Am. Med. Assoc.* **139**, 698–701.

Loosen, P. T. (1985). The TRH-induced TSH response in psychiatric patients: a possible neuroendocrine marker. *Psychoneuroendocrinology* **10**, 237–260.

MacCrimmon, D. J., Wallace, J. E., Goldberg, W. M., and Steiner, D. L. (1979). Emotional disturbance and cognitive deficits in hyperthyroidism. *Psychosom. Med.* **41**, 331–340.

Maes, M., and Meltzer, H. Y. (1995). The serotonin hypotheses of major depression. *In* "Psychopharmacology: The Fourth Generation of Progess" (F. E. Bloom and D. J. Kupfer, eds.), pp. 933–944. Raven Press, New York.

Marangell, L. B., George, M. S., Callahan, A. M., Ketter, T. A., Pazzaglia, P. J., L'Herrou, T. A., Leverich, G. S., and Post, R. M. (1997a). Effects of intrathecal thyrotropin-releasing hormone (protirelin) in refractory depressed patients. *Arch. Gen. Psychiatry* **54**, 214–222.

Marangell, L. B., Ketter, T. A., George, M. S., Pazzaglia, P. J., Callahan, A. M., Parekh, P., Andreason, P. J., Horwitz, B.,

Herscovitch, P., and Post, R. M. (1997b). Inverse relationship of peripheral thyrotropin-stimulating hormone levels to brain activity in mood disorders. *Am. J. Psychiatry* **154**, 224–230.

Marcocci, C., and Chiovato, L. (2000). Thyroid-directed antibodies. In "Werner & Ingbar's The Thyroid: A Fundamental and Clinical Text" (L. E. Braverman and R. D. Utiger, eds.), 8th ed., pp. 414–431. Lippincott Williams & Wilkins, Philadelphia.

Martin, P., Brochet, D., Soubrie, P., and Simon, P. (1985). Triiodothyronine-induced reversal of learned helplessness in rats. *Biol. Psychiatry* **20**, 1023–1025.

Martin, J. V., Williams, D. B., Fitzgerald, R. M., Im, H. K., and von voigtlander, P. F. (1996). Thyroid hormonal modulation of the binding and activity of the GABA$_A$ receptor complex of brain. *Neuroscience* **73**, 705–713.

Mashio, Y., Inada, M., Tanaka, K., Ishii, H., Naito, K., Nishikawa, M., Takahashi, K., and Imura, H. (1982). High affinity 3,5,3'-L-triiodothyronine binding to synaptosomes in rat cerebral cortex. *Endocrinology (Baltimore)* **110**, 1257–1261.

Mason, G. A., Walker, C. H., and Prange, A. J., Jr. (1987). Modulation of gamma-aminobutyric acid uptake of rat brain synaptosomes by thyroid hormones. *Neuropsychopharmacology* **1**, 63–70.

Mason, G. A., Walker, C. H., and Prange, A. J., Jr. (1990). Depolarization-dependent 45Ca uptake by synaptosomes of rat cerebral cortex is enhanced by L-triiodothyronine. *Neuropsychopharmacology* **3**, 291–295.

Mason, G. A., Walker, C. H., and Prange, A. J., Jr. (1993). L-triiodothyronine: Is this peripheral hormone a central neurotransmitter? *Neuropsychopharmacology* **8**, 253–258.

Mason, G. A., Garbutt, J. C., and Prange, A. J., Jr. (1995). Thyrotropin-releasing hormone. In "Psychopharmacology: The Fourth Generation of Progress" (F. E. Bloom and D. J. Kupfer, eds.), pp. 493–503. Raven Press, New York.

Mazurkiewicz, D., and Saggerson, E. D. (1989). Inhibition of adenylate cyclase in rat brain synaptosomal membranes by GTP and phenylisopropyladenosine is enhanced in hypothyroidism. *Biochem. J.* **263**, 829–835.

Mooradian, A. D. (1990). Metabolic fuel and amino acid transport into the brain in experimental hypothyroidism. *Acta Endocrinol. (Copenhagen)* **122**, 156–162.

Morley, J. E. (1981). Neuroendocrine control of thyrotropin secretion. *Endocr. Rev.* **2**, 396–436.

Narihara, R., Hirouchi, M., Ichida, T., Kuriyama, K., and Roberts, E. (1994). Effects of thyroxine and its related compounds on cerebral GABA receptors: Inhibitory action on benzodiazepine recognition site in GABAA receptor complex. *Neurochem. Int.* **25**, 451–454.

Nemeroff, C. B., Kalivas, P. W., Golden, R. N., and Prange, A. J., Jr. (1984). Behavioral effects of hypothalamic hypophysiotropic hormones, neurotensin, substance P and other neuropeptides. *Pharmacol. Ther.* **24**, 1–56.

O'Brien, M. D., and Harris, P. H. (1968). Cerebral-cortex perfusion-rates in myxoedema. *Lancet* **1**, 1170–1172.

Okuno, Y., and Nakayasu, N. (1988). Thyroid function and therapeutic efficacy of thyroxine in depression. *Jpn. J. Psychiatry Neurol.* **42**, 763–770.

Oppenheimer, J. H. (1999). Evolving concepts of thyroid hormone action. *Biochimie* **81**, 539–543.

Oppenheimer, J. H., and Schwartz, H. L. (1997). Molecular basis of thyroid hormone-dependent brain development. *Endocr. Rev.* **18**, 462–475.

Oppenheimer, J. H., Schwartz, H. L., and Surks, M. I. (1974). Tissue differences in the concentration of triiodothyronine nuclear binding sites in the rat: Liver, kidney, pituitary, heart, brain, spleen, and testis. *Endocrinology (Baltimore)* **95**, 897–903.

Orford, M. R., Mazurkiewicz, D., Milligan, G., and Saggerson, E. D. (1991). Abundance of the alpha-subunits of Gi1, Gi2 and Go in synaptosomal membranes from several regions of the rat brain is increased in hypothyroidism. *Biochem. J.* **275**, 183–186.

Orford, M. R., Leung, F. C., Milligan, G., and Saggerson, E. D. (1992). Treatment with triiodothyronine decreases the abundance of the alpha-subunits of Gi1 and Gi2 in the cerebral cortex. *J. Neurol. Sci.* **112**, 34–37.

Pardridge, W. M., Boado, R. J., and Farrell, C. R. (1990). Brain-type glucose transporter (GLUT-1) is selectively localized to the blood-brain barrier. Studies with quantitative western blotting and in situ hybridization. *J. Biol. Chem.* **265**, 18035–18040.

Parry, C. H. (1825). "Collections from the Unpublished Writings of the Late C. H. Parry," Vol. 2. Underwoods, London.

Patten, S. B., Lupin, D. A., Boucher, S. A., and Lamarre, C. J. (1992). Pharmacologic management of refractory depression. *Can. Med. Assoc. J.* **146**, 483–487.

Peake, R. L. (1981). Recurrent apathetic hyperthyroidism. *Arch. Intern. Med.* **141**, 258–260.

Porterfield, S. P., and Hendrich, C. E. (1993). The role of thyroid hormones in prenatal and neonatal neurological development—current perspectives. *Endocr. Rev.* **14**, 94–106.

Prange, A. J., Jr., Wilson, I. C., Rabon, A. M., and Lipton, M. A. (1969). Enhancement of imipramine antidepressant activity by thyroid hormone. *Am. J. Psychiatry* **126**, 457–469.

Prange, A. J., Jr., Wilson, I. C., Knox, A., McClane, T. K., and Lipton, M. A. (1970). Enhancement of imipramine by thyroid stimulating hormone: Clinical and theoretical implications. *Am. J. Psychiatry* **127**, 191–199.

Prange, A. J., Jr., Lara, P. P., Wilson, I. C., Alltop, L. B., and Breese, G. R. (1972). Effects of thyrotropin-releasing hormone in depression. *Lancet* **2**, 999–1002.

Prange, A. J., Jr., Wilson, I. C., Breese, G. R., and Lipton, M. A. (1976). Hormonal alteration of imipramine response: A review. In "Hormones, Behavior, and Psychopathology" (E. J. Sachar, ed.), pp. 41–67. Raven Press, New York.

Reichlin, S. (1998). Neuroendocrinology. In "Williams Textbook of Endocrinology" (J. D. Wilson, D. W. Foster, H. M. Kronenberg, and P. R. Larsen, eds.), 9th ed., pp. 165–248. Saunders, Philadelphia.

Reitan, R. M. (1953). Intellectual functions in myxoedema. Arch. Neurol. Psychiatry **69**, 436.

Reus, V. I., Gold, P., and Post, R. (1979). Lithium-induced thyrotoxicosis. Am. J. Psychiatry **136**, 724.

Robbins, L. R., and Vinson, D. B. (1960). Objective psychological assessment of the thyrotoxic patient and the response to treatment. J. Clin. Endocrinol. **20**, 120.

Roeder, L. M., Hopkins, I. B., Kaiser, J. R., Hanukoglu, L., and Tildon, J. T. (1988). Thyroid hormone action on glucose transporter activity in astrocytes. Biochem. Biophys. Res. Commun. **156**, 275–281.

Roy-Byrne, P. P., Joffe, R. T., Uhde, T. W., and Post, R. M. (1984). Carbamazepine and thyroid function in affectively ill patients. Arch. Gen. Psychiatry **41**, 1150–1153.

Rozanov, C. B., and Dratman, M. B. (1996). Immunohistochemical mapping of brain triiodothyronine reveals prominent localization in central noradrenergic systems. Neuroscience **74**, 897–915.

Rudas, S., Schmitz, M., Pichler, P., and Baumgartner, A. (1999). Treatment of refractory chronic depression and dysthymia with high-dose thyroxine. Biol. Psychiatry **2**, 229–233.

Ruel, J., Faure, R., and Dussault, J. H. (1985). Regional distribution of nuclear T_3 receptors in rat brain and evidence for preferential localization in neurons. J. Endocrinol. Invest. **8**, 343–348.

Sack, D. A., James, S. P., Rosenthal, N. E., and Wehr, T. A. (1988). Deficient nocturnal surge of TSH secretion during sleep and sleep deprivation in rapid-cycling bipolar illness. Psychiatry Res. **23**, 179–191.

Scanlon, M. F., and Toft, A. D. (2000). Regulation of thyrotropin secretion. In "Werner & Ingbar's The Thyroid: A Fundamental and Clinical Text" (L. E. Braverman and R. D. Utiger, eds.), 8th ed., pp. 234–253. Lippincott Williams & Wilkins, Philadelphia.

Schwartz, H. L., and Oppenheimer, J. H. (1978). Nuclear triiodothyronine receptor sites in brain: Probable identity with hepatic receptors and regional distribution. Endocrinology (Baltimore) **103**, 267–273.

Segerson, T. P., Kauer, J., Wolfe, H. C., Mobtaker, H., Wu, P., Jackson, I. M. D., and Lechan, R. M. (1987). Thyroid hormone regulates (TRH) biosynthesis in the paraventricular nucleus of the rat hypothalamus. Science **238**, 78–80.

Sensenbach, W., Madison, L., Eisenberg, S., and Ochs, L. (1954). The cerebral circulation and metabolism in hyperthyroidism and myxedema. J. Clin. Invest. **33**, 1434–1440.

Silverman, D. H. S., Lombardi, C. A., Lu, C. S., Whybrow, P. C., Czernin, J., Phelps, M. E., and Bauer, M. (2001). Effect of thyroid disease on brain metabolism in patients with dementia symptoms. (Abstract). Nucl. Med. **42**, suppl; 225p.

Smallridge, R. C. (2000). Metabolic, physiologic, and clinical indexes of thyroid function. In "Werner & Ingbar's The Thyroid: A Fundamental and Clinical Text" (L. E. Braverman and R. D. Utiger, eds.), 8th ed., pp. 393–401. Lippincott Williams & Wilkins, Philadelphia.

Smith, C. D., and Ain, K. B. (1995). Brain metabolism in hypothyroidism studied with ^{31}P magnetic-resonance spectroscopy. Lancet **345**, 619–620.

Sokoloff, L., Wechsler, R. L., Mangold, R., Balls, K., and Kety, S. S. (1953). Cerebral blood flow and oxygen consumption in hyperthyroidism before and after treatment. J. Clin. Invest. **32**, 202–208.

Sokolov, S. T., Levitt, A. J., and Joffe, R. T. (1997). Thyroid hormone levels before unsuccessful antidepressant therapy are associated with later response to T_3 augmentation. Psychiatry Res. **69**, 203–206.

Spoov, J., and Lahdelma, L. (1998). Should thyroid augmentation precede lithium augmentation—a pilot study. J. Affect. Disord. **49**, 235–239.

Stancer, H. C., and Persad, E. (1982). Treatment of intractable rapid-cycling manic-depressive disorder with levothyroxine. Arch. Gen. Psychiatry **39**, 311–312.

Stein, D., and Avni, J. (1988). Thyroid hormones in the treatment of affective disorders. Acta. Psychiatr. Scand. **77**, 623–636.

Steiner, M., Radwan, M., Elizur, A., Blum, I., Atsmon, A., and Davidson, S. (1978). Failure of l-triiodothyronine (T_3) to potentiate tricyclic antidepressant response. Curr. Ther. Res. **23**, 655–659.

St. Germain, D. (1987). Regulatory effect of lithium on thyroxine metabolism in murine neural and anterior pituitary tissue. Endocrinology (Baltimore) **120**, 1430–1438.

St. Germain, D. L., and Galton, V. A. (1997). The deiodinase family of selenoproteins. Thyroid **7**, 655–668.

Szuba, M. P., Altshuler, L. L., and Baxter, L. R., Jr. (1992). Thyroid function and partial sleep deprivation response. Arch. Gen. Psychiatry **49**, 581–582.

Taylor, J. W. (1975). Depression in thyrotoxicosis. Am. J. Psychiatry **132**, 552–553.

Tejani-Butt, S. M., and Yang, J. (1994). A time course of altered thyroid states on the noradrenergic system in rat brain by quantitative autoradiography. Neuroendocrinology **59**, 235–244.

Tejani-Butt, S. M., Yang, J., and Kaviani, A. (1993). Time course of altered thyroid states on 5-HT1A receptors and 5-HT uptake sites in rat brain: An autoradiographic analysis. *Neuroendocrinology* **57**, 1011–1018.

Tejani-Butt, S. M., Yang, J., Pawlyk, A., and Hahn, C. G. (2000). Receptors and molecular studies. *Neuropsychopharmacology* **23**, S69.

Thorner, M. O., Vance, M. L., Laws, E. R., Horvath, E., and Kovacs, K. (1998). The anterior pituitary. *In* "Williams Textbook of Endocrinology" (J. D. Wilson, D. W. Foster, H. M. Kronenberg, and P. R. Larsen, eds.), 9th ed., pp. 249–340. Saunders, Philadelphia.

Treadway, C. R., Prange, A. J., Jr, Doehne, E. F., Edens, C. J., and Whybrow, P. C. (1967). Myxedema psychosis: Clinical and biochemical changes during recovery. *J. Psychiatr. Res.* **5**, 289–296.

Trzepacz, P. T., McCue, M., Klein, I., Levey, G. S., and Greenhouse, J. (1988). A psychiatric and neuropsychological study of patients with untreated Graves' disease. *Gen. Hosp. Psychiatry* **10**, 49–55.

Tsuruo, Y., Hokfelt, T., and Visser, T. (1987). Thyrotropin releasing hormone (TRH)-immunoreactive cell groups in the rat central nervous system. *Exp. Brain Res.* **68**, 213–217.

Vaidya, V. A., Castro, M. E., Pei, Q., Sprakes, M. E., and Grahame-Smith, D. G. (2001). Influence of thyroid hormone on 5-HT$_{1A}$ and 5-HT$_{2A}$ receptor-mediated regulation of hippocampal BDNF mRNA expression. *Neuropharmacology* **40**, 48–56.

van Doorn, J., Roelfsma, F., and van der Heide, D. (1985). Concentrations of thyroxine and 3,5,3′-triiodothyronine at 34 different sites in euthyroid rats as determined by an isotopic equilibrium technique. *Endocrinology (Baltimore)* **117**, 1201–1208.

Wartofsky, L. (2000). Thyrotoxic storm. *In* "Werner & Ingbar's The Thyroid: A Fundamental and Clinical Text" (L. E. Braverman and R. D. Utiger, eds.), 8th ed., pp. 679–684. Lippincott Williams & Wilkins, Philadelphia.

Weetman, A. P. (2000). Chronic autoimmune thyroiditis. *In* "Werner and Ingbar's The Thyroid: A Fundamental and Clinical Text" (L. E. Braverman and R. D. Utiger, eds.), 8th ed., pp. 721–732. Lippincott Williams & Wilkins, Philadelphia.

Wenzel, K. W., Meinhold, H., Raffenberg, M., Adlkofer, F., and Schleusner, H. (1974). Classification of hypothyroidism in evaluating patients after radioiodine therapy by serum cholesterol, T$_3$-uptake, total T$_4$, fT$_4$-index, total T$_3$, basal TSH and TRH test. *Eur. J. Clin. Invest.* **4**, 141–148.

Wheatley, D. (1972). Potentiation of amitriptyline by thyroid hormone. *Arch. Gen. Psychiatry* **26**, 229–233.

Whybrow, P. C. (1995). Sex differences in thyroid axis function: Relevance to affective disorder and its treatment. *Depression* **3**, 33–42.

Whybrow, P. C., and Bauer, M. (2000a). Behavioral and psychiatric aspects of thyrotoxicosis. *In* "Werner & Ingbar's The Thyroid: A Fundamental and Clinical Text" (L. E. Braverman and R. D. Utiger, eds.), 8th ed., pp. 673–678. Lippincott Williams & Wilkins, Philadelphia.

Whybrow, P. C., and Bauer, M. (2000b). Behavioral and psychiatric aspects of hypothyroidism. *In* "Werner & Ingbar's The Thyroid: A Fundamental and Clinical Text" (L. E. Braverman and R. D. Utiger, eds.), 8th ed., pp. 837–842. Lippincott Williams & Wilkins, Philadelphia.

Whybrow, P. C., and Prange, A. J., Jr. (1981). A hypotheses of thyroid-catecholamine-receptor interaction. *Arch. Gen. Psychiatry* **38**, 106–113.

Whybrow, P. C., Prange, A. J., Jr., and Treadway, C. R. (1969). Mental changes accompanying thyroid gland dysfunction. *Arch. Gen. Psychiatry* **20**, 48–63.

Whybrow, P. C., Coppen, A., Prange, A. J., Jr., Noguera, R., and Bailey, J. E. (1972). Thyroid function and the response to liothyronine in depression. *Arch. Gen. Psychiatry* **26**, 242–245.

Wilson, I. C., Prange, A. J., McClane, T. K., Rabon, A. M., and Lipton, M. (1970). Thyroid-hormone enhancement of imipramine in nonretarded depressions. *N. Engl. J. Med.* **282**, 1063–1067.

Wilson, I. C., Prange, A. J., Jr., and Lara, P. P. (1974). L-Triiodothyronine alone and with imipramine in the treatment of depressed women. *In* "The Thyroid Axis, Drugs, and Behavior" (A. J. Prange, Jr., ed.), pp. 49–62. Raven Press, New York.

22

Gonadal Steroids, Learning, and Memory

Gary Dohanich
Department of Psychology
Tulane University
New Orleans, Louisiana 70118

Although the roles of estrogen, progesterone, and testosterone in the activation and maintenance of reproductive function are well established, emerging evidence indicates that these same steroids influence performance on measures of learning and memory in various species, including humans. These effects are complex and vary with task, gender, and age, as well as the regimens of steroid exposure. Gonadal steroids can affect performance on appetitive and aversive tasks; spatial and nonspatial tasks; conditioning; and acquisition, consolidation, and retention. However, the effects of steroids on learning and memory often are moderate in magnitude and can improve, impair, or not affect performance on various measures of learning and memory. Consequently, the biological and behavioral significance of steroid modulation of cognitive performance remains to be determined. A more important action of gonadal steroids may prove to be their ability to assist neurons in confronting risks encountered thoughout life. These neuroprotective actions could have profound consequences for the prevention and treatment of diseases of aging, including Alzheimer's disease and other well-known pathologies. A better understanding of the mechanisms of steroid action and cognitive function should lead to the development of new steroid treatments to improve neuronal function that has been compromised by trauma, age, or disease.

I. INTRODUCTION

A. Steroids, Learning, and Memory

Steroid hormones are key elements of communication in the body. These remarkable molecules play important roles across the life span, guiding development in young organisms and regulating physiological processes in adults. The attenuation of steroid effects that can accompany age often impairs or eliminates normal functions. A primary feature of endocrine action is the facility of a single hormone to integrate activities in target tissues throughout the body. Estrogen, for example, participates in the regulation of many reproductive processes in mammals, ranging from the induction of mating behaviors to the stimulation of gonadotropin release to the proliferation of the endometrium (Feder, 1981b; Nelson, 2000; Pfaff, 1980; Pfaff et al., 1994). The central and peripheral actions of estrogen afford an organism with a series of coordinated responses necessary for successful reproduction.

However, the effects of gonadal steroids extend beyond the domain of reproduction. Sufficient evidence has accumulated since the 1970s to support the hypothesis that gonadal steroids can influence processes that allow an organism to learn and remember new information. Although this conclusion quickly leads to exciting implications for our understanding of cognitive function and for the treatment of cognitive disability, it also raises questions regarding the nature, mechanism, and significance of the steroid modulation of learning and memory. In order to support the case that a steroid plays a meaningful role in cognition, several central issues must be addressed: adaptive value (the proposed effect of the steroid on learning and memory should have adaptive value to the organism); strength of effect (empirical data supporting the role of the steroid in learning and memory should be sufficiently robust in magnitude and replicability); neural substrate (anatomical and physiological substrates should exist to support the actions of the steroid on learning and memory); and nonmnemonic processes (processes other than those directly mediating steroid effects on learning and memory systems should be identified).

1. Adaptive Value

For a steroid to have a meaningful role in the regulation of cognitive processes, its influence should contribute to the survival of the organism through its reproductive life span. In the case of some steroids, the adaptive value of their effects on learning and memory may not be obvious or even testable. Explanations of adaptive significance can be easy to create but difficult to prove. For example, it is not immediately clear why the endogenous levels of steroids such as estrogen and progesterone should affect the ability of a female to learn and remember information. According to one hypothesis, when estrogen and progesterone levels are high, typical of pregnancy, spatial learning and memory and mobility are reduced in order to limit a female's movement outside the safety of familiar territory (Sherry and Hampson, 1997). Another proposes that spatial learning and memory might suffer when estrogen and progesterone levels are elevated during the time of mating in order to benefit other cognitive functions, such as communication (Desmond and Levy, 1997). However, such explanations of adaptive significance require strong empirical support.

2. Strength of Effect

The reported effects of steroids on cognitive performance can be small in magnitude, difficult to replicate, and even contradictory. Statistical significance implies, but does not prove, biological significance, an obvious point that often is ignored. Further, negative or contradictory data can be banished to the file drawer, inflating the acceptance of an effect. If a hormonal effect can be demonstrated only under highly specific conditions, its generalizability to other experimental or natural situations, as well as to other species, is called into question. There is no rule of thumb for accepting or rejecting a weak or inconsistent finding; only rigorous testing can resolve the value of an experimental result.

3. Neural Substrate

When investigating the putative role of a steroid in learning and memory, we should consider the existence of anatomical and physiological substrates that can support the steroid action. Steroid hormones often exert genomic actions via intracellular receptors that are found in high concentrations in brain regions that control reproduction (McEwen et al., 1978; Pfaff, 1972, 1980; Pfaff and Keiner, 1973). Historically, the number of neurons with estrogen receptors in areas associated with cognition was believed to be low (Pfaff and Keiner, 1973). However, the advent of more sensitive techniques revealed denser distributions of neurons containing estrogen receptors (ERs) and mRNA in the hippocampus and cortex (Shughrue and Merchenthaler, 2000; Weiland et al., 1997). Furthermore, the discovery of multiple subtypes of estrogen receptors, ERα and ERβ, particularly in the hippocampus and cortex, adds another dimension to estrogen action on cognitive processes (Li et al., 1997; Shughrue et al., 1997). In addition to their conventional genomic actions, steroids can affect neuronal activity by other mechanisms that involve steroid membrane receptors and signal transduction pathways (McEwen and Alves, 1999). The detection of steroid receptors in brain regions not involved in reproduction, the discovery of different forms of steroid receptors, and the identification of novel mechanisms of steroid action provide a rich neuroanatomical and neurochemical substrate for steroid modulation of learning and memory.

4. Nonmnemonic Processes

Steroids can affect a wide range of activities in the body that could have important implications when investigating the cognitive effects of hormones. Sensory, motor, regulatory, and affective processes that influence learning and memory performance normally are labeled nonmnemonic to distinguish them from the genuine memory processes that support cognition (Bartus, 2000; Gold and Zornetzer, 1983; Hodges, 1996; Sahgal, 1993). When we study learning and memory, it is vital to remember that we cannot see learning and we cannot see memory, but only performance that may or may not reflect true mnemonic processes. It should be noted, nevertheless, that many of these nonmnemonic processes play important roles in cognition and can be just as important to the acquisition, storage, and retrieval of information as the activities of brain systems that directly mediate learning and memory (Gold and Zornetzer, 1983).

II. LEARNING AND MEMORY

A. Study of Learning and Memory

The biological basis of learning and memory is one of oldest obsessions of psychology, dating back to at least the 1920s. Karl Lashley's unsuccessful attempts to identify the cortical locations where the brain stores its memories led him to conclude that all areas of the cortex contributed equally to every memory (Lashley, 1929, 1950). Lashley's findings, interestingly, were predated by the nineteenth-century theories of Gall and the experiments of Flourens and Goltz (Squire, 1987). Important milestones since Lashley's work include the hypotheses of Hebb (1949), who proposed that synaptic change is the neural basis of memory; the discovery of the selective memory deficits of H.M., a patient who underwent temporal lobe ablations to treat his epilepsy, by Milner and others (Milner, 1959); the development of long-term potentiation as an electrophysiological model of learning and memory by Bliss and Lomo (1973); the use of the invertebrate sea slug *Aplysia* by Kandel and colleagues as a means to study the connectivity and cellular and molecular biology of a simple learning and memory system (Carew *et al.*, 1986); and the development of sophisticated tasks to assess performance in nonhuman species under a variety of experimental conditions (Morris, 1984; Olton *et al.*, 1978). Each of these achievements has important implications for the study of steroids and their influences on cognition. The vast number of experiments devoted to defining the principles of learning and memory has spawned a scientific literature that is both illuminating and dense. The study of cognition continues to be one of the most exciting topics in science—exploring processes and behaviors that members of all species use everyday to interact with their environments, learn from their experiences, and survive as individuals. Humans have taken full advantage of their unmatched cognitive facilities so that our own unique memories come to define our fundamental sense of self.

B. Some Basic Elements of Learning and Memory

There are several fundamental elements common to most forms of learning and memory: pretraining (preacquisition), training (acquisition and learning), consolidation, and retention (memory). Although a reductionistic approach requires that each component be considered individually, these processes should be regarded as an interwoven system that allows the acquisition, encoding, storage, and retrieval of information. During pretraining, a subject explores the learning environment to become familiar with the setting, as well as the demands and rewards of the task, prior to actual training. This pretraining phase can allow a learner to experience the sensorimotor requirements of the task as well as reducing anxiety during the early trials of training itself (Cain, 1998; Morris, 1989). The training phase may be the most difficult to study because, particularly during the early trials, the subject may use several types of memory for successful learning and be most susceptible to the effects of nonmnemonic processes. Consequently, hormonal effects on performance during training may reflect changes in these processes rather than learning itself. It sometimes can be difficult to parcel out the effects of a hormone on learning from its nonmnemonic actions, although pretraining can reduce the influence of these variables on performance (Bartus, 2000; Cain, 1998). As training proceeds, performance normally improves to an asymptotic level over the trials and days of acquisition, as reflected by a learning curve. Consolidation follows training and may occur immediately after each training trial or series of trials. The effects of hormones on consolidation can be determined by treatments administered during this phase, followed by retention tests after periods of elapsed time, a paradigm that also can minimize the effects of hormones on nonmnemonic processes (McGaugh, 2000). Retention can be tested in a variety of ways after performance has reached its asymptote. During retention tests, the memory load can be controlled by the investigator for a given task using such procedures as increasing the time during which information must be held in memory, increasing the number of items that must be held in memory, increasing interference that disrupts memory, or requiring the manipulation of information held in memory (Duff and Hampson, 2000; Rawlins and Deacon, 1993).

The reinforcement structure of a task usually is a key factor for successful learning. Organisms can be motivated to learn and remember a task by the use of positive or negative reinforcements, particularly when the drive state has been elevated by some form of deprivation. For appetitive tasks, typical positive reinforcements include water or food rewards for subjects mildly deprived, for example, to 85–90% of their free-feeding body weights. For aversive tasks, typical negative reinforcements include escaping or avoiding an electric shock in conditioning tasks or a threatening situation in a water maze or a circular platform maze. The type of reward and the level of deprivation, as well as various aspects of the procedure, can affect learning strategies, response patterns, and overall performance (Dale and Roberts, 1986; Hodges, 1996; Spear et al., 1990). When we study the effects of hormones on learning and memory performance, the reinforcement structure can interact with many factors inherent in the task, such as appetite, thirst, pain threshold, and anxiety level. For example, ovariectomy initially increases food intake in some species, an effect that could confound the results from tasks that depend on food deprivation as a reinforcer (Wade, 1975, 1976). Increased body weight associated with ovariectomy also could alter running or swimming abilities. Conversely, food deprivation can disrupt reproductive cycles in some species, undermining attempts to evaluate the effects of the cycle on tasks that require food reward (Daniel et al., 1999).

C. Types of Learning and Memory

Inspired by the pronounced inability of H.M. and other amnesics to remember new factual information while retaining the ability to learn new sensorimotor skills (Squire and Cohen, 1984), researchers divided mnemonic processes into declarative and procedural memories (Squire, 1987). Memory continued to be subdivided in the ensuring years, a strategy fraught with its own problems. There are various tasks used to operationally define different types of learning and memory (Table 1). In the paradigms presented here, the focus is primarily on tasks often used to determine the effects of steroids on learning and memory performance. As we review the effects of gonadal steroids on cognition, it is important to remember that tasks that purport to isolate

TABLE 1
Some Classification Systems of Learning and Memory

Type	Task	Description
Spatial	Place	Extramaze cues to locate reinforcement
		Allocentric strategy
Nonspatial	Cued	Intramaze cues to locate reinforcement
		Allocentric strategy
Nonspatial	Response	Proprioceptive cues to locate reinforcement
		Egocentric strategy
Nonspatial	Object recognition	Intramaze cues to locate reinforcement
		Allocentric strategy
Conditioning	Habituation	Repeated stimulation decreases response
	Sensitization	Facilitating stimulation increases response
	Classical conditioning	Conditioned stimulus elicits conditioned response
	Operant conditioning	Response reinforced appetitively or aversively

a specific memory subtype are often imperfect and that certain tasks may be dependent on the simultaneous use of multiple types of memory.

1. Spatial and Nonspatial Learning and Memory

Tolman (1949) proposed that by learning the relationships between external or internal stimuli and available reinforcements information can be stored as memory for later use during subsequent exposure to the same environment. However, mammals may learn the location of a reward in three-dimensional space by the use of several different strategies and cues (O'Keefe and Nadel, 1978). These include (1) spatially by relationships between distant cues outside the maze and the site of reinforcement (Olton and Collison, 1979), (2) nonspatially by the presence of proximate cues within the maze that mark the location of reinforcement (Kraemer et al., 1983), and (3) nonspatially by the use of proprioceptive cues or responses that guide the subject to the reinforcement (Dale, 1986; Suzuki et al., 1980). All three types of learning and memory depend to some degree on conditioning. An organism in a novel environment can learn and remember the relationship between cues (distant, proximate, or response) and a desired goal in order to guide its later behaviors during a search for a food reward or an escape from an aversive stimulus. The use of distant extramaze cues to locate reinforcements is a form of spatial learning and memory that relies on an allocentric strategy and makes use of information in the subject's environment—for example, remembering that a food pellet is located in the arm of the radial maze opposite from the sink, toward the door, and between the clock and the picture (O'Keefe and Nadel, 1978; Morris et al., 1986). In contrast, a response or egocentric strategy depends on proprioceptive information in the subject that guides the behavior—for example, always turning right to receive a food reward (O'Keefe and Nadel, 1978). Interestingly, gender, age, experience, and hormonal state can influence the use of a particular strategy.

a) Working Memory and Reference Memory

Memory can be subdivided into types based on duration and use (Baddeley, 1986; Olton and Papas, 1979; Olton et al., 1979; Olton, 1983). Working memory is a form of short-term memory that stores information only for the period of time that it remains useful (Baddeley and Hitch, 1974). The retention period for working memory varies according to its definition, lasting less than 1 minute according to some researchers or persisting for many hours as defined by others. In any event, the information stored typically is only useful during a single test session if the features of each trial set change from session to session. Reference memory is a form of long-term memory that stores information in a stable form that continues to be useful across trials over long periods.

Working and reference memories can be defined operationally using several types of cognitive tasks; however, the radial arm maze and the water maze have been the most common applications in experiments using rodents (Fig. 1). The radial arm maze is an appetitive task that takes advantage of the natural foraging strategy of rats; the subject must enter 8–17 different arms to receive a food reward. Working memory (memory for current but temporary information) is the memory of which arms were entered during a radial-arm-maze trial (Olton and Samuelson, 1976). Reference memory (memory for a general principle) is the memory of which arms are always baited over trials (Olton and Papas, 1979). In order to differentiate working and reference memories, the same four arms of the radial maze are baited on all trials and the remaining four arms are never baited. In this paradigm, reentry into an arm previously visited is defined as an error of working memory and entry into an arm that is never baited is defined as an error of reference memory. Alternatively, the water

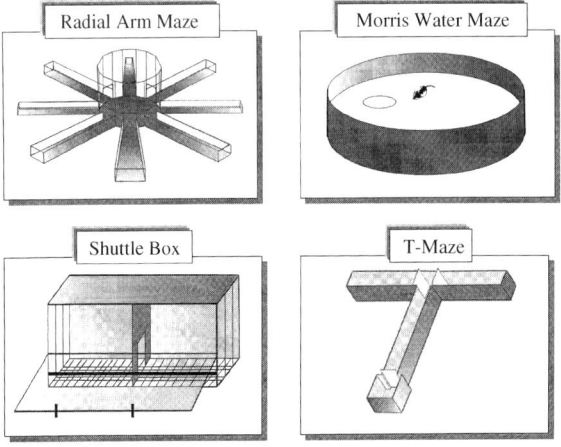

FIGURE 1 Four types of tasks commonly used in the study of steroid effects on learning and memory performance.

maze is an aversive task in which a subject can escape by mounting a small platform hidden beneath the surface of the water (Fig. 1) (Morris, 1981). In the working memory version of the water maze, the subject learns the location of the platform on an information trial at the beginning of a daily session (Morris et al., 1986; Steele and Morris, 1999; Stewart and Morris, 1993). After delays ranging from seconds to hours, retention is measured by the escape latency and path distance to locate the platform on a subsequent trial or trials. Information about the platform location is only useful for 1 day because the platform location is changed daily, requiring repeated acquisition of new information each day. In the reference memory version of the water maze, the subject learns the location of a platform that remains fixed over trials or days of testing, requiring stable place learning (Morris, 1981; Stewart and Morris, 1993). Retention can be tested by determining the length of time that the subject spends in the vicinity of the platform during probe tests in which the platform has been removed from the pool.

These standard versions of the radial arm maze and the water maze often have been modified by researchers, as noted later. In their various forms, neither maze can be considered to be a pure test of either working or reference memory, especially during acquisition of the tasks. The engagement of sensory, motor, and cognitive skills is necessary to complete the water maze successfully. In order to solve the water maze task, subjects must be able to swim, avoid the pool wall where the escape platform is never located, attend to extramaze or intramaze cues, and mount and remain on the platform (Cain, 1998). In the working memory version of the water maze, the subject must learn and remember the position of the escape platform on the first trial of each day to perform successfully on subsequent trials that day (working memory), but the subject also must learn and remember rules that the first trial predicts the location of the platform for the subsequent trials on that day and that the position of the platform will change on the next day (reference memory). Both human and nonhuman mammals learn and store information in a number of ways that depend on the nature and context of the information, as well as on the experience and strategy of the learner. In some cases, the types of learning and memory necessary to solve a task can be parceled out based on performance. In other cases, however, the types of learning and memory may be difficult to differentiate because the integration of multiple processes, including reference and working memories as well as nonmnemonic processes, are required to solve the task.

2. Conditioning

Even before the case of H.M., early behaviorists were parceling out learning and memory into subtypes such as nonassociative (habituation and sensitization) and associative (classical conditioning and operant conditioning). Many believed that learning and memory in most situations could be explained by conditioning theory (Hull, 1943). Conditioning models remain valuable paradigms to study the roles of hormones in certain types of learning and memory (Table 1). The neurobiology of habituation and sensitization has been investigated elegantly at the molecular, cellular, neural, and behavioral levels in invertebrate systems, most notably the gill-withdrawal reflex in the sea slug *Aplysia* (Carew et al., 1983). However, there are few reports of steroid hormone effects on nonassociative learning in the literature. Classical conditioning, a form of associative learning, involves pairing a neutral stimulus with reinforcement to elicit a response until the stimulus alone, now a conditioned stimulus, elicits a conditioned response. The conditioned eye blink response, used successfully to study classical conditioning in mammals, is influenced by the presence of steroid hormones, as described later. Operant conditioning, another form of associative learning, requires a subject to perform a certain response in order to obtain reinforcement and has been studied in paradigms based on positive reinforcement, such as bar pressing for food reward, or negative reinforcement, such as avoiding a mild electric shock. Steroid hormones also have been found to influence operant conditioning performance, as described later. Both classical and operant conditioning often contribute to learning and remembering a conditioned association but conditioning also plays a role in other types of learning and memory, including spatial and nonspatial cognition.

D. Study of Learning and Memory in Primates

The effects of steroids on primates, particularly humans, have received intense interest. Despite the highly advanced cognitive abilities of nonhuman primates and humans, tests of their learning and memory functions sometimes rely on simple tasks believed to tap specific types of cognition. A common test of working memory in nonhuman primates is the nonmatching-to-sample or object discrimination task in which an animal is presented two stimuli and must chose a novel stimulus not presented in the previous trial in order to receive a reward (Table 1) (Gower, 1990). A similar version of this task, sometimes called object recognition, is used in a rodent paradigm (Table 1) (Rothblat and Hayes, 1987). Nonmatching-to-sample and object recognition typically can be configured as nonspatial tasks that depend on visual recognition and working memory or as spatial tasks that depend on place discrimination and working memory. The difficulty of these tasks can be adjusted by manipulations of the retention interval and stimulus similarity. Both tasks have been used to investigate the effects of steroids on learning and memory performance, as described later.

A wide variety of measures have been employed to test the effects of steroids on human cognition. The subtests of the standard Wechsler Adult Intelligence Scale (WAIS) often are used to measure long-term verbal memory (information and vocabulary), verbal reasoning (comprehension), short-term verbal memory (digit span), and psychomotor and visuospatial performance (digit symbol, picture completion, block design, picture arrangement, and object assembly). Additional tests used to determine steroid effects include word, name, and paragraph recall; logical memory; and recurring figures. A true test of working memory, however, is proposed to require the continuous manipulation of information during the task, such as digit ordering (Duff and Hampson, 2000). A thorough review of various tasks used to study human performance is available (Kimura, 1999).

III. OVARIAN HORMONES AND COGNITION IN NONHUMANS

A. Overview

Estrogen and progesterone exhibit the typical four-ring structures of steroid molecules and are synthesized and secreted by several types of tissues in the body, notably the ovarian follicles and corpora lutea, but also neurosecretory cells of the adrenal cortex and fetal placenta (Martin, 1985). Pregnenolone, a 21-carbon steroid derived from cholesterol, is the precursor of all other steroids that are formed as products of various metabolic steroid pathways. After exiting the mitochondria, pregnenolone commonly is converted to progesterone, a 21-carbon structure that can be further metabolized to 21-carbon corticoids or 19-carbon androgens (Feder, 1981a; Martin, 1985; Miller 1988). Some androgens, such as testosterone and androstenedione, can be aromatized to 18-carbon estrogens, including estradiol and its metabolites estrone and estriol. As are many steroid molecules, endogenous forms of estradiol and progesterone are insoluble in water and require binding proteins for transport through aqueous environments such as blood; however, their high lipid solubility allows rapid diffusion across biological membranes (Martin, 1985). In addition to its classic metabolites, progesterone also is converted into a variety of lipid-insoluble metabolites called neurosteroids, such as 5α-pregnan-3α-ol-20-one (THP) and 5-androstan-3β-ol-17-one (DHEAS), known to influence neuronal activity (Baulieu, 1998; Robel et al., 1995; Schumacher et al., 1997).

1. Steroid Mechanisms

Estrogen and progesterone are proposed to modulate cellular function by genomic and nongenomic actions that can operate independently or interactively (Fig. 2). As part of its classic genomic mechanism, estrogen binds to intracellular ERα or ERβ receptors to form homodimer or heterodimer complexes that act at the cellular genome via at least two distinct DNA motifs, estrogen response elements (ERE) or activator protein 1 (AP-1) binding sites (McEwen and Alves, 1999). The activation of these DNA sites by the estrogen-receptor complex, along with the contributions of other transcriptional factors and coregulators, alters the production of mRNA. Proteins synthesized by the genomic route in response to ovarian steroids affect many aspects of cellular physiology, from regulating the concentrations of neurotransmitters to reshaping neuronal structure.

Unlike the slower process characteristic of genomic steroid action that requires minutes to hours, other mechanisms of steroid action be detected within second to minutes (Schmidt et al., 2000). Ultrarapid

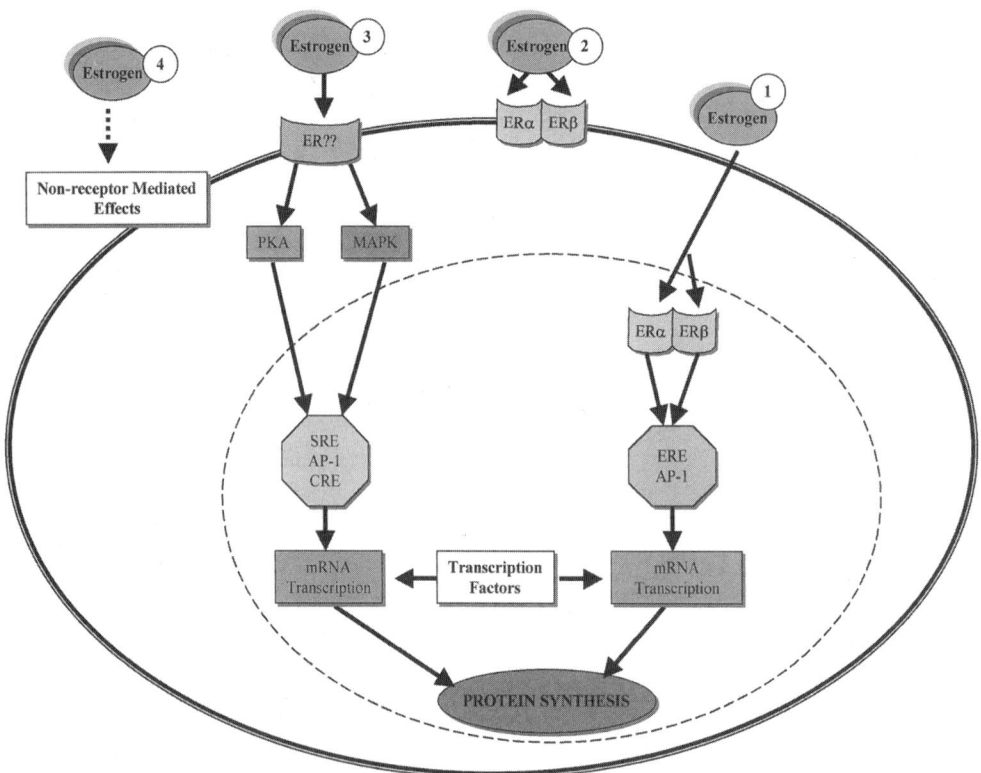

FIGURE 2 Four types of steroid mechanisms postulated to mediate the effects of estrogen on cellular function. ERα, ERβ, estrogen receptors; ER??, unknown estrogen receptor; ERE, estrogen-response element; AP-1, activator protein 1; PKA, protein kinase A; MAPK, mitogen-activated protein kinases; SRE, steroid response element; CRE, cyclic AMP response element. Many additional components and interactions are possible.

effects of steroids on membrane excitability occur within seconds of application and reflect steroid action at the membrane via either receptor- or nonreceptor-mediated events (Joels, 1997; McEwen et al., 1978; Orchinik and McEwen, 1995). Estrogen also regulates cellular events within minutes through various signal transduction systems, probably mediated by the activation of novel membrane receptors or intracellular receptors (Meyer and Habener, 1993; Orchinik and McEwen, 1995). In one proposed model, the binding of steroids to unidentified membrane receptors activates mitogen-activated protein kinases (MAPK) and protein kinase A (PKA), which stimulate or repress transcription through the phosphorylation of AP-1, the cyclic adenosine monophosphate (AMP) responsive element (CRE), and the steroid receptor element (SRE), as well as other transcriptional factors and coregulators (Aronica et al., 1994; Gu and Moss, 1996; Gu et al.,

1996; McEwen and Alves, 1999; Meyer and Habener, 1993; Singh et al., 1999, 2000; Zhou et al., 1996). The identities of the membrane receptors that mediate these actions remain in question, although isoforms of ERα and ERβ receptors cannot be ruled out (Razandi et al., 1999). Consequently, the traditional concept of a steroid and its receptors interacting with a sequence of DNA to form new proteins has been extended dramatically by the discoveries of estrogen receptor subtypes (ERα and six isoforms of ERβ), DNA binding elements (e.g., ERE, AP-1, CRE, and SRE), membrane actions (receptor- and nonreceptor-mediated), and intracellular signal transduction (e.g., MAPK and PKA). Progesterone also uses genomic and nongenomic mechanisms to exert its actions (Rowan and O'Malley, 2000; Schumacher et al., 1997). The effects of progesterone and its neurosteroid metabolites on neuronal membranes appear to be a fundamental mechanism of progestin action in the brain (Baulieu, 1998; Robel et al., 1995; Schumacher et al., 1997). The modulation of the complex cellular biochemistry of neurons by estrogen and progesterone can lead to convergence, divergence, and other interactions of enzyme pathways (Toran-Allerand et al., 1999; Wise et al., 2001). These features provide steroids with an impressive repertoire of tools with which to exert their many actions.

2. Ovarian Steroids and the Study of Cognition

Although the roles of estrogen and progesterone in the activation and maintenance of reproductive function in many species are well established, emerging evidence indicates that these steroids influence performance on various measures of learning and memory in mammals, including humans. These effects are complex and vary with task, gender, age, and the regimens of steroid exposure. Estrogen can affect performance on appetitive and aversive tasks; spatial and nonspatial tasks; conditioning; and acquisition, consolidation, and retention. In most reports, however, the effects of estrogen on performance are moderate in magnitude and their behavioral significance remains to be determined. Progesterone has received limited attention in the area of learning and memory. This steroid often augments the actions of estrogen on reproductive functions and may have similar synergistic effects on cognitive performance when combined with estrogen under certain conditions. The effects of steroids on cognitive performance are described in this chapter in terms relative to comparison groups; that is, learning and memory performance are either improved or impaired by a treatment or condition compared to a control group (e.g., ovariectomized rats versus gonadally intact rats).

As data on the cognitive effects of estrogen and progesterone have accumulated since the 1990s, many researchers and clinicians have become concerned by the complexity of the findings. Estrogen has been found to improve, impair, or not affect performance on various tasks of learning and memory. It is becoming increasingly clear, however, that the cognitive effects of gonadal steroids cannot be reduced to such banalities as "estrogen is good for your memory." Steroid effects are task-dependent and possibly memory-dependent, as pointed out by Sherwin (1994, 1997, 1998) in humans. The same complexities apply to other species.

It also should be noted that the classification of memory types and the underlying neural systems continue to be issues of intense controversy in the general field of learning and memory from which the study of the cognitive effects of steroids is not immune.

A haphazard approach has characterized the study of steroid modulation of cognition, manipulating endogenous and exogenous ovarian steroids to see what happens. In the climate of unfocused hypotheses, inconsistent methodologies, and conflicting findings, attempts have been made to explain the diversity of steroid hormone effects on learning and memory performance within the traditional divisions. As one example, it has been suggested that the effects of ovarian steroids depend on the reward structure of the task, that is, appetitive vs aversive (Markus and Zecevic, 1997). Estrogen enhances performance on some appetitively motivated tasks and impairs performance on some aversively motivated tasks, but not consistently, as described later. A second proposed framework is based on the division of cognitive tasks as hippocampal vs extrahippocampal (Markus and Zecivic, 1997), supported by evidence that 2 weeks of estrogen treatment in ovariectomized rats impaired hippocampally dependent spatial reference memory but enhanced hippocampally independent cued memory in a radial arm maze (Galea et al., 1999a). This hypothesis clearly warrants future attention, especially in light of multiple memory systems models that propose specific learning strategies supported by specific brain regions (Kesner et al., 1993; McDonald and White, 1993, 1994, 1995; O'Keefe and Nadel, 1978; Packard et al., 1989; Packard and McGaugh, 1992). A third context in which to study steroid effects is based on the division of working memory vs reference memory. As noted earlier (Section IIC1a), working memory can be defined as the storage of information that is useful within a single trial and for short durations; reference memory has been defined as the storage of information that is useful over many trials and for long durations. Although this division of memory continues to have its supporters, critics, and indifferents, it provides another model to frame the complex actions of ovarian steroids on learning and memory. Cast in this framework, available data indicate that endogenous or exogenous estrogen enhances performance on tasks that depend primarily on working memory, but usually fails to alter, or even impairs, performance of reference-memory tasks (Daniel et al., 1999; Chesler and Juraska, 2000). Nevertheless, sufficient inconsistencies remain, as described later.

B. Working Memory

Endogenous or exogenous estrogen generally improves performance on tasks that depend on working memory, as measured in radial arm mazes, T mazes, and water mazes, as well as on conditioning tasks in operant chambers and shuttle boxes. Enhancements in performance have been reported during both task acquisition and retention in both male and female rats. Rats exposed to estradiol commit fewer errors during acquisition and display better retention during short and long delays. Estrogen is effective when present at constant levels over a number of days or weeks, treatment paradigms that reflect therapeutic replacement regimens, although evidence demonstrates cognitive enhancements following briefer exposures to estrogen characteristic of the physiological fluctuations of normal reproductive cycles. Some results suggest that the effects of estrogen on cognitive performance may be dependent on steroid dose and duration of the treatment, but there have been no thorough analyses of these parameters.

1. Working Memory and Radial Arm Maze

A number of studies have reported small but significant improvements in radial-arm-maze performance during acquisition and retention trials, particularly when performance depended heavily on spatial working memory (Table 2). In an eight-arm radial maze with all arms baited (Fig. 1; Section IIC1a), estradiol delivered via constant-release Silastic capsules for several weeks following training improved working memory performance in young, gonadectomized male (~3 months of age) and elderly, intact male rats (~24 months of age), when delays of 1–5 hours were

TABLE 2
Ovarian Hormones and Working Memory

Task	Conditions[a]	Species	Effect[b]	Source
Radial arm maze	Silastic E_2	Rat	E	Luine and Rodriguez (1994)
	Silastic E_2	Rat	E	Williams et al. (1994); Williams (1996)
	Silastic E_2	Rat	E	Daniel et al. (1997)
	Silastic E_2	Rat	E	Luine et al. (1998)
	Ovarian E_2 + P	Rat	E	Daniel et al. (1999)
	Silastic E_2	Rat	E	Fader et al. (1999)
	EB 10 μg × 2	Rat	E	Daniel and Dohanich (2000)
	Ovarian E_2 + P	Mouse	E	Wilson et al. (1999)
T maze	EB	Rat	E	Fader et al. (1998)
	Silastic E_2, EB	Rat	E	Gibbs (1999a, 2000)
Water maze	Chronic Poly-E	Rat	E	O'Neal et al. (1996)
	Silastic E_2	Rat	E	Bimonte and Denenberg (1999)
	EB 10 μg × 2	Rat	E	Sandstrom et al. (1999)
	Ovarian E_2 + P	Rat	E	Healy et al. (1999)
	Ovarian E_2 + P	Rat	0	Markowska (1999)
Object recognition	Silastic E_2	Macaque	0	Voytko (2000)
	Silastic E_2, EB	Rat	E	Luine et al. (2001)

[a]Silastic E_2, chronic capsule; Ovarian E_2 + P, intact females; EB, estradiol benzoate; Chronic Poly-E, long-acting depot injection; P, progesterone.
[b]E, enhancement; 0, no effect.

instituted between the fourth- and fifth-arm choices (Luine and Rodriguez, 1994). This effect was dose-dependent in young ovariectomized rats (~3 months of age) in which estradiol levels typical of diestrus (~15 pg/ml), but not proestrus (~90 pg/ml), enhanced spatial working memory performance both during acquisition and on a delay retention task (Luine et al., 1998). Improvements in performance were reported to be more dependent on the duration of estrogen treatment (4 weeks >3 weeks) than on the magnitude of cognitive demand. Similar results were obtained in a series of acquisition experiments conducted in our laboratory. Estradiol delivered by Silastic capsules to produce levels typical of diestrus (~20 pg/ml) for 1 month prior to eight-arm radial maze acquisition, during acquisition, or both, improved performance in young ovariectomized rats trained between 2 and 3 months of age (Daniel et al., 1997). This enhancement was limited to working memory (Fader et al., 1999). These findings agree with earlier reports by Williams and colleagues showing that estradiol delivered via Silastic implants (~40 or ~200 pg/ml) to young or aged ovariectomized rats improved working memory performance during acquisition of a twelve-arm radial maze task with eight arms baited and four arms unbaited (Williams, 1996; Williams et al., 1994). However, after 12 months of chronic estradiol replacement at either plasma level, this improvement was not evident. In agreement with experiments using rats, working memory performance on a radial arm maze also was better in gonadally intact mice than in ovariectomized mice (Wilson et al., 1999).

These studies indicate that exposure of gonadectomized rats to constant physiological levels of estradiol for several weeks enhanced spatial working memory performance, particularly during radial maze acquisition. Gonadally intact female rats displayed differences in sensorimotor function but not acquisition or retention across the estrous cycle in the radial arm maze (Stackman et al., 1997), despite the proliferation of hippocampal CA1 (Cornu Amonnis) spines and synapses reported at proestrus (McEwen and Woolley, 1994; Woolley and McEwen, 1992; Woolley et al., 1990). However, we found that the same short-term estrogen regimen that induced dendritic changes in CA1 (10 μg of estradiol benzoate for 2 days; Gould et al., 1990) improved working memory retention in ovariectomized rats in 1-hour delay trials and increased N-methyl-D-aspartate (NMDA) receptor binding in CA1 (Daniel and Dohanich, 2001).

2. Working Memory and T Maze

Rats learn to alternate visits to the opposite arms of a T maze spontaneously or to obtain food rewards (Fig. 1). It is proposed that the successful alternation over trials depends on the use of allocentric working memory in which an animal remembers the reward location on the previous trial by using extramaze cues placed around the maze. However, T-maze alternations also can be based on other strategies such as egocentric responding, in which an animal learns to turn right and then left on the subsequent trials using internal proprioceptive cues. Young ovariectomized rats treated with systemic injections of estradiol benzoate (5 or 100 μg/kg) or Silastic capsules of estradiol (~20 pg/ml) over days or weeks made more correct alternation responses during the acquisition of a reinforced T-maze task compared to ovariectomized control rats (Dohanich et al., 1994; Fader et al., 1998). In another T-maze design using a delayed matching-to-position task, females were required to return to the same arm where the food reward was found on the previous trial of each trial pair, a fundamentally different paradigm from the nonmatching-to-position requirement of T-maze alternation (Gibbs, 1999a, 2000). Young ovariectomized rats treated with Silastic capsules of estradiol for 2 months reached the performance criterion faster than ovariectomized control rats (Gibbs, 1999a). A similar acceleration in acquisition was found in females ovariectomized at middle age and tested in old age after variable regimens of estrogen and progesterone replacement (Gibbs, 2000). However, in both studies, steroid treatments did not affect performance on trial pairs separated by short delays (5, 10, 30, 60, and 90 seconds), a manipulation that increased the demand on working memory. This lack of a delay effect raises the possibility that estrogen improved T-maze performance by affecting a nonmnemonic factor such as attention or by favoring an egocentric response strategy (Gibbs, 1999a). Interestingly, deficits in the T-maze alternation task (Dohanich et al., 1994; Fader et al., 1998) and in the delayed matching-to-position task (Gibbs, 1999a, 2000) induced by systemic or intrahippocampal administration of the muscarinic receptor antagonist, scopolamine, were prevented by estrogen or estrogen and progesterone replacement.

3. Working Memory and Water Maze

Spatial working memory also can be tested using an aversive task such as the water maze. In this paradigm, rats normally learn to navigate by extramaze cues to escape to a platform hidden just beneath the surface of a pool filled with water made opaque by addition of paint or powdered milk (Fig. 1). In the typical working memory version of the water maze (Section IIC1a; Steele and Morris, 1999), a rat learns the new location of the hidden platform on the first information trial of each day and then retains that information in working memory for subsequent use on a second retention trial, usually presented after delays of minutes to hours. This standard paradigm to study working memory performance has been modified by some investigators, as described later.

In the first study to examine steroid effects on working memory performance in a water maze, estradiol administered as polyestradiol phosphate, a slow-clearing form of estrogen (0.5 mg injection every 3 weeks over 200 days), improved performance following 5-minute, but not 30-minute, delays between the information trial and a retention trial (O'Neal et al., 1996). In this modified version of the standard working memory paradigm, a correct choice was made when a female swam to a hidden escape platform located in the same half of the pool as on the previous information trial. The improvement in working memory performance as indicated by an increase in correct choices was weak, although results indicated that chronic estrogen treatment might maintain performance as females age. In another modified version of the working memory task, an eight-arm radial maze was placed in a pool with seven arms affording escape to removable platforms; reentry into an arm selected previously constituted a working memory error (Bimonte and Denenberg, 1999). Young ovariectomized rats treated for 1 month with Silastic capsules that maintained estradiol levels of approximately 25 pg/ml or 50 pg/ml committed fewer working memory errors than ovariectomized rats without estrogen on the later choices of each trial when the memory load was heaviest. This result reflects a working memory process especially well because successful performance depended on the manipulation of information stored in working memory as each trial proceeded. A similar effect of estradiol replacement on active, but not passive, verbal and spatial working memory performance was reported in female humans (Duff and Hampson, 2000). A third study, presented in abstract form, found that adult ovariectomized rats injected with a regimen of estradiol benzoate that induces dendritic changes in CA1 (10 μg for 2 days) reached a hidden platform in the standard working memory paradigm with shorter latencies and distances after long, but not brief, delay intervals (Sandstrom et al., 1999), a good measure of working memory (Steele and Morris, 1999). The effects of estrogen and progesterone on memory performance paralleled reported changes in CA1 and dentate gyrus spine density.

Several studies documented the cognitive effects of fluctuations in endogenous steroids across the estrous cycle, over the trimesters of pregnancy, and during aging. Using the standard working memory version of the water maze, female rats exhibited the poorest performance locating a movable hidden platform at estrus when estrogen levels were low (Healy et al., 1999). Equivalent levels of performance were found at proestrus, metestrus, and diestrus. Females at estrus required two trials, not one, to learn the location of a hidden platform after the daily information trial. However, there were no delays placed between the information trial (trial 1) and the retention trials (trials 2, 3, 4), a typical feature for evaluating working memory performance (Steele and Morris, 1999). Endogenous estrogen failed to improve working memory performance during pregnancy in rats, as measured in the water maze (Galea et al., 2000). Pregnant females in their first and second trimesters, when estrogen levels are low ($\sim$15 pg/ml) and progesterone levels are high, outperformed pregnant females in their third trimester and nonpregnant females with high estrogen titers ($\sim$40 pg/ml) but low progesterone levels. However, in this study, the position of the hidden platform remained stationary over 4 days of testing at each trimester, a design that more likely measured reference memory performance than working memory performance. In addition, escape latencies and distances were not compared between the first (information) and second (retention) trial of each day when the most sensitive evaluation of working memory performance normally can be made (Steele and Morris, 1999). In a study of aging effects, deficits in working memory performance in the water maze were not evident until 24 months of age, when all females had reached anestrus but well after the onset of acyclicity at 12 and 18 months of age (Markowska, 1999). These results suggest that age, rather than loss of estrogen, may be a more critical factor in working memory deficits.

Although the water maze studies described here used different estrogen regimens and testing methodologies, significant improvements in working memory performance were found. However, in some cases, the reported enhancements were relatively small in magnitude. In our laboratory, using a standard water maze procedure to assess working memory, better performance in female rats usually was associated with the presence of exogenous estrogen or endogenous estrogen and progesterone. Nevertheless, we also found that ovarian steroids failed to improve, and even impaired, working memory performance in some water maze experiments (G. Dohanich, unpublished data). Although it is tempting to conclude that estrogen, with or without progesterone, enhances working memory in an aversively motivated task such as the water maze, the results of three articles and one abstract are insufficient to confirm this hypothesis with confidence.

4. Working Memory and Object Recognition

Another test of working memory is the nonmatching-to-sample or object discrimination task in which an animal is presented two stimuli and must chose the stimulus not presented on the previous trial (Section IID). Ovariectomized macaque monkeys that received estrogen replacement for 5 or 16 months by Silastic capsules ($\sim$170 pg/ml) performed similarly to ovariectomized monkeys with empty capsules ($\sim$25 pg/ml) on the acquisition, retention, and reversal of the object discrimination task (Voytko, 2000). Performance also was not affected by the interval between ovariectomy and testing. Ovariectomy weakly increased sensitivity to the amnesic action of the muscarinic receptor antagonist, scopolamine. Alternatively, ovariectomized rats receiving short-term estrogen treatment were able to recognize the novel object on a nonspatial object recognition task when the intervals between sample and recognition trials were 4 or 12 hours (Luine et al., 2001). Ovariectomized rats that did not receive estrogen treatment discriminated at intervals of 1 or 2 hours, but not 4 or 12 hours. On a spatial-object-placement version of the task, only rats treated with estrogen discriminated between the object's position at intervals of 4 hours, but only after exposure to estrogen for 42, but not 24, hours. Despite the lack of an estrogen effect on object discrimination in a primate, estrogen treatment improved memory on both nonspatial and spatial versions of the task as the demand on memory increased.

5. Summary of Ovarian Steroid Effects on Working Memory Performance

Estrogen improved performance of male and female rats on spatial measures during acquisition and retention, particularly when tasks depended on working memory (Table 2). These effects have been reported using different mazes, tasks, and estrogen conditions, indicating that this steroid can selectively enhance a type of memory operationally defined as working memory. Estrogen treatment enhanced object and place discrimination in female rats but in not female macaques. Nevertheless, the improvements in working memory performance associated with estrogen usually were small and their reliability remains to be confirmed. Furthermore, the roles of nonmmemonic variables have not been addressed adequately. The contribution of progesterone to the improvements induced by estrogen remains understudied, although a synergism with estrogen has been reported (Sandstrom et al., 1999).

C. Reference Memory

Unlike the enhancements of spatial working memory performance by estrogen reported for radial arm mazes, T mazes, and water mazes, endogenous or exogenous ovarian steroids usually fail to improve performance on tasks designed to measure spatial reference memory. The failure of estrogen and progesterone to exert a positive action on procedural or rule learning has been demonstrated to occur in both radial arm mazes and water mazes. In a number of studies, the presence of ovarian hormones in female rats actually impaired performance during acquisition and retention of the water maze, when employed conventionally as a measure of spatial reference memory. Ovarian steroids also sometimes impair acquisition and retention on avoidance conditioning that depends on spatial reference memory as well as on conditioning.

1. Reference Memory and Radial Arm Maze

In order to test spatial reference memory in a conventional radial arm maze, the same arms of the maze are baited on all trials and the remaining arms are never baited for each subject (Section IIC1a). In this paradigm, reentry into an arm previously visited is defined as an error of working memory and entry into an arm that is never baited is defined as an error of reference memory. Only a few studies have examined the effects of estrogen replacement on reference memory in the radial arm maze; none have examined performance over the estrous cycle, and none have asssessed the role of progesterone (Table 3). There are no published reports of changes in reference memory performance in radial arm mazes with 8 or 17 arms in ovariectomized rats treated for days to weeks with Silastic estradiol implants (Fader *et al.*, 1999; Luine *et al.*, 1998; Williams *et al.*, 1994). However, as reported in abstract form, 2 months of treatment with estradiol benzoate (10 µg/day) increased reference memory errors in ovariectomized rats tested on a radial arm maze (Galea *et al.*, 1999a).

2. Reference Memory and Water Maze

The water maze traditionally has been used to test spatial reference memory. Rodents learn to escape to a hidden platform that remains in a fixed position just below the surface of an opaque solution from day to day (Section IIC1a; McNamara and Skelton, 1993; Morris, 1984). Often referred to as place learning, extramaze cues are normally used by rats to locate the place in the water maze where the platform is positioned. The animal must learn the rule to always swim to the same location in order to escape (unlike the working memory

TABLE 3
Ovarian Hormones and Reference Memory

Task	Conditions[a]	Species	Effect[b]	Source
Radial arm maze	Silastic E_2	Rat	0	Williams *et al.* (1994)
	Silastic E_2	Rat	0	Luine *et al.* (1998)
	Silastic E_2	Rat	0	Fader *et al.* (1999)
	EB	Rat	I	Galea *et al.* (1999a)
Water maze	EB + P	Rat	I	Korol *et al.* (1994)
	Ovarian E_2 + P	Rat	I	Frye (1995)
	Ovarian E_2 + P	Rat	I	Galea *et al.* (1995)
	Ovarian E_2 + P	Rat	I	Warren and Juraska (1997)
	Ovarian E_2 + P	Rat	I	Daniel *et al.* (1999)
	Ovarian E_2 + P	Rat	I	Warren and Juraska (2000)
	EB + P	Rat	I	Chesler and Juraska (2000)
	Ovarian E_2 + P	Rat	I	Galea *et al.* (2000)
	Silastic E_2	Rat	0	Singh *et al.* (1994)
	Ovarian E_2 + P	Rat	0	Berry *et al.* (1997)
	E_2, E_2 + P, EB	Rat	E	Pych *et al.* (2000)
	Post-training E_w	Rat	E	Packard *et al.* (1996); Packard and Teather (1997a,b)
	EB	Mouse	I	Fugger *et al.* (1998)
	Ovarian E_2 + P	Mouse	0	Wilson *et al.* (1999)
	Silastic E_2	Mouse	E	Rissanen *et al.* (1999)
Platform maze	Ovarian E_2 + P	Rat	I	Fader *et al.* (1998)

[a]Silastic E_2, chronic capsule; Ovarian E_2 + P, intact females; EB, estradiol benzoate; P, progesterone; posttraining E_w, water-soluble estradiol.
[b]E, enhancement; I, impairment; 0, no effect.

version of the water maze, in which the location of the escape platform is changed from session to session requiring repeated acquisition of new information). Most studies report that reference memory performance in water mazes is impaired by ovarian homones in place learning and subsequent probe trials (Table 3). Gonadally intact female rats exhibited longer escape latencies and, in some cases, longer swim distances to locate a hidden platform than ovariectomized rats, indicating that the presence of the ovaries impairs spatial reference memory (Daniel *et al.*, 1999; Frye, 1995; Korol *et al.*, 1994; Warren and Juraska, 1997). The poorest performance occured when estradiol titers were highest, such as at proestrus in rats (Warren and Juraska, 1997) or when female meadow voles were exposed to males (Galea *et al.*, 1995). Despite the consistency of these findings, it should be noted that the impairment seen at proestrus in rats was limited to several trials (Warren and Juraska, 1997), and another study reported no changes in reference memory performance associated with fluctuating levels of ovarian steroids across the estrous cycle in rats (Berry *et al.*, 1997).

The roles of estrogen and progesterone in reference memory deficits remain unclear. A nonsignificant enhancement of reference memory performance in the water maze was reported in a small sample ($n = 4$) of ovariectomized rats treated with chronic Silastic estradiol capsules (Singh *et al.*, 1994). In experiments from our laboratory, ovariectomy was found to improve reference memory performance as measured in the water maze (Daniel *et al.*, 1999), but estrogen replacement failed to reinstate the reference memory deficits found in gonadally intact female rats (G. Dohanich, unpublished data). In addition, progesterone replacement alone in ovariectomized rats also fails to restore these deficits (Chesler and Juraska, 2000). Taken together, these studies do not support a role for estrogen or progesterone alone in causing reference memory impairments in rats. However, estrogen and progesterone may interact to induce impairments in reference memory as measured in the water maze. When reference memory performance of ovariectomized rats was compared following short-term treatment with estradiol benzoate (10 μg for 2 days), progesterone (500 μg for 1 day), or both, only the combination of estrogen and progesterone induced significant reference memory impairments, as indicated by longer escape latencies and swim distances (Chesler and Juraska, 2000). In addition, the ratio of estrogen to progesterone may be an important factor. Rats in their first and second trimesters of pregnancy, when low estradiol combines with high progesterone, performed better on place learning trials than nonpregnant females, whereas females in their third trimester of pregnancy, when high estradiol combines with low progesterone, performed worse than nonpregnant females (Galea *et al.*, 2000). Although the task used in this study was intended as a measure of working memory performance, features such as a stationary platform throughout each trimester, suggest that the procedure measured reference memory performance according to its traditional definition (Section IIC1a).

Aged pseudopregnant rats performed poorly on the reference memory version of the water maze compared to aged rats in persistent estrus (Warren and Juraska, 2000). Although estradiol levels in these aged females may have been comparable, progesterone titers probably were higher in the pseudopregnant rats. These results again support the hypothesis that the combination or ratio of estradiol and progesterone is associated with impaired performance. However, results presented in abstract form from the same laboratory indicated that acute or chronic replacement of estrogen or estrogen and progesterone improved spatial reference memory performance during acquisition of the water maze task in middle-age ovariectomized rats (Pych *et al.*, 2000).

In the few studies using mice, estradiol have been found to impair, enhance, and not affect reference memory performance. Reference memory impairments following short-term estrogen replacement alone were reported in ovariectomized mice (Fugger *et al.*, 1998). Alternatively, estradiol replacement in ovariectomized mice at plasma levels of 75–100 pg/ml or 300–400 pg/ml improved nonspatial reference memory compared to ovariectomized controls, whereas the lower estradiol level enhanced spatial performance (Rissanen *et al.*, 1999). A third report found no changes in performance following ovariectomy (Wilson *et al.*, 1999). Differences between rats and mice in water maze performance may reflect species-specific strategies. Rats tend to use spatial strategies, whereas mice prefer nonspatial strategies (Frick *et al.*, 2000), although the interaction of strategy and steroid condition remains obscure.

Despite these impairments, estrogen treatment exerts reliable enhancing effects on memory consolidation in the water maze. A single systemic injection or intrahippocampal infusion of a water-soluble form of estradiol administered within 1 hour after a training session in the water maze improved performance on a retention test 24 hours later in both gonadally intact male and gonadectomized female rats (Packard, 1998; Packard *et al.*, 1996; Packard and Teather, 1997a,b). The enhancement in retention by estradiol was blocked by cotreatment with the muscarinic receptor blocker scopolamine and synergized by cotreatment with the muscarinic receptor agonist oxotremorine, implicating the cholinergic system in the consolidation mechanism (Packard *et al.*, 1996; Packard and Teather, 1997a).

3. Reference Memory and Circular Platform Maze

Like the water maze, the circular platform maze is considered to be a spatial task to assess reference memory performance (Barnes, 1979). Rodents are motivated to escape from an aversive environment on the maze surface, an open space illuminated by an intense light. One of 17 holes held constant for each subject over trials affords escape into a small box suspended beneath the maze. Similar deficits in spatial performance as a function of age were found using both mazes (McLay *et al.*, 1999). In agreement with the results reported for water mazes, we found that ovariectomized rats, as well as male rats, displayed significantly shorter escape latencies and visited significantly fewer incorrect holes than intact females in the circular platform maze (Fader *et al.*, 1998).

4. Summary of Ovarian Steroid Effects on Reference Memory Performance

The available evidence supports the hypothesis that ovarian hormones normally impair or fail to affect performance on tasks dependent on spatial reference memory in radial arm mazes, water mazes, and platform mazes. In water mazes, estrogen or progesterone individually seem unable to induce deficits in performance in female rats and a combination of these hormones may be necessary for reference memory deficits to occur. In contrast, a rapidly clearing estradiol can enhance consolidation and retention when administered immediately following place training. The results of the few experiments conducted using female mice have been inconsistent, with estrogen producing impairment, enhancement, or no effect on reference memory performance.

D. Conditioning

Ovarian steroids affect performance on various conditioning tasks (Table 4). Endogenous and exogenous steroids alter acquisition and retention of avoidance responses in which rodents are conditioned to actively avoid a presignaled shock, usually by moving into the safe compartment of a divided shuttle box (active avoidance; Fig. 1) or by passively remaining in the occupied safe compartment (passive avoidance; Fig. 1). These tasks primarily test a rodent's ability to learn and retain a conditioned response to an aversive stimulus, but can require spatial discrimination of the compartments. In addition, ovarian steroids affect performance in both classical and operant conditioning tasks.

1. Active Avoidance

In several early reports, the presence of ovarian hormones was associated with poorer performance of active avoidance tasks (Section IIC2). During proestrus or early estrus when estrogen and progesterone levels were elevated, the performance of female rats in training, retention, or extinction trials was inferior to females at other stages of the cycle, when ovarian hormone levels presumably were lower (Burke and Broadhurst, 1966; Gray, 1977; Ikard *et al.*, 1972). Similar impairments were found in a later series of experiments in which female rats at estrus displayed fewer active avoidance responses than diestrous females with lower estrogen levels, whereas ovariectomized rats treated with estrogen for several days performed poorly compared to ovariectomized rats not receiving estrogen treatment (Diaz-Veliz *et al.*, 1989, 1991, 1995, 2000). On a modified active avoidance T-maze task, estrous mice required more trials to reach acquisition and retention criteria than diestrous mice (Farr *et al.*, 1995). In addition, ovariectomized mice treated with estrogen and progesterone or progesterone alone were impaired compared to ovariectomized controls. These results suggest that inferior performance of this active avoidance task was related to high levels of progesterone, not estrogen (Farr *et al.*, 1995).

In contrast, ovarian steroids also have been reported to improve active avoidance performance in some

TABLE 4
Ovarian Hormones and Conditioning

Task	Conditions[a]	Species	Effect[b]	Reference
Active avoidance	Ovarian E_2 + P	Rat	I	Burke and Broadhurst (1966)
	Ovarian E_2 + P	Rat	I	Ikard et al. (1972)
	Ovarian E_2 + P	Rat	I	Gray (1977)
	EB	Rat	I	Diaz-Veliz et al. (1989, 1991, 1994, 1995, 2000)
	P	Mouse	I	Farr et al. (1995)
	EB + P	Rat	E	Cannizarro et al. (1970)
	Ovarian E_2 + P	Rat	E	Sfikakis et al. (1978, 1984)
	Silastic E_2	Rat	E	Singh et al. (1994)
	E	Rat	E	Fedotova (1999)
	EV	Rat	E	Telegdy and Stark (1973)
	EV	Rat	0	Telegdy et al. (1968)
	Peripregnancy	Rat	0	Kristal et al. (1978)
Passive avoidance	P	Rat	I	van Wimersma Greidanus (1977)
	EV	Rat	I	Rivas-Arancibia and Vasquez-Pereyra (1994)
	EB or P	Rat	I	Mora et al. (1996)
	EB or P	Rat	I	Diaz-Veliz et al. (1997)
	Ovarian E_2 + P	Rat	I	Markus and Zecevic (1997)
	EV	Rat	E	Vasquez-Pereyra et al. (1995)
	Silastic E_2	Rat	0	Gibbs et al. (1998)
	E	Rat	0	Fedotova (1999)
	Silastic E_2	Mouse	0	Fugger et al. (2000)
Classic eye blink	Ovarian E_2 + P	Rat	I	Shors et al. (1998); Wood and Shors (1998)
	Ovarian E_2 + P	Rat	E	Shors et al. (1998)
Operant behavior	Pellet E_2	Rat	I	Lentz et al. (1978)
	Ovarian E_2 + P	Rat	E	Beatty (1973)

[a]Silastic E_2, chronic capsule; Ovarian E_2 + P, intact females; EB, estradiol benzoate; EV, estradiol valerate; P, progesterone.
[b]E, enhancement; I, impairment; 0, no effect.

studies. Ovariectomy decreased the number of active avoidance responses displayed by rats conditioned to a mild electric shock, whereas estradiol replacement by Silastic capsules for 5 or 28 weeks restored avoidance behavior to the levels displayed by gonadally intact females (Singh et al., 1994). Female rats with endogenous or exogenous ovarian steroids out-performed females after ovariectomy or at diestrus in some active avoidance experiments (Cannizarro et al., 1970; Fedotova, 1999; Sfikakis et al., 1978), although not all (Telegdy et al., 1968), whereas the treatment of ovariectomized rats with estrogen and progesterone slowed extinction of an active avoidance pole-jump task (Telegdy and Stark, 1973). On the other hand, hormonal fluctuations associated with pregnancy, preparturition, and postparturition did not affect active avoidance performance in rats (Kristal et al., 1978).

2. Passive Avoidance

Generally, estrogen and progesterone impair performance of passive avoidance in rats (Section IIC2; Table 4). In a modified version of a passive avoidance task, female rats conditioned at proestrus and tested 2 weeks later at proestrus displayed a lower percentage of freezing responses than estrous females or males, indicating poorer acquisition and retention when estrogen and progesterone levels were elevated (Markus and Zecevic, 1997). Deficits in passive avoidance performance at proestrus could not be explained by altered shock sensitivity, state-dependent learning, or nonspecific effects on learning. Interestingly, the impairment in passive avoidance at proestrus occurred only when the conditioned stimulus was the spatial features of the conditioning room rather than an auditory stimulus. Similar deficits in retention were found in gonadally intact rats during proestrus and estrus and in ovariectomized rats treated with estradiol benzoate (10 μg/kg) or progesterone (25 mg/kg) (Diaz-Veliz et al., 1997; Mora et al., 1996; van Wimersma Greidanus, 1977). Ovarian steroids also accelerated the extinction of passive avoidance behavior in gonadally intact male rats (Rivas-Arancibia and Vasquez-Pereyra, 1994).

In a conflicting report (Vasquez-Pereyra et al., 1995), the administration of estradiol valerate 45 minutes before a training trial enhanced short-term retention of a passive avoidance response at a dose of 0.4 mg (10 minutes after training) and long-term retention at a dose of 1.2 mg (24 hours after training). However, in another report, the treatment of ovariectomized rats with estradiol from Silastic capsules over several weeks did not affect retention of a passive avoidance response compared to untreated ovariectomized rats, although deficits induced by a muscarinic antagonist or a benzodiazepine agonist were prevented by estradiol (Gibbs et al., 1998). Gonadally intact females also did not differ from either ovariectomized group, although their response was bimodal, crossing rapidly or slowly into the compartment previously paired with shock. Estrogen treatments also failed to affect passive avoidance retention in hybrid wild-type mice (Fugger et al., 2000). However, knockout mice of this hybrid strain (lacking estrogen receptor ERα) displayed impairments that were reversed by estrogen treatment, suggesting a role of ERα in passive avoidance that involves a novel mechanism of estrogen action.

3. Eye-Blink Conditioning

Using the classically conditioned eye-blink response, Shors and colleagues reported that at proestrus, when estradiol titers are high, female rats learned the response faster that females at estrus or diestrus (Shors et al., 1998). However, this enhancing effect of estrogen can be reversed by exposure to acute stress. Proestrous females, with high levels of estradiol, displayed stronger impairments in eye-blink acquisition when exposed to a stressor than did females at estrus or diestrus (Shors et al., 1998; Wood and Shors, 1998). These results underscore the importance of steroid interactions in learning and memory, particularly combinations that involve ovarian hormones and glucocorticoids.

4. Operant Conditioning

Some of the earliest research on ovarian steroids and conditioning examined the effects of estrogen and progesterone on conditioned operant responding. Gonadally intact female rats displayed better efficiency (more reinforcements per responses) on an appetitive bar-press task (differential reinforcement of low rate-20) compared to males or ovariectomized rats (Beatty, 1973). However, in a subsequent study, no differences were found in response efficiency (DRL-20) between gonadally intact, ovariectomized, or ovariectomized rats with streoid pellets of estradiol, progesterone, or both (Lentz et al., 1978). Ovariectomized rats with estradiol implants did require a longer time to earn 100 reinforcements on one test day than did all other groups. Additional research on ovarian steroid modulation of operant behavior clearly is needed in view of the importance of conditioning on everyday learning and memory.

5. Summary of Ovarian Steroid Effects on Conditioning

Ovarian hormones have been found to impair the acquisition and retention of active avoidance behavior, passive avoidance behavior, operant responding, and eye-blink conditioning in the presence of a stressor. Estrogen also accelerated the extinction of a passive avoidance response. However, several studies report better acquisition and retention of active avoidance, passive avoidance, and eye-blink conditioning in females with endogenous or exogenous estrogen and progesterone. Estrogen also slowed the extinction of a passive avoidance response. The basis for these widely discrepant findings is unknown, although varied methodologies and nonmnemonic variables might account for much of the inconsistency. Clearly, the relationship between ovarian hormones and conditioning remains to be clarified.

E. Learning Strategies

The type of strategy used for a given task may depend not only on the demands of the task but also on the gender and hormonal condition of the individual. When confronted with multiple types of cues, female rats were reported to use extramaze geometry and intramaze landmarks, whereas males attended primarily to extramaze cues, possibly accounting for faster but less flexible performance by males on some spatial tasks (Williams et al., 1990), as well as poorer recovery from brain damage (Roof et al., 1993). However, female humans may rely on landmarks, whereas male humans rely on both landmarks and geometry (Sandstrom et al., 1998). In any event, strategy selection in females may be dependent on estrogen. For example, if female rats were able to use either an allocentric or egocentric strategy, they preferred the allocentric strategy during proestrus or when treated with exogenous estradiol, but an egocentric strategy when estradiol levels were low (Korol et al., 1998). Furthermore, females can shift strategies over the course of the estrous cycle as circulating estradiol levels fluctuate. Consequently, steroids may be able to affect the acquisition and storage of information by biasing the cognitive strategy used during acquisition of various forms of information. Much of the controversy regarding the influence of estrogen on learning and memory may be clarified by careful analysis of these strategies along with the underlying brain systems that are targets of steroid action. The muliple memory systems proposed to regulate spatial, nonspatial, and response learning, as well as fear conditioning, may be used as a valuable model with which to explore the effects of steroids on learning and memory (Kesner et al., 1993; McDonald and White, 1993; Packard et al., 1989; Packard and White, 1990).

F. Ovarian Steroids and Nonmnemonic Effects

Ovarian steroids, of course, affect many physiological and behavioral functions other than reproduction and cognition. As noted earlier, performance on tasks designed to measure learning and memory can lead to the erroneous conclusion that a treatment must be directly modulating mnemonic processes (Section IA4). However, improved or impaired performance could just as

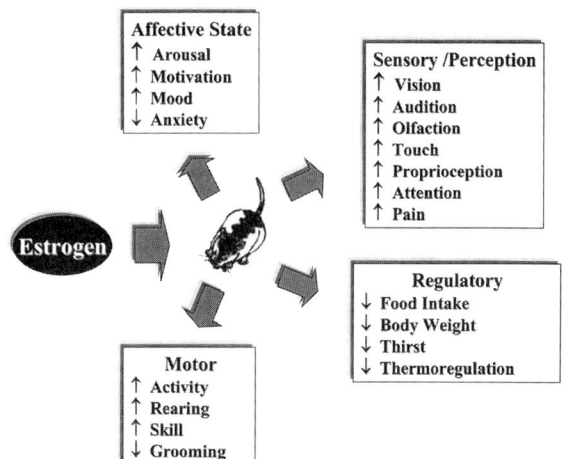

FIGURE 3 The effects of estrogen on functions that might affect learning and memory performance indirectly through their nonmnemonic actions.

well reflect changes in nonmnemonic variables that are related to learning and memory only indirectly. As do many endogenous and exogenous agents, estrogen and progesterone have diverse actions on such functions as arousal and motivation, sensation and perception, thirst and appetite, and motor activity and skill (Fig. 3). The contributions of nonmnemonic processes to treatment effects have been addressed by various behavioral techniques that reduce or account for these variables, such as pretraining experience with cognitive tasks, direct measurement of nonmnemonic factors, and posttraining administration of drugs or hormones. A number of these procedures have been incorporated by investigators in the study of ovarian steroid modulation of learning and memory.

1. Pretraining

Pretraining usually includes exposure to the training or similar environment, experience with the requirements of the task, and even handling by the experimenter (Bucci et al., 1995; Perrot-Sinal et al., 1996; Warren and Juraska, 1997, 2000). In the ideal design, animals should complete trials that feature all components of the task except the actual mnemonic element (Bartus, 2000). The result can be dramatic. For example, several days of nonspatial pretraining swims in a water maze completely counteracted the severe performance deficits associated with the administration of NMDA, or cholinergic receptor antagonists, or a benzodiazepine agonist (Bannerman et al., 1995; Beiko et al., 1997; Cain et al., 1996; Cain, 1997, 1998; Saucier and Cain, 1995; Saucier et al., 1996). In these examples, pretraining was able to eliminate various sensorimotor difficulties sometimes experienced by drug-treated rats, although no single feature of the pretraining experience could account for its effect on performance (Hoh and Cain, 1997).

Although gender differences in water maze performance have been reported (Roof and Havens, 1992), males and females performed similarly when pretraining preceded testing in the same maze (Bucci et al., 1995); age also may have been a factor. In the studies described earlier to determine if reference memory performance varied across the estrous cycle, handled and pretrained females displayed small but significant performance deficits at proestrus (Warren and Juraska, 1997). However, there were no differences in performance across the estrous cycle in females that experienced more extensive handling and pretraining or training on an identical version of the experimental task (Berry et al., 1997). We found that ovariectomized rats that had been trained on a radial arm maze for 20 days still outperformed gonadally intact females on a subsequent water maze task (Daniel et al., 1999). Interestingly, however, this impairment was not evident when gonadally intact females were housed in a complex environment. Clearly, the history of an organism can be a critical variable when assessing steroid effects on cognition.

2. Measurement of Nonmnemonic Effects

Another method that has been used to account for the contributions of nonmnemonic variables in treatment effects is to incorporate a battery of other tasks that measures specific functions. For example, estrogen has been shown to increase locomotor and general activity in a number of species (Axelson et al., 1986; Cushing et al., 1995; Diaz-Veliz et al., 1991; Fahrbach et al., 1985; Kanyt et al., 1999; Thomas et al., 1986). These behaviors could enhance or impede performance in shuttle boxes, operant chambers, or land and water mazes, particularly as a function of the specific measures used to evaluate learning and memory performance. These treatment effects on activity and locomotion can be assessed in running wheels, activity monitors, or by determining running or swimming speeds during maze testing (Geyer, 1990). Along with increased food intake and fat deposition following ovariectomy (McCaffrey and Czaja, 1989; Tartelin and Gorski, 1971; Wade, 1976), reductions in activity levels contribute to increases in the body weight of females. Increased intake at low estrogen levels alters the reward value of food reinforcement in appetitive tasks, as well as affecting running and swimming abilities in land and water mazes. Ovarian hormones also exert complex effects on body temperature and thermoregulation (Simpkins, 1995; Okada et al., 1997). Colonic and skin temperatures can be monitored routinely before, during, or after test sessions (Geller and Adler, 1990). Although changes in thermoregulation induced by ovarian steroids could have important consequences in a water maze, at least one study reported that colonic temperatures as low as 30°C did not affect performance (Panakhova et al., 1984).

An important area of concern when conducting experiments intended to examine treatment effects on cognitive performance is the influence of anxiety. Anxiety that accompanies the stress of a novel situation can exert strong effects on performance, especially during early trials as subjects become familiar with the environment of the maze, the requirements of the task, and even the interactions with the investigator. The presence of anxiety can be problematic, particularly when determining the effects of a treatment on the acquisition of a task. Anxiety levels have been found to vary with gender and hormonal condition (D. Bitran et al., 1991; M. Bitran et al., 1991; Diaz-Veliz et al., 1997; Mora et al., 1996: Nomikos and Spyraki, 1988; Slob et al., 1981), although not in all reports (M. Bitran et al., 1991; Stock et al., 2000). As previously mentioned, extensive handling, exposure to the maze, and appropriate pretraining might reduce the influence of nonmnemonic factors such as anxiety from the stress associated with a new experience. However, it is also possible to measure anxiety directly with a variety of tasks traditionally used to screen putative antianxiety agents. Anxiety levels most often are measured with the plus maze by the proportion of time spent by the subject on the two open arms and the two enclosed arms of the plus-shaped apparatus (Pellow and File, 1986).

In water mazes, clever behavioral procedures have been developed to account for a wide range of nonmnemonic variables that could be affected by an experimental condition. The use of nonspatial cued tasks, in which rodents are tested with visible escape platforms, is an especially valuable technique to account for nonmnemonic variables in water mazes. In this procedure, every feature of a spatial task with a hidden platform is contained in the cued task, except for an intramaze marker that denotes the location of the platform. Differences in performance in the cued task suggest that an experimental treatment affected functions ranging from sensory acuity and motor ability to thermoregulation and motivation. Most water maze studies have not found significant effects of ovarian hormones on cued tasks (Chesler and Juraska, 2000; Daniel et al., 1999; Fugger et al., 1998; Warren and Juraska, 1997, 2000), although there are exceptions (Galea et al., 1999a; Rissanen et al., 1999). A second technique has been to use computerized tracking to assess not only the swimming latency but also the swimming distance to escape to a hidden platform, providing a measure of swim speed that reflects the quality of motor function in treated and control animals. Most water maze studies have not found changes in swim speed that could account for the effects of estrogen and progesterone on reference memory performannce (Chesler and Juraska, 2000; Galea et al., 1995, 2000; Warren and Juraska, 1997, 2000), except for a report in which ovariectomized gerbils treated with Silastic capsules of estradiol had increased escape latencies that could be accounted for by decreased swim speed (Kondo et al., 1997).

3. Posttraining Treatment

Another important methodology to control for the nonmnemonic variables that may be affected by a treatment is to administer cognitive tests only when the compound is not in the body. The posttraining paradigm in which a drug or steroid is administered within 1 hour after training in order to promote or disrupt consolidation is a primary example (McGaugh, 1989). In this model, the steroid is proposed to act during the short period of memory consolidation and clear the system prior to a retention test, usually given 24 hours after treatment. Clearance of the steroid can be confirmed by showing that a treatment given at 2 hours or longer after the end of training fails to affect performance on the retention test. Although this paradigm has been used successfully with many agents with a rapid onset of action and rapid clearance rate, its use with steroids only became possible with the availability of a cyclodextran complex that renders estradiol water-soluble, allowing its rapid action and clearance (Packard et al., 1996; Packard, 1998). Using this procedure, the estradiol-cyclodextran complex enhanced retention when tested 24 hours after the end of a training session if the complex was administered within 1 hour, but not after 2 hours, of training. In our laboratory, we found that the administration of estradiol to 35-day-old ovariectomized rats for 30 days prior to radial arm maze training enhanced performance even though the steroid was not present during training (Daniel et al., 1997). The expression of behavioral effects after the steroid has been removed from the system suggests that the enhancement of working memory cannot be attributed to a direct action of estrogen on nonmnemonic processes, although this effect also may reflect an organizational action of estrogen at the time of puberty (Williams et al., 1990).

Although ovarian steroids affect a wide variety of functions, few experiments have been able to provide evidence of clear links to the effects of these steroids on learning and memory performance. To the contrary, water maze studies that include performance on cued tasks or swim speeds (distance/latency) failed to find clear correlations between the effects of ovarian steroids on cognition and nonmnemonic variables. Nevertheless, the contributions of many variables, such as arousal, attention, motivation, and anxiety, have not been assessed systematically and definitively. Therefore, such factors cannot be dismissed as immaterial to the actions of ovarian steroids on learning and memory performance.

IV. NEUROANATOMY AND NEUROMECHANISMS OF OVARIAN STEROID ACTION

A. Overview

Despite the complexities we have discussed, findings point to ovarian steroids as potential modulators of cognitive performance. Although the neuroanatomy and neuromechanisms that underlie the effects of ovarian steroids on learning and memory have not been resolved, a number of hypotheses have found empirical support. It is reasonable to propose that ovarian steroids modulate the biochemical, electrical, and structural events normally stimulated by learning in the formation of memories. At least four different literatures provide evidence for the anatomical and physiological foundations that may underlie the modulation of learning and memory by ovarian steroids. First, various brain structures contribute to cognitive performance, as indicated by lesion experiments and human case studies. Second, neurotransmitters that subserve these neural systems affect performance when manipulated by pharmacological and molecular techniques, including the administration of selective agonists, antagonists, neurotoxins, and antisense oligonucleotides, as well as the use of genetically modified animals. Third, some neurons that contribute to these pathways contain intracellular receptors that mediate the genomic effects of ovarian steroids. In addition, the actions of ovarian steroids at the neuronal membrane appear to be mediated by novel mechanisms, reflected in rapid electrical and biochemical responses, activation of second messenger systems, and regulation of protein synthesis. Fourth, ovarian steroids alter the structure of neurons and their connections, the neurochemistry of synaptic communication, and the electrical properties of neural circuits implicated in the control of learning and memory.

B. Neuroanatomy

Not surprisingly, functions as important and complex as cognition require the participation of a generous volume of the nervous system. Brain regions empirically implicated in the control of learning and memory processes include, but are not limited to, the hippocampus, basal forebrain, amygdala, striatum, allocortex, and neocortex. Additional subcortical structures include the supramammillary region of the caudal hypothalamus and the monoaminergic nuclei of the midbrain and hindbrain. It is important to note that many of these structures are densely interconnected, providing a sophisticated neural network for information processing, storage, and retrieval (Fig. 4).

Strong evidence accumulated in the 1990s links certain types of memory with specific neuroanatomical systems. The activation of each system is postulated to initiate a characteristic strategy to learn and remember the information necessary to solve a given task. Within this theoretical framework, there is now evidence for at least three separate but interacting memory systems in the brain. The hippocampus and its basal forebrain connections subserve the typical allocentric strategy that depends on the use of extramaze spatial cues (Section IIC1; Kesner et al., 1993; McDonald and White, 1993, 1995; Packard et al., 1989). The dorsal striatum and its connection with the cortex and mesencephalon promote the use of several egocentric strategies that depend on intramaze cues, stimulus–response associations, and propioception (Section IIC1); Kesner et al., 1993; McDonald and White, 1993; Packard et al., 1989; Packard and White, 1990). It has been suggested that the hippocampus holds working memory and that the striatum and neocortex retain reference memory (Packard and White, 1990). The amydala with its various connections to the hippocampus, basal forebrain, diencephalon, and mesencephalon promotes the learning of tasks with strong emotional components such as avoidance behaviors, but the amydala may also modulate other brain regions to add emotional valence to a wide range of memories (McGaugh et al., 1996; Packard et al., 1994; Packard and Teather, 1998). In primates, the prefrontal cortex plays an important role in working memory and decision making, functions postulated to be controlled by separate subdivisions, the dorsolateral–high mesial region and the ventromedial area, respectively (Bechara et al., 1998). There are many elaborate theories that are beyond the scope of this chapter regarding the organization of the brain and its relationship to learning and memory (Eichenbaum et al., 1992; Kesner and Hardy, 1983; O'Keefe and Nadel, 1978).

1. Hippocampus

The hippocampus plays a central role in cognition. Interest in this structure has been inspired by evidence that experimental and neuropathological lesions of the hippocampus and its afferent and efferent projections are associated with learning and memory deficits. A thorough survey of studies that support the role of the hippocampus is beyond the scope of this chapter, but

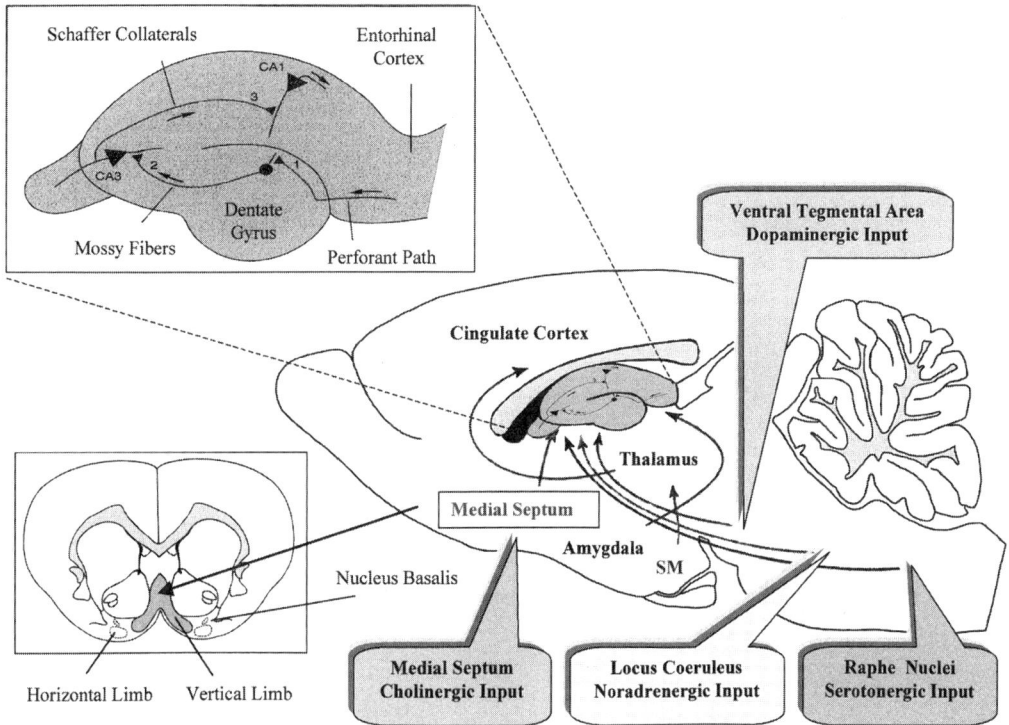

FIGURE 4 Principal brain regions implicated in the control of learning and memory. Only afferents pathways and intrinsic circuitry of the hippocampus are shown for clarity. SM, supramammillary region.

readers are directed to these reviews (Akhondzadeh, 1999; Cohen et al., 1999; Eichenbaum, 1999; Giap et al., 2000; Hasselmo, 1999; Holland and Bouton, 1999; Izquierdo et al., 1999; O'Keefe, 1999; Shapiro and Eichenbaum, 1999; Taube, 1999; Martin et al., 2000; McGaugh, 2000; Rolls, 2000). Damage to the hippocampus of rodents results in a variety of learning and memory impairments, traditionally interpreted as deficits in spatial working memory (Olton, 1983). However, the proposed roles of the hippocampus and its adjacent structures are indeed complex and involve many components and types of cognition, including spatial and nonspatial learning and memory, working and reference memory, and conditioning (Berger et al., 1986; Hampson et al., 1999; Holland and Bouton, 1999; Izquierdo et al., 1999; O'Keefe, 1999; Wan et al., 1994). Damage to the human hippocampus often leads to severe and persistent deficits in forming new episodic and declarative memories without affecting skill and procedural memories, as often experienced in patients suffering from amnesias such as H.M. (Section IIA; Milner, 1959; Penfield and Milner, 1958; Rempel-Clower et al., 1996; Scoville and Milner, 1957; Squire, 1992). Rolls (2000) has suggested that episodic memory may be related to spatial memory if both types of memories are viewed as snapshots of the relationships between spatial and nonspatial elements in a situation.

The subfields of the hippocampus and its adjacent structures receive direct or indirect input from the telencephalic, diencephalic, and mesencephalic regions of the brain (Fig. 4; Amaral, 1987; Amaral and Witter, 1995). The hippocampus requires a number of neurotransmitter systems to carry out its sophisticated functions; primarily glutamatergic, GABAergic (γ-aminobutyric acid), cholinergic, noradrenergic, serotonergic, and dopaminergic afferents, as well as glutamatergic and GABAergic efferents and intrinsic connections. There are four afferent pathways to the hippocampus that have been implicated in learning and memory: the perforant pathway innervates all subfields of the hippocampus from the entorhinal cortex; the septohippocampal pathway sends its projections from the basal forebrain nuclei to all subfields of the hippocampus; the supramammillary pathway travels from the supramammillary area of the caudal hypothalamus to the molecular layer of the hippocampus; and the monoaminergic pathways originate in the locus coeruleus, ventral tegmental area, and raphe nuclei of the midbrain and project mainly to the polymorphic layer of the hippocampus (Amaral, 1987). The principal efferents of the hippocampus project directly from all subfields to subcortical structures, including the basal forebrain nuclei and the mammillary hypothalamus. Similar to its afferent connections, efferents from the hippocampus proper travel to the entorhinal cortex and subicular complex, which communicate with telencephalic sites via their commissural and cortical projections (Amaral, 1987).

The entorhinal cortex and the subicular complex convey information from the neocortex and the amygdaloid complex to the hippocampus proper. The perforant pathway arises from the layers of the entorhinal cortex and projects primarily glutamatergic axons to cell fields throughout the hippocampus via the angular bundle (Kohler, 1985a,b, 1986, 1988; Steward, 1976; Steward and Scoville, 1976), with its strongest projections terminating in the granule cell layer of the dentate gyrus (Claiborne et al., 1986). The intrinsic organization of the hippocampus has important implications for steroid modulation of learning and memory. The perforant pathway is a principal input to the granule cell layer of the dentate gyrus. The dentate gyrus projects its mossy fibers to the CA3 subfield and this intrinsic circuit continues as the neurons of CA3 innervate the CA1 subfield via the Schaffer collaterals, which terminate on the apical dendrites of the stratum radiatum and the basal dendrites of the stratum oriens (Fig. 4; Amaral and Witter, 1995; Li et al., 1994). The electrophysiological phenomena of long- term potentiation and depression, proposed to reflect the changing synaptic efficiency that occurs during learning, can be induced by electrical stimulation of the perforant pathway, the mossy fibers, or the Schaffer collaterals as demonstrated in numerous studies (Bliss and Collingridge, 1993). Pharmacological and molecular manipulations of glutamatergic synapses affect performance on a number of cognitive tasks and affect induction of certain forms of long-term potentiation and depression (Morris, 1989; Steele and Morris, 1999), although the relationship between hippocampal activity and cognition remains controversial (Cain, 1998).

The first brain maps of estrogen receptor distribution visualized by in vivo [^{3}H]estradiol autoradiography revealed few neurons that contained estrogen receptors in the hippocampus (Pfaff and Keiner, 1973; Stumpf et al., 1979). In a later report, this sparse population of neurons with estrogen receptors was found to be localized to specific cells of the hippocampus, particularly the interneurons of the dentate gyrus, CA1, and subiculum (Loy et al., 1988). Other studies soon confirmed the presence of estrogen receptor immunoreactivity (Bettini et al., 1992; DonCarlos et al., 1991; Maggi et al., 1989) and estrogen receptor mRNA in the rat and guinea pig hippocampus (Bettini et al., 1992; Simerly et al., 1990). Estrogen receptor immunoreactivity was found to be distributed in a rostral–caudal gradient in the interneurons of the stratum radiatum of CA1 and the hilus of the dentate gryrus (Weiland et al., 1997). Autoradiography of [^{125}I]estradiol indicated the presence of estrogen receptors in pyramidal neurons of CA1, CA2, and CA3 as well (Shughure and Merchenthaler, 2000).

With the discovery of a new subtype of estrogen receptor, ERβ (Kuiper et al., 1997), the distribution of estrogen receptors in the brain now must be viewed against the backdrop of at least two types of estrogen receptor. The presence of ERα and ERβ immunoreactivity and mRNA has been confirmed and mapped in the rat hippocampus (LaFlamme et al., 1998; Li et al., 1997; Orikasa et al., 2000; Shughrue, 1998; Shughrue et al., 1997). ERα immmunoreactivity was found in the pyramidal cell layer of CA1, CA2, and CA3, whereas ERβ was localized in the pyramidal cells of CA1 and CA2 gyrus, as well as in the glial cells of CA1, CA2, CA3 and the dentate gryus (Azcoitia et al., 1999a). Ultrastructural evidence indicated that ERα immmunoreactivity was localized in the neuronal nuclei, unmyelinated axons, dendritic spines, and astrocytes in CA1 of proestrous rats (Milner et al., 2001). The subcellular distribution of ERα suggests roles in both genomic and nongenomic mechanisms. In addition to their unique distributions, it appears that ERα and ERβ may work through different mechanisms and exert their own specific effects on cellular events (Gustafsson, 2000; Patrone et al., 2000; Paech et al., 1997). Both receptors and their mRNA have been identified in hippocampal neurons of other rodent and primate species (Ivanova and Beyer, 2000; Osterlund et al., 2000a; Pau et al., 1998), as well as during development (Ivanova and Beyer, 2000; Orikasa et al., 2000). ERα immmunoreactivity was found to be weak in the hippocampus and cortex of adult rhesus monkeys (Blurton-Jones et al., 1999). Some discrepancies surround the reported distributions of the receptor types and their mRNA that may be the result of antibody or oligonucleotide specificity, as well as other methodological variables (McEwen and Alves, 1999). Nevertheless, work indicates that the density of ERα may be higher than previously believed in the hippocampus (Orikasa et al., 2000; Shughrue and Merchenthaler, 2000).

2. Basal Forebrain

The basal forebrain nuclei are a continuous field of neurons that extends from the medial septum ventrally as the vertical limb of the diagonal band of Broca, then laterally as the horizontal limbs, and finally laterally and caudally as the nucleus basalis magnocellularis and substantia innominata (Fig. 4; Fibiger, 1982; Mesulam et al., 1983a,b; Woolf, 1991). Electrolytic and neurotoxic (ibotenate, AF64A) lesions of the medial septum or the septohippocampal pathway impaired performance of spatial tasks in radial arm mazes, T mazes, and water mazes (Murray and Fibiger, 1985; O'Keefe, 1979; Olton et al., 1979; Walker and Olton, 1979; Walsh et al., 1998; Wenk et al., 1987). Many of these experiments initially led to the conclusion that medial septal neurons support spatial working memory, but have limited impact on reference memory (Dekker et al., 1991; Jarrard, 1983; Olton and Papas, 1979; Olton et al., 1991). However, the role played by the basal forebrain in spatial memory remains controversial.

Basal forebrain nuclei send cholinergic and GABAergic projections to all subfields of the hippocampus. The septohippocampal pathway originates from the magnocellular neurons of the basal forebrain, primarily the medial septum and the nuclei of the diagonal band of Broca with topographic projections to the ventral and dorsal portions of the hippocampus, respectively (Amaral and Kurz, 1985). Most of these projections travel in the fimbria and dorsal fornix (Lewis and Shute, 1967; Shute and Lewis, 1967) and synapse in the stratum oriens and stratum radiatum of CA2 and CA3 and in the molecular and polymorphic layers of the dentate gyrus. Basal forebrain neurons also innervate areas outside the hippocampus (Woolf, 1991); the medial septum and vertical limb project to the entorhinal, perirhinal, and retrosplenial cortices; the horizontal limb and magnocellular preoptic neurons project to the olfactory bulb, amydala, and the cingulate, piriform, and insular cortices; and the nucleus basalis and substantia innominata project to all four of the neocortices including the prefrontal cortex.

Interest in the role of acetylcholine in learning and memory has been high for many decades, partly based on early observations that muscarinic receptor antagonists, such as scopolamine, had powerful amnesic effects in humans and nonhumans (Bartus and Johnson, 1976; Deutsch, 1971; Drachman and Leavitt, 1974; Watts et al., 1981). Subsequently, the discovery of cholinergic deficits in the brains of patients suffering from Alzheimer's disease has afforded new importance to the role of acetylcholine in cognition and dementia (Davies, 1978; Wilcock et al., 1982). Many basal forebrain neurons use acetylcholine as a neurotransmitter (Mesulam et al., 1983a,b). Immunocytochemistry and tract-tracing techniques revealed that 30–50% of medial septal neurons and 50–75% of diagonal band neurons send cholinergic projections to the hippocampus (Amaral and Kurz, 1985; Wainer et al., 1984).

The cholinergic component of the septohippocampal track imparts a 4–8 Hz rhythm on the hippocampus that has been proposed to facilitate learning by regulating orienting responses, information processing, response inhibition, and voluntary movement (Apartis et al., 1998; Kleshchevnikov, 1999). However, evidence confirms that the theta rhythm is not induced solely by cholinergic inputs from the medial septum but is driven by an interacting network of cholinergic, GABAergic, glutamatergic, and monoaminergic systems contributed by the medial septum, entorhinal cortex, supramammillary region, and monoaminergic nuclei (Denham and Borisyuk, 2000; Kirk, 1998; Leranth et al., 1999; Vertes and Kocsis, 1997; Vertes and McKenna, 2000; Wu et al., 2000).

Although lesion studies supported the role of the medial septum in cognition, the application of neurotoxic lesions to eliminate cholinergic cell bodies has raised controversy about the role of the medial septum in learning and memory. Infusion of 192-immunoglobulin G (IgG)-saporin, a selective cholinergic immunotoxin, into the medial septal nucleus impaired performance on the spatial working memory component of the radial arm maze task (Shen *et al.*, 1996; Walsh *et al.*, 1996), but did not affect spatial reference memory in the radial arm maze (Shen *et al.*, 1996) or in water mazes (Baxter *et al.*, 1995; Baxter and Gallagher, 1996; Berger-Sweeney *et al.*, 1994; Torres *et al.*, 1994). However, subsequent experiments with 192-IgG-saporin indicated that when cell damage was limited specifically to cholinergic neurons in the medial septum, there was no impairment of working memory performance (Chappell *et al.*, 1998). Therefore, some investigators have concluded that cholinergic septal neurons may contribute to, but are not required for, normal working memory (Dornan *et al.*, 1997; Pang and Nocera, 1999). Alternatively, cholinergic neurons of the medial septum, along with other cholinergic nuclei of the basal forebrain, may play a role in attentional processes that assist working memory and promote shifts in learning strategy (Everitt and Robbins, 1997; Janis *et al.*, 1998; Gibbs, 1994; Gibbs, 1999a; Wenk, 1997).

Pharmacological manipulations of the cholinergic systems support a role for acetycholine in learning and memory, but again not without controversy. Generally, muscarinic and nicotinic cholinergic receptor antagonists and cholinergic synthesis inhibitors impair performance on a variety of tasks, most notably those that depend on working memory (Bartus, 2000; Everitt and Robbins, 1997). Although anticholinergic agents impair learning and memory performance under many experimental conditions, these drugs can affect diverse nonmnemonic functions. Therefore, the contribution of nonmnemonic factors affected by anticholinergic agents remains a potential confound in many studies. Alternatively, performance often is enhanced by the administration of muscarinic or nictotinic receptor agonists or inhibitors of the enzyme responsible for the degradation of acetylcholine, acetylcholinesterase. These agents can prevent or overcome cognitive deficits induced by electrolytic and neurotoxic lesions, cholinergic antagonists, aging, and neuropathology.

Many basal forebrain neurons that concentrated radiolabeled estradiol also stained positively for acetylcholinesterase, a weak marker for cholinergic neurons (Fallon *et al.*, 1983). Toran-Allerand later demonstrated that 50–80% of the neurons that were immunoreactive for choline acetyltransferase, a definitive cholinergic marker, contained estrogen receptors in the medial septum, horizontal limb, and nucleus magnocellularis of postnatal rats (Toran-Allerrand *et al.*, 1992). Colocalization of choline acetyltransferase imnunoreactivity or mRNA with estrogen receptors in neurons of the basal forebrain was confirmed in additional studies, despite methodological issues (Gibbs, 1996a; Shughrue *et al.*, 2000). ERα is the predominant receptor type found in basal forebrain neurons (Shughrue *et al.*, 2000) and is colocalized with choline acetyltransferase (Mufson *et al.*, 1999). It is, therefore, not surprising that estrogen can modulate cholinergic neurochemistry in basal forebrain areas, as well as in associated projection sites such as the hippocampus and cortex.

Neurons that release the inhibitory amino acid neurotransmitter GABA also are distributed throughout the basal forebrain (Gritti *et al.*, 1993). GABAergic neurons and cholinergic neurons of the basal forebrain interact bidirectionally in the basal forebrain nuclei (Van der Zee and Luiten, 1994). In addition, both cholinergic and GABAergic neurons project via the septohippocampal pathway to innervate the hippocampus (Amaral and Kurz, 1985). Some cholinergic projections to the hippocampus synapse on GABAergic interneurons, some of which may contain estrogen receptors (Leranth *et al.*, 2000; Murphy and Segal, 1997). Consequently, an estrogen-sensitive circuit comprising GABAergic and cholinergic neurons provides an anatomical substrate for the actions of estrogen on learning and memory processes, as well as on dendritic structure (Daniel and Dohanich, 2001).

3. Supramammillary Area

The supramammillary tract comprises primarily neurons in the suprammamillary area surrounding the mammillary nucleus of the caudal hypothalamus that project to the molecular layer of the hippocampal subfields (Fig. 4; Haglund *et al.*, 1984; Riley and Moore, 1981; Vertes, 1992) as well as to the medial septum. Although the classification of the neurotransmitters used by supramammillary neurons has been difficult, some efferents have been identified as glutamatergic or aspartatergic (Kiss *et al.*, 2000). It has been known for many years that some individuals suffering from alcoholism manifest severe learning and memory deficits known as

Wernicke-Korsakoff's syndrome. The neuropathology associated with this condition is damage to caudal diencephalic neurons (Mair et al., 1979; Mayes et al., 1988; Victor et al., 1971). Experimental lesions of the supramammillary area, often including adjacent sites, impaired acquisition and retention of spatial, but not nonspatial, information, probably by inhibiting the use of allocentric strategies (Neave et al., 1997; Rosenstock et al., 1977; Sziklas and Petrides, 1993, 1998; Sziklas et al., 1996). A significant number of supramammillary neurons were found to be immunoreactive for both the calcium-binding protein calretinin and ERα (Leranth et al., 1999), although this nucleus has received little attention from investigators studying steroid modulation of learning and memory.

4. Monoaminergic Nuclei

Hippocampal projections emerge from the monoaminergic nuclei of the midbrain and hindbrain, ascending to the dentate gyrus (Fig. 4). The densest of these are noradrenergic axons from the locus coeruleus that terminate in the polymorphic layer of the dentate gyrus (Haring and Davis, 1983, 1985a,b; Swanson and Hartman, 1975). Serotonergic neurons from the raphe nucleus also send their axons to the polymorphic layer, terminating primarily on interneurons of the dentate gyrus (Conrad et al., 1974). A much weaker dopaminergic projection originates in the ventral tegmental area and scatters diffuse projections throughout the dentate gyrus (Swanson, 1982). Along with the cholinergic and GABAergic projections from the basal forebrain nuclei, these monoaminergic tracts provide subcortical modulation of hippocampal activity that may facilitate learning (Kirk, 1998). Cholinergic and monoaminergic projections to the neocortex, especially the prefrontal cortex, affect working memory and consolidation, as well as sensory gating and selective attention. Dopaminergic neurons in the substantia nigra, thalamus, and neocortex innervate the striatum. The nigrostriatal pathway originates in the dopamine neurons of the pars compacta of the midbrain substantia nigra, projecting to the dorsal and ventral regions of the striatum. This system plays a critical role in motor function and is implicated in nonspatial memory associated with cued tasks and egocentric strategies that depend on motor responses (Kesner et al., 1993; McDonald and White, 1993; Packard et al., 1989; Packard and White, 1990). Some monoaminergic neurons in the midbrain and hindbrain were reported to contain ERα protein or mRNA (Kritzer, 1997; Leranth et al., 1999; Pau et al., 1998).

C. Regulation of Neurotransmitter Systems by Ovarian Steroids

The evidence presented so far implicates acetylcholine, GABA, glutamate, and the monoamines in the neurochemical control of learning and memory. Ovarian steroids are able to modulate various enzymes, receptors, transporters, and other proteins associated with these systems, providing a neurochemical basis for estrogen and progesterone to alter learning and memory performance.

1. Acetylcholine

Estrogen administered to ovariectomized rats increased the activity of the synthetic enzyme for acetylcholine, choline acetyltransferase, in the horizontal limb and projection sites in the hippocampus and cortex (Luine and McEwen, 1983; Luine, 1985; Singh et al., 1994). Estrogen also increased the number of basal forebrain neurons expressing immunoreactivity for choline acetyltransferase and increased the relative cellular level of its mRNA in ovariectomized rats (Gibbs and Pfaff, 1992; Gibbs et al., 1994; Gibbs, 1996b, 1997; McMillan et al., 1996). Another measure of cholinergic function, high-affinity transport of the precursor choline, also was increased following estrogen treatment in both the frontal cortex and hippocampus of ovariectomized rats, restoring choline uptake to intact levels (O'Malley et al., 1987; Singh et al., 1994). Thus, estrogen receptors are present in many cholinergic neurons and estrogen influences cholinergic neurochemistry in the hippocampus, cortex, and basal forebrain nuclei, brain regions strongly implicated in mammalian learning and memory. However, in our laboratory, we have not detected any consistent changes in muscarinic, M1, or M2 binding associated with estrogen treatment of ovariectomized rats (G. Dohanich, unpublished data).

The effects of estrogen are especially evident when cholinergic systems are challenged. Scopolamine hydrobromide delivered bilaterally to the dorsal hippocampus reduced reinforced T-maze alternation to chance levels in ovariectomized rats previously trained to complete this task (Section IIIB2; Fader et al., 1998). The effects of scopolamine were localized to the hippocampus because scopolamine delivered to the cortical area directly dorsal to the hippocampus failed to affect alternation. Most important, ovariectomized rats treated for 1 week with estradiol benzoate (5 μg/kg daily) prior to intrahippocampal scopolamine administration were not impaired in T-maze alternation. This experiment extended an earlier report that high doses of estradiol benzoate (100 μg/kg for 3 days) counteracted the impairment of reinforced T-maze alternation induced by scopolamine administered by systemic injection (0.2 mg/kg; Dohanich et al., 1994). Similarly, estrogen treatment prevented deficits induced by scopolamine on a matching-to-position T-maze task (Section IIIB2; Gibbs, 1999a). Therefore, estrogen treatment can counteract the amnesic effects of scopolamine, possibly by acting on the hippocampal systems that subserve working memory. Consequently, under strengthened conditions induced by exposure to estrogen, cholinergic systems may be less vulnerable to impairments from amnesic agents such as scopolamine.

Estradiol could act at either the origin or the termination of the septohippocampal pathway because intracellular estrogen receptors are present in neurons of both the medial septum and the hippocampal subfields (Fallon et al., 1983; Gibbs, 1996a; Loy et al., 1988; Maggi et al., 1989; Simerly et al., 1990; Toran-Allerand et al., 1992; Weiland et al., 1996). In order to identify the site of action of estradiol in the mediation of spatial working memory, we studied the behavioral effects of dilute estradiol implants placed in the medial septum or dorsal hippocampus of ovariectomized rats (Fader et al., 2000). Estradiol implants in the medial septum, but not in the hippocampus or cortex, increased the number of correct choices during the acquisition of a radial arm task dependent on working memory. Estradiol implants in the hippocampus, but not the medial septum or cortex, prevented impairments in working memory performance induced by the systemic administration of scopolamine. Consequently, both the medial septum and the hippocampus may play important, although different, roles in estrogen modulation of working memory.

2. Glutamate

Estradiol can regulate glutamatergic transmission in some regions of the brain. The same short-term estrogen treatment that increased CA1 pyramidal cell spines and synapses increased glutamatergic NMDA receptor binding in the CA1 pyramidal layer (Weiland, 1992; Woolley et al., 1997). Immunofluoresence of the NMDA subunit NR1 also was increased by estrogen treatment (Gazzaley et al., 1996) but not receptor binding of the glutamatergic alpha-amino-3-hydroxy-5-methyl-4-isoxazolepropionic acid (AMPA) site (Weiland, 1992; Woolley et al., 1997). Two weeks of estrogen administration to rats ovariectomized for 10 weeks restored NMDA binding, but not AMPA binding, in CA1 and the dentate gyrus to levels found in gonadally intact females (Cyr et al., 2000). In contrast, this same treatment reduced NMDA binding in the frontal cortex and dorsal striatum of ovariectomized rats. The increases in NMDA binding induced by estrogen are proposed to underlie the structural and electrical changes in CA1 associated with elevated estrogen levels (Woolley et al., 1997).

3. γ-Aminobutyric Acid

Estradiol also can regulate GABAergic transmission in the hippocampus. *In vitro* application of estradiol to hippocampal cultures decreased the content of glutamic acid decarboxylase (GAD), the synthetic enzyme for GABA, in pyramidal-cell-layer interneurons (Murphy et al., 1998). A reduced level of GAD, and therefore GABA, should weaken the inhibitory control of interneurons on CA1 pyramidal cells, increasing their excitation and promoting the structural and electrical changes in the hippocampus associated with estrogen. Surprisingly, GAD mRNA was increased in the CA1 pyramidal cell layer after *in vivo* administration of estrogen to ovariectomized rats, although estrogen administered with progesterone prevented the increase in GAD mRNA (Weiland, 1992). Estrogen treatment of male rats did not affect benzodiazepine receptor binding in the hippocampus or cortex (Hruska and Pitman, 1982).

4. Monoamines

A significant number of neurons in the midbrain raphe contain estrogen receptors, providing a mechanism for estrogen to regulate serotonergic neurotransmission (Leranth et al., 1999). Colocalization of ERα- or progestin-receptor immunocytochemistry was reported in raphe neurons that were immunoreactive for tryptophan hydroxylase, an enzyme that synthesizes serotonin (Alves et al., 2000). In rats, serotonin (5-HT) receptor binding increased during proestrus in the hippocampus and striatum (Williams and Uphouse, 1989) and 5-HT$_{2A}$ receptors were increased in cortical areas after estrogen treatment (Fink et al., 1996). The binding of 5-HT$_{1A}$ receptors in the hippocampus of ovariectomized rats was reported to be decreased by 2 weeks of estrogen treatment, although this change was not correlated to decreases in mRNA (Osterlund and Hurd, 1998; Osterlund et al., 2000b). In another report, 4 days of estrogen treatment did not affect the number or affinity of 5HT$_{1A}$ receptors in hippocampus of ovariectomized rats (Clarke and Maayani, 1990). Nevertheless, estrogen treatment facilitated cellular activities regulated by 5-HT$_{1A}$ receptor activation, including the hyperpolarization of CA1 pyramidal cells (Beck et al., 1989), inhibition of hippocampal adenylate cyclase activity (Clarke and Maayani, 1990), and changes in G$_{(i/o)}$-coupled function (Mize and Alper, 2000). The gonadectomy of male or female rats decreased serotonin levels in the hippocampus, an effect that was counteracted by chronic estrogen or testosterone treatments (Bitar et al., 1991).

Immunoreactivity for the estrogen receptor was identified in neurons of the ventral tegmental area and retrorubral field in intact male and female rats (Kritzer, 1997). In an earlier study, dopamine receptor binding in the hippocampus of male rats was reduced by estrogen treatment (Hruska and Pitman, 1982), although dopamine receptor D$_{1A}$ transcription was found to be increased 20% by estrogen in a cotransfected cell line (Lee and Mouradian, 1999). There have been few reports on the regulation of noradrenergic synapses by estrogen; however, the ovariectomy of rhesus monkeys increased immunoreactivity in prefrontal axons for dopamine β-hydroxylase, an enzyme that synthesizes norepinephrine, whereas estrogen or estrogen and progesterone replacement restored dopamine β-hydroxylase immunoreactivity to normal (Kritzer and Kohama, 1999).

D. Structural Change Associated with Ovarian Steroids

It has been known for some time that estrogen exerts powerful effects on neuronal structure, particularly in developing cells and tissues (Toran-Allerand, 1984, 1991), in reproductive regions (Frankfurt, 1994), and during reactive growth following neuronal damage (Harrell et al., 1990; Morse et al., 1992; Stone et al., 1998). One mechanism by which estrogen might influence learning and memory is through the restructuring of dendrites and synapses, particularly in the female hippocampus and cortex. For example, in the dentate gyrus, aged rats ovariectomized for long periods experienced a severe loss of dendritic spines that was restored by short-term, but not long-term, estrogen replacement (Miranda et al., 1999).

The density of apical dendritic spines on pyramidal neurons in the CA1 region was correlated positively with circulating levels of estrogen, as indicated by experiments in which exogenous estrogen was manipulated (Gould et al., 1990; Washburn et al., 1997) or in which estrogen levels varied at different stages of the estrous cycle (McEwen and Woolley, 1994; Woolley et al., 1990; Woolley and McEwen, 1993). Progesterone counteracted estrogen-induced increases following conversion to the neurosteroid tetrahydroprogesterone (Murphy and Segal, 2000). The density of synapses and shapes of boutons in the stratum radiatum of the CA1 region also correlated positively with fluctuation of estrogen levels during the estrous cycle or following estradiol treatment (Woolley and McEwen, 1992; Woolley et al., 1996). Based on increases in NMDA receptor binding (Weiland, 1992; Woolley et al., 1997) and decreases in GAD (Murphy et al., 1998) induced by estrogen in CA1 of the hippocampus, estrogen appears to act on intracellular or possibly other receptors associated with GABAergic interneurons to reduce their inhibition on nearby CA1 pyramidal cells. This hypothesis was supported by evidence that estrogen-induced spine growth was prevented by NMDA receptor blockers (Woolley and McEwen, 1994) or an estrogen receptor antagonist (McEwen et al., 1999). The enhanced activity of these disinhibited pyramidal cells, suggested by their c-Fos response to estradiol (Rudick and Woolley, 2000), is associated with increases in NMDA receptor binding along with changes in the structural and electrical properties of the cells (Woolley et al., 1997). Evidence also indicated that subcortical inputs to CA1 via the fimbria and fornix may contribute to the action of estrogen on spine density (Leranth et al., 2000).

E. Electrical Change Associated with Ovarian Steroids

Endogenous and exogenous estrogen alters the electrical properties of neuronal circuits in cycling female rats. Long-term potentiation is an electrophysiological phenomenon in which strong electrical stimulation of afferents to an area induces long-term changes in synaptic efficiency that have been postulated to represent learning (Bliss and Lomo, 1973). Several studies reported that at proestrus, when endogenous estrogen levels are elevated, or following exposure to exogenous estradiol, long-term potentiation in the CA1 response to Schaffer collateral stimulation was enhanced under both *in vivo* and *in vitro* conditions (Cordoba Montoya and Carrer, 1997; Foy et al., 1999; Good et al., 1999; Warren et al., 1995). The parameters affected by estrogen in these experiments, however, were varied, including postsynaptic amplitude, excitatory postsynaptic potential (EPSP) slope, preinput and pre-output and postinput and post-output curves. Additional *in vitro* studies reported no effect of estrogen on long-term potentiation (LTP) parameters in adult rats (Barraclough et al., 1999; Ito et al., 1999), as well as a suppression of LTP by estrogen in prepubertal females (Ito et al., 1999). The induction of long-term depression in CA1 was found to be decreased at proestrus *in vivo* (Good et al., 1999), but increased in CA1 of the hippocampus taken from ovariectomized rats treated with estradiol (Desmond et al., 2000).

In addition to the effects of estrogen on LTP, hippocampal multiple-unit activity and CA1-population-evoked responses were increased in several earlier studies (Kawakami et al., 1970; Wong and Moss, 1992). Collectively, these data indicate that estrogen modulates structural and electrical activities in the hippocampus. Despite this modulation over the course of the estrous cycle, however, behavioral studies report either impairments in water maze performance when endogenous levels of estradiol and progesterone are elevated or a lack of any change in learning and memory performance over the estrous cycle in water and radial arm mazes (Section III). The relationships between structural, electrical, and cognitive events are likely to be complex and require new avenues of thought (Desmond and Levy, 1997; Joels, 1997; Woolley, 1999).

F. Neuroprotective Effects of Ovarian Hormones

Although much of this section has focused on the putative roles of estrogen and progesterone in learning and memory, the most important action of these hormones may be to promote the survival of neurons. Many events damage neurons throughout life, sometimes leading to grim consequences for cognitive function. Insults to the brain elicit common physiological responses including the formation of free radicals, the release of excitatory amino acids, and an increase in metabolic demand, all of which can lead to cell death, often through apoptosis.

1. Neuroprotection

Estrogen and progesterone have been shown to confer some protection on neurons that are confronted by threats associated with stroke, trauma, hypoglycemia, disease, and aging (Fig. 5) (Wise et al., 2001). Both *in vitro* and *in vivo* studies have documented that estrogen reduces cell damage from oxidative stress (Behl et al., 1995, 1997; Dubal et al., 1998; Goodman et al., 1996; Gridley et al., 1997; Hawk et al., 1998; Mook-Jung et al.,

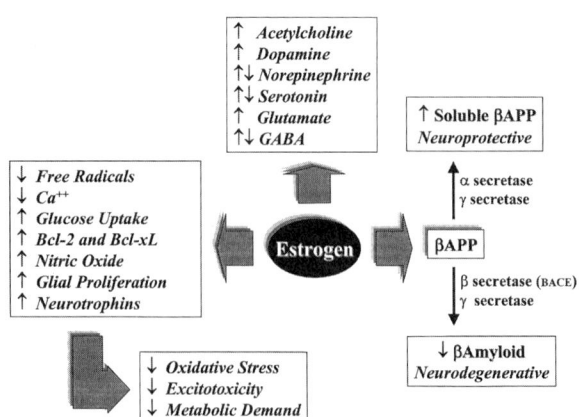

FIGURE 5 Some documented effects of estrogen that might promote neuron survival and slow degenerative processes.

1997; Simpkins et al., 1997; Yang et al., 2000; Zhang et al., 1998), amino acid excitoxicity (Azcoitia et al., 1998, 1999b; Behl et al., 1995, 1997; Goodman et al., 1996; Gridley et al., 1997; Singer et al., 1996; Zaulyanov et al., 1999), increased metabolic load and hypogylcemia (Goodman et al., 1996; Gridley et al., 1997), and amyloid neurotoxicity (Behl et al., 1995, 1997; Bonnefont et al., 1998; Goodman et al., 1996; Green et al., 1996; Gridley et al., 1997; Petanceska et al., 2000; Svensson and Nordberg, 1999; Xu et al., 1998). Progesterone, a much less studied steroid, reduced cell damage, blood–brain barrier leakage, edema, and cognitive deficits following brain trauma (Goodman et al., 1996; Roof et al., 1992, 1993, 1994, 1997; Roof and Hall, 2000), although not in all studies (Behl et al., 1995).

2. Mechanisms of Neuroprotection

Estrogen exerts a wide range of both general and specific effects on the brain that probably contribute to its neuroprotective capabilities (Roof and Hall, 2000). First, it has been known for sometime that estrogen is a strong antioxidant (Mooradian, 1993), able to reduce dangerous free radicals that cause lipid peroxidation and deterioration of cell membranes, especially when combined with another antioxidant (Behl et al., 1995; Goodman et al., 1996; Green et al., 1998; Gridley et al., 1997, 1998; Meng et al., 1999; Vedder et al., 1999). Second, estrogen protection from excitoxic levels of amino acids, often released after brain trauma, has been linked to a rapid receptor-mediated activation of MAPK by estrogen (Singer et al., 1999), kinases also activated by neurotrophic growth factors (Bi et al., 2000; Singh et al., 1999, 2000; Toran-Allerand et al., 1999). Third, estradiol has been shown to facilitate glucose uptake by both the brain and its neurons via increased synthesis of membrane and endothelial glucose transporters (Bishop and Simpkins, 1995; Shi and Simpkins, 1997; Shi et al., 1997), rescuing vulnerable neurons during high metabolic demand or low glucose availability (Lannert et al., 1998; Simpkins, 1995). Hypoglycemia reduced in vivo expression of cyclic AMP responsive element binding protein (CREB) in the hippocampal neurons, which was restored by estrogen replacement (Panickar et al., 1997). Fourth, estrogen is proposed to regulate programmed cell death by receptor-specific mechanisms leading to decreased apoptosis mediated by ERα and increased apoptosis mediated by ERβ (Nilsen et al., 2000). As a putative mechanism, the antiapoptotic proteins, Bcl-2 (Garcia-Segura et al., 1998; Dubal et al., 1999) and Bcl-xL (Pike, 1999) were increased by the presence of estrogen.

Additional mechanisms that could contribute to the neuroprotection offered by estrogen include increases in the primary synthase of nitric oxide (Lopez-Jaramillo and Teran, 1999), shown to be regulated in both brain and peripheral tissues by estrogen (Ceccatelli et al., 1996; McNeill et al., 1999; Okamura et al., 1994a,b; Rachman et al., 1998; Wang and Morris, 1999; Warembourg et al., 1999), and the blunting of intracellular calcium release that contributes to cellular damage caused by oxidative stress, excitotoxicity, and βamyloid (Chen et al., 1998; Goodman et al., 1996). Conjugated estrogen promoted vascular function in rodents by reducing βamyloid accumulation, endothelial cell damage, and inflammation reactions in blood vessel walls in the brain and periphery (Thomas et al., 1999). Finally, hippocampal astroglia have been found to contain ERβ (Azcoitia et al., 1999c), which could provide a mechanism for estrogen to exert neuroprotective actions by stimulating the release of growth factors and other neuroactive agents, as well as by regulating glial proliferation following cell damage (Azcoitia et al., 1999b; Cardona-Gomez et al., 2000; Garcia-Estrada et al., 1999; Garcia-Segura et al., 1999; Granholm, 2000; Mor et al., 1999).

3. Alzheimer's Disease

Evidence that estrogen may delay the onset and reduce the severity of symptoms of Alzheimer's disease, Parkinson's disease, and other dementias has focused strong interest on the role of estrogen in disease and aging. In the case of Alzheimer's disease, there are several putative targets for neuroprotection by estrogen, including its effects on free-radical formation and lipid peroxidation, excitotoxicity, glucose uptake, and apoptosis, as already discussed. The ability of estrogen to curb the disease process probably depends on a multifaceted defense. The most commonly used estrogen preparation for hormone replacement consists of conjugated equine estrogens (Premarin), which have been found to be powerful neuroprotectants of hippocampal, cortical, and basal forebrain neurons against lipid peroxidation, βamyloid neurotoxicity, and glutamate excitotoxicity (Diaz-Brinton et al., 2000).

The proliferation of βamyloid, a 40- to 42-amino-acid protein synthesized from amyloid percursor protein (APP), is highly indicative of Alzheimer's disease (Fig. 5). In individuals without Alzheimer's disease, APP is converted by αsecretase into soluble βamyloid precursor protein (sβAPP), itself neuroprotective. However, a variant enzyme, βsecretase (identified as BACE, β-site APP-cleaving enzyme; Vassar et al., 1999), converts APP into an insoluble and neurotoxic product, βamyloid, that aggregates to form the ubiquitous senile plaques characteristic of Alzheimer's disease (Selkoe, 1996). Individuals who carry the e-4 allele of the apolipoprotein E (ApoE) gene are at greater risk for developing Alzheimer's disease (Cummings et al., 1998). The presence of the ApoE e-4 allele is associated with increased βamyloid deposition, aggregation, and plaque formation.

Estradiol reduced the synthesis of the neurotoxic βamyloid and increased the synthesis of APP and its neuroprotective metabolite sβAPP in vivo and in vitro (Chao et al., 1994; Jaffe et al., 1994; Green et al., 1996; Mook-Jung et al., 1997; Petanceska et al., 2000; Xu et al., 1998). Progesterone also increased the hippocampal expression of APP695, the most common form of APP found in the rat brain (Chao et al., 1994). Interestingly, the neuroprotective effects of estradiol on βamyloid were blocked in two cell lines by the addition of an α7 nicotinic receptor antagonist, indicating direct cholinergic involvement in estrogen neuroprotection (Svensson and Nordberg, 1999). Neurotoxicity from interactions between βamyloid and lipid peroxidation, glucose deficiency, or glutamate excitotoxicity also was reduced in vitro by estrogen (Goodman et al., 1996). Finally, there appears to a link between estrogen and the ApoE e-4 allele that may have important consequences for the risk of developing Alzheimer's disease. The defective protein synthesized from the ApoE e-4 allele may be unable to transport cholesterol for the routine repair of neuronal membranes, an action that may be exacerbated by insufficient levels of estrogen (Birge and Mortel, 1997).

Despite strong evidence that estrogen protects neurons from βamyloid toxicity, results supporting a neuroprotective action of estradiol on cognitive performance following treatment of rodents with βamyloid are scarce. In the only comprehensive study, spontaneous alternation in a Y maze and reference memory performance in a water maze were significantly but equally impaired in gonadally intact female rats and ovariectomized rats following chronic infusion of the neurotoxic 1–42 fragment of βamyloid (Yamada et al., 1999). The results indicate that the presence of endogenous ovarian hormones did not protect the cognitive functions necessary to learn and remember these two tasks. Gonadally intact and ovariectomized rats failed to show significant deficits in a working memory version of the water maze (Section IIC1a) following chronic infusion of βamyloid (1–42). However, the combination of long-term ovariectomy (3 months) and βamyloid (1–42) treatment produced poorer working memory performance than intact females receiving control infusions, indicating that a nonsignificant neurotoxic effect of βamyloid on working memory may be exacerbated by a lack of estrogen (Yamada et al., 1999). The surprising lack of reports on in vivo neuroprotection by estrogen from βamyloid treatment is disturbing and might be accounted for by the difficulty in inducing learning and memory deficits in rats by the adminstration of βamyloid (Cleary et al., 1995; Delobette et al., 1997; Dornan et al., 1993; Harkany et al., 1998; McDonald et al., 1994). Alternatively, evidence that estrogen fails to prevent or reverse learning and memory deficits induced by βamyloid may not reach publication.

The role of estrogen receptors in the neuroprotective actions of estrogen is unresolved. Evidence supports the participation of at least two mechanisms featuring classic intracellular receptors or novel membrane receptors. High concentrations of estradiol increased the number of human SK-N-SH cells surviving in a serum-free medium (Bishop and Simpkins, 1995). Although SK-N-SH cells express estrogen receptor mRNA, equal neuroprotection was conferred by both 17β-estradiol, with high affinity for the intracellular estrogen receptor, and its normally inactive isomer 17α-estradiol, with very low affinity for the intracellular estrogen receptor (Behl et al., 1997; Green et al., 1996, 1997a,b). Furthermore, tamoxifen and ICI 182,780, which block intracellular estrogen receptors, failed to antagonize the neuroprotective effects of either 17β-estradiol or 17α-estradiol (Behl et al., 1995; Diaz-Brinton, 1997; Green et al., 1997a,b; Gridley et al., 1998). Subsequent structure–activity studies indicated that the property that allows a steroid to protect endangered neurons is a phenolic-A ring with three rings of the steroid structure (Behl *et al.*, 1997; Green *et al.*, 1997a,b, 1998; Zaulyanov *et al.*, 1999).

Although these results argue against the mediation of estrogen action by intracellular receptors, other findings support a role for the classic receptor. For instance, low concentrations of estradiol were found to promote survival in a serum-free preparation of fetal hypothalamic neurons, and this action was blocked by tamoxifen (Chowen *et al.*, 1992). Other neuroprotective actions of estrogen, including the stimulation of bcl-2 expression and antiapoptotic effects, also appear to be mediated by intracellular estrogen receptors (Dubal *et al.*, 1999; Nilsen *et al.*, 2000). Although the estrogen-induced stimulation of the MAPK pathway was antagonized by ICI 182,780, suggesting dependence on intracellular receptors (Singer *et al.*, 1999), there is evidence that estradiol can stimulate MAPK through an additional unknown membrane receptor (Singh *et al.*, 1999, 2000; Toran-Allerand *et al.*, 1999).

In summary, a substantial body of evidence strongly supports the effectiveness of estrogen as a neuroprotective steroid, although the role of progesterone is less studied and less compelling. Estrogen prevents neuronal death induced by diverse insults by engaging an assortment of mechanisms that alter lipid metabolism, affect glucose transport, moderate intracellular calcium levels, activate signaling pathways, and stimulate the release of growth factors and the expression of antiapoptotic proteins. These multiple actions of estrogen are effective particularly in counteracting the many insidious cellular events that occur in response to brain trauma. The neuroprotection conferred by estrogen appears to be mediated by multiple receptor mechanisms at intracellular and membrane sites. Ovarian steroids, as well as their natural and synthetic cousins, hold exciting promise in the fight against neurodegeneration.

V. OVARIAN HORMONES AND HUMAN COGNITION

The study of the effects of estrogen and progesterone in human cognition has focused primarily on three female subject populations: premenopausal women without dementia; postmenopausal women without dementia; and postmenopausal women with a diagnosis of dementia, usually Alzheimer's disease. As with nonhuman species, ovarian hormones could influence human cognition by acting directly on memory systems or by affecting nonmnemonic functions. However, the most exciting aspect of ovarian hormone use in humans is as neuroprotection against the threats of age and disease (Section IVE1).

A. Premenopausal Effects of Ovarian Hormones

Moderate fluctuations in cognitive performance have been documented during normal menstrual cycles. Generally, women exhibit poorer spatial performance but better verbal and manual performance during the preovulatory and midluteal phases when estrogen levels are elevated compared to the late luteal and menstrual phases when estrogen levels are lower (Broverman *et al.*, 1981; Hampson, 1990a; Hampson and Kimura, 1988; Komenich *et al.*, 1978; Phillips and Sherwin, 1992b; Wickham, 1958; Zimmerman and Parker, 1973). Estrogen often improves performance on the same verbal and manual tasks in which women outperform men, although estrogen impairs performance on spatial tasks in which men outperform women (Hampson, 1990a,b; Sherwin, 1994). These relationships are maintained when estrogen levels are high but progesterone levels are low such as during the preovulatory phase, indicating that circulating progesterone contributes little to human cognitive performance (Hampson, 1990b). In addition to its enhancement of verbal performance, higher estrogen also is linked to creativity, as measured by performance on tests of divergent thinking and flexibility, abilities that might facilitate learning strategy (Krug *et al.*, 1993).

Despite evidence of correlations between estrogen levels and cognitive performance, questions remain regarding the nature, reliability, magnitude, and importance of these relationships. Menstrual stage affects a number of functions indirectly related to learning and memory performance, ranging from sensory acuity to mood (Bethea *et al.*, 1998; Parlee, 1983). For example, women showed improved visual sensitivity on a discrimination task during the late follicular phase when estrogen is elevated (Friedman and Meares, 1978), an enhancement that could be related to performance on perceptual tasks. As with nonhumans, the effects of ovarian steroids on nonmnemonic factors must be assessed carefully when studying the influences of these steroids on learning and memory performance. Correlations between menstrual stage and cognitive performance have not always been replicated between or within studies (Gordon and Lee, 1993; Resnick et al., 1998). Broad conclusions about the relationships between estrogen and memory type sometimes were not confirmed by performance on different tasks purported to test similar memory types. Finally, the reported effects of estrogen are small to moderate, reflected by the overlapping distributions of performance across menstrual stages, challenging the importance of cycle effects on daily cognitive functioning (Sherwin, 1994). The results from human studies across the menstrual cycle have striking similarities to findings in other species across estrous cycles. Unfortunately, studies on human and nonhuman cognitive performance also are beset by common methodological problems, as noted by Hampson and Kimura (1992). These include the lack of measurements to confirm plasma levels of estradiol at the time of testing, the use of confusing or inconsistent terms to denote reproductive stages, the administration of cognitive tests at inappropriate stages of the cycle, the use of insensitive or inappropriate measures of cognitive performance, the misinterpretation of statistical analyses, and the use of insufficient sample sizes to test modest group differences.

B. Postmenopausal Effects of Ovarian Hormones

With increases in the use of hormone replacement therapy following menopause to maintain bone density (Felson et al., 1993) and cardiovascular function (Ohkura et al., 1995; Stampfer et al., 1991), the effects of hormone replacement therapy on other processes, notably cognitive performance, have received additional attention. Two types of research paradigms are employed commonly—experimental randomized trials in which ovarian hormones or placebos are administered for limited periods to subjects matched on pertinent variables and observational cross-sectional studies in which women already using hormone replacement are compared to a matched sample of nonusers.

Randomized trial studies have been used to examine the effects of estrogen and progesterone replacement on verbal, spatial, and manual performance, as well as on anxiety and affect. In these trials, various estrogen preparations including estradiol, estrone, estriol, progynon, or conjugated equine estrogens (Premarin) have been administered orally, intramuscularly, or transdermally most often to Caucasian women in early menopause who are not suffering from dementia. When compared to a placebo, some of these preparations improved performance on short-term verbal measures—immediate paragraph recall, immediate or delayed paired-associate recall, associate learning, verbal comprehension, digit span, visual search, mental rotation, reaction time, and color naming (Caldwell and Watson, 1952; Duka et al., 2000; Fedor-Freyberg, 1977; Phillips and Sherwin, 1992a; Sherwin, 1988; Sherwin and Gelfand, 1989; Sherwin and Phillips, 1990; Sherwin and Tulandi, 1996; Wolf et al., 1999). Not all randomized trial studies, however, report similar estrogen effects, even on identical measures (Caldwell and Watson, 1952; Ditkoff et al., 1991; Hackman and Galbraith, 1976; Phillips and Sherwin, 1992a; Polo-Kantola et al., 1998; Rauramo et al., 1975; Vanhulle and Demol, 1976).

Cross-sectional studies have failed to clarify the value of estrogen and progesterone in preserving cognitive function when administered to postmenopausal women. Although a number of reports documented better performance by estrogen users on measures such as paragraph recall, proper name recall, digit span, and visual memory and perception (Carlson and Sherwin, 1998; Jacobs et al., 1998; Kampen and Sherwin, 1994; Kimura, 1995; Resnick et al., 1997; Robinson et al., 1994; Steffens et al., 1999; Verghese et al., 2000), hormone replacement did not improve performance on a wide range of other cognitive tests. Several observational studies with small and large samples found no effects of hormone replacement on extensive batteries of cognitive tests, except for measures of verbal fluency and digit span (Barrett-Connor and Kritz-Silverstein, 1993; Carlson and Sherwin, 1998, 2000; Grodstein et al., 2000). In the longitudinal Rancho Bernardo study, men displayed declines in test performance with age that were similar or slightly poorer than women regardless of whether the women were using estrogen or not (Barrett-Connor and Kritz-Silverstein, 1999).

Imaging studies are adding another dimension to the study of steroids and human cognition. During storage of verbal information, estrogen (Premarin, 1.25 mg/day for 3 weeks) increased the activation in the inferior parietal lobule, although, during storage of nonverbal information, estrogen reduced activation in the same region, as determined by function magnetic resonance imaging (Shaywitz et al., 1999). Activation also was increased in the right superior frontal gyrus during retrieval of verbal or nonverbal memory. However, estrogen failed to improve performance on either task. The analysis of cerebral blood flow by positron emission tomography revealed different patterns of regional activation between estrogen users and nonusers while completing verbal and visual tasks (Resnick et al., 1998). Estrogen users demonstrated better performance on cognitive tasks and displayed different activation patterns over a 2-year period in hippocampal and cortical areas (Maki and Resnick, 2000).

Some investigators attribute the discrepant findings to methodological issues ranging from task dissimilarities to varied estrogen regimens to sample sizes (Kimura, 1996; Rice et al., 1997; Sherwin, 1994, 1996, 1997, 1998; Skoog and Gustafson, 1999), whereas others suggest that estrogen simply has little significance for human cognition (Barrett-Connor and Kritz-Silverstein, 1993; Grodstein et al., 2000; Haskell et al., 1997; Skoog and Gustafson, 1999). In some but not all studies (Collins and Landgren, 1995; Duff and Hampson, 2000; Palinkas and Barrett-Connor, 1992; Porter et al., 1996), hormone replacement elevates mood, reduces anxiety, and enhances the quality of life and sense of well-being (Ditkoff et al., 1991; Fedor-Freberg, 1977; Gerdes et al., 1982; Limouzin-Lamothe et al., 1994; Rauramo et al., 1975; Sherwin and Gelfand, 1989). However, the question remains whether these nonmnemonic factors account for, contribute to, or are unrelated to performance on learning and memory tasks. In one randomized trial study, the positive effects of hormone replacement on memory and sense of well-being in postmenopausal women depended on their knowledge of the experiment's purpose (Hogervorst et al., 1999).

Findings from studies of cyclic hormone variation or hormone replacement are remarkably similar across species. Specifically, rats and humans display selective responses to cyclic fluctuations and hormone treatments, with estrogen and progesterone enhancing performance on some tasks (working memory, verbal memory, and motor dexterity) and impairing performance on others (reference memory and spatial memory). However, as pointed out in a review of the literature using meta-analysis (Hogervorst et al., 2000), the reported effects often are small in magnitude and inconsistent across studies. The cognitive tasks vary in many procedural details, demand characteristics, and interpretation, making comparisons across studies problematic. In addition, hormone treatments vary considerably, characterized by different preparations, routes, doses, and durations that rarely exceed several months (Hogervorst et al., 2000).

In a report, women using estrogen or estrogen with progesterone as hormone replacement following menopause outperformed nonusers on a verbal working memory task and a spatial working memory task that required the active manipulation of information during testing. In contrast, all three groups performed equally when tested on working memory tasks that required only passive storage of information (Duff and Hampson, 2000). The authors propose that estrogen exerts an action on neurons of the prefrontal cortex that contain estrogen receptors involved in the active form of working memory assessed by these measures. The results also suggest that estrogen may have stronger effects on more demanding measures of working memory.

C. Protective Actions of Ovarian Hormones

The possibility that ovarian hormones can limit the occurrence, onset, or symptoms of human dementias, in particular Alzheimer's disease, has generated great excitement among scientists, clinicians, and the public. However, although many studies report favorable outcomes from the use of estrogen, the preventative and therapeutic benefits of hormone replacement therapy continue to be studied and debated intensely.

The first reports to indicate the potential therapeutic effects of estrogen featured only a few women with Alzheimer's symptomology who received oral preparations of micronized estradiol (2 mg/day) or Premarin (1.25 mg/day) for 6 weeks (Fillit et al., 1986; Honjo et al., 1989). In both reports, their performance improved on various scales of dementia and cognition, which may have been related to elevated affect. Subsequent attempts to replicate their initial findings met with both failure (Fillit, 1994) and success (Honjo et al., 1993). Similar improvements in cognition and dementia were confirmed in two later reports in which women with Alzheimer's disease were treated for 6 weeks to 45 months with Premarin (Ohkura et al., 1994, 1995). In addition, in a recent randomized trial study, women with Alzheimer's disease received transdermal estradiol patches and displayed improvements in attention and verbal memory compared to women with placebo patches (Asthana et al., 1999). Verbal memory performance correlated with plasma estradiol titers. Despite the promise of these positive findings, randomized trial studies failed to support previous results (Shaywitz and Shaywitz, 2000). In one report, women with Alzheimer's disease graded as mild to moderate performed equally to matched control women on cognitive and mood measures administered 4 and 16 weeks after beginning estrogen treatment (Henderson, 2000). A similar lack of improvement was found in the Alzheimer's Disease Cooperative Study for women with mild to moderate symptoms who were evaluated at 2, 6, 12, and 15 months after the initiation of estrogen treatment (Mulnard et al., 2000).

A number of cross-sectional studies lend support to a role for estrogen in the treatment of Alzheimer's disease. In this methodology, the incidence of Alzheimer's disease is compared between samples of estrogen users and nonusers matched on a range of socioeconomic, demographic, educational, and intellectual variables. In the first search for a possible relationship between Alzheimer's disease and hormone replacement therapy, positive correlations were found between estrogen use self-reported on a health survey and a diagnosis of the disease listed on death certificates (Paganini-Hill and Henderson, 1994). The risk of developing Alzheimer's disease dropped to an odds ratio of 0.69 in women who used estrogen, with the reduced risk associated with increased dose and duration of treatment. Subsequent cross-sectional studies confirmed a reduced risk and, in some reports, a delayed onset of Alzheimer's disease (Baldereschi et al., 1998; Henderson et al., 1994; Kawas et al., 1997; Mortel and Meyer, 1995; Slooter et al., 1999; Tang et al., 1996; Waring et al., 1999). Reductions in risk were related to the duration of hormone replacement therapy (Tang et al., 1996; Waring et al., 1999), although not in all studies (Kawas et al., 1997). Postmenopausal women with dementia responded more favorably to treatment with the acetylcholinesterase inhibitor tacrine if they were using estrogen as hormone replacement therapy (Schneider et al., 1996). Further, Honjo and colleagues (1989) found that plasma estrone levels were significantly lower in women with Alzheimer's disease compared to matched control females, a result later confirmed for both estrone and estradiol (Manly et al., 2000). Nevertheless, a relationship between estrogen use and a reduced risk of Alzheimer's disease was not supported by two other cross-sectional studies (Brenner et al., 1994; Graves et al., 1990).

The possibility that a common oral preparation currently available by prescription has therapeutic value in combating a pathology as devastating as Alzheimer's disease is indeed appealing. However, the benefits of hormone replacement therapy for cognitive function in aging women and men have not been proven. Although there is encouraging evidence from a number of randomized-trial and cross-sectional studies, sufficient contradictory data exist to question the value of replacement therapy to maintain and improve cognitive functions at risk from normal aging or neuropathologies. In an article published in the *American Psychological Association Monitor* (Carpenter, 2001), Barrett-Connor (1991) points out that the superior cognitive performance of women taking estrogen, sometimes in combination with other steroids, might be related to their higher educational attainment and overall health compared to nonusers. She also suggests that reports demonstrating a lack of cognitive effect by estrogen should not be dismissed. In the same article, Sherwin argues that the inconsistency in the human literature is less salient because some studies failed to use cognitive measures sufficiently sensitive to detect the existing differences. In light of the inability of contemporary science to confirm a direct effect of estrogen on mnemonic processes and a neuroprotective action on the brain, recommendations of estrogen use for aging individuals must be made on the bases of its beneficial effects on other processes such as bone growth, cardiovascular function, and psychological affect. Unfortunately, confirming the merit of estrogen use for these functions proved to be a long and arduous venture (Lerner, 1999).

Research that attempts to establish the value of hormone replacement therapy may lead to the development of agents that specifically promote human cognition or neuroprotection such as selective estrogen receptor modulators. A sampling of reviews of the neuroprotective potential of estrogen indicates that the biomedical community remains encouraged about the promise of hormone therapies for brain ailments and motivated to pursue the necessary research. Many point out the need for additional experimental and observational studies with large well-matched samples (Birge, 1996, 1997a,b,c; Farlow and Evans, 1998; Genazzani et al., 1999; Halbreich, 1997; Henderson, 1997a,b, 2000; Kuller, 1996; Lerner, 1999; McEwen et al., 1997; Monk and Brodaty, 2000; Sherwin, 1997; Simpkins et al., 1997; van Duijn, 1999). Long-term cross-sectional studies, such as the 15-year-long Women's Health Initiative Study (WHIMS), are underway (Shumaker et al., 1998).

VI. ANDROGENS AND COGNITION

A. Overview

Testosterone and dihydrotestosterone are synthesized and secreted primarily by the Leydig cells of the male testes, whereas androstenedione and dehydroepiandrosterone (DHEA) are formed by Leydig cells as well as the neurosecretory cells in the zona reticularis of the adrenal cortex of both sexes (Nelson, 2000). Many other tissues and organs express low concentrations of the enzymes involved in *de novo* androgen synthesis and metabolism including neurons and glial cells of the brain (Robel et al., 1995). There are many pathways for androgen metabolism, as well as hundreds of different forms of androgen made by the body. In a principal metabolic route, progesterone derived from pregnenolone is the precursor of the 21-carbon androgen 17α-hydroxyprogesterone that gives rise to the interconvertible androgens, testosterone and androstenedione (Feder, 1981a; Hendricks and Mayer, 1977; Martin, 1976; Nelson, 2000). Testosterone can be reduced at the C-5 position to form the potent peripheral androgen dihydrotestosterone or aromatized to estradiol. Androstenedione also can be aromatized to the weaker estrogen estrone. In an alternative pathway, pregnenolone not converted to progesterone is metabolized to DHEA and its sulfate (DHEAS), which can be aromatized to estriol.

As do other steroids, androgens can exert their actions through intracellular receptors. Androgen receptor mRNA and protein have been identified in the hippocampal and cortical neurons of rodents and primates, as well as in areas involved in reproduction (Abdelgadir et al., 1999; Clancy et al., 1992, 1994; Choate et al., 1998; Doherty and Sheridan, 1981; Handa et al., 1986; Kerr et al., 1995; McGinnis and Katz, 1996; Pomerantz and Sholl, 1987; Puy et al., 1995; Sarrieau et al., 1990; Tohgi et al., 1995; Young and Chang, 1998). Although the regional distributions of androgen receptors and their mRNA vary somewhat among species and experiments, studies report high concentrations of receptor and mRNA in pyramidal cells of rats (Kerr et al., 1995), humans (Tohgi et al., 1995), and fetal monkeys (Pomerantz and Sholl, 1987). The density of neurons with androgen receptor mRNA in the hippocampus and cortex is much higher than the density of neurons with estrogen receptor mRNA (Simerly et al., 1990). However, the receptor subtypes and novel mechanisms identified for estrogen action have not been documented for androgens.

B. Androgen and Nonhuman Cognition

Compared to estrogen, there is a more limited scientific literature on the role of androgen in learning and memory. Many of the existing reports focus on gender differences in performance on a variety of land and water mazes (Section IIC1a). Males were reported to outperform females on a number of spatial and nonspatial tasks (Barrett and Ray, 1970; Beatty, 1979; Berger-Sweeney et al., 1995; Davenport et al., 1970; Dawson, 1972; Dawson et al., 1975; Einon, 1980; Joseph et al., 1978; Roof, 1993; Roof and Havens, 1992; Steenbergen et al., 1990; Williams et al., 1990), although not in all cases (Bucci et al., 1995; Juraska et al., 1984; van Haaren et al., 1987). Various nonmnemonic factors, such as activity, anxiety, and pain sensitivity, have been proposed to account for reported differences by some investigators (Beatty, 1979; Steenbergen et al., 1990; van Haaren et al., 1987; van Hest et al., 1987). Gender differences in water maze performance were found to be preventable if adequate pretraining preceded testing (Bucci et al., 1995).

Motivated by reports of gender differences in performance on various cognitive tasks, investigators manipulated the early hormone environment to determine the consequences of perinatal androgen exposure for learning and memory performance in adulthood (Williams and Meck, 1991; van Haaren et al., 1990). In one of the earliest studies of sexual differentiation of cognitive ability, female rats injected with testosterone on 4 of the first 10 days of life exhibited spatial learning and memory performance similar to that of normal males on the symmetrical maze, whereas the spatial performance of males castrated at birth was similar to that of normal females (Joseph et al., 1978). In a later study, male rats castrated on the first day of life again performed like normal females when tested on a 12-arm radial maze, but performed worse than normal males or females treated with estradiol on the first 9 days of life (Williams et al., 1990). The results suggested that masculinization of spatial learning and memory depends on the conversion of testosterone to estradiol. In addition, it was proposed that early exposure to androgen or estrogen shifted a female's learning strategy from dependence on both landmark and geometry cues to a more efficient but less flexible dependence on only geometry (Williams et al., 1990). Alternatively, in humans, women typically used landmarks to learn to navigate a virtual water maze, whereas men used both landmarks and geometry (Sandstrom et al., 1998). Administration of testosterone during the first week of life improved the performance of female rats but impaired the performance of males in a radial maze and a water maze (Roof, 1993), possibly due to its organizational effects on the development of the dentate gyrus (Roof and Havens, 1992). Similar organizational effects were described earlier in rhesus monkeys when females treated with testosterone during development showed object discrimination equivalent to that of untreated males (Section IID; Clark and Goldman-Rakic, 1989). These studies indicate a relationship between early androgen exposure and later spatial ability.

The ability of androgen, possibly following conversion to estrogen, to affect the development of cognitive abilities wanes after the first 10 days of life. In early experiments, the castration of male rats at different ages prior to puberty and into adulthood, but after the critical postnatal period, did not affect cognitive performance (Commins, 1932; Stone and Commins, 1936). Furthermore, in gonadally intact adult male rodents, exposure to testosterone or other anabolic steroids for 1–3 months did not affect acquisition or retention in the standard reference memory version of the water maze in male rats or voles (Clark et al., 1995; Galea et al., 1995), failed to counteract age-related cognitive deficits in 20-month-old and 31-month-old male rats, and impaired retention in 4.5-month-old and 20-month-old males (Goudsmit et al., 1990). Testosterone and anabolic androgens also failed to affect performance in a working memory version of the radial arm maze task in gonadally intact male rats (Knoth et al., 1993; Smith et al., 1996). On another appetitive spatial task, the gonadectomy of male and female rats in adulthood did not affect performance in a food-rewarded symmetrical maze (Joseph et al., 1978).

For tasks motivated by shock, testosterone was reported to impair the acquisition and retention of active avoidance behavior (Fedotova, 1999; Mora et al., 1983), whereas testosterone and norandrostenolone improved the retention of passive avoidance responses over short-term and long-term intervals (Flood et al., 1995; Vasquez-Pereyra et al., 1995). In a very different test of learning and retention, the castration of male rats impaired their social memory of a familiar conspecific (Sawyer et al., 1984). In avians, testosterone treatments were reported to affect certain components of passive avoidance behavior in chicks (Andrew et al., 1981; Clifton et al., 1982, 1986; M. E. Gibbs et al., 1986) and interfere with vocal learning in song birds (Whaling et al., 1995) whose neurons can metabolize androgen to other active products (Saldana et al., 1999). In general, the administration of androgens to adult rodents and birds well after critical periods of development had no effect or impaired performance on most learning and memory tasks, with better performance only found for social memory and passive avoidance.

In vitro and in vivo studies using rats have not determined the value of testosterone in neuroprotection (Section IVF). Testosterone increased the secretion of the neuroprotective sβAPP and decreased secretion of the neurotoxic βamyloid in cultures of cell lines and cortical neurons (Gouras et al., 2000), an effect that may be related to androgen-induced increases in nerve growth factor and its receptor (Tirassa et al., 1997). In contrast, male rats treated with Silastic pellets of testosterone 1 week before middle cerebral artery occlusion had larger ischemic lesions than control males or males treated with estradiol, suggesting a harmful effect of the androgen when combined with lesions (Hawk et al., 1998).

C. Androgen and Human Cognition

Gender differences in human cognition have intrigued investigators for many years, driven by both scientific and social factors. Typically, studies have identified weak but significant differences between the overlapping distributions of male and female abilities, with women reported to perform better as a group than men on verbal, perceptual, and fine motor tasks, but poorer than men on spatial and quantitative measures (Sherwin, 1994). As suggested by studies in other species, differences in brain structure established during development by the presence or absence of androgen probably account for performance differences between the sexes (Nass and Baker, 1991; Resnick et al., 1986). Cognitive abilities may be more dependent on the prenatal hormone environment than on circulating levels of hormones in adults. Based on evidence from studies of adults, it has been suggested that androgen levels correlate negatively with performance on verbal tasks, but positively with performance on spatial tasks. It also has been proposed that androgen facilitates performance on measures that show a male bias, whereas estrogen facilitates performance on tasks with a female bias. Finally, abnormally high androgen levels in men are hypothesized to impair cognitive performance, whereas low androgen levels in women impair performance. There is some support for each of these proposals.

Hypogonadal men with low levels of circulating testosterone from birth were found to exhibit poorer performance on spatial, but not verbal, measures when compared to eugonadal men, deficits that were not reversed by testosterone supplementation in adulthood (Hier and Crowley, 1982). Hypogonadal men also had general impairments of short-term memory for both spatial and verbal information (Cappa et al., 1988). A report using a sample comprising primarily men with acquired forms of hypogonadism detected a deficit only in verbal fluency that was reversed by testosterone treatment (Alexander et al., 1997). Some spatial and verbal deficits may be specific to idiopathic forms of hypogonadism and result from androgen deprivation from birth (Hier and Crowley, 1982).

Endogenous testosterone levels determined from plasma or saliva samples have been positively correlated with the performance of men on spatial measures (Christiansen and Knussmann, 1987; Christiansen, 1993; Errico et al., 1992) and testosterone supplementation selectively improved spatial performance in elderly men and female-to-male transexuals (Janowsky et al., 1994; van Goozen et al., 1994, 1995). There also is evidence that endogenous and supplemental testosterone impaired performance on some verbal measures (Christiansen and Knussmann, 1987; Christiansen, 1993; Phillips and Sherwin, 1992a; van Goozen et al., 1994, 1995; Wolf et al., 2000), but improved scores on components of the Mini-Mental State Examination (Barrett-Connor and Goodman-Gruen, 1999) and object location (Postma et al., 2000). The relationship between testosterone and spatial ability has been described as curvilinear or U-shaped, with low and high levels of androgen associated with poorer performance on spatial measures than intermediate levels (Barrett-Connor et al., 1999; Moffat and Hampson, 1996). However, several studies report no, or even negative, correlations between testosterone and cognitive abilities (Gouchie and Kimura, 1991; Kampen and Sherwin, 1996; Postma et al., 1999).

The role of testosterone in human cognitive performance remains ill defined (Almeida, 1999). Studies of neural and behavioral differentiation generally agree that perinatal exposure to testosterone improves performance on spatial tasks but impairs performance on verbal measures in adulthood, although these gender differences are small in magnitude and reflect statistical comparisons of overlapping performance distributions. Whether androgens maintain or restore cognitive function or protect the brain from diseases such as Alzheimer's disease in aging men or women is still unproven, but a case for testosterone supplementation for the elderly can be made based on its beneficial effects on other physiological and psychological processes (Almeida, 1999; Kim, 1999; Plouffe and Simon, 1998). For example, testosterone supplementation often elevates mood and libido (Alexander et al., 1997; Wang et al., 1996), possibly by regulating the serotonergic system, which may have important consequences for cognitive performance (Fink et al., 1998, 1999). However, the value of testosterone therapy must be weighed carefully in view of its contraindications and potentially deleterious physiological and psychological effects in both men (Basaria and Dobs, 1999; Conway *et al.*, 2000; Gambineri and Pasquali, 2000; Wang and Swerdloff, 1997) and women (Davis, 1999; Hoeger and Guzick, 1999; Kaunitz, 1997).

VII. CONCLUSION

This chapter has reviewed the primary gonadal steroids that influence cognitive performance. These actions have two consequences, the modulation of learning and memory performance and the promotion of neuronal survival. Both benefits offer promise in our attempts to improve and protect human memory. As we have seen, the effects of steroids on learning and memory performance are not simply a matter of improving our ability to acquire and remember information. The relationships between brain biology and cognitive performance are complex. No one has developed a cohesive model of the interactions between multiple steroid mechanisms, complex neural connectivity, brain biochemistry, and cognitive function.

A. Adaptive Value

At the beginning of the chapter, several questions were posed regarding the importance of steroid modulation of learning and memory performance. The first of these questions concerns the adaptive value of the nonreproductive effects of steroids. The significance of ovarian steroids in learning and memory remains a mystery. In their fertility and parental hypothesis, Sherry and Hampson (1977) suggested that elevated levels of estrogen and possibly progesterone might curtail a female's activities in unfamiliar territory simply by limiting her movement and spatial abilities. Consequently, a female would fare better in the security of her home environment during periods of mating or pregnancy, when gonadal steroid levels are high. However, limitations on movement during periods of high estrogen are counter to the increases in general activity and decreases in anxiety usually associated with elevated estrogen levels. Desmond and Levy (1997) proposed that although spatial ability may be diminished when estrogen is elevated, communication skills are sharpened in both human and nonhuman females, possibly at the expense of spatial processing by the hippocampus and other brain regions. Heightened communication and verbal ability may have more adaptive value than spatial ability near the time of ovulation, when conception is most likely. For example, female rats appear to be more sensitive to ultrasonic communications when sexually receptive (Matochik *et al.*, 1992), whereas female humans may have keener verbal ability and fluency when estrogen levels are elevated. The adaptive significance of a steroid such as testosterone seems less puzzling. Elevations in testosterone typical of mating promote not only diverse reproductive functions, but processes that facilitate dispersal, territoriality, and foraging as components of successful breeding. However, the effects of androgen on spatial abilities in adult organisms are questionable; therefore, the value of these ecological and evolutionary hypotheses can only be determined by sound empirical experiments. Viewed from another perspective, the modulation of learning and memory by gonadal steroids could be related to their regulation of reproductive processes rather than the direct modulation of learning and memory systems. The relationship between cognitive abilities and reproductive behavior may prove to be an interesting avenue of study in the future.

B. Strength of Effect

Weak and inconsistent effects continue to characterize the study of steroid effects on the cognitive performance of both humans and nonhumans, raising concerns about the importance of these nonreproductive actions. Even if reported effects prove to be valid, their significance to everyday cognitive performance may be of little consequence (Sherwin, 1994). On one hand, the diversity of methodologies may contribute to unreliability; on the other hand, effects that can be demonstrated only under highly controlled and highly specific laboratory conditions may have limited importance. Only stronger hypotheses and improved methodologies can resolve these matters definitively. Alternatively, gonadal steroids primarily are hormones of reproduction not cognition, particularly in nonhuman mammals. As such, it may not be surprising that their effects on cognitive function are weak.

C. Neural Substrate

A compelling argument has been made that the neural systems necessary to mediate the effects of gonadal steroids exist in the mammalian brain. A variety of interconnected brain regions and interacting neurotransmitter systems provide the substrate. Much of our discussion has focused on the hippocampus and, in particular, the afferents that provide sensory input and modulate its activity. Although it is clear that the hippocampus plays a significant role in several types of memory processing, the details of its mechanisms continue to be investigated. Models of hippocampal function abound. As a target for steroid regulation, the pyramidal cells, granule cells, and interneurons neurons of the hippocampus either contain estrogen receptors or receive input directly or indirectly from estrogen-concentrating cells in the basal forebrain, entorhinal cortex, amydala, supramammillary nucleus, and midbrain and hindbrain monoaminergic nuclei. A number of neurotransmitter systems contribute to the extrinsic and intrinsic circuitry of the hippocampus and most are affected by the presence of gonadal steroids. The hippocampus is able to alter its structural and electrical properties in response to hormone exposure, although the relevance of these dynamic changes to cognition has not been determined.

D. Nonmnemonic Factors

One of the most important issues in the study of gonadal steroids, learning, and memory performance is the role of processes not directly involved in cognitive processing. We have seen that estrogen can affect diverse biological and psychological functions, any of which or combinations of which can have major consequences for learning and memory performance. The roles of nonmnemonic factors continue to have serious implications for our knowledge of steroid actions in both humans and nonhumans, despite the use of ingenious methods to account for these potential confounds. Although nonmnemonic variables may contaminate the results of an experiment, the identification of the effects of steroids on such processes becomes both necessary and valuable to our understanding.

E. Final Thought

In the first section of this chapter, it was suggested that understanding the nature of gonadal steroid modulation of nonreproductive functions would not be a trivial matter. It may be human nature to expect simple answers to complex questions. However, as in most areas of empirical investigation, there are more questions than answers at the moment. As we find our way through the conundrum of steroids, neurons, and memories, we still must face the practical issues. Are gonadal steroids good for your memory? Sometimes, maybe.

References

Abdelgadir, S. E., Roselli, C. E., Choate, J. V., and Resko, J. A. (1999). Androgen receptor messenger ribonucleic acid in brains and pituitaries of male rhesus monkeys: Studies on distribution, hormonal control, and relationship to luteinizing hormone secretion. *Biol. Reprod.* **60**, 1251–1256.

Akhondzadeh, S. (1999). Hippocampal synaptic plasticity and cognition. *J. Clin. Pharmacol. Ther.* **24**, 241–248.

Alexander, G. M., Swerdloff, R. S., Wang, C., Davidson, T., McDonald, V., Steiner, B., and Hines, M. (1997). Androgen-behavior correlations in hypogonadal men and eugonadal men. *Horm. Behav.* **33**, 85–94.

Almeida, O. P. (1999). Sex playing with the mind. Effects of oestrogen and testosterone on mood and cognition. *Arq. Neuropsiquiatr.* **57**, 701–706.

Alves, S. E., McEwen, B. S., Hayashi, S., Korach, K. S., Pfaff, D. W., and Ogawa, S. (2000). Estrogen-regulated progestin receptors are found in the midbrain raphe but not hippocampus of estrogen receptor alpha (ERalpha) gene-disrupted mice. *J. Comp. Neurol.* **427**, 185–195.

Amaral, D. G. (1987). Memory: Anatomical organization of candidate brain regions. In "Handbook of Physiology" (F. Plum, ed.), Sect. 1, Vol. 5, Part 1, pp. 211–294. American Physiological Society, Bethesda, MD.

Amaral, D. G., and Kurz, J. (1985). An analysis of the origins of the cholinergic and noncholinergic septal projections to the hippocampal formation of the rat. *J. Comp. Neurol.* **240**, 37–59.

Amaral, D. G., and Witter, M. P. (1995). Hippocampal formation. In "The Rat Nervous System" (G. Paxinos, ed.), pp. 443–493. Academic Press, San Diego, CA.

Andrew, R. J., Clifton, P. G., and Gibbs, M. E. (1981). Enhancement of effectiveness of learning by testosterone in domestic chicks. *J. Comp. Physiol. Psychol.* **95**, 406–417.

Apartis, E., Poindessous-Jazat, F. R., Lamour, Y. A., and Bassant, M. H. (1998). Loss of rhythmically bursting neurons in rat medial septum following selective lesion of septohippocampal cholinergic system. *J. Neurophysiol.* **79**, 1633–1642.

Aronica, S. M., Kraus, W. L., and Katzenellenbogen, B. S. (1994). Estrogen action via the cAMP signaling pathway: Stimulation of adenylate cyclase and cAMP-regulated gene transcription. *Proc. Natl. Acad. Sci. U.S.A.* **91**, 8517–8521.

Asthana, S., Raffaele, K. C., Greig, N. H., Schapiro, M. B., Blackman, M. R., and Soncrant, T. T. (1999). Neuroendocrine responses to intravenous infusion of physostigmine in patients with Alzheimer disease. *Alzheimer Dis. Assoc. Disord.* **13**, 102–108.

Axelson, J. F., Zoller, L. C., Tomassone, J. E., and Collins, D. C. (1986). Effects of silastic progesterone implants on activity cycles and steroid levels in ovariectomized and intact female rats. *Physiol. Behav.* **38**, 879–885.

Azcoitia, I., Sierra, A., and Garcia-Segura, L. M. (1998). Estradiol prevents kainic acid-induced neuronal loss in the rat dentate gyrus. *NeuroReport* **9**, 3075–3079.

Azcoitia, I., Sierra, A., and Garcia-Segura, L. M. (1999a). Localization of estrogen receptor beta-immunoreactivity in astrocytes of the adult rat brain. *Glia* **26**, 260–267.

Azcoitia, I., Fernandez-Galaz, C., Sierra, A., and Garcia-Segura, L. M. (1999b). Gonadal hormones affect neuronal vulnerability to exocitoxin-induced degeneration. *J. Neurocytol.* **28**(9), 699–710.

Azcoitia, I., Sierra, A., and Garcia-Segura, L. M. (1999c). Neuroprotective effects of estradiol in the adult rat hippocampus: Interaction with insulin-like growth factor-I signaling. *J. Neurosci. Res.* **58**, 815–822.

Baddeley, A. (1986). Dementia and working memory. *Q. J. Exp. Psychol. A* **38**, 603–618.

Baddeley, A. D., and Hitch, G. J. (1974). Working memory. *In* "The psychology of Learning and Motivation: Advances in Research and Theory" (G. A. Bower, ed.), Vol. 8, pp. 47–90. Academic Press, New York.

Baldereschi, M., Di Carlo, A., and Lepore, V. (1998). Estrogen-replacement therapy and Alzheimer's disease in the Italian Longitudinal Study on Aging. *Neurology* **50**, 996–1002.

Bannerman, D. M., Good, M. A., Butcher, S. P., Ramsay, M., and Morris, R. G. (1995). Distinct components of spatial learning revealed by prior training and NMDA receptor blockade. *Nature (London)* **378**, 182–186.

Barnes, C. A. (1979). Memory deficits associated with senescence: A neurophysiological and behavioral study in the rat. *J. Comp. Physiol. Psychol.* **93**, 74–104.

Barraclough, D. J., Ingram, C. D., and Brown, M. W. (1999). Chronic treatment with oestradiol does not alter in vitro LTP in subfield CA1 of the female rat hippocampus. *Neuropharmacology* **38**, 65–71.

Barrett, R. J., and Ray, O. S. (1970). Behavior in the open field, Lashley III maze, shuttle box, and Sidman avoidance as a function of strain, sex, and age. *Dev. Psychol.* **3**, 73–77.

Barrett-Connor, E. (1991). Postmenopausal estrogen and prevention bias. *Ann. Intern. Med.* **115**, 455–456.

Barrett-Connor, E., and Goodman-Gruen, D. (1999). Cognitive function and endogenous sex hormones in older women. *J. Am. Geriatr. Soc.* **47**, 1289–1293.

Barrett-Connor, E., and Kritz-Silverstein, D. (1993). Estrogen replacement therapy and cognitive function in older women. *JAMA, J. Ann. Med. Assoc.* **269**, 2637–2641.

Barrett-Connor, E., and Kritz-Silverstein, D. (1999). Gender differences in cognitive function with age: The Rancho Bernardo study. *J. Am. Geriatr. Soc.* **47**, 159–164.

Barrett-Connor, E., Goodman-Gruen, D., and Patay, B. (1999). Endogenous sex hormones and cognitive function in older men. *J. Clin. Endocrinol. Metab.* **84**, 3681–3685.

Bartus, R. T. (2000). On neurodegenerative diseases, models, and treatment strategies: Lessons learned and lessons forgotten a generation following the cholinergic hypothesis. *Exp. Neurol.* **163**, 495–529.

Bartus, R. T., and Johnson, H. R. (1976). Short-term memory in the rhesus monkey: Disruption from the anti-cholinergic scopolamine. *Pharmacol. Biochem. Behav.* **5**, 39–46.

Basaria, S., and Dobbs, A. S. (1999). Risks versus benefits of testosterone therapy in elderly men. *Drugs Aging* **15**, 131–142.

Baulieu, E. E. (1998). Neurosteroids: A novel function of the brain. *Psychoneuroendocrinology* **23**, 963–987.

Baxter, M. G., and Gallagher, M. (1996). Intact spatial learning in both young and aged rats following selective removal of hippocampal cholinergic input. *Behav. Neurosci.* **110**, 460–467.

Baxter, M. G., Bucci, D. J., Gorman, L. K., Wiley, R. G., and Gallagher, M. (1995). Selective immunotoxic lesions of basal forebrain cholinergic cells: Effects on learning and memory in rats. *Behav. Neurosci.* **109**, 714–722.

Beatty, W. W. (1973). Effects of gonadectomy on sex differences in DRL behavior. *Physiol. Behav.* **10**, 177–178.

Beatty, W. W. (1979). Gonadal hormones and sex differences in nonreproductive behaviors in rodents: Organizational and activational influences. *Horm. Behav.* **12**, 112–163.

Bechara, A., Damasio, H., Tranel, D., and Anderson, S. W. (1998). Dissociation of working memory form decision making within the human prefrontal cortex. *J. Neurosci.* **18**, 428–437.

Beck, S. G., Clarke, W. P., and Goldfarb, J. (1989). Chronic estrogen effects on 5-hydroxytryptamine-mediated responses in hippocampal pyramidal cells of female rats. *Neurosci. Lett.* **106**, 181–187.

Behl, C., Widmann, M., Trapp, T., and Holsbier, F. (1995). 17-beta estradiol protects neurons from oxidative stress-induced cell death in vitro. *Biochem. Biophys. Res. Commun.* **2165**, 473–482.

Behl, C., Skutella, T., Lezoualc'h, F., Post, A., Widmann, M., Newton, C. J., and Holsboer, F. (1997). Neuroprotection against oxidative stress by setrogens: Structure-activity relationship. *Mol. Pharmacol.* **51**, 535–41.

Beiko, J., Candusso, L., and Cain, D. P. (1997). The effects of nonspatial water maze pretraining in rats subjected to serotonin depletion and muscarinic receptor antagonism: A detailed behavioural assessment of spatial performances. *Behav. Brain Res.* **88**, 201–211.

Berger, T. W., Berry, S. D., and Thompson, R. F. (1986). Role of the hippocampus in classical conditioning of aversive and appetitive behaviors. *In* "The Hippocampus" (R. L. Isaacson and K. H. Pribram, eds.). pp. 203–239. Plenum Press, New York.

Berger-Sweeney, J., Heckers, S., Mesulam, M. M., Wiley, R. G., Lappi, D. A., and Sharma, M. (1994). Differential effects on spatial navigation of immunotoxin-induced cholinergic lesions of the medial septal area and nucleus basalis magnocellularis. *J. Neurosci.* **14**, 4507–4519.

Berger-Sweeney, J., Arnold, A., Gadeau, D., and Mills, J. (1995). Sex differences in learning and memory in mice: Effects of sequence of testing and cholinergic blockade. *Behav. Neurosci.* **109**, 859–873.

Berry, B., McMahan, R., and Gallagher, M. (1997). Spatial learning and memory at defined points of the estrous cycle: Effects on performance of a hippocampal-dependent task. *Behav. Neurosci.* **111**, 267–274.

Bethea, C. L., Pecins-Thompson, M., Schutzer, W. E., Gundlah, C., and Lu, Z. N. (1998). Ovarian steroids and serotonin neural function. *Mol. Neurobiol.* **18**, 87–123.

Bettini, E., Pollio, G., Santagati, S., and Maggi, A. (1992). Estrogen receptor in rat brain: Presence in the hippocampal formation. *Neuroendocrinology* **56**, 502–508.

Bi, R., Broutman, G., Foy, M. R., Thompson, R. F., and Baudry, M. (2000). The tyrosine kinase and mitogen-activated protein kinase pathways mediate multiple effects of estrogen in hippocampus. *Proc. Natl. Acad. Sci. U.S.A.* **97**, 3602–3607.

Bimonte, H. A., and Denenberg, V. H. (1999). Estradiol facilitates performance as working memory load increases. *Psychoneuroendocrinology* **24**, 161–173.

Birge, S. J. (1996). Is there a role for estrogen replacement therapy in the prevention and treatment of dementia? *J. Am. Geriatr. Soc.* **44**, 865–870.

Birge, S. J. (1997a). The role of ovarian hormones in cognition and dementia. *Neurology* **48**(Suppl. 7), S1.

Birge, S. J. (1997b). The role of estrogen in the treatment of Alzheimer's disease. *Neurology* **48**(Suppl. 7), S36–S41.

Birge, S. J. (1997c). Introduction. The role of estrogen in the treatment and prevention of dementia. *Am. J. Med.* **103**(Suppl. 1), 1S–2S.

Birge, S. J., and Mortel, K. F. (1997). Estrogen and the treatment of Alzheimer's disease. The role of estrogen in the treatment and prevention of dementia. *Am. J. Med.* **103**(Suppl. 6), 36S–45S.

Bishop, J., and Simpkins, J. W. (1995). Estradiol enhances brain glucose uptake in ovariectomized rats. *Brain Res. Bull.* **36**, 315–320.

Bitar, M. S., Ota, M., Linnoila, M., and Shapiro, B. H. (1991). Modification of gonadectomy-induced increases in brain monoamine metabolism by steriod hormones in male and female rats. *Psychoneuroendocrinology* **16**, 547–557.

Bitran, D., Hilvers, R. J., and Kellogg, C. K. (1991). Ovarian endocrine status modulates the anxiolytic potency of diazepam and the efficacy of gamma-aminobutyric acid-benzodiazepine receptor-mediated chloride ion transport. *Behav. Neurosci.* **105**, 157–161.

Bitran, M., Hilvers, R. J., and Kellogg, C. K. (1991). Anxiolytic effects of 3 alpha-hydroxy-5 alpha[beta]-pregnan-20-one: Endogenous metabolites of progesterone that are active at the GABAA receptor. *Brain Res.* **203**, 267–274.

Bliss, T. V., and Lomo, T. (1973). Long-lasting potentiation of synaptic transmission in the dentate area of the unanaesthetized rabbit following stimulation of the preforant path. *J. Physiol. (London)* **232**, 357–374.

Bliss, T. V., and Collingridge, G. L. (1993). A synaptic model of memory: Long-term potentiation in the hippocampus. *Nature (London)* **361**, 31–39.

Blurton-Jones, M. M., Roberts, J. A., and Tuszynski, M. H. (1999). Estrogen receptor immunoreactivity in the adult primate brain: Neuronal distribution and association with p75, trkA, and choline acetyltransferase. *J. Comp. Neurol.* **405**, 529–542.

Bonnefont, A. B., Munoz, F. J., and Inestrosa, N. C. (1998). Estrogen protects neuronal cells from the cytotoxicity induced by acetylcholinesterase-amyloid complexes. *FEBS Lett.* **441**(2), 220–224.

Brenner, D. E., Kukull, W. A., Stergachis, A., van Belle, G., Bowen, J. D., McCormick, W. C., Teri, L., and Larson, E. B. (1994). Postmenopausal estrogen replacment therapy and the risk of Alzheimer's disease: A population-based case-control study. *Am. J. Epidemiol.* **140**, 262–267.

Broverman, D. M., Vogel, W., Klaiber, E. L., Majcher, D., Shea, D., and Paul, V. (1981). Changes in cognitive task performance across the menstrual cycle. *J. Comp. Physiol. Psychol.* **95**, 646–654.

Bucci, D. J., Chiba, A. A., and Gallagher, M. (1995). Spatial learning in male and female Long-Evans rats. *Behav. Neurosci.* **109**, 180–183.

Burke, A. W., and Broadhurst, P. L. (1966). Behavioral correlates of the oestrous cycle in the rat. *Nature (London)* **209**, 223–224.

Cain, D. P. (1997). Prior non-spatial pretraining eliminates sensorimotor disturbances and impairments in water maze learning caused by diazepam. *Psychopharmacology (Berlin)* **130**, 313–319.

Cain, D. P. (1998). Testing the NMDA, long-term potentiation, and cholinergic hypotheses of spatial learning. *Neurosci. Behav. Rev.* **22**, 181–193.

Cain, D. P., Saucier, D., Hall, J., Hargreaves, E. L., and Boon, E. F. (1996). Detailed behavioral analysis of water maze acquisition under APV or CNQX: Contribution of sensorimotor disturbances to drug-induced acquisition deficits. *Behav. Neurosci.* **110**, 86–102.

Caldwell, B. M., and Watson, R. I. (1952). An evaluation of psychologic effects of sex hormone administration in aged women: I. Results of therapy after six months. *J. Gerontol.* **7**, 228–244.

Cannizzaro, G., Provenzano, P. M., and Nigito, S. (1970). The effects of castration and of progestin-oestrogen combinations upon avoidance conditioning in female rats. *Pharmacol. Res. Commun.* **2**, 267–276.

Cappa, S. F., Guariglia, C., Papagno, C., Pizzamiglio, L., Vallar, G., Zoccolotti, P., Ambrosi, B., and Santiemma, V. (1988). Patterns of lateralization and performance levels for verbal and spatial taks in congenital androgen deficiency. *Behav. Brain Res.* **31**, 177–183.

Cardona-Gomez, G. P., Trejo, J. L., Fernandez, A. M., and Garcia-Segura, L. M. (2000). Estrogen receptors and insulin-like growth factor-I receptors mediate estrogen-dependent synaptic plasticity. *NeuroReport* **11**, 1735–1738.

Carew, T. J., and Sahley, C. L. (1986). Invertebrate learning and memory: From behavior to molecules. *Annu. Rev. Neurosci.* **9**, 435–487.

Carlson, L. E., and Sherwin, B. B. (1998). Steroid hormones, memory and mood in a healthy elderly population. *Psychoneuroendocrinology* **23**, 583–603.

Carlson, L. E., and Sherwin, B. B. (2000). Higher levels of plasma estradiol and testosterone in healthy elderly men compared with age-matched women may protect aspects of explicit memory. *Menopause* **7**, 168–177.

Carpenter, S. (2001). Does estrogen protect memory? *Monit. Psychol.* **32**, 52–53.

Ceccatelli, S., Grandison, L., Scott, R. E., Pfaff, D. W., and Kow, L. M. (1996). Estradiol regulation of nitric oxide synthase mRNAs in rat hypothalamus. *Neuroendocrinology* **64**, 357–363.

Chao, H. M., Spencer, R. L., Frankfurt, M., and McEwen, B. S. (1994). The effects of aging and hormonal manipulation on amyloid precursor protein APP695 mRNA expression in rat hippocampus. *J. Neuroendocrinol.* **6**, 517–521.

Chappell, J., McMahan, R., Chiba, A., and Gallagher, M. (1998). A re-examination of the role of basal forebrain cholinergic neurons in spatial working memory. *Neuropharmacology* **37**, 481–487.

Chen, J., Adachi, N., Lui, K., and Arai, T. (1998). The effects of 17beta-estradiol on ischemia-inducded neuronal damage in the gerbil hippocampus. *Neuroscience* **87**, 817–822.

Chesler, E. J., and Juraska, J. M. (2000). Acute administration of estrogen and progesterone impairs the acquisition of the spatial Morris water maze in ovariectomized rats. *Horm. Behav.* **38**, 234–242.

Choate, J. V., Slayden, O. D., and Resko, J. A. (1998). Immunocytochemical localization of androgen receptors in brains of developing and adult male rhesus monkeys. *Endocrine* **8**, 51–60.

Chowen, J. A., Torres-Aleman, I., and Garcia-Segura, L. M. (1992). Trophic effects of estradiol on fetal rat hypothalamic neurons. *Neuroendocrinology* **56**, 895–901.

Christiansen, K. (1993). Sex hormone-related variations of cognitive performance in Kung San hunter-gatherers of Namibia. *Neuropsychobiology* **27**, 97–107.

Christiansen, K., and Knussmann, R. (1987). Sex hormones and cognitive functioning in men. *Neuropsychobiology* **18**, 27–36.

Claiborne, B. J., Amaral, D. G., and Cowan, W. M. (1986). A light and electron microscope analysis of the mossy fibers of the rat dentate gyrus. *J. Comp. Neurol.* **246**, 435–458.

Clancy, A. N., Bonsall, R. W., and Micheal, R. P. (1992). Immunohistochemical labeling of androgen receptors in the brain of rat and monkey. *Life Sci.* **50**, 409–417.

Clancy, A. N., Whitman, C., Michael, R. P., and Albers, H. E. (1994). Distribution of androgen receptor-like immunoreactivity in the brains of intact and castrated male hamsters. *Brain Res. Bull.* **33**, 325–332.

Clark, A. S., and Goldman-Rakic, P. S. (1989). Gonadal hormones influence the emergence of cortical function in nonhuman primates. *Behav. Neurosci.* **103**, 1287–1295.

Clark, A. S., Mitre, M. C., and Brinck-Johnsen, T. (1995). Anabolic-androgenic steroid and adrenal steroid effects on hippocampal plasticity. *Brain Res.* **679**, 64–71.

Clarke, W. P., and Maayani, S. (1990). Estrogen effects on 5-HT1A receptors in hippocampal membranes from ovariectomized rats: Functional and binding studies. *Brain Res.* **518**, 287–291.

Cleary, J., Hittner, J. M., Semotuk, M., Mantyh, P., and O'Hare, E. (1995). Beta-amyloid (1–40) effects on behavior and memory. *Brain Res.* **682**, 69–74.

Clifton, P. G., Andrew, R. J., and Gibbs, M. E. (1982). Limited period of actin of testosterone on memory formation in the chick. *J. Comp. Physiol. Psychol.* **96**, 212–222.

Clifton, P. G., Andrew, R. J., and Rainey, C. R. (1986). Effects of gonadal steroids on attack and on memory processing in the domestic chick. *Physiol. Behav.* **37**, 701–707.

Cohen, N. J., Ryan, J., Hunt, C., Romine, L., Wszalek, T., and Nash, C. (1999). Hippocampal system and declarative (relational) memory: Summarzing the data from functional neuroimaging studies. *Hippocampus* **9**, 83–98.

Collins, A., and Landgren, B. M. (1995). Reproductive health, use of estrogen and experience of symptoms in perimenopausal women: A population-based study. *Maturitas* **20**, 101–111.

Commins, W. D. (1932). The effect of castration at various ages upon learning ability of male albino rats. *J. Comp. Psychol.* **14**, 29–53.

Conrad, L. C., Leonard, C. M., and Pfaff, D. W. (1974). Connections to the median and dorsal raphe nuclei in the rat: An autoradiographic and degeneration study. *J. Comp. Neurol.* **156**, 179–205.

Conway, A. J., Handelsman, D. J., Lording, D. W., Stuckey, B., and Zajac, J. D. (2000). Use, misuse and abuse of androgens. The Endocrine Society of Australia consensus guidelines for androgen prescribing. *Med. J. Aust.* **172**, 220–224.

Cordoba Montoya, D. A., and Carrer, H. F. (1997). Estrogen facilitates induction of long term potentiation in the hippocampus of awake rats. *Brain Res.* **778**, 430–438.

Cummings, J. L., Vinters, H. V., Cole, G. M., and Khachaturian, Z. S. (1998). Alzheimer's disease. Etiologies, pathophysiology, cognitive reserve and treatment opportunities. *Neurology* **51**(S1), S2–S17.

Cushing, B. S., Marhenke, S., and McClure, P. A. (1995). Estradiol concentration and the regulation of locomotor activity. *Physiol. Behav.* **58**, 953–957.

Cyr, M., Ghribi, O., and Di Paolo, T. (2000). Regional and selective effects of oestradiol and progesterone on NMDA and AMPA receptors in the rat brain. *J. Neuroendo crinol.* **12**, 445–452.

Dale, R. H. I. (1986). Spatial and temporal response patterns on the eight-arm radial maze. *Physiol. Behav.* **36**, 787–790.

Dale, R. H. I., and Roberts, W. A. (1986). Variations in radial maze performance under different levels of food and water deprivation. *Anim. Learn. Behav.* **14**, 60–64.

Daniel, J. M., and Dohanich, G. P. (2001). Acetylcholine modulates the estrogen-induced increase in NMDA receptor binding CA1 of the hippocampus and the associated improvement in working memory. *J. Neurosci.* **21**, 6949–6956.

Daniel, J. M., Fader, A. J., Spencer, A., and Dohanich, G. P. (1997). Estrogen enhances performance of female rats during acquisition of a radial arm maze. *Horm. Behav.* **32**, 217–225.

Daniel, J. M., Roberts, S. L., and Dohanich, G. P. (1999). Effects of ovarian hormones and environment on radial maze and water maze performance of female rats. *Physiol. Behav.* **66**, 11–20.

Davenport, J. W., Hagquist, W. W., and Rankin, G. R. (1970). The symmetrical maze: An automated closed-field test series for rats. *Behav. Res. Methods Instrum.* **2**, 112–118.

Davies, J. A. (1978). The effect of gamma-butyrolactone on locomotor activity in the rat. *Psychopharmacology* **60**, 67–72.

Davis, S. (1999). Androgen replacement in women: A commentary. *J. Clin. Endocrinol. Metab.* **84**, 1886–1891.

Dawson, J. L. M. (1972). Effects of sex hormones on cognitive style in rats and men. *Behav. Genet.* **2**, 21–42.

Dawson, J. L., Cheung, Y. M., and Lau, R. T. (1975). Developmental effects of neonatal sex hormones on spatial and activity skills in the white rat. *Biol. Psychol.* **3**, 213–229.

Dekker, A. J., Langdon, D. J., Gage, F. H., and Thal, L. J. (1991). NGF increases cortical acetylcholine release in rats with lesions of the nucleus basalis. *NeuroReport* **2**, 577–580.

Delobette, S., Privat, A., and Maurice, T. (1997). In vitro aggregation facilitates ß-amyloid peptide-(25-25)-induced amnesia in the rat. *Eur. J. Pharmacol.* **319**, 1–4.

Denham, M. J., and Borisyuk, R. M. (2000). A model of theta rhythm production in the septal-hippocampal system and its modulation by ascending brain stem pathways. *Hippocampus* **10**, 698–716.

Desmond, N. L., and Levy, W. B. (1997). Ovarian steroidal control of connectivity in the female hippocampus: An overview of recent experimental findings and speculations on its functional consequences. *Hippocampus* **7**, 239–245.

Desmond, N. L., Zhang, D. X., and Levy, W. B. (2000). Estradiol enhances the induction of homosynaptic long-term depression in the CA1 region of the adult, ovariectomized rat. *Neurobiol. Learn. Mem.* **73**, 180–187.

Deutsch, J. A. (1971). The cholinergic synapse and the site of memory. *Science* **174**, 788–794.

Diaz-Brinton, R. (1997). 17 beta-estradiol enhances the outgrowth and survival of neocortical neurons in culture. *Neurochem. Res.* **22**, 1339–1351.

Diaz-Brinton, R., Chen, S., Montoya, M., Hsieh, D., Minaya, J., Kim, J., and Chu, H. (2000). The women's health initiative estrogen replacement therapy is neurotrophic and neuroprotective. *Neurobiol. Aging* **21**, 475–496.

Diaz-Veliz, G., Soto, V., Dussaubat, N., and Mora, S. (1989). Influence of the estrous cycle, ovariectomy, and estradiol replacement upon the acquisition of conditioned avoidance responses in rats. *Physiol. Behav.* **46**, 397–401.

Diaz-Veliz, G., Urresta, F., Dussaubat, N., and Mora, S. (1991). Effects of estradiol replacement in ovariectomized rats on conditioned avoidance responses and other behavior. *Physiol. Behav.* **50**, 61–65.

Diaz-Veliz, G., Urresta, F., Dussaubat, N., and Mora, S. (1994). Progesterone effects on the acquisition of conditioned avoidance responses an other motoric behaviors in intact and ovariectomized rats. *Psychoneuroendocrinology* **19**, 387–394.

Diaz-Veliz, G., Dussaubat, N., and Mora, S. (1995). Effect of oxotremorine on the acquisition of a conditioned avoidance response is modified by the estrous cycle, ovariectomy, and estradiol replacement in rats. *Pharmacol., Biochem. Behav.* **51**, 279–283.

Diaz-Veliz, G., Alarcon, T., Espinoza, C., Dussaubat, N., and Mora, S. (1997). Ketanserin and anxiety levels: Influence of gender, estrous cycle, ovariectomy and ovarian hormones in female rats. *Pharmacol., Biochem. Behav.* **58**, 637–642.

Diaz-Veliz, G., Butron, S., Benavides, M., Dussaubat, N., and Mora, S. (2000). Gender, estrous cycle, ovariectomy, and ovarian hormones influence the effects of diazepam on avoidance conditioning in rats. *Pharmacol., Biochem. Behav.* **66**, 887–892.

Ditkoff, E. C., Crary, W. R., Cristo, M., and Lobo, R. A. (1991). Estrogen improves psychological function in asymptomatic postmenopausal women. *Obstet. Gynecol.* **78**, 991–995.

Dohanich, G. P., Fader, A. J., and Javorsky, D. J. (1994). Estrogen and estrogen/progesterone treatments counteract the effect of scopolamine on T-maze performance in female rats. *Behav. Neurosci.* **108**, 988–992.

Doherty, P. C., and Sheridan, P. J. (1981). Uptake and retention of androgen in neurons of the brain of the golden hamster. *Brain Res.* **219**, 327–334.

DonCarlos, L. L., Monroy, E., and Morrell, J. I. (1991). Distribution of estrogen receptor-immunoreactive cells in the forebrain of the female guinea pig. *J. Comp. Neurol.* **305**, 591–612.

Dornan, W. A., Kang, D. E., McCampbell, A. R., and Kang, E. E. (1993). Bilateral injections of ßA (25–35) + IBO into the hippocampus disrupts acquisition of spatial learning in the rat. *Clin. Neurosci. Neuropathol.* **5**, 165–168.

Dornan, W. A., McCampbell, A. R., Tinkler, G. P., Hickman, L. J., Bannon, A. W., Decker, M. W., and Gunther, K. L. (1997). Comparison of the site specific injections into the basal forebrain on the water maze performance in the male rat after immunolesioning with 192 IgG saporin. *Behav. Brain Res.* **86**, 181–189.

Drachman, D. A., and Leavitt, J. (1974). Human memory and the cholinergic system. A relationship to aging? *Arch. Neurol. (Chicago)* **30**, 113–121.

Dubal, D. B., Kashon, M. L., Pettigrew, L. C., Ren, J. M., Finklestein, S. P., Rau, S. W., and Wise, P. M. (1998). Estradiol protects against ischemic injury. *J. Cereb. Blood Flow Metab.* **18**, 1253–1258.

Dubal, D. B., Shughrue, P. J., Wilson, M. E., Merchenthaler, I., and Wise, P. M. (1999). Estradiol modulates bcl-2 in cerebral ischemia: A potential role for estrogen receptors. *J. Neurosci.* **19**, 6385–6393.

Duff, S. J., and Hampson, E. (2000). A beneficial effect of estrogen on working memory in postmenopausal women taking hormone replacement therapy. *Horm. Behav.* **38**, 262–276.

Duka, T., Tasker, R., and McGowen, J. F. (2000). The effects of a 3-week estrogen hormone replacement on cognition in elderly healthy females. *Psychopharmacology* **149**, 129–139.

Eichenbaum, H. (1999). Neurobiology. The topography of memory. *Nature (London)* **402**, 597–599.

Eichenbaum, H., Otto, T., and Cohen, N. J. (1992). The hippocampus—what does it do? *Behav. Neural. Biol.* **57**, 2–36.

Einon, D. (1980). Spatial memory and response strategies in rats: Age, sex and rearing differences in performance. *Q. J. Exp. Psychol.* **32**, 473–489.

Errico, A. L., Parsons, O. A., Kling, O. R., and King, A. C. (1992). Investigation of the role of sex hormones on alcoholics visuospatial deficits. *Neuropsychologia* **30**, 417–426.

Everitt, B. J., and Robbins, T. W. (1997). Central cholinergic systems and cognition. *Annu. Rev. Psychol.* **48**, 648–649.

Fader, A. J., Hendricson, A. W., and Dohanich, G. P. (1998). Estrogen improves performance of reinforced T-Maze alternation and prevents the amnestic effects of scopolamine administered systemically or intrahippocampally. *Neurobiol. Learn. Mem.* **69**, 225–240.

Fader, A. J., Johnson, P. E. M., and Dohanich, G. P. (1999). Estrogen improves working but not reference memory and prevents amnestic effects of scopolamine on a radial-arm maze. *Pharmacol., Biochem. Behav.* **62**, 711–717.

Fader, A. J., Trapani, J. N., Demers, N., Yoon, A. J., and Dohanich, G. P. (2000). Effects of estradiol administered directly to the dorsal hippocampus or medial septal area on spatial working memory and response to scopolamine injection. *Soc. Neurosci. Abstr.* **26**, 346.17.

Fahrbach, S. E., Meisel, R. L., and Pfaff, D. W. (1985). Preoptic implants of estradiol increase wheel running but not the open field activity of female rats. *Physiol. Behav.* **35**, 985–992.

Fallon, J. H., Hicks, R., and Loughlin, S. E. (1983). The origin of cholecystokinin terminals in the basal forbrain of the rat: Evidence from immunofluorescence and retrograde tracing. *Neurosci Lett.* **37**, 29–35.

Farlow, M. R., and Evans, R. M. (1998). Pharmacologic treatment of cognition in Alzheimer's dementia. *Neurology* **51**(S1), S36–S44.

Farr, S. A., Flood, J. F., Scherrer, J. F., Kaiser, F. E., Taylor, G. T., and Morley, J. E. (1995). Effect of ovarian steroids on footshock avoidance learning and retention in female mice. *Physiol. Behav.* **58**, 715–723.

Feder, H. H. (1981a). Essentials of steroid structure, nomenclature, reactions, biosysnthesis, and measurements. In "Neuroendocrinology of Reproduction" (N. T. Adler, ed.), pp. 19–63. Plenum Press, New York.

Feder, H. H. (1981b). Estrous cyclicity in mammals. *In* "Neuroendocrinology of Reproduction" (N. T. Adler, ed.), pp. 279–348. Plenum Press, New York.

Fedor-Freyburg, P. (1977). The influence of oestrogen on the well being and mental performance in climacteric and postmenopausal women. *Acta. Obstet. Gynecol. Scand.* **64**(Suppl.), 5–69.

Fedotova, Y. O. (1999). Comparative characteristics of learning and behavior processes in conditions of elevated sex hormone levels. *Neurosci. Behav. Physiol.* **29**, 605–607.

Felson, D. T., Zhang, Y., Hannan, M. T., Kiel, D. P., Wilson, P. W. F., and Anderson, J. J. (1993). The effect of postmenopausal estrogen therapy on bone density in elderly women. *N. Engl. J. Med.* **329**, 1141–1146.

Fibiger, H. C. (1982). The organization and some projections of cholinergic neurons of the mammalian forebrain. *Brain Res.* **257**, 327–388.

Fillit, H. (1994). Estrogens in the pathogenesis and treatment of Alzheimer's disease in postmenopausal women. *Ann. N.Y. Acad. Sci.* **743**, 233–238.

Fillit, H., Weinref, H., Cholst, I., Luine, V., McEwen, B. R. A., and Zabriskie, J. (1986). Observations in a preliminary open trial of estradiol therapy for senile dementia- Alzheimer's type. *Psychoneuroendocrinology* **11**, 337–345.

Fink, G., Sumner, B. E., Rosie, R., Grace, O., and Quinn, J. P. (1996). Estrogen control of central neurotransmission: Effect on mood, mental state, and memory. *Cell. Mol. Neurobiol.* **16**, 325–344.

Fink, G., Sumner, B. E., McQueen, J. K., Wilson, H., and Rosie, R. (1998). Sex steroid control of mood, mental state and memory. *Clin. Exp. Pharmacol. Physiol.* **25**, 764–775.

Fink, G., Sumner, B. E., Rosie, R., Wilson, H., and McQueen, J. K. (1999). Androgen actions on central serotonin neurotransmission: Relevance for mood, mental state and memory. *Behav. Brain Res.* **105**, 53–68.

Flood, J. F., Farr, S. A., Kaiser, F. E., La Regina, M., and Morley, J. E. (1995). Age-related decrease of plasma testosterone in SAMP8 mice: Replacement improves age-related impairment of learning and memory. *Physiol. Behav.* **57**, 669–673.

Foy, M. R., Xu, J., Xie, X., Brinton, R. D., Thompson, R. F., and Berger, T. W. (1999). 17beta-estradiol enhances NMDA receptor-mediated ESPSs and long term potentiation. *J. Neurophysiol.* **81**, 925–929.

Frankfurt, M. (1994). Gonadal steroids and neuronal plasticity: Studies in the adult rat hypothalamus. *In* "Hormonal Restructuring of the Adult Brain: Basic and Clinical Perspectives" (V. N. Luine and C. F. Harding, eds.), pp. 45–60. N. Y. Academy of Sciences, New York.

Frick, K. M., Burlingame, L. A., Arters, J. A., and Berder-Sweeney, J. (2000). Reference memory, anxiety and estrous cyclicity in C57BL/6NIA mice are affected by age and sex. *Neuroscience* **95**, 293–307.

Friedman, J., and Meares, R. A. (1978). Comparison of spontaneous and contraceptive menstrual cycles on a visual discrimination task. *Aust. N. Z. J. Psychiatry* **12**, 233–239.

Frye, C. A. (1995). Estrus-associated decrements in a water maze task are limited to acquisition. *Physiol. Behav.* **57**, 5–14.

Fugger, H. N., Cunningham, S. G., Rissman, E. F., and Foster, T. C. (1998). Sex differences in the activational effect of ER-alpha on spatial learning. *Horm. Behav.* **34**, 163–170.

Fugger, H. N., Foster, T. C. Gustafsson, J., and Rissman, E. F. (2000). Novel effects of estradiol and estrogen receptor alpha and beta on cognitive function. *Brain Res.* **17**, 258–264.

Galea, L. A. M., Kavaliers, M., Ossenkopp, K. P., and Hampson, E. (1995). Gonadal hormones and spatial learning in the Morris water-maze in the male and female meadow vole, Microtus pennsylanicus. *Horm. Behav.* **29**, 106–125.

Galea, L. A. M., Paine, T. A., Piaseczna, M. A., and Ormerod, B. K. (1999a). Dissociation of estradiol's effects on learning and memory: Performance enhancement on hippocampal independent and performance inhibition on hippocampal dependent tasks. *Soc. Neurosci. Abstr.* **25**, No. 863.5.

Galea, L. A. M., Ormerod, B. K., Sampath, S., Kostaras, X., Wilkie, D. M., and Phelps, M. T. (2000). Spatial working memory and hippocampal size across pregnancy in rats. *Horm. Behav.* **37**, 86–95.

Gambineri, A., and Pasquali, R. (2000). Testosterone therapy in men: Clinical and pharmacological perspectives. *J. Endocrinol. Invest.* **23**, 196–214.

Garcia-Estrada, J., Luquin, S., Fernandez, A. M., and Garcia-Segura, L. M. (1999). Dehydroepiandrosterone, pregnenolone and sex steroids down-regulate reactive astroglia in the male rat brain after a penetrating brain injury. *Int. J. Dev. Neurosci.* **17**, 145–151.

Garcia-Segura, L. M., Cardona-Gomez, P., Naftolin, F., and Chowen, J. A. (1998). Estradiol upregulates Bcl-2 expression in adult brain neurons. *NeuroReport* **9**, 593–597.

Garcia-Segura, L. M., Naftolin, F., Hutchison, J. B., Azcoitia, I., and Chowen, J. A. (1999). Role of astroglia in estrogen regulation of synaptic plasticity and brain repair. *J. Neurobiol.* **40**, 574–584.

Gazzaley, A. H., Weiland, N. G., McEwen, B. S., and Morrison, J. H. (1996). Differntial regulation of NMDAR1 mRNA and protein by estradiol in the rat hippocampus. *J. Neurosci.* **16**, 6830–6838.

Geller, E. B., and Adler, M. W. (1990). Drugs of abuse and body temperature. *In* "Testing and Evaluaution of Drugs of Abuse" (M. W. Adler and A. Cowan, eds.), pp. 101–119. Wiley-Liss, New York.

Gennzzani, A. R., Spinetti, A., Gallo, R., and Bernardi, F. (1999). Menopause and the central nervous system: Intervention options. *Maturitas* **31**, 103–110.

Gerdes, L. C., Sonnendecker, E. W. W., and Polakow, E. S. (1982). Psychological changes effected by estrogen-progestogen and clonidine treatment in climacteric women. *Am. J. Obstet. Gynecol.* **142**, 98–104.

Geyer, M. A. (1990). Approaches to the characterization of drug effects on locomotor activity in rodents. *In* "Testing and Evaluation of Drugs of Abuse" (M. A. Adler and A. Cowan, eds.), Vol. 6, pp. 81–89. Wiley-Liss, New York.

Giap, H., Teirstein, P., Massullo, V., and Tripuraneni, P. (2000). Barotrauma due to stent deployment in endovascular brachytherapy for restenosis prevention. *Int. J. Radiat. Oncol. Biol. Phys.* **47**, 1021–1024.

Gibbs, M. E., Ng, K. T., and Andrew, R. J. (1986). Effect of testosterone on intermediate memory in day-old chicks. *Pharmacol., Biochem. Behav.* **25**, 823–826.

Gibbs, R. B. (1994). Estrogen and nerve growth factor-related systems in brain: Effects on basal forebrain cholinergic neurons and implications for learning and memory processes and aging. *In* "Hormonal Restructuring of the Adult Brain: Basic and Clinical Perspectives" (V. N. Luine and C. F. Harding, eds.), pp. 165–199. N. Y. Acad. Sci., New York.

Gibbs, R. B. (1996a). Expression of estrogen receptor-like immunoreactivity by different subgroups of basal forebrain cholinergic neurons in gonadectomized male and female rats. *Brain Res.* **720**, 61–68.

Gibbs, R. B. (1996b). Fluctuations in relative levels of choline acetyltransferase mRNA in different regions of the rat basal forebrain across the estrous cycle: Effects of estrogen and progesterone. *J. Neurosci.* **16**, 1049–1055.

Gibbs, R. B. (1997). Effects of estrogen on basal forebrain cholinergic neurons vary as a function of dose and duration of treatment. *Brain Res.* **757**, 10–16.

Gibbs, R. B. (1999a). Estrogen replacement enhances acquisition of a spatial memory task and reduces deficits associated with hippocampal muscarinic receptor inhibition. *Horm. Behav.* **36**, 222–233.

Gibbs, R. B. (1999b). Treatment with estrogen and progesterone affects relative levels of brain-derived neurotrophic factor mRNA and protein in different regions of the adult rat brain. *Brain Res.* **844**, 20–27.

Gibbs, R. B. (2000). Long-term treatment with estrogen and progesterone enhances acquisition of a spatial memory task by ovariectomized aged rats. *Neurobiol. Aging* **21**, 107–116.

Gibbs, R. B., and Pfaff, D. W. (1992). Effects of estrogen and fimbria/fornix transection on p75NGFR and ChAT expression in the medial septum and diagonal band of Broca. *Exp. Neurol.* **116**, 23–29.

Gibbs, R. B., Wu, D., Hersh, L. B., and Pfaff, D. W. (1994). Effects of estrogen replacement on the relative levels of choline acetyltransferase, trkA, and nerve growth factor messenger RNAs in the basal forebrain and hippocampal formation of adult rats. *Exp. Neurol.* **129**, 70–80.

Gibbs, R. B., Burke, A. M., and Johnson, D. A. (1998). Estrogen replacement attenuates effects of scopolamine and lorazepam on memory acquisition and retention. *Horm. Behav.* **34**, 112–125.

Gold, P. E., and Zornetzer, S. F. (1983). The mnemon and its juices: Neuromodulation of memory processes. *Behav. Neural Biol.* **38**, 151–189.

Good, M., Day, M., and Muir, J. L. (1999). Cyclical changes in endogenous levels of oestrogen modulate the induction of LTD and LTP in the hippocampal CA1 region. *Eur. J. Neurosci.* **11**, 4476–4480.

Goodman, Y., Bruce, A. J., Cheng, B., and Mattson, M. P. (1996). Estrogens attenuate and corticosterone exacerbates excitotoxicity, oxidative injury, and amyloid beta-peptide toxicity in hippocampal neurons. *J. Neurochem.* **66**, 1836–1844.

Gordon, H. W., and Lee, P. A. (1993). No difference in cognitive preformance between phases of the mentrual cycle. *Psychoneuroendocrinology* **18**, 521–531.

Gouchie, C., and Kimura, D. (1991). The relationship between testosterone levels and cognitive ability patterns. *Psychoneuroendocrinology* **16**, 323–334.

Goudsmit, E., van de Poll, N. E., and Swaab, D. F. (1990). Testosterone fails to reverse spatial memory decline in aged rats and impairs retention in young and middle-aged animals. *Behav. Neural Biol.* **53**, 6–20.

Gould, E., Woolley, C. S., Frankfurt, M., and McEwen, B. S. (1990). Gonadal steroids regulate dendritic spine density in hippocampal pyramidal cells in adulthood. *J. Neurosci.* **10**, 1286–1291.

Gouras, G. K., Xu, H., Gross, R. S., Greenfield, J. P., Hai, B., Wang, R., and Greengard, P. (2000). Testosterone reduces neuronal secretion of Alzheimer's beta-amyloid peptides. *Proc. Natl. Acad. Sci. U.S.A.* **97**, 1202–1205.

Gower, E. C. (1990). The long-term retention of events in monkey memory. *Behav. Brain Res.* **38**, 191–198.

Granholm, A. C. (2000). Oestrogen and nerve growth factor—neuroprotection and repair in Alzheimer's disease. *Expert. Opin. Invest. Drugs* **9**, 685–694.

Graves, A. B., White, E., and Koepsell, T. D. (1990). A case-control study of Alzheimer's disesase. *Ann. Neurol.* **28**, 766–774.

Gray, P. (1977). Effect of the estrous cycle on conditioned avoidance in mice. *Horm. Behav.* **8**, 235–241.

Green, P. S., Gridley, K. E., and Simpkins, J. W. (1996). Estradiol protects against beta-amyloid (25–35)-induced toxicity in SK-N-SH human neuroblastoma cells. *Neurosci. Lett.* **218**, 165–168.

Green, P. S., Bishop, J., and Simpkins, J. W. (1997a). 17 alpha-estradiol exerts neuroprotective effects on SK-N-SH cells. *J. Neurosci.* **17**, 511–515.

Green, P. S., Gordon, K., and Simpkins, J. W. (1997b). Phenolic A ring requirement for the neuroprotective effect of steroids *J. Steroid Biochem. Mol. Biol.* **63**, 229–235.

Green, P. S., Gridley, K. E., and Simpkins, J. W. (1998). Nuclear estrogen receptor-independent neuroprotection by estratrienes: A novel interaction with glutathione. *Neuroscience* **84**, 7–10.

Gridley, K. E., Green, P. S., and Simpkins, J. W. (1998). Low concentrations of estradiol reduce beta-amyloid (25–35)-induced toxicity, lipid peroxidation and glucose utilization in human SK-N-SH neuroblastoma cells. *Brain Res.* **778**, 158–165.

Gritti, I., Mainville, L., and Jones, B. E. (1993). Codistribution of GABA-with acetylcholine-synthesizing neurons in the basal forebrain of the rat. *J. Comp. Neurol.* **329**, 438–457.

Grodstein, F., Chen, J., Pollen, D. A., Albert, M. S., Wilson, R. S., Folstein, M. F., Evans, D. A., and Stampfer, M. J. (2000). Postmenopausal hormone therapy and cognitive function in healthy older women. *J. Am. Geriatr. Soc.* **48**, 746–752.

Gu, Q., and Moss, R. L. (1996). 17 beta-estradiol potentiates kainate-induced currents via activation of the cAMP cascade. *J. Neurosci.* **16**, 3620–3629.

Gu, Q., Rojo, A. A., Zee, M. C., Yu, J., and Simerly, R. D. (1996). Hormonal regulation of CREB phosphorylation in the anteroventral periventricular nucleus. *J. Neurosci.* **16**, 3035–3044.

Gustafsson, J. A. (2000). An update on estogen receptors. *Semin. Perinatol.* **24**, 66–69.

Hackman, B. W., and Galbraith, D. (1976). Replacement therapy with piperazine oestrone sulfate ("Harmogen") and its effect on memory. *Curr. Med. Res. Opin.* **4**, 303–328.

Haglund, L., Swanson, L. W., and Kohler, C. (1984). The projection of the supramammillary nucleus to the hippocampal formation: An immunohistochemical and anterograde transport study with the lectin PHA-L in the rat. *J. Comp. Neurol.* **229**, 171–185.

Halbreich, U. (1997). Role of estrogen in postmenopausal depression. *Neurology* **48**(S7), S16–S20.

Hampson, E. (1990a). Estrogen-related variations in human spatial and articulatory-motor skills. *Psychoneuroendocrinology* **15**, 97–111.

Hampson, E. (1990b). Variations in sex-related cognitive abilities across the menstural cycle. *Brain Cogn.* **14**, 26–43.

Hampson, E., and Kimura, D. (1988). Reciprocal effects of hormonal fluctuations on human motor and perceptual-spatial skills. *Behav. Neurosci.* **102**, 456–459.

Hampson, E., and Kimura, D. (1992). Sex differences and hormonal influences on cognitive function in humans. In "Behavioral Endocrinology" (J. B. Becker, S. M. Breedlove, and D. Crews, eds.), pp. 357–398. MIT: Press, Cambridge, MA.

Hampson, R. E., Simeral, J. D., and Deadwyler, S. A. (1999). Distribution of spatial and nonspatial information in dorsal hippocampus. *Nature (London)* **402**, 610–614.

Handa, R. J., Reid, D. L., and Resko, J. A. (1986). Androgen receptors in brain and pituitary of female rats: Cyclic changes and comparisons with the male. *Biol. Reprod.* **34**, 293–303.

Haring, J. H., and Davis, J. N. (1983). Acetylcholinesterase neurons in the later hypothalamus project to the spinal cord. *Brain Res.* **268**, 275–283.

Haring, J. H., and Davis, J. N. (1985a). Differential distribution of locus coeruleus projections to the hippocampal formation: Anatomical and biochemical evidence. *Brain Res.* **325**, 366–369.

Haring, J. H., and Davis, J. N. (1985b). Retrograde labeling of locus coeruleus neurons after lesion-induced sprouting of the coeruleohippocampal projections. *Brain Res.* **360**, 384–388.

Harkany, T., O'Mahony, S., Kelly, J. P., Soos, K., Toro, I., Penke, B., Luiten, P. G. M., Nyakas, C., Gulya, K., and Leonard, B. E. (1998). Beta-amyloid (Phe(SO3H)24) 25–35 in rat nucleus basalis induces behavioral dysfunctions, impairs learning and memory and disrupts cortical cholinergic innervation. *Behav. Brain Res.* **90**, 133–145.

Harrell, L. E., Parsons, D. S., and Peagler, A. (1990). The effect of gonadal steroids on the behavioral and biochemical effects of hippocampal sympathetic ingrowth. *Physiol. Behav.* **48**, 507–513.

Haskell, S. G., Richardson, E. D., and Horwitz, R. I. (1997). The effect of estrogen replacement therapy on cognitive function in women: A critical review of the literature. *J. Clin. Epidemiol.* **50**, 1249–1264.

Hasselmo, M. E. (1999). Neuromodulation and the hippocampus: Memory function and dysfunction in a network simulation. *Prog. Brain Res.* **121**, 3–18.

Hawk, T., Zhang, Y. Q., Rajakumar, G., Day, A. L., and Simpkins, J. W. (1998). Testosterone increases and estradiol decreases middle cerebral artery occlusion lesion size in male rats. *Brain Res.* **796**, 296–298.

Healy, S. D., Braham, S. R., and Braithwaite, V. A. (1999). Spatial working memory in rats: No differences between the sexes. *Proc. R. Soc. London* **266**, 2303–2308.

Hebb, D. O. (1949). "The Organization of Behavior." Wiley, New York.

Henderson, V. W. (1997a). The epidemiology of estrogen replacement therapy and Alzeihmer's disease. *Neurology* **48**(S7), S27–S35.

Henderson, V. W. (1997b). Estrogen, cognition, and a woman's risk of Alzheimer's disease. The role of estrogen in the treatment and prevention of dementia. *Am. J. Med.* **103**(Suppl. 3), S11–S18.

Henderson, V. (2000). Oestrogens and dementia. In "Neuronal and Cognitive Effects of Oestrogens" (B. McEwen, ed.), Wiley, West Sussex.

Henderson, V. W., Paganini-Hill, A., Emanuel, C. K., Dunn, M. E., and Buckwalter, J. G. (1994). Estrogen replacement therapy in older women. Comparisons between Alzheimer's disease cases and nondemented control subjects. *Arch. Neurol.* **51**, 896–900.

Henricks, D. M., and Mayer, D. T. (1977). Gonadal hormones and uterine factors. In "Reproduction in Domestic Animals" (H. H. Cole and P. T. Cupps, eds.), pp. 79–117. Academic Press, New York.

Hier, D. B., and Crowley, W. F. (1982). Spatial ability in androgen-deficient men. *N. Engl. J. Med.* **306**, 1202–1205.

Hodges, H. (1996). Maze procedures: The radial-arm and water maze compared. *Brain Res. Cogn. Brain Res.* **3**, 167–181.

Hoeger, K. M., and Guzick, D. S. (1999). The use androgens in menopause. *Clin. Obstet. Gynecol.* **42**, 883–894.

Hogervorst, E., Boshuisen, M., Riedel, W., Willeken, C., and Jolles, J. (1999). 1998 Curt P. Richter Award. The effect of hormone replacement therapy on cognitive function in elderly women. *Psychoneuroendocrinology* **24**, 43–68.

Hogervorst, E., Williams, J., Budge, M., Riedel, W., and Jolles, J. (2000). The nature of the effect of female gonadal hormone replacement therapy on cognitive function in post-menopausal women: A meta-analysis. *Neuroscience* **101**, 485–512.

Hoh, T. E., and Cain, D. P. (1997). Fractioning the nonspatial pretraining effect in the water maze task. *Behav. Neurosci.* **111**, 1285–1291.

Holland, P. C., and Bouton, M. E. (1999). Hippocampus and context in classical conditioning. *Curr. Opin. Neurobiol.* **9**, 195–202.

Honjo, H., Ogino, Y., Naitoh, K., Urabe, M., Kitawaki, J., Yasuda, J., Yamamota, T., Ishihara, S., Okada, H., Yonezawa, T., Hayashi, K., and Nambara, T. (1989). In vivo effects by estrone sulfate on the central nervous system-senile dementia (Alzheimer's type). *J. Steroid Biochem.* **34**, 521–525.

Honjo, H., Ogmo, Y., and Tanaka, K. (1993). An effect of conjugated estrogen to cognitive impairment in women with senile dementia—Alzheimer's type: A placebo-controlled double blind study. *J. Jpn. Menopause Soc.* **1**, 167–171.

Hruska, R. E., and Pitman, K. T. (1982). Distribution and localization of estrogen-sensitive dopamine receptors in the rat brain. *J. Neurochem.* **39**, 1418–1423.

Hull, C. L. (1943). "Principles of Behavior." Appleton-Century-Crofts, New York.

Ikard, W. L., Bennett, W. C., Lundin, R. W., and Trost, R. C. (1972). Acquisition and extinction of the conditioned avoidance response: A comparison between male rats and estrus and non-estrus female rats. *Psychol. Rec.* **22**, 249–254.

Ito, K., Skinkle, K. L., and Hicks, T. P. (1999). Age-dependent, steroid-specific effects of oestrogen on long-term potentiation in rat hippocampal slices. *J. Physiol. (London)* **515**(Pt. 1), 209–220.

Ivanova, T., and Beyer, C. (2000). Ontogenetic expression and sex differences of aromatase and estrogen receptor-alpha/beta mRNA in the mouse hippocampus. *Cell. Tissue Res.* **300**, 231–237.

Izquierdo, I., Schoder, N., Netto, C. A., and Medina, J. H. (1999). Novelty causes time-dependent retrograde amnesia for one-trial avoidance in rats through NMDA receptor- and CaMKII-dependent mechanisms in the hippocampus. *Eur. J. Neurosci.* **11**, 3323–3328.

Jacobs, D. M., Tang, M. X., Stern, Y., Sano, M., Marder, K., Bell, K. L., Schofield, P., Dooneief, G., Gurland, B., and Mayeux, R. (1998). Cognitive function in nondemented older women who took estrogen after menopause. *Neurology* **50**, 368–373.

Jaffe, A. B., Toran-Allerand, C. D., Greengard, P., and Gamdy, S. E. (1994). Estrogen regulates metabolism of Alzheimer amyloid beta precursor protein. *J. Biol. Chem.* **269**, 13065–13068.

Janis, L. S., Glaiser, M. M., Fulop, Z., and Stein, D. G. (1998). Intraseptal injections of 192 IgG saporin produce deficits for strategy selection in spatial-memory tasks. *Behav. Brain Res.* **90**, 23–34.

Janowsky, J. S., Oviatt, S. K., and Orwoll, E. S. (1994). Testosterone influences spatial cognition in older men. *Behav. Neurosci.* **108**, 325–332.

Jarrard, L. E. (1983). Selective hippocampal lesions and behavior: Effects of kainic acid lesions on performance of place and cue tasks. *Behav. Neurosci.* **97**, 873–889.

Joels, M. (1997). Steroid hormones and excitability in the mammalian brain. *Front. Neuroendocrinol.* **18**, 2–48.

Joseph, R., Hess, S., and Birecree, E. (1978). Effects of hormone manipulations and exploration on sex differences in maze learning. *Behav. Biol.* **24**, 364–377.

Juraska, J. M., Henderson, C., and Muller, J. (1984). Differential rearing experience, gender, and radial maze performance. *Dev. Psychobiol.* **17**, 209–215.

Kampen, D. L., and Sherwin, B. B. (1994). Estrogen use and verbal memory in healthy postmenopausal women. *Obstet. Gynecol.* **83**, 979–983.

Kampen, D. L., and Sherwin, B. B. (1996). Estrdiol is related to visual memory in healthy young men. *Behav. Neurosci.* **110**, 613–617.

Kanyt, L., Stolerman, I. P., Chandler, C. J., Saigusa, T., and Pogun, S. (1999). Influence of sex and female hormones on nicotine-induced changes in locomotor activity in rats. *Pharmacol., Biochem. Behav.* **62**, 179–187.

Kaunitz, A. M. (1997). The role of androgens in menopausal hormonal replacement. *Endocrinol. Metab. Clin. North Am.* **26**, 391–397.

Kawakami, M., Terasawa, E., and Ibuka, T. (1970). Changes in multiple unit activity of the brain during the estrous cycle. *Neuroendocrinology* **6**, 30–48.

Kawas, C., Resnick, S., and Morrison, A. (1997). A prospective study of estrogen replacement therapy and the risk of developing Alzheimer's disease: The Baltimore Longitudinal Study of Aging. *Neurology* **48**, 1517–1521; erratum: *Ibid.* **51**, 654 (1998).

Kerr, J. E., Allore, R. J., Beck, S. G., and Handa, R. J. (1995). Distribution and hormonal regulation of androgen receptor (AR) and AR messenger ribonucleic acid in the rat hippocampus. *Endocrinology (Baltimore)* **136**, 3213–3221.

Kesner, R. P., and Hardy, J. D. (1983). Long-term memory for contextual attributes: Dissociation of amygdala and hippocampus. *Behav. Brain Res.* **8**, 139–149.

Kesner, R. P., Bolland, B. L., and Dakis, M. (1993). Memory for spatial locations, motor responses, and objects: Triple dissociation among the hippocampus, caudate nucleus, and extrastriate visual cortex. *Exp. Brain Res.* **93**, 462–470.

Kim, Y. C. (1999). Testosterone supplementation in the aging male. *Int. J. Impotence Res.* **11**, 343–352.

Kimura, D. (1995). Estrogen replacement therapy may protect against intellectual decline in postmenopausal women. *Horm. Behav.* **29**, 312–321.

Kimura, D. (1996). Sex, sexual orientation and sex hormones influence human cognitive function. *Curr. Opin. Neurobiol.* **6**, 259–263.

Kimura, D. (1999). "Sex and Cognition." MIT Press, Cambridge, MA.

Kirk, I. J. (1998). Frequency modulation of hippocampal theta by the supramammillary nucleus and other hypothalamo-hippocampal interactions: Mechanisms and functional implications. *Neurosci. Biobehav. Rev.* **22**, 291–302.

Kiss, J., Csaki, A., Bokor, H., Shanabrough, M., and Leranth, C. (2000). The supramammillo-hippocampal and supramammillo-septal glutamatergic/aspartatergic projections in the rat: A combined [3H]D-aspartate autoradiographic and immunohistochemical study. *Neuroscience* **97**, 657–669.

Kleshchevnikov, A. M. (1999). Synaptic plasticity in the hippocampus during afferent activation reproducing the pattern of the theta rhythm (theta plasticity). *Neurosci. Behav. Physiol.* **29**, 185–196.

Knoth, R., Park, R., Eggebrecht, K., and Clegg, A. (1993). Effects of chronic exposure to testosterone on spatial learning in the rat. *Soc. Neurosci. Abstr.* **23**, 152.11

Kohler, C. (1985a). Intrinsic projections of the retrohippocampal region in the rat brain *J. Comp. Neurol.* **236**, 504–522.

Kohler, C. (1985b). A projection from the deep layers of the entorhinal area to the hippocampal formation in the rat brain *Neurosci. Lett.* **56**, 13–19.

Kohler, C. (1986). Intrinsic connections of the retrohippocampal region in the rat brain II. The medial entorhinal area. *J. Comp. Neurol.* **246**, 149–169.

Kohler, C. (1988). Intrinsic connections of the retrohippocampal region in the rat brain III. The lateral entorhinal area. *J. Comp. Neurol.* **271**, 208–228.

Komenich, P., Lane, D. M., Dickey, R. P., and Stone, S. C. (1978). Gonadal hormones and cognitive performance. *Physiol. Psychol.* **6**, 115–120.

Kondo, Y., Suzuki, K., and Sakuma, Y. (1997). Estrogen alleviates cognitive dysfunction following transient brain ischemia in ovariectomized gerbils. *Neurosci. Lett.* **238**, 45–48.

Korol, D. L., Unick, K., Goosens, K., Crane, C., Gold, P. E., and Foster, T. C. (1994). Estrogen effects on spatial performance and hippocampal physiology in female rats. *Soc. Neurosci. Abstr.* **20**, 143.6.

Korol, D. L., Clark, L. L., and Gold, P. E. (1998). Shifts in preferred learning strategies used by female rats with and without estrogen. *Soc. Neurosci. Abstr.* **24**, 267.6.

Kraemer, P. J., Gilbert, M. E., and Innis, N. K. (1983). The influence of cue type and configuration upon radial-maze performance in the rat. *Anim. Learn. Behav.* **11**, 373–380.

Kristal, M. B., Axelrod, S., and Noonan, M. (1978). Learning in escape/avoidance tasks in female rats does not vary with reproductive condition. *Physiol. Behav.* **21**, 251–256.

Kritzer, M. F. (1997). Selective colocalization of immunoreactivity for intracellular gonadal hormone receptors and tyrosine hydroxylase in the ventral tegmental area, substantia nigra, and retrorubral fields in the rat. *J. Comp. Neurol.* **379**, 247–260.

Kritzer, M. F., and Kohama, S. G. (1999). Ovarian hormones differentially influence immunoreactivity for dopamine beta-hydroxylase, choline acetyltransferase, and serotonin in the dorsolateral prefrontal cortex of adult rhesus monkeys. *J. Comp. Neurol.* **409**, 438–451.

Krug, R., Stamm, U., Pietrowski, R., Fehm, H. L., and Born, J. (1993). Effects of menstrual cycle on creativity. *Psychoneuroendocrinology* **19**, 21–31.

Kuiper, G. G. J. M., Carlsson, B., Grandien, K., Enmark, E., Haggblad, J., Nilsson, S., and Gustafsson, J. (1997). Comparison of the ligand binding specificity and transcript tissue distribution of estrogen receptors alpha and beta. *Endocrinology (Baltimore)* **138**, 863–870.

Kuller, L. H. (1996). Hormone replacement therapy and its potential relationship to dementia. *J. Am. Geriatr. Soc.* **44**, 878–880.

LaFlamme, N., Nappi, R. E., Drolet, G., Labrie, C., and Rivest, S. (1998). Expression and neuropeptidergic characterization of estrogen receptors (ERalpha and ERbeta) throughout the rat brain: Anatomical evidence of distinct roles of each subtype. *J. Neurobiol.* **36**, 357–378.

Lannert, H., Wirtz, P., Schuhmann, V., and Galmbacher, R. (1998). Effects of estradiol (-17beta) on learning, memory and cerebral energy metabolism in male rats after intracerebroventricular administration of streptozotocin. *J. Neural Transm.* **105**, 1045–1063.

Lashley, K. S. (1929). "Brain Mechanisms and Intelligence: A Quantitative Study of Injuries to the Brain." Chicago University Press, Chicago.

Lashley, K. S. (1950). In search of the engram. *Symp. Soc. Exp. Biol.* **4**, 454–482.

Lee, S. H., and Mouradian, M. M. (1999). Up-regulation of D1A dopamine receptor gene transcription by estrogen. *Mol. Cell. Endocrinol.* **56**, 151–157.

Lentz, F. E., Pool, G. L., and Milner, J. S. (1978). Effects of ovariectomy and hormone replacement on DRL behavior in the rat. *Physiol. Behav.* **20**, 477–480.

Leranth, C., Shanabrough, M., and Horvath, T. L. (1999). Estrogen receptor-alpha in the raphe serotonergic and supramammilary area calretinin-containing neurons of the female rat. *Exp. Brain Res.* **128**, 417–420.

Leranth, C., Shanabrough, M., and Horvath, T. L. (2000). Hormonal regulation of hippocampal spine synapse density involves subcortical mediation. *Neuroscience* **101**, 349–356.

Lerner, A. J. (1999). Women and Alzheimer's disease. *J. Clin. Endocrinol. Metab.* **84**, 1830–1834.

Lewis, P. R., and Shute, C. C. (1967). The cholinergic limbic system: Projections to the hippocampal formation, medial cortex, nuclei of the ascending cholinergic reticular system, and the subfornical organ and supra-optic crest. *Brain* **90**, 521–540.

Li, X. G., Somogyi, P., Ylinen, A., and Buzsaki, G. (1994). The hippocampal CA3 network: An in vivo intracellular labeling study. *J. Comp. Neurol.* **339**, 181–208.

Li, X., Schwartz, P. E., and Rissman, E. F. (1997). Distribution of estrogen receptor-beta-like immunoreactivity in rat forebrain. *Neuroendocrinology* **66**, 63–67.

Limouzin-Lamothe, M. A., Mairon, N., Joyce, C. R. B., and Le Gal, M. (1994). Quality of life after menopause: Influence of hormonal replacement therapy. *Am. J. Obstet. Gynecol.* **170**, 618–624.

Lopez-Jaramillo, P., and Teran, E. (1999). Improvement in functions of the central nervous system by estrogen replacement therapy might be related with an increased nitric oxide production. *Endothelium* **6**, 263–266.

Loy, R., Gerlach, J. L., and McEwen, B. S. (1988). Autoradiographic localization of estradiol-binding neurons in the rat hippocampal formation and entorhinal cortex. *Dev. Brain Res.* **39**, 245–251.

Luine, V. N. (1985). Estradiol increases choline acetyltransferase activity in specific basal forebrain nuclei and projection areas of female rats. *Exp. Neurol.* **89**, 484–490.

Luine, V. N., and McEwen, B. S. (1983). Sex differences in cholinergic enzymes of diagonal band nuclei in the rat preoptic area. *Neuroendocrinology* **36**, 475–482.

Luine, V. N., and Rodriguez, M. (1994). Effects of estradiol on radial arm maze performance of young and aged rats. *Behav. Neural Biol.* **62**, 230–236.

Luine, V. N., Richards, S. T., Wu, V. Y., and Beck, K. D. (1998). Estradiol enhances learning and memory in a spatial memory task and effects levels of monoaminergic neurotransmitters. *Horm. Behav.* **34**, 149–162.

Luine, V. N., Gordon, M., and Mohan, C. (2001). Effects of estradiol administration and ovariectomy on spatial and nonspatial memory in rats. Submitted for publication.

Maggi, A., Susanna, L., Bettini, E., Mantero, G., and Zucchi, I. (1989). Hippocampus: A target for estrogen action in the mammalian brain. *Mol. Endocrinol.* **3**, 1165–1170.

Mair, W. P. G., Warrington, E. K., and Weiskrantz, L. (1979). Memory disorder in Korsakoff's psychosis: A neuropathological and neuropsychological investigation of two cases. *Brain* **102**, 749–783.

Maki, P. M., and Resnick, S. M. (2000). Longitudinal effects of estrogen replacement therapy on PET cerebral blood flow and cognition. *Neurobiol. Aging* **21**, 373–383.

Manly, J. J., Merchant, C. A., Jacobs, D. M., Small, S. A., Bell, K., Ferin, M., and Mayeux, R. (2000). Endogenous estrogen levels and Alzheimer's disease among postmenopausal women. *Neurology* **54**, 833–837.

Markowska, A. L. (1999). Sex dimorphisms in the rate of age-related decline in spatial memory: Relevance to alterations in the estrous cycle. *J. Neurosci.* **19**, 8122–8133.

Markus, E. J., and Zecevic, M. (1997). Sex differences and estrous cycle changes in hippocampus-dependent fear conditioning. *Psychobiology* **25**, 246–252.

Martin, C. R. (1976). "Textbook of Endocrine Physiology." Williams & Wilkins, Baltimore, MD.

Martin, C. R. (1985). "Endocrine Physiology." Oxford University Press, New York.

Martin, S. J., Grimwood, P. D., and Morris, R. G. (2000). Synaptic plasticity and memory: An evaluation of the hypothesis. *Annu. Rev. Neurosci.* **23**, 649–711.

Matochik, J. A., White, N. R., and Barfield, R. J. (1992). Variations in scent marking and ultrasonic vocalizations by Long-Evans rats across the estrous cycle. *Physiol. Behav.* **51**, 783–786.

Mayes, A. R., Meudell, P. R., Mann, D., and Pickering, A. (1988). Location of lesions in Korsakoff's syndrome: Neuropsychological and neuropathological data on two patients. *Cortex* **24**, 367–388.

McCaffrey, T. A., and Czaja, J. A. (1989). Diverse effects of estradiol-17beta: Concurrent suppression of appetite, blood pressure, and vascular reactivity in conscious, unrestrained animals. *Physiol. Behav.* **45**, 649–657.

McDonald, M. P., Dahl, E. E., and Overmier, J. B. (1994). Effects of an exogenous ß-amyloid peptide on retention for spatial learning. *Behav. Neural Biol.* **62**, 60–67.

McDonald, R. J., and White, N. M. (1993). A triple dissociation of memory systems: Hippocampus, amygdala, and dorsal striatum. *Behav. Neurosci.* **107**, 3–22.

McDonald, R. J., and White, N. M. (1994). Parallel information processing in the water maze: Evidence for independent memory systems involving dorsal striatum and hippocampus. *Neural Biol.* **61**, 260–270.

McDonald, R. J., and White, N. M. (1995). Hippocampal and nonhippocampal contributions to place learning in rats. *Behav. Neurosci.* **109**, 579–593.

McEwen, B. S., and Alves, S. E. (1999). Estrogen actions in the central nervous system. *Endocr. Rev.* **20**, 279–307.

McEwen, B. S., and Woolley, C. S. (1994). Estradiol and progesterone regulate neuronal structure and synaptic connectivity in adult as well as developing brain. *Exp. Gerontol.* **29**, 431–436.

McEwen, B. S., Krey, L. C., and Luine, V. N. (1978). Steroid hormone action in the neuroendocrine system: When is the genome involved? *Res. Publ. Assoc. Res. Nerv. Ment. Dis.* **56**, 255–268.

McEwen, B. S., Alves, S. E., Bulloch, K., and Weiland, N. G. (1997). Ovarian steroids and the brain: Implications for cognition and aging. *Neurology* **48**(S7), S8–S15.

McEwen, B. S., Tanapat, P., and Weiland, N. G. (1999). Inhibition of dendritic spine induction on hippocampal CA1 pyramidal neurons by a nonsteroidal estrogen antagonist in female rats. *Endocrinology (Baltimore)* **140**, 1044–1047.

McGaugh, J. L. (1989). Dissociating learning and performance: Drug and hormone enhancement of memory storage. *Brain Res. Bull.* **23**, 339–345.

McGaugh, J. L. (2000). Memory—a century of consolidation. *Science* **287**, 248–251.

McGaugh, J. L., Cahill, L., and Roozendaal, B. (1996). Involvement of the amygdala in memory storage: Interaction with other brain systems. *Proc. Natl. Acad. Sci. U.S.A.* **93**, 13508–13514.

McGinnis, M. Y., and Katz, S. E. (1996). Sex differences in cytosolic androgen receptors in gonadectomized male and female rats. *J. Neuroendocrinol.* **8**, 193–197.

McLay, R. N., Freeman, S. M., Harlan, R. E., and Zadina, J. E. (1999). Tests used to assess the cognitive abilities of aged rats: Their relation to each other and to hippocampal morphology and neurotrophin expression. *Gerontology* **45**, 143–155.

McMillan, P. J., Singer, C. A., and Dorsa, D. M. (1996). The effects of ovariectomy and estrogen replacement on trkA and choline acetyltransferase mRNA expression in the basal forebrain of the adult female Sprague-Dawley rat. *J. Neurosci.* **16**, 1860–1865.

McNamara, R. K., and Skelton, R. W. (1993). The neuropharmacological and neurochemical basis of place learning in the Morris water maze. *Brain Res. Brain Res. Rev.* **18**, 33–49.

McNeill, A. M., Kim, N., Duckles, S. P., Kruase, D. N., and Konotos, H. A. (1999). Chronic estrogen treatment increases levels of endothelial nitric oxide synthase protein in rat cerebral microvessels. *Stroke* **30**, 2186–2190.

Meng, Q. H., Hockerstedt, A., Heinonen, S., Wahala, K., Aldercreutz, H., and Tikkanen, M. J. (1999). Antioxidant protection of lipoproteins containing estrogens: In vitro evidence for low- and high-density lipoproteins as estrogen carriers. *Biochim. Biophys. Acta* **1439**, 331–340.

Mesulam, M. M., Mufson, E. J., Levey, A. I., and Wainer, B. H. (1983a). Cholinergic innervation of cortex by the basal forebrain: Cytochemistry and cortical connections of the septal area, diagonal band nuclei, nucleus basalis (substantia innominata), and hypothalamus in the rhesus monkey. *J. Comp. Neurol.* **214**, 170–197.

Mesulam, M. M., Mufson, E. J., Wainer, B. H., and Levey, A. I. (1983b). Central cholinergic pathways in the rat: An overview based on an alternative nomenclature (Ch1–Ch6). *Neuroscience* **10**, 1185–1201.

Meyer, T. E., and Habener, J. F. (1993). Cyclic adenosine 3′, 5-monophosphate response element binding protein (CREB) and related transcription-activating deoxyribonucleic acid-binding proteins. *Endocr. Rev.* **14**, 269–290.

Miller, W. L. (1988). Molecular biology of steroid hormones synthesis. *Endocr. Rev.* **9**, 295–318.

Milner, B. (1959). The memory defect in bilateral hippocampal lesions. *Psychiatr. Res. Rep.* **11**, 43–52.

Milner, T. A., McEwen, B. S., Hayashi, S., Li, C. J., Reagan, L. P., and Alves, S. E. (2001). Ultrastructural evidence that hippocampal alpha estrogen receptors are located at extranuclear sites. *J. Comp. Neurol.* **429**, 355–371.

Miranda, P., Williams, C. L., and Einstein, G. (1999). Granule cells in aging rats are sexually dimorphic in their response to estradiol. *J. Neurosci.* **19**, 3316–3325.

Mize, A. L., and Alper, R. H. (2000). Acute and long-term effects of 17 beta- estradiol on G(i/o) coupled neurotransmitter receptor function in the female rat brain as assessed by agonist-stimulated [35S] GTPgammaS binding. *Brain Res.* **859**, 326–333.

Moffat, S. D., and Hampson, E. (1996). A curvilinear relationship between testosterone and spatial cognition in humans: Possible influences of hand preference. *Psychoneuroendocrinology* **2**, 323–337.

Monk, D., and Brodaty, H. (2000). Use of estrogens for the prevention and treatment of Alzeihmer's disease. *Dementia. Geriatr. Cogn. Disord.* **11**, 1–10.

Mook-Jung, I., Joo, I., Sohn, S., Kwon, H. J., Huh, K., and Jung, M. W. (1997). Estrogen blocks neurotoxic effects of beta-amyloid (1–42) and induces neurite extension on B103 cells. *Neurosci. Lett.* **235**, 101–104.

Mooradian, A. D. (1993). Antioxidant properties of steroids. *J. Steroid Biochem. Mol. Biol.* **45**, 509–511.

Mor, Z. G., Nilsen, J., Horvath, T., Bechmann, I., Brown, S., Garcia-Segura, L. M., and Naftolin, F. (1999). Estrogen and microglia: A regulatory system that affects the brain. *J. Neurobiol.* **40**, 484–496.

Mora, S., Nasello, A. G., Mandelli-Lopes, M., and Diaz-Veliz, G. (1983). LHRH and rat avoidance behavior: Influence of castration and testosterone. *Physiol. Behav.* **30**, 19–22.

Mora, S., Dussaubat, N., and Diaz-Veliz, G. (1996). Effects of the estrous cycle and ovarian hormones on behavioral indices of anxiety in female rats. *Psychoneuroendocrinology* **21**, 609–620.

Morris, R. G. M. (1981). Spatial localization does not depend on the presence of local cues. *Learn. Motivation* **12**, 239–260.

Morris, R. G. M. (1984). Developments of a water-maze procedure for studying spatial learning in the rat. *J. Neurosci. Methods* **11**, 47–60.

Morris, R. G. M. (1989). Synaptic plasticity and learning: Selective impairment of learning in rats and blockade of long-term potentiation in vivo by the N-methyl-D-aspartate receptor antagonist AP5. *J. Neurosci.* **9**, 3040–3057.

Morris, R. G. M., Hagan, J. J., and Rawlins, J. N. P. (1986). Allocentric spatial learning by hippocampectomized rats: A further test of the "spatial mapping" and "working memory" theories of hippocampal function. *Q. J. Exp. Psychol.* **38B**, 365–395.

Morse, J. K. D., Dekosky, S. T., and Scheff, S. W. (1992). Neurotrophic effects of steriods on lesion-induced growth in the hippocampus: II. Hormone replacement. *Exp. Neurol.* **118**, 47–52.

Mortel, K. F., and Meyer, J. S. (1995). Lack of postmenopausal estrogen replacement therapy and the risk of dementia. *J. Neuropsychiatry Clin. Neurosci.* **7**, 334–337.

Mufson, E. J., Cai, W. J., Jaffar, S., Chen, E., Stebbins, G., Sendera, T., and Kordower, J. H. (1999). Estrogen receptor immunoreactivity within subregions of the rat forebrain: Neuronal distribution and association with perikarya containing choline acetyltransferase. *Brain Res.* **849**, 253–274.

Mulnard, R. A., Cotman, C. W., Kawas, C., van Dyck, C. H., Sano, M., Doody, R., Koss, E., Pfeiffer, E., Jin, S., Gamst, A., Grundman, M., Thomas, R., and Thal, L. J. (2000). Estrogen replacement therapy for treatment of mild to moderate Alzheimer disease: A randomized controlled study. Alzheimer's disease cooperative study. *JAMA, J. Am. Med. Assoc.* **283**, 1007–1015.

Murphy, D. D., and Segal, M. (1997). Morphological plasticity of dendritic spines in central neurons is mediated by activation of cAMP response element binding protein. *Proc. Natl. Acad. Sci. U.S.A.* **94**, 1483–1487.

Murphy, D. D., and Segal, M. (2000). Progesterone prevents estradiol-induced dendritic spine formation in cutured hippocampal neurons. *Neuroendocrinology* **72**, 133–143.

Murphy, D. D., Cole, N. B., Greenberger, V., and Segal, M. (1998). Estradiol increases dendritic spine density by reducing GABA neurotransmission in hippocampal neurons. *J. Neurosci.* **18**, 2550–2559.

Murray, C. L., and Fibiger, H. C. (1985). Learning and memory deficits after lesions of the nucleus basalis magnocellularis: Reversal by physostigmine. *Neuroscience* **14**, 1025–1032.

Nass, R., and Baker, S. (1991). Androgen effects on cognition: Congenital adrenal hyperplasia. *Psychoneuroendocrinology* **16**, 189–201.

Neave, N., Nagle, S., and Aggleton, J. P. (1997). Evidence for the involvement of the mammillary bodies and cingulum bundle in allocentric spatial processing by rats. *Eur. J. Neurosci.* **9**, 941–955.

Nelson, R. J. (2000). "An Introduction to Behavioral Endocrinology," Vol. 2. Sinauer Assoc. Sunderland, MA.

Nilsen, J., Mor, G., and Naftolin, F. (2000). Estrogen-regulated developmental neuronal apoptosis is determined by estrogen receptor subtype and the Fas/Fas ligand system. *J. Neurobiol.* **43**, 64–78.

Nomikos, G. G., and Spyraki, C. (1988). Influence of oestrogen on spontaneous and diazepam-induced evploration of rats in an elevated plus maze. *Neuropharmacology* **27**, 691–696.

Nourhashemi, F., Gillette-Guyonnet, S., Andrieu, S., Ghisolfi, A., Ousset, P. J., Grandjean, H., Grand, A., Pous, J., Vellas, B., and Albarede, J. L. (2000). Alzheimer disease: Protective factors. *Am. J. Clin. Nutr.* **71**, 643S–649S.

Ohkura, T., Isse, K., Akazawa, K., Hamamoto, M., Yaoi, Y., and Hagino, N. (1994). Evaluation of estrogen treatment in female patients with dementia of the Alzheimer type. *Endocr. J.* **41**, 361–371.

Ohkura, T., Isse, K., Akazawa, K., Hamamoto, M., Yaoi, Y., and Hagino, N. (1995). Long-term estrogen replacement therapy in female patients with dementia of the Alzheimer's type: 7 case reports. *Dementia* **6**, 99–107.

Okada, M., Hayashi, N., Kometani, M., Nakao, K., and Inukai, T. (1997). Influences of ovariectomy and continuous replacement of 17beta-estradiol on the tail skin temperature and behavior in the forced swimming test in rats. *Jpn. J. Pharmacol.* **73**, 93–96.

Okamura, H., Yokosuka, M., and Hayashi, S. (1994a). Estrogenic induction of NADPH-diaphorase activity in the preoptic neurons containing estrogen receptor immunoreactivity in the female rat. *J. Neuroendocrinol.* **6**, 597–601.

Okamura, H., Yokosuka, M., McEwen, B. S., and Hayashi, S. (1994b). Colocalization of NADPH-diaphorase and estrogen receptor immunoreactivity in the rat ventromedial hypothalmic nucleus: Stimulatory effect of estrogen on NADPH-diaphorase activity. *Endocrinology (Baltimore)* **135**, 1705–1708.

O'Keefe, J. (1979). A review of the hippocampal place cells. *Prog. Neurobiol.* **13**, 419–439.

O'Keefe, J. (1999). Do hippocampal pyramidal cells signal non-spatial as well as spatial information? *Hippocampus* **9**, 352–264.

O'Keefe, J. A., and Nadel, L. (1978). "The Hippocampus as a Cognitive Map." Oxford University Press, Oxford.

Olton, D., Markowska, A., Voytko, M. L., Givens, B., Gorman, L., and Wenk, G. (1991). Basal forebrain cholinergic system: A functional analysis. *Adv. Exp. Med. Biol.* **295**, 353–372.

Olton, D. S. (1983). The use of animal models to evaluate the effects of neurotoxins on cognitive processes. *Neurobehav. Toxicol. Teratol.* **5**, 635–640.

Olton, D. S., and Collison, C. (1979). Intramaze cues and "odor trails" fail to direct choice behavior on an elevated maze. *Anim. Learn. Behav.* **7**, 221–223.

Olton, D. S., and Papas, B. C. (1979). Spatial memory and hippocampal system function. *Neuropsychologia* **17**, 669–681.

Olton, D. S., and Samuelson, R. J. (1976). Remberance of places passed: Spatial memory in rats. *J. Exp. Psychol: Anim. Behav. Processes* **2**, 97–116.

Olton, D. S., Walker, J. A., and Gage, F. H. (1978). Hippocampal connections and spatial discrimination. *Brain Res.* **139**, 295–308.

Olton, D. S., Becker, J. T., and Handelman, G. E. (1979). Hippocampus, space, and memory. *Behav. Brain Sci.* **2**, 313–365.

O'Malley, C. A., Hautmaki, R. D., Kelley, M., and Meyer, E. M. (1987). Effects of ovariectomy and estradiol benzoate on high affinity choline uptake, ACh synthesis, and release from rat cerebral cortical synaptosomes. *Brain Res.* **403**, 389–392.

O'Neal, M. F., Means, L. W., Poole, M. C., and Hamm, R. J. (1996). Estrogen affects performance of ovariectomized rats in a two-choice water-escape working memory task. *Psychoneuroendocrinology* **21**, 51–65.

Orchinik, M., and McEwen, B. S. (1995). Rapid actions in the brain: A critique of genomic and non-genomic mechanisms. *In* "Genomic and Non-genomic Mechanisms" (M. Wehling, ed.), pp. 77–108. CRC Press, Boca Raton, FL.

Orikasa, C., McEwen, B. S., Hayashi, H., Sakuma, Y., and Hayashi, S. (2000). Estrogen receptor alpha, but not beta, is expressed in the interneurons of the hippocampus in prepubertal rats: An in situ hybridization study. *Brain Res. Dev. Brain Res.* **120**, 245–254.

Osterlund, M. K., and Hurd, Y. L. (1998). Acute 17 beta-estradiol treatment down-regulates serotonin 5HT1A receptor mRNA expression in the limbic system of female rats. *Brain Res. Mol. Brain Res.* **55**, 169–172.

Osterlund, M. K., Grandien, K., Keller, E., and Hurd, Y. L. (2000a). The human brain has distinct regional expression patterns of estrogen receptor alpha mRNA isoforms derived from alternative promoters. *J. Neurochem.* **75**, 1390–1397.

Osterlund, M. K., Halldin, C., and Hurd, Y. L. (2000b). Effects of chronic 17 beta-estradiol treatment on the serotonin 5-HT(1A) receptor mRNA and binding levels in the rat brain. *Synapse* **35**, 39–44.

Packard, M. G. (1998). Posttraining estrogen and memory modulation. *Horm. Behav.* **34**, 126–139.

Packard, M. G., and McGaugh, J. L. (1992). Double dissociation of fornix and caudate nucleus lesions on acquisition of two water maze tasks: Further evidence for multiple memory systems. *Behav. Neurosci.* **106**, 436–446.

Packard, M. G., and Teather, L. A. (1997a). Posttraining estradiol injections enhance memory in ovariectomized rats: Cholinergic blockade and synergism. *Neurobiol. Learn. Mem.* **68**, 172–188.

Packard, M. G., and Teather, L. A. (1997b). Intra-hippocampal estradiol infusion enhances memory in ovariectomized rats. *NeuroReport* **8**, 3009–3013.

Packard, M. G., and Teather, L. A. (1998). Amygdala modulation of multiple memory systems: Hippocampus and caudate-putamen. *Neurobiol. Learn. Mem.* **69**, 163–203.

Packard, M. G., and White, N. M. (1990). Lesions of the caudate nucleus selectively impair "reference memory" acquisition in the radial maze. *Behav. Neural. Biol.* **53**, 39–50.

Packard, M. G., Hirsh, R., and White, N. M. (1989). Differential effects of fornix and caudate nucleus lesions on two radial maze tasks: Evidence for multiple memory systems. *J. Neurosci.* **9**, 1465–1472.

Packard, M. G., Cahill, L., and McGaugh, J. L. (1994). Amygdala modulation of hippocampal-dependent and caudate nucleus-dependent memory processes. *Proc. Natl. Acad. Sci. U.S.A.* **91**, 8477–8481.

Packard, M. G., Kohlmaier, J. R., and Alexander, G. M. (1996). Post-training intra-hippocampal estradiol injections enhance spatial memory in male rats: Interaction with cholinergic systems. *Behav. Neurosci.* **110**, 626–632.

Paech, K., Webb, P., Kuiper, G. G., Nilsson, S., Gustafsson, J., Kushner, P. J., and Scanlan, T. S. (1997). Differential ligand activation of estrogen receptors ERalpha and ERbeta at AP1 sites. *Science* **277**, 1508–1510.

Paganini-Hill, A., and Henderson, V. W. (1994). Estrogen deficiency and risk of Alzheimer's disease in women. *Am. J. Epidemiol.* **140**, 256–261.

Palinkas, L. A., and Barrett-Connor, E. (1992). Estrogen use and depressive symptoms in postmenopausal women. *Obstet. Gynecol.* **80**, 30–36.

Panakhova, E., Buresova, O., and Bures, J. (1984). The effect of hypothermia on the rat's spatial memory in the water tank task. *Behav. Neural Biol.* **42**, 191–196.

Pang, K. C. H., and Nocera, R. (1999). Interaction between 192-IgG saporin and intraseptal cholinergic and GABAergic drugs: Role of cholinergicmedial septal neurons in spatial working memory. *Behav. Neurosci.* **113**, 265–275.

Panickar, K. S., Guan, G., King, M. A., Rajakumar, G., and Simpkins, J. W. (1997). 17beta-estradiol attenuates CREB decline in the rat hippocampus following seizure. *J. Neurobiol.* **33**, 961–967.

Parlee, M. B. (1983). Menstrual rhythms in sensory processes: A review of fluctuations in vision, olfaction, audition, taste, and touch. *Psychol. Bull.* **93**, 539–548.

Patrone, C., Pollio, G., Vegeto, E., Enmark, E., de Curtis, I., Gustafsson, J. A., and Maggi, A. (2000). Estradiol induces differential neuronal phenotypes by activating estrogen receptor alpha or beta. *Endocrinology (Baltimore)* **141**, 1839–1845.

Pau, C. Y., Pau, K. Y., and Spies, H. G. (1998). Putative estrogen receptor beta and alpha mRNA expression in male and female rhesus macaques. *Mol. Cell. Endocrinol.* **25**, 59–68.

Pellow, S., and File, S. E. (1986). Anxiolyic and anxiogenic drug effects on exploratory activity in an elevated plus-maze: A novel test of anxiety in the rat. *Pharmacol., Biochem. Behav.* **24**, 525–529.

Penfield, W., and Milner, B. (1958). Memory deficit produced by bilateral lesions in the hippocampal zone. *Arch. Neurol. Psychiatry.* **79**, 475–497.

Perrot-Sinal, T. S., Kostenuik, M. A., Ossenkopp, K. P., and Kavaliers, M. (1996). Sex differences in performance in the Morris water maze and the effects of initial nonstationary hidden platform training. *Behav. Neurosci.* **110**, 1309–1320.

Petanceska, S. S., Nagy, V., Frail, D., and Gandy, S. (2000). Ovariectomy and 17beta-estradiol modulate the levels of Alzheimer's amyloid beta peptides in brain. *Neurology* **54**, 2212–2217.

Pfaff, D. W. (1972). Steroid sex hormones in the rat brain: Specificity of uptake and physiological effects. *UCLA Forum Med. Sci.* **15**, 103–112.

Pfaff, D. W. (1980). "Estrogens and Brain Function." Springer-Verlag, New York.

Pfaff, D. W., and Keiner, M. (1973). Atlas of estradiol-concentrating cells in the central nervous system of the female rat. *J. Comp. Neurol.* **151**, 121–158.

Pfaff, D. W., Schwartz-Giblin, S., and McCarthy, M. M. (1994). Cellular and molecular mechanisms of female reproductive behaviors. *In* "The Physiology of Reproduction" (E. Knobil and J. Neill, eds.), Vol. 2, pp. 107–220. Raven Press, New York.

Phillips, S. M., and Sherwin, B. B. (1992a). Effects of estrogen on memory function in surgically menopausal women. *Psychoneuroendocrinology* **17**, 485–495.

Phillips, S. M., and Sherwin, B. B. (1992b). Variations in memory function and sex steroid hormones across the menstrual cycle. *Psychoneuroendocrinology* **17**, 497–506.

Pike, C. J. (1999). Estrogen modulates neuronal Bcl-xL expression and beta-amyloid-induced apoptosis: Relevance to Alzheimer's disease. *J. Neurochem.* **72**, 1552–1563.

Plouffe, L., and Simon, J. A. (1998). Androgen effects in the central nervous system in the postmenopausal woman. *Semin. Reprod. Endocrinol.* **16**, 135–143.

Polo-Kantola, P., Portin, R., Polo, O., Helenius, H., Irjala, K., and Erkkola, R. (1998). The effect of short-term estrogen replacement therapy on cognition: A randomized, double blind, cross-over trial in postmenopausal women. *Obstet. Gynecol.* **91**, 459–466.

Pomerantz, S. M., and Sholl, S. A. (1987). Analysis of sex and regional differences in androgen receptors in fetal rhesus monkey brain. *Brain Res.* **433**, 151–154.

Porter, M., Penney, G. C., Russell, D., Russell, E., and Templeton, A. (1996). A population based survey of women's experience of the menopause. *Br. J. Obstet. Gynaecol.* **103**, 1025–1028.

Postma, A., Winkel, J., Tuiten, A., and van Honk, J. (1999). Sex differences and menstural cycle effects in human spatial memory. *Psychoneuroendocrinology* **24**, 175–192.

Postma, A., Meyer, G., Tuiten, A., van Honk, J., Kessels, R. P., and Thijssen, J. (2000). Effects of testosterone administration on selective aspects of object-location memory in healthy young women. *Psychoneuroendocrinology* **25**, 563–575.

Puy, L., MacLusky, N. J., Becker, L., Karsan, N., Trachtenberg, J., and Brown, T. J. (1995). Immunocytochemical detection of androgen receptor in human temporal cortex characterization and application of polyclonal and androgen receptor antibodies in frozen and paraffin-embedded tissues. *J. Steroid Biochem. Mol. Biol.* **55**, 197–209.

Pych, J. C., Markham, J. A., and Juraska, J. M. (2000). Chronic and acute replacement of ovarian steroids to aged female rats improves performance on the Morris water maze. *Soc. Neurosci. Abstr.* **26**, No. 651.7.

Rachman, I. M., Unnerstall, J. R., Pfaff, D. W., and Cohen, R. S. (1998). Regulation of neuronal nitric oxide synthase mRNA in lordosis-relevant neurons of the ventromedial hypothalamus following short-term estrogen treatment. *Brain Res. Mol. Brain Res.* **59**, 105–108.

Rauramo, L., Langerspetz, K., Engblom, P., and Punnonen, R. (1975). The effect of castration and peroral estrogen therapy on some psychological function. *Front. Horm. Res.* **8**, 133–151.

Rawlins, J. N. P., and Deacon, R. M. J. (1993). Further developments of maze procedures. *In* "Behavioral Neuroscience" (A. Sahgal, ed.), Vol. 1, pp. 95–106. Oxford University Press, New York.

Razandi, M., Pedram, A., Greene, G. L., and Levin, E. R. (1999). Cell membranes and nuclear estrogen receptors (ERs) originate from a single transcript: Studies of ERα and ERβ expressed in Chinese hamster ovary cells. *Mol. Endocrinol.* **13**, 307–319.

Rempel-Clower, N. L., Zola, S. M., Squire, L. R., and Amaral, D. G. (1996). Three cases of enduring memory impairment after bilateral damage limited to the hippocampal formation. *J. Neurosci.* **16**, 5233–5255.

Resnick, S. M., Berenbaum, S., Gottesman, I., and Bouchard, T. (1986). Early hormonal influences on cognitive functioning in congenital adrenal hyperplasia. *Dev. Psychol.* **22**, 191–198.

Resnick, S. M., Metter, E. J., and Zonderman, A. B. (1997). Estrogen replacement therapy and longitudinal decline in visual memory: A possible protective effect? *Neurology* **49**, 1491–1497.

Resnick, S. M., Maki, P. M., Golski, S., Kraut, M. A., and Zonderman, A. B. (1998). Effects of estrogen replacement therapy on PET cerebral blood flow and neuropsychological performance. *Horm. Behav.* **34**, 171–182.

Rice, M. M., Graves, A. B., McCurry, S. M., and Larson, E. B. (1997). Estrogen replacement therapy and cognitive function in postmenopausal women without dementia. The role of estrogen in the treatment and prevention of dementia. *Am. J. Med.* **103**(Suppl. 5), 26S–35S.

Riley, J. N., and Moore, R. Y. (1981). Diencephalic and brain-stem afferents to the hippocampal formation of the rat. *Brain Res. Bull.* **6**, 437–444.

Rissanen, A., Puolivali, J., van Groen, T., and Riekkinen, P. (1999). In mice tonic estrogen replacement therapy improves non-spatial and spatial memory in a water maze task. *NeuroReport* **10**, 1369–1372.

Rivas-Arancibia, S., and Vazquez-Pereyra, F. (1994). Hormonal modulation of extinction responses induced by sexual steroid hormones in rats. *Life Sci.* **54**, 363–367.

Robel, P., Young, J., Corpechot, C., Mayo, W., Perche, F., Haug, M., Simon, H., and Baulieu, E. E. (1995). Biosynthesis and assay of neurosteroids in rats and mice: Functional correlates. *J. Steroid Biochem. Mol. Biol.* **53**, 355–360.

Robinson, R., Friedman, L., Marcus, R., Tinklenberg, J., and Yesavage, J. (1994). Estrogen replacement therapy and memory in older women. *J. Am. Geriatr. Soc.* **42**, 919–922.

Rolls, E. T. (2000). Memory systems in the brain. *Annu. Rev. Psychol.* **51**, 599–630.

Roof, R. L. (1993). Neonatal exogenous testosterone modifies sex difference in radial arm and Morris water maze performance in prepubescent and adult rats. *Behav. Brain Res.* **53**, 1–10.

Roof, R. L., and Hall, E. D. (2000). Gender differences in acute CNS trauma and stroke: Neuroprotective effects of estrogen and progesterone. *J. Neurotrauma.* **17**, 367–388.

Roof, R. L., and Havens, M. D. (1992). Testosterone improves maze performance and induces development of a male hippocampus in females. *Brain Res.* **572**, 310–313.

Roof, R. L., Duvdevani, R., and Stein, D. G. (1992). Progesterone treatment attenuated brain edema following contusion injury in male and female rats. *Restorative Neurol. Neurosci.* **4**, 425–427.

Roof, R. L., Duvdevani, R., and Stein, D. G. (1993). Gender influences outcome of brain injury: Progesterone plays a protective role. *Brain Res.* **607**, 333–336.

Roof, R. L., Duvdevani, R., Braswell, L., and Stein, D. G. (1994). Progesterone facilitates cognitive recovery and reduces secondary neuronal loss caused by cortical contusion injury in male rats. *Exp. Neurol.* **129**, 64–69.

Roof, R. L., Hoffman, S. W., and Stein, D. G. (1997). Progesterone protects against lipid peroxidation following traumatic brain injury in rats. *Mol. Chem. Neuropathol.* **31**, 1–11.

Rosenstock, J., Field, T. D., and Greene, E. (1977). The role of mammillary bodies in spatial memory. *Exp. Neurol.* **55**, 340–352.

Rothblat, R. A., and Hayes, L. L. (1987). Short-term object recognition in the rat: Nonmatching with trial-unique junk stimuli. *Behav. Neurosci.* **101**, 587–590.

Rowan, B. G., and O'Malley, B. W. (2000). Progesterone receptor coactivators. *Steroids* **65**, 545–549.

Rudick, C. N., and Woolley, C. S. (2000). Estradiol induces a phasic fos response in the hippocampal CA1 and CA3 regions of adult female rats. *Hippocampus* **10**, 274–283.

Sahgal, A. (1993). Practical behavioral neuroscience: Problems, pitfalls, and suggestions. *In* "Behavioural Neuroscience" (A. Sahgal, ed.), Vol. 1, pp 1–8. Oxford University Press, New York.

Saldana, C. J., Clayton, N. S., and Schlinger, B. A. (1999). Androgen metabolism in the juvenile oscine forebrain: A cross-species analysis at neural sites implicated in memory function. *J. Neurobiol.* **40**, 397–406.

Sandstrom, N. J., Kaufman, J., and Huettel, S. A. (1998). Males and females use different distal cues in a virtual environment navigation task. *Brain Res. Cogn. Res.* **6**(4), 351–360.

Sandstrom, N. J., Einstein, G., and Williams, C. L. (1999). Acute estradiol replacement enhances spatial working memory retention in female rats. *Soc. Behav. Neuroendocrinol.* **3**, 205.

Sarrieau, A., Mitchell, J. B., Lal, S., Olivier, A., Quirion, R., and Meaney, M. J. (1990). Androgen binding sites in human temporal cortex. *Neuroendocrinology* **51**, 713–716.

Saucier, D., and Cain, D. P. (1995). Spatial learning without NMDA receptor dependent long-term potentiation. *Nature (London)* **378**, 186–189.

Saucier, D., Hargreaves, E. L., Boon, F., Vanderwolf, C. H., and Cain, D. P. (1996). Detailed behavioral analysis of water maze acquisition under systemic NMDA or muscarinic antagonism: Nonspatial pretraning eliminates spatial learning deficts. *Behav. Neurosci.* **110**, 103–116.

Sawyer, T. F., Hengehold, A. K., and Perez, W. A. (1984). Chemosensory and hormonal mediation of social memory in male rats. *Behav. Neurosci.* **98**, 908–913.

Schmidt, B. M. W., Gerdes, D., Feuring, M., Falkenstein, E., Christ, M., and Wheling, M. (2000). Rapid, nongenomic steroid actions: A new age? *Front. Neuroendocrinol.* **21**, 57–94.

Schneider, L. S., Farlow, M. R., Henderson, V. W., and Pogoda, J. M. (1996). Effects of estrogen replacement therapy on response to tacrine in patients with Alzheimer's disease. *Neurolology* **46**, 1580–1584.

Schumacher, M., Guennoun, R., Robel, P., and Baulieu, E. E. (1997). Neurosteroids in the hippocampus: Neuronal plasticity and memory. *Stress* **2**, 65–78.

Scoville, W. B., and Milner, B. (1957). Loss of recent memory after bilateral hippocampal lesions. *J. Neurol. Neurosurg. Psychiatry* **20**, 11–21.

Selkoe, D. J. (1996). Amyloid beta-protein and the genectis of Alzheimer's disease. *J. Biol. Chem.* **271**, 18295–18298.

Sfikakis, A., Spyraki, C., Sitaris, N., and Varonos, D. (1978). Implication of the estrous cycle on conditioned avoidance behavior in the rat. *Physiol. Behav.* **21**, 441–446.

Sfikakis, A., Malicianos, C., and Constandi, M. (1984). Compensatory adrenal growth and conditioned avoidance response in relation to oestrous cycle and metoclopramide induced constant dioestrus. *Acta Endocrinol. Suppl. (Copenhagen)* **265**, 12–14.

Shapiro, M. L., and Eichenbaum, H. (1999). Hippocampus as a memory map: Synaptic plasticity and memory encoding by hippocampal neurons. *Hippocampus* **9**, 365–384.

Shaywitz, B. A., and Shaywitz, S. E. (2000). Estrogen and Alzheimer disease: Plausible theory, negative clinical trial. *JAMA, J. Am. Med. Assoc.* **283**, 1055–1056.

Shaywitz, S. E., Shaywitz, B. A., Pugh, K. R., Fulbright, R. K., Skudlarski, P., Mencl, W. E., Constable, R. T., Naftolin, F., Palter, S. F., Marchione, K. E., Katz, L., Shankweiler, D. P., Fletcher, J. M., Lacadie, C., Keltz, M., and Gore, J. C. (1999). Effect of estrogen on brain activation patterns in postmenopausal women during working memory tasks. *JAMA, J. Am. Med. Assoc.* **281**, 1197–1202.

Shen, J., Barnes, C. A., Wenk, G. L., and McNaughton, B. L. (1996). Differential effects of selective immunotoxic lesions of medial septal cholinergic cells on spatial working and reference memory. *Behav. Neurosci.* **110**, 1181–1186.

Sherry, D. F., and Hampson, E. (1977). Evolution and the hormonal control of sexually-dimorphic spatial abilities in humans. *Trends Cogn. Sci.* **1**, 50–55.

Sherwin, B. B. (1988). Affective changes with estrogen and androgen replacement therapy in surgically menopausal women. *J. Affec. Dis.* **14**, 177–187.

Sherwin, B. B. (1994). Estrogenic effects on memory in women. *Ann. N. Y. Acad. Sci.* **743**, 213–232.

Sherwin, B. B. (1996). Hormones, mood, and cognitive functioning in postmenopausal women. *Obstet. Gynecol.* **87**, 20S–26S.

Sherwin, B. B. (1997). Estrogen effects on cognition in menopausal women. *Neurology* **48**(Suppl. 7), S21–S26.

Sherwin, B. B. (1998). Estrogen and cognitive functioning in women. *Proc. Soc. Exp. Biol. Med.* **217**, 17–22.

Sherwin, B. B., and Gelfand, M. M. (1989). A prospective one-year study of estrogen and progestin in postmenopausal women: Effects on clinical symptoms and lipoproteins lipids. *Obstet. Gynecol.* **73**, 759–766.

Sherwin, B. B., and Phillips, S. (1990). Estrogen and cognitive functioning in surgically menopausal women. *Ann. N. Y. Acad. Sci.* **592**, 474–475.

Sherwin, B. B., and Tulandi, T. (1996). "Add-back" estrogen reverses cognitive deficits induced by a gonadotropin-releasing hormone agonist in women with leiomyomata uteri. *J. Clin. Endocrinol. Metab.* **81**, 2545–2549.

Shi, J., and Simpkins, J. W. (1997). 17 beta-estradiol modulation of glucose transporter 1 expression in blood-brain barrier. *Am. J. Physiol.* **272**, E1016–1022.

Shi, J., Zhang, Y. Q., and Simpkins, J. W. (1997). Effects of 17beta-estradiol on glucose transporter 1 expression and endothelial cells survival following focal ischemia in the rats. *Exp. Brain Res.* **117**, 200–206.

Shors, T. J., Lewczyk, C., Pacynski, M., Mathew, P. R., and Pickett, J. (1998). Stages of estrous mediate the stress-induced impairment of associative learning in the female rat. *NeuroReport* **3**, 419–423.

Shughrue, P. J. (1998). Estrogen action in the estrogen receptor alpha-knockout mouse: Is this due to ER-beta? *Mol. Psychiatry.* **3**, 299–302.

Shughrue, P. J., and Merchenthaler, I. (2000). Evidence for novel estrogen binding sites in the rat hippocampus. *Neuroscience* **99**, 605–612.

Shughrue, P. J., Lane, M. V., and Merchenthaler, I. (1997). Comparative distribution of estrogen receptor-alpha and -beta mRNA in the rat central nervous system. *J. Comp. Neurol.* **388**, 507–525.

Shughrue, P. J., Scrimo, P. J., and Merchenthaler, I. (2000). Estrogen binding and estrogen receptor characterization (ER alpha and ER beta) in the cholinergic neurons of the rat basal forebrain. *Neuroscience* **96**, 41–49.

Shumaker, S. A., Reboussin, B. A., Espeland, M. A., Rapp, S. R., McBee, W. L., Dailey, M., Bowen, D., Terrell, T., and Jones, B. N. (1998). The Women's Health Initiative Study (WHIMS): A trial of the effect of estrogen therapy in preventing and slowing the progression of dementia. *Controlled Clin. Trials* **19**, 604–621.

Shute, C. C., and Lewis, P. R. (1967). The ascending cholinergic reticular system: Neocortical, olfactory and subcortical projections. *Brain* **90**, 497–520.

Simerly, R. B., Chang, C., Muramatsu, M., and Swanson, L. W. (1990). Distribution of androgen and estrogen receptor mRNA-containing cells in the rat brain: An in situ hydridization study. *J. Comp. Neurol.* **294**, 76–95.

Simpkins, J. W. (1995). Effects of age, reproductive status and ambient temperature on skin temperature regulation in the female rat. *Maturitas* **21**, 97–102.

Simpkins, J. W., Green, P. S., Gridley, K. E., Singh, M., de Fiebre, N. C., and Rajakumar, G. (1997). Role of estrogen replacement therapy in memory enhancement and the prevention of neuronal loss associated with Alzheimer's disease. The role of estrogen in the treatment and prevention of dementia. *Am. J. Med.* **103**(Suppl. 4), S19–S25.

Singer, C. A., Rogers, K. L., Strickland, T. M., and Dorsa, D. M. (1996). Estrogen protects primary cortical neurons from glutamate toxicity. *Neurosci. Lett.* **212**, 13–16.

Singer, C. A., Figueroa-Masot, X. A., Batchelor, R. H., and Dorsa, D. M. (1999). The mitogen-activated protein kinase pathway mediates estrogen neuroprotection after glutamate toxicity in primary cortical neurons. *J. Neurosci.* **19**, 2455–2463.

Singh, M., Meyer, E. M., Millard, W. J., and Simpkins, J. W. (1994). Ovarian steroid deprivation results in a reversible learning impairment and compromised cholinergic function in female Sprague-Dawley rats. *Brain Res.* **644**, 305–312.

Singh, M., Setalo, G., Guan, X., Warren, M., and Toran-Allerand, C. D. (1999). Estrogen-induced activation of mitogen-activated protein kinase in cerebral cortical explants: Convergence of estrogen and neurotrophin signaling pathways. *J. Neurosci.* **19**, 1179–1188.

Singh, M., Setalo, G., Guan, X., Frail, D. E., and Toran-Allerand, C. D. (2000). Estrogen-induced activation of the mitogen-activated protein kinase cascade in the cerebral cortex of estrogen receptor-alpha knock-out mice. *J. Neurosci.* **20**, 1694–1700.

Skoog, I., and Gustafson, D. (1999). HRT and dementia. *J. Epidemiol. Biostat.* **4**, 227–251.

Slob, A. K., Bogers, H., and van Stolk, M. A. (1981). Effects of gonadectomy and exogenous gonadal steroids on sex differences in open field behavior of adult rats. *Behav. Brain Res.* **2**, 347–362.

Slooter, A. J., Bronzova, J., Witteman, J. C., Van Broeckhoven, C., Hofman, A., and van Duijn, C. M. (1999). Estrogen use and early onset Alzheimer's disease: A population-based study. *J. Neurol. Neurosurg. Psychiatry* **67**, 779–781.

Smith, S. T., Stackman, R. W., and Clark, A. S. (1996). Spatial working memory is preserved in rats treated with anabolic-androgenic steroids. *Brain Res.* **737**, 313–316.

Spear, N. E., Miller, J. S., and Jagielo, J. A. (1990). Animal learning and memory. *Annu. Rev. Psychol.* **41**, 169–211.

Squire, L. R. (1987). "Memory and Brain." Oxford University Press, New York.

Squire, L. R. (1992). Memory and the hippocampus: A synthesis from findings with rats, monkeys, and humans. *Psychol. Rev.* **99**, 195–231.

Squire, L. R., and Cohen, N. J. (1984). Human memory and amnesia. *In* "Neurobiology of Learning and Memory" (G. Lynch, J. L. McGaugh, and N. M. Weinberger, eds.), pp. 3–64. Guilford Press, New York.

Stackman, R. W., Blasberg, M. E., Langan, C. J., and Clark, A. S. (1997). Stability of spatial working memory across the estrous cycle of Long-Evans rats. *Neurobiol. Learn. Mem.* **67**, 167–171.

Stampfer, M. J., Colditz, G. A., Willett, W. C. *et al.* (1991). Postmenopausal estrogen therapy and cardiovascular disease. Ten year follow-up from the nurses' health study. *N. Engl. J. Med.* **325**, 756–762.

Steele, R. J., and Morris, R. G. (1999). Delay-dependent impairment of a matching-to-place task with chronic and intrahippocampal infusion of the NMDA- antagonist D-AP5. *Hippocampus* **9**, 118–136.

Steenbergen, H. L., Heinsbroek, R. P., Van Hest, A., and Van de Poll, N. E. (1990). Sex-dependent effects of inescapable shock administration on shuttlebox-escape performance and elevated plus-maze behavior. *Physiol. Behav.* **48**, 571–576.

Steffens, D. C., Norton, M. C., Plassman, B. L., Tschanz, J. T., Wyse, B. W., Welsh-Bohmer, K. A., Anthony, J. C., and Breitner, J. C. (1999). Enhanced cognitive performance with estrogen use in nondemented community-dwelling older women. *J. Am. Geriatr. Soc.* **47**, 1171–1175.

Steward, O. (1976). Topographic organization of the projections from the entorhinal area to the hippocampal formation of the rat. *J. Comp. Neurol.* **167**, 285–314.

Steward, O., and Scoville, S. A. (1976). Cells of origin of entorhinal cortical afferents to the hippocampus and fascia dentata of the rat. *J. Comp. Neurol.* **169**, 347–370.

Stewart, C. A., and Morris, R. G. M. (1993). The watermaze. *In* "Behavioral Neuroscience" (A. Sahgal, ed.), Vol. 1, pp. 107–122. Oxford University Press, New York.

Stock, H. S., Ford, K., and Wilson, M. A. (2000). Gender and gonadal hormone effects in the olfactory bulbectomy animal model of depression. *Pharmacol., Biochem. Behav.* **67**, 183–191.

Stone, C. P., and Commins, W. D. (1936). The effect of castration at various ages upon the learning ability of male albino rats: II. *J. Genet. Psychol.* **48**, 20–28.

Stone, D. J., Rozovsky, I., Morgan, T., Anderson, T. E., and Finch, C. P. (1998). Increased synaptic sprouting in response to estrogen via an apolipoprotein E-dependent mechanism: Implications for Alzheimer's disease. *J. Neurosci.* **18**, 3180–3185.

Stumpf, W. E., and Sar, M. (1979). Steroid hormone target cells in the extrahypothalamic brain stem and cervical spinal cord: Neuroendocrine significance. *J. Steroid Biochem.* **11**, 801–807.

Suzuki, S., Augerinos, G., and Black, A. H. (1980). Stimulus control of spatial behavior on the eight-arm radial maze in rats. *Learn. Motivation* **11**, 1–18.

Svensson, A. L., and Nordberg, A. (1999). Beta-estradiol attenuate amyloid beta-peptide toxicity via nicotinic receptors. *NeuroReport* **10**, 3485–3489.

Swanson, L. W. (1982). The projections of the ventral tegmental area and adjacent regions: A combined fluorescent retrograde tracer and immunofluorescence study in the rat. *Brain Res. Bull.* **9**, 321–353.

Swanson, L. W., and Hartman, B. K. (1975). The central adrenergic system. An immunofluorescence study of the location of cell bodies and their efferent connections in the rat utilizing dopamine-beta-hydroxylase as a marker. *J. Comp. Neurol.* **163**, 467–505.

Sziklas, V., and Petrides, M. (1993). Memory impairments following lesions to the mammillary region of the rat. *Eur. J. Neurosci.* **5**, 525–540.

Sziklas, V., and Petrides, M. (1998). Memory and the region of the mammillary bodies. *Prog. Neurobiol.* **54**, 55–70.

Sziklas, V., Petrides, M., and Leri, F. (1996). The effects of lesions to the mammillary region and the hippocampus on conditional associative learning by rats. *Eur. J. Neurosci.* **8**, 106–115.

Tang, M., Jacobs, D., Stern, Y., Marder, K., Schofield, P., Gurland, B., and Andrews, H. (1996). Effect of oestrogen during menopause on risk and age at onset of Alzheimer's disease. *Lancet* **348**, 429–432.

Tartelin, M. F., and Gorski, R. A. (1971). Variations in food and water intake in the normal and acyclic female rat. *Physiol. Behav.* **7**, 847–852.

Taube, J. S. (1999). Some thoughts on place cells and the hippocampus. *Hippocampus* **9**, 452–457.

Telegdy, G., and Stark, A. (1973). Effect of sexual steroids and androgen sterilization on avoidance and exploratory behavior in the rat. *Acta Physiol. Acad. Sci. Hung.* **43**, 55–63.

Telegdy, G., Hadnagy, J., and Lissak, K. (1968). The effect of gonads on conditioned avoidance behavior of rats. *Acta Physiol Acad Sci. Hung.* **33**, 439–446.

Thomas, D. K., Storlien, L. H., Bellingham, W. P., and Gillette, K. (1986). Ovarian hormone effects on activity, glucoregulation and thyroid hormones in the rat. *Physiol. Behav.* **36**, 567–573.

Thomas, T., Rhodin, J. A., Sutton, E. T., Byrant, M. W., and Price, J. M. (1999). Estrogen protects peripheral and cerebral blood vessels from toxicity of Alzheimer peptide amyloid-beta and inflammatory reaction. *J. Submicrosc. Cytol. Pathol.* **31**, 571–579.

Tirassa, P., Thiblin, I., Agren, G., Vigneti, E., Aloe, L., and Stenfors, C. (1997). High-dose anabolic androgenic steroids modulate concentrations of nerve growth factor and expression of its low affinity receptor (p75-NGFr) in male rat brain. *J. Neurosci. Res.* **47**, 198–207.

Tohgi, H., Utsugisawa, K., Yamagata, M., and Yoshimura, M. (1995). Effects of age on messenger RNA expression of glucocorticoid, thyroid hormone, androgen, and estrogen receptors in postmortem human hippocampus. *Brain Res.* **700**, 245–253.

Tolman, E. C. (1949). There is more than one kind of learning. *Psych. Rev.* **56**, 144–155.

Toran-Allerand, C. D. (1984). Gonadal hormones and brain development: Implications for the genesis of sexual differentiation. *Ann. N. Y. Acad. Sci.* **435**, 101–111.

Toran-Allerand, C. D. (1991). Organotypic culture of the developing cerebral cortex and hypothalamus: Relevance to sexual differentiation. *Psychoneuroendocrinology* **16**, 7–24.

Toran-Allerand, C. D., Miranda, R. C., Bentham, W. D. L., Sohrabji, F., Brown, T. J., Hochberg, R. B., and MacLusky, N. J. (1992). Estrogen receptors colocalize with low-affinity nerve growth factor receptors in cholinergic neurons of the basal forebrain. *Proc. Natl. Acad. Sci. U.S.A.* **89,** 4668–4672.

Toran-Allerand, C. D., Singh, M., and Setalo, G. (1999). Novel mechanisms of estrogen action in the brain: New players in an old story. *Front. Neuroendocrinol.* **20,** 97–121.

Torres, E. M., Perry, T. A., Blokland, A., Wilkinson, L. S., Wiley, R. G., Lappis, D. A., and Dunnett, S. B. (1994). Behavioral histochemical and biochemical consequences of selective immunolesions in discrete regions of the basal forebrain cholinergic system. *Neuroscience* **63,** 95–122.

Van der Zee, E. A., and Luiten, P. G. (1994). Cholinergic and GABAergic neurons in the rat medial septum express muscarinic acetycholine receptors. *Brain Res.* **652,** 263–272.

van Duijn, C. M. (1999). Hormone replacement therapy and Alzheimer's disease. *Maturitas* **31,** 201–205.

van Goozen, S. H., Cohen-Kettenis, P. T., Gooren, L. J., Frijda, N. H., and van den Poll, N. E. (1994). Activating effects of androgens on cognitive performance: Causal evidence in a group of female-to-male transsexuals. *Neuropsychologia* **32,** 1153–1157.

van Goozen, S. H., Cohen-Kettenis, P. T., Gooren, L. J., Frijda, N. H., and van den Poll, N. E. (1995). Gender differences in behavior: Activating effects of cross-sex hormones. *Psychoneuroendocrinology* **20,** 343–363.

van Haaren, F., Wouters, M., and van den Poll, N. E. (1987). Absence of behavioral differences between male and female rats in different radial-maze procedures. *Physiol. Behav.* **39,** 409–412.

van Haaren, F., van Hest, A., and Heinsbroek, R. P. (1990). Behavioral differences between male and female rats: Effects of gonadal hormones on learning and memory. *Neurosci. Biobehav. Rev.* **14,** 23–33.

van Hest, A., van Haaren, F., and van den Poll, N. E. (1987). Behavioral differences between male and female Wistar rats in food rewarded lever holding. *Physiol. Behav.* **39,** 263–267.

Vanhulle, G., and Demol, R. (1976). A double-blind study into the influence of estriol on a number of psychological tests in post-menopausal women. *In* "Consensus on the Menopause Research" (P. A. van Keep, R. B. Greenblatt, and M. Albeaux-Fernet, eds.), pp. 94–99. MTP Press, London.

van Wimersma Greidanus, T. B. (1977). Pregnene-type steroids and impairment of passive avoidance behavior in rats. *Horm. Behav.* **9,** 49–56.

Vasquez-Pereyra, F., Rivas-Arancibia, S., Loaeza-Del Castillo, A., and Schneider-Rivas, S. (1995). Modulation of short term and long term memory by steroid sexual hormones. *Life Sci.* **56,** 255–260.

Vassar, R., Bennett, B. D., Babu-Khan, S., Mendiaz, E. A., Denis, P., Teplow, D. B., Ross, S., Amarante, P., Loeloff, R., Luo, Y., Fisher, S., Fuller, J., Edenson, S., Lile, J., Jarosinski, M. A., Biere, A. L., Curran, E., Burgess, T., Louis, J. C., Collins, F., Treanor, J., Rogers, G., and Citron, M. (1999). Beta-secretase cleavate of Alzheimer's amyloid precursor protein by the transmembrane aspartic protease BACE. *Science* **286,** 735–741.

Vedder, H., Anthes, N., Stumm, G., Wurz, C., Behl, C., and Krieg, J. C. (1999). Estrogen hormones reduce lipid peroxidation in cells and tissues of the central nervous system. *J. Neurochem.* **72,** 2531–2538.

Verghese, J., Kuslansky, G., Katz, M. J., Sliwinski, M., Crystal, H. A., Buschke, H., and Lipton, R. B. (2000). Cognitive performance in surgically menopausal women on estrogen. *Neurology* **55,** 872–874.

Vertes, R. P. (1992). PHA-L analysis of projections from the supramammillary nucleus in the rat. *J. Comp. Neurol.* **326,** 595–622.

Vertes, R. P., and Kocsis, B. (1997). Brainstem-diencephalo-septohippocampal systems controlling the theta rhythm of the hippocampus. *Neuroscience* **81,** 893–926.

Vertes, R. P., and McKenna, J. T. (2000). Collateral projections from the supramammillary nucleus to the medial septum and hippocampus. *Synapse* **38,** 281–293.

Victor, M., Adams, F. D., and Colling, G. D. (1971). "The Wernicke-Korsakoff Syndrome." Blackwell, Oxford.

Voytko, M. L. (2000). The effects of long-term ovariectomy and estrogen replacement therapy on learning and memory in monkeys (*Macaca fasicularis*). *Behav. Neurosci.* **114,** 1078–1087.

Wade, G. N. (1975). Some effects of ovarian hormones on food intake and body weight in female rats. *J. Comp. Physiol. Psychol.* **88,** 183–193.

Wade, G. N. (1976). Sex hormones, regulatory behaviors and body weight. *Adv. Study Behav.* **6,** 201–276.

Wainer, B. H., Bolam, J. P., Freund, T. F., Henderson, Z., Totterdell, S., and Smith, A. D. (1984). Cholinergic synapses in the rat brain: A correlated light and electron microscopic immunohistochemical study employing a monoclonal antibody against choline acetyltransferase. *Brain Res.* **308,** 69–76.

Walker, J. A., and Olton, D. S. (1979). Spatial memory deficit following fimbria-fornix lesions: Independent of time for stimulus processing. *Physiol. Behav.* **23,** 11–15.

Walsh, T. J., Herzog, C. D., Gandhi, C., Stackman, R. W., and Wiley, R. G. (1996). Injection of IgG 192-saporin into the medial septum produces cholinergic hypofunction and dose-dependent working memeory deficits. *Brain Res.* **726,** 69–79.

Walsh, T. J., Gandhi, C., and Stackman, R. W. (1998). Reversible inactivation of the medial septum or nucleus basalis impairs working memory in rats: A dissociation of memory and performance. *Behav. Neurosci.* **112**, 1114–1124.

Wan, R. Q., Pang, K., and Olton, D. S. (1994). Hippocampal and amygdaloid involvement in nonspatial and spatial working memory in rats: Effects of delay and interference. *Behav. Neurosci.* **108**, 866–882.

Wang, C., and Swerdloff, R. S. (1997). Androgen replacement therapy. *Ann. Med.* **29**, 365–370.

Wang, C., Alexander, G., Berman, N., Salehian, B., Davidson, T., McDonald, V., Steiner, B., Hull, L., Callegari, C., and Swerdloff, R. S. (1996). Testosterone replacement therapy improves mood in hypogonadal men—a clinical research center study. *J. Clin. Endocrinol. Metab.* **81**, 3578–3583.

Wang, H., and Morris, J. F. (1999). Effects of oestrogen upon nitric oxide synthase NADPH-diaphorase activity in the hypothalamo-neurohypophysial system of the rat. *Neuroscience* **88**, 151–158.

Warembourg, M., Leroy, D., and Jolivet, A. (1999). Nitric oxide synthase in the guinea pig preoptic area and hypothalamus: Distribution, effect of estrogen, and colocalization with progesterone. *J. Comp. Neurol.* **407**, 207–227.

Waring, S. C., Rocca, W. A., Petersen, R. C., O'Brien, P. C., Tangalos, E. G., and Kokmen, E. (1999). Postmenopausal estrogen replacement therapy and risk of AD: A population-based study. *Neurology* **52**, 965–970.

Warren, S. G., and Juraska, J. M. (1997). Spatial and nonspatial learning across the rat estrous cycle. *Behav. Neurosci.* **111**, 259–266.

Warren, S. G., and Juraska, J. M. (2000). Sex differences and estropausal phase effects on water maze performance in aged rats. *Neurobio. Learn. Mem.* **74**, 229–240.

Warren, S. G., Humphreys, A. G., Juraska, J. M., and Greenough, W. T. (1995). LTP varies across the estrous cycle: Enhanced synaptic plasticity in proestrous rats. *Brain Res.* **703**, 26–30.

Washburn, S. A., Lewis, C. E., Johnson, J. E., Voytko, M. L., and Shively, C. A. (1997). 17alpha-Dihydroequilenin increases hippocampal dendritic spine density of ovariectomized rats. *Brain Res.* **758**, 241–244.

Watts, J., Stevens, R., and Robinson, C. (1981). Effects of scopolamine on radial maze performance in rats. *Physiol. Behav.* **26**, 845–851.

Weiland, N. G. (1992). Estradiol selectively regulates agonist binding sites on the N-methyl-D-aspartate receptor complex in the CA1 region of the hippocampus. *Endocrinology (Baltimore)* **131**, 662–668.

Weiland, N. G., Orikasa, C., Hayashi, S., and McEwen, B. S. (1996). Localization of estrogen receptors in the hippocampus of male and female rats. *Soc. Neurosci. Abstr.* **22**, No. 246.16.

Weiland, N. G., Orikasa, C., Hayashi, S., and McEwen, B. S. (1997). Distribution and hormone regulation of estrogen receptor immunoreactive cells in the hippocampus of male and female rats. *J. Comp. Neurol.* **388**, 603–612.

Wenk, G., Hughey, D., Boundy, V., Kim, A., Walker, L., and Olton, D. (1987). Neurotransmitters and memory: Role of cholinergic, serotonergic, and noradrenergic systems. *Behav. Neurosci.* **101**, 325–332.

Wenk, G. L. (1997). The nucleus basalis magnocellularis cholinergic system: One hundred years of progress. *Neurobiol. Learn. Mem.* **67**, 85–95.

Whaling, C. S., Nelson, D. A., and Marler, P. (1995). Testosterone-induced shortening of the storage phase of song development in birds interferes with vocal learning. *Dev. Psychobiol.* **28**, 367–376.

Wickham, M. (1958). The effects of the menstrual cycle on test performance. *Br. J. Psychol.* **49**, 34–41.

Wilcock, G. K., Esiri, M. M., Bowen, D. M., and Smith, C. C. (1982). Alzheimer's disease. Correlation of cortical choline acetyltransferase activity with the severity of dementia and histological abnormalities. *J. Neurol. Sci.* **57**, 407–417.

Williams, C. L. (1996). Short-term but not long-term estradiol replacement improves radial-arm maze performance of young and aging rats. *Soc. Neurosci. Abstr.* **22**, No. 495.5.

Williams, C. L., and Meck, W. H. (1991). The organizational effects of gonadal steroids on sexually dimorphic spatial ability. *Psychoneuroendocrinology* **16**, 155–176.

Williams, C. L., Barnett, A. M., and Meck, W. H. (1990). Organizational effects of early gonadal secretions on sexual differentiation in spatial memory. *Behav. Neurosci.* **104**, 84–97.

Williams, C. L., Raines, E., and Meck, W. H. (1994). Estradiol replacement improves radial-arm maze performance of perinatal choline supplemented and untreated ovariectomized rats. *Soc. Neurosci. Abstr.* **20**, 151.

Williams, J., and Uphouse, L. (1989). Serotonin binding sites during proestrus and following estradiol treatment. *Pharmacol., Biochem. Behav.* **33**, 615-620.

Wilson, I. A., Puolivali, J., Heikkinen, T., and Riekkinen, P. (1999). Estrogen and NMDA receptor antagonism: Effects upon reference and working memory. *Eur. J. Pharmacol.* **381**, 93–99.

Wise, P. M., Dubal, D. B., Wilson, M. E., Rau, S. W., and Lui, Y. (2001). Estrogens: Trophic and protective factors in the adult brain. *Front. Neuroendocrinol.* **22**, 33–66.

Wolf, O. T., Kudielka, B. M., Hellhammer, D. H., Torber, S., McEwen, B. S., and Kirschbaum, C. (1999). Two weeks of transdermal estradiol treatment in postmenopausal elderly women and its effect on memory and mood: Verbal memory changes are associated with the treatment induced estradiol levels. *Psychoneuroendocrinology* **24**, 727–741.

Wolf, O. T., Preut, R., Hellhammer, D. H., Kudielka, B. M., Schurmeyer, T. H., and Kirschbaum, C. (2000). Testosterone and cognition in elderly men: A single testosterone injection blocks the practice effect in verbal fluency, but has no effect on spatial or verbal memory. *Biol. Psychiatry* **47**, 650–654.

Wong, M., and Moss, R. L. (1992). Long-term and short-term electrophysiological effects of estrogen on the synaptic properties of hippocampal CA1 neurons. *J. Neurosci.* **12**, 3217–3225.

Wood, G. E., and Shors, T. J. (1998). Stress facilitates classical conditioning in males, but impairs classical conditioning in females through activational effects of ovarian hormones. *Proc. Natl. Acad. Sci. U.S.A.* **7**, 4066–4071.

Woolf, N. J. (1991). Cholinergic systems in mammalian brain and spinal cord. *Prog. Neurobiol.* **37**, 475–524.

Woolley, C. S. (1999). Electrophysiological and cellular effects of estrogen on neuronal function. *Crit. Rev. Neurobiol.* **13**, 1–20.

Woolley, C. S., and McEwen, B. S. (1992). Estradiol mediates fluctuations in hippocampal synapse density during the estrous cycle in the adult rat. *J. Neurosci.* **12**, 2549–2554.

Woolley, C. S., and McEwen, B. S. (1993). Roles of estradiol and progesterone in regulation of hippocampal dendritic spine density during the estrous cycle in the rat. *J. Comp. Neurol.* **336**, 293–306.

Woolley, C. S., and McEwen, B. S. (1994). Estradiol regulates hippocampal dendritic spine density via an N-methyl-D-aspartate receptor-dependent mechanism. *J. Neurosci.* **14**, 7680–7687.

Woolley, C. S., Gould, E., Frankfurt, M., and McEwen, B. S. (1990). Naturally occurring fluctuations in dendritic spine density on adult hippocampal pyramidal neurons. *J. Neurosci.* **10**, 4036–4039.

Woolley, C. S., Wenzel, H. J., and Schwartzkroin, P. A. (1996). Estradiol increases the frequency of multiple synapse boutons in the hippocampal CA1 region of the adult female rat. *J. Comp. Neurol.* **373**, 108–17.

Woolley, C. S., Weiland, N. G., McEwen, B. S., and Schwartzkroin, P. A. (1997). Estradiol increases the sensitivity of hippocampal CA1 pyramidal cells to NMDA receptor-mediated synaptic input: Correlation with dendritic spine density. *J. Neurosci.* **12**, 2549–2554.

Wu, M., Shanabrough, M., Leranth, C., and Alreja, M. (2000). Cholinergic excitation of septohippocampal GABA but not cholinergic neurons: Implications for learning and memory. *J. Neurosci.* **20**, 3900–3008.

Xu, H., Gouras, G. K., and Greenfield, J. P. (1998). Estrogen reduces neuronal generation of Alzheimer beta-amyloid peptides. *Nat. Med.* **4**, 447–451.

Yamada, K., Tanaka, T., Zou, L. B., Senzaki, K., Yano, K., Osada, T., Ana, O., Ren, X., Kameyama, T., and Nabeshima, T. (1999). Long term deprivation of oestrogens by ovariectomy potentiates beta-amyloid-induced working memory deficits in rats. *Br. J. Pharamacol.* **128**, 419–427.

Yang, S. H., Shi, J., Day, A. L., Simpkins, J. W., and Robinson, S. E. (2000). Estradiol exerts neuroprotective effects when adminstered after ischemic insult. *Stroke* **31**, 745–750.

Young, W. J., and Chang, C. (1998). Ontogeny and autoregulation of androgen receptor mRNA expression in the nervous system. *Endocrine* **9**, 79–88.

Zaulyanov, L. L., Green, P. S., and Simpkins, J. W. (1999). Glutamate receptor requirement for neuronal death from anoxia-reoxygenation: An in vitro model for assessment of the neuroprotective effects of estrogens. *Cell. Mol. Neurobiol.* **19**, 705–718.

Zhang, Y. Q., Shi, J., Rajakumar, G., Day, A. L., and Simpkins, J. W. (1998). Effects of gender and estradiol treatment on focal brain ischemia. *Brain Res.* **784**, 321–324.

Zhou, Y., Watters, J. J., and Dorsa, D. M. (1996). Estrogen rapidly induces phosphorylation of the cAMP response element binding protein in rat brain. *Endocrinology (Baltimore)* **137**, 2163–2166.

Zimmerman, E., and Parker, M. B. (1973). Behavioral change asociated with the menstrual cycle. *J. Appl. Soc. Psychol.* **3**, 335–344.

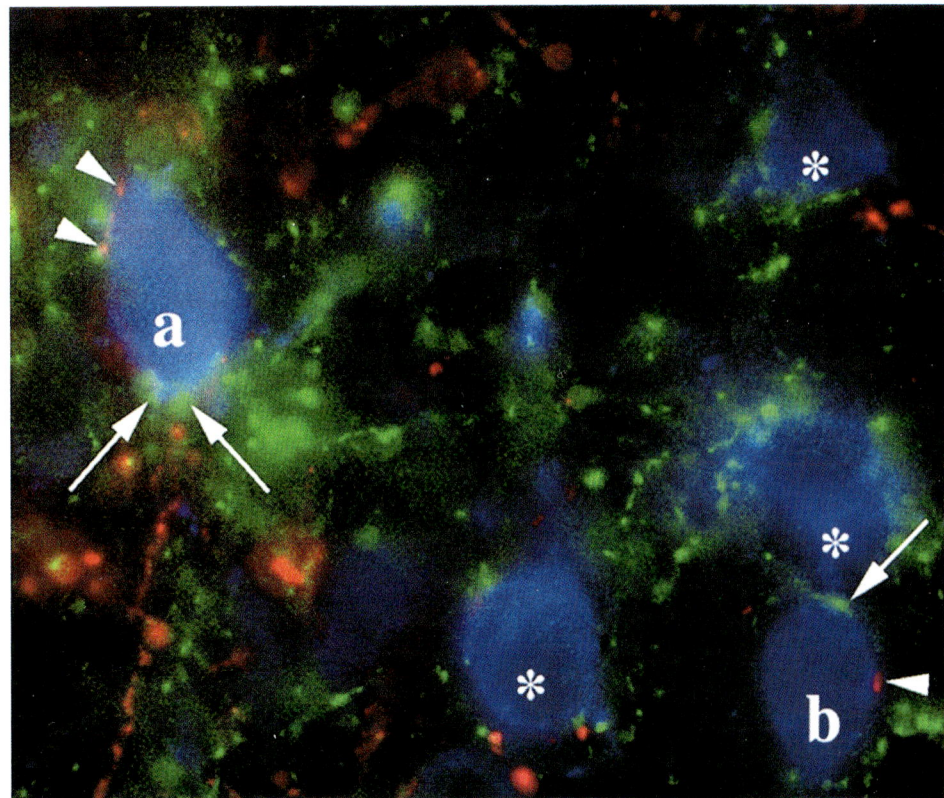

CHAPTER 20, FIGURE 22 Dual innervation of a TRH neuron (blue, a and b) in the paraventricular nucleus by axon terminals containing AGRP (arrows pointing to green fibers) and α-MSH (arrowheads pointing to red fibers). Neurons denoted by asterisks are innervated only by AGRP. (Courtesy of Dr. Csaba Fekete.)

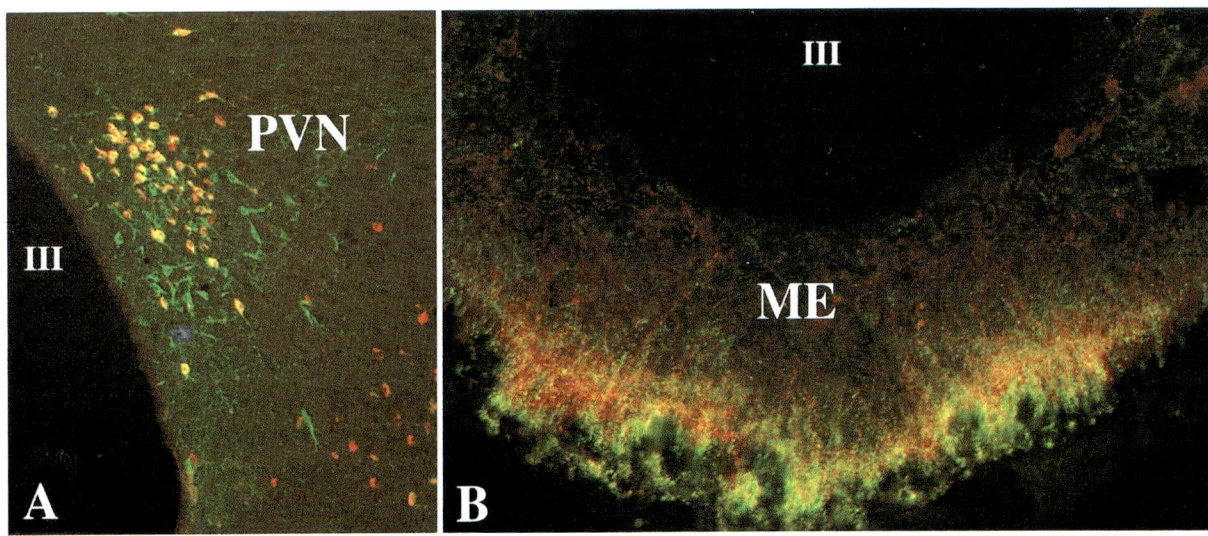

CHAPTER 20, FIGURE 23 (A) Colocalization of CART (green) with TRH (red) in neuronal perikarya in the paraventricular nucleus (PVN) and (B) their axon terminals in the median eminence (ME). Neurons and axon terminals co-containing CART and TRH appear yellow. III = third ventricle.

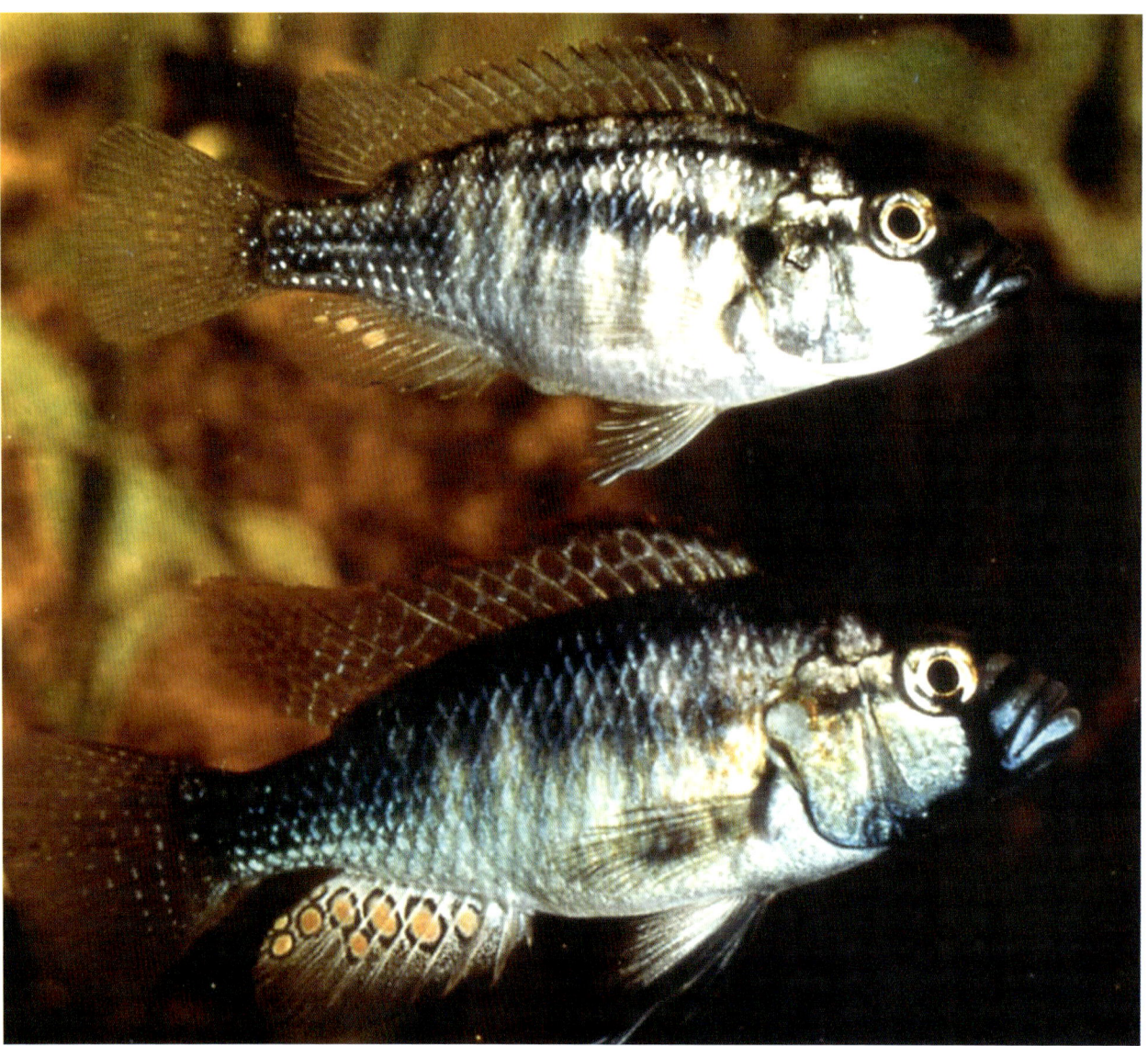

CHAPTER 26, FIGURE 1 Illustration of the body patterns for typical territorial males (Ts) and nonterritorial males (NTs). (Top) NTs lack the robust markings of their territorial counterparts and are colored to maximize camouflage. (Bottom) Ts have distinctive anal fin spots, dark forehead, and lachrymal (eye-bar) stripes and are brightly colored, including orange humeral scales. The overall body color may be either yellow or blue.

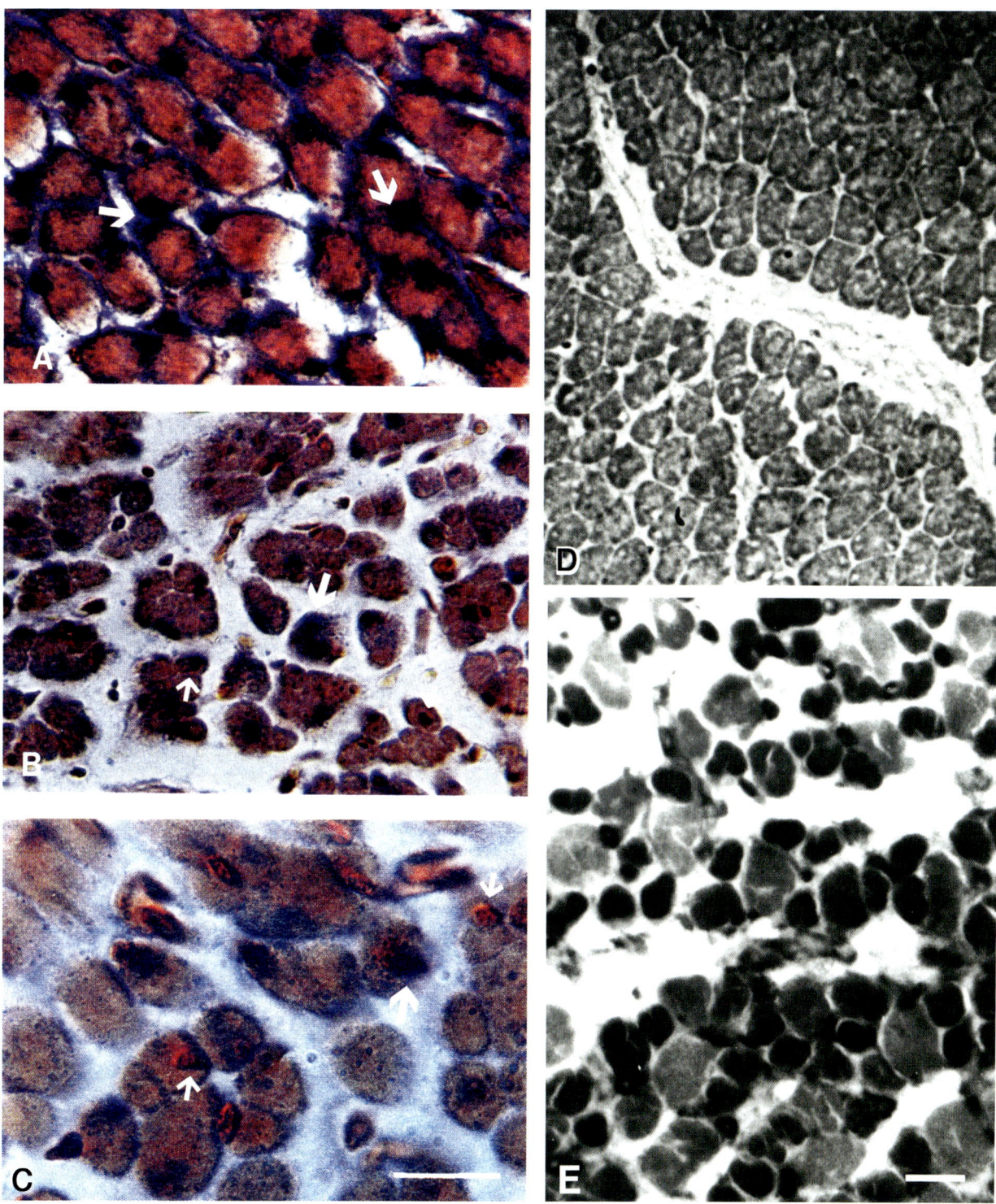

CHAPTER 27, FIGURE 5 Sexually differentiated laryngeal muscle fiber composition. Male laryngeal muscle is homogenous in fiber type as revealed by (D) histochemical staining for ATPase activity. Female laryngeal muscle fibers are heterogeneous in size and ATPase activity with one type that is similar to the male type (medium-size, medium-staining); most female fibers are small and stain darkly. Male muscle fibers are fast twitch, whereas most female muscle fibers are slow twitch, presumably reflecting the preponderance of these small, darkly ATPase staining fibers. Scale bar: 5 µm. From Sassoon *et al.* ©1987 by the Society for Neuroscience. (A, B, C) Laryngeal muscle expresses a tissue-specific myosin heavy chain gene (laryngeal myosin, LM). The LM mRNA transcript is expressed in all muscle fibers in males (arrows) but in only some muscle fibers in females (blue nuclei, large arrows); other nuclei are not associated with accumulation of the LM transcript (red nuclei, small arrows). Scale bar: (A, B) 30 µm; (C) 12 µm. From Catz *et al.* (1992).

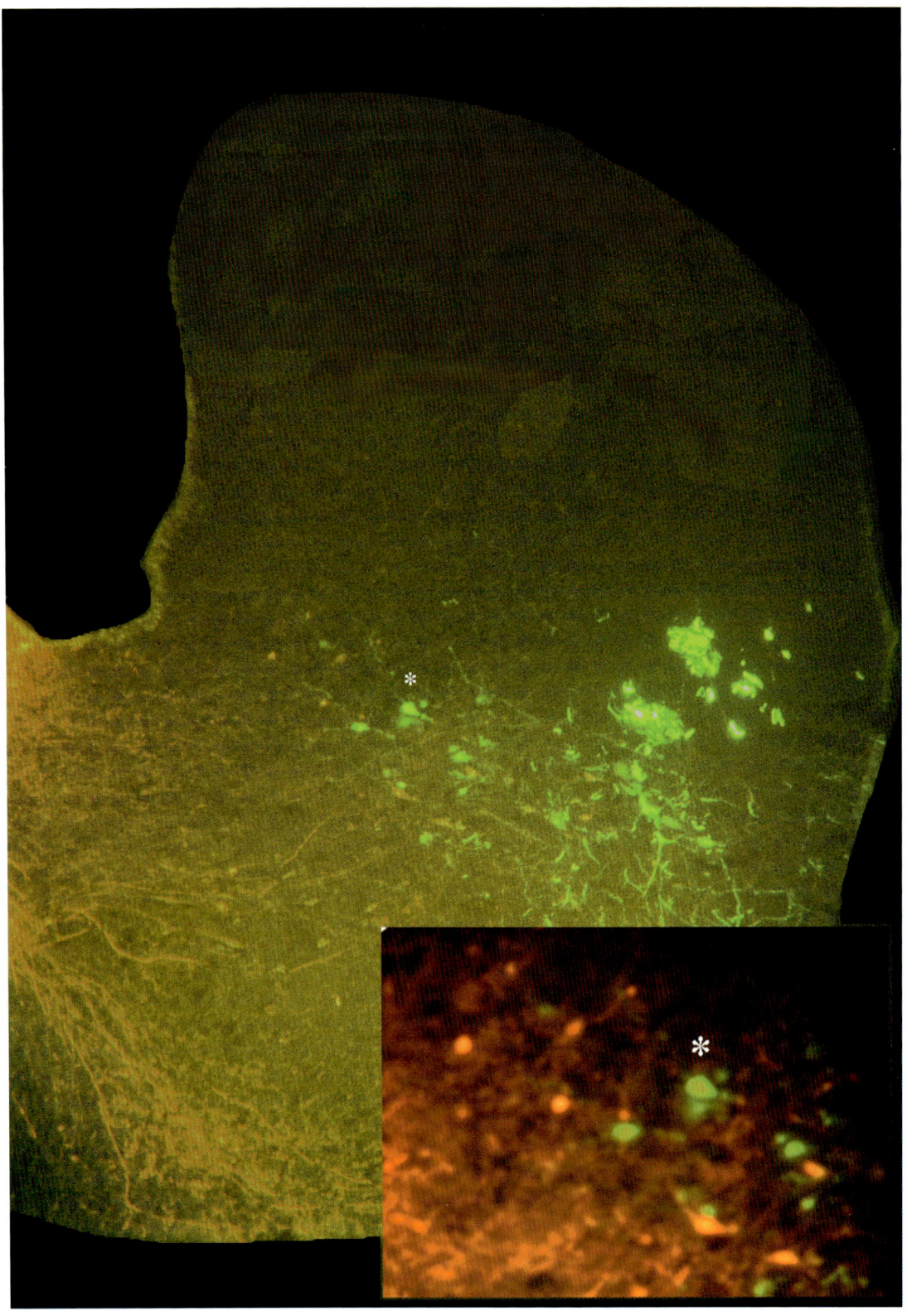

CHAPTER 27, FIGURE 13 Nucleus IX-X includes laryngeal motor neurons and interneurons. Motor neurons (in a horizontal section) were labeled by applying lucifer yellow to the fourth root of the n.IX-X nerve (Simpson *et al.*, 1986). Interneurons (insert at higher magnification) were labeled by contralateral application of fluororuby to n.IX-X (Erik Zornik, unpublished data).

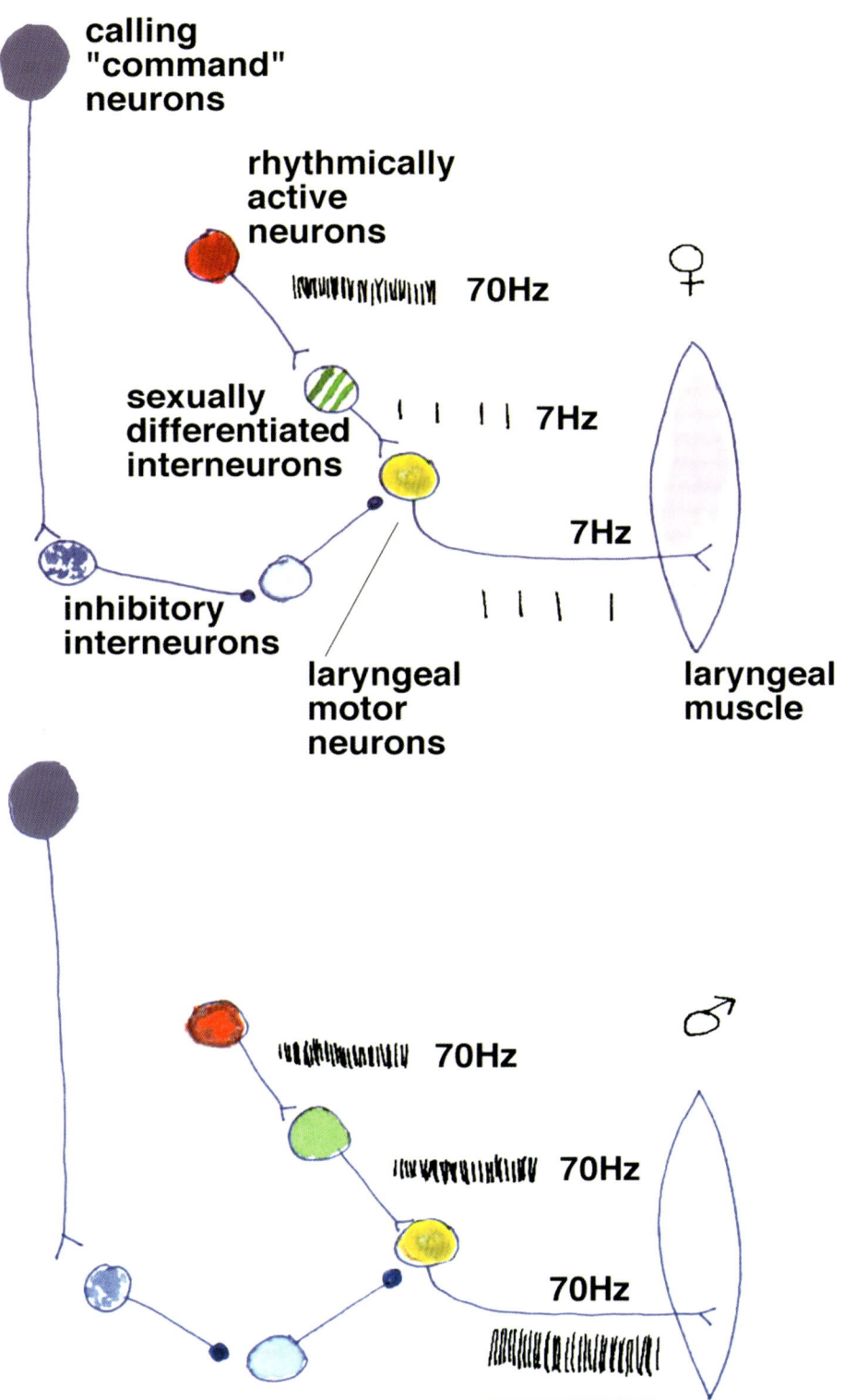

CHAPTER 27, FIGURE 14 A hypothetical scheme for generating a sexually differentiated motor pattern. For simplicity, the circuit is designed to produce different click rates in (A) females (7 Hz) and (B) males (70 Hz). The activity of laryngeal motor neurons (in yellow) is under tonic inhibitory control (light-blue interneurons), relieved by disinhibition in response to activity in calling command interneurons (purple), which may correspond to the DTAM. Excitatory input to laryngeal motor neurons originates with activity in rhythmically active neurons (red) and is shaped into distinct male and female patterns by sexually differentiated interneurons (green stripes: females; solid green: males). Bar: 0.5 s.

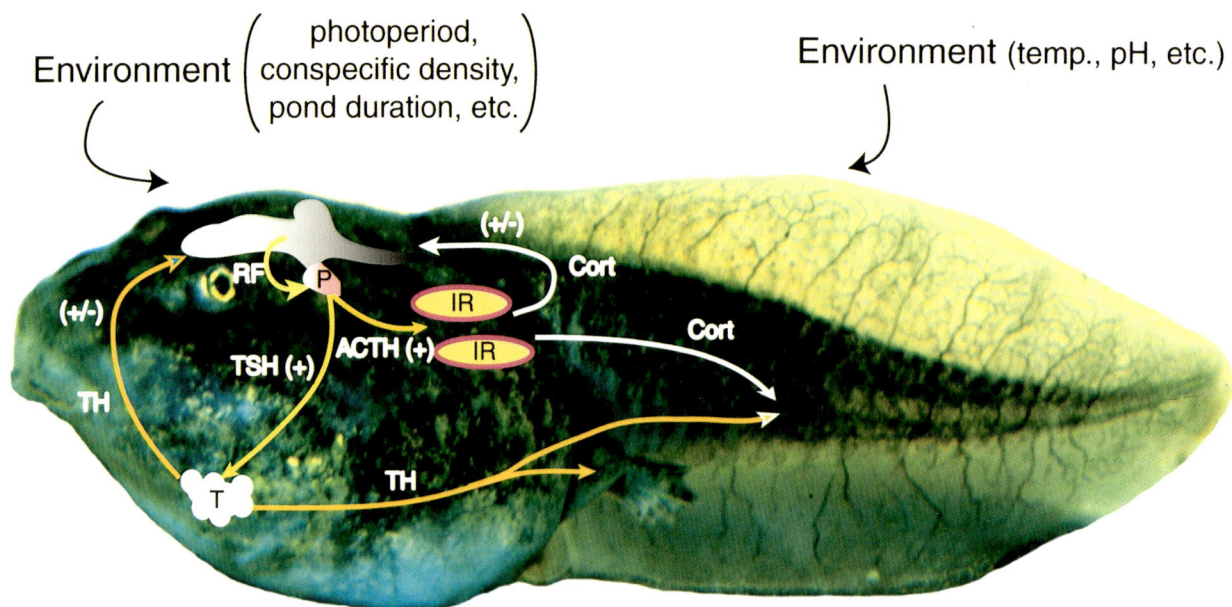

CHAPTER 28, FIGURE 3 Endocrine systems controlling tadpole metamorphosis. P, pituitary gland; RF, releasing factor; IR, interrenal gland; ACTH, adrenocorticotropic hormone; TSH, thyroid stimulating hormone; T, thyroid gland; TH, thyroid hormone; Cort, corticoids. Pluses indicate a stimulatory effect and minuses a negative feedback. In the case of TH and Cort effects on the brain, (+/-) indicates that these hormones promote differentiation of neurosecretory centers (and other brain regions) in addition to their negative feedback effects on neurohormone and pituitary hormone secretion.

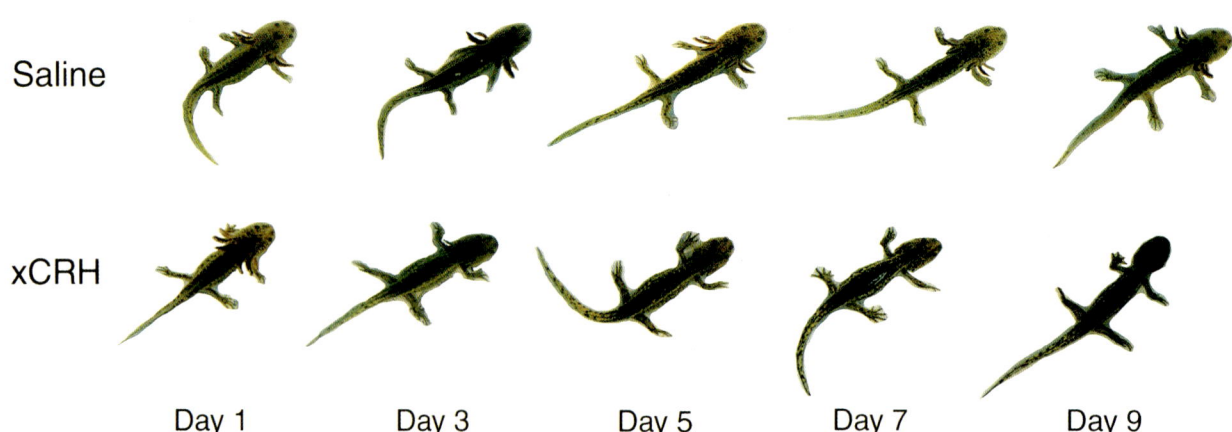

CHAPTER 28, FIGURE 7 Effects of CRH on metamorphosis in Ambystoma tigrinum. Injections of ovine CRH (oCRH, 1 μg, i.p.) or saline (0.6%) were administered daily ($n = 6$). Digital images were captured every other day to access metamorphic progression. Note the gill resorption in larvae receiving oCRH injections.

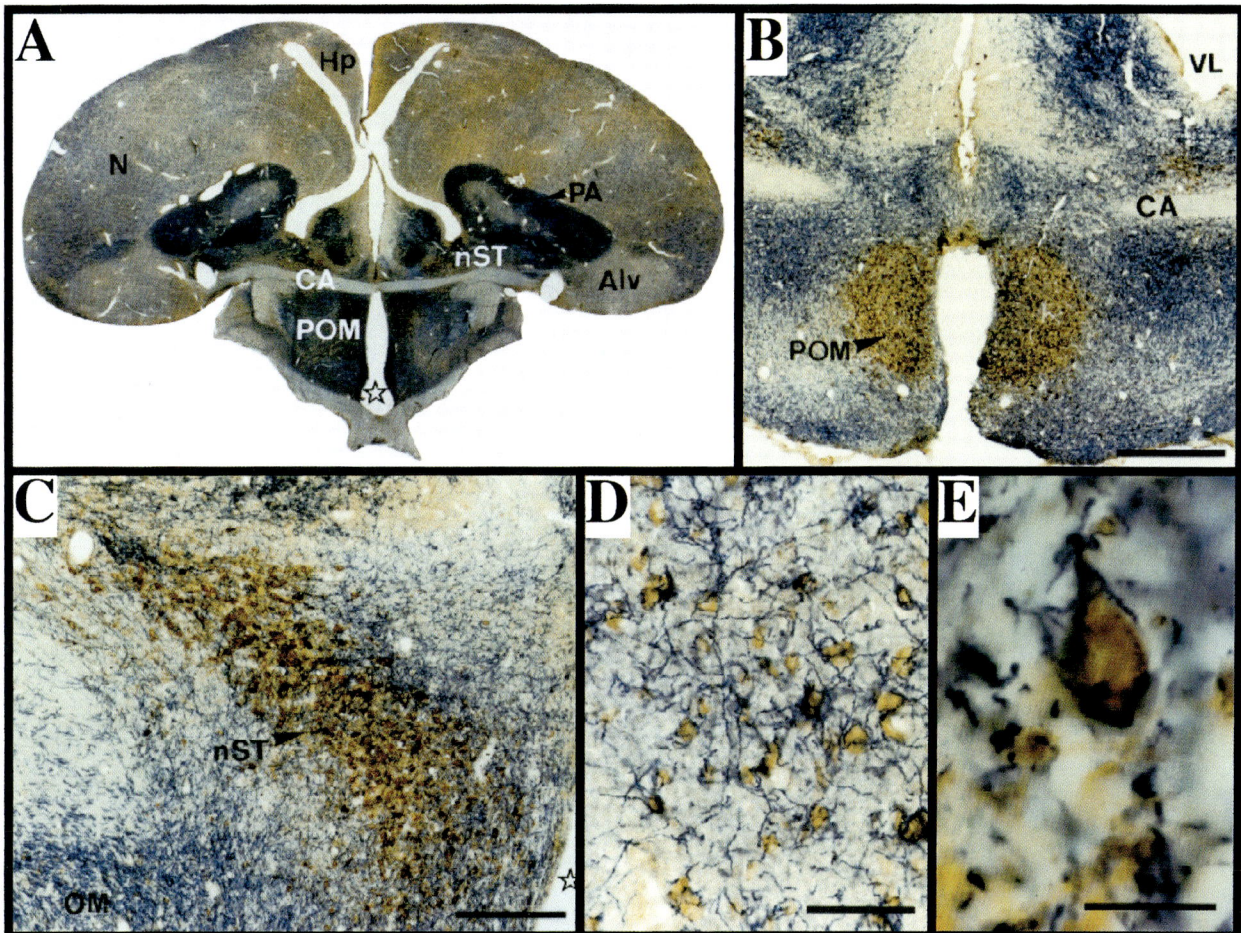

CHAPTER 32, FIGURE 21 Photomicrographs illustrating the interactions between aromatase immunoreactive (ARO-ir) cells (brown chromogen) and tyrosine hydroxylase immunoreactive (TH-ir) fibers (blue chromogen) in the rostral forebrain of male quail. (A) Low magnification of a section at the level of the anterior commissure (CA), illustrating the clusters of ARO-ir cells in the medial preoptic nucleus (POM) and rostral portion of the nucleus striae terminalis (nST). Both clusters are completely surrounded by TH-ir fibers. (B-C) Medium enlargements demonstrating that TH-ir fibers can be observed in close proximity of ARO-ir cells in both the POM (B) and the nST (C). (D) High magnification of the weakly immunoreactive aromatase cells in the neostriatum, illustrating their anatomical relationship with TH-ir fibers. (E) High magnification of one ARO-ir cell from the nST closely associated with TH-ir fibers and punctate structures. Magnification bars: (B) 500 μm, (C) 200 μm, (D) 50 μm, and (E) 20 μm. Modified from Balthazart *et al.* (1998b).

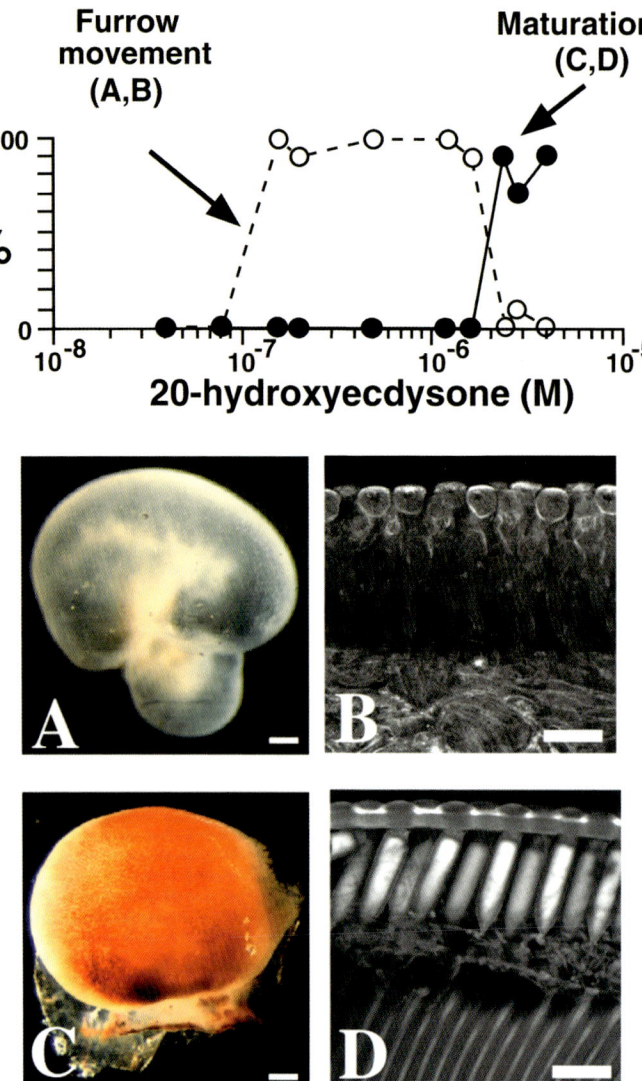

CHAPTER 34, FIGURE 10 Summary of the response of the pupal eye imaginal disc of *Manduca* to treatment with 20E *in vitro*. (Top) The dose–response relationship showing the 20E levels needed to evoke mitosis and movement of the morphogenetic furrow (open circles) and the cellular maturation of the ommatidial units (filled circles). (Bottom) Photomicrographs of the whole eye disc (A,C) and confocal optical sections of the region posterior to the furrow (B,D). In response to low levels of 20E (A,B), furrow movement occurs across the disc and cells behind the furrow differentiate into the cell types of the ommatidium including the sensory neurons. (C,D) High concentrations of 20E induce terminal maturation as manifest by the synthesis of the screening pigments (C) and the formation of the cuticular lens, the crystalline cones, and the elongated photoreceptor rhabdomeres (D). Scale bars: 500 μm (A,C); 25 μm (B,D). Data from Champlin and Truman (1998b).

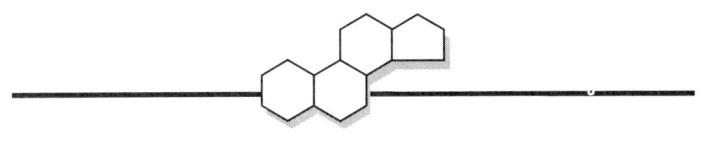

PART II

NONMAMMALIAN HORMONE-BEHAVIOR SYSTEMS

A. Nonmammalian Vertebrates
Chapters 23–33

B. Invertebrates
Chapters 34–44

23

Life History, Neuroendocrinology, and Behavior in Fish

Matthew S. Grober
Center for Behavioral Neuroscience and Department of Biology
Georgia State University
Atlanta, Georgia 30303

Andrew H. Bass
Department of Neurobiology and Behavior
Cornell University
Ithaca, New York 14853

I. INTRODUCTION

Fish make up over half the total number of living vertebrate species and exhibit a level of variation in sexual behavior that is unrivaled among other vertebrates. The early organization (Bass, 1996) and adult reorganization (Grober and Sunobe, 1996; Reavis and Grober, 1999) of neurobiology and behavior generate sexual plasticity in fishes, and these processes can be socially controlled. The major brain areas and neuroendocrine factors that control the development and adult maintenance of reproductive behavior and physiology in fish do not differ substantially from those in mammals (Crews, 1992), suggesting that the examination of fish provides useful insights into the generation of sexual variation in all vertebrates.

II. LIFE HISTORY

The explosive radiation of the percomorph, or advanced, fishes resulted in a tremendous diversity of life histories that has been generated by the invasion of new habitats and characterized by both genotypic adaptation and phenotypic polymorphism. Adaptation to new habitats generates a host of changes in the behavior, anatomy, and physiology of these animals. As a result, percomorph fishes provide a host of natural experiments to investigate the responses of hormones, brain, and behavior to novel environmental challenges. Among fishes, the teleosts include the most commonly recognized fish species (e.g., bass, perch, and flatfish) and represent the most diverse of all vertebrate taxa. In the teleosts, there are at least six classes of reproductive phenotypes (Grober, 1997; Fig. 1): (1) reproductive dysfunction, including permanent infertility and environmentally induced (e.g., social or xenobiotic inhibition) reproductive compromises that result in deficits that vary in both duration and intensity; (2) a single phenotype in a sex, the basic pattern common to most fishes and vertebrates (gonochorism); (3) a single bisexual form that functions as a simultaneous hermaphrodite; (4) multiple phenotypes in a sex that often take the form of two distinct male phenotypes that use different behavioral approaches to acquire mates (known as alternative reproductive tactics); (5) singular reproductive transformations resulting from unidirectional adult sex change; and (6) serial reproductive transformations characterized by back-and-forth (or serial) sex change. This review concentrates on the last three categories.

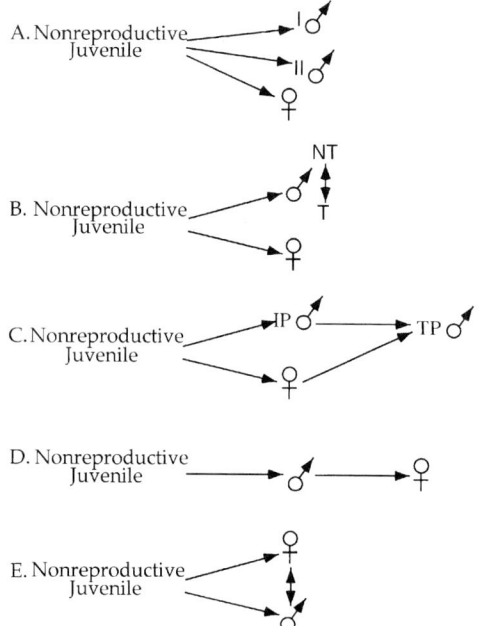

FIGURE 1 A schematic diagram shown the pattern of individual life histories. (A) Fixed alternative mating tactics, such as the midshipman, exhibit two permanent distinct male phenotypes (I, II). Midshipman are gonochoristic with separate nonoverlapping developmental trajectories for each class of males (Bass, 1996). (B) Conditional male mating strategies, such as in cichlids, include reversible changes in status and breeding condition between territorial (T) or nonterritorial (NT). Developmental observations suggest that cichlids are gonochoristic and that the rate of development is socially mediated in males (Fraley and Fernald, 1982). (C) A sex or role changing system (protogyny), found in reef fishes such as bluehead wrasse. Initial-phase males (IP) and female can change into dominant territorial terminal-phase males (TP). Studies suggest that all juveniles go through a female stage before differentiating either as a mature female or male (Shapiro and Rasotto, 1993). (D) Protandrous sex change, as in the anemone fish Amphiprion. The monogamous male may become the larger dominant female in the group. Studies also suggest that gonadal tissue from juveniles passes through an ovarian stage prior to final sexual maturation as either a male or female (Shapiro, 1992). (E) Serially sex-changing, such as in the marine goby. Individuals can repeatedly switch between the sexes. Although no evidence is apparently available for nonreproductive juveniles, adult gobies are known to have an ovotestis (Cole, 1990).

III. CORRELATED CHANGES IN A SUITE OF CHARACTERS

Sexual polymorphism in any given population represents a dynamic interaction between the genetic potential of a species and the environmental–social modulation of this genetic background. For this reason, a holistic approach that examines the system at multiple levels of analysis may be most effective. For example, many fish lay benthic eggs, and this requires one parent to protect the eggs at least until they hatch. Most species exhibit male parental care—the female leaves once the eggs are attached to the bottom and the male is left to care for them. Males attain reproductive success by holding high-quality territories, constituting a mating system known as male resource defense polygyny. A large male that can defend a high-quality territory attracts many females, whereas most males attract very few. This skew in reproductive success can drive the development or evolution of reproductive plasticity (e.g., small sneaker males or sex-role reversal). The generation of this degree of sexual plasticity in turn requires the modification of a host of behavioral, physiological, endocrinological, and anatomical characteristics.

Hence, an important tool in understanding sexual plasticity is delineating the characteristics that are useful for defining sexual phenotype. Even among gonochoristic species, a large number of behavioral, somatic, and gametic characteristics vary in and between the sexes. This is most relevant for studies that use preserved specimens to examine aspects of the mating system or sexual development. Most often these studies rely on the status of one character, the gonad, to determine sexual phenotype or reproductive status. However, the allocation of gonads is not always a good predictor of reproductive behavior or success. For example, the temperate marine goby *Lythrypnus dalli* was initially considered a simultaneous hermaphrodite based on gonadal histology (St. Mary, 1993, 1997). However, behavioral observations indicate that these gobies are sequential hermaphrodites that exhibit only male or female behavior at any one time (Reavis and Grober, 1999; St. Mary, 1993), regardless of the presence of male and female gonads. It has thus become clear that to identify alternative sexual states, we need to examine a group or suite of characters that, together, give us an unambiguous determination of sex and mode of reproduction (Bass, 1992). These characteristics include body size and coloration, gonad anatomy and physiology, genitalia (usually the genital papilla in fish), sex-specific glands (e.g., accessory gonadal structures or testicular glands), signaling structures (e.g., sound-producing mechanisms), behavior, brain chemistry, and endocrinology.

IV. ALTERNATIVE MALE REPRODUCTIVE MORPHS IN MIDSHIPMAN FISH

Perhaps the best-studied system with regard to multiple male reproductive morphs is the plainfin midshipman fish, *Porichthys notatus* (Fig. 1A). Each of the alternative reproductive male morphs in midshipman fish has been defined at multiple levels, from behavioral to subcellular (Bass, 1992, 1996, 1998) (Table 1). A behavior central to the reproductive tactics of midshipman fish is the production of species- and sex-typical vocalizations. Hence, a central theme in all these studies has been to identify how sexual polymorphisms in the peripheral and central nervous system establish male-morph- and female-specific vocal phenotypes. Both the neural basis of sound production and detection (i.e., hearing) have been subjects of extensive investigation. Although sexual polymorphisms for multiple traits have been identified in the vocal motor system, studies of the peripheral and central auditory systems have focused on species-typical traits (Bass *et al.*, 1999; also see Bodnar and Bass, 1997, 1999; McKibben and Bass, 1998, 1999).

A. Spawning and Vocal Behaviors

The plainfin midshipman has a fairly wide geographic distribution along the western coastline of northern California on into Canada (Walker and Rosenblatt, 1988). Bass and Marchaterre (1989a,b) first reported two male reproductive morphs, type I and type II, on the basis of morphological traits including body size, gonad-body size ratios, and sonic muscle and motoneuron size. This was followed by a series of other studies identifying sexual polymorphisms in a large suite of vocal motor traits (Bass, 1992; also discussed later). Brantley and Bass (1994) later showed that each male morph and females have distinct spawning and vocal behaviors. Type I males build nests under rocks in the intertidal and subtidal zones, where they fertilize and then guard eggs deposited on the roof of their nest by females. In contrast, type II males neither build nests nor guard eggs; instead, type II males gain access to gravid females and their eggs by essentially parasitizing the type I male's reproductive tactic—they lie perched outside of or sneak into a type I male's nest and shed sperm in an attempt to compete with the type I male for eggs (Fig. 2).

Type I and II males are clearly polygynous; a single nest may contain several thousand eggs even though a gravid female produces only up to 150–200 eggs each breeding season. Females apparently leave their entire clutch of eggs in a single nest and depart soon after spawning is completed. Only sexually mature adults, embryos, and newly hatched fry are found in nests. Nonreproductive juveniles ranging in age from 5 to 12 months are only found in eel grass beds, where adult morphs are also infrequently found.

Nesting type I males generate three major classes of vocalizations (Brantley and Bass, 1994; Bass *et al.*, 1999). Trains of short-duration (ms range) grunts are produced at intervals of approximately 400 ms during defense of a nest against potential intruder males. Type I males also produce a long-duration in the range of minutes to >1 h) multiharmonic humming sound (Hubbs, 1920) or hum (Ibara *et al.*, 1983). Observations of captive populations of nesting type I males, together with playbacks of natural or computer-synthesized acoustic signals through underwater loudspeakers, show that hums and not grunts can attract females to an artificial nest site (Brantley and Bass, 1994; McKibben and Bass, 1998). A number of parameters influence female recognition and preference for a hum-like signal, including fundamental frequency, intensity, and duration (McKibben and Bass, 1998, 2002). Growls are intermediate in duration (in the range of seconds to minutes) between grunts and hums and have not been studied in captive individuals. Field observations, however, show that growls are only associated with nests containing more than one type I male and are likely to function in some agonistic context (A. Bass, unpublished observations). The fundamental frequency of midshipman hums and grunts is temperature-dependent, but hovers close to 90–100 Hz in their natural habitat (Brantley and Bass, 1994). A type I male's hum may function in one or more contexts, including female choice of individual males, male–male competition, or as a beacon to assist either females, type II males, or other type I males in locating suitable nest sites. Type II males, like females, do not produce grunt trains or hums, but infrequently generate low-amplitude isolated grunts in nonspawning contexts.

TABLE 1
Sexually Polymorphic Traits in Midshipman Fish

	Type I male	Type II male	Female
Behavior			
Nest building	Yes	No	No
Egg-guarding	Yes	No	No
Vocalizations	Hums, grunts, growls	Grunts	Grunts
Fundamental frequency	High	Low	Low
Somatic			
Body size	Large	Small	Intermediate
Gonad size and body-size ratio	Small	Large	Large (gravid); small (spent)
Ventral coloration	Olive-gray	Mottled yellow	Bronze (gravid); mottled (spent)
Vocal motor			
Vocal muscle traits	Large	Small	Small
Vocal neuron traits	Large	Small	Small
Central vocal discharge frequency	High	Low	Low
Neuroendocrine			
Circulating steroids	Testosterone; 11-ketotestosterone	Testosterone	Testosterone; estradiol
Aromatase activity	Low	High	High
GNRH-POA neuron size	Large	Small	Small
GNRH-POA number and body size	Low	High	Low
AVT-POA neuron size	Large	Small	Large
AVT-POA number and body size	Low	High	Low
AVT/isotocin modulation of vocal circuitry	AVT	Isotocin	Isotocin

B. Somatic and Endocrinological Traits

On average, type I males are two- to threefold larger in body size (length and weight) than type II males at the time of sexual maturity. The gonad-to-body-weight ratio (gonosomatic index) is ninefold greater in type II males, who may invest close to 20% of their weight in testes, compared to only 1% in type I males. Gravid females resemble type II males in having a large gonosomatic index, although theirs is even greater. Both gravid females and type II males have a distended and firm belly, reflecting the large size of their gonads. The dorsal body coloration of midshipman, an olive-gray hue, is fairly similar for all three morphs (Fig. 3). During the breeding season, however, the belly of type I males is typically light to dark gray, whereas that of type II males is mottled yellow. Gravid females have a bronze or golden ventral coloration, whereas spent females are more like type II males (Bass and Marchaterre, 1989a; Brantley and Bass, 1994).

Type I males, type II males, and females have contrasting levels of the two principal classes of vertebrate steroid hormones—androgens such as testosterone and estrogens such as 17β-estradiol (Brantley et al., 1993c; Knapp et al., 1999a). Testosterone is detectable in all three morphs, although at progressively lower levels along the continuum: type II males to females to type I males. 17β-Estradiol is detectable among females and a small percentage of type I males, but at much lower levels than testosterone. Teleosts also have a unique form of testosterone known as 11-ketotestosterone. On average, circulating levels of 11-ketotestosterone are about fivefold greater than testosterone in type I males; type II males and females do not have detectable levels. 11-Ketotestosterone levels vary among type I males in accordance with stages of parental care; they are highest for males in nests without any eggs or with eggs

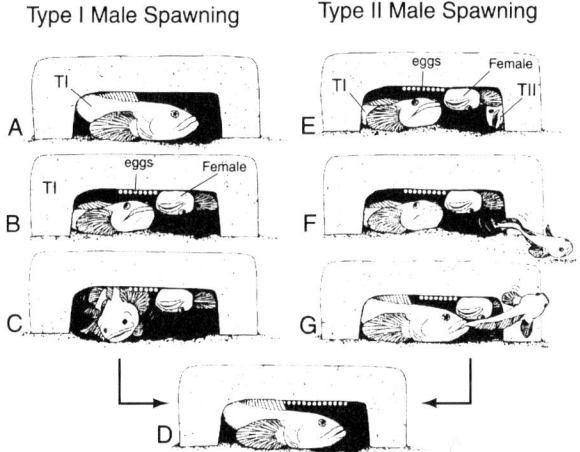

FIGURE 2 Overview of the spawning behavior of type I singing and type II sneaker male midshipman fish *(Porichthys notatus)*. Generalized spawning sequence drawn from photographs of captive, reproductively active individuals in which type I males have taken up residence in artificial nests in aquaria. Left-hand column shows a sequence involving only a type I male and a female. Right-hand column shows spawnings that also involve type II males (TII). A. Type I male (TI) generates advertisement calls (hums) while inside his nest after nightfall. B. After a gravid female enters the nest, the type I male stops humming and they spawn; the female deposits eggs on the nest's roof. C. The type I male rolls and quivers, releasing sperm near the eggs. D. After egg laying is completed, the female leaves the nest and the type I male remains to guard the eggs and hums the next evening to attract another female. E. A type II male inside the nest (far right) sneak-spawns. F. A type II male outside the nest (far right) satellite spawns and releases milt while fanning water toward the nest's opening. G. The nest-guarding type I male attacks a satellite-spawning type II male. D. The type I male remains to guard the eggs after the female and the type II male have departed. Adopted from Brantley and Bass (1994), *Ethology* **96,** 213–232, by permission of Blackwell Wissen Schafts-Verlag Berlin, GmbH.

when compared to males in nests containing mostly hatched embryos (Knapp *et al.,* 1999a). Type I males guard the eggs in their nest while continuing to acoustically court and then spawn with females on successive nights (Brantley and Bass, 1994). Hence, shifting levels of androgens throughout the breeding season may reflect a compromise between investment in paternal care vs courtship and nest defense (Knapp *et al.,* 1999a).

The profile of circulating levels of gonadal steroids resembles that shown for other teleosts with alternative male reproductive tactics (Brantley *et al.,* 1993c). In particular, elevated levels of 11-ketotestosterone characterize the displaying type I male morph vs the nondisplaying type II male morph.

1. Vocal Motor Traits

Sex- and morph-specific vocal behaviors are paralleled by a divergence in neurobiological traits ranging from the size of the sound-producing muscles to the rhythmic firing properties of vocal neurons (Bass, 1992, 1998). The vocal organ of midshipman fish consists of a pair of sonic muscles attached to the lateral walls of their swimbladder. These muscles are the functional analog of the laryngeal and syringeal muscles of terrestrial vertebrates and apparently share a common embryonic origin from occipital head somites (Bass and Baker, 1997). A sixfold greater vocal muscle–body weight ratio in type I males, compared to type II males and females, is paralleled by a fourfold greater muscle-fiber number and fivefold greater muscle-fiber diameter (Brantley *et al.,* 1993b). Dimorphisms in muscle fibers extend to the subcellular level, including the width of Z-lines, which represent the points of overlap of the thin actin filaments of myofibrils; the branching of the sarcoplasmic reticulum, which is the principal site for calcium exchange; the density of mitochondria; and the concentrations of metabolic enzymes (Bass and Marchaterre, 1989a; Walsh *et al.,* 1995). All these traits are greater in magnitude in type I males and probably represent structural and biochemical adaptations related to the metabolic demands of humming.

Each sonic muscle is innervated by a single nerve formed by branches of ventral occipital nerve roots carrying motor axons originating from paired midline vocal-sonic motor nuclei extending from the caudal hindbrain into the rostral spinal cord. Each vocal motor nucleus innervates the ipsilateral sonic muscle. Vocal motoneurons have a round to ovoid-shaped cell body and dendrites that branch throughout both sonic motor nuclei. A single unbranched axon emerges from either the soma or near the base of a primary dendrite and exits the brain via one of the occipital nerves, eventually forming synapses with sonic muscle fibers.

Intracellular recording and staining studies have identified vocal pacemaker neurons that are located ventrolaterally to motoneurons (Bass and Baker, 1990).

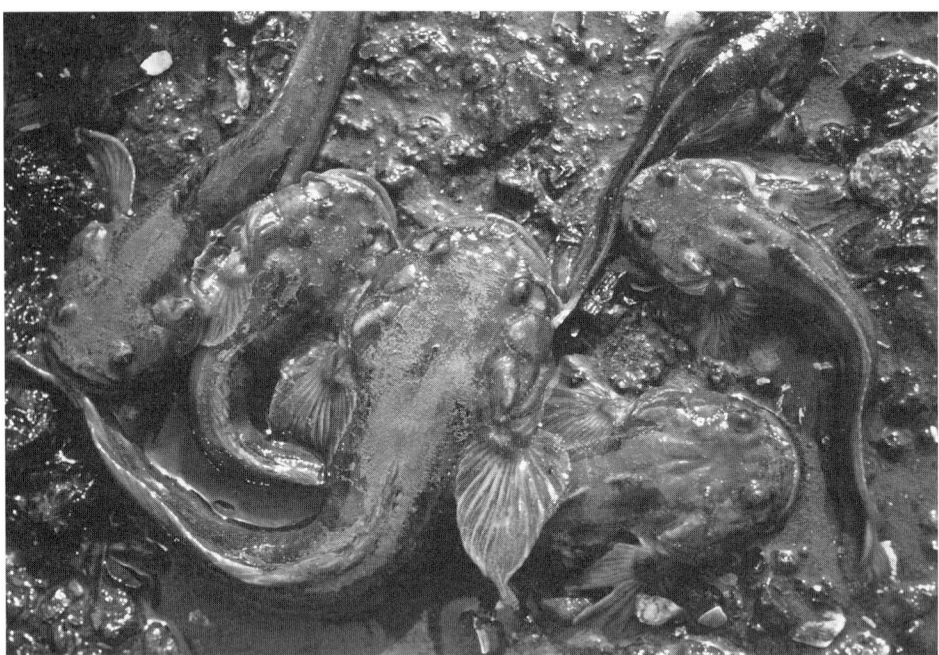

FIGURE 3 Seen from above, the three reproductive morphs of the plainfin midshipman. Type I males (large fish, lower right), type II males (four smaller fish, left and center), and females (topmost fish) appear the same olive-gray. The undersides of the fish differ during breeding season. Type I males are typically light to dark gray on the underside, whereas type II males are mottled yellow. Gravid females have a bronze or golden color on their bellies, and spent females are more like type II males in their appearance. Reprinted from Bass (1996), *Am. Sci.* **84**, 352–363.

The firing frequency of pacemaker neurons is matched 1:1 with that of sonic motoneurons and, in turn, to the fundamental discharge frequency of the vocal motor volley as recorded intracranially from the occipital nerve roots. A single pacemaker neuron innervates the neurons in both motor nuclei, consistent with the hypothesis that their role is to synchronize the firing of motoneurons positioned on both sides of the brain. This in turn, leads to the simultaneous contraction of both sonic muscles at a fundamental discharge frequency that establishes the fundamental frequency of vocalizations. Hence, there is a direct relationship between the rhythmic patterned output of a hindbrain pacemaker-motoneuron circuit and the physical attributes of vocalizations.

The pacemaker-motoneuron circuit fires at a fundamental frequency that is approximately 15–20% higher in type I males than in type II males and females; this parallels sex differences in the fundamental frequency of natural vocalizations (Bass and Baker, 1990, 1991; Brantley and Bass, 1994). The swimbladder itself may contribute to the spectral properties of hums and grunts by influencing the higher-frequency components (harmonics) of the signals.

Intracellular injections of horseradish peroxidase (HRP) show that the somata, dendrites, and axons of vocal neurons are up to threefold larger in magnitude in type I males than in females and type II males (Bass and Baker, 1990); electron microscopic studies show comparable polymorphisms at the level of sonic neuromuscular junctions (Fluet and Bass, 1990). The use of low-molecular-weight tracers (e.g., biocytin and neurobiotin) that are transported transneuronally in the vocal motor system, have permitted a delineation of the entire complement of neurons in the hindbrain vocal circuit of midshipman fish (Bass *et al.*, 1994). Thus, the application of biocytin or neurobiotin crystals to the cut end of a single sonic nerve results in a mapping of the entire bilateral extent of the pacemaker-motoneuron circuitry. The biocytin studies extend and confirm, for a large sample size, our initial demonstration of sexual polymorphisms using intracellular HRP injections

(Bass et al., 1996). These analyses also demonstrate sexual polymorphisms in a previously unidentified group of ventral medullary neurons just rostral to the sonic motor nucleus that extensively link the pacemaker-motoneuron circuitry across the midline (Bass et al., 1996). There are no significant adult sex- or morph-specific differences in motoneuron number after controlling for the effects of body size (Bass and Andersen, 1991; also see Grober et al., 1994). Hence, inter- and intrasexual variation in the organization of the vocal motor system is dependent on a divergence in the morphophysiological properties of individual neurons. Most important, these studies together show that the morphological and physiological traits of a rhythmically active vocal-pattern generator in the hindbrain of type II males and females are similar to one another but strikingly divergent from that of type I males. This pattern of structural traits reflects the divergence in vocal behaviors exhibited by type I males vs type II males and females.

The transneuronal biocytin method for mapping was exploited to trace the ontogeny of the vocal circuit. These studies revealed that sexual maturation of the type I male's mate-calling circuit parallels the ontogeny of its sonic muscle (Brantley et al., 1993b; Bass et al., 1996). Hence, among juvenile type I males, the motoneuron size and volume of the sonic motor nucleus increase most during a stage prior to sexual maturation that parallels a fourfold increase in the number of sonic muscle fibers. A more modest growth phase for motoneurons is coupled to the greatest increase in pacemaker neuron size at a stage coincident with the onset of sexual maturity that parallels a fivefold increase in the size of sonic muscle fibers. Ventral medullary neurons show similar growth increments during both stages. It is important to note that juvenile to type II male and juvenile to adult female transformations are accompanied by no or little change in vocal neuron or muscle size. Transneuronal transport of biocytin and neurobiotin has shown that male dimorphisms in motoneurons may arise very early in development, soon after fry become free swimming (Knapp et al., 1999b). Together, the ontogenetic studies demonstrate alternative growth trajectories for the neurons and muscles that determine morph-specific vocal behaviors.

An individual fish's age can be determined by counting the number of growth increments that appear on its otoliths, much like the rings in the trunk of a tree. The aging of saccular otoliths shows that type I males, type II males, and females overlap in age, although type II males and females can become sexually mature at an earlier age and smaller size (Bass et al., 1996). Together with the delineation of vocal neuron ontogeny, the results support the hypothesis that alternative male morphs in midshipman fish adopt nonsequential, mutually exclusive growth patterns during their first year of life.

C. Neuroendocrine Traits

The two neuropeptides that have been most commonly studied in the context of sexual plasticity among teleost fish, including midshipman fish are gonadotropin-releasing hormone (GnRH) and arginine vasotocin (AVT) (Foran and Bass, 1999; Bass and Grober, 2002).

1. Gonadotrophin-Releasing Hormone

It appears, at least for mammals, that the proper development, adult location, and physiological function of GnRH preoptic cells are necessary for adult reproductive function. Disproportionate variation in any of these parameters often leads to reproductive dysfunction. In contrast to the restrictive organization of GnRH brain nuclei required for normal sexual development in mammals, variability in the adult status of the GnRH centers in the forebrain's preoptic (POA) in fish and may play a role in the production of the wide range of sexual systems (Foran and Bass, 1999; also see Francis et al., 1993; Halpern-Sebold et al., 1986) and, as discussed later, sex reversal (Grober and Bass, 1991).

POA GnRH neurons directly innervate the pituitary in teleosts, unlike most other vertebrates in which a blood portal system mediates the access of GnRH to the anterior pituitary. GnRH can then modulate the release of gonadotropins from the anterior lobe of the pituitary gland, which, in turn, controls the secretion of gonadal steroid hormones. The POA-pituitary-gonadal axis is thus considered to regulate the expression of secondary sex characteristics via the influence of gonadal steroids on sexual differentiation of steroid-sensitive structures such as those of the vocal motor system. Halpern-Sebold et al. (1986) first showed in platyfish, which also have two male morphs that differ in age at sexual maturity, a cascade of GnRH-gonadotropin events along the brain-pituitary axis that are temporally linked to the onset of sexual maturation in each morph. Studies in midshipman fish are consistent with this developmental scenario. Both immunocytochemical and *in situ* hybridization studies have identified the position and extent of GnRH in the forebrain of midshipman fish (Grober *et al.*, 1994, 1995; Foran *et al.*, 1997). There are increases in the number and size of POA-GnRH neurons at the time of juvenile to adult transformations (Fig. 4). However, unlike vocal motor neurons, there is a convergence in GnRH traits among all sexually mature individuals; type I males, type II males, and adult females have a similar GnRH phenotype (number and cell size), consistent with all morphs being sexually mature. Together, the data support the hypothesis that transformations in the organization of the juvenile POA-pituitary-GnRH-gonadotropin axis could initiate a cascade of events leading to sexual maturation.

2. Arginine Vasotocin

Neuropeptides of the vasopressin-oxytocin family (AVT-isotocin in fish) have been implicated in the modulation of a variety of reproductive-related behaviors, including vocalization (Moore, 1992; Boyd, 1997; Goodson and Bass, 2001). As in other vertebrate classes (Moore and Lowry, 1998), AVT-containing neurons are localized to the POA in midshipman fish (Foran and Bass, 1998; Goodson and Bass, 2000a). AVT-immunoreactive (-ir) neurons are larger in type I males and females than in type II males. Unlike the case for GnRH neurons (Grober *et al.*, 1994), AVT cell-size differences among morphs can be explained by differences in body size. However, as is the case for GnRH phenotypes (reanalysis of Grober *et al.*, 1994; data by Foran and Bass, 1999), type II males have more AVT-ir neurons per gram body weight than do type I males (on average almost a sixfold difference).

Ultimately, functional interpretations of the significance of morph- and sex-specific differences in neuropeptide phenotypes rely on neurophysiological studies. A series of studies have now begun to assess AVT influences on the midshipman fish's vocalization circuitry. An immunocytochemical study in midshipman fish has provided a complete mapping of AVT-ir fiber pathways and terminal fields (Goodson and Bass, 2000a). Sites of dense AVT-ir include the anterior hypothalamus (ventral tuberal nucleus) and the midbrain (paralemniscal tegmentum adjacent to the lateral lemniscus). A rhythmic vocal motor output from the hindbrain pacemaker circuitry can also be evoked by electrical stimulation in these same brain regions (which are also linked to the central acoustic circuitry; Bass *et al.*, 2000; Goodson and Bass, 2000a, unpublished observations). Whereas picospritzing AVT into the ventral tuberal hypothalamus of type I males inhibits electrically evoked vocal motor output from this region, a V_1 receptor antagonist facilitates such output

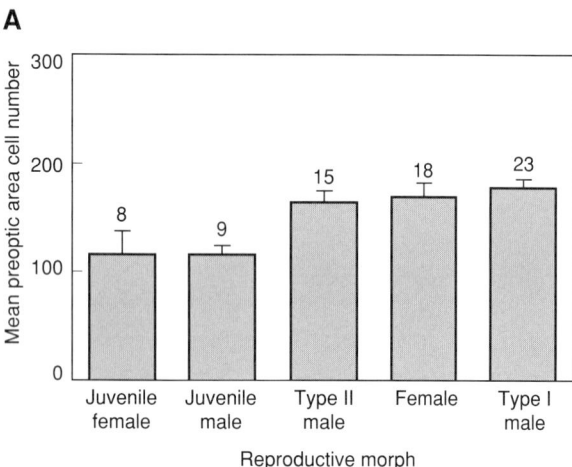

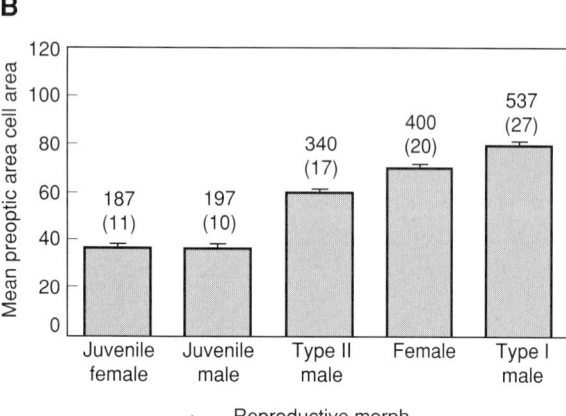

FIGURE 4 Mean GnRH-ir preoptic area (A) cell number and (B) size in the life history stages of midshipman fish, *Porichthys notatus*. Error bars represent the standard error of the mean. The numbers above the error bars in (A) indicate the number of animals. the number of cells measured and number of animals (in parentheses) are also indicated in (B). Modified from Grober *et al.* (1994), with permission.

(Goodson and Bass, 2000b). In contrast, isotocin, another nine-amino-acid peptide that differs from AVT in only one amino acid, is the active substance in type II males and females. Other studies in type I males alone show that both AVT and vasoactive intestinal polypeptide (VIP) influence electrically evoked vocal output from the midbrain tegmentum by reducing the number of vocal motor bursts obtained and increasing response latency; VIP also leads to a reduction in the duration of vocal bursts (Goodson and Bass, 2000a,c). Antagonists have no effect on vocal output evoked from the midbrain, suggesting that AVT and VIP action are not necessary for normal call initiation or vocal motor patterning but rather operate in a condition-dependent manner.

3. Gonadal Steroids and Aromatase

Anatomical and physiological studies of vocal motor traits show that androgens contribute to the masculinization of the type I male vocal circuit among juvenile males; androgens can induce an elevation of the fundamental discharge frequency of the pacemaker-motoneuron circuit and an increase in the size of vocal neurons and muscles in juveniles (Brantley *et al.*, 1993a; Bass, 1995).

One enzyme important to androgen metabolism in the brain is aromatase, which converts testosterone to estrogen. Teleost fishes have the highest known levels of aromatase (Callard *et al.*, 1990). Studies in midshipman fish have identified male morph- and sex-specific patterns of aromatase activity (Schlinger *et al.*, 1999). Aromatase levels were determined for three grossly dissected brain regions: (1) the olfactory bulb and telencephalon, inclusive of the preoptic area; (2) an expansive region including the diencephalon, midbrain, and cerebellum; and (3) a vocal hindbrain region defined approximately by the extent of the ventral medullary-pacemaker-motoneuron circuit identified by Bass *et al.* (1994). The levels are highest in the first two regions, with a modest difference in region 2 between females and type I males. The most striking findings are for the vocal hindbrain where levels are three- to fivefold higher in type II males and females than in type I males. The results suggest that the aromatase-driven conversion of testosterone to estrogen may effectively protect the vocal hindbrain of type II males and females from the masculinizing effects of testosterone on vocal motor traits that characterize type I males. Studies based on the cloning of a partial cDNA sequence for midshipman fish aromatase show the anatomical distribution of brain aromatase and support the biochemical studies of dimorphisms in the vocal hindbrain region (Forlano *et al.*, 2000).

D. Summary Comments

In summary, our studies of adult reproductive morphs in midshipman fish show that (modified from Bass, 1992):

1. Alternative mating tactics among sexually mature males are paralleled by alternative phenotypes for the neurons that determine tactic-specific types of vocal behavior—type I singing males have a suite of vocal motor traits distinct from those of sneak-spawning type II males and of females.

2. Reproductive maturation is not obligatorily linked to the expression of neuronal secondary sex characteristics—sexual maturation of type II male or female morphs does not involve the expression of type-I-male-specific traits.

3. Although type II males and females have morph-specific spawning tactics, they are convergent in a number of traits, including vocal motor phenotype, neurochemical phenotypes (isotocin modulation of vocal motor circuitry), brain aromatase levels, circulating plasma steroids (testosterone), large investment in gonad, absence of parental care, and dependence on type I males for nest construction.

4. Alternative male morphs adopt nonsequential, mutually exclusive growth patterns during their first year of life.

One of the key issues in the midshipman system, and in others including bluegill sunfish and salmon (see Gross, 1996), is whether the male morphs are genetically determined to develop at different rates and thus into different types, or whether there is some social or environmental modulation of the development of variable sexual phenotypes. There is a suggestion that the density of animals during the juvenile phase may determine the type of male that develops in the midshipman fish (Foran, 1998). Similar data have been obtained for a European blenny that exhibits a similar system of two alternative male morphs (Almada *et al.*, 1994, 1995). In the Peacock blenny, two research groups independently began studies on populations of these fish that recruited to sandflats that were modified to support aquaculture. Both populations of this blenny exhibited the same alternative male morph at the same time in response to similar environmental modifications, namely changes in population density. These data are more consistent with phenotypic, environmentally driven plasticity generating the variation in male function rather than a genetic mechanism. One difference between the blenny and the midshipman is that there appears to be a fixed point in the development in the midshipman at which males become fixed in their specific morphology (see Bass *et al.*, 1996). The blenny use one tactic when small (sneaking and female mimicry) and then switch to the alternative tactic when large (aggressive nest holding) (Almada *et al.*, 1994, 1995). Another example of the likely effects of population density on reproductive tactics among males is a Peacock blenny population studied in southern Portugal. Here, large males form nest aggregations that are so dense that the territories are virtually absent, resulting in sex-role reversal with respect to courtship (Almada *et al.*, 1994, 1995). Although males retain the capacity to court when they have no eggs in the nest, they usually assume a passive role in courtship; the females compete aggressively among themselves and actively court males, displaying a female nuptial coloration (Almada *et al.*, 1995). Smaller and younger males adopt female nuptial coloration and female courting behavior toward nest-holder males as a means of entering the nest during or shortly after the spawning of a female (Gonçalves *et al.*, 1996). We know that there are major differences in the physiology of these male morphs and that differences between morphs are mediated in part by androgenic steroids (Oliveira *et al.*, 2001) and forebrain neuropeptides (George *et al.*, 1999).

The midshipman fish story highlights the potential level of sexual plasticity exhibited among fish with multiple male morphs and the multiple levels at which the male morphs diverge from one another and from females. The remainder of this review focuses on fish species that exhibit even more extreme degrees of sexual plasticity, including fish that show adult sex change and thus switch from the entire suite of characters of one sex to those of the other.

V. PRIMACY OF THE BEHAVIOR—BRAIN CASCADE: REVERSIBLE SEX CHANGE IN GOBIES

Of the many fish species that exhibit socially mediated sex reversal (Smith, 1975), the marine goby, *Trimma okinawae,* is one of only a handful of species known to change sex more than once and in either direction (see Fig. 1E) (Kuwamura *et al.*, 1994; Sunobe and Nakazono, 1993). These changes in sexual phenotype are under strict social control and involve rapid changes in the production of sex-specific mating behavior (Sunobe and Nakazono, 1993). Male-typical behavior includes the occupation of a nest, aggression toward other males, and a skipping courtship directed toward females. Female-typical behavior is limited to visiting the nests of males. The presence of these sex-typical behaviors and the anatomy of the gonads, accessory gonadal structure, and genital papillae are used as indicators of complete sex change. The accessory gonadal structure is unique to this family of fish (Gobiidae) and is a reliable characteristic of male sexual identity (Sunobe and Nakazono, 1993). The genital papilla is a sexually dimorphic structure that aids in the delivery of sperm or eggs and also provides a clear indication of sexual state in this species (Grober and Sunobe, 1996).

By using established methods for manipulating small social groups under laboratory conditions (removing or replacing the large male, or both; Sunobe and Nakazono, 1993), we evaluated changes in the gonads, accessory gonadal structure and genital papilla in individuals that experienced male to female (M → F), female to male (F→M), and female to male to female (F→M→F) sexual transformations. During these transitions, behavioral changes are rapid (within minutes to hours of the social trigger), and the time for a complete sex change (behavioral and morphological) depends on the direction and sequence of the change (Grober and Sunobe, 1996). F→M transitions are associated with increased production of male-typical behaviors, whereas M→F transitions involve the loss of these same behavior patterns and the onset of a female-specific behavior (nest visitation). During sex change, the genital papilla and gonads show correlated changes that are consistent with the reproductive behavior of each individual (Grober and Sunobe, 1996). The degree to which the opposite-sex gonad regresses depends on the time since the onset of sex change (Grober and Sunobe, 1996). As predicted by the male-specific activity of the accessory gonadal structure, this organ regresses in females and reexpands in males (Grober and Sunobe, 1996; Sunobe and Nakazono, 1993).

As a first approach to understanding the neuroendocrine mechanisms that control the sex-change process in this species, immunocytochemical methods were used to examine possible changes in the size of AVT-producing cells in the POA following single and serial sex changes. Females, regardless of their prior sexual status, have significantly larger AVT forebrain cells than males and the area of these cells is greatest following M→F transitions, whereas F→M transitions result in a significantly smaller mean cell size. The reversal of a subset of the F→M males back to females results in a return to the larger female-specific mean cell size, and these differences are independent of body size (Grober and Sunobe, 1996). These results are noteworthy for the speed of the changes and their reversibility in fully functional adults. The primary goal for this study was to correlate changes in forebrain AVT cells with changes in a variety of sexual characteristics that were indicative of sex change. As a result, fish were not sampled until they were completely sex reversed (e.g., had spawned successfully as the opposite sex). The advantage of this approach was that it provided an assurance that sex change had occurred. This led to two conclusions: (1) AVT forebrain centers appear to be organized in a sex-specific manner and, 2) sequential transitions between the sexes involve reversible neuroendocrine changes, as well as modifications of a wide range of sex-specific characteristics. The disadvantage of this approach was that it did not provide any indication of how quickly the neurochemistry could change, or an indication of the temporal relationship between behavioral, neurobiological, and gonadal changes. These issues can be addressed in a Caribbean labrid fish, the bluehead wrasse, that also exhibits socially controlled sex change.

VI. TEMPORAL AXIS FOR SOCIAL MODULATION OF AVT PHENOTYPE IN THE BLUEHEAD WRASSE

The bluehead wrasse, *Thalassoma bifasciatum*, has been the subject of intensive study regarding the evolution and ecology of sex change (Warner, 1975; Warner and Hofman, 1980; Warner and Swearer, 1991), and has been the focus of studies addressing how behavior and neuroendocrinology regulate the sex-change process (Godwin *et al.*, 1996; Grober *et al.*, 1991; Grober and Bass, 1991). Populations are composed of two distinct color phases: terminal-phase (TP) males have blue heads, a black-white-black banding behind the head, and green bodies, whereas initial-phase (IP) males and females show a similar yellow coloration (Fig. 5). All individuals first reproduce as either IP males or females. TP individuals (supermales) arise from one of two irreversible processes: (1) sex change in an IP female, or 2) role change in an IP male (see Fig. 1C). In addition to the striking differences in color between IP and TP individuals, there are also dramatic differences in body size, reproductive behavior, and fecundity (Petersen *et al.*, 1992; Warner and Schultz, 1992). TP males aggressively defend breeding sites, gain exclusive access to females, and as a result may mate with up to 100 females per day. IP males show no breeding-site defense and thus are less aggressive than TP males; they mate in large aggregations (∼50 IP males per female) or they sneak-mate with a TP male–IP female pair. This difference in access to females may explain the much higher gonosomatic index (gonad weight/body weight) in IP males, which is probably a response to the intense sperm competition associated with mass spawnings. Finally, IP females show no breeding-site defense and little aggression toward IP fish; and they visit TP-male or IP-mass-spawning sites.

The removal of the TP male from a social group acts as the behavioral trigger for both sex and role change (Warner and Swearer, 1991). Within minutes after the removal of the TP male, the largest IP fish (either male or female) initiates behavioral sex-role change, as evidenced by increased aggression toward other large IP fish and courtship directed toward smaller females (Godwin *et al.*, 1996). The increased aggression probably leads to social dominance, which may be a key factor in the inhibition of sex-role change in subordinates. This functions to limit the number of fish that undergo sex-role change after the loss of a TP male. Gonadal sex reversal in this species follows this rapid behavioral change and can be completed in 7–10 days. This sequence of events highlights the role of social cues

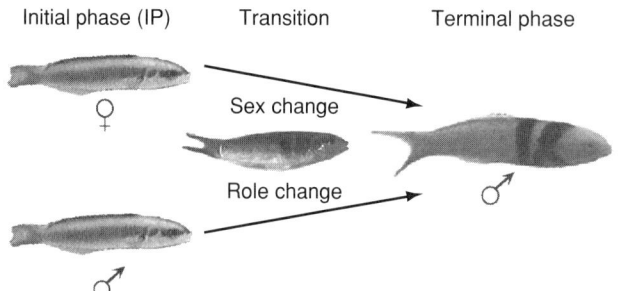

FIGURE 5 Overview of the life history of the bluehead wrasse, *Thalassoma bifasciatum*, a sex-role-changing protogynous fish found in the Caribbean Sea. Both initial-phase (IP) males (via role change) and females (via sex change) can transform into dominant territorial trminal-phase (TP) males. IP males obtain fertilizations by either mating in large aggregations of IP males or sneak-mating during pair spawns of IP females–IP males. This sexual transformation is mediated by social interactions and involves changes in coloration, as well as a host of other sexually polymorphic characteristics.

in the regulation of sexuality in individual members of the social group.

Both sex and role changes in the bluehead wrasse are associated with significant increases in the number of POA GnRH cells (Grober and Bass, 1991), and exogenous androgen implants in IP males and females can trigger increases in GnRH cell number to levels seen in TP males, but have no effect on GnRH cell number in TP males fish (Grober et al., 1991). These early studies have been replicated in other species of sex-changing fish with similar results (Elofsson et al., 1997, for a protandrous fish; Elofsson et al., 1999, for a protogynous fish) and set the stage for work that has examined the temporal relationship between changes in the POA-AVT phenotype and transformations in behavioral phenotypes.

A. Arginine Vasotocin

Studies in the bluehead wrasse used *in situ* hybridization to identify cells that were labeled with a degenerate probe that is complementary to AVT mRNA (Godwin et al., 2000). This technique allows an examination of the regulation of AVT production over the course of sex change. These studies, conducted in the field by manipulating naturally occurring social groups, show that both the number of cells expressing AVT mRNA and the amount of expression per cell increase in a similar manner from females to IP males to TP males. These differences are not due to body size allometry. Rather, TP males appear to have more AVT-mRNA-producing cells and these cells have a higher per cell message production. Godwin et al. (2000) sacrificed fish at 2, 3, and 5 days after removal of the TP male from a social group and quantified the level of AVT mRNA expression in each fish. Compared to unmanipulated females, levels of AVT mRNA expression increase progressively 2 and 3 days after the removal of the TP male. After 3 days, there is a significant increase in mRNA production relative to preremoval levels, resulting in an overproduction of mRNA compared to what is found in established TP males. Moreover, the levels begin dropping after 4 days, suggesting that the increase in AVT mRNA expression can be short-lived and may only be required during the period of social instability, when overproduction of behavior may be critical to acquiring TP male status. The correlation between AVT expression and behavior is striking and suggests a possible causal link between increased AVT mRNA and increases in TP-male-specific behavior patterns. Comparative support for these results comes from work on the Hawaiian congener, *T. duperrey*, in which TP males have significantly more and larger AVT-mRNA-producing cells than either IP sex (Grober, 1998). This difference parallels the results from the bluehead wrasse and suggests that TP males regulate AVT production in a different way than the IP sexes.

Finally, other studies have investigated the effects of exogenous treatment with gonadal steroids on AVT production in the bluehead wrasse. In control fish that were either housed separately or given sham implants, TP males have more peptide-producing cells than either IP sex (McIntyre, 1998). Steroid implants are effective in significantly elevating circulating levels of 11-ketotestosterone. However, these increased hormone levels do not have a significant effect on the number or size of AVT cells in IP males and females. These results indicate that the changes in the brain are not driven by gonadal hormones and support the idea that brain changes precede gonadal transformation. Conversely, elevated levels of 11-ketotestosterone in TP males have a negative effect on AVT peptide production as evidenced by a significant decrease in the number of labeled cells in steroid-treated TP males. This suggests that the higher number of AVT cells in TP males is not a direct result of the increase in androgens that accompanies sex change.

These findings provide an interesting contrast to our earlier work on GnRH (Grober and Bass, 1991; Grober et al., 1991). For both GnRH and AVT, TP males have more and larger cells than IP males and females, indicating a consistent and robust sexual polymorphism in brain areas that are critical for the control of reproductive behavior and physiology. However, androgen implants have much different effects on GnRH than on AVT cells. 11-Ketotestosterone implants increase the number of GnRH cells in both IP sexes to levels characteristic of field-collected TP males, whereas androgen implants have no effect on GnRH cell number in TP males. Both of these results are the exact opposite effect from the other AVT studies discussed. One possible resolution of this contradiction in regulation concerns the function of each peptide and, hence, the temporal nature of its expression. AVT may be primarily involved in producing early changes in behavior, which precede changes in the gonad and thus the ability to produce significant levels of androgens. Conversely, GnRH may primarily be involved in the regulation of gonadal function, and this process occurs later in the sex-change process and may be more sensitive to steroidal regulation.

An integration of available results suggests the following temporal model of socially controlled sex change. Decreases in the amount of aggressive behavior received by the largest subordinate result in rapid changes in brain peptide expression (e.g., AVT; Godwin et al., 2000; NPY, Kramer and Imbriano, 1997). These early changes in the brain permit the production of higher rates of male-typical behavior in the early stages of sex change. The combination of the decreased aggression received and the increased production of male behavior patterns triggers a cascade of changes in the hypothalamic-pituitary-gonadal axis. These would include independent changes in the brain (e.g., the GnRH axis), gonad anatomy and physiology, gonadal steroid levels, and body coloration. This general model conforms quite well to an empirical model that is being testing in ongoing studies of the bluebanded goby. Thus, removal of a dominant male results in rapid increases in aggressive behavior and a cessation of submissive behavior in the dominant female (Reavis and Grober, 1999). These early changes in behavior lead to further changes in forebrain AVT cells (Reavis and Grober, 1999), gonad and accessory gland anatomy (Marxer-Miller et al., 2002), and the structure of the external genitalia (Carlisle et al., 2000). This work can lead to an integrative model of sex change based on early behavioral changes with other systems mapped onto it (e.g., external genitalia, gonad anatomy and physiology, steroid hormones, and neuropeptides; Reavis and Grober, 1999).

VII. SUMMARY

The rapid diversification of the advanced fishes has been associated with the ability in these fishes to express a wide range of sexual phenotypes. These phenotypes can be generated by genetic change over time or the expression of phenotypic variants in response to environmental or social input. Differences between sexual morphs extend to almost all levels of biological organization and can include behavior, coloration, signalling structures, brain chemistry and anatomy, endocrinology, body size, gonad size and anatomy, accessory gonadal structures, and external genitalia. Many or most of these traits are expressed as a suite of characters that are typical of a given sex or sexual morph, and transitions between the morphs involve orderly transitions of the host of associated traits. More generally, there appears to be a high degree of neurochemical and neuroendocrinological conservation associated with the production of sexual polymorphism across the vertebrate taxa (Foran and Bass, 1999; Bass and Grober, 2002). AVT and AVP treatment induces sex-specific reproductive behaviors in a range of vertebrate species, including the spawning reflex in fishes, amplexus in newts, and pair-bonding and parental care in voles (Carter *et al.,* 1995; Egami, 1959; Macey *et al.,* 1974; Moore, 1992). Perhaps the most striking comparison is between our results in fishes, which show a strict correlation between sexual behavior and AVT neurochemistry, and studies showing differences in forebrain peptidergic cell populations in human males who exhibit heterosexual vs homosexual (Swaab and Hofman, 1990) or transsexual (Zhou *et al.,* 1995) behavior.

Acknowledgments

This chapter is dedicated to the memory of Leon Bass and Ronald Grober. We thank the many members of the Bass and Grober labs over the last several years for their input into multiple aspects of this work. The research reported here was supported by NSF (IBN-9723817 to M.S.G. and IBN-9987341 to A.H.B.).

References

Almada, V. C., Gonçalves, E. J., Santos, A. J., and Baptista, C. (1994). Breeding ecology and nest aggregations in a population of *Salaria pavo* (Pisces: Blenniidae) in an area where nest sites are very scarce. *J. Fish Biol.* **45**, 819–830.

Almada, V. C., Gonçalves, E. J., Oliveira, R. F., and Santos, A. J. (1995). Courting females: Ecological constraints affect sex roles in a natural population of the blenniid fish *Salaria pavo. Anim. Behav.* **49**, 1125–1127.

Bass, A. H. (1992). Dimorphic male brains and alternative reproductive tactics in a vocalizing fish. *Trends Neurosci.* **15**, 139–145.

Bass, A. H. (1995). Alternative life history strategies and dimorphic males in an acoustic communication system. Fifth International Symposium on Reproductive Physiology of Fish, *Fish Symp.* **95**, 258–260.

Bass, A. H. (1996). Shaping brain sexuality. *Am. Sci.* **84**, 352–363.

Bass, A. H. (1998). Behavioral and evolutionary neurobiology: A pluralistic approach. *Am. Zool.* **38**, 97–107.

Bass, A. H., and Andersen, K. (1991). Intra- and Inter-sexual dimorphisms in the sound generating motor system in a vocalizing fish: Motor axon number and size. *Brain, Behav. Evol.* **37**, 204–214.

Bass, A. H., and Baker, R. (1990). Sexual dimorphisms in the vocal control system of a teleost fish: Morphology of physiologically identified cells. *J. Neurobiol.* **21**, 1155–1168.

Bass, A. H., and Baker, R. (1991). Adaptive modification of homologous vocal control traits in teleost fishes. *Brain Behav. Evol.* **38**, 240–254.

Bass, A. H., and Baker, R. (1997). Phenotypic specification of hindbrain rhombomeres and the origins of rhythmic circuits in vertebrates. *Brain Behav. Evol.* **50**, 3–16.

Bass, A. H., and Grover, M. S. (2001). Social and neural modulation of sexual plasticity in teleost fish. *Brain Behav. Evol.* **57**, 293–300.

Bass, A. H., and Marchaterre, M. A. (1989a). Sound-generating (sonic) motor system in a teleost fish (*Porichthys notatus*): Sexual polymorphism in the ultrastructure of myofibrils. *J. Comp. Neurol.* **286**, 141–153.

Bass, A. H., and Marchaterre, M. A. (1989b). Sound-generating (sonic) motor system in a teleost fish (*Porichthys notatus*): Sexual polymorphisms and general synaptology of a sonic motor nucleus. *J. Comp. Neurol.* **286**, 154–169.

Bass, A. H., Marchaterre, M. A., and Baker, R. (1994). Vocal-acoustic pathways in a teleost fish. *J. Neurosci.* **14**, 4025–4039.

Bass, A. H., Horvath, B. J., and Brothers, E. (1996). Nonsequential developmental trajectories lead to dimorphic vocal circuitry for males with alternative reproductive tactics. *J. Neurobiol.* **30**, 493–504.

Bass, A. H., Bodnar, D. A., and Marchaterre, M. A. (1999). Complementary explanations for existing phenotypes in an acoustic communication system. In "Neural Mechanisms of Communication" M. Hauser and M. Konishi (eds.), Chapter 17, pp. 493–514. MIT Press, Cambridge, MA.

Bass, A. H., Bodnar, D. A., and Marchaterre, M. A. (2000). Midbrain acoustic circuitry in a vocalizing fish. *J. Comp. Neurol.* **419**, 505–531.

Bodnar, D. A., and Bass, A. H. (1997). Temporal coding of concurrent acoustic signals in auditory midbrain. *J. Neurosci.* **17**, 7553–7564.

Bodnar, D. A., and Bass, A. H. (1999). A midbrain combinatorial code for temporal and spectral information in concurrent acoustic signals. *J. Neurophysiol.* **81**, 552–563.

Boyd, S. K. (1997). Brain vasotocin pathways and the control of sexual behaviors in bullfrogs. *Brain Res. Bull.* **44**, 345–350.

Brantley, R. K., and Bass, A. H. (1994). Alternative male spawning tactics and acoustic signalling in the plainfin midshipman fish, *Porichthys notatus. Ethology* **96**, 213–232.

Brantley, R. K., Marchaterre, M. A., and Bass, A. H. (1993a). Androgen effects on vocal muscle structure in a teleost fish with inter and intrasexual dimorphisms. *J. Morphol.* **216**, 305–318.

Brantley, R. K., Tseng, J., and Bass, A. H. (1993b). The ontogeny of inter- and intrasexual vocal muscle dimorphisms in a sound-producing fish. *Brain, Behav. Evol.* **42**, 336–349.

Brantley, R. K., Wingfield, J., and Bass, A. H. (1993c). Hormonal bases for male teleost dimorphisms: Sex steroid levels in *Porichthys notatus*, a fish with alternative reproductive tactics. *Horm. Behav.* **27**, 332–347.

Callard, G. V., Schlinger, B. S., and Pasmanik, M. (1990). Non-mammalian vertebrate models in studies of brain-steroid interactions. *J. Exp. Zool. Suppl.* **4**, 6–16.

Carlisle, S. L., Marxer-Miller, S. K., Canario, A., Oliveira, R. F., Carneiro, L. A., and Grober, M. S. (2000). Effects of 11-ketotestosterone on genital papilla morphology in the sex changing fish, *Lythrypnus dalli*. *J. Fish Biol.* **57**, 445–456.

Carter, C. S., DeVries, A. C., and Getz, L. L. (1995). Physiological substrates of mammalian monogamy: The prairie vole model. *Neurosci. Behav. Rev.* **19**, 303–314.

Cole, K. S. (1990). Patterns of gonad structure in hermaphroditic gobies (Teleostei: Gobiidae). *Environ. Bio. Fish.* **28**, 125–142.

Crews, D. (1992). Diversity of hormone-behavior relations in reproductive behavior. *In* "Behavioral Endocrinology" (J. B. Becker, S. M. Breedlove, and D. Crews, eds.), pp. 143–186. MIT Press; Cambridge, MA.

Egami, N. (1959). Effect of testosterone on the sexual characteristics of the gobiid fish, *Pterogobius zonoleucus*. *Annot. Zool. Jpn.* **32**, 123–128.

Elofsson, U. O., Winberg, S., and Francis, R. C. (1997). Number of preoptic GnRH-immunoreactive cells correlates with seuxal phase in a protandrously hermaphroditic fish, the dusky anemonefish (*Amphiprion melanopus*). *J. Comp. Physiol. A* **181**, 484–492.

Elofsson, U. O., Winberg, S., and Nilsson, G. E. (1999). Relationships between sex and the size and number of forebrain gonadotropin-releasing homrone-immunoreactive neurons in the ballan wrasse (*Labrus berggylta*), a protogynous hermphrodite. *J. Comp. Neurol.* **410**, 158–170.

Fluet, A., and Bass, A. H. (1990). Sexual dimorphisms in the sound generating motor system of a teleost fish: Ultrastructure of neuromuscular junctions. *Brain Res.* **531**, 312–317.

Foran, C. M. (1998). Phenotypic plasticity in the neuroendocrine axis of a teleost fish with alternative reproductive tactics (*Porichthys notatus*) Ph.D. Thesis, Cornell University, Ithaca, NY.

Foran, C. M., and Bass, A. H. (1998). Preoptic AVT immunoreactive neurons of a teleost fish with two male reproductive morphs. *Gen. Comp. Endocrinol.* **111**, 271–282.

Foran, C. M., and Bass, A. H. (1999). Preoptic GnRH and AVT: Axes for sexual plasticity in teleost fish. *Gen. Comp. Endocrinol.* **116**, 141–152.

Foran, C. M., Myers, D. A., and Bass, A. H. (1997). Modification of gonadotropin releasing hormone (GnRH) mRNA expression in the retinal-recipient thalamus. *Gen. Comp. Endocrinol.* **106**, 251–264.

Forlano, P., Myers, D. A., and Bass, A. H. (2000). Aromatase distribution in the brain of a vocalizing fish with three adult morphs. *Soc. Neurosci. Abstr.* **26**, 1522.

Fraley, N. B., and Fernald, R. D. (1982). Social control of developmental rate in the African cichlid, *Haplochromis burtoni*. *Z. Tierpsychol.*, **60**, 66–82.

Francis, R. C., Soma, K., and Fernald, R. D. (1993). Social regulation of the brain-pituitary-gonadal axis. *Proc. Natl. Acad. Sci. U.S.A.* **90**, 7794–7798.

George, A. A., Watkins, K. K., Carneiro, L. A., Oliveira, R. F., and Grober, M. S. (1999). Courtship in a sexually polymorphic fish: The role of vasotocin and gonadal steroids. *Soc. Neurosci. Abstr.*

Godwin, J. R., Crews, D., and Warner, R. R. (1996). Behavioral sex change in the absence of gonads in a coral reef fish. *Proc. R. Soc. London, Ser. B* **263**, 1683–1688.

Godwin, J., Sawby, R., Warner, R. R., Crews, D., and Grober, M. S. (2000). Hypothalamic arginine vasotocin mRNA abundance variation across sexes and with sex change in a coral reef fish. *Brain, Behav. Evol.* **55**, 77–84.

Gonçalves, E. J., Almada, V. C., Oliveira, R. F., and Santos, A. J. (1996). Female mimicry as a mating tactic in males of the blenniid fish *Salaria pavo*. *J. Mar. Biol. Assoc. U.K.* **76**, 529–538.

Goodson, J. L., and Bass, A. H. (2000a). Vasotocin innervation and modulation of vocal-acoustic ciruitry in the teleost *Porichthys notatus*. *J. Comp. Neurol.* **422**, 363–379.

Goodson, J. L., and Bass, A. H. (2000b). Forebrain peptide modulation of sexually polymorphic vocal motor circuitry. *Nature (London)* **403**, 769–772.

Goodson, J. L., and Bass, A. H. (2000c). Rhythmic midbrain-evoked vocalization is inhibited by vasoactive intestinal. *Brain Res.* **865**, 107–111.

Goodson, J. L., and Bass, A. H. (2001). Social behavior functions and related anatomical characteristics of vasotocin/vasopressin systems in vertebrates. *Brain Res. Rev.* **35**, 246–265.

Grober, M. S. (1997). Conserved neuroendocrine foundations give rise to diverse sexual phenotypes in fish. *In* "Sexual Orientation: Toward Biological Understanding" (L. Ellis and L. Ebertz, eds.), pp. 2–20. Praeger, Westport, CT.

Grober, M. S. (1998). Socially controlled sex change: Integrating ultimate and proximate levels of analysis. *Acta Ethol.* **1**, 3–17.

Grober, M. S., and Bass, A. H. (1991). Neuronal correlates of sex/role change in labrid fishes: LHRH-like immunoreactivity. *Brain, Behav. Evol.* **38**, 302–312.

Grober, M. S., and Sunobe, T. (1996). Serial adult sex change involves rapid and reversible changes in forebrain neurochemistry. *NeuroReport* **7**, 2945–2949.

Grober, M. S., Jackson, I. M. D., and Bass, A. H. (1991). Gonadal steroids affect LHRH preoptic cell number in sex/role changing fish. *J. Neurobiol.* **22**, 734–741.

Grober, M. S., Fox, S., Laughlin, C., and Bass, A. H. (1994). GnRH cell size and number in a teleost fish with two male reproductive morphs: Sexual maturation, final sexual status and body size allometry. *Brain, Behav. Evol.* **43**, 61–78.

Grober, M. S., Myers, T. R., Marchaterre, M. A., Bass, A. H., and Myers, D. A. (1995). Structure, localization and molecular phylogeny of a GnRH cDNA from a sexually polymorphic teleost fish. *Gen. Comp. Endocrinol.* **99**, 85–99.

Gross, M. R. (1996). Alternative reproductive strategies and tactics: Diversity within the sexes. *Trends Ecol. Evol.* **11**, 92–98.

Halpern-Sebold, L. R., Schreibman, M. P., and Margolis-Nunno, H. (1986). Differences between early- and late-maturing genotypes of the platyfish (*Xiphophorus maculatus*) in the morphometry of their immunoreactive luteinizing hormone releasing hormone-containing cells. A developmental study. *J. Exp. Zool.* **240**, 245–257.

Hubbs, C. (1920). The bionomics of *Porichthys notatus* Girard. *Am. Nat.* **54**, 380–384.

Ibara, R. M., Penny, L. T., Ebeling, A. W., van Dykhuizen, G., and Cailliet, G. (1983). The mating call of the plainfin midshipman fish, *Porichthys notatus*. In "Predators and Prey in Fishes" (D. L. G. Noakes eds.), *et al.*, pp. 205–212. Dr. W. Junk Publ., The Hague, The Netherlands.

Knapp, R., Wingfield, J. C., and Bass, A. H. (1999a). Steroid hormones and paternal care in the midshipman fish (*Porichthys notatus*). *Horm. Behav.* **35**, 81–89.

Knapp, R., Marchaterre, M. A., and Bass, A. H. (1999b). Early development of a sexually dimorphic vocal motor system in a vocal fish. *J. Neurobiol.* **38**, 475–490.

Kramer, C. R., and Imbriano, M. A. (1997). Neuropeptide Y (NPY) induces gonad reversal in the protogynous bluehead wrasse, *Thalassoma bifasciatum* (Teleostei: Labridae). *J. Exp. Zool.* **279**, 133–144.

Kuwamura, T., Nakashima, Y., and Yogo, Y. (1994). Sex change in either direction by growth-rate advantage in the monogamous coral goby, *Paragobiodon echinocephalus*. *Behav. Ecol.* **5**, 434–438.

Macey, M. J., Pickford, G. E., and Peter, R. E. (1974). Forebrain localization of the spawning reflex response to exogenous neurohypophysial hormones in the Killifish, *Fundulus heteroclitus*. *J. Exp. Zool.* **190**, 269–280.

Marxer-Miller, S. K., Carlisle, S. L., Canario, A., Carneiro, L., Oliveira, R. F., and Grober, M. S. (2002). Androgens mediate changes in sexually dimorphic characters in a hermaphroditic fish. *Biol. Reprod.* (in review).

McIntyre, K. K. (1998). Arginine vasotocin in the preoptic area of the bluehead wrasse and the effects of 11-ketotestosterone. M.S. Thesis, Arizona State University, Tempe.

McKibben, J. R., and Bass, A. H. (1998). Behavioral assessment of acoustic parameters relevant to signal recognition and preference in a vocal fish. *J. Acoust. Soc. Am.* **104**, 3520–3533.

McKibben, J. R., and Bass, A. H. (1999). Peripheral encoding of behaviorally relevant acoustic signals in a vocal fish: Single tones. *J. Comp. Physiol.* **184**, 563–576.

McKibben, J. R., and Bass, A. H. (2001). Effects of temporal envelope modulation on acoustic signal recognition in a vocal fish. *J. Acoust. Soc. Am.* **109**, 293–294.

Moore, F. L. (1992). Evolutionary precedents for behavioral actions of oxytocin and vasopressin. *Ann. N.Y. Acad. Sci.* **652**, 156–165.

Moore, F. L., and Lowry, C. A. (1998). Comparative neuroanatomy of vasotocin and vasopressin in amphibians and other vertebrates. *Comp. Biochem. Physiol. C* **119**, 251–260.

Olivera, R. F., Carneiro, L. A., Gonçalves, D. M., Canario, A. V. M., and Grober, M. S. (2001). 11-ketotestosterone inhibits the alternative mating tactic in sneaker males of the Peacock blenny, *Salaria pavo*. *Brain Behav. Evol.* **58**, 28–37.

Petersen, C. W., Warner, R. R., Cohen, S., Hess, H. C., and Sewell, A. T. (1992). Variable pelagic fertilization success: Implications for mate choice and spatial patterns of mating. *Ecology* **73**, 391–401.

Reavis, R. H., and Grober, M. S. (1999). An integrative approach to sex change: Social, behavioural and neurochemical changes in *Lythrypnus dalli* (Pisces). *Acta Ethol.* **2**, 51–60.

Schlinger, B. A., Greco, C., and Bass, A. H. (1999). Aromatase activity in hindbrain vocal control region: Divergence between "singing" and "sneaking" males. *Proc. R. Soc. London, Ser. B* **266**, 131–136.

Shapiro, D. Y. (1992). Plasticity of gonadal development and protandry in fishes. *J. Exp. Zool.* **261**, 194–203.

Shapiro, D. Y., and Rasotto, M. B. (1993). Sex differentiation and gonadal development in the diandric, protogynous wrasse, *Thalassoma bifasciatum* (Pisces, Labridae). *J. Zool. Lond.* **230**, 231–245.

Smith, C. L. (1975). The evolution of hermaphroditism in fishes. In "Intersexuality in the Animal Kingdom" (R. Reinboth, ed.), pp. 295–310. Springer-Verlag, Berlin.

St. Mary, C. M. (1993). Novel sexual patterns in two simulatenously hermaphroditic gobies, *Lythrpnus dalli* and *Lythrypnus zebra*. *Copeia* **4**, 1062–1072.

St. Mary, C. M. (1997). Sequential patterns of sex allocation in simultaneous hermaphrodites: Do we need models that specifically incorporate this complexity? *Am. Nat.* **150**, 73–97.

Sunobe, T., and Nakazono, A. (1993). Sex change in both directions by alteration of social dominance in *Trimma okinawae* (Pisces: Gobiidae). *Ethology* **94**, 339–345.

Swaab, D. F., and Hofman, M. A. (1990). An enlarged suprachiasmatic nucleus in homosexual men. *Brain Res.* **537**, 141–148.

Walker, H. J., and Rosenblatt, R. H. (1988). Pacific toadfishes of the genus *Porichthys* (Batrachoididae) with descriptions of three new species. *Copeia,* pp. 887–904.

Walsh, P. W., Mommsen, T. P., and Bass, A. H. (1995). Biochemical and molecular aspects of singing in batrachoidid fishes. *In* "Biochemistry and Molecular Biology of Fishes" (P. W. Hochachka and T. P. Mommsen, eds.), Vol. 4, pp. 279–289. Elsevier.

Warner, R. R. (1975). The adaptive significance of sequential hermaphroditism in animals. *Am. Nat.* **109**, 61–81.

Warner, R. R., and Hoffman, S. G. (1980). Local population size as a determinant of mating system and sexual composition in two tropical reef fishes (*Thalassoma* spp.). *Evolution (Lawrence, Kans.)* **34**, 508–518.

Warner, R. R., and Schultz, E. T. (1992). Sexual selection and male characteristics in the bluehead wrasse, *Thalassoma bifasciatum:* Mating site acquisition, mating site defense, and female choice. *Evolution (Lawrence, Kans.)* **46**, 1421–1442.

Warner, R. R., and Swearer, S. E. (1991). Social control of sex change in the bluehead wrasse. *Biol. Bull. (Woods Holo, Mass.)* **181**, 199–204.

Zhou, J.-N., Hofman, M. A., Gooren, L. J. G., and Swaab, D. F. (1995). A sex difference in the human brain and its relation to transsexuality. *Nature (London)* **378**, 68–70.

24

Weakly Electric Fish: Behavior, Neurobiology, and Neuroendocrinology

Harold H. Zakon
Section of Neurobiology
Institute for Neuroscience
University of Texas
Austin, Texas 78712

G. Troy Smith
Department of Biology
Indiana University
Bloomington, Indiana 47405

I. INTRODUCTION

Weakly electric fish generate weak electric fields from an electric organ in their tails. They sense their own electric organ discharges (EODs) and those of other fish with specialized sensory receptors called electroreceptors. There are two orders of weakly electric fish–the Gymnotiformes, which live in South America, and the Mormyriformes which are found in Africa. These orders are so phylogenetically distant that weakly electric organs and electrosensory capabilities must have evolved independently in each group. Electric fish use this extraordinary sense to locate and identify nearby objects (electrolocation) and to communicate with one another (electrocommunication) (Hopkins 1974).

Electric fish are technically advantageous as experimental subjects for studying the neural and hormonal mechanisms underlying sexual dimorphisms in communication behavior. Electrical signals are stereotyped and easily quantifiable, which allows for the detailed and precise analysis of signal structure. Electric signals are easily synthesized and manipulated, and can be played back to fish; the fish respond to them as they do to naturally emitted signals. Many of these electrical behaviors are influenced by sex steroid hormones. The neural circuits underlying the emission and sensing of the EOD are simple, the circuit elements are known, and most of the cells are accessible for electrophysiological and biophysical analyses. Last, molecular tools are being generated in a number of laboratories that allow an analysis of sex differences in behavior on a molecular level.

Another attractive aspect of studying the breeding biology and communication systems of these fish is the richness and diversity of their behavior and ecology. For example, most species show a strong sexual dimorphism in the EOD, but some show a reverse sexual dimorphism and a few seem to be monomorphic (Westby, 1988; Alves-Gomes and Hopkins, 1997). In gymnotiforms, as far as is known, communication is mainly via electrical signals, whereas other sensory modalities such as vision and olfaction play little or no role. On the other hand, mormyrids have sensitive hearing, and acoustic communication signals are prominent in the courtship of some species (Crawford et al., 1986). Some species lay eggs on vegetation or in the leaf litter and abandon them, whereas others construct nests and tend to their young (Hagedorn and Heiligenberg, 1985). There are differences in habitat choice and gregariousness—in some species individuals are solitary and establish territories in shallow streams; in others, fish school in open water or even gather in large multispecies assemblages (Hopkins, 1981).

Finally, the phylogenies of both orders of weakly electric fish are well worked out, allowing for reasonable speculations about how sexual dimorphisms and other behaviors evolved (Alves-Gomes *et al.*, 1995; Alves-Gomes, 1999).

In this chapter, we discuss electrocommunication, its role in the breeding biology of electric fish, and the regulation of electrocommunication signals by gonadal steroid hormones. We highlight what is common to all electric fish, using exemplars of particular species to illustrate specific points.

A. Electric Organ Discharge as a Communication Signal

Each modality has advantages and disadvantages for communication. Electric signals are restricted to aquatic environments, and they fall off with distance more rapidly than acoustic or visual stimuli (Hopkins, 1999). A major advantage of electric signals is that they provide a private communication channel because many predators cannot sense these signals. Nevertheless, there are electroreceptive predators. Catfish, which grow large and are abundant in the rivers inhabited by electric fish, possess ampullary electroreceptors (see later) allowing them to detect direct current (D.C.) and low-frequency components of EODs. Electric eels, which are gymnotiforms, hunt weakly electric fish by tracking their EODs (Westby, 1988). It is likely that electroreceptive predators have exerted a formidable selection pressure on electric fish to evolve signals that are less detectable to these predators (i.e., to minimize the D.C. and low-frequency components of their EODs) (Stoddard, 1999).

Other aspects of electric signals make them advantageous. Visual signals can only be used in the daytime and are not visible in dense foliage. Acoustic signals are degraded as they pass through the environment by the attenuation of high-frequency components and destructive interference resulting from reflections of sound from leaves or the ground (Hopkins, 1999). Electric signals can be used at night or in light-restricted habitats such as silty streams or the bottoms of large rivers; they can be delivered from a protected location such as a clump of weeds. Most important to this chapter, the temporal fine structure of electric signals is not distorted by the medium, allowing slight variations of EOD waveforms to carry important information (Hopkins and Bass, 1981; McGregor and Westby, 1992; Hopkins, 1999).

II. GENERATION AND RECEPTION OF ELECTRIC SIGNALS

A. Electric-Organ-Discharge Waveform: Pulse or Wave

Despite their dissimilar origins, gymnotiform and mormyriform fish have converged on the same two strategies of EOD generation: pulse- and wave-type EODs. Fish cannot switch between these two EOD types; each species is hardwired to generate one or the other. Pulse species produce brief EOD pulses with long irregular interpulse intervals (Figs. 1–2). Wave fish, on the other hand, generate EODs in which the pulse and the interpulse interval are of comparable durations and the EOD pulses are given with extreme regularity (Fig. 3).

Each EOD type probably confers different advantages for electrolocation (Hopkins, 1999). Pulse-type EODs are energy efficient because they can be produced at low rates at rest and at higher rates when fish are aroused or exploring their environment. Wave-type EODs, conversely, are more costly because they are constantly emitted at a high rate; this may limit wave fish from inhabiting certain habitats such as poorly oxygenated

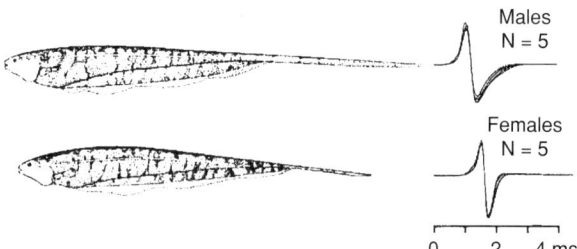

FIGURE 1 Pulse-type EODs from the South American fish the pin-tail knifefish (*Brachyhypopomus pinnicaudatus*). Males (top) possess thicker longer tails than females (bottom) and produce EOD pulses that are longer in duration, especially the second (negative) phase. The EODs are samples from five fish of each sex, scaled in amplitude and overlain. Adapted from Hopkins *et al.* (1990).

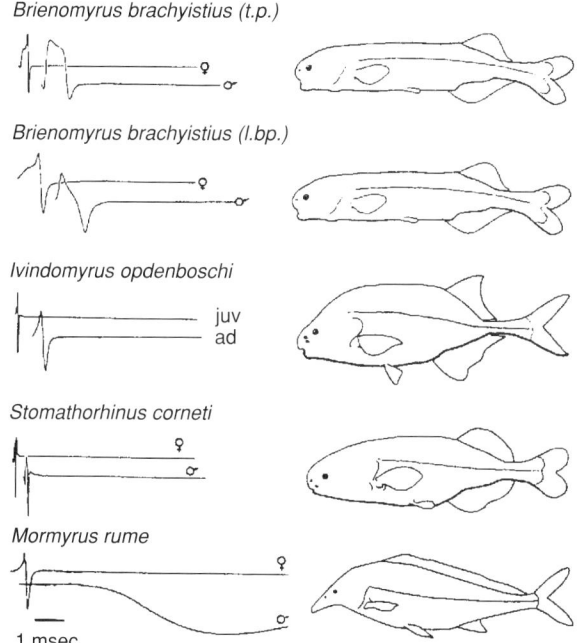

FIGURE 2 Pulse-type EODs from five African electric fish. Note the sexual dimorphism and age difference (*Ivindomyrus opdenboschi*) in EOD pulse shape. Courtesy of C. D. Hopkins.

swamps and streams (Henderson and Crampton, 1997; Crampton, 1998). However, their extreme regularity and higher frequency gives more precise temporal resolution in the sampling of the environment.

The other major selective forces on EOD waveshape come from its use in communication. To ensure repro-

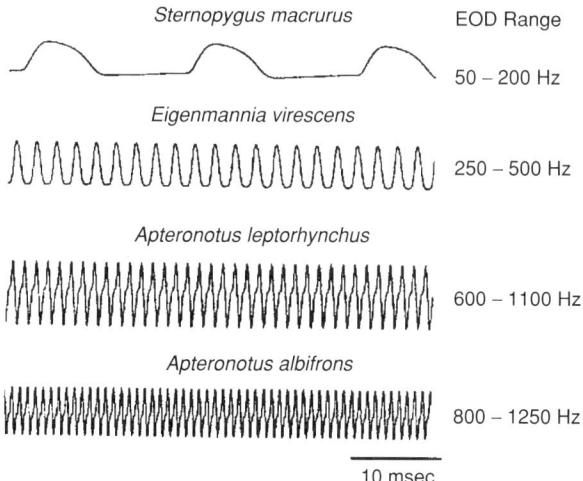

FIGURE 3 Wave-type EODs from four South American species. From Smith (1999).

ductive isolation, EOD waveforms are species-specific (Hopkins and Heiligenberg, 1978; Hopkins, 1981; Kramer, 1990). Subtle variations of the species-specific EOD waveform convey information on sex differences, age differences (larva vs adult), status differences (dominant vs submissive individuals), and individual differences (Hopkins, 1974; Westby and Kirschbaum 1977, 1978; Hagedorn and Zelick, 1989; Crawford, 1992; Carlson, 2000). Before we consider how the EOD waveform conveys this information, it is necessary to first understand how the EOD is generated and received.

B. Neural Circuitry Controlling the Electric Organ Discharge

The neural circuits controlling the EOD are strikingly similar in their organization in gymnotiforms and mormyriforms, although very different in the mechanisms for generating rhythmicity (Grant et al., 1999). Both are organized with intrinsic medullary command neurons that drive nearby follower neurons. The follower neurons send their axons down the spinal cord to innervate electromotorneurons, which are specialized spinal motorneurons. These, in turn, synapse on and activate the electric organ. In both orders, the command neurons receive inputs from diencephalic and midbrain inputs that modulate (gymnotiforms) or contribute to (mormyriforms) the fundamental rhythmicity of the EOD.

In gymnotiforms, the EOD command neurons are a small number (~15–150, depending on species) of pacemaking neurons located in a midline nucleus, called the pacemaker nucleus (PMN) (Fig. 4). These neurons synapse on and drive a second group of neurons in the PMN, called relay cells. Pacemaker neurons are spontaneously oscillating neurons. In at least one species (the brown ghost), their depolarizing potentials are probably initiated by the interactions of a number of intrinsic ionic currents, such as transient and persistent Na^+ currents, a rapidly activating K^+ current, and a Ca^{2+} current (Smith and Zakon, 2000). They fire at highly regular rates in wave fish and at slower and less precise rates in pulse fish (Spiro, 1997). These neurons maintain their rhythmicity even when removed from a fish and placed in a slice chamber (Dye, 1991; Smith and Zakon, 2000).

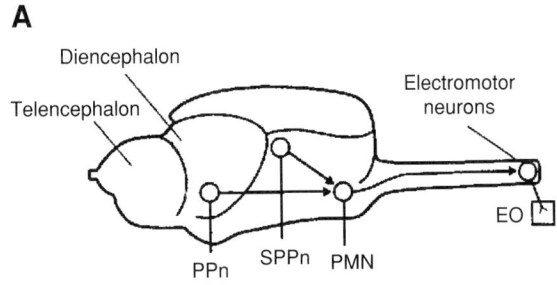

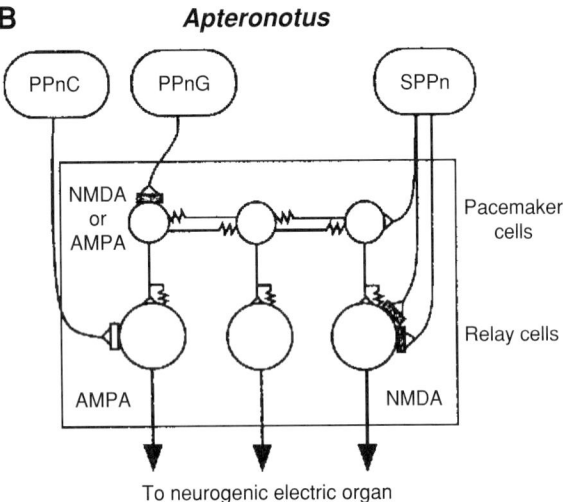

FIGURE 4 Pacemaker nucleus of a South American fish and its inputs. (A) Schematic illustration of the two inputs to the pacemaker nucleus (PMN): the prepacemaker nucleus (PPn) and the sublemniscal prepacemaker nucleus (SPPn). These inputs modulate the firing frequency of the pacemaker neurons in the PMN, which ultimately act on the electric organ (EO). (B) Cell types (pacemaker and relay) on which the inputs from the SPPn and the two divisions of the PPn synapse. NMDA (N-methyl-D-aspartate) and AMPA (α amino-3-hydroxy-5-methyl-4-isoxazolepropionic acid) refer to two classes of glutamate receptors.

Pacemaker neurons are electrotonically and chemically coupled to one another and to the relay cells (Bennett et al., 1967; Elekes and Szabo, 1981). The relay neurons send their axons out of the nucleus and down the spinal cord to innervate electromotoneurons (EMNs) (Bennett et al., 1967). The EMNs then innervate the muscle-derived cells of the electric organ, called electrocytes (except in the Apteronotidae, in which the myogenic electric organ degenerates and axons of the EMNs form the electric organ).

In mormyrids, a similar organization of electrotonically connected command neurons and follower neurons occurs in the medulla, although they are in distinct nuclei (Elekes et al., 1985; Grant et al., 1999). The rhythmic firing of the command neurons is not generated by an intrinsic pacemaking mechanism but, rather, by a complex interaction of synaptic input and intrinsic currents. The command neurons receive input from a number of sources including a strong input from spontaneously firing midbrain premotor neurons. The command neurons integrate this synaptic input and fire two time-locked spikes. Following this characteristic double-action potential, the command cell shows a strong after-hyperpolarization (hypothesized to be due to a Ca^{2+}-activated K^+ conductance or inhibitory feedback), and this delays the generation of the next double-action potential, thereby supplying the essential basal periodicity of spiking rhythmicity (Grant et al., 1999; Carlson and Hopkins, 2000). The command neurons synapse on relay neurons in a neighboring nucleus and these project to the spinal EMNs, and so on.

The morphology of the electrocytes varies greatly between the two orders and even among species in the same order. This is especially true in the mormyriforms, in which these variations are intimately bound up in the generation of species-specific EOD waveforms (Bass, 1986a; Hopkins, 1999). However, their principles of operation are based on the same fundamental features of excitable membranes and current flow. Mainly, electric organs are composed of columns of electrocytes oriented in the same axis and ensheathed in high-resistance connective tissue. This channels the flow of current along the axis of the organ, out into the water, and back into the other end of the electric organ (Bennett and Grundfest, 1959; Bennett, 1961; Bell et al., 1976).

C. Production of Species-Specific Electric-Organ-Discharge Waveforms

1. Pulse Fish

EODs often differ among species in the number and polarity of their phases and by differences in the amplitude and duration of each phase (Figs. 1–2). The number of phases and their polarities are determined by fixed morphological parameters such as the site of innervation, the number of electrically excitable faces, the geometry of the electrocytes, and the location of the electric organ in the body (Bass, 1986a; Caputi,

1999; Hopkins, 1999). Variation in a species, such as sex differences or individual differences, depends on more subtle variation in the duration and amplitudes of each phase, and these depend on modifiable physiological properties such as the duration and amplitude of the action potentials generated by each face.

The simplest EOD is a monophasic pulse. This is generated by an electrocyte with one face that is innervated and generates an action potential and another face that is electrically inexcitable (Keynes and Martins-Ferreira, 1953; Bennett, 1961) (Fig. 5A). Upon depolarization by synaptic input, the innervated face fires an action potential during which positive current (Na^+ ions) enters the innervated face. This causes positive current (probably K^+ ions) to exit the opposite face. In other words, if an electrocyte is innervated on its posterior face, current flows in that face and out the anterior face; the net positive current from all the simultaneously active electrocytes flows headward along the length of the electric organ (into the water and back into the fish's tail). This results in a head-positive pulse.

Both faces of the electrocyte are excitable in those species that produce a diphasic discharge (Fig. 5B). First, upon depolarization by the neurotransmitter, the innervated face fires an action potential during which current flows in one direction. The flow of current through the other membrane depolarizes it, causing it to generate an action potential; current then flows in the opposite direction in the organ. The alternate flow of current headward and then tailward gives the EOD its diphasic shape (Bennett, 1961).

The waveform of the pulse can even be tri- or quatriphasic (Fig. 2). Multiphasic EOD pulses occur in both gymnotiform and mormyriform fish, although the cellular mechanisms responsible for their generation differ in the two groups (Bass, 1986a; Caputi, 1999; Hopkins, 1999).

2. Wave Fish

The production of the EOD in wave-type fish is similar in both orders. It is easiest to consider a wave-type EOD to be a pulse-type EOD with an extremely regular discharge (Fig. 6). If the durations of the EOD pulses are approximately the same as those of the interpulse interval, the EOD is periodic and nearly sinusoidal.

In wave-type fish that possess myogenic electric organs, the EOD pulse is monophasic (i.e., the electrocytes have a single active face). The frequency of a wave-type EOD is determined by the firing frequency of the pacemaker nucleus. However, in order for the waveform to approximate a sine wave, the EO pulse duration must also vary. So, for example, the EOD frequency of *Sternopygus* sp. varies from 50 to 200 Hz and the EO pulse duration varies from 14 to 4 ms (Fig. 6). These two parameters covary so that the fish with the lowest EOD frequency has the longest pulse (Mills and Zakon, 1987; Mills and Zakon, 1991). These two independent parameters may be manipulated by hormonal modulation (see later).

The apteronotidae, the sole group of electric fish without a myogenic EO, also generate wave-type discharges. Some apteronotidae generate EOD frequencies in excess of 1 kHz. Their electromotor system is electrotonically coupled from the PMN to the EMNs (Waxman *et al.*, 1972; Pappas *et al.*, 1975). *Apteronotus* larvae begin life with a myogenic electric organ, but it degenerates within 20 days of hatching, concurrent

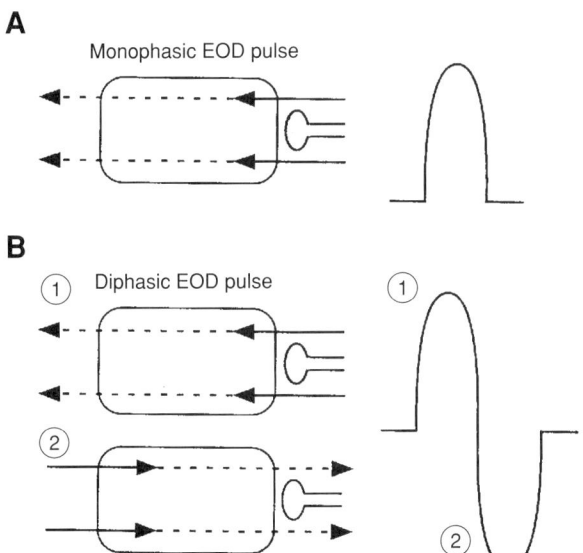

FIGURE 5 Generation of EOD pulses. (A) Monophasic EOD pulse is generated by current flow into the innervated face of an electrocyte and out the opposite face. This generates a pulse as shown at the right. (B) The first phase of a diphasic EOD pulse is generated as in (A). However, if the uninnervated face is excitable, inward current may then flow into it and out the innervated face. This results in the second phase of the EOD as shown at the right.

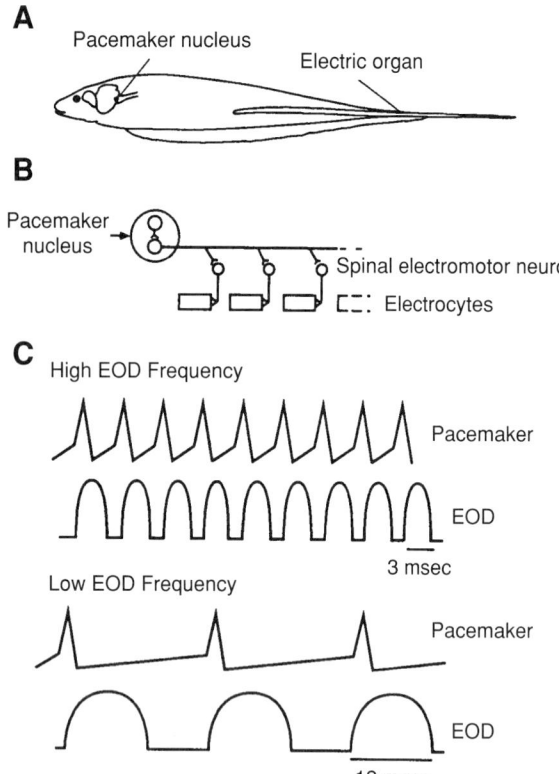

the prepacemaker nucleus (PPn) and the sublemniscal prepacemaker nucleus (SPPn).

Of particular interest is that the inputs from the PPn synapse on relay neurons via glutamate receptors (Fig. 4). When these inputs are active, they depolarize the relay cells, transiently raising their firing frequency and elevating the EOD pulse rate in a pulse fish or the EOD frequency in a wave fish (Fig. 7). This is the basis for a category of social signal called chirps (Dye et al., 1989; Kawasaki and Heiligenberg, 1989). If the glutamatergic input is strong or long-lasting, it can depolarize the relay cells enough to inactivate their

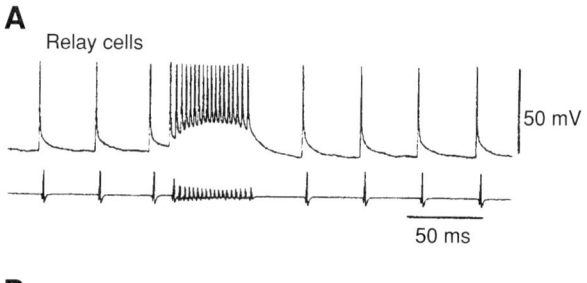

FIGURE 6 Relationship between EOD frequency and electric organ (EO) pulse duration in gymnotiform wave fish. (A) Location of the pacemaker nucleus and the electric organ. (B) Output neurons of the pacemaker nucleus (the relay cells) synapse on electromotor neurons, and these synapse on the cells of the electric organ, the electrocytes. (C) Pacemaker firing frequency and electric organ pulse duration must be precisely correlated to produce a sinusoidal EOD, as in the gold-lined black knifefish (*Sternopygus macrurus*). From McAnelly and Zakon (2000).

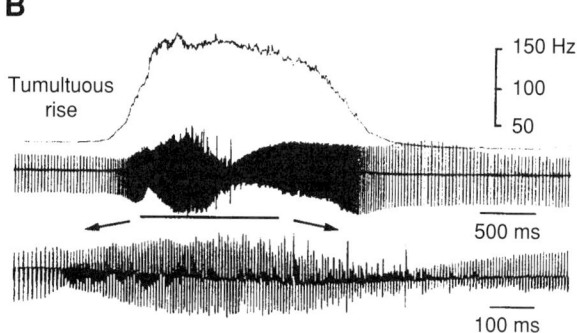

with a developmental increase in EOD frequency (Kirschbaum and Westby, 1975). It is thought that the loss of the myogenic electric organ eliminates the one obligatory chemical synapse in the electromotor circuit that might fail at these high operating frequencies.

3. Social Signals Are Mediated by Neurotransmission via Glutamate Receptors

Electric fish modulate their EOD frequency or pulse rate during social interactions to convey motivational information (see later). The neural mechanisms underlying the generation of these signals is best understood in the pacemaker of gymnotiform fish, where this is accomplished by inputs from two premotor nuclei called

FIGURE 7 Social signals are generated by modulation of the pacemaker. (A) Fish (in this case a South American pulse fish of the genus *Hypopomus*) can be induced to make social signals in an electrophysiological experiment. Relay cells fire a barrage of action potentials as glutamatergic input from the prepacemaker nucleus depolarizes them. The EOD (bottom trace) shows a 1:1 relationship with each pacemaker action potential. During the barrage of action potentials, the EOD show a burst of pulses of decreasing amplitude (due to the inactivation of the Na^+ channels in the electrocytes). (B) During courtship, a male *Hypopomus* makes a social signal referred to as a tumultuous rise, in which EOD frequency is increased by two- or threefold. Recordings of the EOD at two time scales show the increase in frequency. Movements of the fish relative to the recording electrodes cause some of the changes in amplitude in this recording. From Kawasaki and Heiligenberg (1989).

sodium channels and cause them to cease firing (Spiro, 1997). When this happens, no command signals are sent to the spinal cord motorneurons and the EOD transiently ceases as well; this is the basis for a social signal called an interruption (Kawasaki and Heiligenberg, 1989). Chirps can be of different durations in different social circumstances; how the prepacemaker input varies in generating each type of chirp is not known.

D. Reception of the Electric Organ Discharge: The Electroreceptors

Weakly electric fish possess two classes of electroreceptors—ampullary and tuberous receptors. These receptors are distributed over the fish's body, although they are most dense near the head and are innervated by the lateral line nerves. Ampullary receptors are similar in both orders of fish—they are broadly tuned and behave as low-pass filters (∼30–40 Hz to virtually D.C.). Although researchers believe ampullary receptors are used primarily in prey detection, recent data indicate their use in social communication as well (see later) (Metzner and Heiligenberg, 1991).

Tuberous receptors show an extreme amount of variation and plasticity in their filter properties compared to ampullary receptors. Tuberous receptors are tuned to the frequency components of each fish's EOD. The receptors of pulse fish are broadly tuned to capture the wide frequency spectrum of a pulse (Shumway and Zelick, 1988; Hopkins and Heiligenberg, 1978). The tuberous receptors of wave fish are sharply tuned and the receptors of each fish are best tuned to its own EOD frequency (Hopkins, 1976). Because EOD frequency is sexually dimorphic, receptor tuning is as well (Zakon and Meyer, 1983).

There are two types of tuberous receptors in mormyrids. One type, the knollenorgan, is used exclusively for social communication, detecting the pulses of neighboring fish. It fires an action potential on positive zero crossings of the EOD (when the voltage of the EOD goes from negative to positive). Behavioral and physiological evidence suggests that these receptors are used in a two-spike code to determine the durations and phases of the EOD of neighbors (Hopkins and Bass, 1981). That is, knollenorgans on one side of the body fire during positive-to-negative transitions of the EOD, and ones on the other side fire during negative-to-positive transitions. This is due to the geometry of current flow—current emanating from a neighboring fish enters one side of the body and exits the opposite side, depolarizing knollenorgans on the side it enters and hyperpolarizing those on the side it exits. There are neurons in the mormyrid midbrain that are exquisitely sensitive to the duration of an EOD pulse, which can signal the species and sex of the sender (Amagai, 1998; Friedman and Hopkins, 1998).

A comparable receptor type, the pulse marker, occurs in gymnotiforms. Gymnotiform pulse fish have probably evolved a similar two-spike encoding scheme, based on recordings from midbrain electrosensory circuits (Shumway and Zelick, 1988).

The situation in gymnotiform wave fish is more complicated because their tuberous receptors simultaneously sense both their own EOD and that of a neighboring fish. If a nearby fish is of the same sex and close in EOD frequency, their two EODs will beat with each other, which results in predictable changes in the waveform of the combined EOD. If the neighboring fish is of the opposite sex, and therefore has an EOD frequency many tens of hertz distant from the first fish, their EODs add in complex ways (Fleishman, 1992). It is not clear how this information is encoded and read out in the brain.

III. SEX DIFFERENCES AND INDIVIDUAL VARIATION IN ELECTRIC-ORGAN-DISCHARGE WAVEFORM

Most species of weakly electric fish possess sexually dimorphic EODs; in addition, the EOD waveforms of each individual are unique and stable over days (Friedman and Hopkins, 1996). To understand whether these variations are used for communication it is necessary to know if they vary with attributes of the signaler, are perceptible to the receiver, and trigger appropriate behaviors in the receiver.

A. Sexual Dimorphism of the Electric-Organ-Discharge Waveform

Most weakly electric pulse fish possess sexually dimorphic EODs (a few have no apparent sexual dimorphism in EOD waveshape, and it will be intriguing to study their breeding biology (Westby, 1988; C. D. Hopkins, personal communication). In a case of apparent convergence, male pulse fish of both orders produce longer-duration EOD pulses than females (Figs. 1–2). There is no known example of a species in which females produce longer-duration pulses.

In most species of gymnotiform wave fish, EOD frequency is lower in males than in females. There are few species, however, in which it is opposite; the brown ghost *(Apternotus leptorhynchus)* is an example (Fig. 8) (Hagedorn and Heiligenberg, 1985). Because the ancestral and common pattern is for males to have lower EOD frequencies than females, this is a case of reversed sexual dimorphism (Dunlap *et al.*, 1998; Dunlap and Zakon, 1998).

We have no information on the breeding biology or the existence of a sexual dimorphism in the EOD of *Gymnarchus niloticus*, the sole mormyriform wave fish.

That electric fish perceive and respond to these sex differences has been amply demonstrated in numerous species. For example, male fish court female, but not male, EODs or EOD mimics in playback experiments (Hopkins, 1974; Hopkins and Bass, 1981; Crawford, 1991). Conversely, females may respond preferentially to male vs female EOD pulses (Shumway and Zelick, 1988).

There may be species differences in which component of the EOD is used for sex recognition. For example, in the mormyrid *Brienomyrus brachyistius,* the EOD pulse is longer in males (1.2 ms) than in females (0.5 ms). Playback experiments show that the duration of the pulse is the critical variable for sex recognition. On the other hand, male *Pollimyrus adspersus* (formerly classified as *P. isidori;* Crawford, 1997) another mormyrid, ignore the waveform of the EOD pulse, even though it possesses a subtle sexual dimorphism in pulse amplitude (Crawford, 1992). It attends, instead, to sex differences in the regularity of the pattern in which the discharges are delivered. The EOD pulse is exceptionally brief in this species (85–90 μs in both sexes), perhaps too brief in duration for sex differences to be reliably resolved (Crawford, 1991).

What is the function of sex differences in the EOD? It is likely that the male signals are more stimulatory to females than those of females or juveniles. For example, the longer duration of the second phase of the

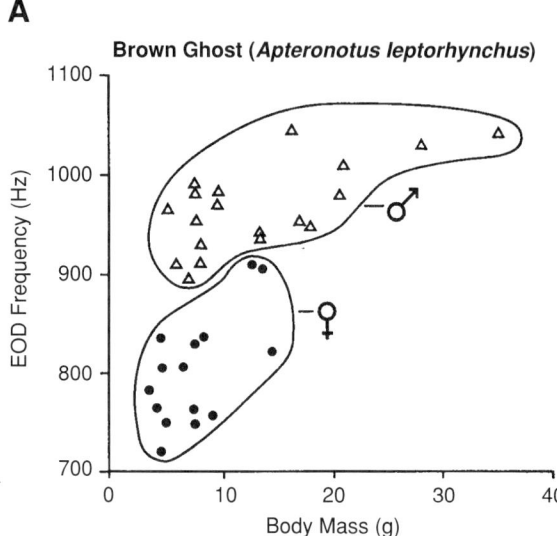

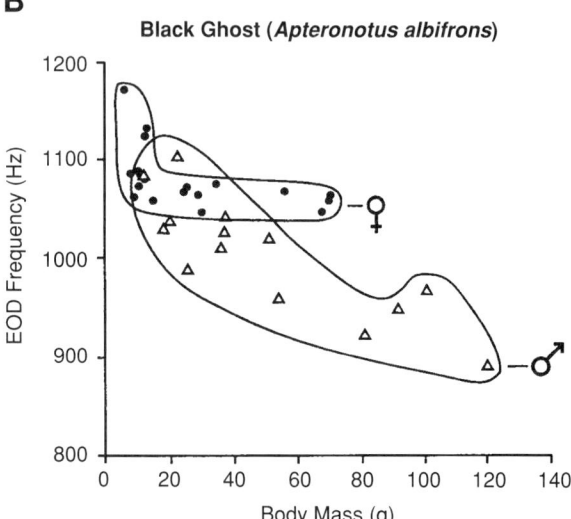

FIGURE 8 EOD frequencies of two related gymnotiform wave fish with sex differences in EOD frequency in opposite directions. (A) Brown ghost females are lower in frequency than males. (B) Black ghost females are higher in frequency than males. From Zakon and Dunlap (1999).

EOD pulse in male pin-tail knifefish (*B. pinnicaudatus*) makes the signal waveform asymmetrical. This results in a brief D.C. component to the signal, which stimulates the ampullary electroreceptors of a female (Metzner and Heiligenberg, 1991). Presumably the more dimorphic the second phase of the EOD is, the more D.C. is generated, and this may be attractive to females. Unfortunately, it should also make the EOD pulse more noticeable to electroreceptive predators such as catfish. Indeed, male pin-tail knifefish are more likely than females to have a wounded or regenerated tail, presumably lost to predation (Hopkins *et al.*, 1990).

B. Individual Differences in Electric-Organ-Discharge Waveform

A detailed analysis of the EOD indicates individual differences in the waveform in every species examined to date. Are these fine variations in EOD waveform perceptible and meaningful to the fish? Weakly electric fish have an exquisite capacity for detecting fine differences in the waveform of real or EOD-like stimuli, as shown by laboratory conditioning experiments (Kramer and Otto, 1991; McGregor and Westby, 1992). A number of demonstrations show that these variations are used in the context of social communication.

The gymnotiform pulse fish *Gymnotus carapo* can be habituated to a situation in which the EOD of one fish is presented from an electrode on the left side of its tank and the EOD of another fish from the right side. When the EOD of a fish is played from the wrong side or the EOD of an unfamiliar fish is presented over either electrode, the fish attacks the electrode (McGregor and Westby, 1992). The total duration of the EOD in this species is 2 ms and the variations in the structure of the EOD waveform are on the order of tens or hundreds of microseconds.

In another experiment, replicate communities of three male and three female *Brienomyrus brachyistius* (a mormyrid pulse fish) were set up and dominance hierarchies were established by the male fish. EOD pulse duration was not initially different among the males. However, after a few weeks, the EOD pulse duration of the dominant males had increased, that of the middle fish was little different from before, and that of the most submissive males decreased (Carlson, 2000).

Do female fish show mate choice and, if so, is it on the basis of the EOD waveform? Female pin-tail knifefish (*B. pinnicaudatus*), a gymnotiform pulse fish, given a choice between a male on one side of the tank and an empty chamber on the other, spent more time near the sexually mature male. However, they actually spent less time near sexually immature males than the empty chamber (Curtis, 1999). This is perhaps not surprising given the propensity of gymnotiform pulse fish to be spread out a few meters from each other in their natural habitat (Hopkins, 1974; Westby, 1988; Crampton, 1998). When females were presented males of different sizes, they preferentially associated with larger males. This choice is indicative of a sexual attraction because the females often spawn with these larger males. The EOD of sexually mature males is longer in duration than that of an immature male, whose EOD is female-like.

Although these experiments illustrate that variation in EOD pulse duration is correlated with social status or breeding conditions, we cannot conclude yet whether these subtle variations convey this information to other fish. It would be extremely interesting to do playback experiments to test this.

Among gymnotiform wave-type fish, there are similar indications that EOD waveform is used for individual discrimination. *Eigenmannia* males have lower EOD frequencies than females. In a tank community of *Eigenmannia*, the largest male possesses the lowest EOD frequency among the males; the largest female has the highest EOD frequency among the females (Hagedorn and Heiligenberg, 1985). The largest fish of both sexes become dominant; they breed with one another and prevent any other fish from breeding.

Similarly, when groups were made with three male and one female brown ghost (*A. leptorhynchus*) the largest male, with the highest EOD frequency (recall that this species has a reversed sexual dimorphism), bred with the female. Without playback experiments it is not possible to know whether it is the electric signals that females base their choices on. There is anecdotal evidence that electrical signals are quite important. Subordinate females have been observed to swim toward a breeding pair of *Eigenmannia*, turn off the EOD completely, and lay their eggs on the periphery of the vegetation in which the dominant pair is breeding. A female who approached them with her EOD on was chased away (Hagedorn and Heiligenberg, 1985).

IV. MODULATION OF ELECTRIC ORGAN DISCHARGES DURING SOCIAL BEHAVIOR

The aspects of the EOD that convey information on species, sex, individual identity, or state of sexual maturity are stable or change slowly. Information transmitted in social encounters about motivational states that change more rapidly, such as aggressiveness or readiness to breed, is signaled by rapid changes in EOD rate.

A. Aggressive Interactions

Agonistic interactions in both wave and pulse fish are accompanied by transient increases in the EOD frequency (in wave fish) or pulse rate (in pulse fish) (Black-Cleworth, 1970; Kramer, 1979).

The mormyrid *Pollimyrus isidori* increase their pulse repetition rate during aggressive encounters from a baseline of tens of pulses per second up to 125 pulses per second for hundreds of milliseconds. Each barrage is followed by a brief silent period. A fish that loses a fight either discharges at a low and regular rate of approximately 10 pulses per second or shuts off its EOD completely. Both sexes behave similarly. This is typical of other mormyrid pulse fish and of gymnotiform pulse fish as well.

The social interactions of gymnotiform wave fish are accompanied by chirps, which are increases in EOD frequency. The parameters of a chirp—mainly duration and frequency excursion—vary depending on the type of social interactions. Agonistic interactions are typically accompanied by brief chirps in which EOD frequency rises by tens of hertz or even 100 Hz, and lasting tens of milliseconds (Fig. 9). It has been documented that agonistic chirps can be further categorized into subtypes based mainly on the extent of the frequency excursion, although the behavioral significance of this is unknown (Engler et al., 2000).

Male glass knifefish (*Eigenmannia virescens*) jockeying for dominance chirp intensely at one another (Hopkins, 1974b; Hagedorn and Heiligenberg, 1985). A dominant male maintains his position by suddenly swimming at other individuals and chirping at them. Males other than the dominant male chirp infrequently. If the dominant male is removed from the tank, other males begin chirping (Hagedorn and Heiligenberg, 1985).

The best-studied example of agonistic chirping is in the brown ghost (*A. leptorhynchus*). Brief agonistic chirps (10–30 ms) are given by brown ghost males and less frequently by females (Zupanc and Maler, 1993;

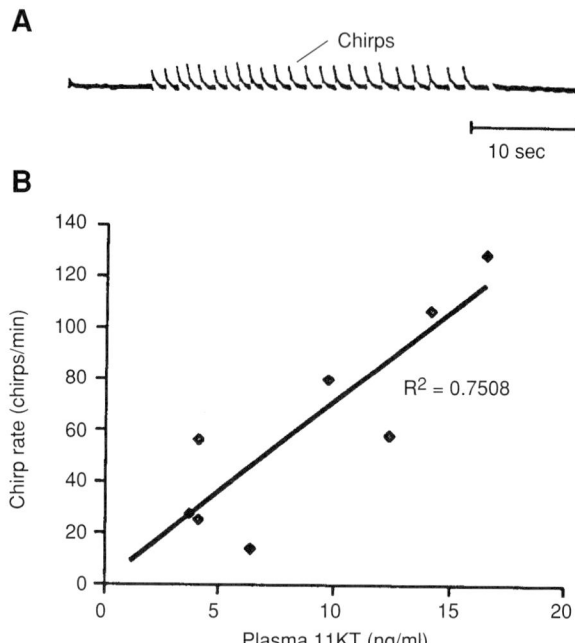

FIGURE 9 Agonistic chirping in brown ghost wave fish. (A) Males maintain a steady EOD frequency, but when presented with an electrical sine wave mimicking an EOD, they make a series of brief (∼20 ms) upward-frequency modulations called chirps. From Dulka and Maler (1994). (B) Chirp rate in males is well correlated with their levels of the androgen 11-ketotestosterone (11 KT) (Dunlap, 2002).

Dulka and Maler, 1994; Dunlap et al., 1998). It is important to note that this sex difference depends, in part, on the circumstances under which the fish are being observed. Chirping is often studied by placing a fish in a perforated plastic tube to constrain its movements, and presenting an electrical sine wave stimulus across the tube. This produces a well-controlled stimulus, but one that has an unnatural geometry. Under these conditions, males chirp robustly, whereas females seldom chirp when stimulus presentations last a minute or less. Females chirp moderately after a longer exposure to a playback stimulus (Triefenbach and Zakon, 2002) and even more intensely in real social encounters (S. Tallarovic, personal communication).

The parameters of the stimulus that a fish is receiving influences chirp rate. For example, when males are studied in a chirp chamber with an EOD mimic near their own EOD frequency, their chirp rate is proportional to stimulus intensity (Dunlap et al., 1998).

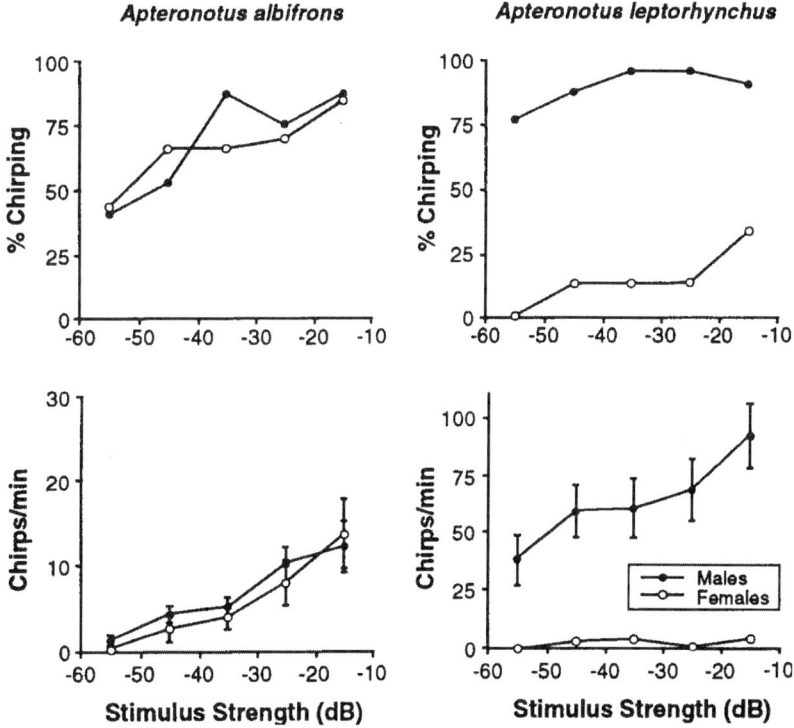

FIGURE 10 Species differences in sex differences in chirping. (A) Brown ghosts (*Apteronotus leptorhynchus*) show a large sex difference in the percentage of individuals that chirped in a minute-long test period, as well as the number of chirps made. (B) Black ghosts (*Apteronotus albifrons*), on the other hand, show no sex difference in these parameters. From Dunlap et al. (1998).

In staged encounters between two fish separated by a mesh barrier, males chirped at other males twice as frequently as they did at females (Dunlap, 2002). When freely swimming fish are presented with EOD mimic stimuli, males with low EOD frequncies (which tend to be the smallest and least mature) chirp more at stimulus frequencies near or below their own EOD frequencies, including female EOD frequencies, but less at stimulus frequencies higher than theirs (which is the range of the larger dominant males). Conversely, males with high EOD frequencies (larger dominant fish), chirp at EOD frequencies across the male range and less at female EOD frequencies (F. Triefenbach, personal communication).

Interestingly, although males make intense (type I; Engler, 2000) agonistic chirps to stimulus frequencies across the species range, they tend to make them more often to stimuli in the female EOD frequency range (Triefenbach and Zakon, 2002). Very long duration chirps, (Engler's type 3 or 4) are only made by males to female EOD frequencies. These are likely to be courtship chirps.

There are interesting species differences in chirping. Black ghosts (*A. albifrons*) show no sex difference in chirping (Dunlap et al., 1998). Black ghosts of both sexes chirp less than male, but more than female, brown ghosts in response to a comparable stimulus (Fig. 10). This is even so when the two species have comparable circulating levels of androgens and similar gonadosomatic indices. Nothing is known about the social interactions of black ghosts and it will be interesting to see how chirps function in social interactions in this species.

In social encounters, submissive wave fish modulate their EOD frequency with long slow rises (Hopkins, 1974; Hagedorn and Heiligenberg, 1985). These are increases of only a few hertz that last for seconds or tens of seconds. This signal is the antithesis of the aggressive signal, as pointed out for animal signals in general by Darwin (1872). When presented with EOD mimic stimuli, female brown ghosts with the highest EOD frequencies (the smallest, least mature females) make more rises than females with the lowest EOD frequencies (larger and more mature). Conversely, male brown ghost with the lowest EOD frequencies (the smallest, least mature males) make more more rises than those with higher EOD frequencies (larger and more mature) (F. Triefenbach, personal communication).

B. Courtship and Spawning

Electric fish breed primarily during the rainy season (Kirschbaum, 1975, 1995), although there are a few possible exceptions to this rule, including the electric eel, which is reported to breed in the dry season (Assunção and Schwassman, 1995), and *Brachyhypopomus occidentalis*, reported to be an acyclical breeder (Hagedorn, 1992). Environmental cues that trigger gonadal recrudescence and reproduction in these species include the pH and conductivity of the water, water level, physical stimulation of rainfall, and food availability (reviewed in Kirschbaum, 1995). For the most part, electric fish are transequatorial in their distribution. Thus, day length and temperature are not reliable zeitgebers for them. However, some species of electric fish also inhabit the temperate zone. One such fish, the pin-tail knifefish, *B. pinnicaudatus*, whose southernmost extent is Uruguay, appears to use daily temperature fluctuations for the regulation of breeding (Silva *et al.*, 1999).

As do olfactory, visual, or acoustic cues in other groups of animals, electrical signals coordinate breeding in weakly electric fish. In both orders of fish, courtship occurs in pairs of fish over a few nights. Typically courtship activity intensifies each night, being the most intense on the night of spawning. Depending on the species, spawning occurs in a single bout or more frequently in a series of bouts. Courtship is accompanied by a variety of stereotyped body postures and movements and variations in the rhythm of the EOD, each sex usually showing a different pattern of EOD modulation.

Among gymnotiform wave fish (*Eigenmannia* and *Apteronotus leptorhynchus*), as courtship commences the male chirps at the female. The female responds by making long rises. As previously mentioned, short chirps such as the male makes on initially encountering females are associated with aggression, and long rises are believed to be a submissive signal. Courtship then continues over a few nights with an intensification of this pattern (Hagedorn and Heiligenberg, 1985).

On the night of spawning, the male chirps incessantly (60–80 chirps/s), although the number of chirps lessens as the chirps become longer (100–200 ms) (Hagedorn and Heiligenberg, 1985). These are courtship chirps. They may be so strong that they result in a transient shutting off of the EOD by the strong depolarization of the relay neurons by the glutamatergic inputs from the PPns (as already discussed). In the presence of a male, the female continues making long rises, now lasting tens of seconds. The male, in turn, often responds to the long rises of the female with renewed bouts of courtship chirping. A number of times during these episodes, the female deposits her eggs (Fig. 11). Female *Apteronouts* make a series of brief (5- to 10-ms) chirps during ovulation. It has been suggested that this signals to the male, who may be patrolling the territory, that ovulation has occurred (Hagedorn and Heiligenberg, 1985).

Comparable electrical displays occur in the gymnotiform pulse fish, such as the pin-tail knife (*B. pinnicaudatus*) and other related species. The male

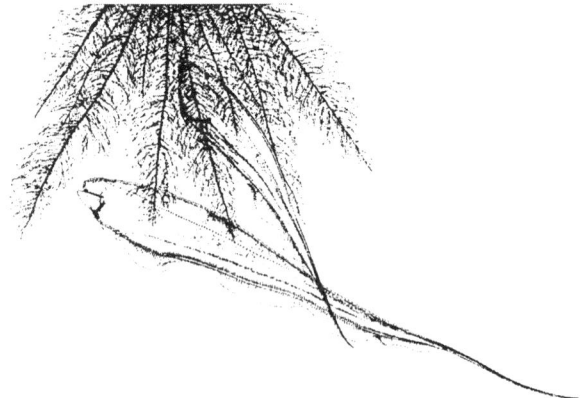

FIGURE 11 Spawning behavior in two glass knifefish (*Eignemannia virsecens*). The gravid female has nestled up into the roots of some water plants and the male hovers below her emitting many long-duration courtshsip chirps. She responds by making long slow rises and releasing her eggs for fertilization. From Hagedorn and Heiligenberg (1985).

swims near his potential nest site, which is a plant, emitting pulses at rates of approximately 50–70 pulses/s. When a female approaches the male, the pair may engage in rate duets in which their rates sometimes shift in parallel and other times mirror each other. The male prods the female with his snout or chases her as his pulse rate increases dramatically in half-second bouts of up to 200 pulses/s (called accelerations by Stoddard, personal communication and tumultuous rises by Kawasaki and Heiligenberg, 1989) (Fig. 7). Eventually the female moves toward his nest plant and he begins making courtship chirps at her (these are distinct from the chirps given in aggressive interactions, called decrement bursts by Hagedorn, 1988). A typical spawning chirp is approximately 25–200 low-amplitude pulses in rapid succession lasting 100–200 ms. Males give long trains of chirps during spawning.

The chirping male enters the plant and backs out. Then the female enters, lays her eggs and backs out. The male reenters the plants, probably fertilizing the eggs. This cycle may be repeated a couple of times until the female leaves.

In the mormyrid pulse fish, courtship and spawning have been well studied in *Pollimyrus isidori*. In this species, and perhaps other mormyrids as well, much of courtship is with acoustic and electric signals (Crawford *et al.*, 1986; Bratton and Kramer, 1989; Crawford, 1991). Early in the spawning cycle, a male establishes a territory and chases away other fish, even females. Eventually he builds one or two nests out of plant material and begins vocalizing.

The resting EOD pattern of *Pollimyrus* is irregular. On the night of spawning, starting on her own territory and continuing throughout the night, the female discharges her EOD very regularly at about 10 pulses per second. During her visits, the male also changes his EOD pattern to a similar regular low-pulse rate and vocalizes profusely (grunt-moan-growl calls); he is electrically silent when he vocalizes. As courtship intensifies, the male and female engage in a series of stereotyped acrobatic swimming movements. During these, they maintain the low regular rhythm of EOD pulses except for a brief moment when they are vent to vent and the male shuts off his EOD. The male ceases vocalizing for the rest of the night, and the pair undergoes a series of spawnings. Following each spawn, the male picks up the eggs in his mouth and transfers them to a nest. After a night of spawning, the male chases the female away.

In playback experiments, Crawford (1991) has shown that the regular EOD pulse rate shown by females during the night of spawning elicits courtship vocalizations form the males, whereas the normal irregular rhythm given by the male (even when used to trigger female EOD pulses) does not.

Hagedorn and Heiligenberg (1985) showed that playing gravid *Eigenmannia* females the signals of a courting male induces them to spawn. Unfortunately, they did not compare this with control electrical signals such as a steady EOD with no chirping. The question of how EOD signals influence the neuroendocrine axis or, conversely, how various hormones initiate the various components of courtship electrical displays is ripe for future investigation.

C. Parental Care

It is generally claimed that gymnotiforms show no parental care and that mormyriforms do. However, because spawning has only been documented in a few species of each group, this is likely to be an overgeneralization. Indeed, spawning has been observed in the laboratory in a representative species of number of families of gymnotiforms (Eigenmannidea, Apteronotidae, and Hypopomidae) and these species make no nests and abandon their eggs once laid. In addition, when the larvae of these or other (*Sternopygus*) species have been found in the field, they have not been associated with an adult fish or anything resembling a nest.

On the other hand, extensive parental care has been documented in the electric eel (*Electrophorus electricus*), which is a gymnotiform fish (Assunção and Schwassman, 1995). Male eels surface and slurp water and air into their mouths, where it mixes with sticky saliva into gobs of foam. They deposit these into a mass of tree roots to form a foam nest at the surface of the water. Spawning has never been observed in eels, but egg masses have been seen in these nests. Eggs are laid in batches in the same nests over months; the later-deposited egg masses, which may contain undeveloped oocytes, are devoured by the larvae from previous batches. Males also protect the young. They vigorously attack when the nest is disturbed and discharge their strong electric organ, although not in immediate proximity to the nest. An intriguing observation was made that, following a disturbance near the nest, the free-swimming larvae clustered over the head of the male and moved in unison with him as he swam into deeper water. Thus, both male (nest building and guarding) and female (supplying egg masses for food) eels contribute to parental care.

Parental care has been observed in species of *Gymnotus*. Although breeding has not been observed in any *Gymnotus* species, dugout nests with young and a male fish hovering over them have been observed in Trinidad for *Gymnotus carapo* (C. D. Hopkins, personal communication). On the other hand, nests made of floating vegetation have been seen for other still unnamed species of *Gymnotus* in Brazil (W. Crampton, personal communication, via C. D. Hopkins). It is interesting to note that the eel, *Electrophorus* and *Gymnotus* are closely related.

As previously mentioned, male *Pollimyrus* make one or two nests of vegetation in advance of spawning. Following each spawn, the male picks up the eggs in his mouth and transfers them to a nest (Crawford *et al.*, 1986; Bratton and Kramer, 1989). After a night of spawning, the male chases the female away. For the next few weeks, the male guards the eggs and protects the fry. He swims around the nest and occasionally pushes against it with his head. If any eggs or larvae fall out, he gently pushes them back in with his head. Once the larvae are free swimming, they school and the male ignores them. They possess a larval electric organ that makes a distinct larval EOD. At approximately 50 days after hatching, the larval electric organ degenerates and an electric organ replaces it. The larval and adult electric organs generate distinct EODs. When the larvae develop the adult EOD, the male begins to behave aggressively toward the larvae and they disperse (Westby and Kirschbaum, 1978).

Last, *Gymnarchus niloticus*, considered to be the most ancient mormyriform fish, is noted to make floating large nests of vegetation and mud. The male actively guards the nest and the larvae remain electrically silent while in the nest (Hopkins, 1986). Whether this is to discourage predation from electroreceptive predators such as catfish or hungry conspecifics is not known.

On the other hand, the mormyrid *Brienomyrus brachyistius* neither builds nests nor shows any parental behavior.

It is perhaps not surprising that, where parental behavior is observed in electric fish, it is seen in the male. This is in keeping with other species of fishes in which males may make substantial investments in their young (Gross and Sargent, 1985; Vincent *et al.*, 1994; Kishida and Specker, 2000). However, nothing is known about the endocrine basis of parental behavior in electric fish.

D. Other Sexually Dimorphic Behaviors

Mormyrid fish discharge irregularly at rest. If a male mormyrid, such as *Pollimyrus*, is presented with an EOD pulse mimic, it responds by quickly (within 12 ms) emitting a pulse after the mimic, whereas a female responds by withholding a pulse for a window of approximately 10–20 ms after the stimulus pulse. This behavior is called the preferred latency response (PLR) in males and preferred latency avoidance (PLA) in females (Lücker and Kramer, 1981). These responses are not observed in high-level social interactions, such as agonistic encounters or courtship, but more often when resting fish are near one another and in electrical contact on their own territories. This is especially true when a female is newly introduced into the tank of an established male.

If two wave-type electric fish with EOD frequencies within 20 Hz of one another meet, their EODs beat and interfere with their ability to electrolocate. Electric fish have evolved a behavior called the jamming avoidance response (JAR), in which a fish shifts its EOD frequency away from that of the other fish to minimize jamming. So, for example, when an *Eigenmannia* is presented with an electrical sine wave a few hertz below its own EOD frequency, it raises its own EOD frequency. Conversely, a sine wave stimulus above its EOD frequency causes it to lower its EOD frequency. Large male fish show, at best, a weak JAR, mature females show a strong JAR only when a stimulus is higher in frequency than their own EOD, and juveniles show a JAR in both directions (Kramer, 1987). The significance of these sex and age differences in not known; however, it has been suggested that these modulations may have a social function as well as or rather than the generally presumed antijamming function. Interestingly, despite strong sexual dimorphisms in other electrical behaviors, brown ghosts (*Apteronotus leptorhynchus*) do not show any sexual dimorphism in the JAR (J. Oestreich, personal communication).

V. STEROID HORMONES AND THE ELECTRIC-ORGAN-DISCHARGE WAVEFORM

A. Endogenous Levels of Gonadal Steroids

Little can be said of circulating levels of hormones in mormyriforms in the field because the sole study (Landsman, 1993) was based on the blood levels of the elephant-nose, *Gnathonemus petersii*, taken in New York 2 days after the fish were captured in Africa. Given the well-known rapid effects of stress on sex steroid levels, the results of this study are ambiguous. However, once in the laboratory and removed from conditions that promote reproductive readiness, the sexual dimorphism of the male EOD pulse waned concurrently with a fall in androgens.

A study indicates that in social groups of three male and three female *Pollimyrus isidori*, in which the males established a dominance hierarchy, levels of 11-keto testosterone (11-KT) were highest (16 ng/ml) in the dominant male, next highest (10 ng/ml) in the next-highest-ranked male, and least (6 ng/ml) in the subordinate male (Carlson and Hopkins, 2000). These fish were in reproductive condition and some of the males even spawned with females during the course of this study. Thus, these hormone levels are indicative of normal levels in the field.

More data are available on gymnotiform wave fish. In the field, androgen levels of male *Sternopygus macrurus* are positively correlated with the degree of testicular development and body size and negatively correlated with EOD frequency (Zakon et al., 1991). However, although all large adult males have high androgen levels and low EOD frequencies, immature males, which have low androgen levels, have either high or low EOD frequencies. Thus, some factor other than androgen level influences EOD frequency in immature males (Zakon et al., 1991). The suggestion that EOD frequency in mature males varies with androgen levels is further supported by a study that noted a tandem increase in 11-KT plasma levels and lowering of EOD frequency in males injected with human chorionic gonadotropin (hCG) (Zakon et al., 1990).

Male brown ghosts in the laboratory also show a positive correlation between plasma 11-KT levels, body size, and EOD frequency; males with low levels (<2.5 ng/ml) have low EOD frequencies (recall that in this species males have higher EOD frequencies than females), whereas those with levels from 5 to 15 ng/ml have the highest EOD frequencies (Zucker, 1997; Dunlap, 2002).

Less is known about sex steroids of females. This is most likely because in all pulse species studied, exogenous estrogens have little or no effect on EOD parameters (see later). Estrogens do affect EOD frequency in wave gymnotiforms, however, so there is some data on females in that order (Meyer, 1983; Meyer et al., 1987; Dunlap et al., 1997). Female *Sternopygus* possess little or no 11-KT and have comparable levels of testosterone (T) to males. The levels of estradiol 17β (E$_2$) in immature females are comparable to those in mature or immature males (<0.5 ng/ml), and gravid females with well-yolked eggs have higher levels (2 ng/ml) (Zakon et al., 1991). In a study of brown ghosts, plasma estrogen levels of 2–6 ng/ml were noted in females; this was significantly greater than in males (Zucker, 1997).

It should be pointed out that in all these studies androgen or estrogen levels are only generally predictive of EOD parameters. They may be high in one group compared to another (dominant vs subordinate, immature vs mature), but EOD parameters do not correlate highly with plasma hormone levels when sampled across individuals in a group. Thus, factors in addition to plasma androgens in males and estrogen in females determine EOD parameters.

The role of endogenous sex steroids in controlling EOD parameters is further supported by the fact that the EOD changes in the expected direction in a number of species following gonadectomy (Meyer, 1983; Zucker, 1997).

B. Exogenous Treatment with Steroid Hormones

There is much data on the effects of exogenous hormones on the EOD waveform. In all species of pulse fish tested, including members of both the gymnotiforms and mormyriforms, the treatment of juveniles of both sexes, castrated males, or females with testosterone or nonaromatizable androgens broadens (masculinizes)

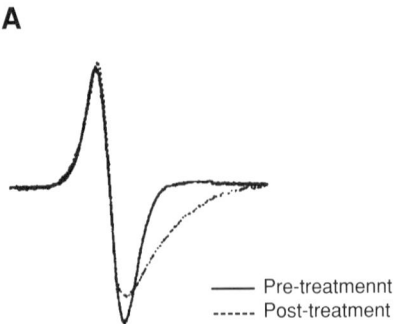

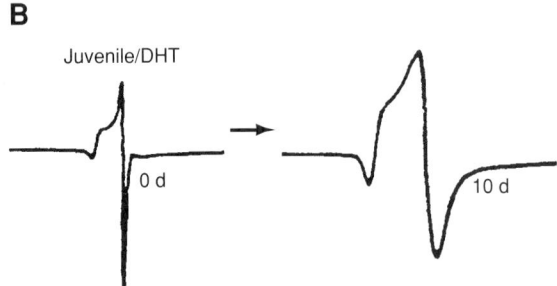

FIGURE 12 Androgens broaden the EOD pulse of both gymnotiform and mormyriform pulse-type fish. (A) EOD pulse of a male pin-tail knifefish (*B. pinnicaudatus*) before and 15 days after implantation with a capsule containing testosterone. From Silva *et al.* (1999). (B) Broadening of the EOD pulse of a juvenile mormyrid *Brienomyrus brachyistius* 10 days after implantation with dihydrotestosterone (DHT). Adapted from Bass and Hopkins (1985).

the pulse and mimics the naturally occurring sexual dimorphism (Bass and Hopkins, 1983; Hagedorn and Carr, 1985; Landsman and Moller, 1988; Freedman *et al.*, 1989; Silva *et al.*, 1999) (Fig. 12). Estrogen does not affect the EOD of pulse-type fish when given alone or in combination with androgens (Hagedorn and Carr, 1985; Landsman and Moller, 1988).

In some cases, the long-term actions of sex steroids affects only a portion of the EOD waveform. For example, in *B. pinnicaudatus* as well as many other species androgen treatment broadens only the second phase of the EOD pulse (Fig. 12A). This suggests that changes in ion currents are restricted to the anterior face of the electrocyte because this is the face that generates the second phase of the EOD (see Fig. 5).

Insofar as there is no obvious change in the rate of EOD in pulse-type fish, it is unlikely that the PMN is influenced by hormone treatment.

In most species of wave gymnotiforms, males have a lower EOD frequency than females. In those species, treatment with androgens resulting in plasma concentrations of a few to 10 ng/ml lowers EOD frequency over a 2-week period (Meyer, 1983; Mills and Zakon, 1987; Dunlap and Zakon, 1998). In addition to lowering EOD frequency, the duration of the EOD pulse is lengthened by androgens as well (Fig. 6). Thus, androgens exert a concerted influence on both the PMN and the electric organ. How androgens coordinate their effects on two different target cell types of the electromotor system reflects the general question of how any hormone or neurotransmitter that acts on multiple sites in a neural network exerts a coordinated action.

In the gold-lined black knifefish (*Sternopygus*), estrogen implants in juvenile fish of both sexes raise (feminize) EOD frequency (Meyer, 1983; Dunlap *et al.*, 1997). In addition, treatment of intact females or castrated fish of both sexes with hCG powerfully increases EOD frequency in *Sternopygus* (Zakon *et al.*, 1990). It is not known whether hCG acts directly on the pacemaker and electrocytes or whether it acts indirectly by releasing another hormone from a nongonadal source.

Although androgens lower EOD frequency in most gymnotiform wave fish, this is not universally true—recall that brown ghost males have a higher EOD frequency than do the females (Meyer *et al.*, 1987). Similarly, 11-KT raises EOD frequency, whereas estrogen and T lower it (Meyer *et al.*, 1987). The effects of T can be blocked by an aromatase inhibitor in this species. In fact, aromatase inhibitors alone raise the EOD frequency of intact females (Zucker, 1997). Thus, it is likely that E_2 is produced by aromatization of T, perhaps in the PMN. Recent data indicate that pacemaker and relay neurons in brown ghosts label with an antibody against piscine aromatase (H. Liu, H. Zakon, A. Bass, unpublished).

On the other hand, the closely related species black ghost shows a pattern similar to other gynotiform wave fish in that the male has a lower EOD frequency than the female and the EOD is lowered by 11-KT and dihydrotestosterone (DHT) treatment (Dunlap *et al.*, 1998). The close phylogenetic relationships between these two species make them good subjects for studying how sexual dimorphisms evolve.

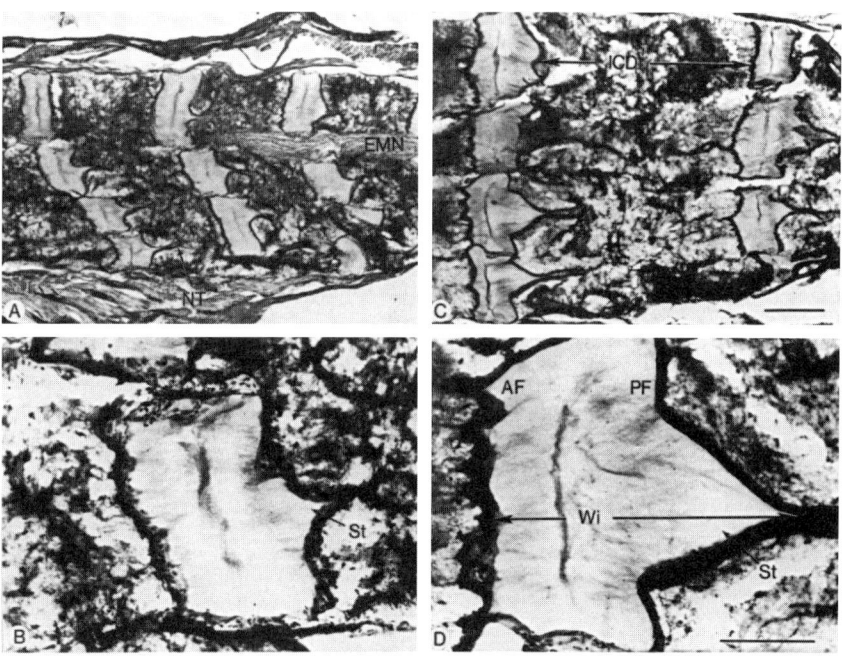

FIGURE 13 Electrocytes from male and female pin-tail knifefish. The right-hand column (A, B) shows electrocytes from a male, and the left-hand column (C, D) shows electrocytes from a female. The top row is at a lower magnification; the bottom row is at a higher magnification. Scale bar in (C), 250 microns; in (D), 100 microns. AF, anterior face; PF, posterior face; WI, width. From Hopkins et al. (1990).

VI. EFFECTS OF HORMONES ON ELECTRIC ORGAN MORPHOLOGY

The size and shape of the electrocytes are sexually dimorphic in a number of species of pulse fish. This is true of both mormyrids and gymnotiforms (Hagedorn and Carr, 1985; Bass et al., 1986; Bass, 1986b). In some cases, this is so pronounced that there is a sex difference in the length or thickness of the tail. In the pin-tail knifefish (B. pinnicaudatus), electrocytes are larger, more widely spaced, and more numerous in males (Hopkins et al., 1990) (Fig. 13). In mormyrids, electrocytes in males are thicker and larger, although this does not result in a visible dimorphism in the tail (Bass et al., 1986; Bass, 1986b; Freedman et al., 1989). Not surprisingly, the treatment of females or sexually immature males with androgens induces these morphological changes in the electrocytes.

In the wave gymnotiform *Sternopygus*, the electrocytes are not sexually dimorphic in size despite the large difference in EOD pulse duration between mature males and females (~3 ms for female and 12 ms for males) (Mills et al., 1992). It is unknown whether *Eigenmannia*, which has a more subtle sex difference in EOD pulse duration, has any sex difference in electrocyte morphology; it is not unexpected because males are larger than females.

The lack of a morphological sex difference in *Sternopygus* demonstrates that sex differences in EOD waveform can come about by changes in the ionic currents of the electrocytes without any accompanying differences in morphology. Thus, it is not certain why morphological differences in electrocyte size occur unless they are actually a mechanism for providing the males with a larger-scale dimorphism in tail size.

VII. INFLUENCE OF HORMONES ON IONIC CURRENTS OF ELECTROMOTOR SYSTEM

A key rationale for studying hormonal modulation of the EOD in weakly electric fish is that they are a superb model system for studying the effects of steroids

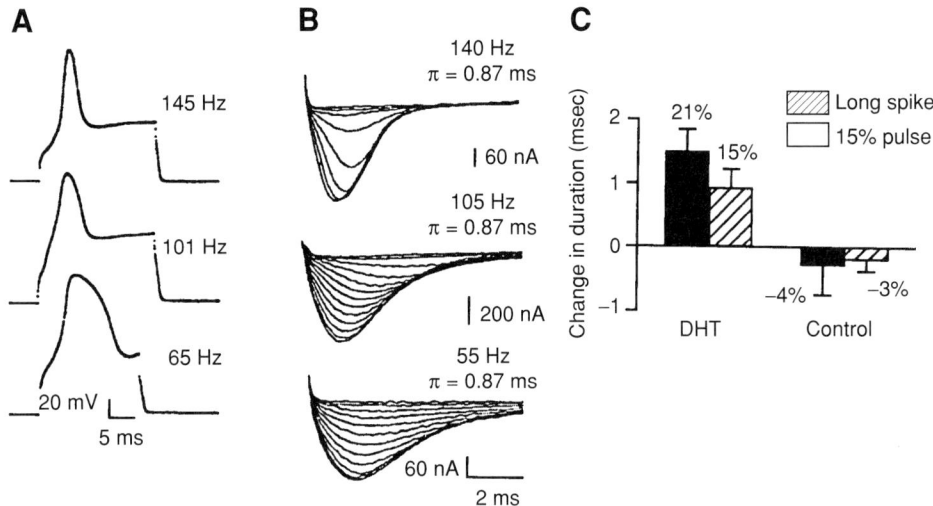

FIGURE 14 Electrocyte action potential duration and Na$^+$ current is individually distinct and influenced by hormones. (A) Intracellular recordings made in electrocytes of high-, mid-, and low-EOD-frequency juvenile *Sternopygus*. Current was injected with one electrode and the voltage responses of the membrane were recorded with another. The number to the right of each trace gives each fish's EOD frequency. Note the systematic individual variation in action potential duration. (B) Voltage clamp recordings from electrocytes from fish with comparable EOD frequencies, as in (A), show that the Na$^+$ current activates and inactivates at different rates. EOD frequency and the exponential time constant of decay of the current (its rate of inactivation) is given to the right of each family of current traces. (C) Androgens broaden the EOD pulse and the electrocyte action potential (labeled long spike). In this experiment, recordings of these two parameters are made before and after treatment with DHT or empty capsules. Note that the control fish show no change in either parameter, but the hormone-treated fish show an increase in both. From Zakon (1999).

on cell membranes (Bass and Volman, 1987; Zakon, 1999). Most information comes from the electrocytes of *Sternopygus macrurus*. The electrocytes of *Sternopygus* generate an action potential that varies from 3 ms in a fish with a high EOD frequency, such as a sexually mature female, to 12 ms in a fish with a low EOD frequency, such as a mature male. Furthermore, the action potential duration is lengthened (masculinized) from days to weeks by chronic androgen treatment (Mills and Zakon, 1991).

Presumably androgens broaden action potentials by influencing the ionic currents of the electrocyte. In order to study this, each ionic current must be studied in isolation under voltage clamp. A number of types of ionic currents are discernable when cells are voltage-clamped—mainly a voltage-dependent Na$^+$ current and a delayed rectifying K$^+$ current (Ferrri and Zakon, 1993). Interestingly, the rates at which the Na$^+$ current turns off (inactivates) and the K$^+$ current turns on (activates) during a long-depolarizing voltage step varies systematically with EOD frequency and EOD pulse duration. Fish with low EOD frequencies have currents that activate and inactivate slowly, those with mid-range EOD frequencies have currents that activate and inactivate faster, and those with the highest EOD frequencies have currents with the fastest rates (Ferrari *et al.*, 1995; McAnelly and Zakon, 2000) (Fig. 14).

Because gonadal steroids influence the duration of the EOD pulse and the electrocyte action potential, it is likely that they do this by influencing one or more of the ionic currents in the electrocytes. The treatment of fish with DHT slows down, whereas treatment with E$_2$ speeds up, the rate of inactivation of the Na$^+$ current (Ferrari *et al.*, 1995; Dunlap *et al.*, 1997). Slowing down the rate of inactivation lengthens, and speeding up inactivation shortens, action potential duration. It is not known whether the rate kinetics of the K$^+$ current is altered by gonadal steroids, although this seems likely.

This raises the question of how the differences in current kinetics are affected by the hormones. Presumably the actions of steroid hormones on these currents is genomic because they take days to manifest. In support of this, electrocytes in this species have nuclear androgen and estrogen receptors (Gustavson et al., 1994; Dunlap et al., 1997). The most likely targets for hormonal regulation are the ion-channel genes themselves or genes for enzymes that could influence the state of the channels, such as kinases.

Studies of the ion currents of the pacemaker neurons are just beginning (Dye, 1991; Smith and Zakon, 2000). Because of technical difficulties, voltage-clamp recordings from pacemaker cells are unachievable. However, the pacemaker nucleus from the brown ghost can be isolated in a slice chamber and the firing frequencies of these cells can be studied in the presence of a variety of pharmacological agents. These studies suggest that Na^+, K^+, and Ca^{2+} currents all contribute to generating the rhythmic command signal for the EOD and to regulating EOD frequency (Smith and Zakon, 2000). In addition, it is possible to voltage-clamp the ionic currents of the EMNs of the brown ghost. The EMNs are similar to pacemaker neurons in that they fire spontaneously at the EOD frequency of the fish they came from. Preliminary studies indicate that the EMNs possess both voltage-dependent Na^+ currents with a strong persistent component and one or more rapidly activating, voltage-dependent K^+ currents. These ionic currents in EMNs are similar to those predicted by pharmacological studies of the PMN (Smith and Zakon, 2000). The role of each of these currents in generating and maintaining the pacemaker frequency of each fish is not yet known. However, it is likely that the persistent Na^+ current is responsible for the depolarizing potentials that support the spontaneous activity that underlies the EOD rhythm. Once the control of oscillatory firing is understood, it will be possible to study the effects of gonadal steroids on these cells.

VIII. RAPID CHANGES IN ELECTRIC-ORGAN-DISCHARGE PARAMETERS

The changes in EOD waveforms induced by exogenous steroids occur over days to weeks. However, changes in EOD waveforms may occur within minutes in freely moving fish. Hagedorn and Heiligenberg (1985) first reported that the EOD of the dominant male *Eigenmannia* in a community tank increases in subjective amplitude (i.e., gets very loud on an audio monitor) on the night of breeding, so much so that it drowns out the signals of other fish. They suggested that the amplitude of the EOD was increasing. This was a radical suggestion at a time when it was believed that the properties of the EOD were determined by fixed aspects of the anatomy and physiology of the electromotor system.

Subsequently, Hagedorn and Zelick (1989) noticed that stressing sexually mature male *Brachyhypopomus occidentalis* causes the sexually dimorphic portion of the EOD pulse to decrease in duration. When two males of comparable size are placed together in a tank with a single hiding place, they compete for it. The winner in this encounter shows a similar shortening in the duration of its EOD pulse and its EOD amplitude falls. Both of these events occur within 2 hours of the interaction.

Under conditions in which accurate calibrated recordings could be made of the EOD of swimming fish, the sexually dimorphic phase of the EOD pulse of male *B. pinnicaudatus* was observed to undergo diurnal variations in duration and amplitude (Franchina and Stoddard, 1998) (Fig. 15). These diurnal excursions occur in isolated males, but are enhanced in individuals exposed to conspecifics behind a mesh barrier. The exposure of a male to another male has a greater effect on the EOD parameters than exposure to a female (Franchina et al., 2001).

The implications of these changes on the behavioral and cellular levels are intriguing. Diurnal fluctuations of EOD amplitude suggest that fish optimize their energy expenditure by generating the largest amplitude discharge only during periods of significant social interaction. The drop in amplitude in the loser's EOD following an aggressive interaction could be a way of being less detectable by or appeasing the winner.

On the cellular level, it is likely that the increase in EOD amplitude is caused by an increase in the magnitude of the electrocyte Na^+ current (McAnelly and Zakon, 1996) (Fig. 15). This can be induced *in vitro* by treating electrocytes (*Sternopygus*) with a membrane-permeant cyclic AMP analog. Further evidence that a cAMP-dependent increase in Na^+ current causes the

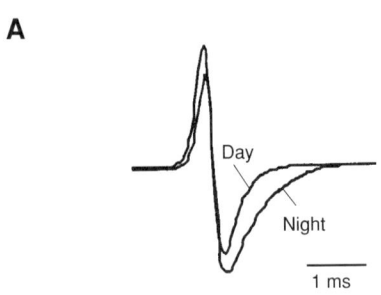
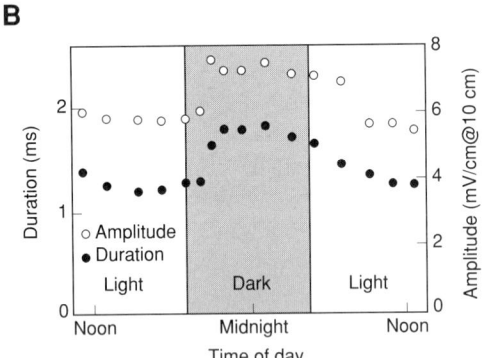
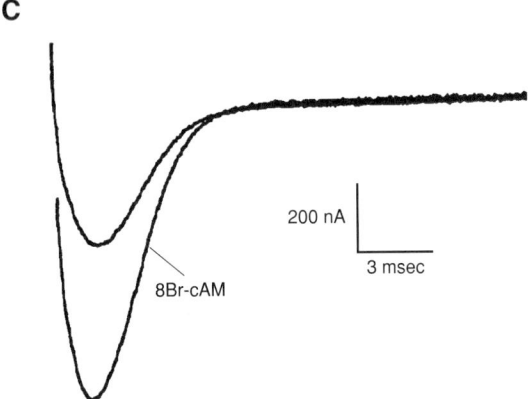

FIGURE 15 Diurnal changes in the EOD of a pulse fish (*B. pinnicaudatus*) and its possible biophysical basis. (A) Traces of EOD waveform during the day and night illustrating the nocturnal increases in amplitude of positive and negative phases of the EOD and duration of the negative phase of the EOD. (B) Measurements of peak-to-peak amplitude and the duration of the second phase of the EOD pulse of a male over 24 hr. (C) Voltage-clamp recordings of the peak Na^+ current from an electrocyte of a wave-fish (*Sternopygus*) before and after treatment with 8-bromo-cyclic AMP. Note that the amplitude of the Na^+ current is enhanced. Such an increase in the Na^+ current is likely to increase the current output of each electrocyte, thereby increasing the amplitude of the EOD. (A) and (B) from Franchina and Stoddard (1998); (C) from McAnelly and Zakon (1996).

increase in EOD pulse amplitude is that EOD amplitude is doubled after injections of cAMP into the electric organ of intact *Sternopygus* (A. Silva and L. McAnelly, personal communication). What factors control the fall in amplitude are not known.

The change in the duration of the sexually dimorphic phase of the EOD is also intriguing because of its rapidity. As is the case with the androgen-induced broadening of the EOD pulse, the effect must be only on the anterior membrane of the electrocyte because this is the membrane that generates the second phase of the EOD pulse. The mechanism by which the rapid effects are initiated and how they interact with the long-term effects of androgens are interesting questions.

IX. HORMONAL MODULATION OF CHIRPING

Because chirping is strongly sexually dimorphic in brown ghosts, it is a good candidate for a behavior regulated by gonadal steroids. Chirping is elicited in intact female brown ghosts implanted with T and DHT and presented with a sine wave near their own EOD frequency. Over the course of 2 weeks, T- and DHT-implanted females chirp more frequently during the test period. However, although androgens caused a significant increase in chirp rate (10–20 chirps/min) over females implanted with empty capsules (2–4 chirps/min), they elicited much less chirping than observed in normal males under the same conditions (>40–60 chirps/minute; Dulka *et al.*, 1995; Dulka, 1997; Dunlap *et al.*, 1998).

A number of explanations could account for the failure of androgen implants in females to fully masculinize chirping behavior. One is that an unknown testicular factor acts in concert with androgens to induce full masculinization. Precedent for this occurs in *Xenopus* in which full masculinizaion of the sexually dimorphic larynx cannot be induced in adult females by androgens, but does occur with testicular transplantation (Watson and Kelley, 1992; Watson *et al.*, 1993). Another is that the nervous systems of the two sexes are organized differently and therefore respond differentially to androgens in adulthood. This is intriguing because fish brains are much more influenced by steroid hormones in an activational than organizational fashion (Zakon, 1999).

Finally, because the females were not gonadectomized, it is possible that estrogen or some other ovarian factor inhibited chirping; estrogen inhibited aggressive behavior in a cichlid fish (Munro and Pitcher, 1985). The effect of E_2 on chirping has not been investigated. It will be interesting to determine whether E_2 actively inhibits chirping or whether it induces female-like chirps, such as those produced during egg-laying.

Despite its influence on basal EOD frequency, 11-KT only marginally induces chirping in females in a chirp chamber (J. Dulka, personal communication). This seems paradoxical given the strong correlation between chirping and plasma 11-KT in staged encounters between two male brown ghosts (Dunlap, 2002) (Fig. 9). In this study, no other steroids were measured so it is possible that 11-KT levels covaried with those of other steroids, such as T and DHT (T and 11-KT levels usually do covary in fish, including gymnotiforms; Zakon et al., 1991) and that these steroids, rather than 11-KT, actually influence chirp rates.

The effects of androgens on chirping may not be directly on the neurons of the PPn, but indirectly via a subpopulation of lateral hypothalamic substance-P-like-containing neurons with projections to the PPn. Substance-P-like immunoreactivity in the PPn is stronger in males than females, and the levels of immunoreactivity can be brought almost to the level of a sexually mature male via T implants in females (Weld and Maler, 1992; Dulka and Maler, 1994; Dulka et al., 1995; Dulka, 1997; Dulka and Ebling, 1999). It is likely that the effects of androgens on the substance-P-like system is entirely due to its up-regulation of the neuropeptide because there are no sex differences in the number of tachykinin receptors in the PPn of males and females (Weld et al., 1994).

Dunlap et al. (2001) showed an influence of social conditions on chirping that is mediated by corticocosterone (CORT). Male brown ghosts were housed either separately or in pairs, but separated by mesh that allowed electrical contact. Each male was tested in a chirp chamber using a standard stimulus every few days. Interestingly, the males housed together chirped at a higher rate than isolated males. Blood samples of paired fish had significantly higher levels of CORT, but no difference in androgen levels. Implanting socially isolated males with CORT caused them to behave like paired males—they chirped at a higher rate to EOD mimic stimuli. It is not known whether CORT acts directly or indirectly via the sparse corticotropin-release factor-positive fibers that project to the PPn (Zupanc et al., 1999).

The neuropeptide arginine vasotocin (AVT), known to activate sex behavior in a variety of other vertebrates, activates chirping in males. If males are already predisposed to chirp to a sine wave stimulus with intense chirps, AVT increases their probability of chirping (Bastian et al., 2001).

Black ghosts, related to brown ghosts, show much less strong sexual dimorphism in and hormonal regulation of chirping. Male and female black ghosts chirp at the same rate to a standard stimulus in a chirp chamber. In keeping with this lack of sexual dimorphism in chirping, T, DHT, and 11-KT have no effect on chirping in gonadectomized fish of either sex, even when the blood androgen levels of the implanted fish were comparable to or slightly above those of brown ghosts (see later) (Dunlap and Zakon, 1998). This is in spite of an effect of these hormones on EOD frequency.

X. HORMONAL PLASTICITY IN ELECTRORECEPTORS

Hormones shift EOD frequency. However, the electroreceptors are so precisely tuned to the EOD frequency in wave-type fish that they would be out of alignment with the EOD if they did not shift as well. Indeed, fish treated with androgens show parallel shifts of electroreceptor tuning (Meyer and Zakon, 1982; Zakon and Meyer, 1983).

A key question is whether the hormones act directly or indirectly on the electroreceptors. That is, hormones might act directly on the PMN to induce a change in EOD frequency, and this change in the frequency at which the electroreceptors are being driven might somehow reset electroreceptor tuning. On the other hand, androgens might act independently at each site to coordinate the electrical activity of these various cell types. As it turns out, androgens still shift electroreceptor tuning in *Sternopygus* in which the pacemaker has been lesioned (Ferrari and Zakon, 1989). Furthermore, androgen receptors have been localized immunocytochemically in electroreceptors. Thus, it seems that electroreceptor tuning is directly influenced by androgens and that the actions of androgens on the electroreceptors, the pacemaker neurons, and the electric organ must be quantitatively matched but independently controlled in each cell type.

A comparable study was done on the mormyrids (Bass and Hopkins, 1984). There the conclusion was that the knollenorgan tuning did not change in fish with transected spinal cords. This result suggests that electroreceptor tuning is influenced by the shape of the EOD pulse in this species.

Unfortunately, other than these older studies, nothing has been done in this field. The question of the biophysical mechanisms by which receptor tuning is derived and shifted by hormone treatment is a fertile one.

XI. CONCLUSION

What general lessons can be learned from studying hormones and behavior in electric fish? First, although electrocommunication signals may be unique to only two orders of fish, they are used in much the same ways as signals in other modalities and are similarly influenced by factors of natural and sexual selection. As with other sexually dimorphic communication signals, the EOD conveys information on the species, age, gender, and individual identity of the signaler and can also transmit information about breeding status, dominance or subordinance, and motivation. As with many other sexually dimorphic communication signals, EODs are often regulated by gonadal steroid hormones through actions on the morphology and physiology of the neurons that control these signals.

Other similarities between systems are apparent in the development and interaction of natural and sexual selection on the behavioral phenotypes. The EOD waveform of pulse fish (and EOD frequency in many wave fish) is similar in juvenile and female gymnotiforms, reminiscent of the plumage similarities of juvenile and female birds. For many sexually dimorphic signals, particularly in species in which males compete for reproductive access to females, male signals are more conspicuous or ornate than those of females. These signals may carry costs, including increased risk of predation and energetic costs. Similarly, in electric fish there is evidence that the electrical signals produced by males are more conspicuous both to conspecific females and to potential predators.

Another striking feature of the electrocommunication system in electric fish is the wealth of species diversity in the biology of these fishes. This diversity includes variations in the magnitude and direction of sex differences in body size, EOD properties, and other electrical behaviors (i.e., chirping); diversity in habitat preferences and associated diversity in physiology and patterning of the EOD; and variation in courtship and parental behavior. This diversity is coupled with numerous striking examples of convergence in the behavior and physiology of these two different orders of fish that independently evolved electrocommunication. These features lend themselves well to comparative studies of the hormonal control of reproductive and communication behavior.

A final highlight of the electrocommunication system is that it has numerous features that allow us to study reproductive communication behavior at multiple levels of analysis. These features include a signal that can be quantitatively analyzed, manipulated, and played back; and a neural circuit that controls the EOD behavior that is well characterized, simple, and accessible enough to allow cellular and even molecular analyses of the mechanisms underlying species, sex, and individual differences in behavior.

References

Alves-Gomes, J. (1999). Systematic biology of gymnotiform and mormyriform electric fishes: Phylogenetic relationships, molecular clocks and rates of evolution in the mitchondrial rRNA genes. *J. Exp. Biol.* **202**, 1167–1183.

Alves-Gomes, J., and Hopkins, C. (1997). Molecular insights into the phylogeny of mormyriform fishes and the evolution of their electric organs. *Brain. Behav. Evol.* **49**, 324–351.

Alves-Gomes, J. A., Orti, G. et al. (1995). Phylogenetic analysis of the South American electric fishes (order gymnotiformes) and the evolution of their electrogenic system: A synthesis based on morphology. *Mol. Biol. Evol.* **12**, 298–318.

Amagai, S. (1998). Time-coding in the midbrain of mormyrid electric fish. II. Stimulus selectivity in the nucleus exterolateralis pars posterior. *J. Comp. Physiol. A* **182**, 131–143.

Assunção, M., and Schwassman, H. (1995). Reproduction and larval development of *Electrophorus electricus* on Marajo Island (Pará, Brazil). *Ichthyol. Explor. Freshwaters* **6**(2), 175–184.

Bass, A. H. (1986a). Species differences in electric organs of mormyrids: Substrates for species-typical electric organ discharge waveforms. *J. Comp. Neurol.* **244**, 313–330.

Bass, A. H. (1986b). A hormone-sensitive communication system in an electric fish. *J. Neurobiol.* **17**, 131–156.

Bass, A. H., and Hopkins, C. D. (1983). Hormonal control of sexual differentiation: Changes in electric organ discharge waveform. *Science* **220**, 971–974.

Bass, A. H., and Hopkins, C. D. (1984). Shifts of frequency tuning in electroreceptors in androgen-treated mormyrid fish. *J. Comp. Physiol. A* **155**, 713–724.

Bass, A. H., and Hopkins, C. D. (1985). Hormonal control of sex differences in the electric organ discharge (EOD) of mormyrid fishes. *J. Comp. Physiol. A* **156**, 587–604.

Bass, A. H., Denizot, J.-P. et al. (1986). Ultrastructural features and hormone-dependent sex differences of mormyrid electric organs. *J. Comp. Neurol.* **254**, 511–528.

Bass, A. H., and Volman, S. F. (1987). From behavior to membranes: testosterone-induced changes in action potential duration in electric organs. *Proc. Natl. Acad. Sci. U.S.A.* **84**, 9295–9298.

Bastian, J., Schneiderjan, S., et al. (2001). Arginine vasotocin modulates a sexually dimorphic communication behavior in the weakly electric fish, *Apteronotus leptorhynchus. J. Exp. Biol.* **204**, 1909–1923.

Bell, C., Bradbury, J. et al. (1976). The electric organ of a mormyrid as a current and voltage source. *J. Comp. Physiol. A* **110**, 65–88.

Bennett, M. V. L. (1961). Modes of operation of electric organs. *Ann. N.Y. Acad. Sci.* **54**, 458–494.

Bennett, M. V. L., and Grundfest, H. (1959). Electrophysiology of electric organ in *Gymnotus carapo. J. Gen. Physiol.* **42**(5), 1067–1104.

Bennett, M. V. L., Pappas, G. D. et al. (1967). Physiology and ultrastructure of electrotonic junctions. IV. Medullary electromotor nuclei in gymnotid fish. *J. Neurophysiol.* **30**, 236–300.

Black-Cleworth, P. (1970). The role of electric discharges in the non-reproductive sopcial behavior of *Gymnotus carapo. Anim. Behav. Monogr.* **3**, 1–77.

Bratton, B., and Kramer, B. (1989). Patterns of the electric organ discharge during courtship and spawning in the mormyrid fish, *Pollimyrus isidori. Behav. Ecol. Sociobiol.* **24**, 349–368.

Caputi, A. (1999). The electric organ discharge of pulse gymnotiforms: The transformation of a simple impulse into a complex spatio-temporal electromotor pattern. *J. Exp. Biol.* **202**, 1229–1241.

Carlson, B. (2000). Androgen correlates of socially induced changes in the electric organ discharge waveform of a mormyrid fish. *Horm. Behav.* **38**, 177–186.

Carlson, B., and Hopkins, C. (2000). Neural mechanisms in the generation of electric signals in mormyrid fish. *Abstr. Soc. Neurosci.* **26**, 1522.

Crampton, W. (1998). Effects of anoxia on the distribution respiratory strategies and electric signal diversity of gymnotiform fishes. *J. Fish Biol.* **53**(Suppl. A), 307–330.

Crawford, J. P. (1997). Hearing and acoustic communication in the mormyrid electric fishes. *Mar. Freshwater Behav. Physiol.* **29**, 1–21.

Crawford, J. D. (1991). Sex recognition by electric cues in a sound-producing mormyrid fish, *Pollimyrus isidori. Brain, Behav. Evol.* **38**, 20–38.

Crawford, J. D. (1992). Individual and sex specificity in the electric organ discharges of breeding mormyrid fish (*Pollimyrus isidori*). *J. Exp. Biol.* **164**, 79–102.

Crawford, J. D., Hagedorn, M. et al. (1986). Acoustic communication in an electric fish, *Pollimyrus isidori* (Mormyridae). *J. Comp. Physiol. A* **159**, 297–310.

Curtis, C. (1999). "Active Female Mate Choice in the Weakly Electric Fish *Brachyhypopomus pinnicaudatus*." Florida International University.

Darwin, C. (1872). "The Expression of Emotion in Man and the Animal." John Murray (publishers):London.

Dulka, J. G. (1997). Androgen-induced neural plasticity and the regulation of electric-social behavior in the brown ghost knifefish: Current status and future directions. *Fish Physiol. Biochem.* **17**, 195–202.

Dulka, J. G., and Ebling, S. (1999). Testosterone increases the number of substance P-like immunoreactive neurons in a specific sub-division of the lateral hypothalamus of the weakly electric, brown ghost knifefish, *Apteronotus leptorhynchus. Brain Res.* **826**, 1–9.

Dulka, J. G., and Maler, L. (1994). Testosterone modulates female chirping behavior in the weakly electric fish, *Apteronotus leptorhynchus. J. Comp. Physiol. A* **174**, 331–343.

Dulka, J. G., Maler, L. et al. (1995). Androgen-induced changes in electrocommunicatory behavior are correlated with changes in substance P-like immunoreactivity in the brain of the electric fish *Apteronotus leptorhynchus. J. Neurosci.* **15**(3), 1879–1890.

Dunlap, K. (2002). Hormonal and body size correlates of electrocommunication behavior during dyadic interactions in a weakly electric fish, *Apteronotus leptorhynchus. Horm. Behav.* **41**(2), 187–194.

Dunlap, K., McAnelly, M. L. et al. (1997). Estrogen modifies an electrocommunication signal by altering the electrocyte sodium current in an electric fish, *Sternopygus. J. Neurosci.* **17**, 2869–2875.

Dunlap, K., Thomas, P. et al. (1998). Diversity of sexual dimorphism in electrocommunication signals and its androgen regulation in a genus of electric fish, *Apteronotus. J. Comp. Physiol. A* **183**, 77–86.

Dunlap, K., Pelczar, P. et al. (2002). Social interactions, and cortisol treatment increase the production of aggressive electrocommunication signals in male electric fish, *Apteronotus leptorhynchus. Horm. Behav.* (in press).

Dunlap, K. D., and Zakon, H. H. (1998). Behavioral actions of androgens and androgen receptor expression in the electrocommunication system of an electric fish, *Eigenmannia virescens. Horm. Behav.* **34**, 30–38.

Dye, J. (1991). Ionic and synaptic mechanisms underlying a brainstem oscillator: An in vitro study of the pacemaker nucleus of *Apteronotus. J. Comp. Physiol. A* **168**, 521–532.

Dye, J. C., Heiligenberg, W. et al. (1989). Different classes of glutamate receptors mediate distinct behaviors in a single brainstem nucleus. *Proc. Natl. Acad. Sci. U.S.A* **86**, 8993–8997.

Elekes, K., and Szabo, T. (1981). Comparative synaptology of the pacemaker nucleus in the brain of the weakly electric fish (gymnotidae). *Adv. Physiol. Sci.* **31**, 107–127.

Elekes, K., Ravaille, M., Bell, C. C., Libouban, S., and Szabo, T. (1985). The mormyrid brainstem—II. The medullary electromotor relay nucleus: An ultrastructural horseradish peroxidase study. *Neuroscience* **15**, 417–429

Engler, G., Fogarty, C. et al. (2000). Spontaneous modulations of the electric organ discharge in the weakly electric fish, *Apteronotus leptorhynchus*: A biophysical and behavioral analysis. *J. Comp. Physio. A* **186**, 645–660.

Ferrari, M. B., and Zakon, H. H. (1989). The medullary pacemaker nucleus is unnecessary for electroreceptor tuning plasticity in Sternopygus. *J. Neurosci.* **9**(4), 1354–1361.

Ferrari, M. B., McAnelly, M. L. et al. (1995). Individual variation in and androgen-modulation of the sodium current in electric organ. *J. Neurosci.* **15**(5), 4023–4032.

Ferrri, M. B., and Zakon, H. H. (1993). Conductances contributing to the action potential of Sternopygus electrocytes *J. Comp. Physiol. A* **173**, 281–292.

Fleishman, L. J. (1992). Communication in the weakly electric fish *Sternopygus macrurus*. I. The neural basis of conspecific EOD detection. *J. Comp. Physiol. A* **170**, 335–348.

Franchina, C., and Stoddard, P. (1998). Plasticity of the electric organ discharge waveform of the electric fish *Brachyhypopomus pinnicaudatus* I. quantification of day-night changes. *J. Comp. Physiol. A* **183**, 759–768.

Franchina, C., Salazar, V. et al. (2001). Plasticity of the electric organ discharge waveform of male *Brachyhypopomus pinnicaudatus*. II. Social effects. *J. Comp. Physiol A* **187**, 45–52.

Freedman, E. G., Olyarchuk, J. et al. (1989). A temporal analysis of testosterone-induced changes in electric organs and electric organ dishcarges of mormyrid fishes. *J. Neurobiol.* **20**, 619–634.

Friedman, M., and Hopkins, C. (1996). Tracking mormyid electric fish in the field using individual differences in electric organ discharges. *Anim. Behav.* **51**, 391–407.

Friedman, M., and Hopkins, C. (1998). Neural substrates for species recognition in the time-coding electrosensory pathway of mormyrid electric fish. *J. Neurosci.* **18**, 1171–1185.

Grant, K., von der Emde, G. et al. (1999). Neural command of electromotor output in mormyrids. *J. Exp. Biol.* **202**, 1399–1407.

Gross, M. R., and Sargent, R. C. (1985). The evolution of male and female parental care in fishes. *Am. Zoo.* **25**, 807–822.

Gustavson, S., Zakon, H. et al. (1994). Androgen receptors in the brain, electroreceptors, and electric organ of a wave-type electric fish. *Abstr. Soc. Neurosci.* **19**, 371.

Hagedorn, M. (1988). Ecology and behavior of a pulse type electric fish, *Hypopomus occidentalis* (Gymnotiformes, Hypopomidae), in a fresh water stream in Panama. *Copeia* **2**, 324–335.

Hagedorn, M. (1992). Social influences on the courtship and breeding of a gymnotiform electric fish. *Proc. IMS/CM2 Int. Aust. Lungfish Breed. Workshop,* Cleveland Metroparks Zoo.

Hagedorn, M., and Carr, C. (1985). Single electrocytes produce a sexually dimorphic signal in South American electric fish *Hypopomus occidentalis* (Gymnotiformes, hypopomidae). *J. Comp. Physiol. A* **156**, 511–523.

Hagedorn, M., and Heiligenberg, W. (1985). Court and spark: Electric signals in the courtship and mating of gymnotid fish. *Anim. Behav.* **32**, 254–265.

Hagedorn, M., and Zelick, R. (1989). Relative dominance among males is expressed in the electric organ discharge characteristics of a weakly electric fish. *Anim. Behav.* **38**, 520–525.

Henderson, P., and Crampton, W. (1997). A comparison of fish diversity and abundance between nutrient-rich and nutrient-poor lakes in the upper Amazon. *J. Trop. Ecol.* **13**(2), 175–198.

Hopkins, C. D. (1974). Electric communication: Functions in the social behaviour of *Eigenmannia virescens. Behaviour* **50**, 270–305.

Hopkins, C. D. (1999). Design features for electric communication. *J. Exp. Biol.* **202**, 1217–1228.

Hopkins, C. D. (1974). Electric communication in the reproductive behaviour of *Sternopygus macrurus* (Gymnotoidei). *Z. Tierpsychol.* **35**, 518–535.

Hopkins, C. D. (1976). Stimulus filtering and electroreception: Tiberous electroreceptors in three species of gymnotoid fish. *J. Comp. Physiol.* **111**, 171–207.

Hopkins, C. D. (1981). On the diversity of electric signals in a community of mormyrid electric fish in West Africa. *Am. Zool.* **21**, 211–222.

Hopkins, C. D. (1986). Behavior of Mormyridae. *In* "Electroreception" (T. H. H. Bullock, ed.), pp. 527–576. Wiley, New York.

Hopkins, C. D., and Bass, A. H. (1981). Temporal coding of species recognition signals in an electric fish. *Science* **212**, 85–87.

Hopkins, C. D., and Heiligenberg, W. F. (1978). Evolutionary designs for electric signals and electroreceptors in gymnotoid fishes of Surinam. *Behav. Ecol. Sociobiol.* **3**, 113–134.

Hopkins, C. D., Comfort, N. *et al.* (1990). Functional analysis of sexual dimorphism in an electric fish, *Hypopomus pinnicaudatus*, order Gymnotiformes. *Brain, Behav. Evol.* **35**, 350–367.

Kawasaki, M., and Heiligenberg, W. (1989). Distinct mechanisms of modulation in a neuronal oscillator generate different social signals in the electric fish *Hypopomus*. *J. Comp. Physiol. A* **165**, 731–741.

Keynes, R. D., and Martins-Ferreira, J. (1953). Membrane potentials in the elecroplates of the electric eel. *J. Physiol. (London)* **119**, 315–351.

Kirschbaum, F. (1975). Environmental factors control the periodical reproduction of tropical electric fish. *Experientià* **3**, 1159–1160.

Kirschbaum, F. (1995). Reproduction and development in mormyriform and gymnotiform fishes. In "Electric Fishes: History and Behavior" (P. Moller, ed.), pp. 267–301. Chapman & Hall, London.

Kirschbaum, F., and Westby, G. W. M. (1975). Development of the electric dishcarge in mormyrid and gymnotid fish (*Marcusenius sp.* and *Eigenmannia virescens*). *Experientia* **31**, 1290–1293.

Kishida, M., and Specker, J. (2000). Paternal mouthbrooding in the black-chinned Tilapia, Sarotherodon melanotheron (Pisces: cichlidae): Changes in gponadal steroids and potential for vitellogenin transfer to larvae. *Horm. Behav.* **37**, 40–48.

Kramer, B. (1979). Electric and motor responses of the weakly electric fish, *Gnathonemus petersii* (Mormyridae), to play-back of social signals. *Behav. Ecol. Sociobiol.* **6**, 67–79.

Kramer, B. (1987). The sexually dimorphic jamming avoidance response in the electric fish *Eigenmannia* (Teleostei, Gymnotiformes). *J. Exp. Biol.* **130**, 39–62.

Kramer, B. (1990). Sexual signals in electric fishes. *Trends Eed. Evol.* **5**(8), 247–250.

Kramer, B., and Otto, B. (1991). Waveform discrimination in the electric fish Eigenmannia: Sensitivity for the phase differences between the spectral components of a stimulus wave. *J. Exp. Biol.* **159**, 1–22.

Landsman, R. (1993). The effects of captivity on the electric organ discharge and plasma hormone levevls in *Gnathonemus petersii* (Mormyriformes). *J. Comp. Physiol. A* **172**, 619–631.

Landsman, R. E., and Moller, P. (1988). Testosterone changes the electric organ discharge and external morphology of the mormyrid fish, *Gnathonemus petersii* (Mormyriformes). *Experientia* **44**, 900–903.

Lücker, H., and Kramer, B. (1981). Development of a sex difference in the preferred latency response in the weakly electric fish, *Pollimyrus isidori* (Cuvier et Valenciennes) (Mormyridae, teleostei). *Behav. Ecol. Sociobiol.* **9**, 103–109.

McAnelly, M. L., and Zakon, H. H. (2000). Co-regulation of voltage-dependent kinetics of Na^+ and K^+ currents. *J. Neurosci.* **20**, 3408–3414.

McAnelly, M. L., and Zakon, H. H. (1996). Protein kinase A activation increases sodium current magnitude in the electric organ of *Sternopygus*. *J. Neurosci.* **16**(14), 4383–4388.

McGregor, P. K., and Westby, G. W. M. (1992). Discrimination of individually characteristic electric organ discharges by a weakly electric fish. *Anim. Behav.* **43**, 977–986.

Metzner, W., and Heiligenberg, W. (1991). The coding of signals in the electric communication of the gymnotiform fish Eigenmannia: From electroreceptors to neurons in the torus semicircularis of the midbrain. *J. Comp. Physiol. A* **169**, 135–150.

Meyer, J. H. (1983). Steroid influences upon the discharge frequency of a weakly electric fish. *J. Comp. Physiol. A* **153**, 29–38.

Meyer, J. H., and Zakon, H. H. (1982). Androgens alter the tuning of electroreceptors. *Science* **217**, 635–637.

Meyer, J. H., Leong, M. *et al.* (1987). Hormone-induced and ontogenetic changes in electric organ discharge and electroreceptor tuning in the weakly electric fish *Apteronotus*. *J. Comp. Physiol. A* **160**, 385–394.

Mills, A. C., and Zakon, H. H. (1991). Chronic androgen treatment increases action potential duration in the electric organ of *Sternopygus*. *J. Neurosci.* **11**(8), 2349–2361.

Mills, A. C., Zakon, H. H. *et al.* (1992). Electric organ morphology of *Sternopygus macrurus*, a wave-type, weakly electric fish with a sexually dimorphic EOD. *J. Neurobiol.* **23**(7), 920–932.

Mills, A. C., and Zakon, H. H. (1987). Coordination of EOD frequency and pulse duration in a weakly electric wave fish: The influence of androgens. *J. Comp. Physiol.* **161**, 417–430.

Munro, A., and Pitcher, T. (1985). Steroid hormones and agonistic behavior in a cichlid teleost, *Aequidens pulcher*. *Horm. Behav.* **19**(4), 353–371.

Pappas, G. D., Waxman, S. G. *et al.* (1975). Morphology of spinal electromotor neurons and presynaptic coupling in the gymnotid *Sternarchus albifrons*. *J. Neurocytol.* **4**, 469–478.

Shumway, C. A., and Zelick, R. D. (1988). Sex recognition and neuronal coding of electric organ dishcarge waveform in the pulse-type weakly electric fish, *Hypopomus occidentalis*. *J. Comp. Physiol. A* **163**, 465–478.

Silva, A., Quintana, L. *et al.* (1999). Water temperature sensitivity of EOD waveform in *Brachyhypopomus pinnicaudatus*. *J. Comp. Physiol. A* **185**, 187–197.

Smith, G., and Zakon, H. (2000). Pharmacological characterization of ionic currents that regulate the rhythm of the medullary pacemaker nucleus in a weakly electric fish. *J. Neurbiol.* **42**, 270–286.

Smith, G. T. (1999). Ionic currents that contribute to a sexually dimorphic communication signal in weakly electric fish. *J. Comp. Physiol. A* **185**, 379–387.

Spiro, J. (1997). Differential activation of glutamate receptor subtypes on a single class of cells enables a neural oscillator to produce distinct behaviors. *J. Neurophysiol.* **78**(2), 835–847.

Stoddard, P. (1999). Predation enhances complexity in the evolution of electric fish signals. *Nature, (London)* **400**, 254–256.

Triefenbach, F. A., and Zakon, H. H. (2002). Signaling responses to sexual and reproductive status cues in the weakly electric fish, *Apteronotus leptorhynchus*. *Anim. Behav.* (in press).

Vincent, A., Ahnesjo, I. *et al.* (1994). Operational sex rations and behavioral sex differences in a pipefish population. *Behav. Ecol. Sociobiol.* **34**(6), 435–442.

Watson, J. T., and Kelley, D. B. (1992). Testicular masculinization of vocal behavior in juvenile female *Xenopus laevis* reveals sensitive periods for song duration, rate, and frequency spectra. *J. Comp. Physiol. A* **171**, 343–350.

Watson, J. T., Robertson, J., Sachdav, U., and Kelley, D. B. (1993). Laryngeal muscle and motor neuron plasticity in *Xenopus laevis*: testicular masculinization of a developing neuromuscular system. *J. Neurobiol.* **24**, 1615–1625.

Waxman, S. G., Pappas, G. D. *et al.* (1972). Morphological correlates of functional differentiation of nodes of Ranvier along single fibres in the neurogenic electric organ of the knife fish *Sternarchus*. *J. Cell Biol.* **53**, 210–224.

Weld, M. M., and Maler, L. (1992). Substance P-like immunoreactivity in the brain of the gymnotiform fish *Apteronotus leptorhynchus*: Presence of sex differences. *J. Chem. Neuroanat.* **5**, 107–129.

Weld, M. M., Kar, S. *et al.* (1994). The distribution of tachykinin binding sites in the brain of an electric fish (*Apteronotus leptorhynchus*). *J. Chem. Neuroanat.*

Westby, G. W. M. (1988). The ecology, discharge diversity and predatory beavhiour of gymnotiforme electric fish in the coastal streams of French Guiana. *Behav. Ecol. Sociobiol.* **22**, 341–354.

Westby, G. W. M., and Kirschbaum, F. (1977). Emergence and development of the electric organ discharge in the mormyrid fish, *Pollimyrus isidori*. I. The larval discharge. *J. Comp. Physiol. A* **122**, 251–271.

Westby, G. W. M., and Kirschbaum, F. (1978). Emergence and development of the electric organ discharge in the mormyrid fish, *Pollimyrus isidori*. II. Replacement of the larval by the adult discharge. *J. Comp. Physiol. A* **127**, 45–59.

Zakon, H. H. (1999). Sex steroids and weakly electric fish: A model system for activational mechanisms of hormone action. *In* "Sexual Differentiation of the Brain" (A. Matsumoto, ed.). CRC Press, Boca Raton, FL.

Zakon, H. H., and Dunlap, K. D. (1999). Sex steroids and communication signals in electric fish: A tale of two species. *Brain, Behav. Evol.* **54**, 61–69.

Zakon, H. H., and Meyer, J. H. (1983). Plasticity of electroreceptor tuning in the weakly electric fish, *Sternopygus macrurus*. *J. Comp. Physiol. A* **153**, 477–487.

Zakon, H. H., Yan, H.-Y. *et al.* (1990). Human chorionic gonadotropin-induced shifts in the electrosensory system of the weakly electric fish, *Sternopygus*. *J. Neurobiol.* **21**, 826–833.

Zakon, H. H., Thomas, P. *et al.* (1991). Electric organ discharge frequency and plasma sex steroid levels during gonadal recrudescence in a natural population of the weakly electric fish *Sternopygus macrurus*. *J. Comp. Physiol. A* **169**, 493–499.

Zucker, M. S. (1997). Hormonal basis of sexual dimorphism in and steroid sensitivity of the electric organ discharge frequency of the gymnotiform fish, *Apteronotus leptorhynchus*., University of Texas at Austin.

Zupanc, G., and Maler, L. (1993). Evoked chirping in the weakly electric fish *Apteronotus leptorhynchus*: A quantitative biophysical analysis. *Can. J. Zool.* **71**, 2301–2310.

Zupanc, G., Jorschke, I. *et al.* (1999). Corticotropin releasing factor in the brain of the gymnoiform fish, *Apteronotus leptorhynchus*: Immunohistochemical studies combined with neuronal tract tracing. *Gen. Comp. Endocrinol.* **114**, 349–364.

25

Hormonal Pheromones in Fish

Norm Stacey
Department of Biological Sciences
University of Alberta
Edmonton, Alberta, Canada T6G 2E9

Peter Sorensen
Department of Fisheries, Wildlife and Conservation Biology
University of Minnesota
St. Paul, Minnesota 55108

*F*ish, the most diverse and ancient group of vertebrates, commonly employ released hormones and metabolites as external chemical signals that mediate behavioral and physiological synchrony between conspecifics. Although little is known about how these systems evolved, it appears that they primarily reflect specialization of the neural (olfactory) systems of receiving organisms to detect naturally released hormonal products. However, in at least some instances specialization appears to have occurred to produce particular types of hormonal products in greater quantity. Thus, in some species of fish, the same (or similar) suites of hormonal compounds may be functioning as both internal and external chemical signals. It is thought likely that most hormonal pheromones are recognized (function as) mixtures of multiple components that may on occasion include nonhormonal products. The most thoroughly studied example of a fish hormonal pheromone system is that of the goldfish, for which five hormonal products with specific pheromonal function have been identified. The African catfish, Atlantic salmon, and Arctic char represent somewhat less understood model species from a variety of taxonomic groups. Further, electrophysiological recording from the olfactory epithelia of well over a hundred species of fish show that most detect hormonal products, although how these odorants are used has not been elucidated. Apparent parallels between how hormonal products function within and outside the body are discussed.

I. INTRODUCTION

Fish are the most ancient group of vertebrates and the most abundant in species and biomass—of over 25,000 described species, more than 95% are teleosts (modern bony fish), which inhabit an extraordinary range of aquatic habitats (Nelson, 1994). Living in water, a universal solvent that readily transmits body metabolites and is frequently dimly lit, fish have come to employ intraspecific chemical signals (pheromones) in most aspects of their lives (Liley, 1982; Liley and Stacey, 1983; Smith, 1992; Sorensen, 1992a,b; Sorensen and Caprio, 1997; Sorensen and Stacey, 1999). Moreover, research since the 1980s has revealed that reproductive synchrony among a very large number of fishes is commonly mediated by hormonal pheromones (sex pheromones comprising hormonal compounds).

Fish exhibit a seemingly endless array of reproductive strategies and behaviors, in which the regulatory roles of hormones and pheromones are poorly understood. For instance, although most fish are gonochorists (sexes are separate), many exhibit hermaphroditism that can be simultaneous (both genders are functional at the same time), protandrous (male function develops first), protogynous (Price, 1984; Warner, 1984; Kuwamura and Nakashima, 1998), or even bidirectional (Munday et al., 1998). Descriptions of fish chemical ecology suggest that sex pheromones are ancient and have assumed many diverse functions in all the major groups examined, including lampreys, sharks, and sturgeons (Bjerselius *et al.,* 1995a; L. E. Rasmussen, personal communication; Kasumyan, 1993). Although hormonal pheromones have yet to be definitively identified in any of these ancient species, there is reason to believe that the sea lamprey, *Petromyzon marinus,* employs a novel mixture of sulfated sex steroids in a manner similar to that described in teleost fish (Bjerselius *et al.,* 1995a). If these systems in extant primitive species are representative of pheromonal function in ancient fishes and pheromone systems are as dynamic as other aspects of fish biology, there have been tremendous diversification and specialization in fish pheromone systems. It therefore is surprising that our current understanding of fish sex pheromones indicates they are relatively simple in chemical composition and, with few exceptions (e.g., Kawabata, 1993), are hormonally derived.

Reproduction in animals is regulated by a complex endogenous network of neuronal and nonneuronal chemical signaling systems that operate at numerous levels to synchronize behavioral and gonadal functions in the individual. In the case of fish hormonal pheromones, we argue that the key components of this endogenous network—steroids and prostaglandins—extend into the environment where they act as potent exogenous signals that synchronize reproductive functions between and among conspecifics. Although findings that hormonal products can have additional functions as external pheromonal signals may at first seem novel, it actually is relatively common for chemical signals to serve multiple (but often related) functions at the autocrine, paracrine, and endocrine levels in the vertebrate body. Further, some (e.g., Carr, 1988) have suggested that there is good evolutionary reason to suggest conservation of chemical signals.

Hormonal pheromones appear to function as a special class of sexual signals. Typically, vertebrate sexual signals are generated by gonadal sex steroids that modify the structure or function of somatic effectors. Fish, for example, generate a great variety of sexually dimorphic signals by using sex steroids to alter morphological and behavioral phenotype in a manner that transmits visual, electrical, acoustic, or chemical information (Liley and Stacey, 1983; Stacey, 1987; Borg, 1994; Bass, 1993; Zakon *et al.,* 1995). A feature common to these and similar signaling systems in tetrapods is that the important reproductive information carried by an individual's steroid hormone production is transmitted only indirectly to conspecifics, through somatic effectors that may require many days to become functional and, therefore, can transmit only relatively tonic information about the signaler's past hormonal status. In contrast, fish hormonal pheromone systems transmit rapid information about a signaler's current hormonal status by serving as a direct link between the signaler's endocrine system and the nervous system(s) of conspecifics (Fig. 1). Such differences between direct (hormonal pheromone) and indirect (effector-mediated) signaling systems have profound implications for both the frequency and amplitude of pheromonal signals and thus alter the very nature of sex pheromone function. Fish are not unique among vertebrates in using released hormonal products as sex pheromones (e.g., the volatile androgen, androstenone, in the pig; Melrose *et al.,* 1971; Dorries *et al.,* 1997); however, the evidently widespread occurrence of hormonal pheromones among the fishes has three important implications for our understanding of hormone-brain-behavior (HBB) interactions in vertebrates.

First, the study of hormonal pheromones promises to provide important insights into the functioning of the olfactory system (cranial nerve one), a system that is poorly understood but whose biochemical, cellular, and anatomical features have been highly conserved throughout vertebrate evolution (Sorensen and Caprio, 1997). As in insects, it is clear that substantial portions of the vertebrate olfactory system are devoted to pheromonal detection and processing, the mechanisms of which can probably be clarified through the study of identified, biologically relevant ligands and receptors. Because of the specificity with which they interact with their olfactory receptors (Sorensen *et al.,* 1988, 1990), hormonal pheromones should provide powerful tools for deciphering how the nervous system encodes odor information (Sorensen *et al.,* 1998). In particular, these pheromones can be used to address specific questions as to how the brain encodes complex information about chemical identity. In addition, because many steroids and prostaglandins simultaneously function both as endogenous hormones and as exogenous pheromones, characterizing the receptors that mediate multiple responses to these chemical signals could provide important insights as to how hormonal pheromone systems have evolved. Last, because sensitivity to some

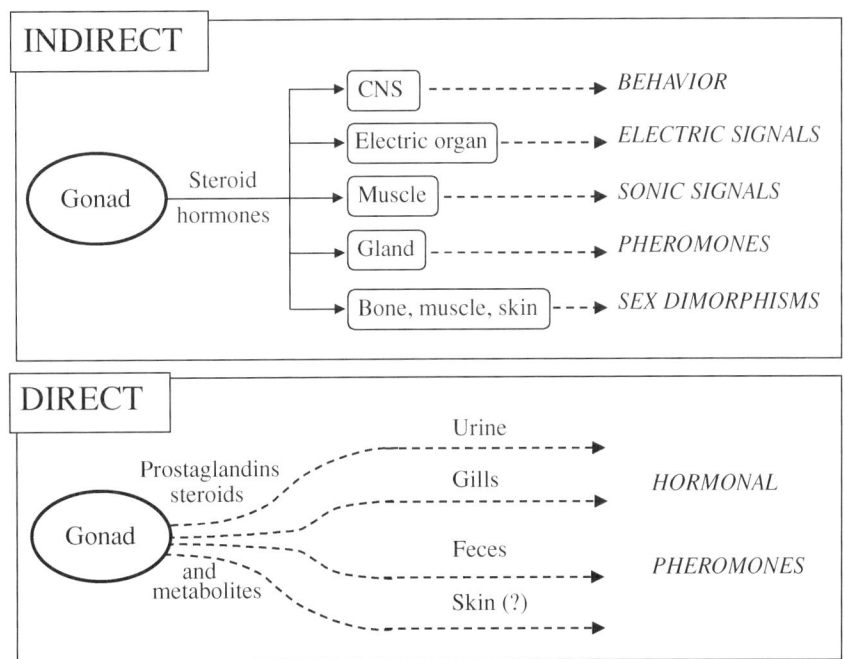

FIGURE 1 Steroid hormones typically generate sexual signals indirectly by altering the structure and function of nongonadal target organs. Hormonal pheromones generate sexual signals directly after release via a number of routes. From Stacey and Cardwell (1997), with permission.

hormonal pheromones is known to be sexually dimorphic and to be influenced by hormonal sex steroids (e.g., Cardwell et al., 1995), hormonal pheromones provide a new model for investigating the endocrine gating of sensory input (see Section V).

Second, because hormonal pheromones are derived from a homologous and evolutionarily conserved vertebrate endocrine system, they should serve as invaluable model systems for comparative and evolutionary studies of how pheromones arise and the HBB systems with which they coevolve. Although comparative studies have been informative in examining the evolution of some insect pheromonal systems (Loefstedt et al., 1986), we believe similar studies of fish have great promise because of evidence for homologous hormonal pheromones in a number of speciose higher teleost taxa (Stacey and Cardwell, 1995, 1997; Stacey et al., 1995) that exhibit considerable diversity in mating systems.

Third, the existence of hormonal pheromones challenges our classical concept that sex hormone actions are limited to reproductive synchrony in the individual. Moreover, in cases in which the action of a hormonal pheromone is to increase synthesis (and presumably release) of hormones detectable by conspecifics (e.g., Dulka et al., 1987a), there is the basis for a pheromonally mediated endocrine feedback system involving at least two individuals and potentially many more (Fig. 2). Because such intraspecific pheromonal processes provide the raw material through which sexual selection can act to modify social behavior and reproductive function, it is reasonable to expect that hormonal pheromones have had profound influences on the way that HBB relationships have evolved in the fishes.

In this review we survey the understanding of fish hormonal pheromones, emphasizing the role of these compounds as pheromones in the context of their hormonal origins. Although we review published information for all fish species in which the evidence for hormonal pheromones seems clear, much of our discussion deals with goldfish (Carassius auratus), the best-understood example of hormonal pheromone function. This review is broad in scope because our interests lie in how hormonal pheromone systems, which integrate so many aspects of fish biology, could have evolved and presently function.

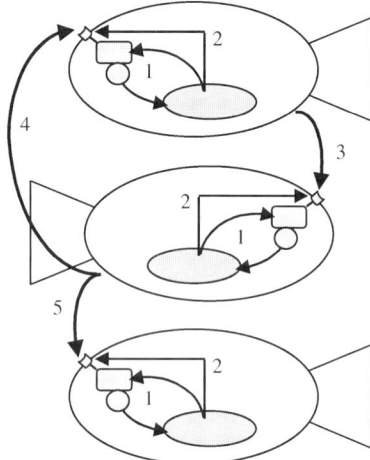

FIGURE 2 Hormonal regulation of reproduction in all fish involves endogenous interactions in the brain-pituitary-gonadal axis (1). In fish that employ hormonal pheromones, this regulation can also include endogenous steroidal control of olfactory function (2), and exogenous actions on the behavior and physiology of conspecifics through released hormonal pheromones (3). In turn, endocrine response of the conspecific detecting the pheromone could exert feedback effects on the pheromone producer (4) as well as effects on additional conspecifics (5).

II. HORMONES, PHEROMONES, OLFACTION, AND BEHAVIOR

A. Olfactory Signals and Pheromones: General Concepts and Definitions

Briefly stated, pheromones are chemical signals that pass between individuals of the same species (Sorensen and Wyatt, 2000). Odors are predisposed to function as social signals not only because of their ubiquitous nature, but also because they are discriminated with great sensitivity and specificity by the vertebrate olfactory system and are capable of being dispersed and detected in dark or noisy environments. In addition, because organisms can detect only a portion of the myriad compounds that surround them, pheromonal stimuli can have a covert quality. Not surprisingly, the vast majority of invertebrates and vertebrates have evolved to employ pheromones that mediate diverse social phenomena, not all of which are reproductive in nature (see Sorensen and Wyatt, 2000).

Darwin (1887) first recognized that odorous compounds released by organisms exert specific effects on conspecifics; however, Bethe (1932) first gave them a name—ectohormones. Bethe (1932) contrasted the external actions of ectohormones to internal actions of endohormones, a term that he suggested replace the term hormone. Bethe's terminology fell out of use; Karlson and Luscher (1959) revived the concept of external chemical signals, suggesting they be called pheromones (from the Greek *pherin*, "to transfer," and *hormon* "to excite"). Karlson and Luscher defined pheromones as "substances that are excreted to the outside of an individual and received by a second individual of the same species in which they release a specific reaction, for example a definite behaviour or developmental process" [p. 55]. The term has since been subject to controversy, especially among mammalian biologists who have identified few pheromones but are concerned about evidence that mammalian pheromones can be chemically complex and modified by experience (see Sorensen,1992a; Sorensen and Stacey, 1999). Attempting to resolve some of these difficulties, we (Sorensen and Stacey, 1999) have proposed that a sex pheromone be defined as "a substance, or mixture of substances, which is released by an individual and which evokes a specific and adaptive reproductive response in conspecifics, the expression of which does not require specific learning" [p. 17]. Our definition is intended to incorporate only odorous cues directly associated with the act of reproduction; thus, migratory cues employed by maturing fish to locate spawning grounds are not considered reproductive pheromones. Notably, our definition leaves open the possibilities that pheromones can be mixtures, that responses to them can be modified by experience, and that they need not be species-specific.

B. Hormonal Pheromones

Since clear evidence for hormonal sex pheromones was first published (Colombo *et al.*, 1980, 1982; Van Den Hurk and Lambert, 1983), research on dozens of fish species has demonstrated that they release sex pheromones made up partially or wholly of hormones or hormonal metabolites. We term these hormonally derived stimuli hormonal pheromones, acknowledging that at least in some cases they might be components of mixtures containing nonhormonal components (Stacey and Sorensen, 1991; Sorensen and Stacey, 1999). The possibility that nonhormonal odorants are important sexual signals in fish is not addressed in detail in this review because very little information exists on this topic. Indeed, with the possible exception of L-amino acids, which have been suggested to stimulate gamete release in the rose bitterling *(Rhodeus ocellatus),* a species that releases its gametes into freshwater molluscs (Kawabata, 1993), and tetrodotoxin, which has been suggested to serve as a sexual signal in the puffer fish *(Fugu rubripes;* Matsumura, 1985), all sex pheromones described in fish are steroids, prostaglandins, or their metabolites. That fish should commonly employ hormonal products in their pheromonal signals makes good sense, and we expect it to be true for most fishes; however this in no way precludes a role for other types of compounds. Indeed, we believe any unique body metabolite that is produced by sexually active fishes should be considered a candidate for sex pheromonal function.

The discovery of hormonal pheromones has simplified many issues related to intraspecific chemical communication in fish, insofar as it has been possible to replace some fuzzy concepts of conspecific odors of unknown chemical nature with clear examples of known pheromonal compounds whose production, release, detection, and biological functions can be quantified. On the other hand, such advances necessitate new terminology if we are to prevent confusion when discussing this new information (Sorensen and Stacey, 1999). The new terms we propose are of two types—those related to the nature of the pheromones themselves and those related to their presumed functions.

1. Special Terminology Related to Pheromones and Their Composition

Studies of fish hormonal pheromones have produced numerous examples in which hormones and their metabolites have been shown to be released, to stimulate the olfactory system, or to induce a specific reproductive response. However, despite clear evidence for biological activity of water-borne hormonal compounds in fish, it is important to realize that in no case are we confident that we know the complete chemical identity of a natural fish pheromone. The reason for this is that the net result of hormone synthesis, metabolism, and release is likely to be a complex mixture of changing proportions (Scott *et al.,* 1991b; Scott and Sorensen, 1994). The following terminology, originally proposed by Sorensen and Stacey (1999), is intended to clarify discussion of pheromonal mixtures and other issues related to pheromonal composition.

1. **Hormonal product:** Hormonal products are hormones, their precursors, and metabolites that are released to the water in urine or feces or across the gills (Scott and Vermeirssen, 1994; Vermeirssen and Scott, 1996), but are not known to be detected by conspecifics or to function as pheromones.

2. **Hormonal odorant:** Hormonal odorants are released hormones, their precursors, and metabolites that stimulate olfactory neurons of conspecifics, but have no known pheromonal function.

3. **Pheromonal stimulus:** A pheromonal stimulus is an odorant (a compound that stimulates the olfactory system) or mixture of odorants that elicits biological response, but is known not to be the entire natural pheromone or has not been examined to determine if this is the case.

4. **Single-component hormonal pheromone:** A single-component hormonal pheromone is a pheromone that acts through only one olfactory receptor mechanism. If the receptor mechanism is highly specific, the pheromone may consist of only one hormonal compound; if it is less specific, the pheromone may be a mixture containing both a primary (most potent) component see (item 6) and redundant (less potent) components that interact with the same receptor mechanism.

5. **Multiple-component pheromone:** A multiple-component pheromone is a pheromone containing more than one primary component, each acting through its own olfactory receptor mechanism. A multiple-component pheromone may be obligate (i.e., a precise mixture is required to elicit full biological activity) or facultative (i.e., a mixture is not required, although typically present and containing components that modulate one another's activity). It may also contain nonhormonal components. Most insect pheromones are obligate mixtures, but this possibility has not been directly addressed in fish (Sorensen *et al.,* 1998).

6. **Primary component:** A primary component is a hormonal compound that induces biological response on its own and acts via its own olfactory

receptor. Obligate multiple-component pheromones have biological activity only if the primary components are present. In facultative multiple-component pheromones, all components with stimulatory effects on an organism's biology are, by definition, primary components because they all have their own independent actions. In goldfish, the steroid 17,20β-dihydroxy-4-pregnen-3-one (17,20β-P) is an example of a primary component in a facultative multiple-component mixture released by preovulatory females (Sorensen et al., 1987, 1990, 1995a; see Section IV.D.1.d.ii).

7. **Secondary component:** Secondary components, found only in obligate multiple-component pheromones, are single components that act via their own olfactory receptor and are required for full activity of an obligate multiple-component pheromone, but do not induce a response on their own.

8. **Inhibitory component:** Inhibitory components may be found in a facultative pheromonal mixture, reduce response(s) to the primary component(s), and act via their own olfactory receptor. In the goldfish, preovulatory steroid pheromone (see Section IV.D.1.d.ii), androstenedione (AD) appears to be an example of such an inhibitory component (Stacey, 1991).

For several reasons, we exclude from our definitions and discussion the terms "releaser" and "primer," proposed by Wilson and Bossert (1963) to differentiate pheromones that have rapid behavioral effects on behavior from pheromones that have slower physiological effects. First, although these terms could be helpful if used to describe pheromonal effects, they have been applied to the pheromones themselves, resulting in the conception that a pheromone must be either a primer or a releaser. However, as noted by Wilson and Bossert (1963), "it is quite possible for the same pheromone to be both a releaser and a primer," and this certainly is the case with many hormonal pheromones in fish (see Section IV.D.1.d). Second, because all pheromones exert their effects through physiological mechanisms, the proposed distinction between releasers and primers is contradictory.

Our proposed terminology is difficult to apply to fish hormonal pheromones because in no case do we know the chemical identity of any natural fish pheromone. Nonetheless, we hope that the adoption of such terminology will clarify the discussion of and increase awareness of the potential diversity of pheromone types.

2. Evolution and the Terminology of Pheromone Function

Traditionally, discussions of pheromonal function include the term "chemical communication," and imply situations in which an individual not only is specialized for the production and release of a pheromone (which itself may be specialized), but also benefits from a conspecific receiver's adaptive response. In the case of many insects and mammals, in which there are clear specializations for pheromone production and clear benefits to pheromone receivers and donors, such discussions are not problematic. In the case of fish hormonal pheromones, however, it often is unclear whether the donor is specialized for pheromone production or even if it benefits from the receiver's response.

For these reasons, we have proposed a theoretical framework and associated terminology to distinguish what we perceive to be distinctly different stages in the evolution of hormonal pheromone function (Stacey and Sorensen, 1991; Sorensen and Stacey, 1999) (Fig. 3). Briefly, we propose that hormonal pheromone systems should readily arise in fish because they commonly release hormonal products that have the potential to transmit valuable information to conspecifics. Moreover, we propose that a hormonal pheromone originates when evolutionary change in an individual enables it to detect and respond adaptively to a hormonal product released by conspecifics. This initial stage in pheromone evolution, which we term chemical spying, is characterized by a specialized receiver that benefits from its pheromonal response. In addition, the donor may or may not benefit from the receiver's response, but, it is important to note, remains in an unspecialized state with respect to pheromone production and release. With the transition to chemical spying, the detected hormonal product now can be termed either a pheromonal stimulus (in reference to its action on the receiver) or a pheromonal cue (in reference to the donor's unspecialized state) (Fig. 3).

Theoretically, chemical spying is stable if there is no mechanism whereby the receiver's response can act as a selective force for specialization of the donor (see Sorensen and Stacey, 1999). To cite an extreme example, Pacific herring (*Clupea harengus pallasi*) spawn

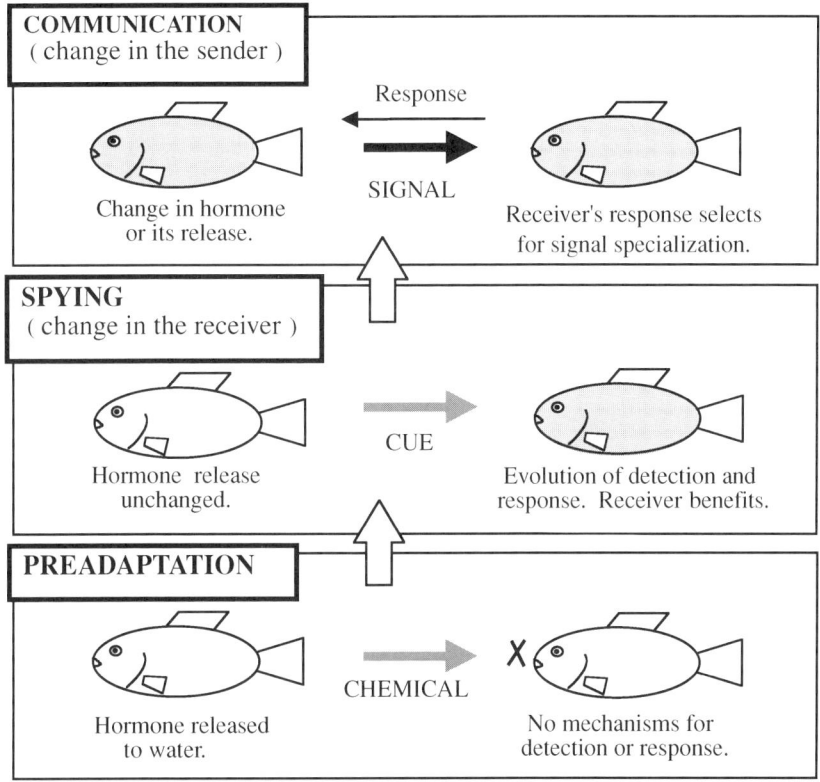

FIGURE 3 Proposed stages in the evolution of hormonal pheromones. From Stacey and Sorensen (1991), "Biochemistry and Molecular Biology of Fishes," pp. 109–135, © 1991 with permission from Elsevier Science, and from Stacey and Sorensen (1991), with permission.

en masse in dense schools that can extend along kilometers of shoreline. Males and females do not coordinate their sexual activities, but independently deposit gametes on benthic substrates, the prolonged motility of the released sperm and the dense bisexual aggregations ensuring a high rate of fertilization (Stacey and Hourston, 1982; Carolsfeld et al., 1992). The spawning in both sexes is rapidly triggered by exposure to the male's milt (sperm and seminal fluid), which contains a partially characterized pheromone (Sherwood et al., 1991; Carolsfeld et al., 1992, 1997). We believe the herring pheromone represents an example of chemical spying; because in this species' mating system males do not fertilize the eggs of the females they stimulate to spawn, there appears to be no mechanism whereby a male's reproductive success can be influenced by the quality of his pheromone production.

In other cases, however, the receiver's response directly benefits the individual donor and thereby has the potential to act as a selective force for donor specializations that could involve modified pheromone production or release. With specialization of the donor, chemical spying progresses to chemical communication and the pheromonal cue now is termed a pheromonal signal (Fig. 3).

Admittedly, we know too little about hormonal pheromone function in any species to be confident in applying terms such as chemical spying and pheromonal signal. However, we find that such specific vocabulary clarifies our thinking on important questions of hormonal pheromone function and evolution. To cite just one example, it often is assumed that sex pheromones of reproductively sympatric species are specific, such that maladaptive reproductive responses to heterospecific odors are avoided. Although species specificity of sex pheromones is poorly understood in fish (Sorensen and Stacey, 1999), selection for such specificity might be expected to be common for fish hormonal pheromones, given the evidently limited chemical diversity of fish steroids and prostaglandins and the numerous natural situations in which a number of species interact closely. If so, this selection is expected to take many forms, depending on factors such as whether maladaptive responses to heterospecifics involve the donors or receivers of the species involved and whether the participants are engaged in chemical spying or chemical communication (Sorensen and Stacey, 1999).

C. Sense of Smell

Olfactory ablation and electrophysiological recording experiments demonstrate that fish, like other vertebrates, detect pheromonal signals exclusively via their olfactory system (cranial nerve 1) (Sorensen and Caprio, 1997). This is significant for several reasons. First, the olfactory system is an ancient sensory system associated with telencephalic regions mediating social behaviors. The neural components of this olfactory system have been highly conserved during vertebrate evolution (Hildebrand and Shepherd, 1997; Sorensen and Caprio, 1997), allowing fish to serve as relevant models of vertebrate olfactory function. Second, the olfactory system is unique among sensory systems in that it comprises primary sensory neurons, olfactory receptor neurons (ORNs), that regenerate throughout the life of the animal and project directly to the brain (olfactory bulb). Third, olfactory responsiveness of fish to some hormonal pheromones is sexually dimorphic and influenced by circulating steroid hormones (Cardwell et al., 1995), implying the existence of a dynamic interplay between the olfactory and reproductive endocrine systems. Fourth, responsiveness to food odors (amino acids), and presumably to hormonal pheromones as well (Rosenblum et al., 1991), is mediated by membrane-bound receptors located on the ORNs (Buck and Axel, 1991; Ngai et al., 1993a,b; Cao et al., 1998; Speca et al., 1999; see Section II.C.2.a). Thus, the finding that many hormonal pheromone stimuli are unmodified hormones whose internal actions are also mediated by membrane-bound receptors, raises the intriguing possibility that external olfactory receptors for hormonal pheromones may be similar or identical to internal hormone receptors in the brain, gonad, and other tissues.

1. Anatomy of the Olfactory System

A major question about fish hormonal pheromones is how the nervous system detects and deciphers this chemosensory information. Indeed, this complex question has not been answered for any well-defined, biologically relevant chemosensory signal in any vertebrate (see Xu et al., 2000). Consequently, we discuss the olfactory system only as it pertains to fish hormonal pheromones, which offer special promise toward understanding the vertebrate olfactory system because they are well-defined chemical signals whose function is presumably associated with relatively well-defined (innate) neural pathways (Sorensen et al., 1998).

In fish, as in other vertebrates, the olfactory system comprises three neuroanatomical components—the olfactory epithelium, the olfactory bulbs, and the olfactory terminal fields in the telencephalon and hypothalamus (Fig. 4). The olfactory epithelium covers

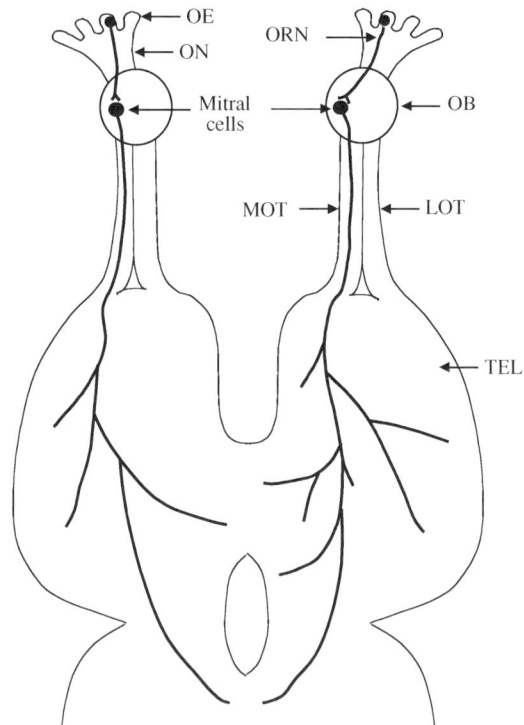

FIGURE 4 Highly schematic representation of the fish olfactory system in horizontal section. (For details of olfactory projections to the brain, see Dulka 1993). LOT, lateral olfactory tract; MOT, medial olfactory tract; OB, olfactory bulb; OE, olfactory epithelium; ON, olfactory nerve; ORN, olfactory receptor neuron; TEL, telencephalon.

the surface of the olfactory rosette, located in the paired nasal capsules, and contains both nonsensory supporting cells and the ORNs that respond to odorous information. Although the morphology of the olfactory rosette is enormously variable among fishes (see Zeiske et al., 1992), with few exceptions (e.g., sharks and lamprey) the olfactory epithelium of fish, like that of most other vertebrates, contains two principal classes of ORNs—ciliated and microvillous—of which several subtypes have now been described in fish (Hansen and Zeiske, 1998; Hansen et al., 1999; Morita and Finger, 1998). As in all vertebrates, the functional significance of these two classes of ORNs is as yet unclear in fish, although correlative studies suggest that only the microvillar neurons carry pheromonal information (see Section II.C.2.a). Both ciliated and microvillar ORNs are found intermingled (Morita and Finger, 1998) in the fish olfactory epithelium, although weakly defined zones may exist. This situation contrasts with that of tetrapods, many of which have two olfactory epithelia—the main olfactory epithelium, which contains largely ciliated receptor cells, and the vomeronasal system, which contains largely microvillar cells (Eisthen, 1992; Dulka, 1993).

From the olfactory epithelium, ORNs project via the olfactory nerves to the olfactory bulbs (Fig. 4), in which the ORN axons form the outermost of four bulbar layers, which also include, from superficial to deep, the glomerular layer, the mitral cell layer, and the internal (granule cell) layer (Satou, 1990). Although a few ORNs and the terminal nerve (see Section II.C.2.c) project directly from the olfactory epithelium through the olfactory bulb to the brain, the dendritic processes of the overwhelming majority of ORNs terminate in the bulbs. In the bulbs, ORNs with common receptors converge and synapse on mitral cell apical dendrites in the bulbar glomeruli, which comprise dense aggregations of the neuropils of mitral and granule cells. Granule cells function as local interneurons in the bulb and possess many inhibitory dendrodendritic synapses with both mitral cells and ruffed cells, the latter constituting another class of output neuron that does not synapse with ORNs and whose precise function is unknown. Granule cells also receive input from centrifugal nerve fibers projecting from the brain to the bulb. The nature of these interconnections is complex and not well understood, at least as it pertains to pheromonal processing.

Both ruffed and mitral cells project to the brain through the medial olfactory tract (MOT) and lateral olfactory tract (LOT), nerve bundlets comprising many thousands of neurons, and terminate in specific terminal fields in the telencephalon and hypothalamus (Dulka, 1993; Fig. 4). Little is understood about how natural odor information (including hormonal pheromones) is processed, although there is strong reason to believe that olfactory glomeruli process information associated with specific odorant receptors (see Section II.C.2.b). It appears that in fish, as in other vertebrates, the olfactory bulb represents odor identity with a spatial mapping system that is supplemented by a temporal coding scheme, as observed in insects (Laurent, 1999), although this has not been systematically examined.

The fish olfactory system evidently employs some type of spatial map to represent natural odor and pheromone identity. As reviewed by Dulka (1993), neurophysiological studies of common carp (*Cyprinus carpio*) and goldfish reveal a lateral–medial subdivision of olfactory function that appears to originate in the olfactory bulb; for example, output neurons in the medial portion of the bulb tend to project to the MOT, and lateral fibers project to the LOT. In addition, olfactory tract stimulation studies in cod (*Gadus morhua;* Doving and Selset, 1980) and lesion studies in goldfish (Stacey and Kyle, 1983; Dulka and Stacey, 1991), crucian carp (*Carassius carassius;* Hamdani et al., 2000), and African catfish (*Clarias gariepinus;* Resink et al., 1989a) demonstrate that responses to food are mediated by the LOT, whereas responses to pheromones are mediated exclusively by the MOT. These studies are consistent with extracellular recordings in goldfish (Sorensen et al., 1991) showing that activity of the LOT is induced only by amino acids (putative feedings cues), whereas activity of the MOT is induced by all known odorants including identified hormonal pheromones (sex steroids and prostaglandins).

In fish, the LOT and MOT have different projection patterns to the telencephalon (see Dulka, 1993; Fig. 4). Upon entering the brain, the MOT appears to divide into two distinct rami. One ramus projects to the ventral regions of the telencephalon, which receive input only from the MOT and are associated with reproductive behavior in both goldfish (Kyle et al., 1982) and salmon (*Oncorhynchus nerka*) (Satou et al., 1982). The other MOT ramus projects to the anteroventral preoptic region (POA) (Levine and Dethier, 1985). The POA, which receives input from both the LOT and MOT, is associated with the control of male behavior (Kyle et al., 1987) and gonadotropin release (Peter et al., 1986). Both forebrain regions contain considerable aromatase activity (Gelinas and Callard, 1997). What little is known about forebrain processing of pheromonal information, and potential endocrine modulation of these functions, is discussed briefly in Sections IV.D.1.d.iv and V, respectively.

2. Olfactory Basis of Hormonal Pheromone Detection

Although studies of the goldfish, zebrafish, trout, and African catfish demonstrate that components of the fish olfactory system detect and respond to hormonal pheromones, no system is well understood. The following synopsis thus draws from many sources.

a) Olfactory Receptor Neurons Most of what is known about detection of hormonal pheromones is derived from electroolfactogram (EOG) studies demonstrating that the olfactory epithelium of many fish responds to water-borne steroids and prostaglandins with extreme specificity and sensitivity (picomolar response thresholds). Several behavioral studies have shown that this extracellular recording technique, which integrates the responses of many neurons, accurately reflects the olfactory sensitivity and specificity of the goldfish olfactory system when odor concentration is taken into account (Sorensen et al., 1988, 1990). Additional support comes from neural recordings from the olfactory epithelium (Sorensen and Caprio, 2000) and from mitral cells in the olfactory bulb (Hanson, 2001; L. R. Hanson and P. W. Sorensen, unpublished results). Multiunit neural recordings from the goldfish epithelium have also shown that pheromone-sensitive ORNs are widely dispersed throughout the olfactory epithelium, relatively few in number, and most abundant near the central raphe (Sorensen and Caprio, 2000, and unpublished results).

Microvillous ORNs of fish appear to transduce pheromone responses. The most compelling evidence comes from goldfish studies (Zippel et al., 1997), which first sectioned the olfactory nerves to induce degeneration of the olfactory epithelium and general loss of EOG responsiveness and then over the following weeks correlated ORN regeneration with the recovery of odor responses at the olfactory and whole-animal level. Ciliated ORNs regenerated first, and their appearance was accompanied by recovery of EOG responses to amino acids and of behavioral response to food odor (Zippel et al., 1997); however, recovery of EOG and behavioral responsiveness to sex steroid and prostaglandin pheromones did not occur until a week later, when microvillous ORNs appeared in the olfactory epithelium. In mammals, in which microvillous ORNs are the dominant cell type in the vomeronasal organ, they also are believed to mediate pheromonal responses (Dorries et al., 1997; Morita and Finger, 1998); however, as with fish (Dulka, 1993), the evidence is indirect and the functional significance unclear.

Hormonal pheromone receptors have yet to be cloned. However, the goldfish steroid pheromone $17,20\beta$-P binds with low capacity and high affinity to a membrane preparation of goldfish olfactory epithelium (Rosenblum et al., 1991). Binding is highly specific, as expected of an olfactory receptor, and also similar to that expected from ovarian membranes on which this steroid functions as a maturation-inducing hormone (Nagahama et al., 1995; see Section II.D.1). Biochemical similarities between the two receptor types have yet to be explored, however. Unfortunately, nothing is known of signal transduction mechanisms associated with pheromone sensitivity in fish, although studies of amino acid stimulation in catfish have established the presence of G-protein-mediated adenylate cyclase and phospholiapse C systems in fish ORNs (Sorensen and Caprio, 1997).

Interestingly, presumptive fish olfactory receptors with unknown chemosensitivies have now been cloned several times using probes based on G-protein-linked receptors found in mammalian olfactory epithelia. Two distinct classes of olfactory receptors are known in fish (Dryer and Berghard, 1999): a V2R (vomeronasal) type that resembles a mGluR-type (metabotropic glutamate) receptor found in the mammalian vomeronasal system and is believed to mediate responses to pheromones (Cao et al., 1998; Naito et al., 1998) and a G-olf (G-protein associated olfactory) type based on the original seven-transmembrane type of receptors isolated in the rat by Buck and Axel (1991). Interestingly, the V2R-type receptor appears to be found in microvillous cells

(Cao et al., 1998), and one has been functionally cloned in goldfish (Speca et al., 1999) and found to bind the amino acid L-arginine with high specificity, intensifying the mystery of the roles of ciliated and microvillous ORNs. The G-olf receptors have been characterized in several species and, although they have not been functionally expressed in fish, Ngai et al. (1993a,b) estimate fish typically possess approximately 100 of them, compared to over a thousand in mammals. As with mammals, *in situ* hybridization using probes for the G-olf receptors indicates that each fish ORN expresses one or perhaps a few of them. Thus, fish ORNs are likely to be quite specialized for the detection of particular classes of odorants, although this has yet to be demonstrated.

There is considerable evidence for sexual dimorphism in the olfactory epithelium of fish. Males of some deep-sea fish possess much larger olfactory epithelia than do females (Baird et al., 1990), presumably a result of intense selection for mate detection. Although ultrastructural differences in the olfactory systems of male and female mammals have also been noted (Dorries, 1992), the differences do not appear so pronounced. Further, although the functional relevance of this dimorphism is not clear in mammals, EOG recording indicates that this olfactory dimorphism in fish is androgen-dependent and specifically related to particular prostaglandin-derived hormonal pheromones (Cardwell et al., 1995; Sorensen and Goetz, 1993). Whether androgen-induced sensitivity to these hormonal pheromones is associated with changes in ORN type, receptor expression, changes in signal transduction pathways, or other processes has not been examined (see Section IV.D.1.d.iv). Presumably, the olfactory system is an endocrine target in all vertebrates, and fish hormonal pheromone systems appear to have excellent potential to address this intriguing phenomenon.

b) Olfactory Bulb The glomeruli of the vertebrate olfactory bulb appear to be the functional units that encode molecular features of odor cues and pass this information to the brain (Xu et al., 2000). This notion is largely derived from mammals, in which ORNs with common receptors have been demonstrated to project to common glomeruli (Ressler et al., 1994), and glomeruli have been demonstrated to discriminate specific molecular features of odorants (Mori et al., 1999). Together, these findings suggest that individual glomeruli mediate responses to particular types of chemical stimuli, and together form a chemotopic map of odor identity (Buck, 1996). Complicating this situation are findings suggesting that at least some mammalian receptors interact with many odorants; thus, it appears that odorant identity may in some instances be encoded by complex combinatorial patterns of glomerular activation across the olfactory bulb (Aranada et al., 2000). Some evidence also exists for this hypothesis in fish (see later), for which the situation is further complicated by the fact that many projection neurons synapse with ORNs associated with more than one glomerulus (Satou, 1990; Sorensen and Caprio, 1997). Little is understood about how any biologically relevant odors are encoded in any vertebrate; however, the distinct possibility remains that some odors of special significance, such as pheromones, may be discriminated by specialized receptors and associated neural pathways, known as labeled lines. Indeed, it is well established for insects that the macroglomerular complex in the antennal lobe contains highly specialized nerve fibers dedicated to processing pheromonal information (see Sorensen et al., 1998). We discuss studies that support the idea that the fish brain may process hormonal pheromone information in a loosely analogous manner later.

In fish, studies of both the goldfish and zebrafish (*Danio rerio*) reveal that odor coding also involves a bulbar map that may involve both complex combinatorial codes for food odors and simpler labeled lines for hormonal pheromones. Although the clearest evidence for such labeled lines comes from the finding that pheromonal information is carried by the MOTs alone (e.g., Stacey and Kyle, 1983; Dulka and Stacey, 1991), other studies describe specialized chemosensitivities of glomeruli from which the pheromone-sensitive projection neurons found in the MOT presumably originate.

For example, in our field potential electroencephalogram (EEG) recordings from the surface of the male goldfish bulb (Hanson et al., 1998), amino acids consistently produce large responses across the entire bulb, whereas hormonal pheromones elicit small, spatially restricted responses. An apparently comparable situation was observed in zebrafish when presumptive pheromonal and nonpheromonal odorants were used to activate the bulbar projections of ORNs that had been loaded with voltage- and calcium-sensitive dyes (Friedrich and Korsching, 1997, 1998). Zebrafish ORNs that responded to amino acids, bile acids, and nucleotides exhibited overlapping activity patterns involving multiple glomeruli. In contrast, ORNs that responded to prostaglandin F2α (PGF2α) and 17α,20β-dihydroxy-4-pregnen-3-one-20β-sulfate (17,20β-P-S), two hormonal odorants that induce EOG responses in zebrafish (see Section III.B.2), induce a focus of activity in the medial bulb (Friedrich and Korsching, 1998).

Single-unit recordings from mitral cells in the goldfish olfactory bulb (Zippel et al., 1999, 2000; Hanson, 2001) reveal specialized glomeruli (and associated projection neurons) that process hormonal pheromone information; however, these goldfish data describe a more complex scenario than that suggested by the dye studies of zebrafish ORN function (Friedrich and Korsching, 1998). The complex electrophysiological response characteristics of pheromone-sensitive goldfish-bulb-output neurons have been described by two research groups (Zippel and Sorensen) and appear to be different from those of amino-acid-sensitive neurons. Several important points emerge from these ongoing single-unit studies.

First, both Zippel et al. (2000) and we (Hanson, 2001) describe numerous mitral cells that respond both to hormonal pheromones and to other odorant classes. This finding suggests to us that the brain processes some pheromonal information in the context of nonpheromonal odors and supports our finding that the behavioral responsiveness of goldfish to hormonal pheromones is influenced by background (body) odor (Sorensen et al., 2000).

Second, approximately 5% of the mitral cells we have recorded convey only information associated with a single class of hormonal pheromones, suggestive of a labeled line. Such highly specialized mitral cells could be associated with the pheromone-responsive ORNs identified by Freidrich and Korsching (1998), who may have visualized them simply because they respond most strongly to pheromonal cues. We propose that in goldfish these highly specialized mitral cells, which we never observe when testing food odors (amino acids), drive fundamental (i.e., instinctual) responses to pheromones, whereas the less specialized pheromone-sensitive units provide additional supplemental information as it relates to background odor. This proposal is consistent with reports in insects and mammals in which seemingly innate behavioral responses can be modulated by experience and associated odorous stimuli (see Sorensen et al., 1998).

Zippel et al. (1999) do not report clear chemosensory specialization in any bulbar unit, although their multiunit recordings are much less likely to distinguish such specialized units because of the complex spontaneous firing patterns of olfactory bulb projection neurons. However, Zippel et al. (2000) report (without providing anatomical data) that ruffed cells in the goldfish olfactory bulb respond to hormonal pheromones, suggesting this cell type has a role in pheromonal responses. In conclusion, preliminary data from goldfish and zebrafish suggest that pheromonal information is processed in the olfactory bulb both by highly specialized glomeruli that detect a single class of pheromone and by less specialized glomeruli that detect blends of pheromonal and nonpheromonal odorants.

In contrast to the situation for goldfish and zebrafish, Hara and Zhang (1997) report that a number of salmonid species exhibit EOG responses to PGF2α and a sex steroid (etiocholanolone glucuronide, ETIO-G), but do not exhibit visually discernible bulbar EEG responses to hormonal pheromones. Hara and Zhang (1997) interpret this apparent absence of a pheromone-induced EEG response as evidence for an extra-bulbar pathway. However, in the absence of direct neuroanatomical data suggesting what these pathways are, we feel the reported absence of pheromone-induced EEG response in salmonids (Hara and Zhang, 1997) should be viewed with caution. Indeed, our recent bulbar EEG recordings from male goldfish demonstrate that, although we can record EEG responses to hormonal pheromones (Hanson, 2001), they are few in number and so small that their detection requires sophisticated frequency analysis rather than simple integration. In any case, no matter what the explanation for Hara and Zhang's (1997) observation, it demonstrates that hormonal pheromones are discriminated by unconventional neural pathways in the olfactory bulb.

c) Terminal Nerve The terminal nerve (TN; nervus terminalis = cranial nerve 0) is an extra-bulbar neural pathway whose fibers in many vertebrates associate with the olfactory nerves and tracts, and extend anteriorly to the nasal cavity and posteriorly to both the preoptic and hypothalamic areas and, in teleost fish, to the retina (Demski, 1993). Demski and

Northcutt (1983) proposed that the TN is a chemosensory system specialized for mediating responses to sex pheromones and cited a variety of supporting observations. For example, TN fibers connect the olfactory epithelium to specific telencephalic nuclei implicated in reproduction (von Bartheld and Meyer, 1986; Kyle et al., 1987); some TN neurons are immunoreactive for gonadotropin-releasing hormone (GnRH) (Eisthen and Northcutt, 1996); and electrical stimulation of either the optic nerve or the MOT induces sperm release in goldfish (Dulka and Demski, 1986). However, when the olfactory epithelium of goldfish was exposed to hormonal pheromones and other odorants that goldfish are known to detect, single-unit extracellular recordings failed to detect any change in TN activity, whereas bulbar units responded to many odors (Fujita et al., 1991). In contrast, tactile stimulation of the body inhibited the spontaneous activity of many TN neurons. Although the functions of the TN and the GnRH it contains remain enigmatic, patch clamp studies (Eisthen et al., 2000) demonstrate that GnRH can modulate ion channel functions of salamander olfactory receptor neurons, providing indirect evidence that the TN could exert neuromodulatory effects on ORNs, perhaps associated with physical activity of mating. The precise relevance of these findings to fish olfaction is unclear, however, because TN ablation studies in several fish species have failed to detect effects on reproduction (Kobayashi et al., 1994, 1997a; Yamamoto et al., 1997).

D. Hormones and Reproductive Behavior in Fish

The hormonal regulation of reproductive behaviors in fishes has been studied since the early twentieth century; however, considering the incredible reproductive diversity of fishes, relatively little is known. Here, we briefly update this topic and refer the reader to reviews of earlier literature on hormone–behavior interactions (Liley, 1969; Liley and Stacey, 1983; Stacey, 1987; Borg, 1994) and plasma hormone levels (Fostier et al., 1983; Borg, 1994).

1. Gonadal Steroid Hormones

As in tetrapods, steroidogenesis and gametogenesis in fish are controlled primarily by the pituitary gonadotropins, GTH I and GTH II, homologous to tetrapod follicle-stimulation hormone (FSH) and luteinizing hormone (LH), respectively (Sohn et al., 1999). During the reproductive cycle, GTH stimulation of gonadal recrudescence typically results in sexually dimorphic plasma concentrations of 17β-estradiol (E_2) and 11-ketotestosterone (11-KT)—in males, E_2 is often undetectable and 11-KT is typically much higher than in females (Borg, 1994). E_2 stimulates the synthesis and follicular uptake of vitellogenins (Specker and Sullivan, 1994) and regulates pituitary GTH II secretion both in vivo (Kobayashi and Stacey, 1990; Khan et al., 1999) and in vitro (Trudeau et al., 1993). In males, the role of 11-KT is less clear, but there is evidence it regulates gonadal sex differentiation (Piferer et al., 1993), male sex dimorphisms (Borg, 1994), GTH secretion (Antonopoulou et al., 1999), and spermatogenesis (Miura et al., 1996). The function of 11-KT in females is unknown (Borg, 1994).

In most fishes examined, the plasma testosterone (T) concentrations of females are equivalent to or greater than those in males (Borg, 1994). T influences GTH secretion in male and female fish (Kobayashi and Stacey, 1990; Trudeau et al., 1993; Antonopoulou et al., 1999; Khan et al., 1999) and also induces male secondary sex characters; however, in cases in which the potency of exogenous T and 11-KT have been compared, 11-KT typically is the more potent androgen (Borg, 1994). In skin of brown trout (Salmo trutta), for example, the fact that 11-KT is more potent than T in stimulating epidermal changes (Pottinger and Pickering, 1985) is problematic because the nuclear androgen receptor from brown trout skin binds T with considerably more affinity than 11-KT (Pottinger, 1987). The reproductive role of T in fish also has been unclear because the effects of exogenous T could be exerted through T receptors or following conversion to 11-KT or E_2; indeed, fish exhibit particularly high concentrations of aromatase (Pasmanik and Callard, 1985). Also, the kidney of the male stickleback (Gasterosteus aculeatus), an androgen target most sensitive to 11-KT (Borg et al., 1993), is reported to have a membrane receptor for 11-KT (Jakobsson et al., 1996).

The respective roles of T and 11-KT in fish reproduction could be clarified by findings (Sperry and Thomas, 1999a,b) that two species from the highly derived order Perciformes—a sciaenid (spotted seatrout, Micropogonias undulatus) and a serranid (kelp bass, Paralabrax clathratus)—each have two distinct nuclear androgen receptors (AR_1 and AR_2). AR_1, found primarily in the brain, binds only T with high affinity, whereas AR_2, found primarily in gonadal tissue, binds a number of androgens with high affinity, including 5α-dihydrotestosterone (DHT), T, and 11-KT. Fish may commonly possess these two androgen receptors (Sperry and Thomas, 1999a) because the binding characteristics of AR_1 in the derived perciforms are similar to those of androgen receptors in the more primitive orders Cypriniformes (goldfish, *Carassius auratus*; Pasmanik and Callard, 1988) and Salmoniformes (rainbow trout, *Oncorhynchus mykiss*; Slater *et al.*, 1995), whereas the binding of the perciform AR_2 is similar to that of androgen receptors in coho salmon (*Oncorhynchus kisutch*; Fitzpatrick *et al.*, 1994).

Both male and female fish produce 17,20β-P and related steroids near the time of final gonadal maturation and spawning. In females, 17,20β-P appears to be the maturation-inducing steroid (MIS) in a variety of species (Nagahama *et al.*, 1995), although the related 17α,20β,21-trihydroxy-4-pregnen-3-one (17,20β,21-P; also termed 20β-S; e.g., Trant and Thomas, 1989) serves this role in others (Thomas, 1994; Thomas and Das, 1997). In males, the role of 17,20β-P is less clear, although it has been shown to increase milt production and sperm motility in salmonids (Miura *et al.*, 1992). In spotted seatrout (*Cynoscion nebulosus*), membrane 17,20β,21-P receptors in the testis and on sperm indicate a role for this steroid in sperm function (Thomas *et al.*, 1997).

2. Hormones and Male Behavior

The temporal relationship between plasma androgens and spawning suggests that, as in other vertebrates, androgens regulate the expression of male reproductive behaviors in fish. On a seasonal basis, plasma T and 11-KT generally are low or undetectable during the part of the nonbreeding season prior to testicular recrudescence, increase with testicular growth, spermatogenesis, and the development of male secondary characters, and reach peak levels prior to or at the time of spawning, at which point both androgens typically decrease and 17,20β-P briefly increases (Borg, 1994). However, this simple pattern is complicated by the fact that male sex hormones also are strongly influenced by sociosexual stimuli, such as territorial actions with other males (Cardwell and Liley, 1991; Liley and Kroon, 1995; Cardwell *et al.*, 1996), the presence of a reproductively active female (Kyle *et al.*, 1985; Sorensen *et al.*, 1989; Oliveira *et al.*, 1996), and factors associated with nesting and paternal care (Pankhurst, 1995; Pankhurst *et al.*, 1999; Knapp *et al.*, 1999). In addition, in species with alternative male mating strategies, androgen profiles of the male morphs differ (Brantley *et al.*, 1993).

Male reproductive behaviors are reduced or abolished by castration and restored in castrates (Liley, 1969; Liley and Stacey, 1983; Borg, 1994) or induced in juveniles (Cardwell *et al.*, 1995) and females (Stacey and Kobayashi, 1996; Kobayashi and Nakanishi, 1999) by exogenous androgens. In the few cases in which the relative behavioral potencies of T and 11-KT have been compared, 11-KT is the more potent androgen—for example, bluegill sunfish (*Lepomis macrochirus*; Kindler *et al.*, 1991); threespine stickleback (*Gasterosteus aculeatus*; Borg and Mayer, 1995); and goldfish (Stacey and Kobayashi, 1996). The functional relationship between 11-KT and male reproductive behaviors and the typically low 11-KT levels in females suggest that this steroid (and its precursors and metabolites) are good candidates for generating a gender-specific odor that indicates presence of a sexually active male.

Peak plasma concentrations of 17,20β-P and related 21-carbon steroids are closely associated with spawning in a number of species—for example, African catfish (Schoonen *et al.*, 1988), white sucker (*Catostomus commersoni*; Scott *et al.*, 1984), and rainbow trout (*Oncorhynchus mykiss*; Liley *et al.*, 1986)—suggesting these steroids might influence male behavior. In the only reported test of this possibility, Mayer *et al.* (1994) used castrate rainbow trout to compare the behavioral effectiveness of 17,20β-P and 11-ketoandrostenedione (11-KA), assuming the latter is converted in the blood to 11-KT, as in Atlantic salmon (*Salmo salar*; Mayer *et al.*, 1990). Although Mayer *et al.* (1994) found that 17,20β-P was more effective than 11-KA in restoring male behaviors, further studies have failed to confirm this behavioral effect of 17,20β-P (N. R. Liley, personal communication).

3. Hormones and Female Behavior

The hormonal control of female reproductive behavior has been examined in relatively few species, but appears likely to be determined by the mode of reproduction employed. For example, sexual receptivity in the ovoviviparous guppy (*Poecilia reticulata*) is regulated by estrogenic steroids, whereas spawning of oviparous species may be commonly regulated by prostaglandins (Liley and Stacey, 1983; Kobayashi and Stacey, 1993; Sorensen *et al.*, 1995b).

The female guppy becomes receptive to male courtship for several days after parturition, coincident with maximal ovarian steroidogenesis and production of a sex pheromone (Meyer and Liley, 1982; see Section IIIA). Ovarian estrogen appears to synchronize female behavior and attractiveness with ovarian function because exogenous estrogen restores both the receptivity of ovariectomized females (Liley, 1972) and pheromone production by hypophysectomized females (Meyer and Liley, 1982). The endocrine control of sexual behavior in the female guppy thus appears comparable to typical internally fertilizing tetrapods in that exogenous estrogen restores behavioral deficits induced by ovariectomy. In contrast, the spawning of externally fertilizing female fishes appears to be induced not by ovarian estrogen, but by PGF2α (Stacey, 1981; Liley and Stacey, 1983).

PGF2α injection induces female spawning behavior (behaviors normally associated with oviposition) in nonovulated females of several perciform and cypriniform species—for example, cichlid, (*Cichlosoma bimaculatum*; Cole and Stacey, 1984), paradise fish (*Macropodus opercularis*; Villars *et al.*, 1985), and *Puntius* spp. (Liley and Tan, 1985; Cardwell *et al.*, 1995). However, the clearest evidence that PGF2α is the endogenous regulator of female behavior comes from the goldfish, in which female sexual activity normally is restricted to the brief postovulatory period when ovulated oocytes are in the oviduct, and the plasma concentration of PGF2α increases dramatically (Sorensen *et al.*, 1995b). The period of spawning activity can be extended by preventing egg release, terminated by stripping out the ovulated eggs, and restored in stripped fish or induced in nonovulated fish by intraovarian injection of ovulated eggs or egg substitutes (Stacey and Liley, 1974; Stacey, 1976; Sorensen *et al.*, 1995b). Ovulated eggs appear to induce spawning by stimulating prostaglandin (PG) synthesis because the effect of ovulated eggs or egg substitutes is blocked by the prostaglandin synthesis inhibitor indomethacin and restored in indomethacin-treated fish by PGF2α injection (Stacey, 1976; Sorensen *et al.*, 1995a). PGF2α appears to act in the brain (Stacey and Peter, 1979) through a mechanism independent of sex steroids because behavioral response is unaffected by ovariectomy or steroid replacement therapy (Kobayashi and Stacey, 1993) and is equivalent in males and females (Stacey, 1981; Stacey and Kyle, 1983 (Fig. 5).

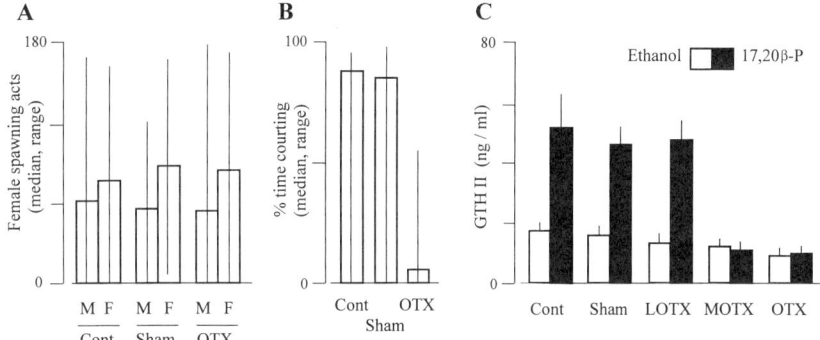

FIGURE 5 Effects of olfactory tract (OT) lesions on reproductive function in goldfish. (A) Injection of PGF$_{2\alpha}$ (100 ng/g) induces female spawning behavior that is equivalent both between males (M) and females (F), and among control (Cont), sham-operated (Sham) and bilaterally OT-sectioned fish (OTX). (B) Bilateral OT section reduces courtship behavior of male goldfish. (C) The GTH II increase induced by exposure to water-borne 17,20β-P is blocked by OTX and bilateral section of the medial OTs (MOTX), but not by bilateral section of the lateral OTs (LOTX). (A) and (B) redrawn from Stacey and Kyle (1983), *Physiol. Behav.* **30**, 621–628, © 1983, with permission from Elsevier Science; (C) redrawn from Dulka and Stacey (1991), *J. Exp. Zool.* **257**, 223–229, © 1991, Wiley-Liss Inc., a subsidiary of John Wiley & Sons, Inc.

In summary, the available evidence indicates that, at least in goldfish, PGF2α produced in the reproductive tract acts as a short-latency short-duration hormone that synchronizes female sexual activity with the presence of ovulated eggs. Furthermore, given that PGF2α injection induces female behavior in several other egg-laying species and that PGF2α and other F-series PGs appear to function as pheromones in many fishes (see Section IV.A), we suspect postovulatory PGF2α synthesis is a widespread mechanism regulating female sex behaviors in oviparous fishes.

III. DEVELOPMENT OF HORMONAL PHEROMONE STUDIES

To understand a pheromone's function, we require internally consistent information on (1) the control, source, and timing of pheromone synthesis; (2) the mechanism(s) of pheromone release; (3) the sensitivity and specificity of pheromone detection; (4) the nature and biological function of the pheromone-induced response; and (5) the nature of the interaction (spying or communication) between pheromone donor(s) and receiver(s) (Fig. 3). From this perspective, no hormonal pheromone is well understood. For goldfish hormonal pheromones, however, there is considerable information on all but the aspect 5.

A. Fish Reproductive Pheromones

In fish, conspecific odors influence diverse functions including schooling, migration, fright (alarm) reactions, parent–young interactions, and behavioral and physiological reproductive responses (Pfeiffer, 1982; Liley, 1982; Liley and Stacey, 1983; Van Weerd and Richter, 1991; Smith, 1992; Stacey et al., 1986; Solomon, 1990). However, there is good evidence for chemical identity only for reproductive pheromones (and possibly fright substance; Pfeiffer et al., 1985).

Early studies clearly show that male or female holding water of many species induces conspecific behavioral and physiological responses indicative of reproductive function (see reviews in Liley, 1982; Liley and Stacey, 1983; Stacey et al., 1986). Particularly convincing are studies of oviparous species—for example, goldfish (Partridge et al., 1976), salmonids (*Oncorhynchus* spp.; Honda, 1982), and frillfin goby (*Bathygobius soporator*; Tavolga, 1956)—in which males are more responsive to water from ovulated females than from nonovulated females, suggesting that production of a postovulatory pheromone coincides with female sexual receptivity. Similarly strong evidence for male sex pheromones comes from species in which the male is territorial and parental, and defends a nest site to which the female is attracted for spawning. Thus, in one goby (*Gobius niger* or *G. jozo*; Colombo et al., 1982) and several belontiid (gourami) species (Lee and Ingersoll, 1979), the finding that female attraction to male odor occurred only in ovulated (sexually receptive) females or increased when females had ovulated provides strong evidence that female response is sexual in nature and not simply a general social attraction.

External structures specialized for pheromone production and release appear to be rare in fish. In one of only several known examples, ovulated females of the peacock blenny (*Salaria pavo* = *Blennius pavo*) are attracted to the male's cryptic nest both by male-specific visual cues and by chemical cues evidently produced by the male's specialized anal fin appendages. In laboratory tests, females are attracted to the odor of mature males and to extracts of the anal fin appendages, but not to the odor of mature males lacking appendages (Ide, 1993; Laumen et al., 1974; Zeeck and Ide, 1996).

Many fish appear to produce sex pheromones in the gonads or reproductive tract (Stacey et al., 1986), the clearest evidence being that fluids or washes from dissected ovaries induce reproductive responses in males of a number of species—for example, *B. soporator* (Tavolga, 1956), pondsmelt (*Hypomesus olidus*; Okada et al., 1978); rainbow trout (Honda, 1980a), and loach (*Misgurnus anguillicaudatus*; Honda, 1980b)—whereas extracts of dissected testes induce conspecific sexual responses in pondsmelt (Okada et al., 1978) and Pacific herring (*Clupea harengus pallasi*; Stacey and Hourston, 1982; Carolsfeld et al., 1997). In many other studies, however, the evidence for sex pheromones of gonadal origin is equivocal because test odors were prepared from hand-stripped gonadal fluids (seminal plasma and the fluid bathing ovulated eggs) that are assumed to contain urine. Urine uncontaminated by gonadal fluids can be a rich source of sex pheromones (e.g., Colombo et al., 1982; Scott et al., 1994), and, at least in marine species where urine is concentrated to conserve water, gonadal sex steroids and their metabolites can reach high concentrations (Scott et al., 1991a,b).

The first report that a hormone might function as a pheromone in fish appears to be that of Amouriq (1965; see also other papers reviewed by Liley, 1969), who found that a synthetic estrogen mimics the increase in locomotory behavior exhibited by male guppies in response to female holding water. Johansen (1985) also found that both female holding water and E_2 (but not other steroids) induce similar shifts of temperature preference in male guppies. Female guppies do produce a pheromone that attracts males and stimulates their courtship behaviors, its production being maximal shortly after parturition (when the female is sexually receptive) and evidently dependent on the action of estrogen on the ovary (Crow and Liley, 1979). However, neither ovarian extracts nor estrogens induce the male behavioral responses induced by female holding water (Meyer and Liley, 1982).

B. Early Studies of Hormonal Pheromones

The hypothesis that released hormones are obvious pheromonal candidates in fish (Doving, 1976) found its first clear support in the black goby (*Gobius niger* = *G. jozo*), and the zebrafish (*Danio rerio*) in which evidence for putative steroidal pheromones was sought in studies of *in vitro* steroidogenesis and bioassays of physiology and behavior.

1. Black Goby (Gobius niger = G. jozo)

Reproduction in *G. jozo* appears typical of many gobiid species (Miller, 1984) in which the male is territorial and parental and uses visual and chemical signals to attract ovulated females to his nest site (also see Section IV.H.1). As with many other gobies (Miller, 1984), male *G. jozo* possess a specialized nonspermatogenic portion of the testis, the mesorchial gland, which contains a high concentration of interstitial (Leydig) cells producing primarily 5β-reduced androgen conjugates, in particular etiocholanolone-glucuronide (ETIO-G) and etiocholanolone sulphate (Colombo et al., 1977). When ovulated, female *G. jozo* are attracted not only to male urine (Colombo et al., 1982) but also to ETIO-G (Colombo et al., 1980), which can induce oviposition in the absence of a male. The apparent testicular specialization of *G. jozo* for steroidal pheromone production likely evolved in response to mate selection by females based on male steroid production. Such steroidal hormonal pheromones might be common among gobiid fish, because we (Murphy and Stacey, 2002; Murphy et al., 2001) have found that the round goby (*Neogobius melanostomus*), which employs a mating system similar to *G. jozo*, exhibits sensitive EOG responses to a variety of conjugated and unconjugated steroids, including ETIO-G (see Section IV.H.1).

The gobiid mesorchial gland and the seminal vesicles of the African catfish (see Section I.V.F.1) appear to be the only clear examples of structural specialization for enhanced production of hormonal pheromone signals. However, such specializations may be quite common because similar testicular structures are found not only in other gobies (Asahina et al., 1989; Fishelson, 1991), but also in many other fishes (Lahnsteiner and Patzner, 1990; Rasotto, 1995) in which the possibility of hormonal pheromone use has not been investigated.

2. Zebrafish (Danio rerio)

Unlike *Gobius*, zebrafish are neither egg guarders nor territorial. As with many cyprinids, small groups of males pursue ovulated females and compete for fertilization access as eggs are scattered among aquatic vegetation. Hormonal pheromones have been proposed to stimulate ovulation and to attract males to females (Van Den Hurk and Resink, 1992).

In mixed-sex groups, female zebrafish exhibit a 4- to 5-day ovulatory cycle, which ceases if they are removed from conspecifics. However, provided they are not anosmic, isolated females resume ovulation when exposed to holding water from males and, to a lesser extent, from females (Van Den Hurk et al., 1987b; Van Den Hurk and Resink, 1992). Isolated females also resume ovulation in response to whole testicular homogenate or a subfraction containing steroid conjugates, but not in response to a subfraction containing only unconjugated steroids or a glucuronide subfraction treated with β-glucuronidase (Van Den Hurk et al., 1987b). Although zebrafish testes synthesize a variety of steroid glucuronides *in vitro*, the two of these that have been tested (testosterone-glucuronide, T-G; androsterone-glucuronide) did not induce ovulation of isolated females (Van Den Hurk et al., 1987a).

As in many fish (Stacey et al., 1986), male zebrafish discriminate between odors of ovulated and nonovulated females and become unresponsive to ovulated females when made anosmic (Van Den Hurk and Lambert, 1983). Using time spent near an odor source as a bioassay, Van Den Hurk and Lambert (1983) showed that intact males (but not anosmic males or females) respond more to ovarian extracts from ovulated females than to extracts from females in mid-cycle. Males also respond both to extracts containing steroid glucuronides and to a mixture of 17β-estradiol-17β-glucuronide (E$_2$-17G) and T-G; these were ineffective when tested alone (Van Den Hurk and Lambert, 1983) and are known to be synthesized by the zebrafish ovary (Lambert et al., 1986).

Despite this evidence that male and female zebrafish respond both physiologically and behaviorally to steroid glucuronides, our EOG studies provide no evidence that zebrafish detect these compounds. Zebrafish do exhibit olfactory responses to F2-series prostaglandins, as do all of the more than 70 other cyprinid species we have examined with EOG recording (Stacey and Cardwell, 1995, 1997). However, when tested with over 100 steroids (including E$_2$ and T glucuronides) at 1 nM (0.001 μM) concentrations, zebrafish exhibited consistent responses only to 17,20β-P-S, which also is the only steroid detected by two congeners (D. albolineatus and D. malabaricus). Michel and Lubomudrov (1995), who examined EOG response of zebrafish to high concentrations (0.01–100 μM) of three steroids (E$_2$, 17,20β-P, and progesterone), found that the last two steroids induced small responses but no clear concentration–response relationship. Although the results of our EOG studies fail to support earlier proposals (Van Den Hurk and Resink, 1992) regarding pheromonal glucuronides in zebrafish, they are entirely consistent with studies of odor-induced olfactory bulb activity in zebrafish showing that PGF2α and 17,20β-P-S induce bulbar activity, whereas E$_2$-17G and T-G do not (Friedrich and Korsching, 1998).

C. Studies of Pheromone Production, Release, and Detection

Early hormonal pheromone studies examined pheromone production principally by identifying the products of in vitro steroidogenesis. Other work has focused more on determining concentrations of hormones and hormonal products in blood, urine, and water to characterize the sensitivity and specificity of the olfactory system to these putative pheromonal compounds.

1. Hormonal Pheromone Production In Vivo

In studies of G. niger (= G. jozo) (see Section III.B.1), in vitro gonadal steroidogenesis (Colombo et al., 1977) evidently was successful in identifying pheromonal steroids (Colombo et al., 1982). In general, however, hormone concentrations in blood and urine, are expected to provide a more reliable picture of the suite of released hormonal compounds containing pheromonal odorants. In the few cases in which the dynamics of hormone change have been followed simultaneously in plasma and water (Stacey et al., 1989; Scott and Sorensen, 1994), plasma concentrations serve as a realistic indicator of release.

2. Hormonal Pheromone Release

Ideally, studies of pheromone production should address both the route(s) and the rate of pheromone release. In general, the release of steroids and prostaglandins to the water is not well understood in fish, although the available information suggests that the majority of conjugated steroids and some prostaglandins are released in urine or bile, whereas unconjugated steroids probably are released across the gills (Scott and Liley, 1994; Scott and Vermeirssen, 1994; Appelt and Sorensen, 1995; Vermeirssen and Scott, 1996). Urine can be released in pulses (Curtis and Wood, 1991) and can contain high concentrations of conjugated steroids in both marine (Scott et al., 1991b; Scott and Canario, 1992) and freshwater species (Rocha and Reis-Henriques, 1996). Moreover, because the unconjugated and conjugated forms of a steroid can be released by different routes (Scott and Vermeirssen, 1994) and detected by different olfactory receptor mechanisms (Sorensen et al., 1995b), they have the potential to generate distinct pheromonal stimuli with distinct functions. Therefore, understanding the route of release is extremely important in understanding a pheromonal function.

Information on the rate of release of a hormonal product, in combination with information on release route and olfactory potency, determines whether the active space is restricted to the immediate vicinity of a donor fish or whether detection at a distance is possible. Although this aspect of hormonal pheromone function is very poorly understood, information on hormonal pheromone release and detection in goldfish (Sorensen and Stacey, 1990) has been used to develop theoretical models of pheromone dispersion and detection in marine fishes living at different depths (Jumper and Baird, 1991; Baird et al., 1996).

Studying pheromone production and release can be straightforward when the pheromonal stimuli are known (e.g., Stacey et al., 1989; Van Der Kraak et al., 1989). However, when a number of compounds are being measured to determine which is likely to have pheromonal function, the situation can be complex, primarily because fish produce and release a great variety of hormonal products into the water (e.g., Parks and Leblanc, 1998). For example, reports of unusually high concentrations of a steroid in blood or urine have prompted speculation about pheromone function (Scott and Canario, 1992; Rocha and Reis-Henriques, 1996), although there is no reason why pheromonal stimuli should be the major components of released hormonal mixtures. Indeed, 17,20β-P, a potent primary component of a facultative multicomponent goldfish pheromone (see Section IV.D.1.d.ii), is a relatively minor component of a mixture of released steroids (Sorensen and Scott, 1994).

3. Hormonal Pheromone Detection by the Olfactory Organ

Our understanding of the nature and function of hormonal pheromones has benefited tremendously from the use of underwater EOG recording, an extracellular technique that measures transepithelial voltage changes thought to represent summed multireceptor responses to olfactory ligands (Ottoson, 1971; Hara, 1994). EOG recordings have two important applications in hormonal pheromone studies. First, they can readily determine the sensitivity and specificity of a species' olfactory organ to a large suite of hormonal odorants. In goldfish, for example, results of EOG recordings in which 17,20β-P is detected with great sensitivity and specificity by the olfactory epithelium are entirely consistent with results of physiological bioassay (Sorensen et al., 1987, 1990). Second, when combined with quantitative studies of pheromone release (Stacey et al., 1989), the results of such EOG studies enable predictions about the active space of a pheromone (e.g., Sorensen and Stacey, 1990; Baird et al., 1996; Sorensen et al., 2000) (Table 1).

TABLE 1
Active Space of Pheromonal Compounds Released by Periovulatory Goldfish[a]

Compound	Release mode	Duration (hr)[b]	Active space at peak release
AD	Gill	6	Female slowly swimming: medium filament[c]
			Female quickly swimming: none
17,20β-P	Gill	12	Female slowly swimming: wide filament[d]
			Female quickly swimming: medium filament
17,20β,21-P	Gill	3	Female slowly swimming: thin filament[e]
			Female quickly swimming: none
17,20β-P-S	Urine	9	~16 35-cm diameter spheres/hr
17,20β,21-P-S	Urine	9	~16 10-cm diameter spheres/hr
17,20β-P-G	Urine	9	~16 3-cm diameter spheres/hr
15K-PGF2a	Urine	Variable[f]	~16 50-cm diameter spheres/hr

[a] Active space is determined by olfactory detection threshold, release rate, and release mode (gill or urine) (see Sorensen et al., 2000).
[b] Time the compound is detected by a non-swimming fish.
[c] Total active space 5–10 liter/hr.
[d] Total active space >30 liter/hr.
[e] Total active space 1–5 liter/hr.
[f] Determined by the time required to complete oviposition.

EOG recording also can be used in cross-adaptation studies that evaluate the discriminatory ability of olfactory receptor neurons by comparing the EOG response to a test compound before and during adaptation to an adapting compound. If a test compound induces the same EOG response before and during adaptation, it is assumed to act through an olfactory receptor mechanism separate from that mediating response to the adapting compound (e.g., Caprio and Byrd, 1984; Sorensen et al., 1995b). Thus, for a species that detects a number of related hormonal odorants, EOG cross-adaptation can reveal whether these odorants function as a single-component pheromone with numerous redundant components, or as a multiple-component pheromone. Such EOG cross-adaptation studies indicate that goldfish olfactory receptor neurons discriminate three steroid and two prostaglandin odors (see Section IV.D.1.d). Studies of steroid discrimination in the round goby (Murphy et al., 2001) demonstrate a good correspondence between the results of EOG cross-adaptation and behavioral bioassay (see Section IV.H.1).

For species in which hormonal pheromone studies already are in progress, EOG recording can be particularly useful for integrating information on pheromone production and release into the design of physiologically meaningful behavioral or physiological bioassays. Moreover, for species in which hormonal pheromones have not been studied, EOG recording can assess the likelihood that hormonal pheromone systems are present by quickly determining olfactory sensitivity to a large number of hormones and hormone metabolites. Assuming that such olfactory responsiveness generally is indicative of pheromonal function, we have used such EOG screening to survey the distribution and diversity of putative hormonal pheromones in a variety of freshwater fishes (Sorensen et al., 1992; Stacey et al., 1994a, 1995; Stacey and Cardwell, 1995, 1997). In addition to E- and F-series prostaglandins, our test odorants include all unconjugated, glucuronidated, and sulfated forms of most commercially available steroids that we suspect to be potential candidates for pheromonal function (e.g., see Murphy et al., 2001). Naturally, we expect this approach will commonly generate false negatives (e.g., Section IV.H.2) because some hormonal pheromones undoubtedly are novel hormonal products that are not commercially available. Nonetheless, although fewer than 150 species have been subjected to EOG screening, it already is clear that hormonal pheromones are widespread among freshwater fishes. Of equal importance is the fact that, whereas there are great differences among higher taxa in the hormonal products detected, the patterns of detected compounds among related in lower taxa are remarkably similar (Stacey et al., 1994a; Stacey and Cardwell, 1995, 1997; see Section IV.D.2). If this is also true for other higher taxa that have not been examined, it is possible that intensive study of a few key species could provide insight into the hormonal pheromones of large numbers of fishes.

IV. BIOLOGY OF HORMONAL PHEROMONES

Because of the strong relationship between phylogeny and olfactory response to hormonal products, we review current information on hormonal pheromones from a phylogenetic perspective (after Nelson, 1994).

A. Phylogenetic Distribution of Hormonal Pheromones in Fishes

All five classes in Subphylum Vertebrata consist entirely or partially of fishes, a paraphyletic group that excludes tetrapods and contains at least 24,000 gill-breathing aquatic species whose limbs, if present, are in the shape of fins. Virtually all information about fish hormonal pheromones comes from Class Actinopterygii, the ray-finned fishes. In addition, a variation on the actinopterygian hormonal pheromones occurs in sea lamprey (*Petromyzon marinus*; Class Cephalaspidomorpha), in which bile steroids, rather than sex steroids, appear to function as attractants during spawning migrations (Li and Sorensen, 1991; Li et al., 1995; Bjerselius et al., 1995a). There appear to be no studies of hormonal pheromones in Classes Myxini (hagfishes), Chondrichthyes (sharks and rays), or Sarcopterygii (lobe-fin fishes).

Class Actinopterygii contains two extant subclasses, Chondrostei (sturgeons and paddlefishes) and the Neopterygii, which contains the apparently monophyletic Division Teleostei (with more than 95% of living fishes), as well as minor groups of uncertain affinity (e.g., bowfin and gars). Although systematic

TABLE 2
Evidence for Hormonal Pheromones in Orders of Euteleost Fish[a]

Order	Number of extant species	Number of species examined	Common names	Example genera	Evidence for hormonal pheromones	
					PGs	Steroids
Ostariophysin Orders						
Cypriniformes	2662	>80	Cyprinids	*Carassius, Danio*	+	+
Characiformes	1343	>20	Characins	*Astyanax, Colossoma*	+	+
Siluriformes	2405	>10	Catfishes	*Clarias, Ictalurus*	+	+
Gymnotiformes[b]	62	1	Knifefishes	*Apteronotus*	+	
Osmeriformes[c]	236	1	Smelts	*Plecoglossus*	+	
Salmoniformes	66	9	Salmonids	*Salmo, Oncorhynchus*	+	+
Cyprinodontiformes[d]	807	1	Rivulines	*Aplocheilus*	+	
Scorpaeniformes[e]	1271	1	Sculpins	*Cottocomephorus*		+
Perciformes	9293	10	Cichlids, gobies	*Haplochromis, Neogobius*	+	+

[a] Systematic terminology from Nelson (1994).
[b] J. G. Dulka, unpublished results.
[c] See Kitamura *et al.* (1994b).
[d] N. E. Stacey (unpublished results).
[e] See Katsel *et al.* (1992).

relationships among teleosts are poorly understood, Nelson (1994) recognizes three primitive and minor subdivisions—Osteoglossomorpha (mooneyes, old world knifefish, etc.), Elopomorpha (tarpon and eels), and Clupeomorpha (herrings)—as well as Subdivision Euteleostei, which contains nearly 95% of all teleosts. Because almost all hormonal pheromone studies deal with euteleostean species, the occurence of hormonal pheromones in the primitive teleost subdivisions is unclear. The failure of EOG recordings to detect olfactory responses in two chondrostean sturgeons (Kitamura *et al.*, 1994b; Stacey and Cardwell, 1995, 1997) and in the osteoglossomorph goldeye (*Hiodon alosoides*; Stacey and Cardwell, 1995) might simply reflect the small number of hormonal test odors used in these studies. It is unfortunate, considering the good evidence for a sex pheromone in Pacific herring (*Clupea harengus pallasi*; e.g., Carolsfeld *et al.*, 1997a,b), that EOG recordings have not been conducted on any clupeomorph species. Nonetheless, EOG recording using a large array of hormonal test odors has demonstrated olfactory sensitivity to steroids and prostaglandins in the primitive elopomorph *Megalops cyprinoides* (Stacey and Cardwell, 1995, 1997), indicating that hormonal pheromones are not restricted to euteleost species.

The Subdivision Euteleostei has 32 recognized orders (Nelson, 1994), in 11 of which at least one species has been examined for EOG responses to hormonal compounds (Stacey *et al.*, 1994a; Stacey and Cardwell, 1995, 1997) (Table 2). Species from the three orders that did not exhibit EOG responses (Gadiformes, Gasterosteiformes, and Scorpaeniformes) all were tested with a relatively small number of compounds. The eight orders that exhibited EOG responses, plus one order (Scorpaeniformes) likely to contain species using hormonal pheromones (see Katsel *et al.*, 1992; see Section IV.I), represent four of the nine recognized euteleost superorders (Nelson, 1994). Considering that evidence for hormonal pheromones has been sought in less than 1% of extant fishes, most of which are from only two orders (Cypriniformes and Characiformes; Table 2), the diversity of positive higher taxa suggests that hormonal pheromones will be found to be widespread among fishes.

B. Lamprey and Hagfish

Both hagfish and lamprey (the two extant groups of jawless fishes) have well-developed olfactory systems (Zeiske *et al.*, 1992), but only lamprey (Order

Petromyzontiformes) have been examined for pheromones. Among the approximately 40 species of lamprey, virtually all pheromone research has been directed toward the sea lamprey (*Petromyzon marinus*), which invaded the North American Great Lakes in the 1930s and has had enormous impact on Great Lakes fishes (Sorensen and Vrieze, 2001). Like many lamprey species, sea lamprey have an extended larval phase that may last up to 20 years, followed by an oceanic parasitic phase that culminates in sexual maturation and migration into rivers, where spawning occurs.

Spawning-stream selection has been relatively well studied and is mediated by larval pheromones, a key component of which is a unique set of bile steroids (Li *et al.*, 1995; Bjerselius *et al.*, 1995a; Sorensen and Vrieze, 2001). Once in rivers, however, male and female lamprey appear to locate one another using sex pheromones (Teeter, 1980; Li, 1994; Bjerselius *et al.*, 2000). The male pheromone (which attracts females) coincides with spermiation and can be induced within just a few days by GnRH injection, suggesting an endocrine origin (Li, 1994; Bjerselius *et al.*, 1995a). Further support for this possibility comes from EOG studies showing that the pheromone is in the urine and probably made up of several fractions, at least one of which is sulfated and steroidal (P. W. Sorensen and R. Bjerselius, unpublished results). Interestingly, although several synthetic sulfated sex steroids stimulate the olfactory system (Li, 1994), none of these are expected to occur in the urine, indicating that the pheromone might be a novel steroid. This would not be surprising because sea lamprey appear to possess novel, uncharacterized sex steroid pathways (Kime and Rafter, 1981). An early report (Adams *et al.*, 1987) that T is a pheromone in male sea lamprey has not been confirmed by EOG studies (W. Li and P. W. Sorensen, unpublished), which show lamprey do not detect T or any known derivative.

C. Primitive Fishes (Noneuteleost Actinopterygeans)

Almost nothing is known of possible hormonal pheromones in primitive fishes. Although male sturgeon (*Acipenser gueldenstaedti* and *A. stellatus*) are reported to respond to a releaser pheromone from females (Kasumyan, 1993), the nature of this pheromone is unknown. Kitamura *et al.* (1994b) failed to detect EOG response to F2 prostaglandins in immature sturgeon (bester, *Huso huso* × *Acipenser ruthenus*). Also, using as test odors several dozen steroids and prostaglandins (including those known to be detected by goldfish and other species), we observed no olfactory responses in immature sturgeon (*Acipenser* sp.) treated with androgen to enhance potential PG responses. The same suite of test odors also failed to induce olfactory responses in the more derived goldeye (*Hiodon alosoides*). However, when tested with a larger suite of test hormones, a tarpon (*Megalops cyprinoides*; Subdivision Elopomorpha) responded to nanomolar concentrations of 13,14-dihydro-15-keto-PGF2α and two steroids, 17,20β-P-S and 5β-pregnan-3α,17α,20β-triol (Stacey and Cardwell, 1997).

D. Order Cypriniformes

The Order Cypriniformes (carps and minnows, 2600 species) is one of three large orders within the Superorder Ostariophysi (Subdivision Euteleostei), which comprises nearly 6500 mainly freshwater species (Table 2). Much of our information on hormonal pheromones comes from studies of ostariophysin fishes, many of which are ecologically and economically important. Order Cypriniformes comprises two superfamilies, the Cyprinoidea, containing Family Cyprinidae, and the Cobitoidea, containing the Families Catostomidae (suckers), Cobitidae (loaches), Gyrinochelidae (algae eaters), and Balitoridae (river loaches) (Table 3).

1. Goldfish

More is known about hormonal pheromone function in goldfish than in any other teleost. This is not because goldfish pheromones are extraordinary or even unusual, but simply because progress understanding them has been facilitated by the fact that this species is a well-understood model of fish reproductive neuroendocrinology and behavior (Peter, 1983; Peter *et al.*, 1986; Stacey, 1981; Trudeau, 1997). It is a legitimate concern that this leading model species for hormonal pheromone research has undergone centuries of domestication that might have altered its hormonal pheromone systems. However, although no study has addressed this issue directly, investigations of

TABLE 3
EOG Responses to F-Series Prostaglandins and Steroids in Order Cypriniformes[a]

Superfamily	Family	Subfamily	Number of species examined	PGF	Steroids		
					21-Carbon	19-Carbon	18-Carbon
Cyprinoidea	Cyprinidae	Cyprininae	>40	++[b]	++	+[c]	+
		Gobioninae	1	++	++	−[d]	−
		Danioninae	15	++	+	+	+
		Acheilognathinae	5	++	−	−	−
		Leuciscinae	8	++	++	−	−
		Cultrinae	1	++	++	++	−
		Alburninae	1	++	++	−	−
		Psylorhynchinae	0				
Cobitoidea	Gyrinocheilidae		1	++	−	−	−
	Catostomidae		5	++	−	−	−
	Cobitidae		4	++	−	−	−
	Balitoridae		1	++	−	−	−

[a] Systematic terminology from Rainboth (1991).
[b] All tested species in the taxon responded to at least one compound in this category.
[c] Some of the tested species in the taxon responded to at least one compound in this category.
[d] No tested species in the taxon responded to any compounds in this category.

hormonal pheromones in the closely related wild Crucian carp (*Carassius carassius*; Bjerselius et al., 1995b) and the feral common carp (*Cyprinus carpio*; Irvine and Sorensen, 1993; Stacey et al., 1994b) indicate hormonal pheromone functions very similar to those of goldfish (Section IV.D.2).

The goldfish mating system is typical of other nonterritorial nonparental species in the Family Cyprinidae, and appears identical to that of the common carp, with which it will hybridize (Taylor and Mahon, 1977). Goldfish (and common carp) are temperate species that undergo vitellogenesis during the winter months and typically ovulate large numbers of oocytes several times over a protracted spring–summer spawning season. Female goldfish under ideal conditions can ovulate as frequently as once a week, although there appears to be no regular spawning cycle (Kobayashi et al., 1988); in temperate climates, females might ovulate only a single batch of several hundred eggs each year. Female goldfish ovulate several hours before dawn, at which time small groups of males compete for access to the ovulated female as she repeatedly enters aquatic vegetation to oviposit adhesive eggs over a period of several hours. In such a scramble-competition mating system (Emlen and Oring, 1977), we believe that intense sperm competition, in which males are under intense pressure to anticipate ovulation and compete for spawning access to females, is the major factor shaping the evolution of the goldfish hormonal pheromone system.

It perhaps is not surprising then that evolutionary selection has favored males capable of responding to female odors, given that goldfish are sexually monomorphic and often spawn in socially chaotic groups in dim and turbid water. Indeed, the reproductive functions of males appear much more dependent on olfactory input than do those of females. As discussed in Section IV.D.1.d, sectioning the medial olfactory tracts abolishes male endocrine responses to female odors and almost completely inhibits male sexual behavior, but appears to have no effect on female gonadal development, ovulation, or spawning behavior (Dulka and Stacey, 1991; Kobayashi et al., 1994, 1997a; Stacey and Kyle, 1983; Figure 5).

a) Males, Hormones, and Reproduction Endocrine changes during the annual spawning cycle of male goldfish appear typical of other fishes that spawn more than once in a breeding season (Borg, 1994). Plasma concentrations of GTH II, T, and 11-KT begin to increase a month or more prior to spawning and reach peak levels during the spawning season (Kobayashi et al., 1986b). Although these hormonal changes associated with seasonal temperature and photoperiod are marked, the most dramatic hormonal changes in males occur in response to sexual interaction. For example, if males are held with females undergoing their preovulatory GTH II surge, they dramatically increase plasma GTH II prior to the occurrence of ovulation (Kobayashi et al., 1986c; Stacey et al., 1989). In addition, males that have not been exposed to females during the preovulatory GTH II surge increase plasma GTH II when allowed to spawn with ovulated or PGF2α-injected females (Kyle et al., 1985; Zheng and Stacey, 1997). As discussed in detail in Section IV.D.1.d, there is extensive evidence that changes in male hormones are induced by female hormonal pheromones.

Preovulatory and postovulatory female stimuli that increase GTH II in male goldfish also increase their plasma sex steroids. Thus, both T and 17,20β-P appear to increase in concert with the GTH II increase induced by the presence of preovulatory females (Kobayashi et al., 1986d). Similarly, when male common carp are held with females during their preovulatory GTH II surge, males with high plasma androgens start producing 17α-hydroxyprogesterone (17-P) and 17,20β-P (Barry et al., 1990).

b) Females, Hormones, and Reproduction Changes in the endocrine system of female goldfish experiencing ovarian growth and ovulation are dramatic and have been described in some detail (Kagawa et al., 1983; Kobayashi et al., 1986b, 1987). Briefly, as ovarian growth proceeds from winter to early spring, plasma concentrations of GTH II rise slowly, stimulating increased E_2 synthesis, which in turn stimulates vitellogenesis. When vitellogenesis is complete, E_2 synthesis decreases and T synthesis increases (Kagawa et al., 1984), perhaps due to reduction in $P450_{arom}$ gene expression in follicular granulosa cells as in salmonids (Young et al., 1997). Gonadotropin levels during this stage are influenced both by the stimulatory effect of increasing temperatures (Kobayashi et al., 1986b) and by the inhibitory effects of plasma E_2 and T (Kobayashi and Stacey, 1990, 1993).

Later, upon completion of vitellogenesis, a variety of exogenous and endogenous cues (see later) trigger a preovulatory surge of GTH II (Stacey et al., 1979a), stimulating a shift in steroid synthesis pathways from 19- and 18-carbon steroids to 21-carbon steroids (Nagahama et al., 1986). The follicular thecal cells then synthesize 17-P, which in turn is metabolized by the granulosa cells to 17,20β-P, the major MIS of goldfish (Nagahama, 1990). Acting through oocyte membrane receptors, 17,20β-P stimulates the resumption and completion of meiosis (Nagahama, 1994).

Although the mechanisms that induce ovulation are not fully understood, there is evidence in fish that MISs induce ovulation (follicular rupture) by stimulating the synthesis of follicular prostaglandin F2α (PGF2α) (Goetz and Garczynzki, 1997). Further, after ovulation has occurred and the eggs are in the oviduct, it appears that PGF2α synthesis persists, perhaps as a consequence of interactions between the ovulated eggs and oviduct (Sorensen et al., 1995b). Increased concentrations of plasma PGFs can be measured in recently ovulated female and induced in nonovulated female goldfish by injecting egg substitutes into their oviducts (P. W. Sorensen, unpublished data).

c) Regulation of Ovulation Possibly because the goldfish mating system lacks pairing, territoriality, and postfertilization parental investment, the timing of ovulation plays a large role in determining the reproductive success of both females and males. For females, the precise timing of ovulation is extremely important because of seasonal availability of spawning substrate and conditions for offspring development. For males, the timing of ovulation is important because females ovulate infrequently and competition among males is intense. Female goldfish have evolved four mechanisms that modulate the timing and occurrence of ovulation: sensitivity to increased water temperature, sensitivity to aquatic vegetation (spawning substrate), sensitivity to a steroid pheromone, and ovarian steroid feedback.

Although female goldfish with postvitellogenic follicles seldom ovulate when held in cool water (12°C), they typically ovulate within a few days if temperature is raised to 20°C (Yamamoto et al., 1966; Stacey et al., 1979a,b). Further, if aquatic vegetation is added, this stimulus alone frequently stimulates ovulation within a few days and, if accompanied by an increase in water temperature (simulating springtime flooding), ovulation rates are especially high (Stacey et al., 1979a,b). There also is preliminary evidence for a pheromonal role in ovulation. If females are held in isolation under conditions in which ovulation occurs infrequently (cool without vegetation), the addition of waterborne 17,20β-P to the aquaria significantly increases the proportion of females ovulating (Sorensen and Stacey, 1987). Although the olfactory stimulus of water-borne 17,20β-P can induce ovulation, it is not a necessary cue—females rendered anosmic by olfactory tract section ovulate and spawn normally (Kobayashi et al., 1994). The ovulatory response to 17,20β-P could be the mechanism responsible for synchronized ovulation among group-housed females (Kobayashi et al., 1988), and may have evolved as a predator swamping strategy.

The effectiveness of exogenous cues as ovulatory triggers might suggest endogenous cues from the ovary are unimportant; however, there also is evidence that T stimulates ovulation. For example, when repeated spontaneous ovulations occurred in all-female groups held at 20°C with spawning substrate, plasma T levels were significantly higher in the several days preceding ovulation than in the several days following, whereas plasma E_2 exhibited the opposite trend (Kobayashi et al., 1988). Furthermore, when ovariectomized females were implanted with E_2 or T, held for 3 months at 12°C, and then warmed to 20°C to induce a photoperiodically synchronized preovulatory GTH II surge, 9 of 12 T-treated females responded, whereas only one E_2-treated female and none of the control females responded (Kobayashi et al., 1989). Together, these findings suggest that increasing plasma T plays a priming role for the preovulatory GTH II surge, but determines the timing of ovulation only if exogenous factors already are present.

d) Female Hormonal Pheromones Female goldfish release a changing mixture of hormonal products as they undergo vitellogenesis, ovulate, and spawn. At least three types of female hormonal products are discriminated by males and function as discrete pheromones that affect male behavior and reproductive physiology. It is not clear if any are specialized products, and at least one of them (the preovulatory pheromone) functions as a mixture whose specific composition and biological activity changes with time. The three pheromones are released in a sequential fashion by females during the course of their spawning cycle. One, of unknown chemical identity, is produced and released well in advance of ovulation (the female maturational pheromone), another is released hours prior to ovulation and spawning (the steroidal preovulatory pheromone), and the last is released by ovulated spawning fish (the prostaglandin postovulatory pheromone) (Fig. 6). One component of the preovulatory pheromone, 17,20β-P (Fig. 7), also influences conspecific females. The preovulatory steroidal pheromone and postovulatory prostaglandin pheromone induce qualitatively similar effects on plasma GTH II concentration in males (e.g., Sorensen et al., 1989); however, these pheromones are detected by separate olfactory receptor mechanisms (Sorensen et al., 1988, 1990, 1995a) and exert their effects through different central mechanisms (Zheng and Stacey, 1996, 1997; discussed in Section IV.D.1.d.iv). The pheromones released by female goldfish are the best characterized of any vertebrate; nonetheless, our understanding is rudimentary.

i) Female maturation pheromone. Yamazaki and Watanabe (1979) first suggested that during vitellogenesis, when plasma E_2 concentrations are at their peak, female goldfish release a chemical cue that is recognized by males. Because goldfish are physically isomorphic, such a female-specific cue could benefit males by enabling them to associate with mature females that will soon ovulate and spawn. Initial evidence for this pheromone came from the observation that if gonadectomized fish were fed food containing either T or E_2, those fed T developed a more complex olfactory epithelium and chased those fed E_2 (Yamazaki and Watanabe, 1979). Yamazaki (1990) confirmed this result and suggested that E_2-treated fish released a stimulatory cue in their urine. We (P. W. Sorensen and M. Kobayashi, unpublished) repeated Yamazaki and Watanabe's (1979) initial study using water collected from gonadectomized fish implanted with E_2 implants. Notably, this cue cannot be either E_2 or a simple glucuronidated or sulfated form of E_2 because EOG recordings indicate that male goldfish do not detect these compounds (Sorensen et al., 1987; P. W. Sorensen, unpublished data); however, males might detect other E_2 metabolites not yet tested in EOG recordings. The complete identity of this cue, the precise timing of its release

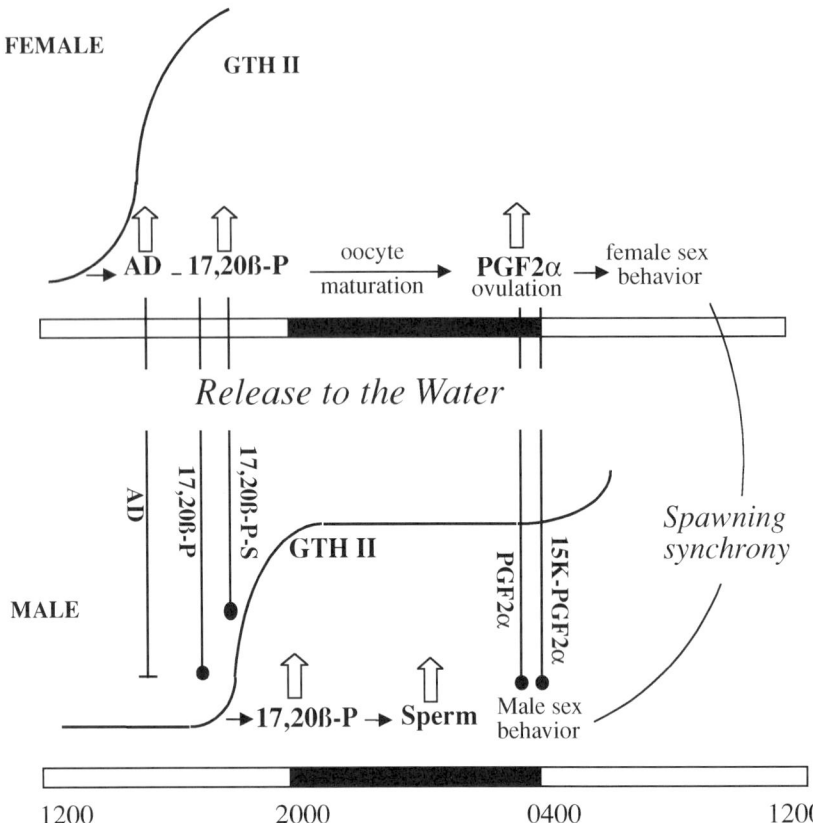

FIGURE 6 Model of the goldfish hormonal pheromone system. An afternoon to evening surge in female GTH II stimulates steroidogenesis and the release of many steroids, but especially androstenedione (AD), into the water. Early in the surge, AD suppresses any responses that males might otherwise exhibit to the small amounts of 17,20β-P being released at that time. Later, the quantities of AD released by females drop as 17,20β-P comes to dominate the released preovulatory steroid mixture, causing the preovulatory pheromone to increase GTH II in exposed males; still later, a urinary metabolite of 17,20β-P (17,20β-P-S) comes to dominate the mixture. By the end of the night, males have greatly increased levels of sperm (because of 17,20β-P-induced GTH II release) and the females have ovulated. With ovulation, female steroid production and release drops and circulating PGF2α increases dramatically. PGF2α acts as a hormone to stimulate female reproductive behavior and is metabolized and cleared to the water where, together with its principal metabolite 15-keto-prostaglandin F2α (15K-PGF2α), it functions as a sex pheromone with strong behavioral effects on males. Redrawn from Sorensen et al. (1998), Curr. Opin. Neurobiol. 8, 458–467, © 1998, with permission from Excerpta Medica Inc.

relative to other cues, and its true behavioral function need to be ascertained.

ii) The preovulatory steroid pheromone. During the female goldfish's preovulatory GTH II surge, which immediately precedes ovulation and spawning, rapid changes in steroid synthesis occur. These changes are reflected both in plasma steroids and in the patterns with which they are metabolized and released to the water (Scott and Sorensen, 1994; Sorensen and Scott, 1994). When the release rate of 17,20β-P from spontaneously ovulating females was studied, it was found to be high and closely correlated with circulating levels, suggesting a possible lack of specialization (Stacey et al., 1989). Two studies that have examined release

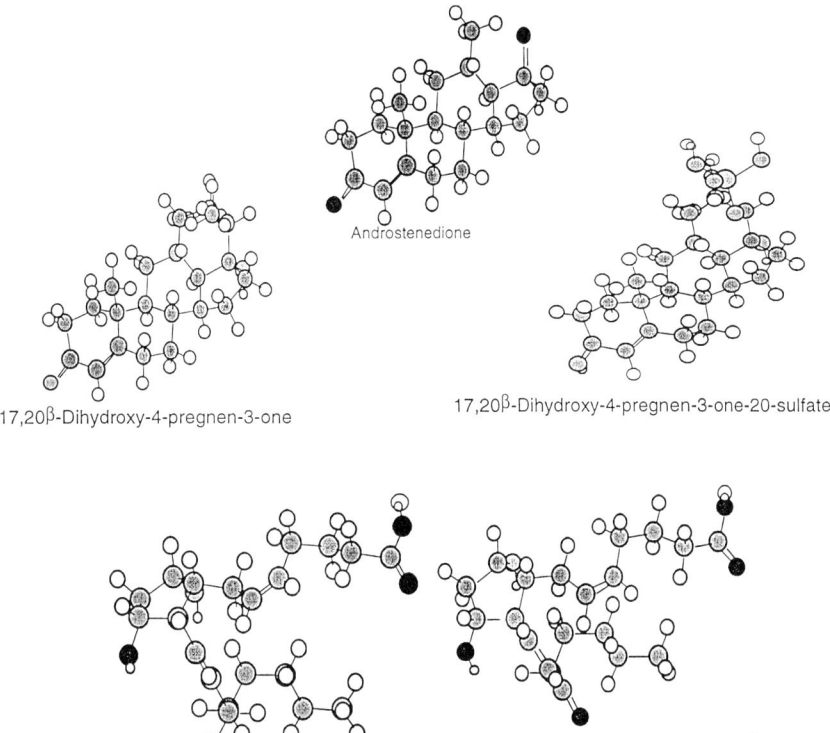

FIGURE 7 Hormonal products that are known to be released by female goldfish and to possess pheromonal activity in the species.

patterns of both 19-carbon and 21-carbon steroids in goldfish induced to ovulate with human chorionic gonadotropin (hCG) describe release rates of 17,20β-P equivalent to those seen in spontaneously ovulating fish (Stacey et al., 1989) and a shift from release of 19-carbon steroids to release of 21-carbon steroids as fish approach ovulation (Scott and Sorensen, 1994; Sorensen and Scott, 1994); AD and free, sulfated, and glucuronidated forms of T reached a peak rate within 6 hours of hCG injection, whereas the release of free and conjugated 17,20β-P and 17,20β,21-P peaked about 9 hours after injection and then declined (Sorensen and Scott, 1994). These changes in release follow those seen in plasma (Moriwaki et al., 1991), although they are slightly later than that measured in spontaneously ovulating fish (Stacey et al., 1989). Although free steroids appear to be released almost exclusively across the gills in goldfish, both glucuronidated and sulfated forms are released in the urine (Sorensen et al., 2000). These changing profiles of sex steroid production and release, coupled with their different release mechanisms, have implications for their function as pheromones.

Of approximately three dozen steroids known to be released by ovulatory goldfish, three have been identified as primary pheromonal components that are detected by the olfactory epithelium of both male and female goldfish with high sensitivity and specificity— 17,20β-P, 17,20β-P-S, and AD (Sorensen et al., 1990, 1995a; Stacey, 1991). EOG recording and accompanying bioassays demonstrate that the olfactory system is remarkably sensitive (picomolar detection thresholds) to each of these steroids, and that this sensitivity is highly specific. Indeed, minor changes in steroid structure (e.g., altering the orientation of a single hydroxyl group) dramatically decrease both olfactory and biological responses to them (Sorensen et al., 1990, 1995a) (Fig. 8).

The preovulatory steroid pheromone is a complex mixture. Early in the female GTH II surge, release of the three components is low and AD is dominant (Scott and Sorensen, 1994). Release then increases rapidly, with

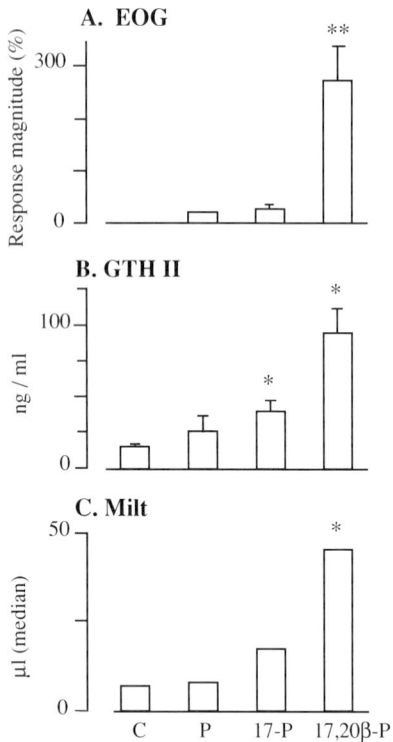

FIGURE 8 Olfactory, endocrine, and gonadal responses of male goldfish exposed to one of three 21-carbon steroids (progesterone, P; 17α-hydroxyprogesterone, 17-P; 17,20β-P) or a control vehicle (C = 10^{-8} M methanol or ethanol). (A) EOG responses to 10^{-8} M steroids expressed as a percentage of response to 10^{-5} M L-serine. (B) Serum GTH II concentrations of males after being exposed for 1 hr to 5×10^{-10} M steroid concentration. (C) Milt (sperm and seminal fluid) volumes of males after 8 hr of steroid exposure. * and **, significantly different from control ($P < 0.05$ and $P < 0.01$, respectively). Adapted from Sorensen *et al.* (1990).

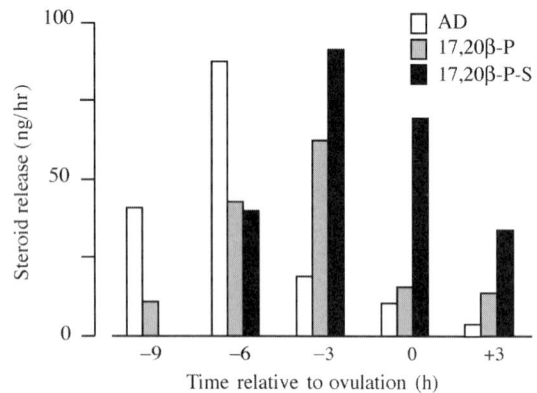

FIGURE 9 Relative release profiles of the three steroids that make up the goldfish preovulatory pheromone. Adapted from Scott and Sorensen (1994).

release of AD peaking first and then falling as release of both 21-carbon steroids peaks together before ovulation (Scott and Sorensen, 1994) (Fig. 9). At ovulation, release of all three steroids decreases, with 17,20β-P-S dominating for a few hours (Fig. 9) until release patterns revert to basal levels, which again are dominated by AD (Scott and Sorensen, unpublished results). Here we consider the actions of 17,20β-P first, because it appears to be the primary active component and is best understood. Later, we consider the actions of the differing mixtures in which it is found.

It appears that the principal function of 17,20β-P is to increase male steroidogenesis and milt production, thereby giving exposed males increased fertility by the time of spawning (Dulka *et al.*, 1987a; Sorensen *et al.*, 1989, 1990; Zheng *et al.*, 1997; Fig. 6). Even momentary exposure to low (picomolar) concentrations of 17,20β-P stimulates a neuroendocrine reflex that evokes large increases in GTH II release, which in turn trigger increases in circulating steroid levels and milt production (Dulka *et al.*, 1987a). These changes in response to 17,20β-P, which can be detected as an increased volume of stripped milt within 4–6 hours of exposure (Dulka *et al.*, 1987a; Zheng and Stacey, 1996), mimic those seen in male fish exposed to the odor of ovulatory females (Stacey *et al.*, 1989) and presumably serve to give exposed males increased releasable sperm in the sperm ducts by the time the female ovulates.

In addition to these endocrine changes, exposure to 17,20β-P mildly increases male sexual arousal (swimming and searching behavior), presumably a response that allows males to remain close to mature ovulatory females so that they have an advantage when the females ovulate (DeFraipont and Sorensen, 1993; Poling *et al.*, 2001). Indeed, these behavioral changes are distinguished by the fact that they persist for up to 12 hours even in the absence of females (Sorensen *et al.*, 1989; Poling *et al.*, 2001). It also is significant that 17,20β-P (like all free steroids) is released via the gills; thus, free sex steroids probably function as tonic close-range cues that are closely associated with the immediate physical presence of a female and may give the signal a species-specific character (Sorensen *et al.*, 2000). Evidence demonstrates that steroidal mixtures with 17,20β-P as the dominant component appear to have the same actions as 17,20β-P alone, suggesting that the precise mixture composition is not important, although this has not been documented fully.

Two studies have directly demonstrated the importance of pheromonal 17,20β-P to male reproductive success. First, DeFraipoint and Sorensen (1993) found that males exposed to this pheromone are more behaviorally competitive than unexposed males for access to spawning females and produce more sperm with greater motility. Second, using microsatellite DNA fingerprinting, Zheng et al. (1997) showed that, in competitive spawning, a male exposed overnight to 17,20β-P fertilizes dramatically more eggs than an unexposed control male. Although pheromone-exposed males were more behaviorally competitive than control males, confirming the results of DeFraipont and Sorensen (1993), their increased fertility in spawning also must be due at least in part to increased sperm quality because they also had significantly greater paternity than control males in competitive *in vitro* fertilization (Zheng *et al.*, 1997).

The pheromonal function of 17,20β-P is augmented by a variety of redundant steroidal components (defined in Section II.B.1, item 4) that appear to act through the same receptor mechanism but lack a functional identity. For example, 17-P, 17,20β,21-P, and 17,20β-P-20β-glucuronide are all released by female goldfish in significant quantities concurrently with 17,20β-P (Sorensen and Scott, 1994), but, although they are detected by male goldfish (albeit with much less sensitivity) and have biological activity (Sorensen *et al.*, 1991, 1995a), they appear to act via the same receptor mechanism as 17,20β-P and exert exactly the same kinds of effects (i.e., they function as 17,20β-P analogs). Because these redundant cues are considerably less potent olfactory stimulants than the principal component (17,20β-P), their combined pheromonal effect is not expected to be great, distinctive, or even necessary, and therefore they probably serve simply to amplify the effect of 17,20β-P. Notably, at least two authors have misinterpreted the implications of the existence of these redundant cues and suggested that they imply the system is either less specific or more complex than is actually the case (Moore, 1994; Zippel *et al.*, 2000). When considering pheromone function, it is extremely important to consider receptor sensitivity in the context of specificity and what the animal is therefore likely to perceive. Indeed, this consideration has led us to our conclusion that the preovulatory pheromone naturally functions as a blend of just a few (probably three) perceived principal components. We now discuss the nature of these blends.

Early in the female GTH II surge, when steroid release rates are relatively low, AD (which EOG cross-adaptation has shown to be detected by a unique receptor mechanism; Sorensen *et al.*, 1991) is released in relatively greater quantities than 17,20β-P and little 17,20β-P-S is present. The presence of AD in this blend (which is secreted through the gills) exerts dramatic inhibitory effects (Fig. 6), resulting in a facultative mixture. Thus, although 17,20β-P is highly stimulatory on its own, adding AD so that it becomes the most abundant component (as is the case at the onset of the female GTH II surge) causes 17,20β-P to lose both its endocrinological and behavioral activity (Stacey, 1991; K. R. Poling and P. W. Sorensen, unpublished results). We suspect that males have evolved the ability to detect and respond to AD (this mixture) because it prevents them from responding prematurely or inappropriately to transient wisps of 17,20β-P released by females that are not close to ovulating. Notably, inhibitory-modulatory components have also been characterized in mammalian ovulatory pheromones (Stern and McClintock, 1998), in which they play similar roles synchronizing endocrine cycles.

17,20β-P-S, the third steroid in the preovulatory pheromone, becomes the dominant component late in the preovulatory period, as the release rates of AD and other 19-carbon steroids decline (Scott and Sorensen, 1994; Sorensen and Scott, 1994). This derivative of 17,20β-P, which is presumably produced by the up-regulation of sulfotransferase activity to promote metabolism, appears to function as a primary stimulatory component in the changing steroidal mixture. Notably, 17,20β-P-S is secreted independently of free steroids, via the urine (Sorensen *et al.*, 2000). EOG recording shows that 17,20β-P-S is detected with high sensitivity (picomolar thresholds) and specificity (independent receptor sites) by the goldfish olfactory epithelium (Sorensen *et al.*, 1995a) and is processed by neural circuitry independent of that for 17,20β-P in the olfactory bulb (Hanson, 2001). 17,20β-P-S is released in the urine and stimulates both the male endocrine system and behavior (see later) (Sorensen *et al.*, 2000). Urinary release is important because goldfish release urine in distinct controlled pulses that lend it the potential (as yet unstudied for steroids) to serve a specialized behavioral function (Appelt and Sorensen, 1999).

At present, we feel that 17,20β-P-S is best viewed as a single-component urinary pheromone whose behavioral and endocrine actions complement those of the 17,20β-P pheromone with which it eventually mixes; thus, we consider it part of the preovulatory pheromone family. Poling *et al.* (2001) have demonstrated that exposure to nanomolar concentrations of 17,20β-P-S elicits immediate dramatic increases in male sexual behavior that are more intense but briefer in duration (15 min vs hours) than responses to 17,20β-P. These differences in male behavioral response are consistent with the idea that because these cues are released in different manners they should have different functions; that is, 17,20β-P-S need not necessarily be signaling the immediate presence of a female because it is released as occassional (once a minute or so) pulses that should be detectable at a distance from the female (Appelt and Sorensen, 1999; Sorensen *et al.*, 2000). As with exposure to 17,20β-P, exposure to 17,20β-P-S increases blood GTH II concentration and milt volume in males (Sorensen *et al.*, 1995a; Poling *et al.*, 2001). Interestingly, ongoing experiments suggest that a mixture of 17,20β-P and 17,20β-P-S have greater behavioral activity than either steroid alone (K. R. Poling and P. W. Sorensen, unpublished), although there is no indication of synergism with respect to endocrine action (Sorensen *et al.*, 1995a). Several sulfated progestins are released together with 17,20βP-S (Sorensen and Scott, 1994; Sorensen *et al.*, 1995a) and presumably function as redundant components, amplifying the actions of this special urinary cue that probably has important functions as a social stimulant.

In conclusion, it is now clear that the goldfish preovulatory pheromone is a complex mixture whose precise composition and function changes with time during the female ovulatory GTH II surge. Early in the surge, the steroid mixture has little activity, but as its composition shifts from being dominated by AD, to 17,20β-P, and finally to 17,20β-P-S, it assumes both endocrine- and behavioral-stimulating abilities with long-lasting actions and then shifts to a cue with stronger and more immediate effects on behavior. Presumably, one reason males have evolved to discriminate this mixture is that it permits them to synchronize their reproductive system, sperm production, and behavior with the female's reproductive cycle. Another reason (which has not been studied) is that the mixture could impart taxa-specific character to the cue, components of which are likely to be released by any reproductively active species of fish.

Several potentially confusing and important issues remain to be resolved with respect to the preovulatory pheromone. First, a complicating factor is that male goldfish (see Section IV.D.1.e) also release AD, one of the key elements of preovulatory pheromone, so the distinction between male and female cues becomes confusing to those studying fish—although perhaps not to the fish because the external space influenced by gill steroids is small (Sorensen *et al.*, 2000). Another unresolved issue is whether and how AD and 17,20β-P-S affect female goldfish, which detect these steroids as well as males do (Sorensen *et al.*, 1995a) and which also respond to 17,20β-P (Sorensen and Stacey, 1987). Also to be resolved are the complexity of the real pheromonal mixture and whether goldfish are able to distinguish small changes in mixture composition. In spite of these uncertainties, the goldfish preovulatory pheromone is perhaps the best understood among the vertebrates, is easily studied, and seems general enough to make us suppose that many other species of fish are probably using released sex steroids in much the same manner.

iii) Postovulatory prostaglandin pheromone. At the time of ovulation (about 12 hours after onset of the GTH II surge and late in the scotophase; Fig. 6), female goldfish become sexually active and attractive to males (Stacey and Liley, 1974; Stacey *et al.*, 1979a,b; Sorensen *et al.*, 1995b). Female behavioral activity in goldfish is directly associated with the presence of recently ovulated eggs (Stacey and Liley, 1974; Stacey, 1981; Sorensen *et al.*, 1995b), which are known to exert their effects on behavior by stimulating an increase in circulating F prostaglandin (Stacey, 1976; Sorensen *et al.*, 1995b; see Section II.D.3) (Fig. 10). It is extremely important to male goldfish that they locate females at the time of ovulation (if not before), both because ovulated females must spawn within a few hours (before oocytes become nonviable) and because male competition for access to females is intense. A PG-derived hormonal pheromone serves this purpose. So important is the PG pheromone that males without functional olfactory systems typically fail to spawn (Stacey and Kyle, 1983).

As with the preovulatory steroid pheromone, the postovulatory PG pheromone appears to be

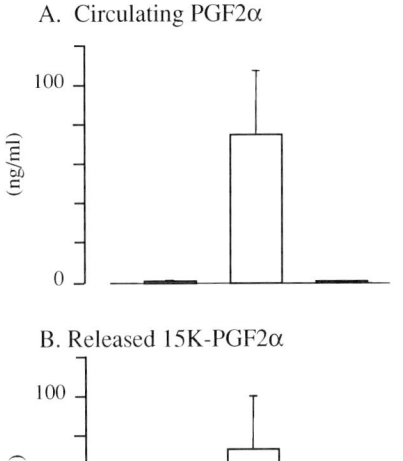

FIGURE 10 Quantities of F prostaglandins found in the blood of periovulatory goldfish and in the water in which they were held. (A) Plasma concentrations of PGF2α (ng/ml). (B) Water concentrations of 15K-PGF2α expressed as release rate (ng/hr). For these experiments, vitellogenic female goldfish were injected with hCG (10 I.U./g body weight) to induce ovulation. Pre-OV, hCG-injected females 2–4 hr prior to ovulation; OV, females that were sampled within an hour of having ovulated and had not been offered the opportunity to spawn; Spent, fish that were sampled up to 4 hr after ovulation and had released all of their eggs during the course of spawning with males. Values were calculated using mass spectrometry. P. W. Sorensen, A. R. Brash, and F. W. Goetz (unpublished results).

a mixture of several compounds, the most important being PGF2α and its metabolite, 15-ketoprostaglandin (15K-PGF2α). Biochemical studies have clearly demonstrated that these products are released in great quantity (100 ng/hr) by recently ovulated goldfish, as well as by nonovulated fish that have been injected with PGF2α or have had eggs placed into the oviduct (Sorensen et al., 1988, 1995b; P. W. Sorensen, unpublished). Both PGs are released exclusively in the urine, 15K-PGF2α in the greatest quantities (Appelt et al., 1995). Interestingly, females alter their urination rate when sexually active, suggesting that active signaling may be occurring (Appelt and Sorensen, 1999).

EOG recording has demonstrated that PGF2α and 15K-PGF2α are detected with great sensitivity (nanomolar and picomolar thresholds, respectively) and specificity by the male olfactory epithelium, which possesses two independent receptor mechanisms for these compounds. EOG sensitivity and specificity have been confirmed by behavioral assays (Sorensen et al., 1988). Interestingly, unlike steroids, sensitivity to PGs is sexually dimorphic in goldfish and carp (Irvine and Sorensen, 1993; Sorensen and Goetz, 1993), males being more sensitive than females (Fig. 11). Finally, waterborne PGs induce clear behavioral responses, which we discuss in detail next.

Several studies have described strong male behavioral responses to PGs added to aquarium water (Sorensen et al., 1986, 1988, 1989). In particular, groups of mature male goldfish exposed to low concentrations (0.1 nM) of PGs actively inspect and actively chase one another (Sorensen et al., 1988, 1989) (Fig. 12). These responses to PGs differ from those elicited by 17,20β-P in three ways. First, the level of activity elicited by PGs is far greater than that elicited by 17,20β-P; however, response to PGs persists (in the absence of a female releasing the cue) for only 10–20 min, whereas males exposed to 17,20β-P are active for many hours (Sorensen et al., 1989; DeFraipont and Sorensen, 1993; Poling et al., 2001). Second, such water-borne PGs have little if any effect on male behavior unless they are injected into the aquarium as a stream (like urine) and in the presence of other fish (P. W. Sorensen, unpublished). Third, water-borne PGs rarely stimulate GTH II release in isolated males, whereas males typically increase blood GTH II concentrations in the presence of a PG-releasing female (Kyle et al., 1985; Zheng and Stacey, 1996, 1997). Thus, unlike 17,20β-P, behavioral and endocrine response to PGs is highly dependent on the social context in which it is encountered (see Section IV.D.1.d.iv).

The true behavioral function of the PG pheromone has not been clearly identified, although it could have several functions, which need not be mutually exclusive. For instance, it might serve to alert males that ovulation has occurred, to identify females in groups, or to attract males from a distance to groups that contain ovulated females. Designing a model female that can release pheromones in controlled pulsatile fashion could help to distinguish among these possibilities.

How and why goldfish use a mixture of two PGS is also unresolved. Information indicates that males

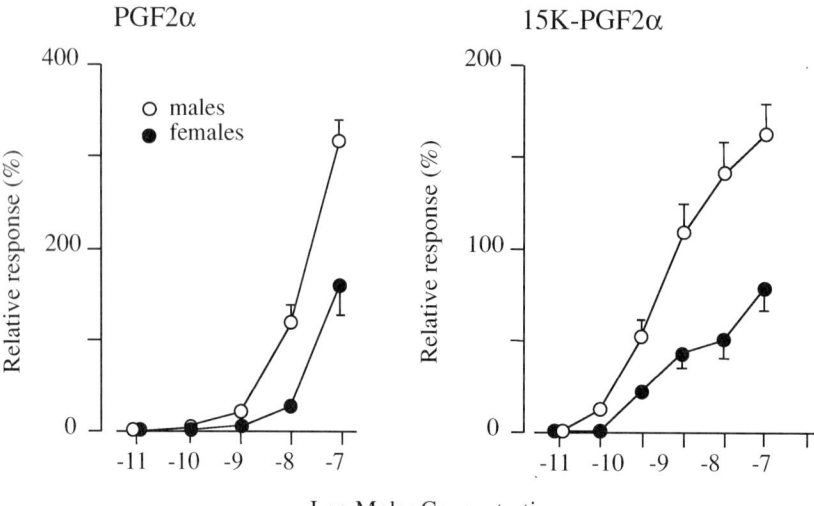

FIGURE 11 Electroolfactogram responses (mean and standard error) of sexually mature male goldfish and sexually recrudescing female goldfish to PGF2α and 15K-PGF2α. Responses are expressed as a percentage of responses elicited by 10^{-5} M L-serine (a food odor). From Sorensen and Goetz (1993), *J. Lipid Mediators* **6**, 385–393, © 1993, with permission from Elsevier Science.

exhibit equivalent behavioral responses if exposed to PGF2α, 15K-PGF2α, or a mixture of the two (Sorensen et al., 1988, 1989). Pehaps the most plausible reason that males have evolved to discriminate two PGs is that this redundancy (which is associated with different receptor mechanisms with different sensitivities) may assist them in locating the source of the pheromone.

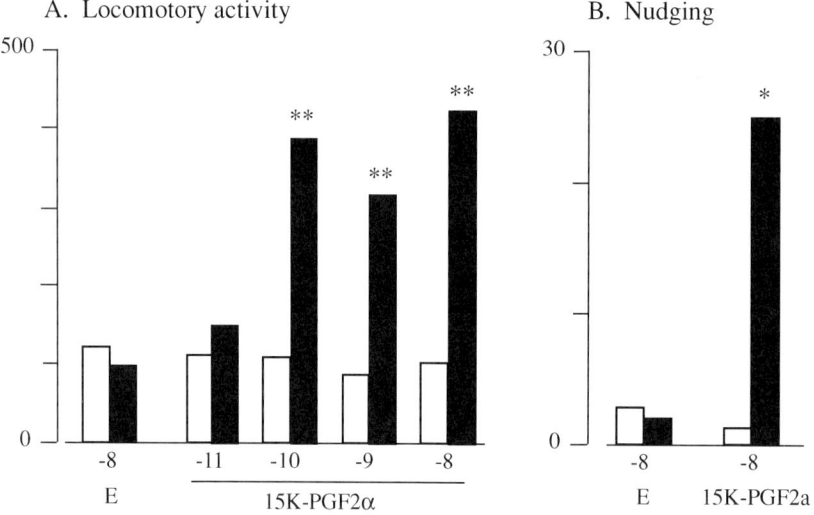

FIGURE 12 (A) Locomotory activity and (B) nudging behavior of all-male groups of goldfish for 15 min prior to (open bars) and during (filled bars) continuous addition (10 ml/min) of ethanol control (E) or several concentrations of 15K-PGF2α to their aquaria. * and **, significantly different from preexposure ($P < 0.05$) and $P < 0.01$, respectively). Adapted from Sorensen et al. (1988).

The question of whether the PG pheromone is species-specific is difficult to address because none of the identified hormonal products are unusual. Sorensen et al. (2000) review possible bases for specificity. First, although the active space of these cues is relatively large (about 100 liters; Table 1), release occurs in urinary pulses with a frequency of only about one per minute unless the female is spawning. Second, male goldfish apparently perceive the PG pheromone in the background odor within which it occurs, because their responses are inhibited if they are simultaneously exposed to the odor of heterospecifics (Sorensen et al. 2000); heterospecific visual or behavioral cues could have similar effects. These possibilities warrant study.

That goldfish simultaneously use PGF2α as a subcellular (autocrine) factor stimulating ovulation, a hormone synchronizing female sexual behavior with ovulation (Sorensen et al., 1995b), and exogenously as a pheromone synchronizing male courtship with female behavior (Sorensen and Goetz, 1993) is remarkable. Certainly this observation speaks both to the existence of strong evolutionary pressure to conserve signaling mechanisms and to the likelihood that many species have evolved similar types of cues. Indeed, as discussed in Section IV.D.2, there is strong evidence that the pheromones of many species employ PGs, presumably because of their common association with ovulation and the key role that ovulation plays in fish reproductive biology.

iv) Central mechanisms of pheromone action. Despite numerous studies demonstrating that released steroids, PGs, and their metabolites have pheromonal functions in a variety of fish species, only in goldfish do we have information on the central neural mechanisms mediating hormonal pheromone effects. As discussed in Sections IV.D.1.d.ii and IV.D.1.d.iii, the preovulatory steroid pheromone (17,20β-P) and the postovulatory PG pheromone released by female goldfish both can increase GTH II and milt volume in males, although the PG pheromone does so only in the context of appropriate social cues (Kyle et al., 1985; Dulka et al., 1987a; Sorensen et al., 1989; DeFraipont and Sorensen, 1993; see later). It is clear that different neural mechanisms at both the peripheral and central levels underlie responsiveness to these pheromones, whose actions may differ to a greater extent than we realize (Sorensen et al., 1988; Dulka et al., 1992; Zheng and Stacey, 1996, 1997).

To understand the different mechanisms mediating effects of pheromonal 17,20β-P and PGs on GTH II and milt, it is necessary to appreciate that these pheromones exert their effects in quite different social contexts. For example, males in a social group containing a preovulatory female must typically encounter wisps of 17,20β-P (and other steroids of the preovulatory pheromone) in darkness, hours before spawning begins, and therefore are unlikely to maintain continuous physical or olfactory contact. Consistent with this concept, males increase GTH II concentration and milt volume if exposed to 17,20β-P even for a brief period (Dulka et al., 1987a) or when isolated from conspecifics (Stacey and Sorensen, 1986; Sorensen et al., 1989). In contrast, males encountering pheromonal PGs immediately and dramatically increase social contact and, if they encounter a female releasing this cue, attempt (because this female normally is ovulated) to maintain physical contact throughout the ensuing courtship and spawning period. Thus, under normal conditions, endocrine and testicular responses to pheromonal PGs occur while the male simultaneously receives additional physical, chemical, and behavioral cues from the receptive female. Accordingly, we (Sorensen et al., 1989) find that exposure to a PG mixture (PGF2α and 15K-PGF2α) does not increase GTH II in isolated males, but does increase GTH II in all-male groups in which the mixture increases social interactions, suggesting that PG-induced social behavior between fish, but not necessarily mating behavior per se, is a prerequisite for the endocrine response. Experiments have yet to be performed that separate the effects of social interaction with the PG pheromone. In the discussion in this section, we use PG pheromone to describe the entire set of olfactory and other stimuli perceived by males during interaction with a sexually active (ovulated or PGF2α-injected) female.

The first indication that pheromonal 17,20β-P and PGF activate different endocrine mechanisms in male goldfish was the observation that 17,20β-P exposure was equally effective at any time of day, whereas PG pheromone was most effective at night (Dulka et al., 1987b). Also, although the latency to GTH II increase was similarly short (15–20 min) for the two pheromones (Kyle et al., 1985; Dulka et al., 1987a),

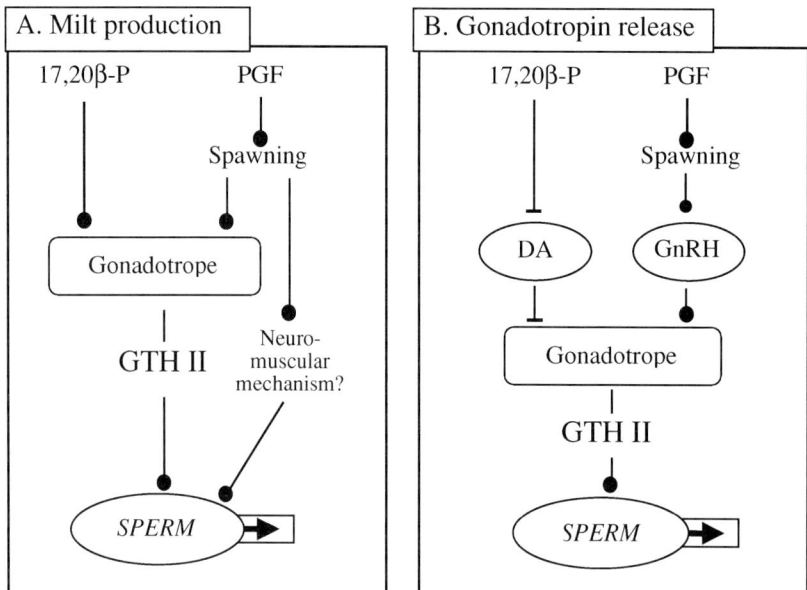

FIGURE 13 Schematic model illustrating the differential effects of pheromonal 17,20β-P and PGF on (A) milt (sperm and seminal fluid) production and (B) gonadotropin release in the goldfish.

the latency to PG-pheromone-induced milt increase was shorter (<1 h; Kyle et al., 1985) than the latency to 17,20β-P-induced milt increase (3–6 hr; Dulka et al., 1987a). The 17,20β-P effect on milt appeared to be GTH-II-dependent because the milt response was blocked by acute hypophysectomy (Dulka et al., 1987a). The possibility that the actions of the PG pheromone are not directly linked to GTH II increases was suggested both by the fact that exposure to spawning females could stimulate dramatic behavior and milt increases in males prior to measurable increases in the GTH II (Kyle et al., 1985) and by the fact that PG-pheromone-induced milt increase is not blocked in hypophysectomized fish (Zheng and Stacey, 1996).

That pheromonal 17,20β-P increases milt only through GTH II is indicated by the fact that pretreatment with hCG, to swamp the system abolishes the effect of subsequent 17,20β-P exposure (Zheng and Stacey, 1996); in contrast, hCG-pretreated fish are still able to increase milt volume in response to the PG pheromone. Finally, the time course of PG-pheromone-induced milt increase is similar at 20°C (the normal spawning temperature) and 10°C, whereas the time course of the 17,20βP-induced milt response is greatly extended at the lower temperature, as is the response to

hCG treatment (Zheng and Stacey, 1996). In summary, although both pheromonal 17,20β-P and PG increase both blood GTH II concentration and milt volume, 17,20β-P appears to increase milt by stimulating GTH II release, whereas PG pheromone also can increase milt through an extra-pituitary pathway (Fig. 13). The nature of this extra-pituitary pathway is unknown, but may involve central mechanisms known to stimulate testicular and sperm-duct contractions in goldfish (Demski and Dulka, 1984; Dulka and Demski, 1986).

Pheromonal 17,20β-P and PG differ not only in the way they regulate milt volume, but also in the mechanisms by which they induce GTH II release. Control of GTH II release in goldfish is controlled by hypothalamic neurons that innervate the gonadotropes and release stimulatory GnRH or inhibitory dopamine (DA), which acts through DA type 2 (D2) receptors (Peter et al., 1986; Trudeau, 1997). Pheromonal 17,20β-P evidently increases GTH II release by reducing tonic DA release in the pituitary because the pituitary dihydroxyphenylacetic acid (DOPAC; the primary DA metabolite in goldfish) to DA ratio decreases within 20 min of pheromone exposure (Dulka et al., 1992). Also, D2 receptor agonists (bromocryptine and LY171555) block 17,20β-P-induced GTH-II and milt increase, but do not affect these responses to PG pheromone (Zheng and Stacey, 1997).

The role of GnRH in mediating these pheromone effects on GTH II release is less clear. A GnRH antagonist (Ac-Δ^3-Pro^1,4FD-Phe^2,D-Trp^{3,6}) blocked GTH II responses to both pheromones and blocked the milt response to 17,20β-P but not to PG (Zheng and Stacey, 1997), indicating that GnRH mediates the action of both pheromones and providing additional support for the extra-pituitary mechanism mediating PG-pheromone-induced milt increase. These results do not eliminate the possibility that GnRH could play different roles (permissive vs dynamic) in mediating the actions of the two pheromones. Nonetheless, it seems clear that only pheromonal 17,20β-P induces GTH II release by modulating dopaminergic function (Fig. 13).

e) Male Hormonal Pheromones   Given the preceding evidence that periovulatory females release potent steroid and PG pheromones influencing male reproductive functions, it would seem only prudent to expect that hormonal products released by males also have pheromonal effects on conspecifics. The possibility of female response to male pheromones has received little attention, although we find no evidence that the occurrence of ovulation is influenced by the presence of males (Stacey *et al.*, 1979b). Water-borne 17,20β-P increases the occurrence of ovulation (Sorensen and Stacey, 1987), but we believe this phenomenon occurs normally in response to the odor of preovulatory females, given that release of 17,20β-P by females is far greater than by males (Sorensen and Scott, 1994). Indeed, it seems likely that male competition has removed selective pressures for female goldfish to evolve mechanisms that monitor male presence. On the other hand, we expect that a male's success in sperm competition depends not only on mechanisms that increase his absolute fertility by monitoring cues from ovulatory females, but also on mechanisms that increase his relative fertility by monitoring cues from male competitors. Although there is good evidence that the male goldfish exhibits apparently adaptive reproductive responses to other males (Stacey, 1991; Stacey *et al.*, 2001), it is unclear whether these responses are mediated by pheromones.

The results of several simple experiments indicate that males can increase or decrease their milt production in response to male conspecifics (Fig. 14). For example, if one male in a group is injected with hCG, all males increase their milt volume (Stacey, 1991; Stacey

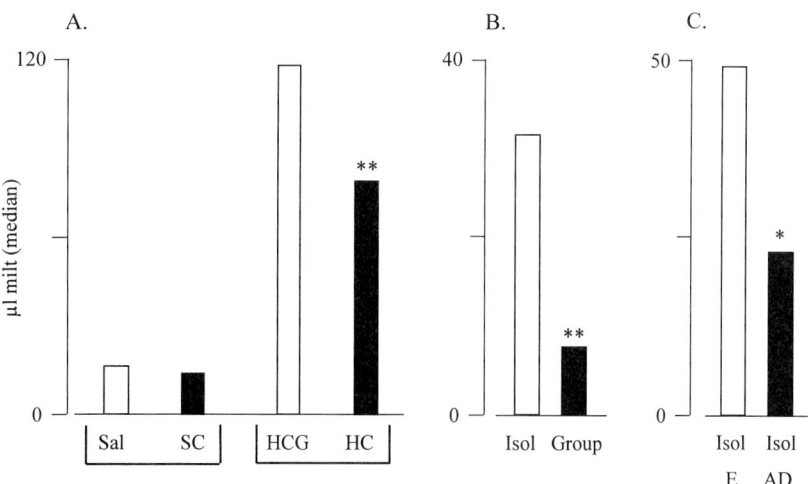

FIGURE 14   Stimulatory and inhibitory effects on milt production among male goldfish. (A) Males held overnight (HC) with a male injected with hCG (5 IU/g) (HCG) have significantly larger milt volumes than males (SC) held with a saline-injected male (Sal). (B) Males isolated overnight (Isol) have significantly larger milt volmes than males held in groups. (C) Milt production of isolated males is inhibited by water-borne androstenedione (AD, 10 nM). E, ethanol control. From Stacey (1991).

et al., 2001), suggesting that males normally detect and respond to other males in which GTH II is increased above basal levels. Similarly, if a male is exposed to 17,20β-P (to increase his GTH II levels) and added to a group, milt volumes of the grouped males increase (E. J. Fraser and N. E. Stacey, unpublished results). On the other hand, if a male is removed from a group and held in isolation, his milt volume also increases dramatically (Stacey, 1991; Stacey *et al.*, 2001), suggesting that males tonically inhibit their milt production in the presence of males with basal GTH II concentrations. In both the hCG-male effect and the isolation effect, milt volume increases appear different than those resulting from exposure to pheromonal 17,2β-P and PGF2α—the latencies are longer and they are not accompanied by an increase in GTH II (Stacey *et al.*, 2001; E. J. Fraser and N. E. Stacey, unpublished results).

We have been unsuccessful so far in all attempts to demonstrate that hCG-injected males (which have elevated plasma 17,20β-P; Kobayashi *et al.*, 1986a) release a stimulating odor or that grouped males release an inhibiting odor (E. J. Fraser and N. E. Stacey, unpublished results). However, because males do not increase milt volume if they are isolated in aquaria containing AD (Stacey, 1991; N. E. Stacey, unpublished results; Fig. 14), we suspect that the isolation effect is a response to removal from a tonic inhibitory AD pheromone that probably has a very small active space. Indeed, Poling *et al.* (2001) have shown that exposing all-male groups to AD induces apparently agonistic behaviors that are qualitatively and temporally distinct from responses to 17,20β-P and 17,20β-P-S. The fact that males release far greater quantities of AD than do females (Sorensen and Scott, 1994) suggests that these behavioral responses to AD exposure are normal components of male–male interactions.

Admittedly, the hCG-male effect and isolation effect are not well characterized and possibly not mediated by hormonal pheromones. Nonetheless, we feel they are as important to an understanding of male goldfish reproduction as are the well-characterized female pheromones. From our understanding, we propose that in the spawning season males regulate their milt production in response to antagonistic stimuli from male conspecifics. In the absence of cues from preovulatory or ovulated females, a male maintains basal GTH II and steroids and is both a source and a receiver of unknown

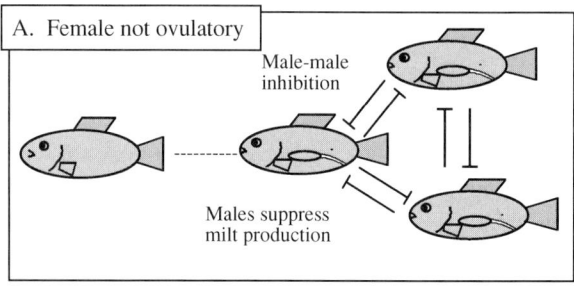
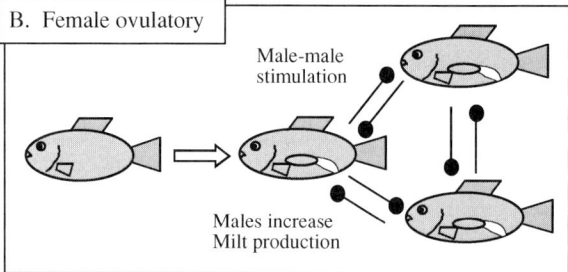

FIGURE 15 Proposed inhibitory and stimulatory effects on milt production among male goldfish. (A) In the absence of ovulatory cues from females, males reduce their milt production in response to inhibitory cues from conspecifics. (B) Males increase milt production in response to ovulatory cues and thereby emit cues that stimulate milt production in conspecifics. From Stacey *et al.* (2001), *Comp. Biochem. Physiol.*, © 2001 with permission from Elsevier Science.

cues that inhibit milt production (Fig. 15A). However, when exposed to the female preovulatory pheromone, a male increases his GTH-II concentration and milt volume, and thereby becomes the source of unknown cues that stimulate milt production in additional males (Fig. 15B). Together with evidence for pheromonally mediated ovulatory synchrony among females (Sorensen and Stacey, 1987; Kobayashi *et al.*, 1988), these stimulatory male–male interactions could provide a pheromonal explanation for synchronized spawning under natural conditions.

2. Other Cypriniform Fishes

Common carp, Crucian carp, and goldfish—all from the Subtribe Cyprini (Rainboth, 1991)—appear to possess similar hormonal pheromone systems. EOG studies of goldfish and common carp (Irvine and Sorensen, 1993) indicate the two species have a remarkably similar pattern of sensitivity to a variety of steroids and prostaglandins. Also, 17,20β-P induces in carp GTH II and testicular responses equivalent to those observed in goldfish (Stacey et al., 1994b). As with goldfish and common carp, Crucian carp detect both 17,20β-P and PGF2α (Bjerselius and Olsen, 1993). When placed in a stream channel in which the flow is divided longitudinally to enable a choice between unscented water and water containing a detectable concentration of 17,20β-P, male (but not female) Crucian carp exhibit a mild avoidance of 17,20β-P (Bjerselius and Olsen, 1993), the same response exhibited by male goldfish (Bjerselius et al., 1995c). The biological significance of this behavior is puzzling and warrants further study.

Whereas goldfish and common carp (and possibly Crucian carp) respond to a similar suite of hormonal compounds, more distantly related cypriniforms vary greatly in olfactory responsiveness (Stacey and Cardwell, 1995, 1997). In the loach (Misgurnus anguillicaudatus; Family Cobitidae), as in goldfish, PGs released by ovulated females function as a potent pheromone that stimulates male sexual activities. The suite of courtship and spawning behaviors that males direct toward ovulated females is similar to that directed toward nonovulated females that have been injected with PGF2α, 15-keto-PGF2α, or 13,14-dihydro-15-keto-PGF2α; as in goldfish (Stacey and Kyle, 1983), these male behaviors are virtually absent in anosmic males (Kitamura et al., 1994a). EOG studies (Kitamura et al., 1994a) show that, although male loach detect PGF2α (1 nM detection threshold), they are much more sensitive to 15-keto-PGF2α and 13,14-dihdro-15-keto-PGF2α (1 pM detection threshold). In hCG-injected female loach, PG release to the water is negligible prior to ovulation, but then increases dramatically, 13,14-dihydro-15-keto-PGF2α being released in the greatest quantities (Ogata et al., 1994).

Although all cypriniforms examined detect F2-series prostaglandins, none of the study species from Superfamily Cobitoidea detect any of a large number of conjugated and nonconjugated steroids (Kitamura et al., 1994b; Stacey and Cardwell, 1995, 1997; Table 3). Considering the small number of cobitoid species examined by EOG recording, it is unclear whether the olfactory systems of all cobitoids are likely to be insensitive to steroidal compounds. Such insensitivity seems likely for gyrinocheilids and catostomids. Gyrinocheilidae is a monogeneric family (four species), and the five studied sucker species represent the three recognized subfamilies (Ictobinae, Ictiobus; Cycleptinae, Myxocyprinus; Catostominae, Catostomus, Moxostomus) (Cardwell et al., 1992; Sorensen et al., 1992) of Family Catostomidae). However, for the large Families Cobitidae and Balitoridae, further species must be examined. Nonetheless, the present EOG information on steroid sensitivity is consistent with the division of Order Cypriniformes into cyprinoid and cobitoid superfamilies (Nelson, 1994).

In contrast to the situation with Superfamily Cobitoidea, detection of steroidal compounds is widespread among higher taxa of the Cyprinoidea (Family Cyprinidae) (Table 3). Of the eight recognized cyprinid subfamilies (Rainboth, 1991; Nelson, 1994), at least one species from all but the minor Subfamily Psylorhynchinae (two genera, five species) have been examined by EOG recording (Table 3). Of the seven subfamilies examined, only Acheilognathinae (bitterlings) failed to exhibit olfactory responsiveness to tested steroidal compounds (but see Section IV.H.2). As discussed more fully elsewhere (Stacey et al., 1995; Stacey and Cardwell, 1995, 1997), patterns of olfactory response to steroids are surprisingly consistent among cyprinid species in lower taxa (tribe, subtribe, genus). Because a reasonable number of their species have been examined, two tribes from Subfamily Cyprininae serve as good examples. Species from Tribe Labeonini respond to a very limited range of steroids. Of fifteen species examined, all responded to 17,20β-P-S and eleven (e.g., Epalzeorhynchus, Lobocheilus, and Osteochilus) detected no other test steroid. The other four species (the only Labeo species examined) also detect a variety of unconjugated steroids through a second, broadly tuned olfactory receptor mechanism that seems most sensitive to 17-P (Stacey et al., 1995). Unlike the relatively simple patterns of EOG responsiveness in Tribe Labeonini, species in Tribe Systomini (e.g., Cyclocheilichthys, Hampala, and Puntius) have complex patterns of responsiveness due to detection of a wide range of 19- and 21-carbon steroids. Because cross-adaptation studies have been conducted on only a few of these species (e.g., Puntius schwanenfeldi; Cardwell et al., 1995), it is unclear whether species in Tribe Systomini have diverse hormonal pheromone systems or simply minor differences in specificity of very broadly tuned but shared olfactory receptor mechanisms.

E. Order Characiformes

The Order Characiformes reaches its highest diversity in South America (where cypriniforms are absent), the remaining species occuring in Central America, the southwestern United States, and Africa. Although we have examined far fewer characiform species than cypriniform species, and almost all of these from Family Characidae, the patterns of EOG responsiveness are broadly comparable insofar as the compounds detected are most similar among the lowest taxa (Cardwell and Stacey, 1995). As with Cypriniformes and other ostariophysins, all characiforms tested detect PGFs, and some detect 21-carbon steroids such as 17,20β-P (*Acestorhynchus* sp., Subfamily Characinae) and 11β,21-P (*Chalceus* sp., Subfamily Bryconinae). The tribe Tetragonopterinae (tetras; Family Characidae) is similar to the characiform Danioninae and Labeonini (Stacey *et al.*, 1995; Stacey and Cardwell, 1995, 1997) in having highly specific responses to steroids. Of fourteen tetra species tested, three detected no steroids and the remainder detected only 17β-estradiol-3-sulfate (E_2-S), a steroid not known to be detected by any cypriniform species.

One tetra that detects E_2-S is *Astyanax mexicanus*, a common species that ranges from Texas to central Brazil and has established a number of hypogean (cave-dwelling) populations (the Mexican blind cavefish) in limestone caves. Hypogean *A. mexicanus* have remarkable EOG responses to PGF2α (0.1 pM detection threshold; 30 to 50 mV response magnitude at 10 nM) (Cardwell and Stacey, 1995), leading us to hypothesize that olfactory hypersensitivity had evolved as a compensatory response to lost visual function. Surprisingly, however, sighted, epigean (surface-dwelling) conspecifics exhibit equivalent olfactory responsiveness (Cardwell and Stacey, 1995), suggesting extreme olfactory sensitivity may have evolved for unknown reason in surface waters and preadapted this fish for cave existence.

F. Order Siluriformes

Hormonal pheromones have been extensively studied in the African catfish (*Clarias gariepinus*, Family Clariidae; Van Den Hurk and Resink, 1992). However, for the other 33 families in this worldwide order, there is almost no information, despite the fact that olfaction has been extensively studied in the channel catfish (*Ictalurus punctatus*; Sorensen and Caprio, 1997). Indeed, the channel catfish provides one of the few examples in which a fish sex pheromone has found practical application (Timms and Kleerekoper, 1972).

1. African Catfish (*Clarias gariepinus*)

Clarias typically spawn as male–female pairs, the eggs being scattered and fertilized on submerged vegetation, often at night and in turbid water (Lambert *et al.*, 1986). There is circumstantial evidence that these spawning interactions are facilitated by an ovarian pheromone that synchronizes ovulation (Resink *et al.*, 1989d) and strong evidence that male hormonal pheromones attract the female (reviewed in Van Den Hurk and Resink, 1992).

The pheromones of male *Clarias* evidently are steroid glucuronides synthesized in the seminal vesicle (SV), an unpaired lobular accessory gland that empties its secretions into the caudal unpaired portion of the sperm duct (Van Den Hurk and Resink, 1992); sperm bathed in SV fluid have increased duration of motility when diluted in water, as occurs at ejaculation (Van Den Hurk *et al.*, 1987c). SV lobules contain branching tubules, lined with a secretory epithelium and separated by a complex interstitial tissue containing cells that have the ultrastructural and steroidogenic features of the interstitial (Leydig) cells of the testis (Van Den Hurk *et al.*, 1987c). Steroidogenesis in the interstitial cells, followed by glucuronidation in interstitial and epithelial cells, probably produces the steroid glucuronides present in SV fluid (Resink *et al.*, 1989b).

When ovulated, female *Clarias* tested in a two-choice maze prefer the odor of a male (visually isolated from the female) over the odor of a visually isolated female; this preference is abolished if the olfactory tracts are bilaterally sectioned (Resink *et al.*, 1987). Ovulated females also prefer intact males over males from which the SV has been removed (an operation that reduces the olfactory potency of male odor as determined by EOG recording; Resink *et al.*, 1989c) and are less attracted to intact males than to males that are castrated, an operation that increases both SV size (Resink *et al.*, 1987) and the olfactory potency of male odor (Resink *et al.*, 1989c).

These female responses to male odors are consistent with further studies showing that ovulated females are attracted to SV fluid and to SV fluid fractions containing steroid glucuronides, but are not attracted to fractions from which steroid glucuronides have been removed (Resink et al., 1989b). Bilateral lesion of the medial olfactory tract abolished female attraction to SV fluid fractions containing steroid glucuronides, whereas lateral olfactory lesions had no effect (Resink et al., 1989a). Interestingly, females responded in the maze only if males (visually isolated and with SVs removed) were placed in each choice chamber, suggesting cues additional to SV odors are required.

Using the same behavioral assay, Resink et al. (1989b) showed that a mixture of seven synthetic glucuronides, containing all but one (5β-androstan-$3\alpha,17\beta$-diol-11-one) of the major glucuronides in SV fluid (Schoonen et al., 1988), attracted ovulated females in a dose-dependent manner. EOG recordings (Resink et al., 1989c) indicate that only two steroids in this mixture have the olfactory potency probably required of a pheromonal steroid (5β-pregnan-$3\alpha,17\alpha$-diol-20-one-3-glucuronide, 10 pM threshold; 5β-androstan-3a,11β-diol-17-one = 11β-hydroxy-ETIO-G, 1 nM threshold). Preliminary analysis of holding water from mature males and females suggests only 5β-pregnan-$3\alpha,17\alpha$-diol-20-one-3-glucuronide is released in amounts sufficient to be detectable (Van Weerd et al., 1991).

Despite the considerable evidence that female *Clarias* respond behaviorally to steroid glucuronides released by males, many important aspects of pheromonal function in this species remain to be investigated. For example, it is not known whether the attraction response of ovulated females requires an obligate mixture or whether (as in goldfish; Sorensen et al., 1987, 1990) single compounds are effective. More generally, research has been focused on the SV as an odor source. However, evidence for a pheromone in postovulatory ovarian fluid (Resink et al., 1989d), the steroidogenic capacity of male *Clarias* skin (Ali et al., 1987), and extensive evidence for olfactory-mediated effects of adult odor on gonadal development of conspecifics (Van Weerd and Richter, 1991) all suggest additional sources and functions of pheromones in this species. EOG studies, which so far have been used only to determine olfactory potency of steroid glucuronides in SV fluid (Resink et al., 1989c), could readily be used to determine whether *Clarias* detects other conjugated steroids, free steroids, or PGs.

2. Other Siluriforms

Considering their ecological and economic importance, and the fact that catfish have become a model species for olfactory research (Sorensen and Caprio, 1997), it is unfortunate that little is known about the hormonal pheromones of species other than *Clarias*. In preliminary EOG studies of catfish species from Africa (several *Synodontis* spp.; Family Mochokidae) and South America (*Hypostomus* sp., Family Loricariidae; *Pimelodella picta* and *Pseudoplatystoma corruscans*, Family Pimelodidae), we find that all are sensitive to F2-series prostaglandins and one or more unconjugated steroids. However, it is unknown what functions these hormonal odorants might mediate and whether detection of hormonal products occurs in the other 30 families of siluriforms.

G. Salmonid Fishes (Order Salmoniformes; Family Salmonidae)

Although the salmonids are a relatively small taxon (approximately 70 species in 11 genera), they have attracted much attention due to their dramatic migratory life history and commercial importance. The salmonids include three subfamilies: Salmoninae (salmon and trout; approximately 30 species in seven genera); Coregoninae (whitefish); and Thymallinae (grayling). With the exception of a single EOG study (Hara and Zhang, 1997) showing that lake whitefish (*Coregonus clupeaformis*) detect F prostaglandins, all evidence for hormonal pheromones comes from studies of three salmonin genera (*Salmo, Salvelinus,* and *Oncorhynchus*). Unfortunately, pheromone research effort devoted to the Salmoninae has been spread across many taxa, with the result that a coherent story has yet to emerge for any one species, and that novel and potentially important findings await replication. We organize our review of the salmonids around genera and stimulus types, a scheme that has proven appropriate for the cypriniforms, which show little variation among congeners.

1. Genus Salmo

Although a great deal of the evidence for hormonal pheromones in salmonids comes from a *Salmo* species, the Atlantic salmon (*S. salar*), there are data for only one other congener, the closely related brown trout (*S. trutta*), with which *S. salar* will hybridize (Hurrell and Price, 1991). Male Atlantic salmon often mature precociously as parr (Beall and de Gaudemar, 1999), a life-history stage that has served as a model for pheromone studies. Yet to be addressed is whether such precocious maturity influences olfactory or endocrine function in any special manner. Nevertheless, endocrine, EOG, and behavioral studies indicate that precociously mature males use both steroids and prostaglandins as sex pheromones and also describe two aspects of hormonal pheromone function not observed in any other species: (1) rapid seasonal changes in olfactory responsiveness to a steroid (Moore, 1991), and (2) rapid urine-induced increase in olfactory responsiveness to a steroid (Moore and Scott, 1992). Key aspects of studies describing these phenomena are reviewed here in the context of the four odor cues identified for this group.

a) Urine Several studies have now shown that exposure to urine from male and ovulated female Atlantic salmon increases milt volume and plasma concentrations of GTH II, 17,20β-P, and T in male parr (Waring and Moore, 1995; Waring et al., 1996). Mature male brown trout have also been found to exhibit GTH II and milt increases when exposed to urine from either brown trout or Atlantic salmon (Olsen et al., 2000). This apparent lack of pheromonal species-specificity is consistent with observations of hybridization between these closely related species that normally segregate temporally. Evidence now exists that PG might be an active component of urinary cues for both Atlantic salmon and brown trout (see Section IV.G.1.d). Somewhat less clear is the role of sex steroids.

b) Testosterone Moore and Scott (1991) report that, as measured by EOG recording, the olfactory system of hatchery-raised, precociously mature male Atlantic salmon parr is extremely sensitive to T, but not to a variety of other 18-, 19-, or 21-carbon steroids. They also report that olfactory sensitivity to T changes near the time of spawning; prior to spermiation, fish did not detect T, but when they were spermiated their olfactory system became extremely sensitive and then declined in sensitivity rapidly afterward. Another EOG study of the olfactory sensitivity of Atlantic salmon parr reports that sensitivity to T is altered by exposure to extreme pH, but the study does not reexamine the effects of season (Moore, 1994). In a related report, Moore (1991) states that spermiated male parr are attracted to waterborne T, but details of this study have never been presented. Waring et al. (1996) report that exposure to T did not effect milt volume or hormone concentrations and present no new behavioral data. Although both sexes of Atlantic salmon have high titers of circulating T (Stuart-Kregor et al., 1981; So et al., 1985), T concentration in urine is low (3–4 ng/ml), equivalent in mature males and females and in ovulated females (Moore and Waring, 1996). Although urinary T-G is greatly increased in ovulated females (>100 ng/ml; Moore and Waring, 1996), Atlantic salmon parr do not detect this conjugate (Moore and Scott, 1992).

Unlike Atlantic salmon, male brown trout have consistently been found not to detect T using EOG recording, even when they are treated with androgens (Essington and Sorensen, 1996) or captured while on spawning redds and fully spermiated (P. W. Sorensen and K. H. Olsen, unpublished). Using a membrane-binding assay, Pottinger and Moore (1997) report the presence of low-capacity high-affinity T binding sites in the olfactory epithelia of brown trout; however, both male and female trout have equivalent levels, and similar binding activity is also seen in the brain of both male and female rainbow trout (see later). Regrettably, the mechanism regulating the brief window of EOG sensitivity to T in Atlantic salmon parr therefore remains enigmatic. Moreover, such a dramatic change in olfactory responsiveness is in marked contrast to the situation in several cyprinids, in which steroid-induced EOG responses of juvenile and mature fish differ only slightly (Irvine and Sorensen, 1993) or are equivalent (Cardwell et al., 1995). However, studies of parr–smolt transformation in *S. salar* (Morin et al., 1997) have found modest changes in EOG responses to L-alanine.

c) 17,20β-P-Sulfate In another EOG study, Moore and Scott (1992) report that the olfactory epithelium of mature male Atlantic salmon parr becomes extremely sensitive to 17,20β-P-S immediately following brief exposure to female urine. Remarkably, although the fish were totally insensitive to this steroid prior to urine exposure, only a 5-second exposure to a 1:100,000 dilution of ovulatory urine was sufficient to sensitize their epithelia to the extent that large responses to 17,20β-P-S were seen down to a detection threshold of approximately 1 pM (Moore and Scott, 1992). Some responses to other stimuli such as T and T-S were also reported in sensitized epithelia, but details are lacking. Only urine from ovulated fish evoked this response (but only one urine sample was tested), and sensitization persisted for up to 48 hours in the five parr tested. There is no precedent in the olfactory literature for such a rapid sensitization of the olfactory epithelium in any vertebrate, and the authors do not present a physiological explanation for their observations. Further, although 17,20β-P-S is in high concentration (>100 ng/ml) in urine of ovulated Atlantic salmon (Moore and Waring, 1996), its pheromonal function remains unknown. Although 17,20β-P-S exposure occasionally elicits increases in plasma GTH II in mature male parr, it has not been found to affect milt volume or plasma steroid concentrations (Waring and Moore, 1995; Waring et al., 1996).

In marked contrast to Moore and Scott (1992), Sorensen and colleagues (Essington and Sorensen, 1996; P. W. Sorensen and K. H. Olsen, unpublished) have been unable to measure any olfactory responses to 17,20β-P-S using EOG recording in either mature male Atlantic salmon parr or brown trout. In three separate attempts using small groups of androgen-treated brown trout, sexually mature brown trout collected during the act of spawning, and precociously mature Atlantic salmon parr, we have failed to measure EOG responses to even 10 nM concentrations of 17,20β-P-S, 17,20β-P, T, or T-S, either before or after exposure to various urines from both male and ovulated female salmon, as well as ovulatory fluid. We have, however, consistently been able to record EOG responses to other nonpheromonal stimuli such as amino acids and bile acids (Essington and Sorensen, 1996). EOG responses to urine itself have been confirmed, however.

d) Prostaglandins Moore and Waring (1996) propose that the endocrine priming action of urine from ovulated females is induced by urinary PGs. Using EOG recording, they have discovered that precociously mature Atlantic salmon parr are somewhat sensitive (10 nM threshold) to 15K-PGF2α and highly sensitive to PGF2α and PGF1α (Moore and Waring, 1995), the latter acting through a common receptor mechanism (Moore and Waring, 1996). Interestingly, their data suggested that EOG sensitivity to PGs appeared to peak dramatically during the spawning season. Hara and Zhang (1997) have confirmed that immature brown trout detect these compounds as well. The analysis of female salmon urine shows it contains moderate levels of immunoreactive PGFs (Moore and Waring, 1996). Finally, Moore and Waring have shown that mature male Atlantic salmon parr exposed to 0.1 nM PGF2α or PGF1α increase plasma GTH II, androgens, and 17,20β-P, the same suite of endocrine responses induced by exposure to urine from ovulated females. These PG-mediated endocrine responses are blocked by exposure to the carbamate pesticide, carbofuran, which reduces olfactory responsiveness to PGF2α (Waring and Moore, 1997). Together, these findings suggest that PGs originating from ovulated females can function as pheromones with endocrine actions in this species. It is important to note that a biochemical characterization of PG metabolism has yet to be accomplished for any salmonid.

Brown trout also appear to employ PGFs as pheromones. EOG recordings show brown trout are highly sensitive to both PGF2α and PGF1α, although no evidence of any sexual dimorphism or seasonal effect has been noted (Essington and Sorensen, 1996; Hara and Zhang, 1997; P. W. Sorensen and K. H. Olsen, unpublished). Similarly, Olsen et al. (2000) have found that exposing male brown trout to PGF2α stimulates GTH II release and milt production. Considering that the spawning habits of brown trout and Atlantic salmon are extremely similar, it is curious that brown trout do not exhibit the seasonal changes in olfactory sensitivity to PGs described in Atlantic salmon. Yet to be determined for any *Salmo* is the biochemical identity of the urinary pheromone, the PGs it contains, and the biological significance of the proposed PG pheromone, which must function in the fast-flowing waters these species inhabit.

2. Genus Salvelinus

EOG recordings show that PGF2α is detected by the olfactory system of arctic char (*Salvelinus alpinus*), lake char (*S. namaycush*), and brook char (*S. fontinalis*) (Essington and Sorensen, 1996; Sveinsson and Hara, 2000; Hara and Zhang, 1997). As for *Salmo* sp., all *Salvelinus* species examined also appear somewhat sensitive to PGF1α. With the possible exception of ETIO-G, which is detected by all salmonids tested (Essington and Sorensen 1996; Hara and Zhang, 1997) and T-G in brook char (Essington and Sorensen, 1996), chars have not been found to detect any sex steroids or their metabolites. In striking contrast to the Atlantic salmon, EOG responsiveness to PGF2α does not appear to be influenced by gender or maturational state in arctic char (Sveinsson and Hara, 2000) or brook char (Essington and Sorensen, 1996).

Using a combination of behavioral studies and immunoassay, Sveinsson and Hara (1995), demonstrate that male arctic char release immunoreactive PGFs to the water and that these compounds can attract ovulated females—a scenario dramatically different than that proposed for *Salmo*. Such differences between these genera are very surprising given the nearly identical reproductive biology and endocrinology of these groups and the fact that brook char and brown trout will freely hybridize when give the opportunity (Sorensen *et al.*, 1995c).

3. Genus Oncorhynchus

One of the first examples of sex pheromone function in a salmonid fish was the finding (Emanuel and Dodson, 1979) that female rainbow trout (*Oncorhynchus mykiss*) release sexual attractants in their urine. Nonetheless, the identities of the pheromonal cues used by this important salmonid genus remain enigmatic (Olsen and Liley, 1993). Although an early report by Pottinger and Moore (1997) found both that immature rainbow trout detect T, as measured by EOG recording, and that their epithelia possess a small number of high-affinity membrane-binding sites for T, this work has yet to be confirmed. Indeed, in contrast to *Salmo* and *Salvelinus* species, several EOG studies of *Oncorhynchus* species have consistently failed to detect responses to tested prostaglandins and sex steroids (with the exception of ETIO-G, already mentioned)—rainbow trout (Kitamura *et al.*, 1994b; Hara and Zhang, 1997; P. W. Sorensen, unpublished results), amago salmon (*O. rhodurus*; Kitamura *et al.*, 1994b), and mature male chinook salmon (*O. tshawytscha*; A. H. Dittman and P. W. Sorensen, unpublished results). Thus, despite the facts that urine from ovulated rainbow trout exerts a rapid and consistent endocrine priming effect on males (Scott *et al.*, 1994; Vermeirssen *et al.*, 1995) and the urine from ovulated masu salmon (*O. masou*) contains high concentration of PGF2α (Yambe *et al.*, 1999), it seems unlikely that PGF2α is an active priming component of ovulated trout urine. In fact, Yambe *et al.* (1999) present evidence that a urinary pheromone employed by masu salmon does not have the chemical characteristics of known sex steroids or PGs. Also puzzling is Dittman and Quinn's (1994) observation that chinook salmon are repelled by 17,20β-P because the olfactory system of this species does not detect this steroid (A. H. Dittman and P. W. Sorensen, unpublished results). It is likely, as Yambe *et al.* (1999) speculate, that this group of fishes employs novel hormonal products that have not been identified.

4. Conclusions

Although there is now a great deal of evidence that various salmonid species employ hormonal products as sex pheromones, a lack of clear, consistent and comparative studies appears to have lead to a rather unfocused story that is difficult to understand. However, it does appear that PGs have a role in urinary pheromones in both *Salmo* and *Salvelinus* and that this function is different from that in *Oncorhynchus* and other fish such as goldfish. Much less clear is the possible role of sex steroids as pheromones and the possibility that peripheral olfactory function varies with endocrine state in this group. Detailed studies that include biochemical fractionation of crude body odors, electrophysiological techniques with greater power than EOG, and controlled behavioral assays in natural settings are urgently needed to resolve these important and fascinating problems.

H. Order Perciformes

The systematic relationships of the perciform fishes is unresolved (Johnson and Patterson, 1993); however, the more than 9000 species recognized as Order Perciformes account for 40% of extant teleost fishes and constitute the most speciose of all vertebrate orders (Nelson, 1994). Perciforms are the dominant vertebrate group in the oceans and many tropical freshwaters and include many species of ecological, scientific, and economic importance—white bass and perch (*Morone* spp.; Family Moronidae), freshwater perches (*Perca* spp.; Family Percidae), porgies (*Sparus* and *Pagrus* spp.; Family Sparidae), tilapia (Family Cichlidae), wrasses (Family Labridae), mackerels and tunas (Family Scombridae), and gobies (*Gobius* and *Neogobius*; Family Gobiidae).

Considering the widespread importance of the perciform fishes, it is unfortunate that so little is known about their hormonal pheromones. Our early EOG studies (Stacey et al., 1994a), using only several dozen steroids and prostaglandins as test odors, failed to detect olfactory responses in several perciforms. However, we have reported EOG responses to steroids in the African mouthbrooding cichlid (*Haplochromis burtoni*; Family Cichlidae; Robison et al., 1998) and observed responses to steroids in several other African cichlids (N. E. Stacey and J. R. Cardwell, unpublished results) and to F2 prostaglandins in a darter (*Etheostoma* sp.; Family Percidae; N. E. Stacey, unpublished results). The round goby (*Neogobius melanostomus*) is the only perciform species in which hormonal pheromone studies have progressed beyond the preliminary stages (Murphy et al., 2001; Murphy and Stacey, 2002), although studies are in progress on the ruffe (*Gymnocephalus cernuus*; Family Percidae; e.g., Murphy et al., 2000).

1. Round Goby (Neogobius melanostomus; Family Gobiidae)

A native of the Caspian and Black Seas, the round goby (*Neogobius melanostomus*) has been introduced in ship ballast to the Great Lakes, from which it may soon spread to the Mississippi system (MacInnis and Corkum, 2000). Spawning in *Neogobius* is similar to that of many other gobiids (Miller, 1984), insofar as males establish territories, engage in visual and acoustic communication to attract females to their nest site (e.g., Moiseyeva and Rudenko, 1976), and care for single or multiple batches of eggs (MacInnis and Corkum, 2000). Given the evidence that the steroid ETIO-G has pheromonal function in the black goby (*G. jozo*; Colombo et al., 1980, 1982; see Section III.B.1), we used EOG recording to assess the potential use of hormonal pheromones by *Neogobius* (Murphy et al., 2001), information that might lead to development of a method of biological control for this potentially damaging exotic (e.g., MacInnis and Corkum, 2000).

In EOG recordings using a large suite of synthetic hormones at nanomolar concentrations, male and female *Neogobius* do not exhibit olfactory responses to PGs, but exhibit sexually isomorphic responses to more than a dozen free and conjugated 18-, 19- and 21-carbon steroids (including ETIO-G) (Murphy et al., 2001). EOG cross-adaptation studies (see Section III.C.3) suggest that these steroid hormonal odorants act on four classes of olfactory receptor mechanisms, termed the estrone (E_1), 17β-estradiol-3β-glucuronide (E_2-3G), etiocholanolone (ETIO), and dehydroepiandrosterone-3-sulfate (DHEA-S) classes, according to the most potent known ligand for each. The natural steroid ligands are unknown, however, because steroid release by *Neogobius* has not been studied.

Despite the clear evidence that *Neogobius* detect a number of steroidal odorants, we understand very little about the putative hormonal pheromone system of *Neogobius* because neither males nor females displayed overt reproductive behaviors when exposed to any of the detectable steroids (Murphy et al., 2001). However, when males were exposed to ETIO, E_1, or E_2-3G or when females were exposed to ETIO, the frequency of ventilation (opercular and buccal pumping) increased significantly during the first few minutes of exposure and returned to preexposure levels (i.e., adapted) within 12–15 min of constant exposure (Fig. 16). This sex dimorphism in ventilatory behavior evidently is androgen-dependent because females implanted with methyl-testosterone (MT) exhibit male-typical patterns of response within several weeks (Murphy and Stacey, 2001; see Section V).

These transient, ventilation increases induced by steroid odorants in *Neogobius* may facilitate odor detection by increasing water flow through the olfactory organ, as has been proposed in other benthic fish, such as the flounders *Lepidopsetta bilineata* and *Platichthys stellatus* (Nevitt, 1991). Regardless, such ventilation change provides a simple bioassay to determine if steroids discriminated at the sensory level (as indicated by EOG cross-adaptation studies) also are discriminated behaviorally.

For example, when they are adapted to 10 nM E_1 in their aquarium water, male round gobies do not increase ventilation if the E_1 concentration is increased by 10% (to 11 nM) (Fig. 16C) or if they are exposed to 1 nM E_2 (Fig. 16D), which EOG recordings indicate is detected by the same olfactory receptor mechanism as E_1 (Murphy et al., 2001). However, males adapted to 10 nM E_1 consistently increase ventilation when exposed to 1 nM ETIO or E_2-3G (Fig. 16E–F) which EOG recordings indicate are detected by olfactory receptor mechanisms different than that detecting E_1 (Murphy et al., 2001). Ironically, although we know nothing of

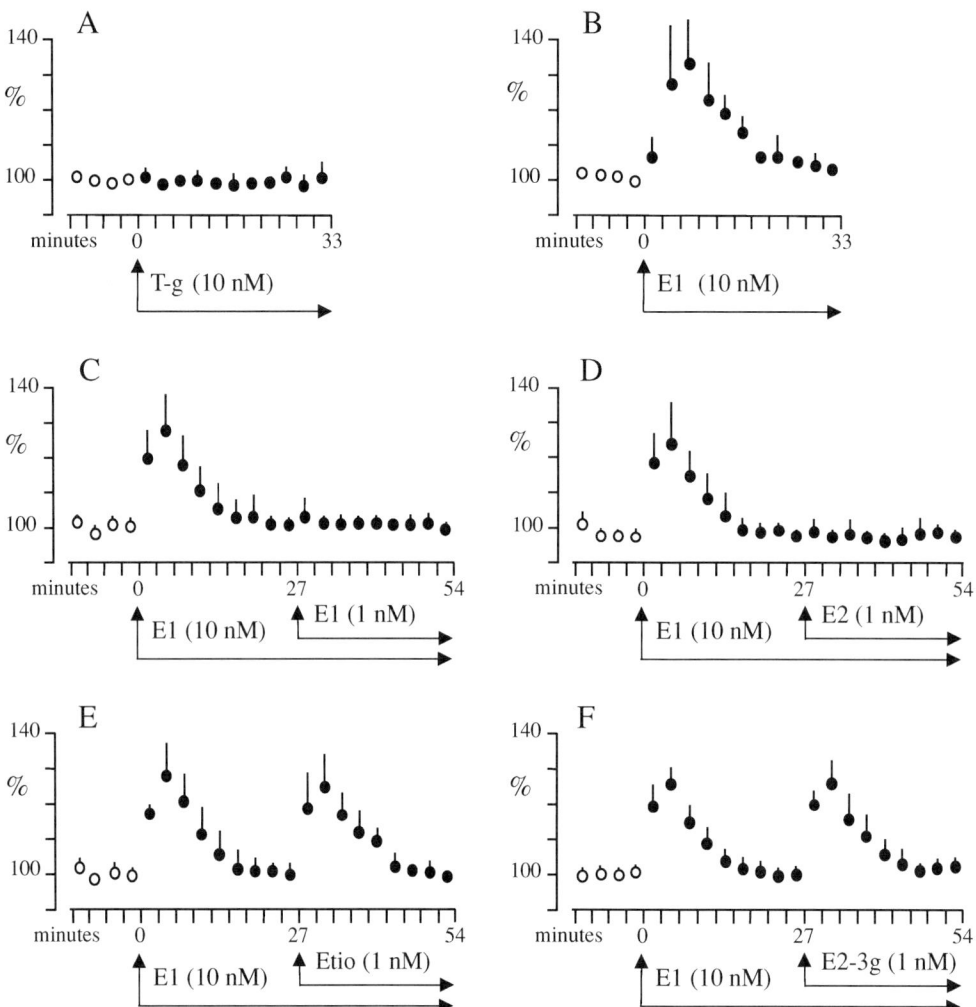

FIGURE 16 Ventilation response to steroid odorants in male round gobies (*Neogobius melanostomus*). (A) Ventilation is unaffected by exposure to testosterone glucuronide (T-G; arrow), which does not induce EOG response. (B) It increases transiently in response to estrone (E1), which does induce EOG response. (C) Once adapted to 10 nM E1, males do not respond to a 10% increase in E1. (D) Nor do this respond to exposure to 1 nM estradiol (E2D), which interacts with the same olfactory receptor mechanism as estrone (Murphy et al., 2001). E–F. In contrast, E1-adapted males respond to both etiocholanolone (Etio), estradiol-3-glucuronide (E2-3g), steroids that interact with a different olfactory receptor mechanism than E1 (Murphy et al., 2001).

the putative pheromonal functions of steroid odoants in *Neogobius*, the ventilation response to these compounds has provided the clearest evidence that EOG cross-adaptation studies can give us insight into how odor information is processed centrally.

2. Eurasian Ruffe (*Gymnocephalus cernuus*; Family Percidae)

The ruffe is a small Asian percid that has been accidently introduced into North American freshwaters, where potentially detrimental effects on native fauna have generated interest in its biology. Because both alarm and sex pheromones have been characterized in ruffe (Maniak et al., 2000; Murphy et al., 2000; P. W. Sorensen and C. A. Murphy, unpublished results), its chemical signaling system is the best understood of the percids, the dominant family of freshwater fishes in eastern North America. The ruffe's reproductive biology is quite different from that of the goby and closely resembles that of most other percids. It spawns only once in the spring, does not employ a specific spawning substrate, is sexually monomorphic, and, as with the goldfish, employs a promiscuous mating system in which males engage in scramble competition (Emlen and Oring, 1977) for access to females at the time of spawning. Although ruffe reproduction involves a hormonal pheromone system, it appears to be very different from those of the goldfish and round goby.

Behavioral bioassays using holding water clearly demonstrate that female ruffe release a behaviorally active pheromone (or pheromones) during final oocyte maturation, but cease doing so after ovulation (P. W. Sorensen and C. A. Murphy, unpublished results). Thus, despite the similar reproductive strategies of male goldfish and ruffe, male goldfish rely heavily on chemical cues (PG pheromones; Sorensen et al., 1988) to identify receptive females, whereas male ruffe evidently employ other sensory cues.

Based on our behavioral observations of ruffe (P. W. Sorensen and C. A. Murphy, unpublished results), we initially questioned whether $17,20\beta$-P or $17,20\beta,21$-P, the proposed MIS for other perciforms (e.g., spotted seatrout, *Cynoscion nebulosus*; Family Sciaenidae; Thomas and Trant, 1989) might, as in goldfish, be functioning as the ruffe preovulatory pheromone. Accordingly, we used EOG recording to test the olfactory sensitivity of male ruffe to many steroids (and PGs), including all those known to be detected by other fishes, and found that none elicited notable responses. However, EOG recordings (N. E. Stacey, unpublished results) demonstrating that PGF2α is detected by a darter (*Etheostoma* sp.; Subfamily Percinae, Tribe Etheostomatini) indicate that species closely related to ruffe (Subfamily Percinae, Tribe Percini) might employ postovulatory hormonal pheromones.

Reasoning that the ruffe preovulatory pheromone might be a novel metabolite of the MIS, we (P. W. Sorensen and C. A. Murphy, unpublished results) next injected females with $17,20\beta$-P or $17,20\beta,21$-P and found that these treatments stimulated the release of an unknown sulfated urinary pheromone. EOG screening studies have been extremely helpful in broadly characterizing the patterns of hormonal detection in many fish taxa (Stacey and Cardwell, 1995, 1997; Stacey et al., 1995). However, our experiments in ruffe (P. W. Sorensen and C. A. Murphy, unpublished results) emphasize that, because of the extreme specificity of fish hormonal pheromone receptor mechanisms, EOG screening studies can generate misleading false negatives (e.g., Section III.C.3) unless they test the natural ligand or a close mimic. For example, we would have concluded in this paper that a number of species in the cypriniform Tribe Labeonini (Section IV.D.2) detected no steroids had Scott and Canario (1992) not discovered the importance of sulfation in steroid metabolism of fishes and kindly provided us with $17,20\beta$-P-S as an EOG test odor.

I. Unidentified Pheromones in Other Fish

Many species of fish not discussed have been shown through various bioassays to exhibit reproductive responses to conspecific odors that are only partially characterized or wholly unknown (see Liley, 1982; Stacey et al., 1986). In cases in which such species do not respond to hormonal compounds in EOG recordings, however, we cannot exclude the existence of hormonal pheromones. Given the specificity of olfactory receptors that detect hormonal compounds and how little is known about hormone metabolism in fish, it is expected that the hormonal pheromones of many species are undescribed hormonal products. The ruffe (Section IV.H.2) is an excellent example. Although we expect that the vast majority of fishes employ sex pheromones and that most of these pheromones are hormonally derived, there is no reason why some sex pheromones should not contain nonhormonal compounds. Indeed, there already is evidence that this is the case in several species (Matsumura, 1985; Kawabata et al., 1992; Kawabata, 1993). In general, we believe fish evolve to employ preexisting chemicals that have biological relevance; hormonal compounds routinely fall into this category and so might other cues. It must be kept in mind that in situations in which fish use pheromones for functions other than reproduction (Liley, 1982; Solomon, 1990; Smith, 1992), the pheromones are unlikely to be hormonally derived. This being the case, the possibility of nonhormonal sex pheromones cannot be ignored.

V. HORMONAL MODULATION OF HORMONAL PHEROMONE FUNCTION

An important aspect of hormonal pheromone function is that organismal responsiveness should be restricted to appropriate reproductive stages. Although this topic has received relatively little attention, we expect that such temporal restriction of responsiveness might be achieved in three ways, which need not be mutually exclusive. First, there might be peripheral gating, whereby olfactory sensitivity is modulated by altering either the function of existing ORNs or by stimulating the development of new ORNs. Second, there might be central gating, whereby responsiveness is modulated by regulating those central mechanisms that mediate pheromone action. Third, responsiveness might be modulated in an indirect fashion by altering those behaviors that determine the likelihood of encountering pheromones. Although we are unaware of any evidence supporting the third possibility, there is some support for the possibility that androgenic hormones modulate pheromonal responsiveness through both peripheral and central actions.

The clearest evidence for androgen-mediated responsiveness of peripheral olfactory sensitivity comes from studies of the tinfoil barb (*Puntius schwanenfeldi*; Family Cyprinidae, Subfamily Systomini), in which 15K-PGF2α-induced EOG responses of wild adult males were greatest in individuals with breeding tubercles, an androgen-dependent secondary sex character (Cardwell et al., 1995). To determine if androgen mediates responsiveness to 15K-PGF2α, the most potent PGF odorant in *Puntius*, Cardwell et al. (1995) implanted unsexed juveniles (25% of pubertal weight) with MT, 11-KA, DHT, or blank pellets and found that by day 18 postimplant EOG response to 15K-PGF2α was increased in MT and 11-KA fish, but unchanged in DHT fish. This androgen effect was odor-specific, insofar as MT implant did not affect EOG responses to 17α, 21-dihydroxyprogesterone (17,21-P) or 11-KT (Fig. 17), the two steroid odorants to which *P. schwanenfeldi* is most sensitive (Cardwell et al., 1995; J. R. Cardwell, unpublished results). MT treatment of juveniles also increased sexual behaviors directed toward PGF2α-injected juvenile fish (Cardwell et al., 1995), suggesting the enhanced EOG responses were representative of increased olfactory input, although central androgen actions were probably also involved. Sorensen and Bowdin (1994) have confirmed that androgen treatment similarly sensitizes the olfactory epithelium of goldfish to PGs.

The dramatic effect of androgen on EOG response to PGs in *Puntius*, and the apparent absence of effect on EOG response to steroids, is consistent with information from other species in which PG-induced EOG responses are greater in males than in females, but gender has little if any influence on steroid-induced responses (Sorensen et al., 1987, 1990; Bjerselius and Olsen, 1993; Irvine and Sorensen, 1993; Sorensen and Goetz, 1993; Murphy et al., 2001; P. W. Sorensen and N. E. Stacey, unpublished results). Indeed, the only inconsistency in this pattern are reports that EOG responsiveness of Atlantic salmon to T is sexually dimorphic and associated with sexual maturity (Moore, 1991; Moore and Scott, 1991, 1992; see Section IV.G.1.b).

Although the etiology of androgen-induced olfactory sensitivity to PGs is unknown, several mechanisms can be postulated. New PG olfactory receptors might be expressed on existing ORNs or signal transduction mechanisms associated with existing inactive receptors might be activated. Too little is known about specific control of olfactory receptor expression or transduction to speculate about these possibilities. However, it also is possible that new ORNs might be produced in response to androgen binding in the basal cells of the olfactory epithelium. The facts that nuclear androgen receptors have been characterized in fish olfactory epithelium (Pottinger and Moore, 1997), that ORNs can regenerate in approximately 3 weeks in goldfish held at 20°C (Zippel et al., 1993), and that ORN generation might proceed more rapidly in *Puntius* held at 27°C, support this possibility.

The clearest evidence that androgens can act on central mechanisms to modulate responses to hormonal pheromones comes from studies in which the olfactory epithelia of males and females are equally sensitive to sex steroids, but only males exhibit behavioral responses. These studies used androgen-treated females as proxies for androgen-treated males, assuming that androgens induce heterotypical behavior in females through the same mechanism(s) by which they induce homotypical behavior in males. This approach is not only feasible (because of the adult sexual bipotentiality of the brain of many fish; Kobayashi et al., 2000), but attractive because testicular regeneration in fish can make castration and steroid replacement therapy impractical.

Two studies have examined the effects of androgens on central mechanisms underlying responsiveness to hormonal pheromones. The first employed goldfish. Male and female goldfish exhibit equivalent EOG responses to 17,20β-P regardless of sexual maturity (Sorensen et al., 1987). However, 17,20β-P exposure

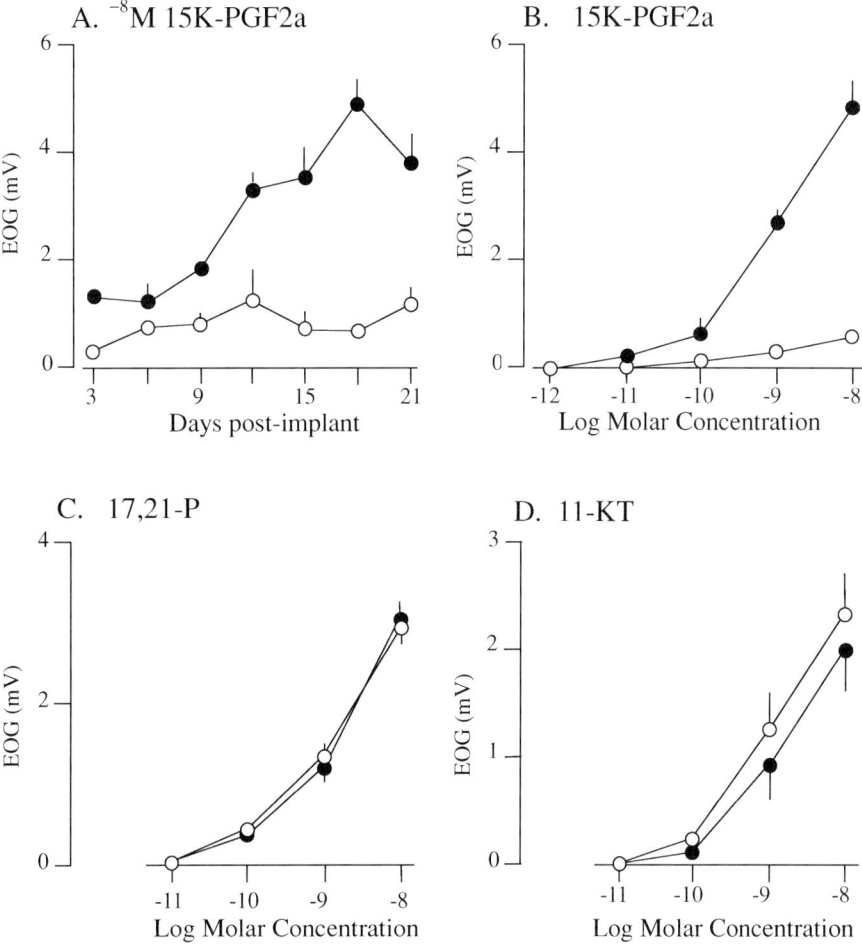

FIGURE 17 Effect of methyl-testosterone (MT) implants on EOG response to prostaglandin and steroids in juvenile *Puntius schwanenfeldi*. (A) Time course of MT-induced increase in EOG response to 10 nM 15K-PGF2α. When tested at 18 days postimplant. (B) EOG responsiveness to 15K-PGF2α is increased, whereas (C) responsiveness to 17α,21-dihydroxy-progesterone (17,21-P) and (D) 11-ketotestosterone (11-KT) is unaffected. Open circles, control bees way pellets; closed circles, MT-containing pellets. From Cardwell et al. (1995), *J. Comp. Physiol. A* **176**, 55–61, © 1995 Springer-Verlag, with permission.

induces different endocrine responses in males and females. Whereas males respond with GTH II increases at all times of day (Dulka et al., 1987b), females appear to respond only at night (Sorensen and Stacey, 1987). Further, females implanted with 11-KT respond to this pheromone in a male-typical manner, suggesting that this androgen acts through a central mechanism(s) (Kobayashi et al., 1997b). In the second study, using round gobies (*Neogobius melanostomus*), it has been found that although the olfactory epithelia of male and female detect sex steroids equally well, only males respond behaviorally to the three sex steroids assayed by Murphy et al. (2001; see Section IV.H.1). Further, male-typical behavioral responsiveness can be induced in females within just 2 weeks by implanting them with MT (Murphy and Stacey, 2002). Exactly where androgens exert their effects on either the goldfish or goby have not been examined.

VI. SUMMARY

Although it has been clear since the early 1900s that fish commonly use chemical signals to coordinate many aspects of their reproductive behavior, it was not until the 1970s that anyone imagined either the significance of these cues or that they might be hormonal products (Doving, 1976; Colombo et al., 1980). The field has progressed rapidly since that time, with five hormonal pheromones being extensively characterized for the goldfish and others being clearly demonstrated in approximately half a dozen other species of fish. In addition, because the majority of the nearly 200 species of fish tested for olfactory sensitivity to hormones respond to at least one, it is reasonable to expect that the vast majority of fish possess hormonal pheromone systems and that the functions of many of these systems differ greatly from the very few we know. Despite this progress, only in the goldfish are we moving toward a rudimentary understanding of a species' hormonal pheromones that encompasses their gonadal origins, biochemical identities, olfactory potencies and specificities, and biological activities. Nevertheless, it is reassuring that many key elements of the goldfish story have now been replicated in the goldfish and closely related species and that, by most measures, the goldfish is an appropriate model for further study.

The study of fish hormonal pheromones is fascinating and relevant for many reasons. An understanding of these cues is only now providing valuable insight into how internal and external chemical signaling systems have coevolved and interact to coordinate reproduction functions in and among individuals. Further, at least in goldfish, the study of hormonal pheromones has established them as new and powerful tools for deciphering not only how the olfactory system encodes odor information, but also how the brain regulates important behavioral and neuroendocrinological function. They also provide unique opportunities to address how vertebrate endocrine function can influence basic neural function. Identified hormonal pheromones also have clear potential to function as tools to unlock many of the mysteries surrounding olfactory and endocrine receptor function and identity. Finally, it is important to recognize that hormonal pheromones probably serve as signals essential to the lives of many commercially and ecologically important fishes and that these systems need to be understood if we are to protect the world's fishes from pollutants, overexploitation, and ecosystem degradation.

Acknowledgments

Norm Stacey gratefully acknowledges many years of support from the Natural Sciences and Engineering Research Council of Canada (N.S.E.R.C.). Peter Sorensen thanks the Alberta Heritage Foundation for Medical Research (the first funding agency to gamble on this topic), the Minnesota Agricultural Experiment Station, Minnesota Sea Grant, the National Institutes of Health (NIH/DC03792), and the National Science Foundation (NSF/IBN9723798), all of which have generously supported research on fish hormonal pheromones over the past 2 decades.

References

Adams, M. E., Teeter, J. A., Katz, Y., and Johnsen, P. B. (1987). Sex pheromones of the sea lamprey (*Petromyzon marinus*): Steroid studies. *J. Chem. Ecol.* **13**, 387–395.

Ali, S. A., Schoonen, W. G. E. J., Lambert, J. G. D., Van Den Hurk, R., and Van Oordt, P. G. W. J. (1987). The skin of the male African catfish, *Clarias gariepinus*: A source of steroid glucuronides. *Gen. Comp. Endocrinol.* **66**, 415–424.

Amouriq, L. (1965). Origine de la substance dynamogene emise par *Lebistes reticulatus* femelle (Poisson Poeciliidae, Cyprinodontiformes). *C. R. Hebd. Seances Acad. Sci.* **260**, 2334–2335.

Antonopoulou, E., Swanson, P., Mayer, I., and Borg, B. (1999). Feedback control of gonadotropins in Atlantic salmon, *Salmo salar*, male parr. *Gen. Comp. Endocrinol.* **114**, 142–150.

Appelt, C. W., Sorensen, P. W., and Kellner, R. G. (1995). Female goldfish appear to release pheromonally active F-prostaglandins in urinary pulses. In "Proceedings of the Fifth International Symposium on the Reproductive Physiology of Fish" (F. W. Goetz and P. Thomas, eds.). Fish Symp. 95, p. 270. University of Texas at Austin.

Appelt, C. W., and Sorensen, P. W. (1999). Freshwater fish release urinary pheromones in a pulsatile manner. In "Advances in Chemical Signals in Vertebrates" (R. E. Johnston, D. Müller-Schwarze, and P. W. Sorensen, eds.), pp. 247–256. Kluwer Academic/Plenum Press, New York.

Aranada, R. C., Kini, A. D., and Firestein, S. (2000). The molecular receptive range of an odorant receptor. *Nat. Neurosci.* **3**, 1248–1255.

Asahina, K., Suzuki, K., Hibiya, T., and Tamaoki, B. (1989). Structure and steroidogenic enzymes of the seminal vesicles of the urohaze-goby (*Glossogobius olivaceus*). *Gen. Comp. Endocrinol.* **74**, 385–391.

Baird, R. C., Jumper, G. Y., and Gallaher, E. E. (1990). Sexual dimorphism and demography in two species of oceanic midwater fishes (Stomiiformes: Sternoptychidae) from the eastern Gulf of Mexico. *Bull. Mar. Sci.* **47**, 561–566.

Baird, R. C., Johari, H., and Jumper, G. Y. (1996). Numerical simulation of environmental modulation of chemical signal structure and odor dispersal in the open ocean. *Chem. Senses* **21**, 121–134.

Barry, T. P., Santos, A. J. G., Furukawa, K., Aida, K., and Hanyu, I. (1990). Steroid profiles during spawning in male common carp. *Gen. Comp. Endocrinol.* **80**, 223–231.

Bass, A. H. (1993). From brains to behavior: Hormonal cascades and alternative mating tactics. *Rev. Fish Biol. Fish.* **3**, 181–186.

Beall, E., and de Gaudemar, B. (1999). Plasticity of reproductive behaviour in Atlantic salmon *Salmo salar* (Salmonidae) in relation to environmental factors. *Cybium* **23**, 9–28.

Bethe, A. (1932). Vernachlassigte hormone. *Naturewissenschaften* **20**, 177–181.

Bjerselius, R., and Olsen, K. H. (1993). A study of the olfactory sensitivity of crucian carp (*Carassius carassius*) and goldfish (*Carassius auratus*) to $17\alpha,20\beta$-dihydroxyprogesterone and prostaglandin F2α. *Chem. Senses* **18**, 427–436.

Bjerselius, R., Sorensen, P. W., and Li, W. (1995a). Spermiated sea lamprey release a potent sex pheromone. *In* "Proceedings of the Fifth International Symposium on the Reproductive Physiology of Fish" (F. W. Goetz and P. Thomas, eds.), Fish Symp. 95, p. 271. University of Texas at Austin.

Bjerselius, R., Olsen, K. H., and Zheng, W. (1995b). Endocrine, gonadal and behavioral responses of male crucian carp (*Carassius carassius*) to the hormonal pheromone $17\alpha,20\beta$-dihydroxy-4-pregnen-3-one. *Chem. Senses* **20**, 221–230.

Bjerselius, R., Olsen, K. H., and Zheng, W. B. (1995c). Behavioral and endocrinological responses of mature male goldfish to the sex pheromone $17\alpha,20\beta$-dihydroxy-4-pregnen-3-one. *J. Exp. Biol.* **198**, 747–754.

Bjerselius, R., Li, W., Teeter, J. H., Seelye, J. G., Johnsen, P. B., Maniak, P. J., Grant, G. C., Polkinghorne, C. N., and Sorenson, P. W. (2000). Direct behavioural evidence that unique bile acids released by larval sea lamprey (*Petromyzon marinus*) function as a migratory pheromone. *Can. J. Fish. Aquat. Sci.* **57**, 557–569.

Borg, B. (1994). Androgens in teleost fishes. *Comp. Biochem. Physiol. C* **109**, 219–245.

Borg, B., and Mayer, I. (1995). Androgens and behaviour in the three-spined stickleback. *Behaviour* **132**, 1025–1036.

Borg, B., Antonopoulou, E., Andersson, E., Carlberg, T., and Mayer, I. (1993). Effectiveness of several androgens in stimulating kidney hypertrophy, a secondary sexual character, in castrated male threespine stickleback, *Gasterosteus aculeatus*. *Can. J. Zool.* **71**, 2327–2329.

Brantley, R. K., Wingfield, J. C., and Bass, A. H. (1993). Sex steroid levels in *Porichthys notatus*, a fish with alternative reproductive tactics, and a review of the basis for male dimorphism among teleost fishes. *Horm. Behav.* **27**, 332–347.

Buck, L. B. (1996). Information coding in the vertebrate olfactory system. *Annu. Rev. Neurosci.* **19**, 517–544.

Buck, L., and Axel, R. (1991). A novel, multigene family may encode odorant receptors: A molecular basis for odor recognition. *Cell (Cambridge, Mass.)* **65**, 171–187.

Cao, Y., Oh, B. C., and Stryer, L. (1998). Cloning and localization of two multigene receptor families in goldfish olfactory epithelium. *Proc. Natl. Acad. Sci. U.S.A.* **95**, 11987–11992.

Caprio, J., and Byrd, R. P., Jr. (1984). Electrophysiological evidence for acidic, basic, and neutral amino acid olfactory receptor sites in catfish. *J. Gen. Physiol.* **84**, 403–422.

Cardwell, J. R., and Liley, N. R. (1991). Androgen control of social status in males of a wild population of stoplight parrotfish, *Sparisoma viride* (Scaridae). *Horm. Behav.* **25**, 1–18.

Cardwell, J. R., and Stacey, N. E. (1995). Hormonal sex pheromones in characiform fishes: An evolutionary case study. *In* "Fish Pheromones: Origins and Modes of Action" (A. V. M. Canario and D. M. Power, eds.), pp. 47–55. University of Algarve Press, Faro, Portugal.

Cardwell, J. R., Dulka, J. G., and Stacey, N. E. (1992). Acute olfactory sensitivity to prostaglandins but not to gonadal steroids in two sympatric species of *Catostomus* (Pisces: Cypriniformes). *Can. J. Zool.* **70**, 1897–1903.

Cardwell, J. R., Stacey, N. E., Tan, E. S. P., McAdam, D. S. O., and Lang, S. L. C. (1995). Androgen increases olfactory receptor response to a vertebrate sex pheromone. *J. Comp. Physiol. A* **176**, 55–61.

Cardwell, J. R., Sorensen, P. W., Van Der Kraak, G. J., and Liley, N. R. (1996). Effect of dominance status on sex hormone levels in laboratory and wild spawning male trout. *Gen. Comp. Endocrinol.* **101**, 333–341.

Carolsfeld, J., Sherwood, N. M., Kyle, A. L., Magnus, T. H., Pleasance, S., and Kreiberg, H. (1992). Characterization of a spawning pheromone from Pacific herring. *In* "Chemical Signals in Vertebrates" (R. L. Doty and D. Müller-Schwarze, eds.), Vol. 6, pp. 343–348. Plenum Press, New York.

Carolsfeld, J., Tester, M., Kreiberg, H., and Sherwood, N. M. (1997a). Pheromone-induced spawning of Pacific herring: I. Behavioral characterization. *Horm. Behav.* **31**, 256–268.

Carolsfeld, J., Scott, A. P., and Sherwood, N. M. (1997b). Pheromone-induced spawning of Pacific herring. 2. Plasma steroids distinctive to fish responsive to spawning pheromone. *Horm. Behav.* **31**, 269–276.

Carr, W. E. S. (1988). The molecular nature of chemical stimuli in the aquatic environment. *In* "Sensory Biology of Aquatic Animals" (J. Atema, R. R. Fay, A. N. Popper, and W. Tavolga, eds.), pp. 3–27. Springer-Verlag, New York.

Cole, K. S., and Stacey, N. E. (1984). Prostaglandin induction of female spawning behavior in *Cichlosoma bimaculatum* (Pisces, Cichlidae). *Horm. Behav.* **18**, 235–248.

Colombo, L., Belvedere, P. C., and Pilati, A. (1977). Biosynthesis of free and conjugated 5β-reduced androgens by the testis of the black goby, *Gobius jozo* L. *Boll. Zool.* **44**, 131–144.

Colombo, L., Marconato, A., Belvedere, P. C., and Frisco, C. (1980). Endocrinology of teleost reproduction: A testicular steroid pheromone in the black goby, *Gobius jozo* L. *Boll. Zool.* **47**, 355–364.

Colombo, L., Belvedere, P. C., Marconato, A., and Bentivegna, F. (1982). Endocrinology of teleost reproduction. In "Proceedings of the Second International Symposium on the Reproductive Physiology of Fish" (C. J. J. Richter and H. J. T. Goos, eds.), pp. 84–94. Pudoc, The Netherlands.

Crow, R. T., and Liley, N. R. (1979). A sexual pheromone in the guppy, *Poecilia reticulata* (Peters). *Can. J. Zool.* **57**, 184–188.

Curtis, B. J., and Wood, C. M. (1991). The function of the urinary bladder *in vivo* in the freshwater rainbow trout. *J. Exp. Biol.* **155**, 567–583.

Darwin, C. (1887). "The Descent of Man and Selection in Relation to Sex," 2nd rev. ed. John Murray, London.

DeFraipont, M., and Sorensen, P. W. (1993). Exposure to the pheromone 17α,20β-dihydroxy-4-pregnen-3-one enhances the behavioral spawning success, sperm production, and sperm motility of male goldfish. *Anim. Behav.* **46**, 245–256.

Demski, L. S. (1993). Terminal nerve complex. *Acta. Anat.* **148**, 81–95.

Demski, L. S., and Dulka, J. G. (1984). Functional-anatomical studies on sperm release evoked by electrical stimulation of the olfactory tract in goldfish. *Brain Res.* **291**, 241–247.

Demski, L. S., and Northcutt, R. G. (1983). The terminal nerve: A new chemosensory system in the vertebrates. *Science* **202**, 435–437.

Dittman, A. H., and Quinn, T. P. (1994). Avoidance of a putative pheromone, 17α,20β-dihydroxy-4-pregnen-3-one, by precociously mature chinook salmon (*Oncorhynchus tshawytscha*). *Can. J. Zool.* **72**, 215–219.

Dorries, K. M. (1992). Sex differences in olfaction in mammals. In "The Science of Olfaction" (M. Serby and K. Chobor, eds.), pp. 245–253. Springer, New York.

Dorries, K. M., Adkins-Regan, E., and Halpern, B. P. (1997). Sensitivity and behavioral responses to the pheromone androstenone are not mediated by the vomeronasal organ in domestic pigs. *Brain, Behav. Evol.* **49**, 53–62.

Doving, K. (1976). Evolutionary trends in olfaction. In "The Structure-Activity Relationships in Olfaction" (G. Benz, ed.), pp. 149–159. IRL Press, London.

Doving, K. B., and Selset, R. (1980). Behavior patterns in cod released by electrical stimulation of olfactory tract bundlets. *Science* **207**, 559–560.

Dryer, L., and Berghard, A. (1999). Odorant receptors: A plethora of G-protein-coupled receptors. *Trends Pharmacol. Sci.* **20**, 413–417.

Dulka, J. G. (1993). Sex pheromone systems in goldfish: Comparisons to vomeronasal systems in tetrapods. *Brain, Behav. Evol.* **42**, 265–280.

Dulka, J. G., and Demski, L. S. (1986). Sperm duct contractions mediate centrally evoked sperm release in goldfish. *J. Exp. Zool.* **237**, 271–279.

Dulka, J. G., and Stacey, N. E. (1991). Effects of olfactory tract lesions on gonadotropin and milt responses to the female sex pheromone, 17α,20β-dihydroxy-4-pregnen-3-one, in male goldfish. *J. Exp. Zool.* **257**, 223–229.

Dulka, J. G., Stacey, N. E., Sorensen, P. W., and Van Der Kraak, G. J. (1987a). A sex steroid pheromone synchronizes male-female spawning readiness in goldfish. *Nature (London)* **325**, 251–253.

Dulka, J. G., Sorensen, P. W., and Stacey, N. E. (1987b). Socially-stimulated gonadotropin release in male goldfish: Differential circadian sensitivities to a steroid pheromone and spawning stimuli. In "Proceedings of the Third International Symposium on the Reproductive Physiology of Fish" (D. R. Idler, L. W. Crim, and J. M. Walsh, eds.), p. 160. Memorial University Press, St. John's, Newfoundland.

Dulka, J. G., Sloley, B. D., Stacey, N. E., and Peter, R. E. (1992). A reduction in pituitary dopamine turnover is associated with sex pheromone-induced gonadotropin increase in goldfish. *Gen. Comp. Endocrinol.* **86**, 496–505.

Eisthen, H. L. (1992). Phylogeny of the vomeronasal system and of receptor cell types in the olfactory and vomeronasal epithelia of vertebrates. *Microsc. Res. Tech.* **23**, 1–21.

Eisthen, H. L., and Northcutt, R. G. (1996). Silver lampreys (*Ichthyomyzon unicuspis*) lack a gonadotropin-releasing hormone- and FMRF amide-immunoreactive terminal nerve. *J. Comp. Neurol.* **370**, 159–172.

Eisthen, H. L., Delay, R. J., Wirsig-Wiechmann, C. R., and Dionne, V. E. (2000). Neuromodulatory effects of gonadotropin releasing hormone on olfactory receptor neurons. *J. Neurosci.* **20**, 3947–3955.

Emanuel, M. E., and Dodson, J. J. (1979). Modification of the rheotropic behavior of male rainbow trout (*Salmo gairdneri*) by ovarian fluid. *J. Fish. Res. Board Can.* **36**, 63–68.

Emlen, S. T., and Oring, L. W. (1977). Ecology, sexual selection, and the evolution of mating systems. *Science* **197**, 215–223.

Essington, T. E., and Sorensen, P. W. (1996). Overlapping sensitivities of brook trout and brown trout to putative hormonal pheromones. *J. Fish Biol.* **48**, 1027–1029.

Fishelson, L. (1991). Comparative cytology and morphology of seminal vesicles in male gobiid fishes. *Jpn. J. Ichthyol.* **38**, 17–30.

Fitzpatrick, M. S., Gale, W. L., and Schreck, C. B. (1994). Binding characteristics of an androgen receptor in the ovaries of coho salmon, *Oncorhynchus kisutch*. *Gen. Comp. Endocrinol.* **95**, 399–408.

Fostier, A., Jalabert, B., Billard, R., Breton, B., and Zohar, Y. (1983). The gonadal steroids. *Fish Physiol.* **9A**, 277–372.

Friedrich, R. W., and Korsching, S. I. (1997). Combinatorial and chemotopic odorant coding in the zebrafish olfactory bulb visualized by optical imaging. *Neuron* **18**, 737–752.

Freidrich, R. W., and Korsching, S. I. (1998). Chemotopic, combinatorial, and noncombinatorial odorant representations in the olfactory bulb revealed using a voltage-sensitive axon tracer. *J. Neurosci.* **18**, 9977–9988.

Fujita, I., Sorensen, P. W., Stacey, N. E., and Hara, T. J. (1991). The olfactory system, not the terminal nerve, functions as the primary chemosensory pathway mediating responses to sex pheromones in goldfish. *Brain, Behav. Evol.* **38**, 313–321.

Gelinas, D., and Callard, G. (1997). Immunolocalization of aromatase- and androgen receptor-positive neurons in the goldfish brain. *Gen. Comp. Endocrinol.* **106**, 155–168.

Goetz, F. W., and Garczynski, M. (1997). The ovarian regulation of ovulation in teleost fish. *Fish Physiol. Biochem.* **17**, 33–38.

Hamdani, E.-H., Stabell, O. B., Alexander, G., and Doving, K. B. (2000). Alarm reaction in the Crucian carp is mediated by the medial bundle of the medial olfactory tract. *Chem. Senses* **25**, 103–109.

Hansen, A., and Zeiske, E. (1998). The peripheral olfactory organ of the zebrafish, *Danio rerio*: An ultrastructural study. *Chem. Senses* **23**, 39–48.

Hansen, A., Zippel, H. P., Sorensen, P. W., and Caprio, J. (1999). Ultrastructure of the olfactory epithelium in intact, axotomized, and bulbectomized goldfish, *Carassius auratus*. *Microsc. Res. Tech.* **45**, 325–338.

Hanson, L. R. (2001). Neural coding of identified sex pheormones in the goldfish, *Carassius auratus*. Ph.D. Thesis, University of Minnesota, St. Paul.

Hanson, L. R., Sorensen, P. W., and Cohen, Y. (1998). Sex pheromones and amino acids evoke distinctly different spatial patterns of electrical activity in the goldfish olfactory bulb. *Ann. N. Y. Acad. Sci.* **855**, 521–524.

Hara, T. J. (1994). The diversity of chemical stimulation in fish olfaction and gustation. *Rev. Fish Biol. Fish.* **4**, 1–35.

Hara, T. J., and Zhang, C. (1997). Topographic bulbar projections and dual neural pathways of the primary olfactory neurons in salmonid fishes. *Neuroscience* **82**, 301–313.

Hildebrand, J. G., and Shepherd, G. M. (1997). Mechanisms of olfactory discrimination: Converging evidence for common principles among phyla. *Annu. Rev. Neurosci.* **20**, 595–631.

Honda, H. (1980a). Female sex pheromone of rainbow trout, *Salmo gairdneri*, involved in courtship behavior. *Bull. Jpn. Soc. Sci. Fish.* **46**, 1109–1112.

Honda, H. (1980b). Female sex pheromone of the loach, *Misgurnus anguillicaudatus*, involved in courtship behavior. *Bull. Jpn. Soc. Sci. Fish.* **46**, 1223–1225.

Honda, H. (1982). On the female sex pheromones and courtship behavior in the salmonids, *Oncorhynchus masou* and *O. rhodurus*. *Bull. Jpn. Soc. Sci. Fish.* **48**, 47–49.

Hurrell, R. H., and Price, D. J. (1991). Natural hybrids between Atlantic salmon, *Salmo salar* L, and trout, *Salmo trutta*, in a Swedish river. *J. Fish Biol.* **39**, 343–348.

Ide, V. (1993). Auserbeitung und Durchfuhrung von Biotests zum Nachweis von Pheromonen bei Blenniiden. Diplom Thesis, University of Oldenburg.

Irvine, I. A. S., and Sorensen, P. W. (1993). Acute olfactory sensitivity of wild common carp, *Cyprinus carpio*, to goldfish sex pheromones is influenced by gonadal maturity. *Can. J. Zool.* **71**, 2199–2210.

Jakobsson, S., Mayer, I., Schulz, R. W., Blankenstein, M. W., and Borg, B. (1996). Specific binding of 11-ketotestosterone in an androgen target organ, the kidney of the male three-spined stickleback, *Gasterosteus aculeatus*. *Fish. Physiol. Biochem.* **15**, 459–467.

Johansen, P. H. (1985). Female pheromone and the behavior of male guppies (*Poecilia reticulata*) in a temperature gradient. *Can. J. Zool.* **63**, 1211–1213.

Johnson, G. D., and Patterson, C. (1993). Percomorph phylogeny: A survey of acanthomorphs and a new proposal. *Bull. Mar. Sci.* **52**, 554–626.

Jumper, G. Y., Jr., and Baird, R. C. (1991). Location by olfaction: A model and application to the mating problem in the deep-sea hatchetfish *Argyropelecus hemigymnus*. *Am. Nat.* **138**, 1431–1458.

Kagawa, H., Young, G., and Nagahama, Y. (1983). Changes in plasma steroid hormone levels during gonadal maturation in goldfish, *Carassius auratus*. *Bull. Jpn. Soc. Sci. Fish.* **49**, 1783–1787.

Kagawa, H., Young, G., and Nagahama, Y. (1984). In vitro 17β-estradiol and testosterone production by ovarian follicles of the goldfish, *Carassius auratus*. *Gen. Comp. Endocrinol.* **54**, 139–143.

Karlson, P., and Luscher, M. (1959). 'Pheromones': A new term for a class of biologically active substances. *Nature (London)* **183**, 55–56.

Kasumyan, A. O. (1993). Behavioral reaction of ascipenserid males to female releaser postovulatory pheromone. *Dokl. Akad. Nauk SSSR* **333**, 402–404.

Katsel, P. L., Dmitrieva, T. M., Valeyev, R. B., and Kozlov, Y. P. (1992). Sex pheromones of male yellowfin Baikal sculpin

(*Cottocomephorus grewingki*): Isolation and chemical studies. *J. Chem. Ecol.* **18**, 2003–2010.

Kawabata, K. (1993). Induction of sexual behavior in male fish (*Rhodeus ocellatus ocellatus*) by amino acids. *Amino Acids* **5**, 323–327.

Kawabata, K., Tsubaki, K., Tazaki, T., and Ikeda, S. (1992). Sexual behavior induced by amino acids in the rose bitterling *Rhodeus ocellatus ocellatus*. *Nippon Suisan Gakkaishi* **58**, 839–844.

Khan, I. A., Hawkins, M. B., and Thomas, P. (1999). Gonadal stage-dependent effects of gonadal steroids on gonadotropin II secretion in the Atlantic croaker (*Micropogonias undulatus*). *Biol. Reprod.* **61**, 834–841.

Kime, D., and Rafter, J. (1981). Biosynthesis of 15-hydroxylated steroids by gonads of the river lamprey, *Lampetra fluviatilis, in vitro*. *Gen. Comp. Endocrinol.* **44**, 69–76.

Kindler, P. M., Bahr, J. M., and Philipp, D. P. (1991). The effect of exogenous 11-ketotestosterone, testosterone, and cyproterone acetate on prespawning and parental care behaviors of male bluegill. *Horm. Behav.* **25**, 410–423.

Kitamura, S., Ogata, H., and Takashima, F. (1994a). Activities of F-type prostaglandins as releaser sex pheromones in cobitide loach, *Misgurnus anguillicaudatus*. *Comp. Biochem. Physiol. A* **107**, 161–169.

Kitamura, S., Ogata, H., and Takashima, F. (1994b). Olfactory responses of several species of teleost to F-prostaglandins. *Comp. Biochem. Physiol. A* **107**, 463–467.

Knapp, R., Wingfield, J. C., and Bass, A. H. (1999). Steroid hormones and paternal care in the plainfin midshipman fish (*Porichthys notatus*). *Horm. Behav.* **35**, 81–89.

Kobayashi, M., and Nakanishi, T. (1999). 11-Ketotestosterone induces male-type sexual behavior and gonadotropin secretion in gynogenetic crucian carp, *Carassius auratus langsdorfii*. *Gen. Comp. Endocrinol.* **115**, 178–187.

Kobayashi, M., and Stacey, N. E. (1990). Effects of ovariectomy and steroid hormone implantation on serum gonadotropin levels in female goldfish. *Zool. Sci.* **7**, 715–721.

Kobayashi, M., and Stacey, N. E. (1993). Prostaglandin-induced female spawning behavior in goldfish (*Carassius auratus*) appears independent of ovarian influence. *Horm. Behav.* **27**, 38–55.

Kobayashi, M., Aida, K., and Hanyu, I. (1986a). Effects of HCG on milt amount and plasma levels of steroid hormones in male goldfish. *Bull. Jpn. Soc. Sci. Fish.* **52**, 755.

Kobayashi, M., Aida, K., and Hanyu, I. (1986b). Annual changes in plasma levels of gonadotropin and steroid hormones in goldfish. *Bull. Jpn. Soc. Sci. Fish.* **52**, 1153–1158.

Kobayashi, M., Aida, K., and Hanyu, I. (1986c). Gonadotropin surge during spawning in male goldfish. *Gen. Comp. Endocrinol.* **62**, 70–79.

Kobayashi, M., Aida, K., and Hanyu, I. (1986d). Pheromone from ovulatory female goldfish induces gonadotropin surge in males. *Gen. Comp. Endocrinol.* **63**, 451–455.

Kobayashi, M., Aida, K., and Hanyu, I. (1987). Hormone changes during ovulation and effects of steroid hormones on plasma gonadotropin levels and ovulation in goldfish. *Gen. Comp. Endocrinol.* **67**, 24–32.

Kobayashi, M., Aida, K., and Hanyu, I. (1988). Hormone changes during the ovulatory cycle in goldfish. *Gen. Comp. Endocrinol.* **69**, 301–307.

Kobayashi, M., Aida, K., and Hanyu, I. (1989). Induction of gonadotropin surge by steroid hormone implantation in ovariectomized and sexually regressed female goldfish. *Gen. Comp. Endocrinol.* **73**, 469–476.

Kobayashi, M., Amano, M., Kim, M.-H., Furukawa, K., Hasegawa, Y., and Aida, K. (1994). Gonadotropin-releasing hormones of terminal nerve origin are not essential to ovarian development and ovulation in goldfish. *Gen. Comp. Endocrinol.* **95**, 192–200.

Kobayashi, M., Amano, M., Kim, M.-H., Yoshiura, Y., Sohn, Y. C., Suetake, H., and Aida, K. (1997a). Gonadotropin-releasing hormone and gonadotropin in goldfish and masu salmon. *Fish Physiol. Biochem.* **17**, 1–8.

Kobayashi, M., Furukawa, K., Kim, M.-H., and Aida, K. (1997b). Induction of male-type gonadotropin secretion by implantation of 11-ketotestosterone in female goldfish. *Gen. Comp. Endocrinol.* **108**, 434–445.

Kobayashi, M., Stacey, N. E., Aida, K., and Watabe, S. (2000). Sexual plasticity of behavior and gonadotropin secretion in goldfish and gynogenetic crucian carp. *In* "Proceedings of the Sixth International Symposium on the Reproductive Physiology of Fish" (B. Norberg, O. S. Kjesbu, G. L. Taranger, E. Andersson, and S. O. Stefansson, eds.), pp. 117–124. John Grieg AS, Bergen.

Kuwamura, T., and Nakashima, Y. (1998). New aspects of sex change among reef fishes: Recent studies in Japan. *Environ. Biol. Fish.* **52**, 125–135.

Kyle, A. L., Stacey, N. E., and Peter, R. E. (1982). Ventral telencephalic lesions: Effects on bisexual behavior, activity and olfaction in the male goldfish. *Behav. Neural Biol.* **36**, 229–241.

Kyle, A. L., Stacey, N. E., Peter, R. E., and Billard, R. (1985). Elevations in gonadotropin content and milt volume as a result of spawning in the goldfish. *Gen. Comp. Endocrinol.* **57**, 10–22.

Kyle, A. L., Sorensen, P. W., Stacey, N. E., and Dulka, J. G. (1987). Medial olfactory tract pathways controlling sexual reflexes and behavior in teleosts. *Ann. N. Y. Acad. Sci.* **519**, 97–107.

Lahnsteiner, F., and Patzner, R. A. (1990). Functions of the testicular gland of blenniid fish: Structural and histochemical investigations. *Experientia* **46**, 1005–1007.

Lambert, J. G. D., Van Den Hurk, R., Schoonen, W. G. E. J., Resink, J. W., and Van Oordt, P. G. W. J. (1986). Gonadal steroidogenesis and the possible role of steroid glucuronides as sex pheromones in two species of teleosts. *Fish Physiol. Biochem.* **2**, 101–107.

Laumen, T. J., Pern, U., and Blum, V. (1974). Investigations on the function and hormonal regulation of the anal appendices in *Blennius pavo* (Risso). *J. Exp. Zool.* **190**, 47–56.

Laurent, G. (1999). A systems perspective on early olfactory coding. *Science* **286**, 723–728.

Lee, C. T., and Ingersoll, D. W. (1979). Social chemosignals in five *Belonttiidae* (Pisces) species. *J. Comp. Physiol. Psychol.* **93**, 1171–1181.

Levine, R. L., and Dethier, S. (1985). The connections between the olfactory bulb and the brain in the goldfish. *J. Comp. Neurol.* **237**, 427–444.

Li, W. (1994). The olfactory biology of adult sea lamprey (*Petromyzon marinus*). Ph.D. Dissertation, University of Minnesota, St. Paul.

Li, W., and Sorensen, P. W. (1991). Highly independent olfactory receptor sites for conspecific bile acids in the sea lamprey, *Petromyzon marinus*, *J. Comp. Physiol. A* **180**, 429–438.

Li, W., Sorensen, P. W., and Gallaher, D. D. (1995). The olfactory system of migratory adult sea lamprey (*Petromyzon marinus*) is specifically and acutely sensitive to unique bile acids released by conspecific larvae. *J. Gen. Physiol.* **105**, 569–587.

Liley, N. R. (1969). Hormones and reproductive behavior in fishes. *Fish Physiol.* **3**, 73–116.

Liley, N. R. (1972). The effects of estrogens and other steroids on the sexual behavior of the female guppy, *Poecilia reticulata*. *Gen. Comp. Endocrinol., Suppl.* **3**, 542–552.

Liley, N. R. (1982). Chemical communication in fish. *Can. J. Fish. Aquat. Sci.* **39**, 22–35.

Liley, N. R., and Kroon, F. J. (1995). Male dominance, plasma hormone concentrations, and availability of milt in male rainbow trout (*Oncorhynchus mykiss*). *Can. J. Zool.* **73**, 826–836.

Liley, N. R., and Stacey, N. E. (1983). Hormones, pheromones, and reproductive behavior in fish. *Fish Physiol.* **9B**, 1–63.

Liley, N. R., and Tan, E. S. P. (1985). The induction of spawning behavior in *Puntius gonionotus* (Bleeker) by treatment with prostaglandin F2α. *J. Fish Biol.* **26**, 491–502.

Liley, N. R., Breton, B., Fostier, A., and Tan, E. S. P. (1986). Endocrine changes associated with spawning behavior and social stimuli in a wild population of rainbow trout (*Salmo gairdneri*). I. Males. *Gen. Comp. Endocrinol.* **62**, 145–156.

Loefstedt, C., Herrebout, W. M., and Du, J.-W. (1986). Evolution of the ermine moth pheromone tetradecyl acetate. *Nature (London)* **323**, 621–623.

MacInnis, A. J., and Corkum, L. D. (2000). Fecundity and reproductive season of the round goby, *Neogobius melanostomus*, in the upper Detroit River. *Trans. Am. Fish. Soc.* **129**, 136–144.

Maniak, P. J., Lossing, R. D., and Sorensen, P. W. (2000). Injured Eurasian ruffe, *Gymnocephalus cernuus*, release an alarm pheromone that could be used to control their dispersal. *J. Great Lakes Res.* **26**, 183–195.

Matsumura, K. (1985). Tetrodotoxin as a pheromone. *Nature (London)* **378**, 563–564.

Mayer, I., Borg, B., and Schulz, R. (1990). Conversion of 11-ketoandrostendione to 11-ketotestosterone by blood cells of six fish species. *Gen. Comp. Endocrinol.* **77**, 70–74.

Mayer, I., Liley, N. R., and Borg, B. (1994). Stimulation of spawning behavior in castrated rainbow trout (*Oncorhynchus mykiss*) by 17α,20β-dihydroxy-4-pregnen-3-one, but not by 11-ketoandrostenedione. *Horm. Behav.* **28**, 181–190.

Melrose, D. R., Reed, H. G. B., and Patterson, R. C. S. (1971). Androgen steroids associated with boar odour as an aid to the detection of oestrus in pig artificial insemination. *Br. Vet. J.* **127**, 497–502.

Meyer, J. H., and Liley, N. R. (1982). The control of production of a sexual pheromone in the guppy, *Poecilia reticulata*. *Can. J. Zool.* **60**, 1505–1510.

Michel, W. C., and Lubomudrov, L. M. (1995). Specificity and sensitivity of the olfactory organ of the zebrafish, *Danio rerio*. *J. Comp. Physiol. A* **177**, 191–199.

Miller, P. J. (1984). The tokology of Gobiid fishes. In "Fish Reproduction: Strategies and Tactics" (G. W. Potts and R. W. Wootton, eds.), pp. 119–153. Academic Press, New York.

Miura, C., Miura, T., Yamashita, M., Yamauchi, K., and Nagahama, Y. (1996). Hormonal induction of all stages of spermatogenesis in germ-somatic cell coculture from immature Japanese eel testis. *Dev. Growth Differ.* **38**, 257–262.

Miura, T., Yamauchi, K., Takahashi, H., and Nagahama, Y. (1992). The role of hormones in the acquisition of sperm motility in salmonid fish. *J. Exp. Zool.* **261**, 359–363.

Moiseyeva, Y. B., and Rudenko, V. I. (1976). The spawning of the round goby, *Gobius melanostomus*, under aquarium conditions in winter. *J. Ichthyol.* **8**, 690–692.

Moore, A. (1991). Behavioral and physiological responses of precocious male Atlantic salmon (*Salmo salar* L.) parr to testosterone. In "Proceedings of the Fourth International Symposium on the Reproductive Physiology of Fish" (A. P. Scott, J. P. Sumpter, D. E. Kime, and M. S. Rolfe, eds.), pp. 194–196. Fish Symp. 91, Sheffield.

Moore, A. (1994). An electrophysiological study of the effects of pH on olfaction in mature male Atlantic salmon (*Salmo salar*) parr. *J. Fish Biol.* **45**, 493–502.

Moore, A., and Scott, A. P. (1991). Testosterone is a potent odorant in precocious male Atlantic salmon (*Salmo salar* L.) parr. *Philos. Trans. R. Soc. London, Ser. B* **332**, 241–244.

Moore, A., and Scott, A. P. (1992). 17α,20β-dihydroxy-4-pregnen-3-one-20-sulphate is a potent odorant in precocious male Atlantic salmon parr which have been pre-exposed to the urine of ovulated females. *Proc. R. Soc. London, Ser. B* **249**, 205–209.

Moore, A., and Waring, C. P. (1995). Seasonal changes in olfactory sensitivity of mature male Atlantic salmon (*Salmo salar* L.) parr to prostaglandins. In "Proceedings of the Fifth International Symposium on the Reproductive Physiology of Fish" (F. W. Goetz and P. Thomas, eds.), Fish Symp. 95, pp. 273. University of Texas at Austin.

Moore, A., and Waring, C. P. (1996). Electrophysiological and endocrinological evidence that F-series prostaglandins function as priming pheromones in mature male Atlantic salmon (*Salmo salar*) parr. *J. Exp. Biol.* **199**, 2307–2316.

Mori, K., Nagao, H., and Yoshiaha, Y. (1999). The olfactory bulb: Coding and processing of odor molecule information. *Science* **286**, 711–715.

Morin, P.-P., Hara, T. J., and Eales, J. G. (1997). Thyroid function and olfactory responses to L-alanine during induced smoltification in Atlantic salmon, *Salmo salar*. *Can. J. Fish. Aquat. Sci.* **54**, 596–602.

Morita, Y., and Finger, T. E. (1998). Differential projections of ciliated and microvillous olfactory receptor cells in the catfish, *Ictalurus punctatus*. *J. Comp. Neurol.* **398**, 539–550.

Moriwaki, T., Kobayashi, M., Aida, K., and Hanyu, I. (1991). Changes in plasma gonadotropin and steroid hormone levels during ovulation induced by HCG treatment in female goldfish. *Nippon Suisan Gakkaishi* **57**, 41–43.

Munday, P. L., Caley, M. J., and Jones, G. P. (1998). Bi-directional sex change in a coral-dwelling goby. *Behav., Ecol. Sociobiol.* **43**, 371–377.

Murphy, C. A., and Stacey, N. E. (2002). Methyl-testosterone induces male-typical ventilatory behavior in response to putative steroidal pheromones in female round gobies (*Neogobius melanostomus*). *Horm. Behav.* (in press).

Murphy, C. A., Maniak, P. J., and Sorensen, P. W. (2000). Functional and biochemical characterization of a novel sex pheromone in the Eurasian ruffe, *Gymnocephalus cernuus*. In "Proceedings of the 9th International Zebra Mussel and Aquatic Nuisance Species Conference" (Duluth, MN, April 16–30, 1999), p. 211. The Professional Edge, Pembroke, Ontario.

Murphy, C. A., Stacey, N., and Corkum, L. D. (2001). Putative steroidal pheromones in the round goby, *Neogobius melanostomus*: Olfactory and behavioral responses. *J. Chem. Ecol.* **27**, 443–470.

Nagahama, Y. (1990). Endocrine control of oocyte maturation in teleosts. In "Progress in Comparative Endocrinology" (A. Epple, C. G. Scanes, and M. H. Stetson, eds.), pp. 385–392. Wiley-Liss, New York.

Nagahama, Y. (1994). Molecular biology of oocyte maturation in fish. In "Perspectives in Comparative Endocrinology" (K. G. Davey, R. E. Peter, and S. S. Tobe, eds.), pp. 193–198. National Research Council, Ottawa.

Nagahama, Y., Goetz, F. W., and Tan, J. D. (1986). Shift in steroidogenesis in the ovarian follicles of the goldfish (*Carassius auratus*) during gonadotropin-induced oocyte maturation. *Dev., Growth Differ.* **28**, 555–561.

Nagahama, Y., Yoshikuni, M., Yamashita, M., and Tanaka, M. (1995). Regulation of oocyte maturation in fish. *Fish Physiol.* **13**, 393–439.

Naito, T., Saito, Y., Yumamoto, J., Nozaki, Y., Tomura, K., Hazama, M., Nakanishi, S., and Breener, S. (1998). Putative pheromone receptors related to Ca sensing receptor in *Fugu*. *Proc. Natl. Acad. Sci. U.S.A.* **95**, 5178–5181.

Nelson, J. S. (1994). "Fishes of the World," 3rd ed. Wiley, New York.

Nevitt, G. A. (1991). Do fish sniff? A new mechanism of olfactory sampling in pleuronectid flounders. *J. Exp. Biol.* **157**, 1–18.

Ngai, J., Dowling, M. M., Buck, L., Axel, R., and Chess, A. (1993a). The family of genes encoding odorant receptors in the channel catfish. *Cell (Cambridge, Mass.)* **72**, 657–666.

Ngai, J., Chess, A., Dowling, M. M., Necles, N., Macagno, E. R., and Axel, R. (1993b). Coding of olfactory information: Topography of odorant receptor expression in the catfish olfactory epithelium. *Cell (Cambridge, Mass.)* **72**, 667–680.

Ogata, H., Kitamura, S., and Takashima, F. (1994). Release of 13,14-dihydro-15-keto-prostaglandin F2α, a sex pheromone, to water by cobitid loach following ovulatory stimulation. *Fish. Sci.* **60**, 143–148.

Okada, H., Sakai, D. K., and Sugiwaka, K. (1978). Chemical stimulus on the reproductive behavior of the pondsmelt. *Sci. Rep. Hokkaido Fish Hatchery* **33**, 89–99.

Oliveira, R. F., Almada, V. C., and Canario, A. V. (1996). Social modulation of sex steroid concentrations in the urine of male cichlid fish *Oreochromis mossambicus*. *Horm. Behav.* **30**, 2–12.

Olsen, K. H., and Liley, N. R. (1993). The significance of olfaction and social cues in milt availability, sexual hormone status, and spawning behavior of male rainbow trout (*Oncorhynchus mykiss*). *Gen. Comp. Endocrinol.* **89**, 107–118.

Olsen, K. H., Bjerselius, R., Petersson, E., Jarva, E., Mayer, I., and Hedenskog, M. (2000). Lack of species-specific primer effects of odours from female Atlantic salmon, *Salmo salar*, and brown trout, *Salmo trutta*. *Oikos* **88**, 213–220.

Ottoson, D. (1971). The electro-olfactogram. In "Handbook of Sensory Physiology" (L. M. Biedler, ed.), pp. 95–131. Springer-Verlag, New York.

Pankhurst, N. W. (1995). Hormones and reproductive behavior in male damselfish. *Bull. Mar. Sci.* **57**, 569–581.

Pankhurst, N. W., Hilder, P. I., and Pankhurst, P. M. (1999). Reproductive condition and behavior in relation to plasma levels of gonadal steroids in the spiny damselfish *Acanthochromis polyacanthus*. *Gen. Comp. Endocrinol.* **115**, 53–69.

Parks, L. G., and Leblanc, G. A. (1998). Involvement of multiple biotransformation processes in the metabolic elimination of testosterone by juvenile and adult fathead minnows (*Pimephales promelas*). *Gen. Comp. Endocrinol.* **112**, 69–79.

Partridge, B. L., Liley, N. R., and Stacey, N. E. (1976). The role of pheromones in the sexual behavior of the goldfish. *Anim. Behav.* **24**, 291–299.

Pasmanik, M., and Callard, G. V. (1985). Aromatase and 5-alpha-reductase in the teleost brain, spinal cord, and pituitary gland. *Gen. Comp. Endocrinol.* **60**, 241–251.

Pasmanik, M., and Callard, G. V. (1988). A high abundance androgen receptor in goldfish brain: Characteristics and seasonal changes. *Endocrinology (Baltimore)* **123**, 1162–1171.

Peter, R. E. (1983). The brain and neurohormones in teleost reproduction. *Fish Physiol.* **9B**, 97–135.

Peter, R. E., Chang, J. P., Nahorniak, C. S., Omeljaniuk, R. J., Sokolowska, M., Shih, S. H., and Billard, R. (1986). Interactions of catecholamines and GnRH in regulation of gonadotropin secretion in teleost fish. *Recent Prog. Horm. Res.* **42**, 513–548.

Pfeiffer, W. (1982). Chemical signals in communication. *In* "Chemoreception in Fishes" (T. J. Hara, ed.), pp. 307–326. Elsevier, Amsterdam.

Pfeiffer, W., Riegelbauer, G., Meier, G., and Scheibler, B. (1985). Effect of hypoxanthine-3(N)-oxide and hypoxanthine-1(N)-oxide on central nervous excitation of the black tetra *Gymnocorymbus ternetzi* (Characidae, Ostariophysi, Pisces) indicated by dorsal light response. *J. Chem. Ecol.* **11**, 507–524.

Piferer, F., Baker, H., and Donaldson, E. M. (1993). Effects of natural, synthetic, aromatizable and nonaromatizable androgens in inducing male sex differentiation in genotypic female chinook salmon (*Oncorhynchus tshawytscha*). *Gen. Comp. Endocrinol.* **91**, 51–65.

Poling, K. R., Fraser, E. J., and Sorensen, P. W. (2001). The three steroidal components of the goldfish preovulatory pheromone signal evoke different behaviors in males. *Comp. Biochem. Physiol. B* **129**, 645–651.

Pottinger, T. G. (1987). Androgen binding in the skin of mature male brown trout, *Salmo trutta* L. *Gen. Comp. Endocrinol.* **66**, 224–232.

Pottinger, T. G., and Moore, A. (1997). Characterization of putative steroid receptors in the membrane, cytosol and nuclear fractions from the olfactory tissue of brown and rainbow trout. *Fish Physiol. Biochem.* **16**, 45–63.

Pottinger, T. G., and Pickering, A. D. (1985). The effects of 11-ketotestosterone and testosterone on the skin structure of brown trout, *Salmo trutta* L. *Gen. Comp. Endocrinol.* **59**, 335–342.

Price, D. J. (1984). Genetics of sex determination in fishes—a brief review. *In* "Fish Reproduction: Strategies and Tactics" (G. W. Potts and R. J. Wootton, eds.), pp. 77–90. Academic Press, London.

Rainboth, W. J. (1991). Cyprinids of South East Asia. *In* "Cyprinid Fishes: Systematics, Biology and Exploitation" (I. J. Winfield and J. S. Nelson, eds.), pp. 156–210. Chapman & Hall, London.

Rasotto, M. B. (1995). Male reproductive apparatus of some Blennioidei (Pisces: Teleostei). *Copeia*, pp. 907–914.

Resink, J. W., Van Den Hurk, R., Van Zoelen, R. F. O. G., and Huisman, E. A. (1987). The seminal vesicle as source of sex attracting substances in the African catfish, *Clarias gariepinus*. *Aquaculture* **63**, 115–128.

Resink, J. W., Voorthuis, P. K., Van den Hurk, R., Vullings, H. G. B., and Van Oordt, P. G. W. J. (1989a). Pheromone detection and olfactory pathways in the brain of the female African catfish, *Clarias gariepinus*. *Cell Tissue. Res.* **256**, 337–345.

Resink, J. W., Schoonen, W. G. E. J., Alpers, P. C. H., File, D. M., Notenbloom, C. D., Van Den Hurk, R., and Van Oordt, P. G. W. J. (1989b). The chemical nature of sex attracting pheromones from the seminal vesicle of the African catfish, *Clarias gariepinus*. *Aquaculture* **83**, 137–151.

Resink, J. W., Voorthuis, P. K., Van Den Hurk, R., Peters, R. C., and Van Oordt, P. G. W. J. (1989c). Steroid glucuronides of the seminal vesicle as olfactory stimuli in African catfish, *Clarias gariepinus*. *Aquaculture* **83**, 153–166.

Resink, J. W., Van Den Berg, T. W. M., Van Den Hurk, R., Huisman, E. A., and Van Oordt, P. G. W. J. (1989d). Induction of gonadotropin release and ovulation by pheromones in the African catfish, *Clarias gariepinus*. *Aquaculture* **83**, 167–177.

Ressler, K. J., Sullivan, S. L., and Buck, L. B. (1994). Information coding in the olfactory system: Evidence for a stereotyped and highly organized epitope map in the olfactory bulb. *Cell. (Cambridge, Mass.)* **79**, 1245–1255.

Robison, R. R., Fernald, R. D., and Stacey, N. E. (1998). The olfactory system of a cichlid fish responds to steroidal compounds. *J. Fish Biol.* **53**, 226–229.

Rocha, M. J., and Reis-Henriques, M. A. (1996). Plasma and urine levels of C_{18}, C_{19} and C_{21} steroids in an asynchronous fish, the tilapia *Oreochromis mossambicus* (Teleostei, Cichlidae). *Comp. Biochem. Physiol. C* **115**, 257–264.

Rosenblum, P. M., Sorensen, P. W., Stacey, N. E., and Peter, R. E. (1991). Binding of the steroidal pheromone $17\alpha,20\beta$-dihydroxy-4-pregnen-3-one to goldfish (*Carassius auratus*) olfactory epithelium membrane preparations. *Chem. Senses* **16**, 143–154.

Satou, M. (1990). Synaptic organization, local neural circuitry, and functional segregation of the teleost olfactory bulb. *Prog. Neurobiol.* **34**, 115–142.

Satou, M., Oka, Y., Fujita, I., Koyama, T., Shiga, M., Kasunoki, T., Matsushima, T., and Ueda, K. (1982). Effects of brain lesions and electrical activity on sexual behavior in hime salmon (land locked red salmon, *Oncoryhnchus nerka*). *Zool. Mag.* **91**, 459–468.

Schoonen, W. J. E. J., Lambert, J. G. D., and Van Oordt, P. G. W. J. (1988). Quantitative analysis of steroids and steroid glucuronides in the seminal vesicle fluid of feral spawning and feral and cultivated non-spawning African catfish, *Clarias gariepinus*. *Gen. Comp. Endocrinol.* **70**, 91–100.

Scott, A. P., and Canario, A. V. M. (1992). $17\alpha,20\beta$-Dihydroxy-4-pregnen-3-one-20-sulphate: A major new metabolite of the teleost oocyte maturation-inducing steroid. *Gen. Comp. Endocrinol.* **85**, 91–100.

Scott, A. P., and Liley, N. R. (1994). Dynamics of excretion of $17\alpha,20\beta$-dihydroxy-4-pregnen-3-one-20-sulphate, and of the glucuronides of testosterone and 17β-oestradiol, by urine of reproductively mature male and female rainbow trout (*Oncorhynchus mykiss*). *J. Fish Biol.* **44**, 117–129.

Scott, A. P., and Sorensen, P. W. (1994). Time course of release of pheromonally active steroids and their conjugates by ovulatory goldfish. *Gen. Comp. Endocrinol.* **96**, 309–323.

Scott, A. P., and Vermeirssen, E. L. M. (1994). Production of conjugated steroids by teleost gonads and their role as pheromones. *In* "Perspectives in Comparative Endocrinology" (K. G. Davey, R. E. Peter, and S. S. Tobe, eds.), pp. 645–654. National Research Council, Ottawa.

Scott, A. P., MacKenzie, D. S., and Stacey, N. E. (1984). Endocrine changes during natural spawning in the white sucker, *Catostomus commersoni*. II. Steroid hormones. *Gen. Comp. Endocrinol.* **56**, 349–359.

Scott, A. P., Sherwood, N. M., Canario, A. V. M., and Warby, C. M. (1991a). Identification of free and conjugated steroids, including cortisol and 17α-20β-dihydroxy-4-pregnen-3-one, in the milt of Pacific herring, *Clupea harengus pallasi*. *Can. J. Zool.* **69**, 104–110.

Scott, A. P., Canario, A. V. M., Sherwood, N. M., and Warby, C. M. (1991b). Levels of steroids, including cortisol and $17\alpha,20\beta$-dihydroxy-4-pregnen-3-one, in plasma, seminal fluid and urine of Pacific herring (*Clupea harengus pallasi*) and North Sea plaice (*Pleuronectes platessa* L.). *Can. J. Zool.* **69**, 111–116.

Scott, A. P., Liley, N. R., and Vermeirssen, E. L. M. (1994). Urine of reproductively mature female rainbow trout, *Oncorhynchus mykiss* (Walbaum), contains a priming pheromone which enhances plasma levels of sex steroids and gonadotrophin II in males. *J. Fish Biol.* **44**, 131–147.

Sherwood, N. M., Kyle, A. L., Kreiberg, H., Warby, C. M., Magnus, T. H., Carolsfeld, J., and Price, W. S. (1991). Partial characterization of a spawning pheromone in the herring *Clupea harengus pallasi*. *Can. J. Zool.* **69**, 91–103.

Slater, C. H., Fitzpatrick, M. S., and Schreck, C. B. (1995). Characterization of an androgen receptor in salmonid lymphocytes: Possible link to androgen-induced immunosuppression. *Gen. Comp. Endocrinol.* **100**, 218–225.

Smith, R. J. F. (1992). Alarm signals in fish. *Rev. Fish Biol. Fish.* **2**, 33–63.

So, Y., Idler, D. R., Truscott, B., and Walsh, D. M. (1985). Progestogens, androgens, and their glucuronides in the terminal stages of oocyte maturation in land-locked Atlantic salmon. *J. Steroid Biochem.* **23**, 583–591.

Sohn, Y. C., Yoshiura, Y., Suetake, H., Kobayashi, M., and Aida, K. (1999). Isolation and characterization of goldfish thyrotropin β subunit gene including 5'-flanking region. *Gen. Comp. Endocrinol.* **115**, 463–473.

Solomon, D. J. (1990). A review of chemical communication in freshwater fish. *J. Fish Biol.* **11**, 363–376.

Sorensen, P. W. (1992a). Hormones, pheromones, and chemoreception. *In* "Fish Chemoreception" (T. J. Hara, ed.), pp. 199–228. Chapman & Hall, London.

Sorensen, P. W. (1992b). Hormonally-derived sex pheromones in goldfish: A model for understanding the evolution of sex pheromone systems in fish. *Biol. Bull. (Woods Hole, Mass.)*. **183**, 173–177.

Sorensen, P. W., and Bowdin, L. (1994). Olfactory responsiveness of female goldfish to sex pheromones is enhanced by exposure to elevated levels of circulating androgenic sex hormones. *Chem. Senses* **19**, 555–556.

Sorensen, P. W., and Caprio, J. (1997). Chemoreception. *In* "The Physiology of Fishes" (D. H. Evans, ed.), 2nd ed., pp. 375–405. CRC Press, Boca Raton, FL.

Sorensen, P. W., and Caprio, J. (2000). Restricted distribution and chemospecificity of pheromone-sensitive olfactory receptor neurons in the goldfish olfactory epithelium. *Chem. Senses* **25**, 670 (Abst. 263).

Sorensen, P. W., and Goetz, F. W. (1993). Pheromonal and reproductive function of F-prostaglandins and their metabolites in teleost fish. *J. Lipid Mediators* **6**, 385–393.

Sorensen, P. W., and Scott, A. P. (1994). The evolution of hormonal sex pheromones in teleost fish: Poor correlation between the pattern of steroid release by goldfish and olfactory sensitivity suggests that these cues evolved as a result of chemical spying rather than signal specialization. *Acta Scand. Physiol.* **152**, 191–205.

Sorensen, P. W., and Stacey, N. E. (1987). 17α,20β-dihydroxy-4-pregnen-3-one functions as a bisexual priming pheromone in goldfish. *Am. Zool.* **27**, 412.

Sorensen, P. W., and Stacey, N. E. (1990). Identified hormonal pheromones in the goldfish: The basis for a model of sex pheromone function in fish. *In* "Chemical Signals in Vertebrates" (D. MacDonald, D. Müller-Schwarze, and S. E. Natynczuk, eds.), Vol. 5, pp. 302–311. Oxford University Press, Oxford.

Sorensen, P. W., and Stacey, N. E. (1999). Evolution and specialization of fish hormonal pheromones. *In* "Advances in Chemical Signals in Vertebrates" (R. E. Johnston, D. Müller-Schwarze, and P. W. Sorensen, eds.), pp. 15–47. Kluwer Academic/Plenum Press, New York.

Sorensen, P. W., and Vrieze, L. A. (2001). Recent progress understanding the chemical ecology and potential application of the sea lamprey migratory pheromone. *J. Great Lakes Res.* (in press).

Sorensen, P. W., and Wyatt, J. (2000). Pheromones. *In* "The Corsini Encyclopedia of Psychology and Behavioral Science" (W. E. Craighead and C. B. Nemeroff, eds.), 3rd ed., pp. 1193–1195. Wiley, New York.

Sorensen, P. W., Stacey, N. E., and Naidu, P. (1986). Release of spawning pheromone(s) by naturally ovulated and prostaglandin-injected, nonovulated female goldfish. *In* "Chemical Signals in Vertebrates" (D. Duvall, D. Müller-Schwarze, and R. M. Silverstein, eds.), Vol. 4, pp. 149–154. Plenum Press, New York.

Sorensen, P. W., Hara, T. J., and Stacey, N. E. (1987). Extreme olfactory sensitivity of mature and gonadally-regressed goldfish to a potent steroidal pheromone, 17α,20β-dihydroxy-4-pregnen-3-one. *J. Comp. Physiol. A* **160**, 305–313.

Sorensen, P. W., Hara, T. J., Stacey, N. E., and Goetz, F. W. (1988). F prostaglandins function as potent olfactory stimulants that comprise the postovulatory female sex pheromone in goldfish. *Biol. Reprod.* **39**, 1039–1050.

Sorensen, P. W., Chamberlain, K. J., and Stacey, N. E. (1989). Differing behavioral and endocrinological effects of two female sex pheromones on male goldfish. *Horm. Behav.* **23**, 317–332.

Sorensen, P. W., Hara, T. J., Stacey, N. E., and Dulka, J. G. (1990). Extreme olfactory specificity of the male goldfish to the preovulatory steroidal pheromone 17α,20β-dihydroxy-4-pregnen-3-one. *J. Comp. Physiol. A* **166**, 373–383.

Sorensen, P. W., Hara, T. J., and Stacey, N. E. (1991). Sex pheromones selectively stimulate the medial olfactory tracts of male goldfish. *Brain Res.* **558**, 343–347.

Sorensen, P. W., Irvine, I. A. S., Scott, A. P., and Stacey, N. E. (1992). Electrophysiological measures of olfactory sensitivity suggest that goldfish and other fish use species-specific mixtures of hormones and their metabolites as sex pheromones. *In* "Chemical Signals in Vertebrates" (R. Doty and D. Müller-Schwarze, eds.), Vol. 6, pp. 357–364. Plenum Press, New York.

Sorensen, P. W., Scott, A. P., Stacey, N. E., and Bowdin, L. (1995a). Sulfated 17α,20β-dihydroxy-4-pregnen-3-one functions as a potent and specific olfactory stimulant with pheromonal actions in the goldfish. *Gen. Comp. Endocrinol.* **100**, 128–142.

Sorensen, P. W., Brash, A. R., Goetz, F. W., Kellner, R. G., Bowdin, L., and Vrieze, L. A. (1995b). Origins and functions of F prostaglandins as hormones and pheromones in the goldfish. *In* "Proceedings of the Fifth International Symposium on the Reproductive Physiology of Fish" (F. W. Goetz and P. Thomas, eds.), Fish Symp. 95, pp. 244–248. University of Texas at Austin.

Sorensen, P. W., Cardwell, J. R., Essington, T., and Weigel, D. E. (1995c). Reproductive interactions between brook and brown trout in a small Minnesota stream. *Can. J. Fish. Aquat. Sci.* **52**, 1958–1965.

Sorensen, P. W., Christensen, T. A., and Stacey, N. E. (1998). Discrimination of pheromonal cues in fish: Emerging parallels with insects. *Curr. Opin. Neurobiol.* **8**, 458–467.

Sorensen, P. W., Scott, A. P., and Kihslinger, R. L. (2000). How common hormonal metabolites function as relatively specific pheromonal signals in goldfish. *In* "Proceedings of the Sixth International Symposium on the Reproductive Physiology of Fish" (B. Norberg, O. S. Kjesbu, G. L. Taranger, E. Andersson, and S. O. Stefansson, eds.), pp. 125–128. John Grieg AS, Bergen.

Speca, D. J., Lin, D. M., Sorensen, P. W., Isacoff, E. Y., Ngai, J., and Dittman, H. (1999). Functional identification of a goldfish odorant receptor. *Neuron* **23**, 487–498.

Specker, J. L., and Sullivan, C. V. (1994). Vitellogenesis in fishes: Status and perspectives. *In* "Perspectives in Endocrinology" (K. G. Davey, R. E. Peter, and S. S. Tobe, eds.), pp. 304–315. National Research Council, Ottawa.

Sperry, T. S., and Thomas, P. (1999a). Characterization of two nuclear androgen receptors in Atlantic croaker: Comparison of their biochemical properties and binding specificities. *Endocrinology (Baltimore)* **140**, 1602–1611.

Sperry, T. S., and Thomas, P. (1999b). Identification of two nuclear androgen receptors in kelp bass (*Paralabrax clathratus*) and their binding affinities for xenobiotics: Comparison with Atlantic croaker (*Micropogonias undulatus*) androgen receptors. *Biol. Reprod.* **61**, 1152–1161.

Stacey, N. E. (1976). Effects of indomethacin and prostaglandins on spawning behavior of female goldfish. *Prostaglandins* **12**, 113–128.

Stacey, N. E. (1981). Hormonal regulation of female reproductive behavior in fish. *Am. Zool.* **21**, 305–316.

Stacey, N. E. (1987). Roles of hormones and pheromones in fish reproductive behavior. In "Psychobiology of Reproduction: An Evolutionary Perspective" (D. Crews, ed.), pp. 28–69. Prentice-Hall, Englewood Cliffs, NJ.

Stacey, N. E. (1991). Hormonal pheromones in fish: Status and prospects. In "Proceedings of the Fourth International Symposium on the Reproductive Physiology of Fish" (A. P. Scott, J. P. Sumpter, D. S. Kime, and M. S. Rolfe, eds.), pp. 177–181. Fish Symp. 91, Sheffield.

Stacey, N. E., and Cardwell, J. R. (1995). Hormones as sex pheromones in fish: Widespread distribution among freshwater species. In "Proceedings of the Fifth International Symposium on the Reproductive Physiology of Fish" (F. W. Goetz and P. Thomas, eds.), Fish Symp. 95, pp. 244–248. University of Texas at Austin.

Stacey, N. E., and Cardwell, J. R. (1997). Hormonally-derived pheromones in fish: New approaches to controlled reproduction. In "Recent Advances in Marine Biotechnology" (M. Fingerman, R. Nagabhushanam, and M.-F. Thompson, eds.), Vol. 1, pp. 407–454. Oxford-IBH, New Delhi.

Stacey, N. E., and Hourston, A. H. (1982). Spawning and feeding behavior of captive Pacific herring, *Clupea harengus pallasi*. *Can. J. Fish. Aquat. Sci.* **39**, 489–498.

Stacey, N. E., and Kobayashi, M. (1996). Androgen induction of male sexual behaviors in female goldfish. *Horm. Behav.* **30**, 434–445.

Stacey, N. E., and Kyle, A. L. (1983). Effects of olfactory tract lesions on sexual and feeding behavior of goldfish. *Physiol. Behav.* **30**, 621–628.

Stacey, N. E., and Liley, N. R. (1974). Regulation of female spawning behavior in the female goldfish. *Nature (London)* **247**, 71–72.

Stacey, N. E., and Peter, R. E. (1979). Central action of prostaglandins in spawning behavior of female goldfish. *Physiol. Behav.* **22**, 1191–1196.

Stacey, N. E., and Sorensen, P. W. (1986). $17\alpha,20\beta$-dihydroxy-4-pregnen-3-one: A steroidal primer pheromone which increases milt volume in the goldfish. *Can. J. Zool.* **64**, 2412–2417.

Stacey, N. E., and Sorensen, P. W. (1991). Function and evolution of fish hormonal pheromones. In "Biochemistry and Molecular Biology of Fishes" (P. W. Hochachka and T. P. Mommsen, eds.), Vol. 1, pp. 109–135. Elsevier, Amsterdam.

Stacey, N. E., and Sorensen, P. W. (1999). Pheromones, fish. In "Encyclopedia of Reproduction" (E. Knobil and J. D. Neill, eds.), Vol. 1, pp. 748–755. Academic Press, San Diego.

Stacey, N. E., Cook, A. F., and Peter, R. E. (1979a). Ovulatory surge of gonadotropin in the goldfish, *Carassius auratus*. *Gen. Comp. Endocrinol.* **37**, 246–249.

Stacey, N. E., Cook, A. F., and Peter, R. E. (1979b). Spontaneous and gonadotropin-induced ovulation in the goldfish, *Carassius auratus* L.: Effects of external factors. *J. Fish Biol.* **15**, 349–361.

Stacey, N. E., Kyle, A. L., and Liley, N. R. (1986). Fish reproductive pheromones. In "Chemical Signals in Vertebrates" (D. Duvall, D. Müller-Schwarze, and R. M. Silverstein, eds.), Vol. 4, pp. 117–133, Plenum Press, New York.

Stacey, N. E., Sorensen, P. W., Van Der Kraak, G. J., and Dulka, J. G. (1989). Direct evidence that $17\alpha,20\beta$-dihydroxy-4-pregnen-3-one functions as a goldfish primer pheromone: Preovulatory release is closely associated with male endocrine responses. *Gen. Comp. Endocrinol.* **75**, 62–70.

Stacey, N. E., Cardwell, J. R., Liley, N. R., Scott, A. P., and Sorensen, P. W. (1994a). Hormonal sex pheromones in fish. In "Perspectives in Endocrinology" (K. G. Davey, R. E. Peter, and S. S. Tobe, eds.), pp. 438–448. National Research Council, Ottawa.

Stacey, N. E., Zheng, W. B., and Cardwell, J. R. (1994b). Milt production in common carp (*Cyprinus carpio*): Stimulation by a goldfish steroid pheromone. *Aquaculture* **127**, 265–276.

Stacey, N. E., Cardwell, J. R., and Murphy, C. (1995). Hormonal pheromones in freshwater fishes: Preliminary results of an electro-olfactogram survey. In "Fish Pheromones: Origins and Modes of Action" (A. V. M. Canario and D. M. Power, eds.), pp. 47–55. University of Algarve Press, Faro, Portugal.

Stacey, N. E., Fraser, E. J., Sorensen, P. W., and Van Der Kraak, G. J. (2001). Milt production in goldfish: Regulation by multiple social stimuli. *Comp. Biochem. Physiol. C* **130**, 467–476.

Stern, K., and McClintock, M. K. (1998). Regulation of ovulation by human pheromones. *Nature (London)* **392**, 177–179.

Stuart-Kregor, P. A. C., Sumpter, K. P., and Dodd, J. M. (1981). The involvement of gonadotrophin and sex steroids in the control of reproduction in the parr and adults of Atlantic salmon, *Salmo salar* L. *J. Fish Biol.* **18**, 59–72.

Sveinsson, T., and Hara, T. J. (1995). Mature males of arctic charr, *Salvelinus alpinus*, release F-type prostaglandins to attract conspecific mature females and stimulate their spawning behaviour. *Environ. Biol. Fishes* **42**, 253–266.

Sveinsson, T., and Hara, T. J. (2000). Olfactory sensitivity and specificity of arctic charr, *Salvelinus alpinus*, to a putative male pheromone, prostaglandin F2α. *Physiol. Behav.* **69**, 301–307.

Tavolga, W. N. (1956). Visual, chemical and sound stimuli as cues in the sex discriminatory behavior of the gobiid fish, *Bathygobius soporator*. *Zoologica* **41**, 49–64.

Taylor, J., and Mahon, R. (1977). Hybridization of *Cyprinus carpio* and *Carassius auratus*, the first two exotic species in the lower Laurentian Great Lakes. *Environ. Biol. Fishes* **1**, 205–208.

Teeter, J. (1980). Pheromone communication in sea lampreys (*Petromyzon marinus*): Implications for population management. *Can. J. Fish. Aquat. Sci.* **37,** 2123–2132.

Thomas, P. (1994). Hormonal control of final oocyte maturation in sciaenid fishes. In "Perspectives in Comparative Endocrinology" (K. G. Davey, R. E. Peter, and S. S. Tobe, eds.), pp. 619–662. National Research Council of Canada, Ottawa.

Thomas, P., and Das, S. (1997). Correlation between binding affinities of C21 steroids for the maturation-inducing steroid membrane receptor in spotted seatrout ovaries and their agonist and antagonist activities in an oocyte maturation bioassay. *Biol. Reprod,* **57,** 999–1007.

Thomas, P., and Trant, J. M. (1989). Evidence that $17\alpha,20\beta,21$-trihydroxy-4-pregnen-3-one is a maturation-inducing steroid in spotted seatrout. *Fish Physiol. Biochem.* **7,** 185–191.

Thomas, P., Breckenridge-Miller, D., and Detweiler, C. (1997). Binding characteristics and regulation of the $17,20\beta,21$-trihydroxy-4-pregnen-3-one (20beta-S) receptor on testicular and sperm plasma membranes of spotted seatrout (*Cynoscion nebulosus*). *Fish Physiol. Biochem.* **17,** 109–116.

Timms, A. M., and Kleerekoper, H. (1972). The locomotor response of male *Ictalurus punctatus,* the channel catfish, to a pheromone released by the ripe female of the species. *Trans. Am. Fish. Soc.* **102,** 302–310.

Trant, J. M., and Thomas, P. (1989). Isolation of a novel maturation-inducing steroid produced in vitro by ovaries of Atlantic croaker. *Gen. Comp. Endocrinol.* **75,** 397–404.

Trudeau, V. L. (1997). Neuroendocrine regulation of gonadotrophin II release and gonadal growth in goldfish. *Rev. Reprod.* **2,** 55–68.

Trudeau, V. L., Murthy, C. K., Habibi, H. R., Sloley, B. D., and Peter, R. E. (1993). Effects of sex steroid treatments on gonadotropin-releasing hormone-stimulated gonadotropin secretion from the goldfish pituitary. *Biol. Reprod.* **48,** 300–307.

Van Den Hurk, R., and Lambert, J. G. D. (1983). Ovarian steroid glucuronides function as sex pheromones for male zebrafish, *Brachydanio rerio. Can. J. Zool.* **61,** 2381–2387.

Van Den Hurk, R., and Resink, J. W. (1992). Male reproductive system as sex pheromone producer in teleost fish. *J. Exp. Zool.* **261,** 204–213.

Van Den Hurk, R., Van Zoelan, G. A., Schoonen, W. G. E. J., Resink, J. W., Lambert, J. G. D., and Van Oordt, P. G. W. J. (1987a). Do testicular steroid glucuronides of zebrafish, *Brachydanio rerio,* evoke ovulation in female conspecifics? *Gen. Comp. Endocrinol.* **66,** 19.

Van Den Hurk, R., Schoonen, W. G. E. J., Van Zoelen, G. A., and Lambert, J. G. D. (1987b). The biosynthesis of steroid glucuronides in the testis of zebrafish, *Brachydanio rerio,* and their pheromonal function as ovulation inducers. *Gen. Comp. Endocrinol.* **68,** 179–188.

Van Den Hurk, R., Resink, J. W., and Peute, J. (1987c). The seminal vesicle of the catfish, *Clarias gariepinus*: A histological, histochemical and enzyme-histochemical, ultrastructural, and physiological study. *Cell Tissue Res.* **247,** 573–582.

Van Der Kraak, G. J., Sorensen, P. W., Stacey, N. E., and Dulka, J. G. (1989). Periovulatory female goldfish release three potential pheromones: $17\alpha,20\beta$-dihydroxyprogesterone, $17\alpha,20\beta$-dihydroxyprogesterone-glucuronide, and 17α-hydroxyprogesterone. *Gen. Comp. Endocrinol.* **73,** 452–457.

Van Weerd, J. H., and Richter, C. J. J. (1991). Sex pheromones and ovarian development in teleost fish. *Comp. Biochem. Physiol. A* **100,** 517–527.

Van Weerd, J. H., Sukkel, M., Lambert, J. G. D., and Richter, C. J. J. (1991). GCMS-identified steroids and steroid glucuronides in ovarian growth-stimulating holding water from adult African catfish, *Clarias gariepinus. Comp. Biochem. Physiol.* **98,** 303–311.

Vermeirssen, E. L. M., and Scott, A. P. (1996). Excretion of free and conjugated steroids in rainbow trout (*Oncorhynchus mykiss*): Evidence for branchial excretion of the maturation-inducing steroid $17\alpha,20\beta$-dihydroxy-4-pregnen-3-one. *Gen. Comp. Endocrinol* **101,** 180–194.

Vermeirssen, E. L. M., Scott, A. P., Sumpter, J. P., and Prat, F. (1995). A pheromone in female trout urine. In "Proceedings of the Fifth International Symposium on the Reproductive Physiology of Fish" (F. W. Goetz and P. Thomas, eds.), Fish Symp. 95, pp. 249–251. University of Texas at Austin.

Villars, T. A., Hale, N., and Chapnick, D. (1985). Prostaglandin F2α stimulates reproductive behavior of female paradise fish (*Macropodus opercularis*). *Horm. Behav.* **19,** 21–35.

von Bartheld, C. S., and Meyer, D. L. (1986). Tracing of single fibers of the nervus terminalis in the goldfish brain. *Cell Tissue Res.* **245,** 143–158.

Waring, C. P., and Moore, A. (1995). F-series prostaglandins have a priming pheromonal effect on mature male Atlantic salmon parr. In "Proceedings of the Fifth International Symposium on the Reproductive Physiology of Fish" (F. W. Goetz and P. Thomas, eds.), Fish Symp. 95, pp. 255–257. University of Texas at Austin.

Waring, C. P., and Moore, A. (1997). Sublethal effects of a carbamate pesticide on pheromonal mediated endocrine function in mature male Atlantic salmon (*Salmo salar* L.) parr. *Fish Physiol. Biochem.* **17,** 203–211.

Waring, C. P., Moore, A., and Scott, A. P. (1996). Milt and endocrine responses of mature male Atlantic salmon (*Salmo salar*

L.) parr to water-borne testosterone, 17,20β-dihydroxy-4-pregnen-3-one-20-sulfate, and the urines from adult female and male salmon. *Gen. Comp. Endocrinol.* **103**, 142–149.

Warner, R. R. (1984). Mating behavior and hermaphroditism in coral reef fishes. *Am. Sci.* **72**, 128–136.

Wilson, E. O., and Bossert, W. H. (1963). Chemical communication among animals. *Recent Prog. Horm. Res.* **19**, 673–716.

Xu, F., Greer, C. A., and Shepherd, G. M. (2000). Odor maps in the olfactory bulb. *J. Comp. Neurol.* **422**, 489–495.

Yamamoto, K., Nagahama, Y., and Yamazaki, F. (1966). A method to induce artificial spawning of goldfish all through the year. *Bull. Jpn. Soc. Sci. Fish.* **32**, 977–983.

Yamamoto, N., Oka, Y., and Kawashima, S. (1997). Lesions of gonadotropin-releasing hormone-immunoreactive terminal nerve cells: Effects on the reproductive behavior of male dwarf gouramis. *Neuroendocrinology* **65**, 403–412.

Yamazaki, F. (1990). The role of urine in sex discrimination in the goldfish *Carassius auratus*. *Bull. Fac. Fish. Hokkaido Univ.* **41**, 155–161.

Yamazaki, F., and Watanabe, K. (1979). The role of sex hormones in sex recognition during spawning behavior of the goldfish, *Carassius auratus* L. *Proc. Indian Natl. Sci. Acad., Part B* **45**, 505–511.

Yambe, H., Shindo, M., and Yamazaki, F. (1999). A releaser pheromone that attracts males in the urine of mature female masu salmon. *J. Fish Biol.* **55**, 158–171.

Young, G., Todo, T., Kobayashi, T., Guan, G., and Nagahama, Y. (1997). Steroidogenesis by the salmonid ovarian follicle: The two-cell type model revisited. In "Advances in Comparative Endocrinology" (S. Kawashima and S. Kikuyama, eds.), pp. 1443–1449. Monduzzi Editore, Bologna.

Zakon, H., Ferrari, M. B., and Schaefer, J. (1995). Behavior, brains and biophysics: Steroidal modulation of communication signals in electric fish. In "Proceedings of the Fifth International Symposium on the Reproductive Physiology of Fish" (F. W. Goetz and P. Thomas, eds.), Fish Symp. 95, pp. 264–266. University of Texas at Austin.

Zeeck, E., and Ide, V. (1996). The role of sex pheromones in the reproductive behavior of *Blennius pavo* (Riso). In "Fish Pheromones: Origins and Modes of Action" (A. V. M. Canario and D. M. Power, eds.), pp. 33–38. University of Algarve Press, Faro, Portugal.

Zeiske, E., Theisen, B., and Breucker, H. (1992). Structure, development, and evolutionary aspects of the peripheral olfactory system. In "Fish Chemoreception" (T. J. Hara, ed.), pp. 13–39. Chapman & Hall, London.

Zheng, W., and Stacey, N. E. (1996). Two mechanisms for increasing milt volume in male goldfish. *J. Exp. Zool.* **276**, 287–295.

Zheng, W., and Stacey, N. E. (1997). A steroidal pheromone and spawning stimuli act *via* different neuroendocrine mechanisms to increase gonadotropin and milt volume in male goldfish (*Carassius auratus*). *Gen. Comp. Endocrinol.* **105**, 228–235.

Zheng, W., Strobeck, C., and Stacey, N. E. (1997). The steroid pheromone 17α,20β-dihydroxy-4-pregnen-3-one increases fertility and paternity in goldfish. *J. Exp. Biol.* **200**, 2833–2840.

Zippel, H. P., Lago-Schaaf, T., and Caprio, J. (1993). Ciliated olfactory receptor neurons in goldfish (*Carassius auratus*) partially survive nerve axotomy, rapidly regenerate and respond to amino acids. *J. Comp. Physiol. A* **173**, 537–547.

Zippel, H. P., Sorensen, P. W., and Hansen, A. (1997). High correlation between microvillous olfactory receptor cell abundance and sensitivity to pheromones in olfactory nerve-sectioned goldfish. *J. Comp. Physiol. A* **180**, 39–52.

Zippel, H. P., Reschke, C., and Korff, V. (1999). Simultaneous recordings from two physiologically different types of relay neurons, mitral cells and ruffed cells, in the olfactory bulb of goldfish. *Cell. Mol. Biol.* **45**, 327–337.

Zippel, H. P., Gloger, M., Luthje, L., Nasser, S., and Wilke, S. (2000). Pheromone discrimination ability of olfactory bulb mitral and ruffed cells in the goldfish (*Carassius auratus*). *Chem. Senses* **25**, 339–349.

26

Social Regulation of the Brain: Status, Sex, and Size

Russell D. Fernald

Program in Neuroscience
Stanford University
Stanford, California 94305

*I*t is self-evident that the brain controls behavior, but can behavior also control the brain? Evidence has revealed that social behavior can cause changes in certain brain structures in adult animals. Such alterations can be dramatic and reversible and are typically related to reproductive behavior. How does behavior sculpt the brain and how are these changes controlled? Our studies link organismal behavior with molecular events by using a fish model system in which social behaviors regulate reproduction. This African cichlid fish exihibits complex observable behaviors centered around the existence of two distinct classes of males, those with territories and those without. We show that a variety of neural and endocrine changes result from changes in social status. Surprisingly, we also demonstrate that body growth rate is regulated by social status and immediate social history. Discovering how social information is transduced into physiological processes via cellular and molecular changes presents a major challenge for future research.

I. INTRODUCTION

Among social animals, the behavior of one individual or of a group of individuals can strongly influence the behavior of other animals, as first systematically described by Konrad Lorenz (1935). The nature of such influential interactions depends on the species, the situation, and the actual behavioral interaction. The most reliable predictor of these encounters is the social status of the individuals involved. For example, a dominant animal threatened by a nondominant animal behaves differently than does a dominant animal threatened by another dominant individual. Similarly, behavior by a female produces quite different reactions in males depending on their social status. It is fair to say that in every social system that has been observed, the behavior of individuals depends in part on their social status and in part on their physical environment. This universal dependence of behavior on context is the primary scientific framework used to interpret behavior during social interactions.

But how does an animal know its own status and behave appropriately? And how does an individual recognize an opportunity to change status upward or acquiesce to an imposed change in status downward? Clearly, in the short term, physiological processes allow the animal to act and, in the long term, cellular and molecular processes accommodate to changes in its external reality or social status. Some of the required physiological and molecular changes must precede behavioral change, but others are a consequence of that change. How are these internal changes regulated by social interaction? There must be a transduction of social information into internal change—but how? To a great extent, this must depend on how the animal perceives and interprets events in its world.

Von Uexküll (1909) first realized that every animal species experiences life differently, living in what he called its *Umwelt*, or unique perceptual world. A bat using sonic echoes to probe the world in darkness surely perceives its surroundings differently than does a giraffe, which relies on its eyes, nose, and ears, or a weakly electric fish that relies almost entirely on faint electrical signals for information. Each animal species has a particular complement of sensory capabilities that fundamentally restricts the physical stimuli it can use to make behavioral decisions. This constraint on the perceived world necessarily limits the possible behavioral responses of any animal. Writing at the beginning of the twentieth century, Von Uexküll could not possibly have anticipated the discovery of magnetic, electric, or pressure senses; nor could he have imagined seeing into the infrared and ultraviolet or even that light detection exists at some remarkable places other than the eye (Arikawa *et al.*, 1996). These discoveries make his writing all the more prescient, and the many interesting unusual animal umwelts reveal the many ways that natural selection has shaped animal perceptions. The range of sensory capabilities are matched by variations in animal form and function that also reflect adaptations to the environment.

In evolutionary change, the ultimate arbiter of successful adaptations is behavior. An animal that survives does so because it behaves successfully during the multitude of interactions with other animals and with its environment. Yet behavior, in turn, depends on intricate physiological, cellular, and, ultimately, molecular adaptations. A major challenge in biology is to understand the linkages across these levels of analysis as an animal interacts with its world. How is behavior controlled via physiological processes and, correspondingly, how does behavior influence physiological, cellular, or molecular events? Here I summarize evidence from experiments designed to discover the mechanisms that underlie the synergistic interactions between behavior and physiology in a model system uniquely suited for this inquiry.

II. MODEL SYSTEM

To understand how behavior influences the brain and vice versa, our laboratory studies a cichlid fish (*Haplochromis burtoni*) native to Lake Tanganyika in central Africa. In its natural habitat, there are two kinds of males—those with territories and those without (Fernald and Hirata, 1977a,b). Territorial males (Ts), which make up only approximately 10–15% of the males, are brightly colored with a blue or yellow body color, a dramatic black stripe through the eye, vertical black bars on the body, a black spot on the tip of the gill cover, and a large red patch just behind it (Fig. 1). In contrast, nonterritorial males (NTs) are cryptically colored, making them difficult to distinguish from the substrate and from females, which are similarly camouflaged—that is, the nonterritorial males appear nearly identical to females. The animals live in a lek-like social system in which the brightly colored territorial males vigorously defend contiguous territories arrayed over a food supply (Fernald, 1977). The number of territorial males is limited by the size of the available food supply.

This species has an elaborate social system that depends on signaling among animals. Social communication in *H. burtoni* depends primarily on visual signals (Fernald, 1984). Territorial males are very active, performing at least 19 distinct behavioral acts during fast-paced social encounters (Fernald, 1977). They divide their time among digging a pit in the center of their territory, fighting with neighbors at common territorial boundaries, chasing nonterritorial animals away, and soliciting and courting females. Solicitation and courtship behaviors are easily identified because the males display bright coloration patterns toward the courted female. Courtship includes leading the female toward the territory and during courting quivering his spread, brightly colored anal fin in front of the female. Females led into the territory feed by nipping at and sifting through the bottom cover.

Interestingly, nonterritorial males mimic this female behavior accurately enough that the territorial males allow them to eat in the territory. Soon enough, however, the deception is discovered and the female impersonator is chased off. If a genetic female responds to

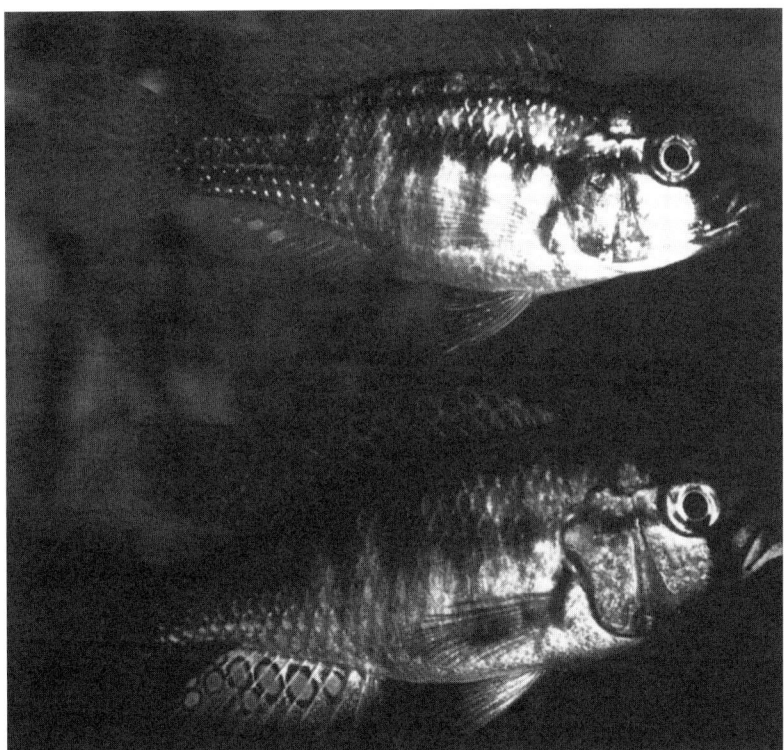

FIGURE 1 Illustration of the body patterns for typical territorial males (Ts) and nonterritorial males (NTs). (Top) NTs lack the robust markings of their territorial counterparts and are colored to maximize camouflage. (Bottom) Ts have distinctive anal fin spots, dark forehead, and lachrymal (eye-bar) stripes and are brightly colored, including orange humeral scales. The overall body color may be either yellow or blue. **See insert for a color version of this figure.**

the entreaties of a male, he leads her into his pit and continues the elaborate courtship movements, swimming to the front of the female and rapidly quivering his entire body with his anal fin spread in her view. As the pair disappears into the spawning pit out of direct view of the territory, other animals exploit this opportunity to feed energetically. The spawning male repeatedly interrupts his courtship behavior to chase intruders off his limited food supply. If physiologically ready and adequately stimulated, the female lays her eggs at the bottom of the pit, collecting them in her mouth almost immediately. After she lays several eggs, the male swims in front of her, again displaying the anal fins spots, his body quivering. The female then nips at the male's anal fin as though she mistakes his spots for uncollected ova; so, while attempting to collect the spots, the female ingests the milt ejected near them from the male and ensures fertilization. After several bouts of this alternating behavior, the female may go to the territory of another male to lay more eggs or depart from the territorial arena with the fertilized eggs to brood them (Fernald, 1984).

This brief description of the natural behavior of *H. burtoni* reveals the extensive role social interactions play in its daily life. It is important to note that, under the appropriate conditions, the behavior of *H. burtoni* in the laboratory matches exactly that found in the field (Fernald, 1977), making this a useful species for studying the influence of social behavior on the brain. Clearly, the behavior is guided by visual signals and the social scene largely governs the behavior of individual animals. Each behavioral act influences the next, both in the observed individual and in the animals involved in the interaction. During these encounters, information is exchanged between individuals that influences the next behavioral interaction of these animals. How do animals exchange key information and what are the consequences of that exchange?

III. DIFFERENCES BETWEEN TERRITORIAL AND NONTERRITORIAL MALES

As young *H. burtoni* grow, the social behavior of conspecifics regulates their behavioral and gonadal development and even their growth in a differentiated fashion (Fraley and Fernald, 1982). For the first 7–8 weeks of life, living in a group facilitates growth of males, compared to broodmates reared in total isolation with visual contact (Fig. 2). However, after this time, group-reared males that do not acquire and defend territories grow more slowly than those with territories. Males that do form territories develop their color patterns faster, weigh more, and have larger and more highly developed gonads than do animals reared under any other conditions (Fig. 2B). Concomitantly, group-reared fish show early-developing agonistic and aggressive behavioral patterns (chase, tailbeat, and fin spread) and chromatic patterns (eyebar and opercular spot) more than 2 weeks before these features appear in animals reared in physical isolation.

The absolute growth rate of *H. burtoni* under optimal conditions is dramatic and has resulted in novel developmental strategies over evolutionary time. These include the addition of new cells to the lens, retina, and brain (Fernald and Wright, 1983; Fernald, 1983, 1989; Johns and Fernald, 1981). Such social control of maturation and growth is found in many species (e.g., Borowsky, 1973; Schultz *et al.*, 1991) and takes a variety of forms. In *H. burtoni*, however, there are some unique effects of this social regulation of growth, most important being that it is not limited to early development.

Juvenile males raised with adults present, which is the natural condition, show suppressed gonadal maturation relative to those reared without adults (Davis and Fernald, 1990). As well as having smaller testes, these animals have smaller gonadotropin-releasing-hormone

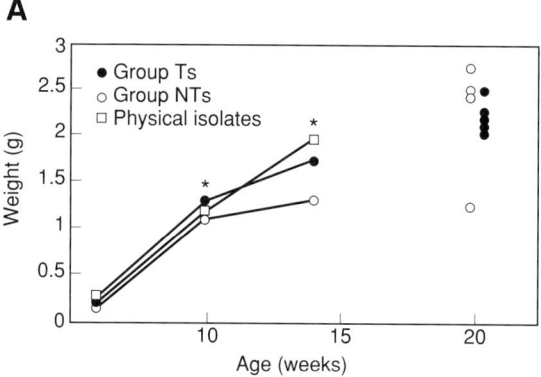

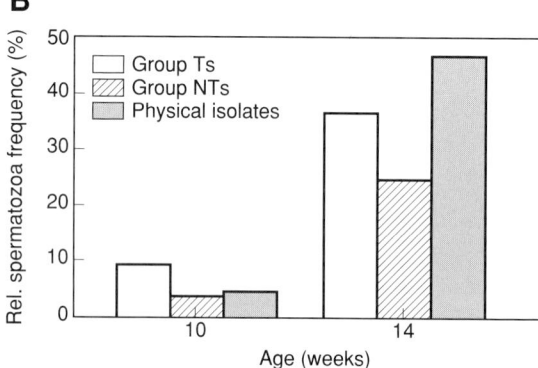

FIGURE 2 Development and maturation in group-reared (open and filled circles) and physically isolated (diamonds) juvenile *H. burtoni*. (A) Growth rates expressed as body weight for the different categories. Asterisks indicate that group-reared territorial fish (filled circles) weigh significantly more after 10 and 14 weeks than their nonterritorial (open circles) tankmates. Differences in standard lengths are not significant (data not shown). Note that after 20 weeks, size differences are no longer evident. (B) Relative estimates of mature spermatozoa in cross sections of the central testicular lobule. Note the rapid increase in physically isolated males between week 10 and week 14. After Fraley and Fernald (1982); Davis and Fernald (1990).

(GnRH)-containing neurons in the preoptic area, a region in the ventral telencephalon adjacent to the hypothalamus (Fig. 3). These neurons project to the pituitary (Bushnik and Fernald, 1995), where they release GnRH. The somata sizes of GnRH-containing neurons differ eightfold in volume depending on the social conditions. Because GnRH is the main signaling peptide that regulates reproductive maturity, the social control of maturation acts by changing structures in the brain. Thus, the social control of maturation is reflected via changes in structures in the brain.

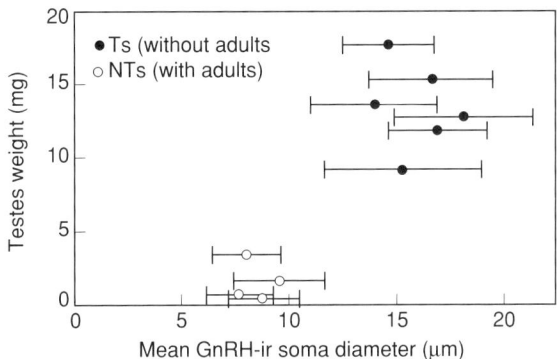

FIGURE 3 Demonstration of social regulation of the reproductive axis in juvenile *H. burtoni*. Testes weights of 20-week-old early-maturing (without adults present) territorial males (filled circles) and maturation-suppressed (with adults present) nonterritorial males (open circles) plotted against the respective average soma diameters for the largest 30% of preoptic GnRH-immunoreactive (GnRH-ir) neurons (± standard deviation). Neuron sizes are independent of body size in this experiment. Note the striking differences in cell size as well as testes weight between the two groups. After Davis and Fernald (1990).

What are the salient sensory cues that a juvenile male fish perceives that influence its initial social state? In the laboratory, if juvenile males are reared alone, they develop into territorial males with all the defining characteristics from large gonads to prominent lachrymal stripes. This shows that every male has the potential for social dominance, that this is the default developmental pathway, and that any genetic influence on dominance is negligible in comparison to social cues.

We have begun to dissect these social cues by sensory modality to determine the ones responsible for suppressing nonterritorial males and have discovered that, in addition to visual cues, tactile stimuli play a part (M. R. Davis and R. D. Fernald, unpublished observations). Thus, if a cohort of young fish are raised in the same aquarium as an older established community, the young males remain nonterritorial, as previously stated. If, however, the two groups are separated by a fine mesh net, one that allows visual and chemical contact and even permits threat displays across the barrier, they quickly learn that the would-be bullies on the other side of the tank are unable to chase and bite them. Freed from the threat of aggression by the big territorial males, the younger fish form their own communities, where again some 10% of the males escape maturational suppression and become territorial. In turn, these suppress the maturation of the remaining 90% of the males on their side of the net. Because both the older and younger communities have visual and chemical access to one another, these findings indicate that biting and nipping behaviors form some part of the suppressive signal imparted to nonterritorial fish.

Our studies have shown (Muske and Fernald, 1987a,b), that the territorial males differ not only in their social displays, but also in the prominence of those signals to other viewers. Becoming and remaining socially dominant produces long-term physiological changes, just as losing social dominance influences the physiological state. Given the importance of the correct production and recognition of social signals, there must be mechanisms responsible for their development and for their transduction into physiological system.

IV. SOCIAL CONTROL OF SEX AND SIZE

In the natural environment of *H. burtoni*, there are costs and benefits associated with territoriality. The obvious benefits are that territorial males have a reliable food supply and that they are the only males that spawn. The costs are that the bright flashy colors and active behaviors of dominant males make them conspicuous to birds of prey. Indeed, predation of territorial males occurs at a significantly higher rate than does that of females or nonterritorial males (Fernald and Hirata, 1977b). When a T is removed, the vacated space provides an opportunity for a NT to switch social state. Within a few seconds, such NTs produce an eyebar and exhibit aggressive behaviors. What endogenous changes accompany this outward transformation and how are they related to one another?

A. Social Regulation of Reproduction

To understand whether social status also regulates reproduction in adult animals, adult males were converted from territorial (T) to nonterritorial (NT) or vice versa and their reproductive axis examined. To do this, Ts were moved into communities with larger Ts; as a result, they became NTs (T → NT). Correspondingly, NTs were moved to new communities consisting of females and smaller males that they could dominate, as a

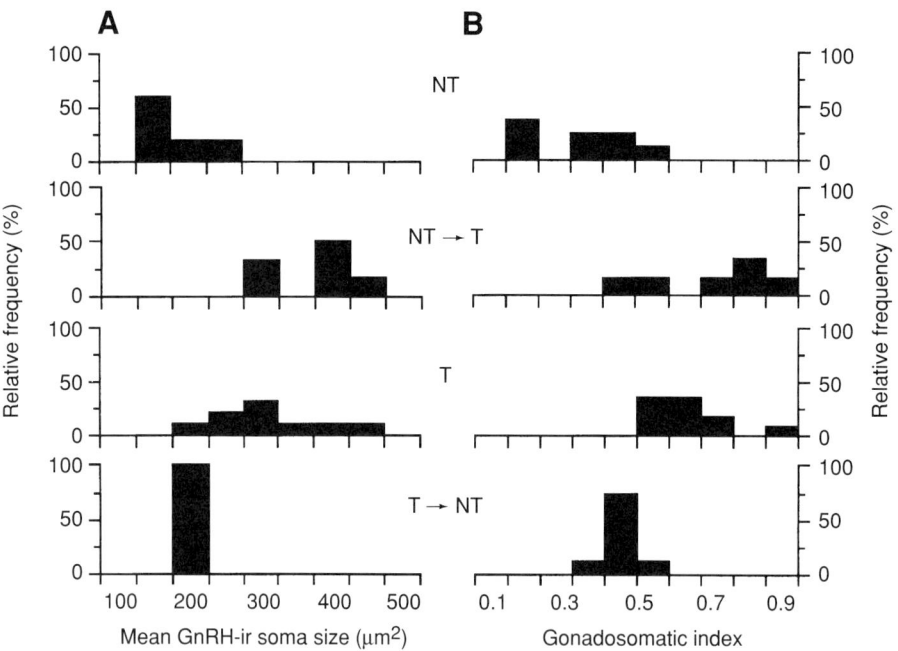

FIGURE 4 The effect of social change on (A) GnRH cell size and (B) GSI as shown in frequency histograms measured in the four possible social classes of animals. (A) Mean soma sizes of POA GnRH-IR (GnRH-ir) neurons. (B) Gonadosomatic indices (GSI). Percentage of individuals are plotted for each social category (NT, T, NT → T, T → NT). There are significant differences in soma sizes as well as GSI between animals that were Ts and ascended NT → Ts when compared to animals that were NTs and descended T → NTs. Modified after Francis et al. (1993).

result of which they became Ts (NT → T). In each case, the subjects remained in the altered social setting for 4 weeks, after which the size of GnRH containing cells was measured (Francis et al., 1993).

To quantify the consequences of this change in social status on reproductive competence, we measured changes in the gonad size and in the mean soma sizes of the preoptic area (POA) GnRH-immunoreactive (GnRH-IR) (Fig. 4). The mean value of both the soma size of POA GnRH-IR neurons (Fig. 4A) and gonadosomatic index (GSI) (Fig. 4B) were significantly larger in both NT → Ts and control Ts than in T → NTs and NTs. In two other GnRH-IR cell groups, one located in the terminal nerve region and the other in the mesencephalon, there was no difference in mean soma sizes between Ts and NTs (Davis and Fernald, 1990). Thus the change in POA GnRH-containing neurons is not a general property of cells expressing GnRH but rather is confined to those in the hypothalamic-pituitary-gonadal (HPG) axis.

These data show that following social change, endogenous changes occur that equip a newly dominant male for his new social and reproductive status. Conversely, animals subjected to a downgrade in social status (T → NT) lost both GnRH cell size and gonad size, producing a match to their new social state. Clearly, social status determines both the soma size of POA irGnRH neurons and GSI, and these effects are reversible. The relatively larger testes and GnRH-IR neurons characteristic of Ts is a consequence of their social dominance and when this dominance advantage is lost, both neurons and testes shrink.

Because the precipitating event in these studies was the experimentally manipulated change in social status, it is clear that in these teleosts changes in social status can initiate changes in endocrine state. However, such changes in social and endocrine systems interleave so fluently that they suggest a complex nexus of interactions rather than a linear chain of control. GnRH-containing neurons in the hypothalamus of adult Ts

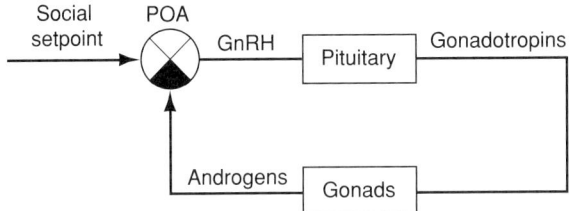

FIGURE 5 Schematic illustration showing the regulation of GnRH release in male *H. burtoni* via a social setpoint. Our data show that neurons in the preoptic area (POA) integrate both social and hormonal signals to regulate GnRH release. In this model, the setpoint for the GnRH level is determined by social signals, and the maintenance of the GnRH level at this setpoint is achieved by negative feedback from gonadal androgens. Modified from Soma *et al.* (1996).

both influence and are influenced by circulating gonadal hormones. We know this because castration of Ts caused GnRH neurons to increase in size (Soma *et al.*, 1996). This neuronal hypertrophy in castrated animals was prevented either by testosterone (T) or by 11-ketotestosterone (11-KT) treatment. Estradiol (E_2) treatment did not reduce GnRH cell size in castrated animals. These results (Fig. 5) indicate that androgens reduce the size of GnRH cells through negative feedback. Because E_2 had no effect, androgen influence on GnRH cell size appears to be independent of aromatization. These data are consistent with the hypothesis that the setpoint for hypothalamic GnRH cell size is determined by social cues and that this setpoint is maintained via negative feedback by gonadal androgens. Territorial males have large GnRH-containing neurons despite high circulating androgens, not because of them.

The castration experiment was performed on Ts. Enlarged GnRH neurons resulted, and although the mean soma sizes were even slightly bigger than those in control Ts, their large size is in concert with the social dominance of the animal. To test whether GnRH neuronal cell size and social state can be dissociated, the castration experiment was replicated, this time using NTs. Following surgery to remove gonadal tissue, the fish were returned to the social settings from which they came, ensuring that they remained nonterritorial. Behavioral observations confirmed that these animals were indeed NTs. Two weeks later, the fish were sacrificed and their brains were examined for the sizes of the GnRH neurons in the POA. The number of animals that survived the surgical intervention followed by restoration to the community tank was small, and thus the results are preliminary. They suggest, however, that the GnRH neurons grew to be insignificantly different from those seen in Ts (R. D. Yu and Fernald, unpublished observations). Thus, through experimental manipulation it appears that GnRH neuronal soma size and social behavior can be uncoupled.

In *H. burtoni*, the regulation of growth and development may be adaptive in their natural habitat, where territorial space is limited. In the shore pools where these animals live, only a fraction of the males can breed at any time. As already noted, these breeding males appear to be particularly vulnerable to avian predators (Fernald and Hirata, 1977b), and hence territorial ownership may be relatively brief. Thus, there may be a selective advantage for males to have a retarded growth rate until they have an opportunity to become territorial, whereupon they grow rapidly.

Interestingly, following our original observation, we have analyzed in more detail the rate at which social interactions influence the GnRH cell size. We have discovered that the rate of cell size change is a function of the direction of the social transition (White *et al.*, 2002). Animals moving from nonterritorial to territorial status achieve the changes in GnRH-containing cell size (cf. Fig. 3) in just 7 days, whereas animals moving from territorial to nonterritorial may require 4 weeks until completion. This result is intuitively satisfying because there is such a distinct selective advantage to being a T. Preliminary analysis of the behavior of animals that are moving in either direction is quite instructive. Many Ts that have lost status continue to act territorial, even if only in concealed locations and at times when they are not being scrutinized by the new dominant male.

In sum, these data suggest that external social signals are transduced into at least two different pathways in *H. burtoni* males. One of these is hormonal, determining the reproductive state of the animal, and the other behavioral. Although in intact animals the two pathways correspond and the hormonal cues maintain the necessary physiological state associated with social state, it is possible to dissociate the circuitry by experimental intervention (e.g., castration of nonterritorial males).

Further support that the two systems can be dissociated comes from work in *H. burtoni* females in which the social circuit appears to be muted or missing, although the endocrine circuitry shows plasticity parallel to that seen in males.

In contrast to males, female *H. burtoni* do not appear to have differences in social status. They spend most of their time at the fringes of the dominant male's territory where they school with nonterritorial males. As previously described, they move into territorial waters only to feed or spawn. This absence of social difference among females prompted the questions: Are GnRH neurons in female *H. burtoni* plastic, similar to males, and, if so, what regulates changes in cell size? As already described, a ripe female lays her eggs and then takes them into her mouth for fertilization and brooding. The brood is carried for approximately 2 weeks before being released. The changes in female appearance that accompany these reproductive states are due to physiological rather than social events. Thus, differences in body color, which in males reflects reproductive status, do not occur in females. Instead, a female that is ready to spawn has an enlarged abdomen, due to the presence of ripe eggs. Later, after spawning, females with distinctively large mouth cavities filled with fry are not ready to spawn and avoid males.

Because females do not engage in the aggressive social interactions that regulate male GnRH cell size, it is possible that they might not show the same plastic changes. GnRH cell size would then be sexually dimorphic, increasing in females simply as a function of development and becoming stable at maturity. This would contrast with the life-long potential for plasticity seen in males. Alternatively, because GnRH cell size in males is correlated with both social and reproductive status, cell size in females might fluctuate according to the female reproductive cycle.

To study possible changes in cell size in female *H. burtoni*, we analyzed cell size as a function of reproductive state in females (White and Fernald, 1993). Although there is some contribution of body size to the cell size changes, body size differences do not account for all of the observed changes. Soma sizes in spawning females are typically twice as large as those in females carrying broods, whereas postreproductive fish have the largest neuronal soma sizes. These changes occur within the 2 weeks it takes to brood a clutch and the differences in GnRH neuronal soma size are comparable to those seen between dominant and subordinate males.

Taken together, these data have provided considerable insight into how social signals regulate reproductive physiology. The other major influence on the social behavior of *H. burtoni* is changes in its physical environment.

B. Environmental Influences on Social Status and Size

The shore pools of Lake Tanganyika, the natural habitat of *H. burtoni*, are relatively unstable. Winds and the presence of large animals such as hippopotami cause considerable changes in the local conditions animals face (Fernald and Hirata, 1977b). Only a fraction of the males can breed at any time, and these animals are particularly vulnerable to avian predators. As a consequence, reproductive opportunities may arise as frequently as they vanish because territorial ownership may be relatively brief. To untangle the causal relationship between environmental state and social status, we kept animals in stable and fluctuating habitats and assessed the consequences on the reproductive axis and body size.

In *H. burtoni*, habitat complexity influences the fraction of the male population that can sustain territories (Hofmann *et al.*, 1999). Moreover, the stability of the habitat affects the duration of territorial tenure because in a fluctuating habitat, in which the three-dimensional layout changes frequently, males hold territories for a significantly shorter time than in a stable habitat. Even a stable habitat results in a significant level of change in social status (Hofmann *et al.*, 1999). To our surprise, we found that this intrinsic instability is caused by differential growth rates. Specifically, NTs and NT → Ts grow faster than Ts and T → NTs (Fig. 6). It seems likely that after establishing a territory, animals allocate energy simultaneously toward reproduction and growth to maintain a competitive advantage over other Ts. Indeed, animals that lose a territory slow their growth rate and may even shrink (Hofmann *et al.*, 1999). A possible mechanism regulating differential growth is the control of somatostatin release in the pituitary. Because this neurohormone inhibits the release of growth hormone (GH), it is a likely site of control (Brazeau *et al.*, 1973; Gillies, 1997). This is supported by our data showing that somatostatin-containing neurons in the POA change size (Fig. 6) when social status and,

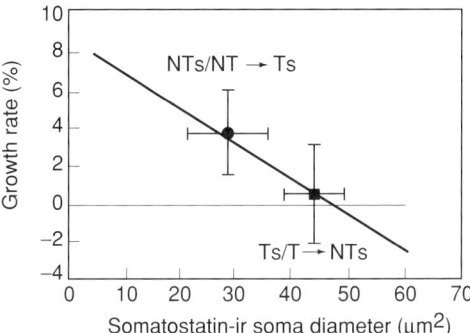

FIGURE 6 Relationship between growth rates and the mean somatostatin-IR (Somatostatin-ir) soma size in *H. burtoni*. NTs and NT → T males (filled circle; mean ± standard deviations) have smaller soma cross-sectional areas and grow faster than Ts and T → NTs (filled square; mean ± standard deviations). After Hofmann and Fernald (2000).

consequently, growth rate change (Hofmann and Fernald, 2000). The somata of these neurons are significantly larger in Ts and T → NTs than in NTs and NT → Ts. It is unknown whether larger neurons produce more somatostatin to be released into the pituitary or whether they represent an accumulation of somatostatin as its release is inhibited. Preliminary evidence from measurements of circulating GH (Hofmann et al., 1999) suggests that the latter may be the case, thus inhibiting the release of GH from the pituitary in NTs and NT → Ts. This surprising result makes likely the social regulation of insulin-like growth factor I (IGF-I), which mediates many of the somatic effects of GH and whose release is controlled by GH (Mommsen, 1998).

Why do animals that have lost a territory (T → NTs) slow down their growth rate and even shrink? Behavioral stressors may play a role. As shown by Fox et al. (1997), in *H. burtoni* status switches in both directions can be accompanied by elevated levels of the major stress hormone cortisol, with the T → NT change showing the most pronounced increase. NT → Ts with increased cortisol levels usually did not maintain territoriality. Fish descending in rank consistently showed high levels of cortisol that could, in turn, cause somatic growth to be down-regulated. As has been shown in another cichlid, the tilapia *Oreochromis mossambicus*, chronic administration of cortisol leads to a reduction in body weight and reproductive parameters such as gamete size and levels of sex steroids (Foo and Lam, 1993). Although the regulatory interactions between GH and cortisol are very complex (Thakore and Dinan, 1994; van Weerd and Komen, 1998), *in vivo* experiments have demonstrated an inhibitory effect of glucocorticoids on somatic growth in many vertebrates including fish (e.g., Pickering, 1990).

Could cortisol also be involved in the growth rate differences between established Ts and NTs? Fox et al. (1997) showed that cortisol levels in Ts and NTs do not differ as long as the fish community remains unstable. However, in a situation of relatively high social stability, Ts have significantly lower levels of circulating cortisol than NTs. Under such a stable situation, NTs still grow faster than Ts. Therefore, growth may not be effectively inhibited by cortisol in those animals. Rather, we hypothesize that other factors may become significant when animals maintain a particular social behavior for many weeks (e.g., feeding habits, behavioral activity, and energy expenditure).

V. CONCLUSION

In *H. burtoni* males, the brain is continually being remodeled by social behavior throughout life. Such neural renovations make sense because there are limited resources and a clear selective advantage for males that can respond quickly to reproductive opportunities. The external phenotypic plasticity allows males to allocate physiological resources to reproduction or growth, depending on social and environmental circumstances. Our studies of this model system reveal remarkably intricate interrelationships between habitat structure, behavior, and the brain. It seems likely that such connections exist in other species and await discovery.

References

Arikawa, K., Suyama, D., and Fujii, D. (1996). Light on butterfly mating. *Nature (London)* **382**, 119.

Borowsky, R. (1973). Social control of adult size in males of *Xiphophorus variatus*. *Nature (London)* **245**, 332–335.

Brazeau, P., Vale, W., Burgus, R., Ling, N., Butcher, M., Rivier, J., and Guillemin, R. (1973). Hypothalamic polypeptide that inhibits the secretion of immunoreactive pituitary growth hormone. *Science* **179**, 77–79.

Bushnik, T. L., and Fernald, R. D. (1995). The population of GnRH-containing neurons showing socially mediated size changes project to the pituitary in a teleost, *Haplochromis burtoni. Brain, Behav. Evol.* **46**, 371–377.

Davis, M. R., and Fernald, R. D. (1990). Social control of neuronal soma size. *J. Neurobiol.* **21**, 1180–1188.

Fernald, R. D. (1977). Quantitative observations of *Haplochromis burtoni* under semi-natural conditions. *Animal Behav.* **25**, 643–653.

Fernald, R. D. (1983). Neural basis of visual pattern recognition in fish. *In* "Advances in Vertebrate Neuroethology" (J. P. Ewert, R. R. Capranica, and D. J. Ingle, eds.), pp. 569–580. Plenum Press, New York.

Fernald, R. D. (1984). Vision and behavior in an African cichlid fish. *Am. Scientist* **72**, 58–65.

Fernald, R. D. (1989). Retinal rod neurogenesis. *In* "Development of the Vertebrate Retina" (B. L. Finley and D. R. Sengelaub, eds.), pp. 31–42. Plenum Press, New York.

Fernald, R. D., and Hirata, N. R. (1977a). Field study of *Haplochromis burtoni*: Quantitative behavioral observations. **25**, 964–975.

Fernald, R. D., and Hirata, N. R. (1977b). Field study of *Haplochromis burtoni*: Habitats and co-habitants. *Envir. Biol. Fishes* **2**, 299–308.

Fernald, R. D., and Wright, S. E. (1983). Maintenance of optical quality during crystalline lens growth. *Nature (London)* **301**, 618–620.

Foo, J. T. W., and Lam, T. J. (1993). Retardation of ovarian growth and depression of serum steroid levels in the tilapia *Oreochromis mossambicus* by cortisol implantation. *Aquaculture* **115**, 133–143.

Fox, H. E., White, S. A., Kao, M. H. F., and Fernald, R. D. (1997). Stress and dominance in a social fish. *J. Neurosci.* **17**, 6463–6469.

Fraley, N. B., and Fernald, R. D. (1982). Social control of developmental rate in the African cichlid, *Haplochromis burtoni*. *Zeitschrift für Tierpsychologie* **60**, 66–82.

Francis, R. C., Soma, K., and Fernald, R. D. (1993). Social regulation of the brain-pituitary-gonadal axis. *Proc. Nat. Acad. Sci. U.S.A.* **90**, 7794–7798.

Gillies, G. (1997). Somatostatin: The neuroendocrine story. *Trends Pharmacol. Sci.* **18**, 87–95.

Hofmann, H. A., and Fernald, R. D. (2000). Social status controls somatostatin-neuron size and growth. *J. Neurosci.* **20**, 1248–1252.

Hofmann, H. A., Benson, M. E., and Fernald, R. D. (1999). Social status regulates growth rate: Consequences for life-history strategies. *Proc. Natl. Acad. Sci. U.S.A.* **95**, 14171–14176.

Johns, P. R., and Fernald, R. D. (1981). Genesis of rods in teleost fish retina. *Nature (London)* **293**, 141–142.

Lorenz, K. (1935). Der Kumpan in der Umwelt des Vogels. *J. Ornitho.* **80**, No. 2.

Mommsen, T. P. (1998). Growth and metabolism. *In* "The Physiology of Fishes" (D. H. Evans, ed.), pp. 65–97. CRC Press, Boca Raton, FL.

Muske, L. E., and Fernald, R. D. (1987a). Control of a teleost social signal. I. Neural basis for differential expression of a color pattern. *J. Comp. Physiol. A* **160**, 89–97.

Muske, L. E., and Fernald, R. D. (1987b). Control of a teleost social signal. II. Anatomical and physiological specializations of chromatophores. *J. Comp. Physiol. A* **160**, 99–107.

Pickering, A. D. (1990). Stress and the suppression of somatic growth in teleost fish. *Prog. Clin. Biol. Res.* **342**, 473–479.

Schultz, E. T., Clifton, L. M., and Warner, R. R. (1991). Energetic constraints and size-based tactics: The adaptive significance of breeding-schedule variation in a marine fish, *Micrometrus minimus* (Embiotocidae). *Am. Nat.* **138**, 1408–1430.

Soma, K. K., Francis, R. C., Wingfield, J. C., and Fernald, R. D. (1996). Androgen regulation of hypothalamic neurons containing gonadotropin-releasing hormone in a cichlid fish: Integration with social cues. *Horm. Behav.* **30**, 216–226.

Thakore, J. H., and Dinan, T. G. (1994). Growth hormone secretion: The role of glucocorticoids. *Life Sci.* **55**, 1083–1099.

van Weerd, J. H., and Komen, J. (1998). The effects of chronic stress on growth in fish: A critical appraisal. *Comp. Biochem. Physiol.* **120**, 107–112.

von Uexküll, J. (1909). "Umwelt und Innenwelt der Tiere." Springer, Berlin.

White, S. A., and Fernald, R. D. (1993). Gonadotropin-releasing hormone-containing neurons change size with reproductive state in female *Haplochromis burtoni*. *J. Neurosci.* **13**, 434–441.

White, S. A., Kasten, T. L., Bond, C. T., Adelman, J. P., and Fernald, R. D. (1995). Three gonadotropin-releasing hormone genes in one organism suggest novel roles for an ancient peptide. *Proc. Natl. Acad. Sci. U.S.A.* **92**, 8363–8367.

White, S. A., Nguyen, T., and Fernald, R. D. (2002). Social regulation of gene expression during changes in social status. *J. Neurosci.* (Submitted for publication.)

Hormonal Regulation of Motor Output in Amphibians: Xenopus laevis Vocalizations as a Model System

Darcy B. Kelley
Department of Biological Sciences
Columbia University
New York, New York 10027

I. INTRODUCTION

Sexually differentiated motor patterns are common to many vertebrate reproductive systems. Their occurrence is due to the action of gonadal steroids during development and in adult life. Understanding how sex-specific motor programs are generated requires uncovering the mechanisms for motor program production and for hormonal regulation of the sensory, neural, and muscular elements that produce these behaviors. The complexity of most vertebrate systems poses a steep challenge. However, the vocal behaviors of the South African clawed frog, *Xenopus laevis*, have proved to be a highly useful model system in addressing these issues. These frogs are native to southern Africa and are entirely aquatic. Their vocal repertoire is rich and sex-specific, but the mechanisms of vocal production are relatively simple. Steroid hormones regulate the sexual differentiation of vocal elements and are required for vocal displays in adulthood. These features permit us to dissect the cellular and molecular mechanisms used in sexually differentiated motor control and to place these elements within the behavioral context of the animal's natural habitat.

II. VOCAL REPERTOIRE

Xenopus laevis is an anuran (frogs and toads), a member of a large genus of approximately 29 species; all *Xenopus* are aquatic throughout their life span. This latter feature is secondary; *Xenopus* is believed to be derived from an ancestral terrestrial anuran because it retains many common features (Trueb, 1996). The preferred habitat for *Xenopus laevis* is murky ponds filled with decaying vegetable matter. Frogs call at night and this characteristic, together with lack of visibility in the ponds, probably accounts for the very complex vocal repertoire used in social communication.

X. laevis uses eight distinct vocalizations in social interactions (Fig. 1). Five of these are exclusive to males, one is shared and one is exclusive to females. The basic vocal unit is a click, a brief burst of sound with a relatively wide range of component frequencies. Male clicks are generally distinguishable from female clicks by having the majority of sound energy at approximately 2 kHz; for females clicks, most sound energy is at approximately 1 kHz. An exception is the click in growling (Fig. 1C), a male-specific vocal behavior, at approximately 1 kHz.

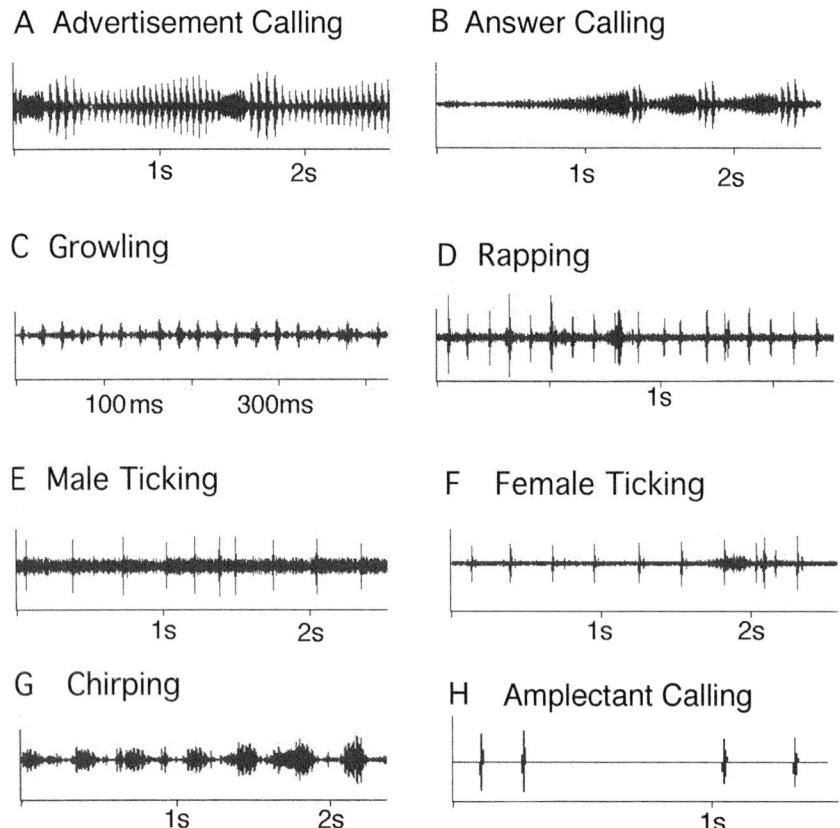

FIGURE 1 The vocal repertoire of *Xenopus laevis*. Male-specific vocal behaviors include the (A) advertisement, (B) answer, and (H) amplectant calls, (C) growling and (G) chirping. Female-specific calls includes (D) rapping; (E, F) both sexes tick. Each call is represented by an oscillogram (sound amplitude over time). The fundamental unit of all calls is the click, a brief sound burst containing many frequencies. Male and female clicks differ in frequency (higher in males), except for the clicks of growling, which overlap the female frequency range. Each call has a distinctive rate and temporal pattern. Advertisement and answer calls contain clicks that vary progressively in amplitude (intensity modulation); clicks in other calls are not intensity modulated. Calls made by females are illustrated in D and F.

Each vocalization is distinguished by its rate of click production and its temporal pattern (Kelley and Tobias, 1999). The simplest and slowest trill (series of clicks) is ticking (Russell, 1954), with an interclick interval (ICI) of approximately 230 ms. Both males and females tick (Fig. 1E–F), although ticking is much more prominent in the vocal repertoire of females. Females also produce a rapid (80-ms ICI) trill, rapping (Fig. 1D) (Tobias et al., 1998); males do not rap. The male-specific vocalizations are growling, chirping, and the amplectant, advertisement, and answer calls. Growling is a rapid (19 ms ICI) trill. Chirping consists of brief series of 2–5 clicks at a 20 ms ICI separated by approximately 500 ms intervals. The amplectant call is a slow (~180 ms ICI) and brief (2–3 clicks) trill. All of these simple calls are monotonous; they do not have an internal temporal structure nor are their component clicks modulated in intensity.

The most complex calls are the advertisement and answer calls (given exclusively by males). The advertisement call consists of a series of alternating fast and slow trills; the ICI for the fast trill is 18 ms, whereas that of the slow trill portion is 36 ms. Each advertisement call consists of approximately 195 ms of a fast and approximately 805 ms of a slower trill, which can be produced without pause for over an hour; bouts of calling are often preceded by an introductory slow trill (Wetzel and Kelley, 1983). Clicks comprising both the slow- and the fast-trill portions are intensity modulated; the amplitude of the fast trill can increase progressively as the trill proceeds. The answer call is a modification of the advertisement call in which the duration of the fast trill is lengthened (280 ms), the duration of the slow trill is shortened (265 ms), and the intensity modulation is increased dramatically (Tobias et al., 1998). All of these calls can be recorded from natural ponds in South Africa and can be elicited reliably in the laboratory, thus permitting analyses of their roles in social communication and of the cellular mechanisms of vocal production.

III. VOCAL COMMUNICATION

To determine the role played by these behaviors in social communication, we have surveyed their association with other behavioral interactions. This correlation can only be accomplished under conditions of high visibility such as in clear artificial ponds or in laboratory observation tanks. Our studies suggest that all of the male's calls are used in male–male communication and some also in male–female communication (Kelley et al., 2001). In females, ticking and rapping appear to be exclusively directed at males; we have not yet identified any vocal behaviors used in female–female interactions. The male advertisement call and female rapping are positively phonotactic signals. Females approach a calling male or a broadcast of recorded advertisement calling (Picker, 1983). Males approach a rapping female or a loudspeaker broadcasting rapping (Tobias et al., 1998).

Rapping stimulates, while ticking suppresses, male vocalizations (Fig. 2). Both calling by an actual female and a broadcast version of calling are effective. These opposite effects of the two calls are conveyed entirely by click rate. If presented at the rapping rate (80 ms ICI), artificial rapping made up of clicks taken from a tape of ticking is as effective as natural rapping in suppressing vocalizations (Tobias et al., 1998). The vocal stimulation effect is present at ICIs up to 99 ms; suppression occurs at intervals from 117 to 230 ms (Kelley et al., 2001), the range of ICIs for natural ticking. Female vocal behaviors thus have the ability to either enhance or suppress vocalizations in males, depending on the rate of click production. Both effects are dramatic; rapping, for example, acts as an acoustic aphrodisiac both in stimulating calling and in approach.

In addition to its role in vocal suppression, female ticking also functions as a release call, inducing the male to release the female from amplexus (clasping). In sexually active male–male pairs, however, growling is the vocalization most closely associated with the clasped male (Kelley et al., 2001). When both males are sexually active, ticking is not confined to amplexus. When only one male is active in clasping, the clasped male ticks and this is the only situation in which ticking occurs. The evidence thus suggests that both growling and ticking function as release calls in male–male pairs. The final call type is the amplectant call given by a male clasping either a female or another male. We have few clues as to the functional significance of this low-intensity call; it might serve to augment receptivity in females.

IV. HORMONAL CONTROL OF VOCAL BEHAVIORS IN ADULTS

Much of the vocal communication between frogs is tied to reproductive state. In the laboratory, sexual activity can be stimulated by injection of human chorionic gonadotrophin (hCG). This effect was the basis of an early test for human pregnancy because hCG is similar to frog gonadotrophin. In intact adults, hCG administration increases levels of circulating gonadal steroids and induces ovulation and oviposition in females and sperm release in males (Kelley, 1996). Advertisement calling in males is increased by hCG injection, abolished by castration, and reinstated by exogenous androgens, testosterone or dihydrotestosterone (Fig. 3). hCG does not increase calling in castrated males if given alone. However, in castrated males the effects of hCG and androgen on calling are synergistic, even at high androgen levels, suggesting that additional targets of hCG exist.

The effects of gonadal steroids on most other male vocal behaviors have not been examined. An exception is growling; unlike advertisement calling castration

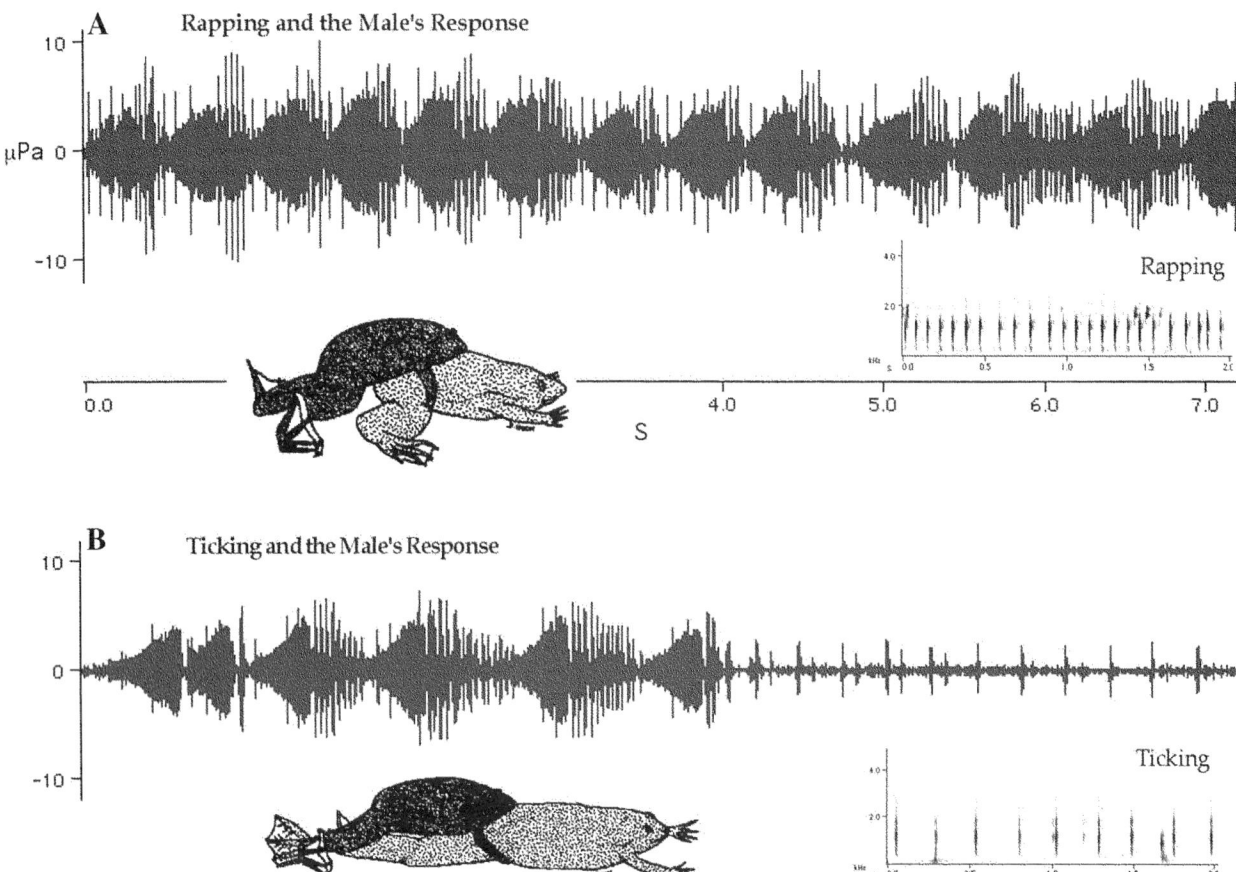

FIGURE 2 Rapping stimulates and ticking suppresses male calling. The upper portion of each panel illustrates male–female duets as oscillograms; the lower panel illustrates the female vocalization as a sound spectrogram. Original illustration by Barbara Goun.

does not abolish growling (S. Horng, unpublished). Our understanding of the endocrine control of ticking and rapping is also incomplete. Ticking is enhanced by ovariectomy and suppressed in intact females by hCG injection. One consequence of hCG injection is that females ovulate and then oviposit as the eggs transit the oviducts. Oviposition is associated with rapping (Tobias et al., 1998). Neither estrogen nor progesterone, alone or in combination, suppresses ticking. Exogenous androgens and prostaglandin E2 (PGE2) do suppress ticking (Weintraub et al., 1985). Androgen is an estrogen precursor in the ovary and can be detected in the circulation of intact females after hCG injection. The cells that line the oviduct express the biosynthetic enzyme for prostaglandin synthesis and the PGE2 effect might thus mimic endocrine events associated with oviposition (Kelley et al., 1987). Both hormones associated with ovulation and oviposition could mediate in the suppression of the female's release call. The injection of PGE2, however, does not induce rapping (A. Yamaguchi and M. L. Tobias, unpublished).

V. MECHANISMS OF SOUND PRODUCTION: CARTILAGENOUS AND MUSCULAR ELEMENTS

The vocal organ in Xenopus laevis is the larynx, a box-like structure of muscle and cartilage located immediately dorsal to the heart (Fig. 4). The larynx is connected via the glottis to the buccal cavity anteriorly and via paired tracheae to the lungs posteriorly. All calls are produced and responded to underwater and thus actual respiration does not accompany vocalizations. Instead,

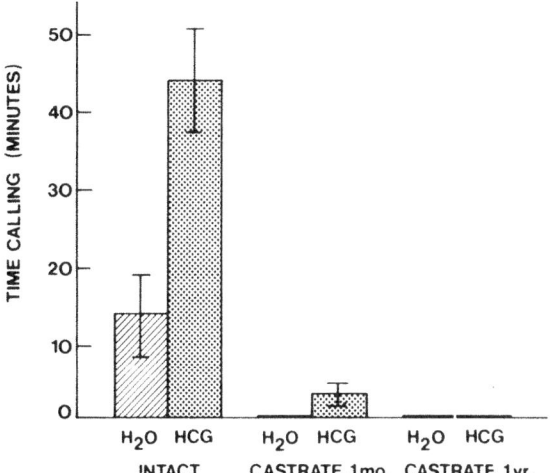
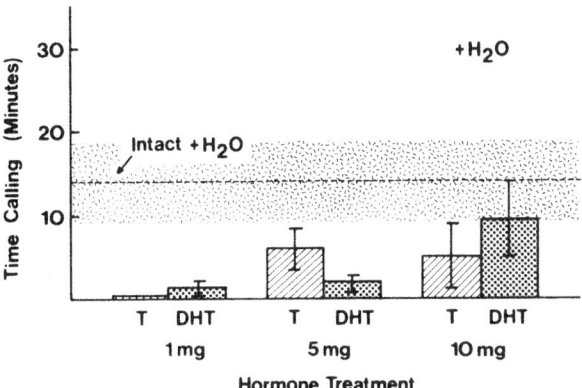
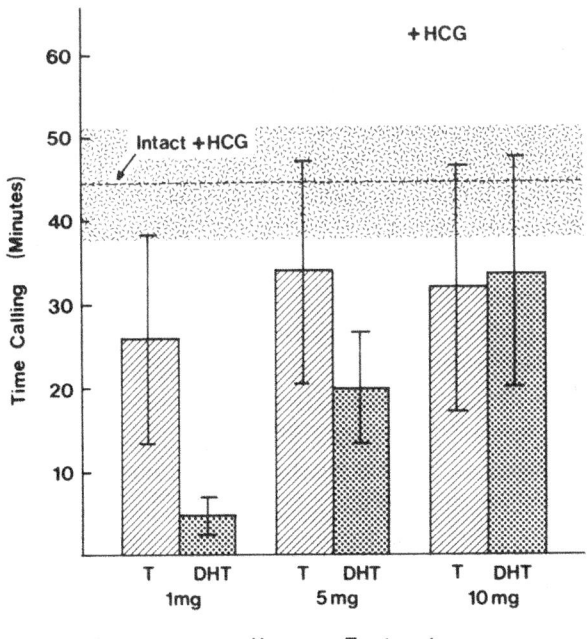

FIGURE 3 Hormonal control of advertisement calling in male Xenopus laevis. Castration abolished calling, which is reinstated by androgen treatment (T, testosterone; DHT, dihydrotestosterone). Gonadotrophin (hCG) treatment synergizes with androgen in the reinstatement of calling, even though males are gonadectomized (lower panel). From Wetzel and Kelley (1983).

the larynx contains highly modified portions of the arytenoid cartilages that function as sound-producing discs. In the related species Xenopus borealis, in which the larynx is sufficiently transparent, actual click production accompanies the pulling apart of the discs, which are otherwise tightly opposed (Yager, 1982), and it is thought that this sound-production mechanism is common to the genus, including *Xenopus laevis*.

The movement of the arytenoid discs is the result of the contraction of the intrinsic laryngeal bipennate muscles (Fig. 4). These pairs of muscles flank the lateral and dorsal aspects of the larynx and insert via a tendon onto the arytenoid discs. A band of elastic cartilage that partially encircles the discs probably contributes to their close apposition. A layer of secreted extracellular material on the medial surfaces of the discs may be essential to the implosion thought to account for sound production. When the bipennate muscles contract, they generate tension on the tendon. When that tension exceeds the forces that hold the discs together, the arytenoid discs open and a click is produced (see Fig. 6, later). As the laryngeal muscles relax, the discs close again. Our understanding of the biomechanics of sound production is not complete, especially in species other than *X. borealis* in which the actual movements of the discs have not been observed.

VI. SEX DIFFERENCES

A. Laryngeal Muscle

1. Molecules and Physiology

The laryngeal bipennate muscles differ markedly in males and females. Histochemical techniques, assays for adenine triphosphatase (ATPase) and succinic dehydrogenase (SDHase), reveal that male muscle is homogeneous—fibers stain lightly for acid stable ATPase (Fig. 5D) and intensely for SDHase. Using these assays, female muscle contains three fiber types–one

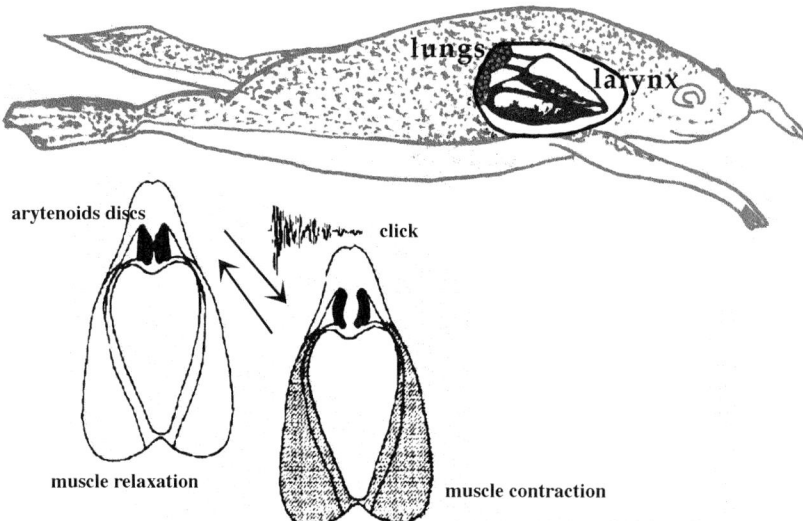

FIGURE 4 Vocal production in *Xenopus laevis*. The larynx, or vocal organ, is located just dorsal to the heart and connects to the buccal cavity via the glottis anteriorly; posteriorly the larynx connects to the lungs via paired tracheae. The mouth is closed during vocalizations. Click production is due to contraction of intrinsic laryngeal bipennate muscles connected, via a tendon, to the arytenoid discs. Original illustration by Julio Perez. From *Anuran Communication*, edited by Michael J. Ryan, published by the Smithsonian Institution Press, Washington, DC; copyright © 2001. Used by permission of the publisher.

similar to the male profile, one that stains intensely for both ATP and SDH, and a third type that has little ATPase or SDHase activity (Fig. 5E). Most fibers (75%) are in the second category. The ATPase activity reflects the enzymatic action of the myosin heavy chain (MHC). Preincubation at different pH conditions can be used to distinguish ATPase activity associated with fast-twitch fibers from that associated with slow-twitch fibers. The activity of SDHase, a mitochondrial enzyme, is correlated with resistance to fatigue. The histochemical results suggest that in males laryngeal muscle fibers are entirely fast-twitch and fatigue-resistant. In females, most muscle fibers are slow-twitch and fatiguable.

MHC composition is a major determinant of the contractile properties of individual muscle fibers. Each MHC is the product of a separate gene, and we thus sought to determine whether differences in the male and female larynx represent differences in MHC gene expression. Because the requirements for ATPase activity are stringent, the conservation of 5′ sequence for different MHC genes is very high. We thus used a 3′ fragment from two different *Xenopus* MHC clones to screen the laryngeal library. This approach yielded a MHC mRNA fragment (312 nucleotides of coding and 144 nucleotides of 3′-UTR) expressed much more abundantly in male than in female adult laryngeal muscle (Catz et al., 1992). This transcript appears to be expressed only in laryngeal muscle and is thus called laryngeal myosin (LM). In sequence it is 79% identical (at the amino acid level) to rat β-cardiac MHC and to human embryonic MHC and 78% identical to chicken embryonic MHC. The transcript is localized over the nuclei of laryngeal muscle fibers (Fig. 5A–C). Every nucleus in male laryngeal muscle is labeled with the LM probe (Fig. 5A). In female muscle, only approximately 20% of muscle fibers are LM positive; the size distribution of these fibers suggests that these are some of the female's fast-twitch muscle fibers (Fig. 5B–C). We do not know whether the LM isoform is coexpressed with other MHC isoforms. It is likely, however, that LM makes a significant contribution to contractile properties of laryngeal fibers, especially in males.

Using the *vox in vitro* preparation, muscle-contraction characteristics can be observed directly and correlated with vocal production (Fig. 6). This preparation consists of the isolated larynx and its motor innervation (Tobias and Kelley, 1987). Laryngeal nerves can

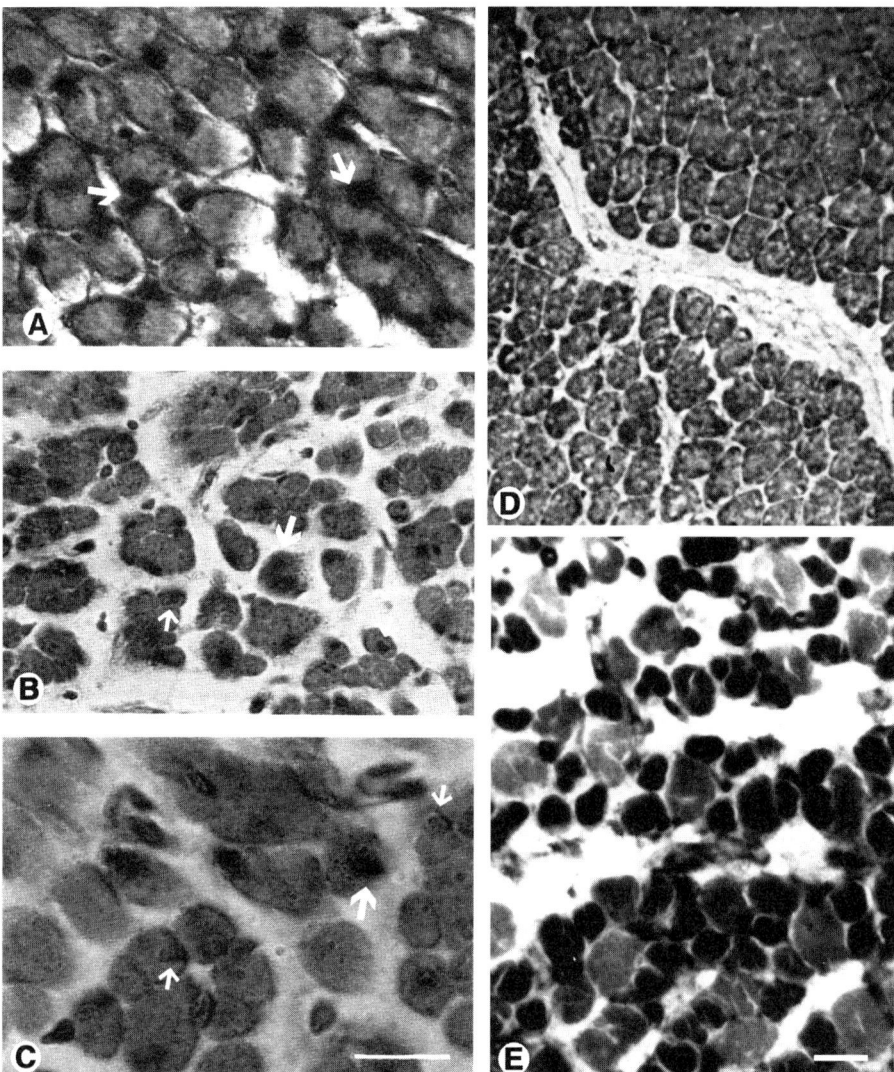

FIGURE 5 Sexually differentiated laryngeal muscle-fiber composition. Male laryngeal muscle is homogeneous in fiber type as revealed by (D) histochemical staining for ATPase activity. Female laryngeal muscle fibers are heterogeneous in size and ATPase activity, with one type that is similar to the male type (medium-size, medium-staining); most female fibers are small and stain darkly. Male muscle fibers are fast twitch, whereas most female muscle fibers are slow twitch, presumably reflecting the preponderance of these small, darkly ATPase-staining fibers. Scale bar: 5 μm. From Sassoon et al., © (1987) by the Society for Neuroscience. (A, B, C) Laryngeal muscle expresses a tissue-specific myosin heavy chain gene (laryngeal myosin, LM). The LM mRNA transcript is expressed in all muscle fibers in males (arrows), but in only some muscle fibers in females (large arrows); other nuclei are not associated with accumulation of the LM transcript (small arrows). Scale bar (A, B): 30 μm; (C): 12 μm. From Catz et al. (1992). **See insert for a color version of this figure.**

be stimulated electrically and the resultant muscle activity recorded via electromyogram (EMG) electrodes. The result of muscle contraction and relaxation can be recorded using a tension transducer attached to the tendon just distal to the arytenoid discs.

The *vox in vitro* preparation reveals that the physiological properties of laryngeal muscle are as sexually differentiated as its histochemical profile (Fig. 6). The most dramatic difference between male and female laryngeal muscle is the rate at which each produces

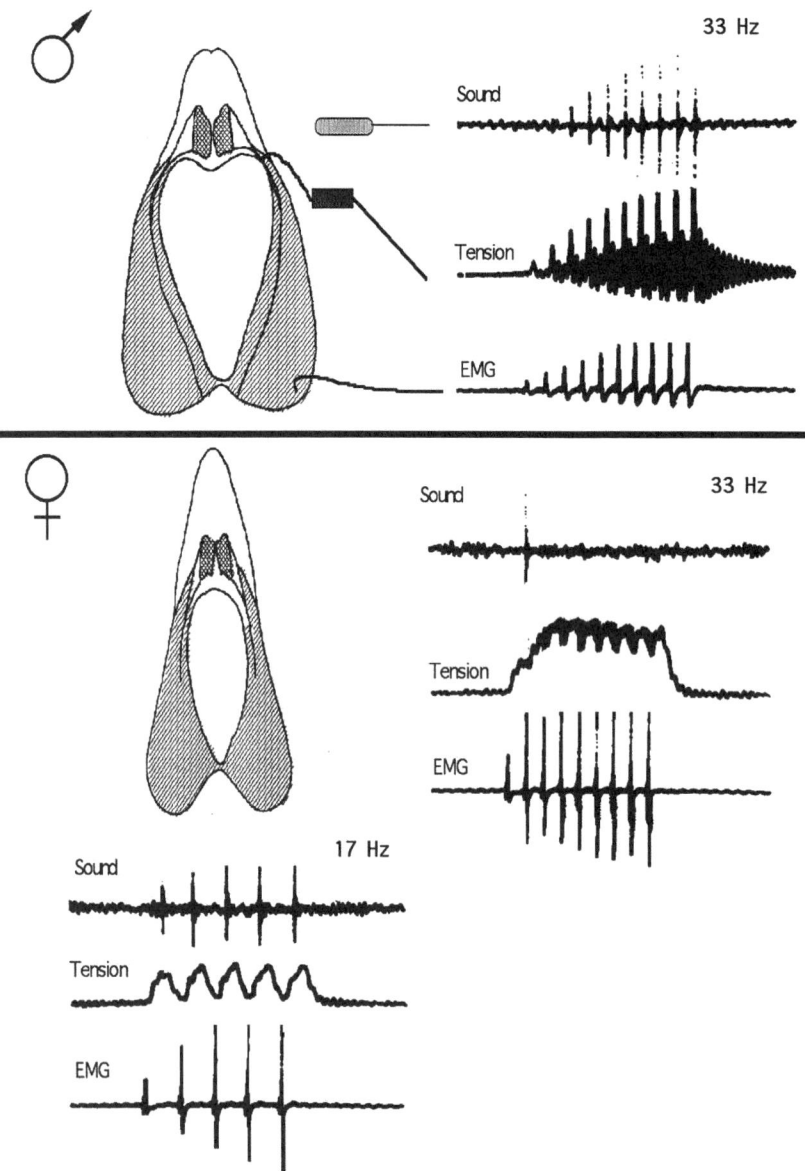

FIGURE 6 The *vox in vitro* preparation (Tobias and Kelley, 1987). The isolated larynx produces clicks closely resemembling those in actual vocal behaviors in response to stimulation of the laryngeal nerves. This preparation permits recoding of electrical acivity from laryngeal muscle fibers (electromyogram, EMG), tension recordings from the tendons that insert into the arytenoid discs and sound recordings. Male muscle can contract and relax rapidly (33–100 Hz), whereas female muscle tetanizes at these rapid rates of nerve stimulation, blocking click production after the discs open. From Kelley and Tobias (1999).

discrete tension transients. Males can produce discrete tension transients at interstimulus intervals (ISIs) as low as 10 ms. Females, however, can only produce discrete tension transients at ISIs greater than 30 ms. In females, nerve stimulation at 29 pulses per second (pps; interpulse interval, IPI, 35 ms) permits discrete tension transients, whereas stimulation at 33 pps (IPI 30 ms) produces only sustained tension (Fig. 6, lower panel).

2. Relation to Click Production

If both nerves are stimulated at appropriate rates a small microphone adjacent to the arytenoid discs can be used to record click production. The isolated larynx can produce trills that resemble the actual click trains of male and female vocalizations (Fig. 6). This feature permits unusually close correlations between muscle contraction characteristics and click production. Actual sound production by the isolated vocal organ is unusual for vertebrates (additional examples are sound production by the swim bladders of some fish; Bass et al., 1999). This experimental-favorable preparation in *Xenopus laevis* reflects the highly modified system of sound production, uncoupling respiration from vocalization, that accompanied the transition to underwater life.

When suprathreshold, each tension transient produces a click. Thus, when female laryngeal nerves are stimulated at 33 pps, a single click is produced when the threshold tension value is reached; no clicks are produced during maintained tension (Fig. 6). For males, each discrete tension transient produces a click at stimulation rates up to 100 pps; beyond this value, tension is maintained and no clicks are produced. By and large, muscle contraction in the larynx is isometric. Muscle fibers attach to the cartilagenous skeleton and to a relatively immobile tendon, and muscle length thus does not change dramatically during contraction. Under these conditions, muscle-fiber contractions can produce isometric twitches (discrete tension transients) that can summate at higher rates of stimulation, and at even higher rates can produce unfused or fused tetanus (maintained tension). Male and female muscle fibers differ markedly in the threshold for muscle tetanus (>30 pps for female; >100 pps for males). During muscle tetanus, clicks cannot be produced because the arytenoid discs are held open. Only when the rate of nerve stimulation is reduced below the threshold for tetanus can muscle fibers relax and the discs close. Each click is produced, then, by a cycle of muscle contraction and relaxation. If muscle fibers do not relax, as in tetanus, clicks cannot be produced.

The ability to rapidly contract and relax is thus integral to the production of rapid click trains by the male vocal organ. In addition, because trills are prolonged, it is essential that the overall fatigue of laryngeal muscle be minimal. The presence of intense SDHase activity (and the very high density of mitochondria) suggest that male laryngeal muscle is also highly fatigue-resistant. Fatigue-resistant fast-twitch muscle fibers (type IIA) have been identified in mammalian systems. These, however, exhibit tetanus at rates as low as 20 Hz, whereas *Xenopus laevis* laryngeal muscle does not exhibit tetanus at 100 Hz. These values for mammalian muscle are taken from individual muscle units, all of the muscle fibers innervated by a single motor axon. We do not know whether the behavior of the entire laryngeal muscle that we measure in the *vox in vitro* preparation reflects the properties of homogeneous populations of motor units or, instead, the successive recruitment of different sorts of motor units. We assume in the *in vitro* preparation that trains of nerve stimuli of constant amplitude drive the same population of laryngeal axons. However, *in vivo*, recordings from the laryngeal nerve (see later) reveal that the fast trills of males are driven by the synchronous activity of laryngeal axons. The slower trills of females and of males are produced by asynchronous neural activity. These observations raise the possibility that laryngeal motor units can act successively; populations might alternate in producing muscle contraction, thus reducing the fatigue factor.

B. Laryngeal Motor Neuron: The Neuromuscular Synapse

The *vox in vitro* preparation allows us to directly examine neuromuscular transmission at the laryngeal synapse of males and females (Tobias and Kelley, 1988). Under physiological conditions (recording in physiological saline solution) the male neuromuscular synapse is subthreshold for action potential production (Fig. 7A). A single shock delivered to the laryngeal nerve produces an excitatory postsynaptic potential in the postsynaptic muscle cell, but not an action potential. Trains of stimuli are required for action potential production at male synapses; even during repetitive stimulation, some subthreshold events can be recorded. The male synapse is thus low safety factor, in the sense that transmission is not reliable. The amplitude of the evoked response increases until the action potential is produced, indicating an underlying facilitation of synaptic transmission. This pattern of responses to nerve stimulation suggests that male synapses are weak and that EMG potentiation can be

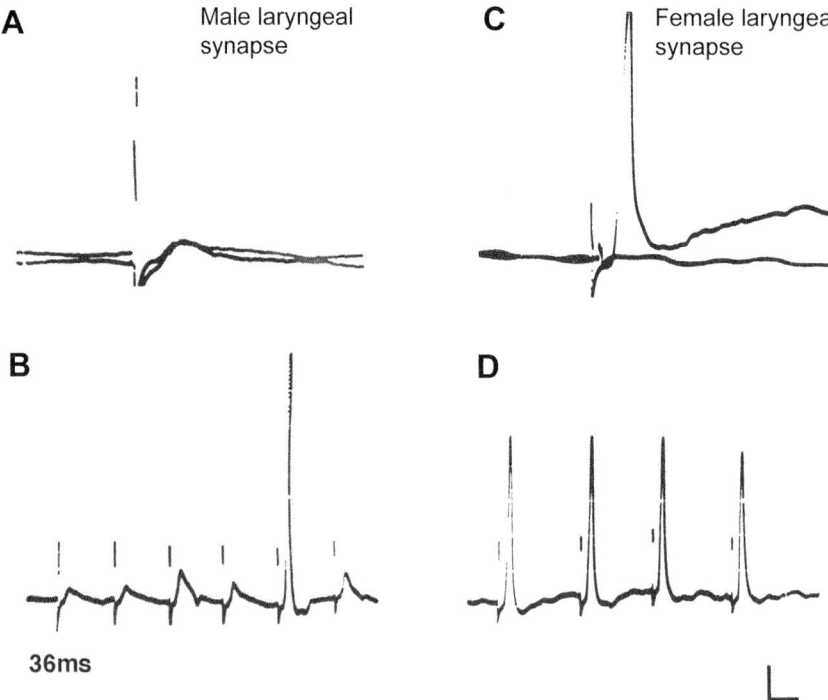

FIGURE 7 Sexually differentiated laryngeal neuromuscular synapses studied in normal Ringer's solution. (A) The dominant type of synapse in males is type II; in response to a nerve stimulus, this fiber type produces subthreshold responses (excitatory postsynaptic potentials). Repeated stimulation is required for muscle action-potential production; even during trains, synaptic failures occur. (B) Some male synapses (type I) have multiple inputs, at least one of which is suprathreshold for action potential production. (C) The predominant type of synapse in female laryngeal muscle is one in which transmission is suprathreshold for muscle action-potential production (type III). Scale bars for right-hand panels, bottom three traces and left-hand panel: 10 mV (vertical), 20 ms (horizontal); left-hand panel, upper trace: 10 mV, 5 ms. From Tobias and Kelley, © (1988) by the Society for Neuroscience.

produced by the facilitation of synaptic strength during repetitive activity of the laryngeal nerve. In females, on the other hand, laryngeal synapses are typically strong or high safety factor. In physiological saline, each shock to the laryngeal nerve produces an action potential in the postsynaptic muscle fiber (Fig. 7C).

To look more closely at synaptic transmission, we examined male and female synapses under conditions (lowered calcium and increased magnesium concentrations in the saline) in which postsynaptic action potentials were blocked just in females (Tobias et al., 1995). These conditions permit the observation of subthreshold events in females and allow measurement of the quantal content of laryngeal synapses. Using the method of failures developed by DelCastillo and Katz (1954), quantal content values for male laryngeal synapses were shown to be considerably greater than for female synapses with little overlap in values between the sexes (Fig. 8). Sex differences in synaptic efficacy could be due to characteristics of neurotransmitter release (presynaptic) or to the response, triggered by acetylcholine, of the muscle fiber. We examined postsynaptic contributions by measuring miniature endplate potentials (MEPPs), depolarizations of the muscle membrane at the synapse due to the spontaneous release of a vesicle of neurotransmitter. MEPP amplitudes and rise times did not differ in the sexes, suggesting that the postsynaptic muscle fiber is equally sensitive to neurotransmitter. For this reason, and because the quantal content is very sensitive to calcium concentration in the

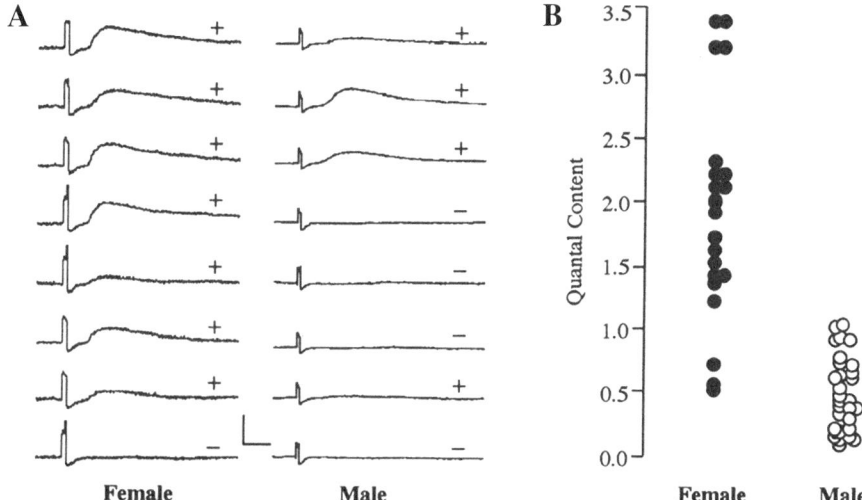

FIGURE 8 Quantal contents of laryngeal synapses are sexually differentiated. Synaptic transmission at the laryngeal synapse was examined using the method of failures, in which male and female larynges were bathed in a low-calcium high-magnesium saline that just blocked action potential production in females. Quantal contents differ markedly and are lower in males; because spontaneous miniature endplate potential are equivalent in the sexes, we believe the sex difference in transmission is presynaptic. Scale bar: 10 mV (vertical), 5 ms (horizontal). From Tobias *et al.*, © 1995 by the Society for Neuroscience.

saline (which affects vesicle release but not postsynaptic receptors), we believe that the sex difference in transmission at the vocal synapse is presynaptic in origin. One interpretation of these results is that, per action potential invading the synaptic terminal, the probability that a synaptic vesicle containing acetylcholine will be released is less in males than in females.

Males rely on facilitation to augment vesicle release to the point at which a muscle action potential is triggered. Females do not require facilitation under physiological conditions. By examining the synapse under conditions in which synaptic transmission was reduced (decreased calcium or curare-containing saline), we can compare facilitation at male and female laryngeal neuromuscular junctions (Ruel *et al.*, 1998). Somewhat surprisingly (given that both release itself and facilitation are calcium-dependent), we did not observe any marked difference in facilitation indices between the sexes, either in response to paired pulses (Fig. 9A), a classic neurophysiological preparation, or to trains of stimuli (Fig. 9B), a condition mimicking the vocal production. The only sex difference in facilitation observed was that the response of female synapses to trains of stimuli reached maximal values (plateaued) after 2–4 stimuli; male synapses did not plateau (Fig. 9B). However, the facilitation index (ratio of the responses to the first and last stimuli in the train) did not differ between the sexes (Fig. 9C). We conclude that sex differences in release itself, rather than facilitated release, account for sex differences underlying EMG potentiation at the vocal synapse.

Extracellular recordings from the male larynx reveal that the amplitude of the electromyogram increases during trains of nerve stimulation; progressive increases in click amplitude (intensity modulation) accompany this pattern of EMG potentiation (Fig. 6). The underlying mechanism is the facilitation of the male's weak neuromuscular synapses that accompanies repetitive activity of the laryngeal motor neuron axons. Progressive increases in click amplitude are an acoustically appealing feature of the male's advertisement and answer calls (see discussion later).

C. Vocal Nerve Activity

Given the very powerful filtering properties of the neuromuscular synapse, it was possible that peripheral constraints accounted entirely for sex differences in

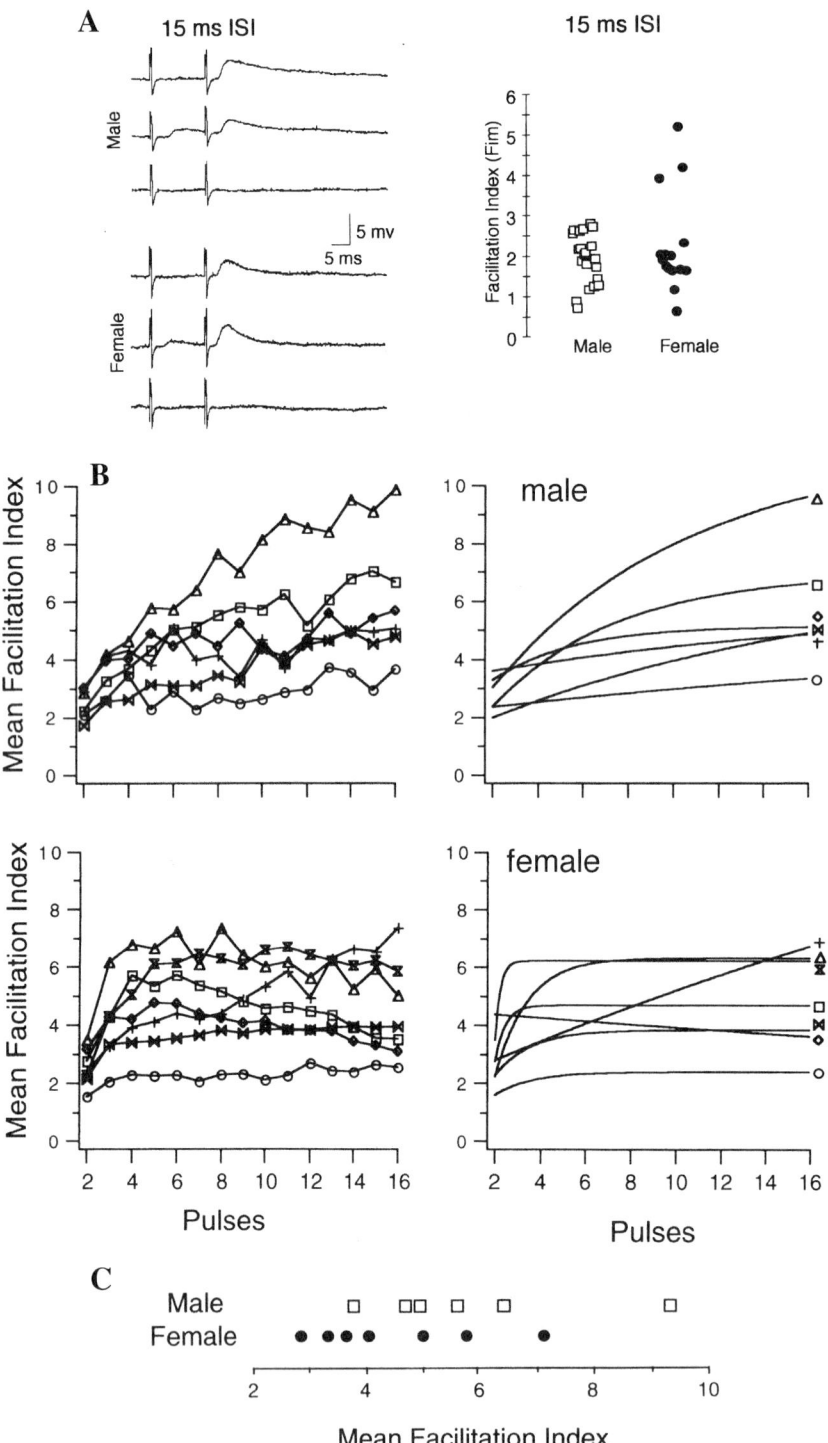

FIGURE 9 Facilitation at the neuromuscular synapse is not sexually differentiated. Synapses were examined in reduced calcium (A) or curare-containing (B) saline, and subjected (A) to paired-pulse facilitation or (B) to trains of stimulation that mimic nerve activity during vocal production. In neither paradigm was there a sex difference in facilitation (C). From Ruel *et al.* (1998), *J. Comp. Physiol. A* **182**, 38–39, copyright Springer-Verlag.

vocal behaviors. For example, we might imagine that laryngeal motor neurons fire rapidly under states of heightened sexual activity and more slowly in states of reduced sexual activity and that these two patterns are sculpted into distinct male and female trills by features of the laryngeal synapse. To test this idea directly, we recorded from the laryngeal nerves and bipennate muscles of vocalizing male and female frogs (Yamaguchi and Kelley, 2000). Nerve recordings enabled us to examine the pattern of activity of laryngeal motor neurons and the degree of synchrony in neuronal activity. Muscle recordings (EMGs) enabled us to assess the potential contributions of the neuromuscular synapse to actual call production.

Recordings of activity in the laryngeal nerve (the nerve compound action potential, CAP) revealed that sex-specific patterns closely match actual vocal patterns (Fig. 10A). Thus male and female specific vocal behaviors are generated in the central nervous system (CNS). Measurements of nerve CAP durations associated with different call types revealed a close relation to call rate (Fig. 10B)—the more rapid the trill, the shorter the CAP duration. The very rapid trills produced only by males have short CAP durations. For slower trills, however, such as the male amplectant call and female ticking, CAP durations do not differ by sex. The duration of the nerve CAP reflects the degree of synchrony of axon activity; highly synchronized CAPs are short. A short synchronous CAP is required for rapid trills because, in the cycle of click production, the muscle must contract and relax completely before the next trill can be produced. Slower trills, on the other hand, can be produced either with short- or long-duration CAPs because the ICI is sufficiently long to permit click production in either case. The association between CAP duration and ICI is very tight for rapid trills, but much looser for slower trills (Fig. 10B).

Synchronizing the activity of laryngeal motor neurons produces the short CAPs associated with male-specific rapid calls. Motor neuron synchrony could be achieved at the level of the neurons themselves via recurrent excitatory synapses or, even more effectively, via electrical coupling. Electrical coupling of motor neurons has been described for another sexually differentiated motor nucleus, the spinal nucleus of the bulbocavernosus in male rats (Matsumoto *et al.*, 1988). Alternatively, highly synchronized synaptic input to laryngeal motor neurons, perhaps even a subpopulation, might be responsible for the highly coordinated activity that produces growling, advertisement, and answer calls.

Recordings from the laryngeal nerve of singing males also reveal a progressive increase in CAP amplitude during the fast-trill portion of the advertisement call (Fig. 10A). The amplitude of these highly synchronized CAPs reflects the number of laryngeal motor neurons that produce action potentials; a progressive increase in amplitude is the result of progressive recruitment of vocal motor neurons. Creating progressively louder clicks during the fast trill *in vivo* is the result of a program of motor neuron recruitment from the CNS. *In vitro*, the laryngeal synapse also facilitates with repetitive nerve activity; the cell body is not attached to the axon in the *vox in vitro* preparation and the shocks to the nerve activate all laryngeal axons. Thus, there are two independent ways to produce EMG potentiation and progressively louder clicks (intensity modulation)—recruitment in the CNS and facilitation at the vocal synapse. In support of this idea, the EMG potentiation in the *in vivo* preparation is enhanced relative to CAP potentiation in the nerve (Fig. 10C).

VII. PROGRESSIVE INCREASES IN CLICK AMPLITUDE ARE ATTRACTIVE TO FEMALES

The multiple mechanisms that ensure intensity modulation suggest that this acoustic feature is important for communication. One possibility is that intensity modulation functions in mate choice; both modulated calls, advertisement and answer calls, attract females (Fig. 11A). We tested the contribution of intensity modulation to phonotaxis by comparing female responses to artificially generated calls with and without progressive increases in click loudness during the fast trill (Fig. 11C–D). Tape-recorded calls were broadcast from underwater loudspeakers located at opposite ends of a rectangular tank and the female's response (distance travelled relative to her initial position) was recorded (D. Ikelheimer, M. L. Tobias, S. Nowicke, and D. B. Kelley, unpublished). The same female was tested with computer-generated modulated and unmodulated *X. laevis* trills and with the male call from another species,

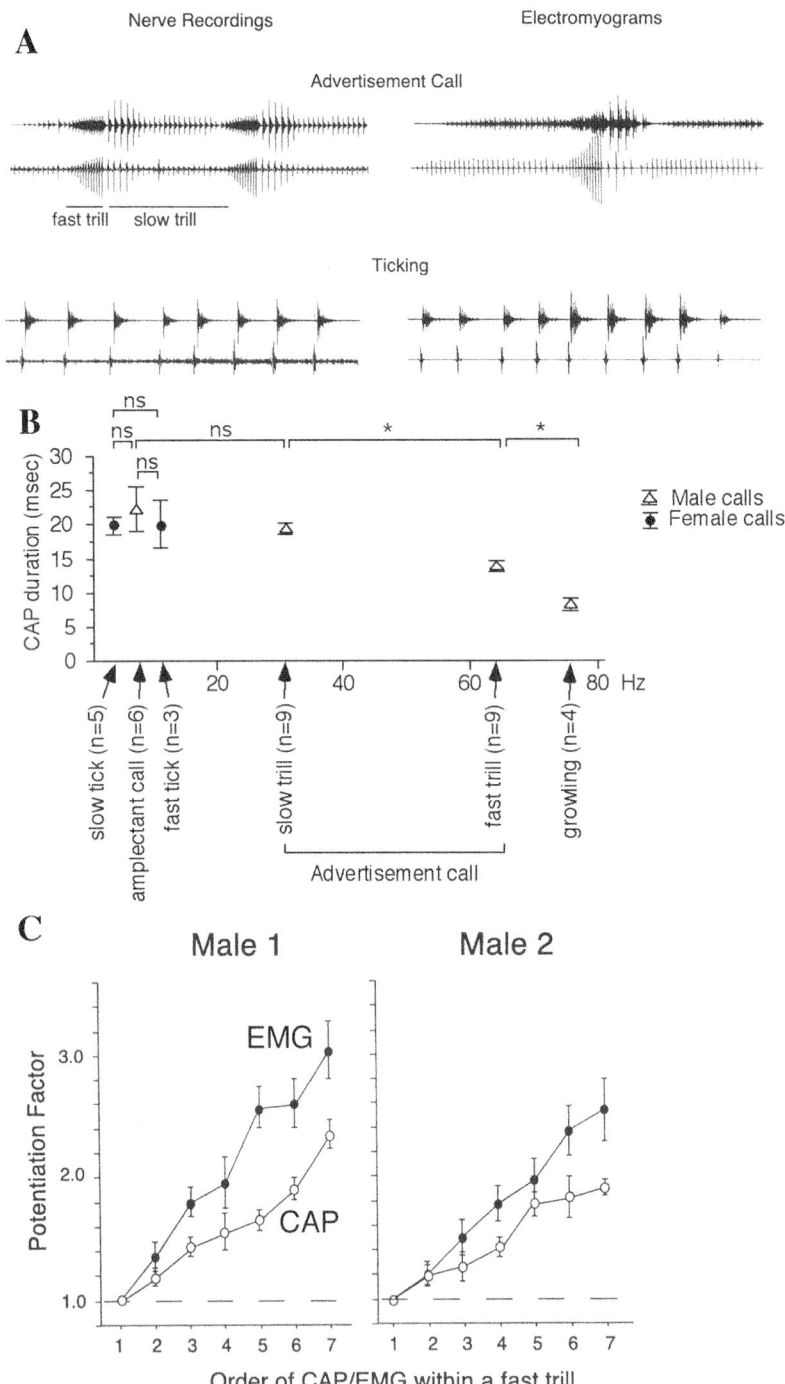

FIGURE 10 Recordings from the laryngeal nerve of singing frogs. (A) For males and females, nerve compound action potentials (CAPs) and EMG activity (lower traces) match sound production (upper traces). Vocal patterns are thus generated in the central nervous system (CNS). (B) Fast trills are associated with short-nerve CAPs and slow trills with longer (asynchronous) CAPs. We have suggested that two different kinds of motor units (corresponding to the laryngeal synapse types in Fig. 7) might contribute selectively to fast and slow calls and be sexually differentiated. (C) The laryngeal synapse amplifies the recruitment of motor units that originates in the CNS. The vocal system thus uses several mechanisms to insure progressive increases in the amplitude of clicks during male advertisement and answer calls. From Yamaguchi and Kelley, © 2000 by the Society for Neuroscience.

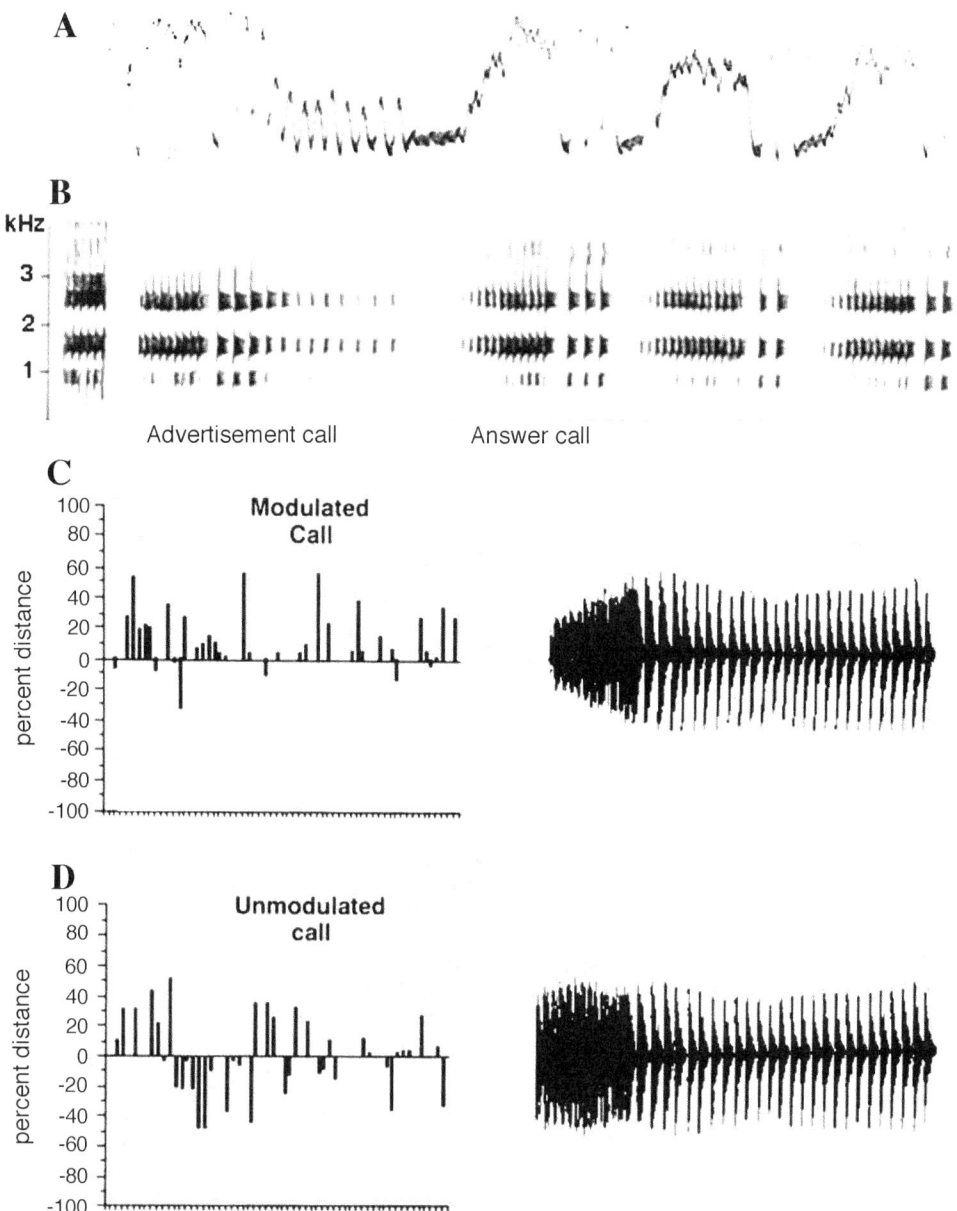

FIGURE 11 Intensity modulation is an attractive feature of the male's call. (A and B) The amplitude envelope of an advertisement and three answer calls. Intensity modulation is enhanced in the answer call. Female responses to computer generated calls (C) with amplitude modulation and (D) without intensity modulation. Females that had swum toward the modulated call swam away from the unmodulated call. From D. Ikelheimer, M. L. Tobias, S. Nowicke, and D. B. Kelley, unpublished study.

X. borealis (not shown). The modulated trill was more attractive than the unmodulated trill and both were more effective than the *X. borealis* advertisement call in eliciting phonotaxis (not shown). If amplitude modulation enhances male reproductive success, the redundant neural mechanisms underlying the call feature have been under strong selective pressure.

Why intensity modulation is attractive to females is not clear. The male's answer call is even more strongly intensity-modulated than the advertisement call (Fig. 11A). The duration of the fast trill is lengthened relative to the advertisement call, thus providing greater potential for the progressive modulation of click amplitude. The answer call is very reliably produced in response to rapping (Tobias et al., 1998). Females rap when they are about to oviposit, a situation that places a premium on locating a partner for amplexus (Tobias et al., 1998). Intensity modulation of the advertisement call might provide strong cues to the species of the caller, especially since calls of sympatric species (like *X. gilli*) lack intensity modulation. In addition, intensity modulation might enhance the female's ability to locate the calling male.

VIII. GENERATING VOCALIZATIONS IN VERTEBRATES

How are the distinct temporal patterns of the call types produced in the CNS? Robert Schmidt (1968) developed an isolated-brain-stem preparation in *Rana pipiens* to address this question. For the most part, only male frogs have been examined. The ventral CNS from the preoptic area (POA) rostrally to the first spinal nerve caudally can be maintained for days in oxygenated saline. Stimulation of the POA evokes actual advertisement calling in intact males and laryngeal nerve (N.IX-X) correlates (i.e., CAPs) of advertisement calling in the isolated preparation. In the intact animal, these correlates are accompanied by rapid contractions of glottal muscles. Recordings from the N.IX-X reveal spontaneous periodic activity correlated with pulmonary and buccal respiration (Schmidt, 1992). When the POA is stimulated, activity that correlates with that observed during vocalization can be recorded in the laryngeal motor nucleus (n.IX-X) and in a more rostral nucleus, the pretrigeminal nucleus of the dorsal tegmental area of the medulla (DTAM)—the locations of these brain regions are illustrated in Fig. 12.

A combination of lesion and stimulation studies in the isolated-brain-stem preparation led Schmidt (1992) to propose a model for the generation of calling that involves two independent generators—DTAM and the pulmonary respiration generator (PPG). The PPG is coextensive with n.IX-X and appears to have two subdivisions—an expiratory generator in the anterior half and an inspiratory generator in the posterior half. Both are reciprocally connected to their contralateral counterparts at the level of n.IX-X; the connection produces strong excitatory interactions. Lesions of the posterior half of n.IX-X abolish pulmonary-respiration correlates without abolishing vocal correlates. These are evoked by the stimulation of the POA or DTAM. In contrast, maintaining the anterior extent of n.IX-X is essential for producing vocal correlates. When DTAM is isolated from n.IX-X (and from the contralateral DTAM), POA stimulation still evokes complex slow waves. An intact connection with the PPG was required, however, for the fully pulsed activity correlated with vocal production.

The PPG is spontaneously active, ryhthmic, and relatively slow (1 pulse per 2 seconds). Activity generated by DTAM is not spontaneous, but can be evoked by POA stimulation or stimulation in DTAM itself; the evoked activity is rapid and matches laryngeal nerve activity correlated with calling. When the PPG is lesioned, the vocal phase evoked by POA or DTAM stimulation is lengthened, suggesting that the PPG inhibits activity triggered from DTAM. This effect is diminished if contralateral connections are severed, suggesting reciprocal excitatory interactions between PPGs. Schmidt believed that all vocalizations of *Rana pipiens* were produced by a single generator and were shaped into different forms by sensory and endocrine input.

The close connection between the generation of breathing and vocal behavior in *Rana* supports previous suggestions that vocal behaviors are an elaboration of intense breathing activated by touch. A complementary view, advanced by Bass and Baker (1997), is that rhythmic activity of many kinds, ranging from eye movements to electric organ discharges—and including both breathing and calling—are driven by rhythmic activity of specialized interneurons in all vertebrates. These cells are located in the caudal hindbrain in regions derived from rhombomeres 7 and 8. They are capable of oscillatory activity, either spontaneous or evoked by presynaptic inputs. For *R. pipiens*, the interneurons that are coextensive with n.IX-X would represent this specialized group. If so, it would be preferable to refer to these interneurons as rhythmically active (rather than pattern generating) and to consider their inputs to respiration and to vocalization circuits separately. In rodents, a group of spontaneously active neurons that drive respiration have been identified (Feldman, 1995;

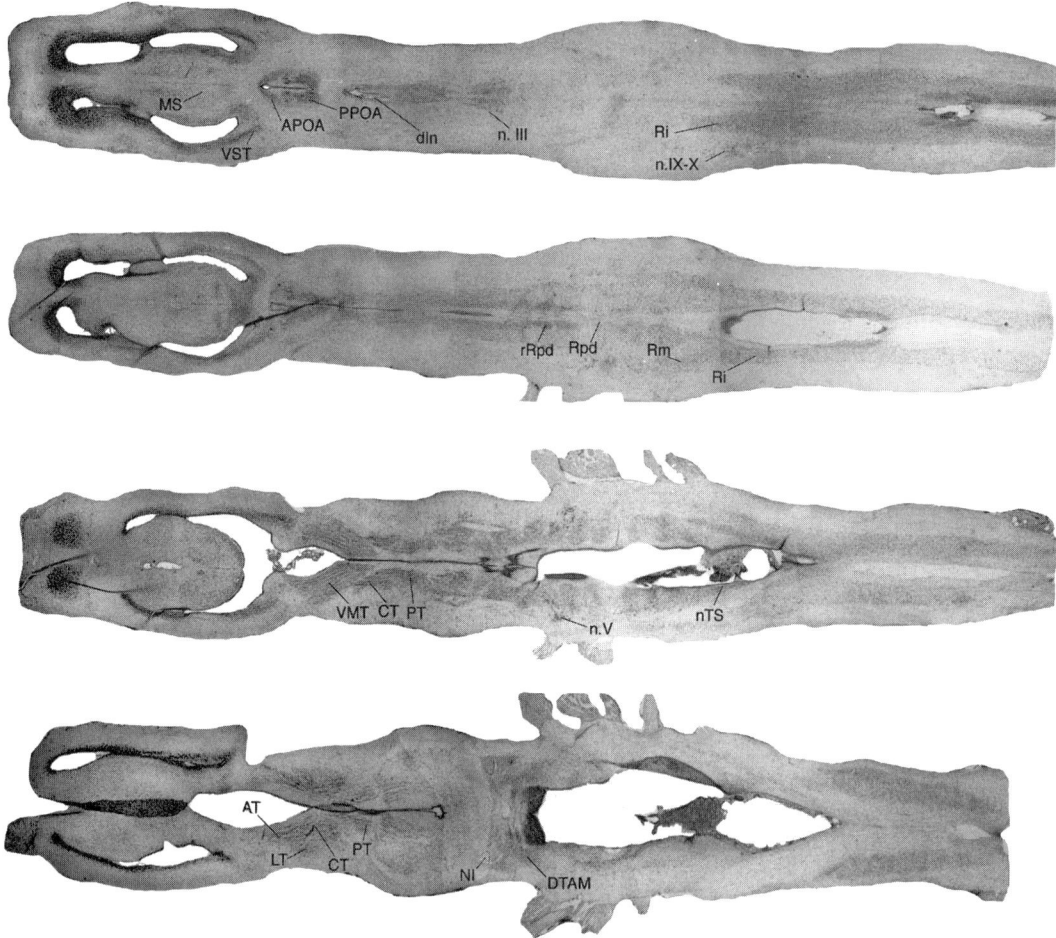

FIGURE 12 Brain regions associated with anuran vocal production; cresyl-violet-stained horizontal sections through the CNS of a male *X. laevis*; the most dorsal section is at the top, anterior is to the right. Laryngeal motor neurons are located in cranial nerve IX-X (n.IX-X). These receive input from the adjacent Ri and the pre-trigeminal nucleus of the DTAM. Nucleus DTAM is reciprocally connected to the VST. APOA, anterior preoptic area; AT, anterior thalamic nucleus; CT, central thalamic nucleus; DTAM, dorsal tegmental area of the medulla; LT, lateral thalamic nucleus; NI, nucleus isthmi; PPOA, posterior preoptic area; PT, posterior thalamic nucleus; Ri, inferior reticular formation; VST, ventral striatum.

Smith *et al.*, 2000). These cells are located in the pre-Botzinger complex that lies at the rostral tip of nucleus ambiguus corresponding to the frog n.IX-X and derived from rhombomeres 7 and 8. They are responsible for the fictive breathing rhythm that can be recorded from the hypoglossal nerve rootlets in isolated slices of neonatal medulla. Cells of the pre-Botzinger complex project to premotor neurons responsible for translating their rhythm into the coordinated activity of the various motor pools active during inspiration and expiration. These premotor neurons make up the ventral respiratory group that is coextensive with nucleus ambiguus (n.IX-X).

What about DTAM? Located ventral to the cerebellum, this nucleus is not spontaneously active. Schmidt (1992) suggests that DTAM is homologous to the parabrachial nucleus of other vertebrates. The parabrachial complex is located in the dorsal tegmentum at the level of the brachium conjunctivum, a major fiber tract for the cerebellum. The vocalization-related roles of the parabrachial nucleus have been examined in several birds, echolocating bats, cats, and squirrel monkeys (Jurgens, 1976; Rubsamen and Schweizer, 1986; Wild and Arends, 1987; Farley et al., 1992; Reinke and Wild, 1997, 1998; Schuller et al., 1997; Wild et al., 1997). The parabrachial nuclei project to the nucleus ambiguus (the mammalian nucleus containing laryngeal motoneurons); in bats the connection is reciprocal (Rubsamen and Schweizer, 1986). In pigeons, the ascending projections of parabrachial nuclei have been mapped to dorsal thalamus, hypothalamus, and septum; descending projections include the nucleus ambiguus (Wild and Arends, 1987; Wild et al., 1990). In cats, the parabrachial nuclei contain neurons whose activity nuclei is related to vocal output and respiration (Stocker et al., 1997). In squirrel monkeys, the parabrachial region is interposed between cingulate cortex and periaqueductal gray and the nucleus ambiguus (Jurgens and Pratt, 1979). The parabrachial complex contains a number of subnuclei, including the Kolliker–Fuse nucleus and parabrachial nuclei proper; the former is catecholaminergic, whereas the latter are cholinergic. The circuitry underlying vocalization from the midbrain to caudal medulla thus appears to be remarkably well conserved across vertebrates. On the basis of DTAM's connectivity and neurotransmitter phenotype (see later), Schmidt's suggestion that DTAM is homologous to a parabrachial nucleus is well supported. However, unlike R. pipiens, patterned activity in the parabrachial nucleus related specifically to vocalization has not been described in other vertebrates.

A. Sexually Differentiated Vocal Patterns in *Xenopus laevis*

The connections of laryngeal motor neurons in *Xenopus laevis* closely resemble those in other vertebrate vocal systems. The laryngeal motor nucleus contains motor neurons that innervate the larynx and interneurons in approximately equal numbers (Fig. 13); glottal motoneurons are located at the anterior pole of the nucleus (Simpson et al., 1986). Laryngeal motor neurons send a single axon to their target muscle; they are not reciprocally connected. Injection of the retrograde tracer horseradish peroxidase-wheat germ agglutining (HRP-WGA) into n.IX-X reveals labeled cells in adjacent, more medial reticular formation and in DTAM, bilaterally (Wetzel et al., 1985). The latter connection is reciprocal and due to n.IX-X interneurons. DTAM

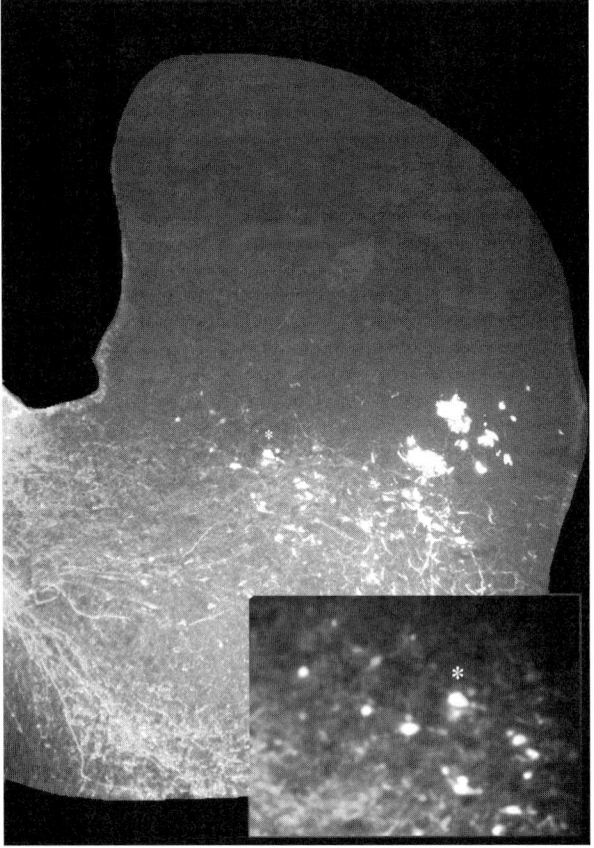

FIGURE 13 Nucleus IX-X includes laryngeal motor neurons and interneurons. Motor neurons (in a horizontal section) were labeled by applying lucifer yellow to the fourth root of the n.IX-X nerve (Simpson et al., 1986). Interneurons (insert at higher magnification) were labeled by contralateral application of fluororuby to n. IX-X. (Erik Zornik, unpublished data.) **See insert for a color version of this figure.**

also projects to reticular formation adjacent to n.IX-X. The injection of HRP into DTAM reveals reciprocal connections with the contralateral DTAM and projections from more anterior brain nuclei, including some thalamic nuclei, the ventral striatum, and the POA (via thalamus).

These observations provide neuroanatomical support for Schmidt's model for the generation of anuran vocalizations. Some differences are expected because *Xenopus lavis* vocalizes underwater. Thus, despite the fact that glottal motor neuron axons travel with those innervating laryngeal bipennate muscle, we do not record respiratory correlates from laryngeal nerve axons in vocalizing males and females. The absence of respiratory correlates probably reflects the inhibition of this activity while the animal is under the surface of the water and is calling. Activity can be recorded when frogs rise to the surface and breathe (A. Yamaguchi, personal communication). We expect to find neurons in or anterior to n.IX-X that generate spontaneous oscillatory activity; these neurons could be a subpopulation of n.IX-X interneurons and be scattered throughout the rostral–ventral extent of the nucleus, a pattern that corresponds to the rhythm generators identified by Schmidt. Another possibility is that n.IX-X interneurons are premotor, but not intrinsically oscillatory, and that a separate rhythm generator can be identified, perhaps at the rostral pole of n.IX-X in a position comparable to the pre-Botzinger complex of mammals.

How is contraction of the bipennate muscles on both sides of the larynx coordinated? This is an important issue in vocal production because, despite the fact that movement of the aryenoid disks is coupled biomechanically via the cartilaginous skeleton of the larynx, both sets of bipennate muscles must contract simultaneously to produce clicks. Because motor neuron axons do not cross the midline, coordination is presumably effected by interneurons, some of which could recieve input from motor neuron collaterals. Candidates include DTAM interneurons, interneurons in the nucleus (n.IX-X interneurons) or interneurons in the adjacent inferior reticular formation (n.Ri). The latter (particularly the lateral nucleus of Ri) project to n.IX-X bilaterally; mapping the projections of n.IX-X interneurons in the nucleus will require intracellular injections of tracer. Nucleus DTAM projects to n.IX-X both ipsilaterally and contralaterally. Projections include motor neurons and interneurons.

A major issue is how the temporal patterns of the different calls are generated. Males, for example, produce six call types, each with a distinctive temporal, rate, and amplitude structure. One possibility is that motor neurons are dedicated to the production of only certain call types. Intracellular recordings from the *vox in vitro* preparation (Tobias and Kelley, 1988) reveal that male laryngeal motor neurons make two kinds of synapses on muscle fibers, type II (weak) and type I (strong). Each laryngeal motor neuron innervates many muscle fibers; a plausible scenario is that synapse types are the same for each motor neuron, and we can thus classify laryngeal motor units as belonging to, at minimum,

two categories, weak and strong. Slow calls, such as the amplectant call, are probably produced by strong motor units, whereas rapid calls are produced initially by strong units and then by both types as recruitment and facilitation proceed (Yamaguchi and Kelley, 2000). Strong motor units fire synchronously and may be coupled either electrically or via strong excitatory connections to synergist motor neurons. These two types of motor unit may be intermingled in n.IX-X or segregated anatomically in the nucleus; this issue can only be addressed by impaling individual axons in the laryngeal nerve, identifying the type of synapse made, and backfilling the responsible motor neuron.

Another possibility (not mutually exclusive with the one just outlined) is that the responsibility for generating different patterns is primarily that of the prevocal interneurons. This idea comes from respiratory pattern generation in mammals, in which all interneurons in the ventral respiratory group are thought to be driven by the rhythmic output of the pre-Botzinger nucleus, but each is thought to have different electrophysiological properties and to connect to separate motor neuron pools. A model incorporating this and other features of vocal circuitry is illustrated in Fig. 14. Which vocal behavior is actually produced would depend on hormonal state and on sensory stimulation. The most extreme example here comes from auditory input. Male calling is stimulated by rapping and silenced by ticking (Tobias *et al.*, 1998). These two sorts of inputs must, at some point in the auditory–vocal pathway, access excitatory and inhibitory interneurons, respectively.

1. Vocal Effectors

Male and female brains generate very different vocal ouputs in *Xenopus laevis*. This difference is produced by the endocrine milieu in which young frogs develop. Under the influence of testosterone and estrogen, and following priming by hormones secreted by the thyroid and pituitary glands, the developmental trajectory of laryngeal motor neurons, muscle fibers, and laryngeal cartilages diverge (Kelley, 1996). This sexually differentiated program is described elsewhere (see Breedlove, Jordan and Kelley, Chapter 65). Briefly, sex differences in cell number in n.IX-X and the larynx are due to androgen action. Androgen acts as a mitogen for laryngeal myoblasts and chondroblasts; under the influence of the testes, juvenile males add approximately

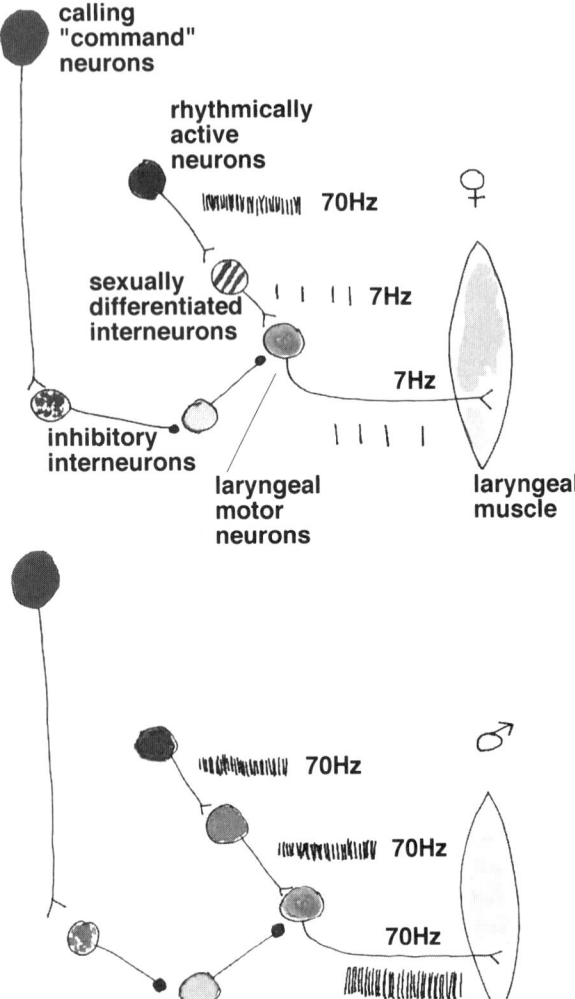

FIGURE 14 A hypothetical scheme for generating a sexually differentiated motor pattern. For simplicity, the circuit is designed to produce different click rates in (A) females (7 Hz) and (B) males (70 Hz). The activity of laryngeal motor neurons is under tonic inhibitory control (light interneurons), relieved by disinhibition in response to activity in calling command interneurons, which may correspond to the DTAM. Excitatory input to laryngeal motor neurons originates with activity in rhythmically active neurons and is shaped into distinct male and female patterns by sexually differentiated interneurons (stripes, females; solid, males). Bar: 0.5 s. **See insert for a color version of this figure.**

150 muscle fibers daily until the adult complement is reached at 6 months after metamorphosis is complete (Marin et al., 1990). In females, muscle fiber addition is slower and not dependent on the gonads. The end result is a larynx with 10 times more muscle fibers in males than in females. Adult males have approximately two times more neurons in n.IX-X than adult females (Kelley, 1996). Again, this difference depends on gonadal androgen; in males, the testes are responsible for rescuing n.IX-X cells from ontogenetic cell death (Kay et al., 1999). Both actions of androgen depend for their timing on thyroid hormone (TH) secretion, which opens the critical period for androgen-induced cell proliferation and initiates ontogenetic cell death in n.IX-X (Cohen and Kelley, 1996; Robertson and Kelley, 1996). Androgen secretion is also responsible for switching muscle fiber type in males from slow to fast and for expression of the fast, larynx-specific myosin heavy chain gene (Catz et al., 1992). These actions require a brief exposure to prolactin, stimulated by TH secretion (Edwards et al., 1999). All of these effects of androgen are developmental and permanent (see Breedlove, Jordan, and Kelley, Chapter 65, for a discussion of organizational effects of steroids).

Androgen secretion in adulthood activates advertisement calling in males; this effect is a temporary (activational) one (Wetzel, 1983). Not all male vocal behaviors are androgen-dependent; growling, for example, is not affected by castration. Another activational effect is the control of synaptic strength by estrogen; ovariectomy weakens the strong synapses of adult females and estrogen strengthens the weak synapses of male and female juveniles. Estrogen cannot, however, be the only factor controlling synaptic strength in males because they normally are not exposed to any estrogen (Kelley, 1996) and yet have some (~20%) strong synapses.

To what extent do these hormone-induced sex-specific features account for differences in the vocal periphery and the CNS circuitry that generate vocal behaviors? We provided androgen implants or testis transplants to females at various stages of postmetamorphic development (including adulthood) and correlated effects on vocal behaviors with changes in muscle fiber numbers and type (Watson and Kelley, 1992; Watson et al., 1993). The number of laryngeal muscle fibers was determined by counts from micrographs. Muscle fiber types were assayed via physiological recordings, histochemical assays, and in situ hybridization using the LM probe. Testis transplants into females masculinized laryngeal fiber number and type at every developmental

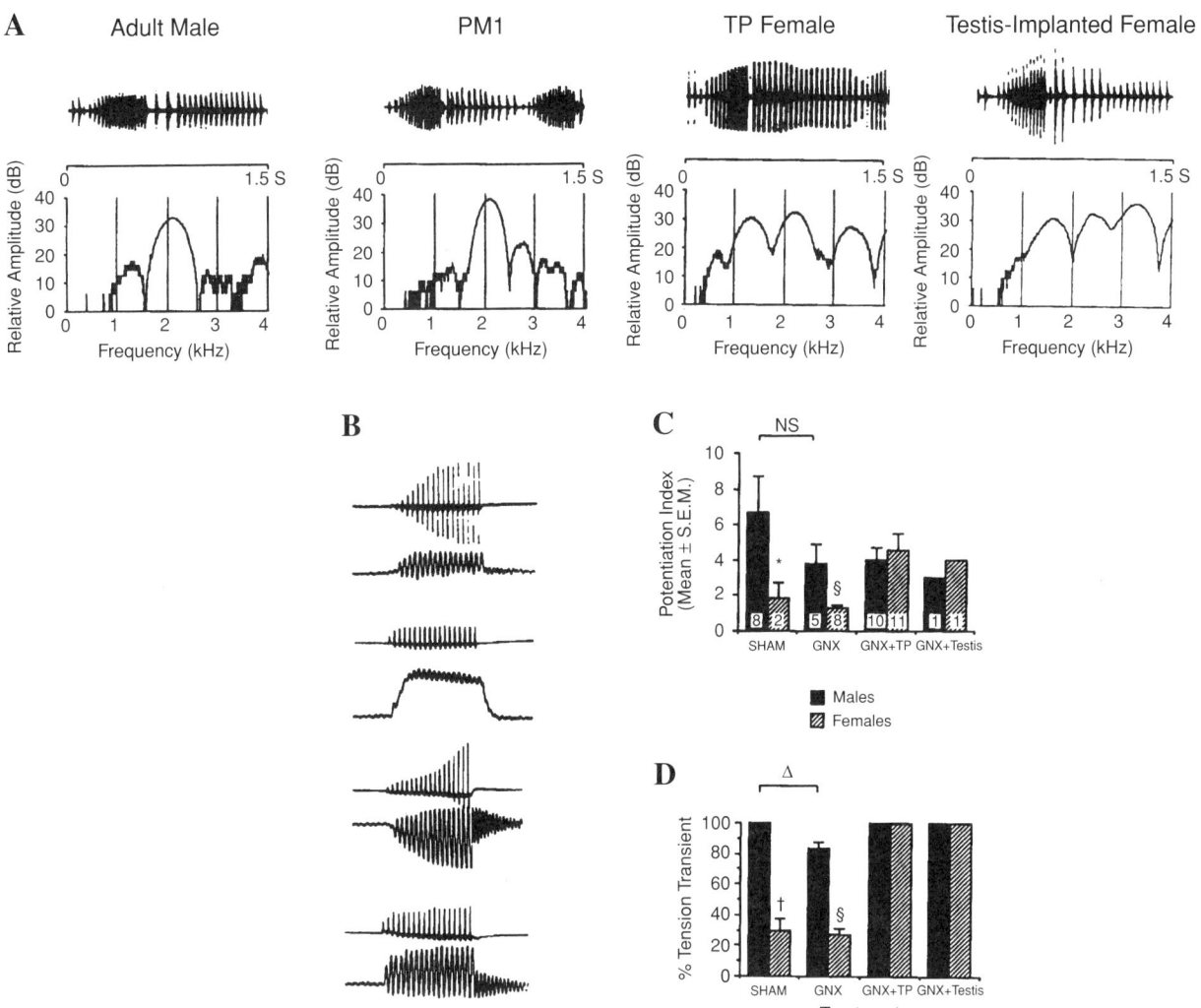

FIGURE 15 Vocal behavior of female *Xenopus laevis* can be masculinized by a testis transplant or prolonged androgen treatment. (A) All females that called after androgen treatment produced alternating fast and slow trills characteristic of advertisement calling. Call rates and click frequencies were completely masculine only in females that received transplants early in postmetamorphic development. (B) Laryngeal tension records from (top to bottom) a gonadally intact adult male, a long-term castrated adult male, an androgen-implanted female, and a testis-transplanted female. Both EMG potentiation (reflecting synaptic facilitation) and tension transients (reflecting fiber-type composition) could be masculinized by long-term treatments. From Watson and Kelley (1992), *J. Comp. Physiol. A.* **171**, 343–350, copyright Springer-Verlag.

stage (Fig. 15). The masculinization of muscle fiber number was partial; that is, even several years after the transplant, the number of laryngeal muscle fibers was less than that of untreated males or males with transplants. In contrast, masculinization of muscle fiber type was complete; testis-transplanted females displayed an entirely fast-twitch complement of muscle fibers and the ability to produce complete tension transients at rapid rates of nerve stimulation, mimicking those of male fast trills. EMG potentiation was also masculinized, suggesting that synaptic efficacy was male-like (most probably due to ovariectomy, however, rather than androgen exposure). In contrast to the efficacy of the testis transplants, implants of androgen had no effect on muscle fiber numbers in adult females.

We can determine whether the CNS produced masculine vocal patterns in these animals by examining the songs of implanted and transplanted frogs with masculinized peripheral vocal systems. All females that received testis transplants at juvenile stages produced advertisement calls as adults. Songs were indistinguishable in duration and trill rates from those of males. In contrast, provision of androgen to adult females (via transplants or implants) was less effective in the percentage of females calling (30 vs 100% for juveniles). Those females that did call produced alternating fast and slow trills, and the fast trills were intensity modulated. Unlike hormonally intact females, then, testis-transplanted females do express male-typical patterned neural output. The duration of treatment was long, and we do not know what cellular changes in the CNS accompany this shift in vocal behaviors. Both sexes may have the neural machinery required for advertisement calling, with access to the motor neuron output being somehow blocked in females; androgen treatment would then overcome that blockade.

A testis transplant masculinizes cell numbers in adult females and is twice as effective as an androgen implant in permitting advertisement calling. Testis transplants increase layngeal muscle fiber and motor neuron axon numbers; androgen implants do not. Even untreated females have enough motor neurons, interneurons, and laryngeal muscle fibers to produce rapping and ticking. Why should having more cells facilitate the expression of advertisement calling? One possibility is that the androgen rescue of n.IX-X cells and stimulation of muscle fiber addition is selective for the weak motor units that underlie facilitation and, perhaps, for the premotor neurons that translate rhythmic activity of the generator interneurons into alternating fast and slow trills. In this scenario, the developmental default phenotype exhibited in the absence of the gonads, would be the survival of the strong motor units required to generate slow calls such as ticking and the amplectant call. The weak motor neurons would only survive if androgen were present and would only have muscle fibers to drive if androgen had induced muscle fiber addition. Motor neurons rescued from ontogenetic cell death by androgen would preferentially synapse on muscle fibers added during the early juvenile stages and those synapses would be maintained in their weak state into adult life. The first part of this scenario could be tested by determining whether muscle fibers with weak synapses in males were those formed after metamorphosis and muscle fibers with strong synapses were formed without androgen action.

Even adult females can generate the advertisement call pattern provided that they receive a testis transplant and that sufficient time is allowed for masculinization of cell number to occur (Fig. 15). In this preparation, the number of axons in the laryngeal nerve increases suggesting that the number of motor neurons increases. These new laryngeal motor neurons cannot be derived from those generated early in development because these undergo ontogenetic cell death and are removed beginning at metamorphosis. The production of a masculine vocal pattern by these genetic females also suggests that the requisite interneurons are present and functional. The plasticity revealed by the testis transplant suggests that adult females maintain a population of responsive cells that can be recruited into functional vocal circuits even in adulthood, provided that the correct endocrine milieu is recreated. These responsive cells could be neuronal stem cells that respond to testicular secretion with proliferation and differentiation or postmitotic interneurons that can be induced to transform into premotor interneurons or laryngeal motor neurons.

IX. SUMMARY AND CONCLUSION

The vocal system of *Xenopus laevis* permits us to address, experimentally, the question of how the CNS, motor neurons, and muscle effectors generate distinct patterns of activity in the sexes. During development, the vocal system becomes sexually differentiated under the influence of steroid hormones secreted by the gonads. These same hormones are required for the activation of some vocal patterns and for the strength of connections between the vocal CNS and the muscular periphery. Male- and female-specific patterns of activity that correspond closely to actual vocal behaviors can be recorded from the laryngeal nerve. This characteristic now permits us to begin to determine how different vocal patterns are generated at the level of individual motor neurons and interneurons. The separation of vocalization from respiration in *Xenopus laevis* also permits us to test current concepts of how brain-stem rhythms are generated and translated into motor programs for specific behaviors.

References

Bass, A., Bodnar, D., and Marchaterre, M. (1999). Complementary eplanations for existing phenotypes in an acoustic communication system. *In* "The Design of Animal Communication" (M. Hauser and M. Konishi, eds.), pp. 493–514. MIT Press, Cambridge, MA.

Bass, A. H., and Baker, R. (1997). Phenotypic specification of hindbrain rhombomeres and the origins of rhythmic circuits in vertebrates. *Brain, Behav. Evol.* **50**(Suppl. 1), 3–16.

Catz, D. S., Fischer, L. M. *et al.* (1992). Sexually dimorphic expression of a laryngeal-specific, androgen-regulated myosin heavy chain gene during *Xenopus laevis* development. *Dev. Biol.* **154**(2), 366–276.

Cohen, M. A., and Kelley, D. B. (1996). Androgen-induced proliferation in the developing larynx of *Xenopus laevis* is regulated by thyroid hormone. *Dev. Biol.* **178**(1), 113–123.

Del Castillo, J., and Katz, B. (1954). Quantal components of the end-plate potential. *J. Physiol. (Lond.)* **124**, 560–573.

Edwards, C. J., Yamamoto, K. *et al.* (1999). Prolactin opens the sensitive period for androgen regulation of a larynx-specific myosin heavy chain gene. *J. Neurobiol.* **41**(4), 443–451.

Farley, G. R., Barlow, S. M. *et al.* (1992). Factors influencing neural activity in parabrachial regions during cat vocalizations. *Exp. Brain Res.* **89**(2), 341–351.

Feldman, J. L. (1995). Neurobiology of breathing control. Where to look and what to look for. *Adv. Exp. Med. Biol.* **393**, 3–5.

Jurgens, U. (1976). Projections from the cortical larynx area in the squirrel monkey. *Exp. Brain Res.* **25**(4), 401–411.

Jurgens, U., and Pratt, R. (1979). The cingular vocalization pathway in the squirrel monkey. *Exp. Brain Res.* **34**(3), 499–510.

Katz, B., and Miledi, R. (1967). The release of acetylcholine from nerve endings by graded electric pulses. *Proc. R. Soc. Lond. B* **167**, 23–38.

Kay, J. N., Hannigan, P. *et al.* (1999). Trophic effects of androgen: Development and hormonal regulation of neuron number in a sexually dimorphic vocal motor nucleus. *J. Neurobiol.* **40**(3), 375–385.

Kelley, D. B. (1996). Sexual differentiation in *Xenopus laevis*. *In* "The Biology of Xenopus" (R. Tinsley and H. Kobel, eds.), pp. 143–176. Oxford University Press, Oxford.

Kelley, D. B., and Tobias, M. L. (1999). Vocal communication in *Xenopus laevis*. *In* "The Design of Animal Communication" (M. D. Hauser and M. Konishi, eds.) pp. 9–35. MIT Press, Cambridge, MA.

Kelley, D. B., Weintraub, A. S., and Bockman, R. S. (1987). Oviductal prostaglandin synthesis and female sexual receptivity in *Xenopus laevis*. *Adv. Prostaglandin, Thromboxane Leukotriene Res.* **17B**, 1133–1135.

Kelley, D. B., Tobias, M. L., and Horng, S. (2001). Producing and perceiving frogs songs; dissecting the neural bases for vocal behaviors in *Xenopus laevis*. *In* "Anuran Communication" (M. Ryan, ed.), pp. 156–166. Smithsonian Institution Press, Washington, DC.

Marin, M. L., Tobias, M. L. *et al.* (1990). Hormone-sensitive stages in the sexual differentiation of laryngeal muscle fiber number in *Xenopus laevis*. *Development (Cambridge, UK)* **110**(3), 703–711.

Matsumoto, A., Arnold, A. P. *et al.* (1988). Androgenic regulation of gap junctions between motoneurons in the rat spinal cord. *J. Neurosci.* **8**(11), 4177–4183.

Picker, M. D. (1983). Hormonal induction of the aquatic phonotactic response of *Xenopus*. *Behaviour* **86**, 74–90.

Reinke, H., and Wild, J. M. (1997). Distribution and connections of inspiratory premotor neurons in the brainstem of the pigeon (*Columba livia*). *J. Comp. Neurol.* **379**(3), 347–362.

Reinke, H., and Wild, J. M. (1998). Identification and connections of inspiratory premotor neurons in songbirds and budgerigar. *J. Comp. Neurol.* **391**(2), 147–163.

Robertson, J. C., and Kelley, D. B. (1996). Thyroid hormone controls the onset of androgen sensitivity in the developing larynx of *Xenopus laevis*. *Dev. Biol.* **176**(1), 108–123.

Rubsamen, R., and Schweizer, H. (1986). Control of echolocation pulses by neurons of the nucleus ambiguus in the rufous horseshoe bat, *Rhinolophus rouxi*. II. Afferent and efferent connections of the motor nucleus of the laryngeal nerves. *J. Comp. Physiol. A* **159**(5), 689–699.

Ruel, T. D., Kelley, D. B. *et al.* (1998). Facilitation at the sexually differentiated laryngeal synapse of *Xenopus laevis*. *J. Comp. Physiol. A* **182**(1), 35–42.

Russell, W. (1954). Experimental studies of the reproductive behavior of *Xenopus laevis*. I. The control mechanisms for clasping and unclasping, and the specificity of hormone action. *Behaviour* **7**, 113–188.

Sassoon, D. A., Gray, G. E. *et al.* (1987). Androgen regulation of muscle fiber type in the sexually dimorphic larynx of *Xenopus laevis*. *J. Neurosci.* **7**(10), 3198–3206.

Schmidt, R. S. (1968). Preoptic activation of frog mating behavior. *Behaviour* **30**, 239–257.

Schmidt, R. S. (1992). Neural correlates of frog calling: Production by two semi-independent generators. *Behav. Brain Res.* **28**(1–2), 17–30.

Schuller, G., Fischer, S. *et al.* (1997). Significance of the paralemniscal tegmental area for audio-motor control in the moustached bat, *Pteronotus p. parnellii*: The afferent or efferent connections of the paralemniscal area. *Eur. J. Neurosci.* **9**(2), 342–355.

Simpson H. B., Tobias, M. L., and Kelley, D. B. (1986). Origin and identification of fibers in the cranial nerve IX-X complex of *Xenopus laevis*: Lucifer Yellow backfills in vitro. *J. Comp. Neurol.* **244**, 430–444.

Smith, J. C., Butera, R. J. *et al.* (2000). Respiratory rhythm generation in neonatal and adult mammals: The hybrid pacemaker-network model. *Respir. Physiol.* **122**(2–3), 131–147.

Stocker, S. D., Steinbacher, B. C., Jr. *et al.* (1997). Connections of the caudal ventrolateral medullary reticular formation in the cat brainstem. *Exp. Brain Res.* **116**(2), 270–282.

Tobias, M. L., and Kelley, D. B. (1987). Vocalizations by a sexually dimorphic isolated larynx: Peripheral constraints on behavioral expression. *J. Neurosci.* **7**(10), 3191–3197.

Tobias, M. L., and Kelley, D. B. (1988). Electrophysiology and dye-coupling are sexually dimorphic characteristics of individual laryngeal muscle fibers in *Xenopus laevis*. *J. Neurosci.* **8**, 2422–2429.

Tobias, M. L., Kelley, D. B. *et al.* (1995). A sex difference in synaptic efficacy at the laryngeal neuromuscular junction of *Xenopus laevis*. *J. Neurosci.* **15**, 1660–1668.

Tobias, M. L., Viswanathan, S. *et al.* (1998). Rapping, a female receptive call, initiates male-female duets in the South African clawed frog. *Proc. Natl. Acad. Sci. U.S.A.* **95**(4), 1870–1875.

Trueb, L. (1996). Historical constraints and morphological novelties in the evolution of the skeletal system of pipid frogs (Anura:Pipidae). In "The Biology of Xenopus" (Tinsley, R. C., and Kobel, H. R., eds.), pp. 349–378. Clarendon Press, Oxford.

Watson, J. T., and Kelley, D. B. (1992). Testicular masculinization of vocal behavior in juvenile female *Xenopus laevis* reveals sensitive periods for song duration, rate, and frequency spectra. *J. Comp. Physiol. A* **171**(3), 343–350.

Watson, J. T., Robertson, J. *et al.* (1993). Laryngeal muscle and motor neuron plasticity in *Xenopus laevis*: Testicular masculinization of a developing neuromuscular system. *J. Neurobiol.* **24**(12), 1615–1625.

Weintraub, A., Kelley, D. B., and Bockman, R. S. (1985). Prostaglandin E2 induces receptive behaviors in female *Xenopus laevis*. *Horm. Behav.* **19**, 386–399.

Wetzel, D. M., and Kelley, D. B. (1983). Androgen and gonadotropin control of the mate calls of male South African clawed frogs, *Xenopus laevis*. *Horm. Behav.* **17**, 388–404.

Wetzel, D. M., Haerter, U. L. *et al.* (1985). A proposed neural pathway for vocalization in South African clawed frogs, *Xenopus laevis*. *J. Comp. Physiol. A* **157**(6), 749–761.

Wild, J. M., and Arends, J. J. (1987). A respiratory-vocal pathway in the brainstem of the pigeon. *Brain Res.* **407**(1), 191–194.

Wild, J. M., Arends, J. J. *et al.* (1990). Projections of the parabrachial nucleus in the pigeon (*Columba livia*). *J. Comp. Neurol.* **293**(4), 499–523.

Wild, J. M., Li, D. *et al.* (1997). Projections of the dorsomedial nucleus of the intercollicular complex (DM) in relation to respiratory-vocal nuclei in the brainstem of pigeon (*Columba livia*) and zebra finch (*Taeniopygia guttata*). *J. Comp. Neurol.* **377**(3), 392–413.

Yager, D. (1982). A novel mechanism for underwater sound production in *Xenopus laevis*. *Am. Zool.* **122**, 887.

Yamaguchi, A., and Kelley, D. B. (2000). Generating sexually differentiated vocal patterns: Laryngeal nerve and EMG recordings from vocalizing male and female African clawed frogs (*Xenopus laevis*). *J. Neurosci.* **20**, 1559–1567.

Endocrinology of Complex Life Cycles: Amphibians

Robert J. Denver, Karen A. Glennemeier, and Graham C. Boorse

Department of Biology
University of Michigan
Ann Arbor, Michigan 48109

I. INTRODUCTION TO COMPLEX LIFE CYCLES

Amphibians exhibit considerable diversity in behavioral, physiological, and life history strategies. They are geographically widespread, occupying a diverse range of habitats. Amphibians that undergo metamorphosis have two very different life stages that are affected differently by environmental factors. Most anuran (frog) larvae are aquatic, and tadpoles are found in a wide variety of habitats, ranging from water-filled crevices in rocks, logs, or leaves to larger ponds or streams. Most then undergo morphological, biochemical, and physiological transformation into adults, which are sensitive to different environmental variables than larvae, due to this shift in habitat (Duellman and Trueb, 1994). Some amphibians have lost the larval form and develop directly into the adult morphology (direct development); others do not metamorphose but reproduce in the aquatic habitat while retaining the larval morphology (paedomorphosis).

Amphibians that undergo a metamorphosis exhibit strong variation, both between and within species, in the duration of the larval period (Wilbur and Collins, 1973; Werner, 1986). Larvae encounter diverse ecological conditions during development. Variation in abiotic factors (e.g., water availability, temperature, and photoperiod) as well as biotic factors (e.g., intra- and interspecific competition, and predation) can interact in complex ways to influence larval growth and development (Semlitsch, 1987a; Sredl and Collins, 1992; Rowe and Dunson, 1995; Taylor and Scott, 1997). The timing of metamorphosis is a central amphibian life history trait that probably reflects the quality and relative permanence of the larval habitat. Species that breed in predictable habitats (i.e., permanent or semipermanent lakes and ponds) tend to have longer larval periods. Species that breed in unpredictable habitats (i.e., ephemeral pools) generally have much shorter larval periods (see Fig. 1).

Amphibian larvae exhibit plasticity in the timing of metamorphosis and can capitalize on favorable conditions for growth as long as such conditions last (up until a genetically determined upper limit to the length of the larval period; see Newman, 1992). Such plasticity may permit amphibian larvae to match their phenotype (morphology, physiology, and metamorphic timing) to prevailing environmental conditions. Animals capable of phenotypic plasticity may have a higher probability of surviving in unpredictable habitats than those with a genetically fixed phenotype (Stearns, 1989; Newman, 1992).

Among the most extreme evolutionary modifications of the ancestral complex life history is paedomorphosis.

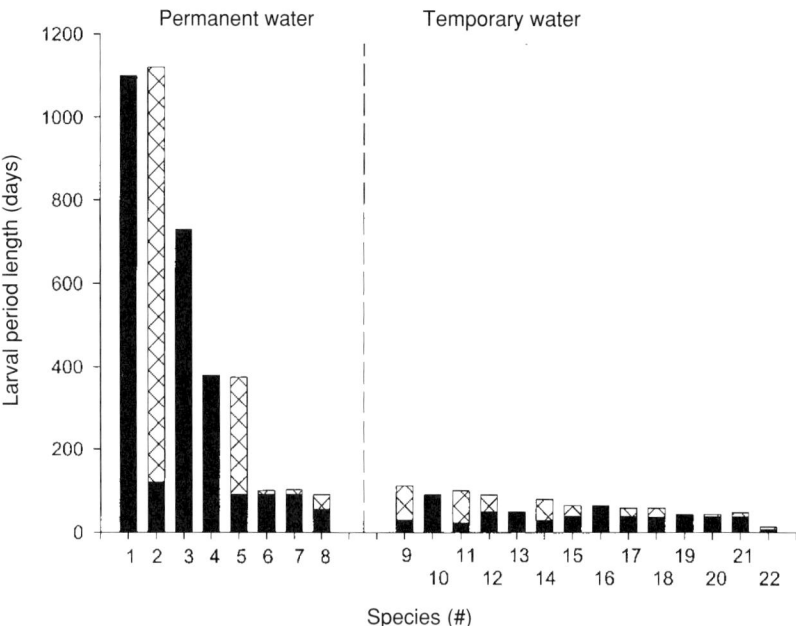

FIGURE 1 The duration of larval periods of selected amphibian species as a function of habitat permanence. Filled bars indicate the minimum duration and hatched bars the maximum duration of the larval period for those species for which information is available. This figure is based partly on information compiled by Low (1976) and Duellman and Trueb (1994) and Denver (1997b). (1) *Rana fuscigula* (Wager, 1965), (2) *R. catesbeiana* (Stebbins, 1951; Bruneau and Magnin, 1980), (3) *R. fasciata fuellborni* (Stewart, 1967), (4) *Ascaphus truei* (Noble and Putnam, 1931; Stebbins, 1951), (5) *R. clamitans* (Stebbins, 1951), (6) *R. grayi* (Wager, 1965), (7) *R. boylei* (Stebbins, 1951), (8) *R. pipiens* (Stebbins, 1951), (9) *R. temporaria* (Miaud et al., 1999; Brady and Griffiths, 2000), (10) *R. sylvatica* (Stebbins, 1951), (11) *Spea (Scaphiopus) hammondii* (Morey and Janes, 1994; R. J. Denver, unpublished data), (12) *Bufo americanus* (Wilbur, 1987), (13) *Pixicephalus adspersus* (Stewart, 1967), (14) *B. boreus* (Hayes et al., 1993), (15) *Hyla arenicolor* (Stebbins, 1951), (16) *H. pseudopuma* (Crump, 1989a), (17) *B. punctatus* (Stebbins, 1951), (18) *B. woodhousei* (Mayhew, 1968; Blair, 1972), (19) *S. bombifrons* (Stebbins, 1951), (20) *B. rangeri* (Stewart, 1967), (21) *B. cognatus* (Stebbins, 1951), and (22) *S. couchi* (Newman, 1988).

Most amphibian larvae undergo a metamorphosis to an adult form before becoming sexually mature. Some species of urodele amphibians (e.g., salamanders and newts) exhibit paedomorphosis, in which reproductive maturity is attained while in a larval or branchiate form. Paedomorphosis refers to the retention of juvenile characteristics in sexually mature adults (Gould, 1977). Many terms have been used describe sexual reproduction while retaining larval characteristics. We choose to use the term "paedomorphosis" for our discussion because it describes retention of larval traits in a sexually mature form, but does not describe the process by which this state is achieved. Other terms such as "neoteny" (deceleration of somatic development) and "progenesis" (acceleration of sexual maturation) describe processes by which paedomorphic development occurs (for more on terminology, see Gould, 1977; McKinney and MacNamara, 1991; Reilly et al., 1997).

Paedomorphosis can either be obligate or facultative depending on the species. Obligate paedomorphs never undergo metamorphosis and remain in an aquatic habitat their entire lives (e.g., *Necturus; Proteus; Amphiuma;* and *Ambystoma mexicanum,* axolotl). The primary focus of our discussion is on facultative paedomorphs, with limited treatment of obligate paedomorphs. Facultatively paedomorphic species can either become paedomorphic and remain in the aquatic habitat or metamorphose and move into the terrestrial environment where they become sexually mature (e.g., *Ambystoma tigrinum, A. talpoideum, A. gracile,* and *Notophthalmus viridescens*; Duellman and Trueb, 1994). The developmental decision to become paedomorphic or to metamorphose may depend on the prevailing environmental conditions rather than the animal's genotype (Harris, 1987; Semlitsch, 1987a; Licht, 1992; Jackson and Semlitsch, 1993) and may be controlled by the interplay of antagonistic hormonal pathways (see Sections IV and V).

II. EVOLUTIONARY ECOLOGY OF AMPHIBIANS

A. Metamorphosis

Amphibians exhibit considerable inter- and intraspecific variation in the duration of the larval period. The rate of development generally is inversely related to larval growth rate and therefore to size at metamorphosis, which can have profound effects on individual fitness. Both a longer larval period and a smaller size at metamorphosis can delay adult reproductive maturity, decrease size at first reproduction, and in some cases decrease adult survival to first reproduction (Berven and Gill, 1983; Smith, 1987; Semlitsch *et al.,* 1988). All of these factors decrease the chance of contributing offspring to the next generation. A longer time to metamorphosis may also increase larval exposure time to aquatic predators (Wilbur, 1980; Werner, 1986) or decrease the chance of metamorphosing before a quickly drying pond disappears (Newman, 1992).

1. Environmental Factors That Influence the Duration of the Larval Period

The upper and lower limits of the length of the larval period are determined by genetic factors that are subject to natural selection. The plasticity of larval period length within these limits is also subject to natural selection and is influenced at both the proximate and ultimate levels by the environment. Although metamorphic timing is determined by both genetic and environmental factors, its expression depends on the development and activity of endocrine glands and the actions of the hormones that these glands produce (see later).

Wilbur and Collins (1973) suggested that there is a threshold of minimum body size that must be reached before metamorphosis is possible and that larval growth rates determine the timing of metamorphosis after this minimum size has been attained. Werner (1986) added mortality risk in the larval and adult habitats to the list of factors that ultimately influence metamorphosis. Environmental factors that influence growth rate or mortality risk therefore should alter the timing of metamorphosis. The effects of specific environmental factors may differ depending on the animal's stage of growth or development. For example, the same factor may be inhibitory to growth if present early in the larval phase or stimulatory to development if present during metamorphosis (e.g., population density, food availability, pond drying, or predation; reviewed by Denver, 1997b). Thus, body size and stage of development may interact in complex ways to determine the phenotypic response to specific environmental variables.

The predictability of rainfall (and, thus, pond duration) profoundly influences amphibian life history strategies. Species that breed in habitats that are permanent and predictable (i.e., lakes, streams, and permanent ponds) generally have longer larval periods, whereas those that breed in habitats that are unpredictable and ephemeral (i.e., temporary ponds) exhibit rapid development (Fig. 1). A short development time is of particular importance in adaptation to a desert environment in which rainfall is unpredictable and ponds are of short duration (Low, 1976; Newman, 1992).

2. Evolution of the Timing of Metamorphosis

The larval stage often is more vulnerable than the adult stage and may be characterized by a higher degree of uncertainty with regard to individual mortality (Duellman and Trueb, 1994). Tadpoles (and eggs) are more vulnerable than adults to predation, due to their small size and relative lack of mobility (Duellman and Trueb, 1994). Competition for resources may also be especially high among larvae, due to rapid growth rates (and, thus, high energy demands) and high densities of conspecifics. Such competition may increase larval mortality rates (Wilbur and Collins, 1973; Smith, 1983). Because of their aquatic habitat, larvae are also especially vulnerable to changes in rainfall or humidity levels and the duration of ponds.

When survivorship in one life-cycle stage is much less certain than in another, we expect to see, among other responses, the minimization of the time spent in the more vulnerable stage (Low, 1976). This expectation is confirmed in habitats with unpredictable rainfall and standing water levels, such as those found in arid regions. Desert amphibians generally exhibit rapid rates of development, with some larvae entering metamorphosis in as little as 8 days after hatching (*Scaphiopus couchii*; see Newman, 1992). Spadefoot toads (genus *Scaphiopus*) typically inhabit arid regions and breed in temporary ponds of unpredictable duration. The length of the larval stage in Couch's spadefoot toads typically ranges from 8 to 15 days, compared to a range of 30 to >1000 days for species found in more permanent aquatic habitats (Fig. 1).

The larval stage is typically more vulnerable and uncertain than the adult stage—why haven't all anurans evolved to minimize the time spent in the larval stage? The answer probably involves the trade-off between development rate and size at metamorphosis. Tadpoles that develop rapidly are typically smaller than those that develop more slowly, with a longer period for growth. Small size at transformation may reduce reproductive potential (Berven and Gill, 1983; Smith, 1987; Semlitsch *et al.*, 1988), a cost that limits the benefit of rapid development in an unpredictable larval habitat. In addition to the costs of rapid metamorphosis, physical constraints may also limit growth and development. For example, Wilbur and Collins (1973) proposed that larvae must reach a minimum body size in order to metamorphose.

a) Phenotypic Plasticity Phenotypic plasticity in development time allows larvae to develop either slowly or rapidly, depending on environmental conditions. Phenotypic plasticity refers generally to phenotypic variation induced by environmental change, and a plastic reaction norm, as described by Stearns (1989), refers to the relationship between phenotypic variation and the environment when the phenotype varies as a continuous function of the environmental signal.

Phenotypic plasticity is especially pronounced in desert-dwelling species (and those of other ephemeral, unpredictable habitats). By artificially altering pond duration, Newman (1988) found that *S. couchii* larvae developed faster (and metamorphosed at a smaller size) in short-duration ponds than in long ones. Newman (1988, 1992) concluded that phenotypic plasticity may have developed in these desert anurans as a result of the fitness trade-off between rapid and slow development under various environmental circumstances.

Other species, both desert and nondesert, that breed in unpredictable habitats show developmental plasticity in response to pond drying (see Table 1). Not all species that have been examined respond to pond drying, which may reflect the relative permanence of the ancestral habitat of the species under study. For example, *R. utricularia*, which breeds in more permanent water, did not show accelerated development rate in response to pond drying (Wilbur, 1987; note that *B. americanus* showed a pond-drying response in the same study). Tadpoles of other ranid species showed developmental responses to pond desiccation (see Table 1). Of those that have been studied, more species than not

TABLE 1
Amphibian Species That Accelerate Metamorphosis in Response to Pond Desiccation[a]

Species	Source
Ambystoma spp.	
A. talpoideum	Semlitsch and Gibbons (1985); Semlitsch (1987a); Semlitsch and Wilbur (1988)
Bufo spp.	
B. americanus	Wilbur (1987)
B. maculatus	Spieler (2000)
Hyla spp.	
H. pseudopuma	Crump (1989a)
Rana spp.	
R. blairi	Parris (2000)
R. sphenocephala	Parris (2000)
R. temporaria	Loman (1999); Laurila and Kujasalo (1999); Merila *et al.* (2000)
Scaphiopus spp.	
S. couchii	Newman (1989); Morey and Janes (1994)
S. hammondii	Denver *et al.* (1998)

[a] Pond desiccation refers to experimental paradigms that include outdoor experiments with cattle tanks and artificial ponds and observations in natural ponds and aquaria maintained in laboratories in which the water level was manipulated. See Brady and Griffiths (2000) for conflicting results.

appear capable of responding to habitat permanence by altering their rates of development (but see Brady and Griffiths, 2000; Spieler, 2000).

To identify the proximate environmental cue(s) that tadpoles of the western spadefoot toad (*S. hammondii*) use to accelerate development in response to pond drying, we manipulated water levels in aquaria in which tadpoles were reared (Denver *et al.*, 1998). Under these laboratory conditions, tadpoles accelerate metamorphosis as the water volume is reduced. Tadpoles can grade their developmental response with respect to the rate of water volume reduction. Furthermore, tadpoles responded to the release from ecological stress (the refilling of the aquarium) by capitalizing on the improved growth conditions. The physiological response to experimental water-volume reduction results in the activation of the endocrine axes that drive metamorphosis (Denver, 1998).

Intraspecific competition may also affect larval development rates. Several studies have shown that resource limitation influences amphibian development, but that the direction of this influence depends on the developmental stage at which the limitation is initiated. For example, increased competition for resources, present early in the larval period, has been shown to decrease larval growth rate, survivorship, and size at metamorphosis and to increase the length of the larval period (Brockelman, 1969; Wilbur and Collins, 1973; Wilbur, 1976, 1977; Smith, 1987; Berven and Chadra, 1988; Scott, 1990). Similarly, D'Angelo and colleagues (1941) showed that starvation before the early limb development stage retarded metamorphosis in both *R. sylvatica* and *R. pipiens*; however, starvation after this stage accelerated metamorphosis. We observed a similar, developmental-stage-dependent phenomenon in *S. hammondii* tadpoles (Denver *et al.*, 1998), and Morey and Reznick (2000) reported nearly identical results in three species of spadefoot toads, *S. couchii, S. hammondii, and S. intermontanus*. These studies suggest that there is a critical period of development for responding positively to limited resources that may reflect a minimum required size or developmental stage for metamorphosis (see also Crump, 1989b; Newman, 1994).

Abiotic factors such as temperature, photoperiod, dissolved oxygen content (DOC), and pH also influence the length of the larval period in amphibians (Wassersug and Seibert, 1975; Gutierrez *et al.*, 1984; Feder and Moran, 1985; Wright *et al.*, 1986; Burns *et al.*, 1987; Edwards and Pivorun, 1991). Increased temperature is well known as accelerating larval growth and development (Hayes *et al.*, 1993). However, temperature can interact in complex ways with other factors such as resource level and density to affect time to and size at metamorphosis (Marian and Pandian, 1985; Beachy, 1995; Newman, 1998).

As mentioned, the environment has a strong influence on the timing of metamorphosis. The physiological bases for plasticity in the timing of metamorphosis are discussed in Section III and placed into an ecological context in Section V.

B. Facultative Paedomorphosis

In facultatively paedomorphic species, both paedomorphic and metamorphic individuals often coexist in the same population in nature and each morph is probably associated with discrete fitness-related consequences. Several hypotheses have been proposed for the maintenance of these alternate morphologies (see Whiteman, 1994, for review), but evidence supports the paedomorphic advantage hypothesis, which predicts that paedomorphosis evolves in relatively permanent aquatic habitats. In such conditions, paedomorphs experience an advantage in one or more fitness components that lead to increased lifetime reproductive success. In support of this hypothesis, paedomorphs are more prevalent in stable aquatic conditions, such as permanent water (Semlitsch, 1987a) and low larval population density (Harris, 1987; Semlitsch, 1987a); paedomorphs may also be favored in habitats where predation risk is low (Jackson and Semlitsch, 1993) (Fig. 2).

Age at maturation is a central life history trait. Paedomorphs undergo sexual maturation earlier than metamorphs (Ryan and Semlitsch, 1998). For example, in Alpine newts (*Triturus alpestris*), metamorphs typically require several years to mature (Miaud *et al.*, 2000), whereas paedomorphs can mature at 1 year of age (Denoel and Joly, 2000). The primary advantages of earlier maturation are greater probability of survival to first reproduction, shortened generation time, and potential increases in lifetime reproductive success (Stearns, 1991; Roff, 1992).

In addition, paedomorphs are present at the breeding site as soon as they mature, allowing them to reproduce

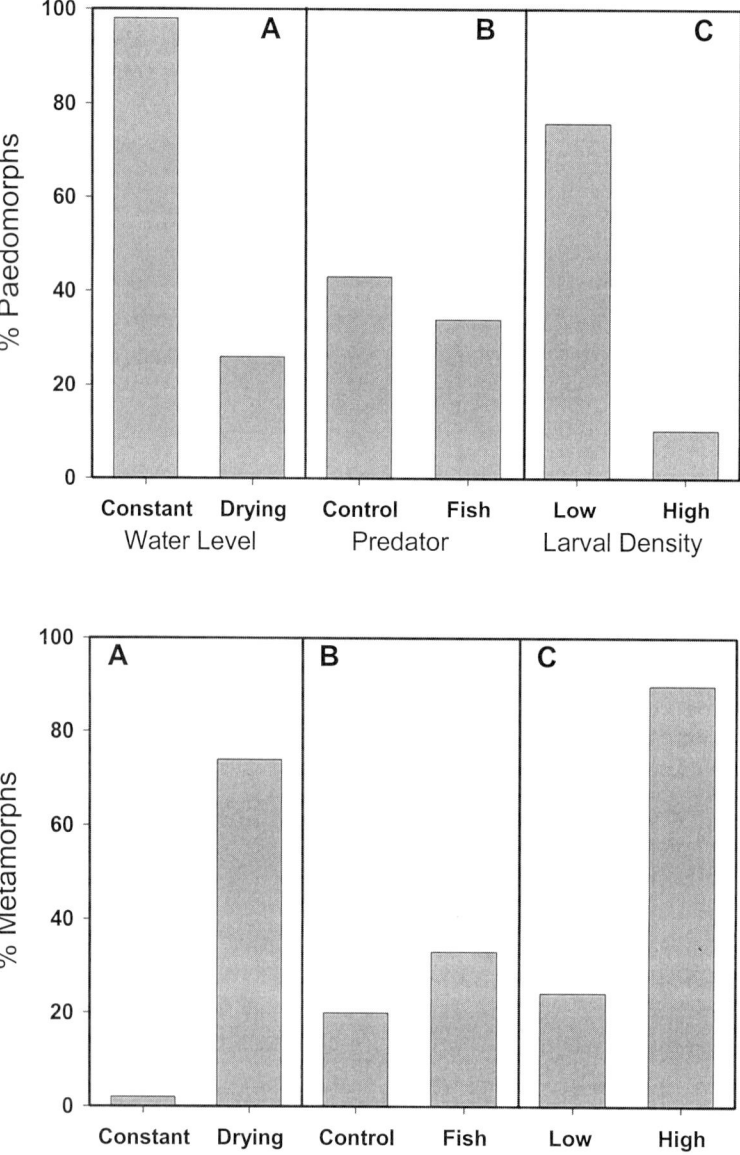

FIGURE 2 Percentages of paedomorphs (top graph) and metamorphs (bottom graph) observed in the facultatively paedomorphic salamanders (A–B) *Ambystoma talpoideum* and (C) *Notophthalamus viridescens dorsalis* exposed to different environmental conditions. Larvae were reared under conditions of (A) constant or decreasing (drying) water level, (B) presence or absence of a fish predator, or (C) high or low population density. Data modified from (A) Semlitsch (1987a); (B) Jackson and Semlitsch (1993); (C) Harris (1987).

earlier than migrating metamorphs for any given breeding season. Paedomorphs are capable of courtship, sperm transfer, insemination, and oviposition prior to the arrival of terrestrial adults migrating to the breeding pond (Scott, 1993; Krenz and Sever, 1995). Because competition and other density-dependent factors influence growth and survival in many amphibian species (Harris, 1987; Semlitsch, 1987b; Taylor and Scott, 1997), early reproduction by paedomorphic adults may allow their offspring time to grow prior to the hatching of larvae from terrestrial adults. Because of the earlier growth opportunities, larvae from paedomorphic adults may have a competitive advantage due to their larger size compared with larvae of terrestrial metamorphic adults. Early growth and survival benefits can later translate into enhanced adult performance and thus greater fitness (Semlitsch et al., 1988). Paedomorphs retain the ability to undergo metamorphosis. However, this transition typically only occurs in the spring after the breeding season (Semlitsch, 1985; Whiteman, 1994).

The paedomorphic advantage model predicts metamorphosis is maintained in a population by selection acting primarily during the occasional years of unfavorable aquatic conditions. Higher proportions of metamorphs are generated during aquatic conditions such as low water levels (Semlitsch, 1987a), high conspecific density (Harris, 1987), and the presence of a fish predator (Jackson and Semlitsch, 1993) (Fig. 2). The transition to a terrestrial habitat not only allows larvae to escape deteriorating aquatic conditions, but also permits metamorphic adults to colonize newly formed pools during subsequent breeding seasons. Such pools may be free from predators and yield higher larval growth rates (Whiteman et al., 1996).

Larvae receive input from their environment and choose a life history strategy that has the highest relative fitness for the prevailing ecological conditions (i.e., they exhibit developmental plasticity). The proximate mechanisms by which facultative paedomorphic salamanders select a particular life history trajectory are the subject of Section IV.

III. ENDOCRINOLOGY OF METAMORPHOSIS

A. Overview

Hormones orchestrate the diverse morphological and physiological changes that occur during metamorphosis (see Fig. 3). Gudernatch (1912) first showed that the vertebrate thyroid gland contained a factor that could induce precocious metamorphosis if fed to tadpoles. This compound, later identified as 3,5,3'5'-tetraiodothyronine, thyroxine (Kendall, 1915; Harrington, 1926; Harrington and Barger, 1927), and referred to as thyroid hormone (TH), is now known to be the primary hormone controlling amphibian metamorphosis. Although hormones produced by the anterior pituitary gland and the interrenal glands (the amphibian homologs of the mammalian adrenal cortex) can influence the rate of metamorphosis, exogenous

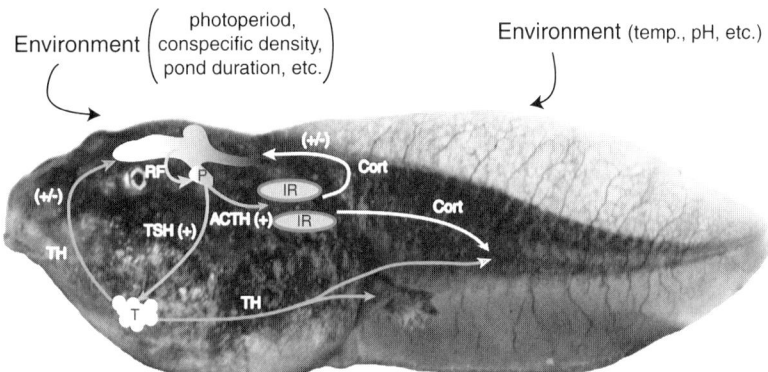

FIGURE 3 Endocrine systems controlling tadpole metamorphosis. ACTH, adrenocorticotropic hormone; Cort, corticoids; IR, interrenal gland; P, pituitary gland; RF, releasing factor; T, thyroid gland; TH, thyroid hormone; TSH, thyroid-stimulating hormone. Pluses indicate a stimulatory effect and minuses a negative feedback. In the case of TH and Cort effects on the brain, (+/−) indicates that these hormones promote differentiation of neurosecretory centers (and other brain regions) in addition to their negative feedback effects on neurohormone and pituitary hormone secretion.
See insert for a color version of this figure.

TH alone can induce the entire suite of tissue transformations (see Kikuyama *et al.*, 1993; Shi, 1996). Furthermore, chemical or surgical thyroidectomy results in metamorphic stasis (Dodd and Dodd, 1976; Kikuyama *et al.*, 1993).

The work of William Etkin laid much of the foundation for our understanding of the endocrine control of metamorphosis. Etkin (1968) proposed a model for the hormonal changes that occur during amphibian metamorphosis. He also coined the terms in common use among amphibian endocrinologists for describing the stages of anuran development: premetamorphosis, when the larvae grows but little or no morphological change occurs and plasma TH concentrations are low; prometamorphosis, when hind-limb growth accelerates and plasma TH concentration rises; and metamorphic climax, the final and most rapid phase of morphological change when thyroid activity is at its peak (see Dodd and Dodd, 1976; White and Nicoll, 1981; Table 2).

The following section describes the cast of endocrine characters that interact to control metamorphosis. For each endocrine axis involved in metamorphosis we first examine its developmental schedule. This allows predictions of when the endocrine system is sufficiently developed to allow the animal to become competent to respond to the external environmental. We also examine the multiple levels at which the activity and functioning of each endocrine axis can be regulated. In Section V on integration, we address how the endocrine system determines the timing of metamorphosis and mediates environmental effects on amphibian development.

B. Thyroid Hormone

1. Role in Amphibian Development

Perhaps the most striking characteristic of amphibian metamorphosis, from the perspective of hormonal control, is that a single signaling molecule, produced by a highly restricted group of cells (the thyroid epithelial cells), can orchestrate the entire suite of molecular, biochemical, and morphological changes. Depending on the tissue, TH can induce cell proliferation, death, differentiation, or migration. Target cells for TH are known to activate both similar and different sets of genes according to the concentration of this single signaling molecule. Specific tissues exhibit different dose sensitivities to TH, and the challenge for investigators studying the molecular basis of TH action during metamorphosis is to determine how and why individual tissues respond differently to the hormone and exhibit differential dose responses.

2. Thyroid Gland Development and Hormone Production

The thyroid gland develops early in the amphibian embryo when the anlage consists of a thickening of the pharyngeal epithelium; these cells are capable of synthesizing small iodoproteins (reviewed by Dodd and Dodd, 1976; Regard *et al.*, 1978). The gland matures functionally at the time of hatching, when it separates into two distinct lobes and is essentially completely developed by late premetamorphosis to early prometamorphosis (Nieuwkoop and Faber, 1956; Saxén *et al.*, 1957a,b; Kaye, 1960; Dodd and Dodd, 1976; Regard *et al.*, 1978). Multiple measures of thyroid activity, including radioiodine uptake, gland ultrastructure, and plasma concentrations or tissue content of THs, show that thyroid activity increases markedly during prometamorphosis (Table 2), peaks at metamorphic climax, and declines thereafter to reach an adult level of activity (Kaye, 1960; Dodd and Dodd, 1976; Regard *et al.*, 1978; Kikuyama *et al.*, 1993). Ultrastructural analyses show a dramatic increase in thyroid follicular cell height during prometamorphosis, with a peak at metamorphic climax that corresponds to the peak in plasma concentrations (and tissue content) of THs (see Dodd and Dodd, 1976; Regard *et al.*, 1978).

When Etkin proposed his endocrine-based model for metamorphosis, investigators at the time did not have sensitive and quantitative methods for determining plasma TH concentrations. Early methods relied on the determination of protein-bound iodide to estimate plasma TH titers (Just, 1972). Subsequently, sensitive and specific radioimmunoassays (RIAs) were developed that allowed determinations of plasma thyroxine (T_4; the primary product of the thyroid gland) and 3,5,3′-triiodothyronine (T_3; derived from T_4 by monodeiodination in target tissues; see Fig. 4) concentrations during metamorphosis. These studies confirmed earlier studies and the predictions of Etkin by demonstrating low to nondetectable plasma TH concentrations during premetamorphosis, increasing concentrations during prometamorphosis, and a dramatic peak at

TABLE 2
Comparison of Three Staging Tables for Postembryonic Feeding Stages of Anuran Larvae[a]

N-F staging[b] for X. laevis	Major common diagnostic features and morphological changes	T-K staging[c]	Gosner staging[d]	Etkin terminology[e]
1–45	Nonfeeding stages (comparable to Shumway stages[f] 1–24)		1–25	
46		I	26	Premetamorphosis
47–48	Feeding begins	II	27	
49–50		III	28	
51		IV	29	
		V	30	
52	Foot-paddle stages			
		VI	31	
53		VII	32	
		VIII	33	
54		IX	34	
		X	35	
55	Hind-limb stages	XI	36	Prometamorphosis
		XII	37	
56		XIII	38	
57–58		XIV–XVI	39–40	
59	Tadpole reaches maximum length	XVII	40	
60		XVIII	41	
		XIX		
61		XX		
62	Rapid tail resorption begins, front limbs erupt[g]	XXI	42	Climax
63		XXII	43	
64		XXIII	44	
65	Stump of tail remains	XXIV	45	
66	Tail completely resorbed, juvenile frog	XXV	46	

[a] Table is derived from similar tables published by Nieuwkoop and Faber (1956), Dodd and Dodd (1976) and Kikuyama et al. (1993) with the addition of Gosner staging. Note that the table is modified somewhat with respect to the table published by Kikuyama et al. (1993), with deference to the comparison between X. laevis and the staging of R. pipiens (Taylor and Kollros, 1946) made by Nieuwkoop and Faber (1956). Comparison of Taylor and Kollros (1946) with Gosner (1960) staging tables is based on that of Gosner (1960).
[b] Nieuwkoop and Faber (1956).
[c] Taylor and Kollros (1946).
[d] Gosner (1960).
[e] Etkin (1968).
[f] Shumway (1940).
[g] The front limbs erupt in X. laevis at stage 58 and continue to grow and develop through metamorphic climax. In other amphibians, such as ranids or pelobatids (e.g., Scaphiopus), the front limbs develop internally and then erupt at metamorphic climax.

metamorphic climax (Leloup and Buscaglia, 1977; Miyauchi et al., 1977; Regard et al., 1978; Mondou and Kaltenbach, 1979; Suzuki and Suzuki, 1981; Weil, 1986; Niinuma et al., 1991b).

Because of the difficulty of obtaining blood from small tadpoles for analysis by RIA, only those species with tadpoles large enough to obtain a serum sample were analyzed. Thus, most blood measurements

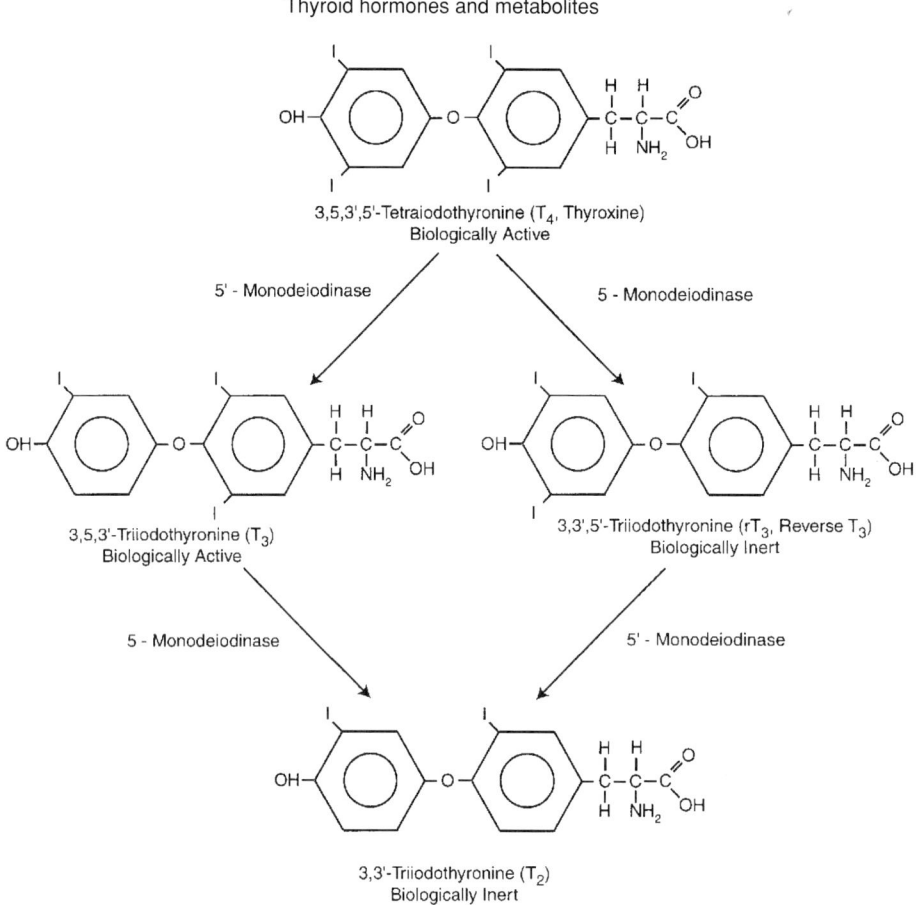

FIGURE 4 Thyroid hormone structure and metabolism. Arrows indicate deiodination by tissue monodeiodinases, resulting in bioactivation or bioinactivation of the substrate.

have been done on ranid species (e.g., *Rana catesbeiana* and *Rana clamitans*); however, Leloup and Buscaglia (1977) and Tata et al. (1993) have measured THs in plasma pools of *X. laevis* (see also Buscaglia et al., 1985, for measures of plasma T_3 and T_4 in other *Xenopus* spp.). In species with small tadpoles, developmental changes in TH content of whole bodies and individual tissues have been determined. These analyses have shown that changes in whole-body TH content in the smaller species essentially parallel changes observed in the plasma of tadpoles of the larger species—*Bufo japonicus* (Niinuma et al., 1991b), *Spea hammondii* (Denver, 1993, 1997a, 1998), *X. laevis* (R. J. Denver, unpublished data), *Bufo marinus* (Weber et al., 1994). The peak in whole-body T_3 and T_4 coincides with peak uptake of ^{131}I in *Bufo japonicus* (Niinuma et al., 1991b). Thus, it is likely that determination of whole-body hormone content provides a reasonable estimate of physiological changes in TH production in species for which blood samples are unobtainable.

3. Control of Thyroid Hormone Secretion, Metabolism, and Transport

a) Pituitary Control The increase in thyroid gland growth and biosynthetic activity during prometamorphosis is dependent on the pituitary hormone thyrotropin (thyroid-stimulating hormone, TSH). The development of the thyroid gland is arrested in hypophysectomized tadpoles, resulting in the failure to metamorphose (Regard and Mauchamp, 1971, 1973; Dodd and Dodd, 1976). This condition can be reversed by injecting TSH (Regard and Mauchamp, 1971, 1973). It is likely that the early development of the thyroid gland does not depend on TSH because its development occurs before immunoreactive TSH cells are present in the anterior pituitary, which occurs at NF stage 42 in *X. laevis* and at similar stages in ranid frogs (Moriceau-Hay et al., 1982; Tanaka et al., 1991; Gracia-Navarro et al., 1992). However, it cannot be ruled out that small amounts of TSH sufficient to support thyroid development are produced earlier than these stages, but cannot be detected due to limitations in the sensitivity of the immunohistochemical detection methods.

Although functional thyroid follicles are present at stages that precede the prometamorphic rise in TH production, the rate of hormone synthesis is coordinate with the development of the pituitary gland and the production of TSH (Kaye, 1960; Dodd and Dodd, 1976; Buckbinder and Brown,1993; Denver, 1996). The amphibian thyroid gland develops sensitivity to TSH during late embryogenesis (just prior to hatching), as can be demonstrated by the increased radioiodine uptake by thyroids following TSH injection (see Kaye, 1960). There have been no direct measures of circulating TSH (by RIA) in amphibians. However, evidence for an increase in circulating TSH at the early limbbud stage (T-K stage III) in *R. pipiens* tadpoles was provided by Kaye (1961).

Thyrotropin is composed of two subunits, α and β, that are derived from two separate genes. The α subunit is common among the glycoprotein hormones (i.e., the gonadotropins (GtHs), luteinizing hormone (LH) and follicle-stimulating hormone (FSH), and TSH); whereas, the β subunit confers hormonal specificity on the molecule (Pierce and Parsons, 1981). The cDNAs for TSHβ subunit have now been isolated from three amphibian species—two anurans, *X. laevis* (Buckbinder and Brown, 1993) and *R. catesbeiana* (Okada et al., 2000), and one urodele, *Hynobius retardatus* (Kanki and Wakahara, 2000; partial cDNA). Deduced amino acid sequences of the amphibian TSHβ subunits show that they exhibit 40–73% sequence similarity to known vertebrate TSHβ molecules. Northern blot analysis of the developmental expression of pituitary α glycoprotein subunit and TSHβ subunit mRNAs in *X. laevis* tadpoles did not detect the expression of these genes at NF stage 52 but showed a dramatic increase in expression by stage 57 (stages between 52 and 57 were not analyzed; Buckbinder and Brown, 1993). A similar developmental schedule of TSHβ mRNA expression was demonstrated in the bullfrog (Okada et al., 2000). Thus, TSH biosynthesis is coordinated with thyroid gland development and hormone secretion, and the stimulatory action of pituitary TSH is necessary for thyroid gland growth and hormone biosynthesis.

b) Thyroid Hormone Conversion The major product of the amphibian thyroid gland is T_4, with minor amounts of T_3 produced (see Rosenkilde, 1978; Buscaglia et al., 1985; Fig. 4). The result is that the plasma T_4 concentration tends to be an order of magnitude greater than T_3 (Regard et al., 1978; Larras-Regard et al., 1981). The only case in which this relationship may not hold is for *X. laevis*, in which the reported plasma T_3:T_4 ratio is very similar and may even exceed 1 at metamorphic climax (Leloup and Buscaglia, 1977; Buscaglia et al., 1985). Measures of the tissue content of T_4 and T_3 in various species show that the two hormones are present in roughly similar amounts (Niinuma et al., 1991b; Weber et al., 1994; Denver, 1997a, 1998). Although a comprehensive analysis of both blood concentrations and tissue contents of THs has not been done for any species, it is likely that the higher T_3:T_4 ratio in tissues compared with T_3:T_4 ratios in blood reflects high tissue 5'-monodeiodinase activity.

Tissue monodeiodinases convert T_4, the product of the thyroid gland, to T_3 by removing one iodine atom at the 5'-position (see Fig. 4). T_3 is often referred to as the biologically active form of TH because the TH receptors (TRs) possess 10 times greater affinity for T_3 than for T_4 (see Leonard and Visser, 1986; Oppenheimer et al., 1995). Similarly, T_3 exhibits 3–10 times greater biological activity than T_4 in amphibia as it does in other vertebrates (Wahlborg et al., 1964; Lindsay et al., 1967; Rosenkilde, 1978; Frieden, 1981; White and Nicoll, 1981). Thus, data support the view that, although T_4 is the primary product of the thyroid gland, T_3 derived from conversion in the target tissues is the biologically active form of the hormone. T_4 can also be inactivated by conversion to reverse T_3 (3,3',5'-triiodothyronine; rT_3) and diiodothyronine (T_2); neither compound binds to the TRs. Similarly, T_3 can be inactivated by deiodination (Fig. 4).

The tissue deiodinases catalyze two basic reactions—a 5'-monodeiodination (outer ring) that results in bioactivation and a 5-monodeiodination (inner ring) that results in the bioinactivation of the substrate, T_4, or T_3 (Fig. 4). Three types of vertebrate deiodinases have been described that differ in their substrate specificity, kinetics, and sensitivity to inhibitors. Thus, the isozymes were originally identified by operational definitions based on their biochemical and pharmacological characteristics and not as specific polypeptides. However, cloning of cDNAs for subunits of each of these enzymes allows the assignment of biochemical attributes to specific proteins (see St. Germain, 1994).

Tadpoles possess both 5- and 5′-deiodinase activities; although, the enzymes exhibit primarily type II and type III activities, with no evidence for an enzyme with type I characteristics (Becker et al., 1997). Complementary DNAs for two enzymes, presumably corresponding to these two different activities, have been cloned in *R. catesbeiana*; an amphibian type III enzyme was first cloned in *X. laevis* (St. Germain et al., 1994). In *R. catesbeiana*, these two enzymes exhibit tissue-specific and developmental stage-specific expression patterns. For simplicity, in the following discussion we abbreviate the type II enzyme as D2 and the type III enzyme as D3.

During metamorphosis, coincident with rising plasma titers of T_3 and T_4, there is an increase in both D2 and D3 activities in target tissues (Buscaglia et al., 1985; Galton, 1991; Brown et al., 1996; Becker et al., 1997; Kawahara et al., 1999). In bullfrog tadpoles the D2 and D3 enzymes exhibit differential tissue expression. For example, D2 enzyme activity (and mRNA) is expressed in the tail, intestine, hind limb, forelimb, eye, and skin, but no D2 could be detected in the liver or kidney of bullfrog tadpoles at any stage (Galton, 1988; Galton and Hiebert, 1988; Becker et al., 1997). This finding contrasts sharply with many other vertebrates in which both the liver and kidney possess high 5′-deiodinase activities, and both organs are thought to be the primary sources of circulating T_3 (St. Germain and Galton, 1997). By contrast with D2, D3 enzyme activity (and mRNA) is expressed in liver and kidney as well as the tail, intestine, hind limb, forelimb, eye, skin (*R. catesbeiana*, Becker et al., 1997; *X. laevis*, Wang and Brown, 1993; Brown et al., 1996), and brain (*X. laevis* head, Brown et al., 1996; brain, Denver et al., 1997).

In tissues in which both enzymes are expressed, D2 and D3 exhibit comparable ontogenetic expression profiles (Becker et al., 1997). In the bullfrog tadpole, the expression patterns of each of these genes correlate well with the schedule of metamorphic changes in particular organs. For example, D2 activity is highest in hind limbs during prometamorphosis, at which time the limbs are differentiating, and declines at metamorphic climax. In the tail, which is the last organ to undergo metamorphic transformation (resorption), D2 activity is very low until metamorphic climax. The D3 activity exhibited similar ontogenetic profiles (Becker et al., 1997). These findings led Becker et al. (1997) to hypothesize that the coexpression of the two enzymes during metamorphosis generates a push–pull mechanism, thereby providing for tight control of intracellular T_3 concentrations in tissues at times of maximum metamorphic changes. However, although these findings in the bullfrog were partially corroborated in *X. laevis* for D3 mRNA expression, species differences were also evident (Kawahara et al., 1999). D3 mRNA in *X. laevis* showed similar ontogenetic profiles to *R. catesbeiana* in the tail, intestine, and liver, but the hind limb and kidney showed patterns of expression that were directly opposite. D2 mRNA expression in *X. laevis* has not been analyzed. The meaning of such species differences in expression patterns is unknown, but must be understood in order to derive general principles regarding the roles that the deiodinases play in regulating tissue responsiveness to TH during metamorphosis.

The regulation of deiodinase gene expression is poorly understood. Conflicting results for the regulation of D2 activity have been published. Buscaglia et al. (1985) reported that in *X. laevis* treated with the goitrogen perchlorate D2 activity remained at low premetamorphic levels. Replacement with T_3 or T_4 in these animals induced D2 activity, suggesting that TH positively regulates 5′-deiodination. By contrast, Becker et al. (1997) reported that in bullfrog tadpoles treated with the goitrogen methimazole D2 activity was elevated and replacement with T_4, but not T_3, down-regulated this activity. D3 enzyme activity and mRNA are clearly up-regulated by T_3. The cDNA for the *X. laevis* D3 gene was twice isolated as a T_3-regulated gene in differential screens of the tail and brain (Wang and Brown, 1993; Denver et al., 1997). Response kinetics and the resistance of up-regulation of the mRNA to protein synthesis inhibition suggest that it is a direct T_3 response gene. This gene is up-regulated in the tail, brain, intestine and hind limb, but is down-regulated in the liver (Wang and Brown, 1993; Denver et al., 1997; Kawahara et al., 1999). This pattern of T_3 responsiveness fits the ontogenetic expression profiles for the gene when it is up-regulated during late prometamorphosis to metamorphic climax in each of the tissues in which it responds positively to the hormone but down-regulated in the liver (Kawahara et al., 1999). Clearly, the roles of THs and other physiological and environmental factors in the regulation of deiodinase gene expression and enzyme activity require further study.

What is the evidence for a physiological role for tissue deiodinases in the control of metamorphosis? Several investigators have treated tadpoles with iopanoic acid (IOP), which blocks D2 and D3 activities in tadpoles (Buscaglia et al., 1985; Galton, 1989; Becker et al., 1997). The hypothesis tested was: If conversion of T_4 to T_3 is important for the metamorphic process, then IOP should block metamorphosis. As predicted, treatment with IOP inhibited metamorphosis, and this blockade could be overcome by replacement with T_3 but not T_4 (Galton, 1989; Becker et al., 1997). These findings support the view that T_3 is the biologically active hormone and its generation from T_4 is essential to metamorphosis. Similarly, the importance of the degradation of THs to the coordination of metamorphic transformations is supported by studies with transgenic frogs. The overexpression of a D3 green-fluorescent-protein (GFP) fusion protein in transgenic X. laevis resulted in metamorphic stasis and resistance to exogenous TH (Huang et al., 1999). At a finer level, D3 has been implicated in the modulation of T_3-dependent development of the visual system in tadpoles (Marsh-Armstrong et al., 1999). Taken together, the data point to a central role for tissue deiodinases in modulating tissue responsiveness to T_3 through their exertion of tight control over intracellular concentrations of the hormone.

c) Thyroid Hormone Transport in Blood Once synthesized, T_4 diffuses out of thyroid follicular cells and into the bloodstream, where it becomes reversibly bound to plasma proteins. The plasma proteins serve to transport the hormone from the site of production to its target tissues. Several vertebrate plasma-binding proteins that bind T_4 and T_3 with varying affinities have been identified. Thyroxine-binding globulin (TBG) is found only in large eutherian mammals, and it binds T_4 with high affinity and low capacity (Power et al., 2000). Transthyretin (TTR; also known as prealbumin) is found in all vertebrates and it binds T_4 with moderate affinity and intermediate capacity. Both TBG and TTRs can also bind T_3, although in most cases with 10 times lower affinity than T_4 (Power et al., 2000); however, the situation in amphibia is the reverse—see later). The two primary sites for TTR expression in vertebrates are the liver and the choroid plexus (although it is expressed at other sites; see Power et al., 2000). In most mammals TTR is expressed in both tissues, in reptiles it appears to be expressed only in the choroid plexus, and in teleosts and amphibians it is expressed primarily in the liver (see Power et al., 2000; although see Funkenstein et al., 1999, for TTR expression in the skin and other tissues of the teleost fish, *Sparus aurata*). An essential function of TTR is its interaction with retinol binding protein, which acts as a carrier for all-*trans*-retinol in the blood. The functional significance of this interaction is not known, but it is intriguing that T_3 and 9-*cis*-retinoic acid (which is a metabolite of all-*trans*-retinol) serve as ligands for the TR–retinoid-X receptor (TR-RXR) heterocomplex. Evidence supports the hypothesis that the TR-RXR heterodimer is the active complex that binds to promoters of TH target genes and activates transcription in the presence of TH (see later). Serum albumin also binds T_3 and T_4 in many species with low affinity and high capacity. Power et al. (2000) suggest that albumin might be the principal T_4-binding protein in amphibia.

By contrast with other tetrapods, but similar to teleost fishes, amphibian TTRs exhibit much greater affinity for T_3 than for T_4 (Yamauchi et al., 1993, 1998, 1999, 2000). The functional significance of the apparent evolutionary transformation of TTR from a T_3-binding to a T_4-binding protein is not known (see Power et al., 2000). In *R. catesbeiana*, the binding affinity of TTR for T_3 is 100–360 times greater than for T_4 (Yamauchi et al., 1993, 2000). Bullfrog TTR exhibits low nanomolar affinity for T_3—using TTR purified from plasma, 0.67 nM (Yamauchi et al., 1993); using whole plasma or recombinant TTR, 8–9 nM (Yamauchi et al., 2000). By contrast, the affinity of recombinant *X. laevis* TTR for T_3 is much lower than the bullfrog protein (550 nM; Yamauchi et al., 2000). However, a similar relationship between the affinities of TTR for T_3 and T_4 exists in *X. laevis* (affinity for T_4, 13 μM; Yamauchi et al., 2000). Circulating TTR protein is present in bullfrog and *X. laevis* tadpoles during premetamorphosis and prometamorphosis, but declines at metamorphic climax (Yamauchi et al., 1998, 2000).

What might be the functional significance of the developmental expression pattern of TTR in tadpoles? TTR expression is high during prometamorphosis when thyroid activity is increasing (see previous discussion) and plasma T_4 and T_3 concentrations are rising. Based on the free hormone hypothesis (Mendel, 1989; Ekins, 1990), we predict that TTR at this stage of development reduces the free fraction of hormone in the blood and thus limits the availability of the hormone to target tissues. On the other hand, TTR serves as a sink for the hormone in the blood, thus maintaining increasing plasma concentrations of THs before thyroid gland activity accelerates in response to rising titers of plasma TSH. At metamorphic climax, when plasma T_3 and T_4 concentrations are maximal, TTR concentration in the blood declines. The continued rise in plasma TH concentrations (without a high-affinity plasma protein binder to slow hormone clearance) probably results in an increased free hormone fraction (at least for T_3) in the blood. At the same time, the rate of clearance of T_3 from the circulation probably increases. However, because the thyroid synthetic rate is so high at metamorphic climax, total T_3 concentrations continue to rise. Thus, we predict that not only does the hormone production rate increase at metamorphic climax, but also the proportional availability of T_3 to the target tissues. To our knowledge T_3 or T_4 clearance rates have not been calculated in tadpoles at different stages of development. Based on TTR expression profiles we predict that clearance rates are lower during prometamorphosis than during premetamorphosis or metamorphic climax. Furthermore, given the lower affinity of TTR for T_4 compared with T_3, we predict that the clearance rate for T_4 is higher than T_3.

d) Cellular Uptake of Thyroid Hormone It was once thought that, because of their lipophilicity, THs entered cells by simple diffusion across plasma membranes. However, the highly polar nature of the alanine side chain precludes free membrane passage of the iodothyronines (Friesema et al., 1999). It is clear that THs can be actively taken up by cells via plasma membrane transporters (Hennemann et al., 1998). The saturable, carrier-mediated uptake of THs has been demonstrated in rat liver cells (Rao et al., 1976; Krenning et al., 1981), cultured fibroblasts (Cheng et al., 1980), human and rat red blood cells (RBCs; Docter et al., 1982; Zhou et al., 1992), rat thymus cells, and tadpole RBCs (Galton et al., 1986; Yamauchi et al., 1989).

Findings point to an important role for amino acid permeases in the uptake of THs by cells (see Ritchie et al., 1999). The T_3-inducible gene IU12 from *X. laevis* intestine (Shi and Brown, 1993; Liang et al., 1997) encodes a subunit of a heterodimeric amino acid permease complex (Torrents et al., 1998). Findings by Ritchie and colleagues (1999) show that this permease complex efficiently transports T_3 and T_4 when expressed in the *Xenopus* oocyte expression system, but is inhibited by reverse T_3. The fact that the IU12 is a T_3-inducible gene suggests that it might play a role in mediating T_3 uptake by cells during tadpole metamorphosis (see Liang et al., 1997). Other TH transporters that have been identified include organic anion transporters such as Ntcp and oatp1-3 (Abe et al., 1998; Friesema et al., 1999). The possibility for specific receptors for TTR also has been demonstrated, although this means of hormone uptake requires further investigation (see Divino and Schussler, 1990; Schussler, 2000).

e) Cytosolic Thyroid Hormone Binding Proteins Upon entering cells, and before binding to nuclear receptors (see later), THs encounter a series of intracellular binding proteins. These cytoplasmic TH binding proteins (CTHBPs) are represented by several classes of multifunctional proteins. These proteins represent a variety of enzymatic activities in the cell. For example, two genes were cloned in *X. laevis* that are CTHBPs. One is a cytosolic aldehyde dehydrogenase that catalyzes the formation of retinoic acid (an important developmental signaling molecule that signals via nuclear receptors; see later; Yamauchi and Tata, 1994), and the other is homologous to mammalian M2 pyruvate kinase (Shi et al., 1994). Protein disulfide isomerase (PDI) and related proteins catalyze the formation of disulfide bonds in and between proteins, and human PDI possesses a high-affinity binding site for TH (Cheng et al., 1987; Yamauchi et al., 1987). We cloned a cDNA encoding a PDI-like protein as a T_3-responsive gene in the *X. laevis* brain (Denver et al., 1997).

It has been suggested that the functional significance of hormone binding to these CTHBPs is to serve to transport THs in the cytoplasm to the nucleus where the TRs are located. Alternatively, they could serve as chelators to limit the cellular free-TH concentration or act as buffer proteins in the maintenance of intracellular levels of TH (see Shi, 2000). However, in considering a role for these proteins in TH transport, the possibility that TH might serve a regulatory role for the enzymatic activities of these proteins should not be overlooked. As an example, the human M2 pyruvate kinase functions as a kinase in its tetrameric form, but only binds TH in its monomeric form. The binding of TH results in a shift toward the monomeric form and thus the inhibition of the kinase activity (Ashizawa and Cheng, 1992). Thus we predict that TH serves to inhibit this enzymatic pathway.

4. Mechanisms of Thyroid Hormone Action: Thyroid Hormone Receptors

Tadpoles become competent to respond to exogenous TH at the time of hatching (Tata, 1968). This establishment of competence to respond to the hormone probably depends on the expression of TRs (see Shi et al., 1996). TRs are ligand-activated transcription factors that belong to the steroid hormone receptor superfamily (Mangelsdorf and Evans, 1995). There are two TR genes, termed α and β, in all vertebrates (Lazar, 1993). Owing to its pseudotetraploidy, X. laevis possesses four TR genes, two α and two β (Brooks et al., 1989; Yaoita et al., 1990). The two X. laevis TRα genes each appears to give rise to a single unique protein, whereas alternative mRNA splicing of TRβ transcripts can give rise to two different receptor isoforms for each TRβ gene (Yaoita et al., 1990; Shi, 2000).

The TRα genes are first expressed shortly after hatching in X. laevis, and their expression rises during premetamorphosis and remains high throughout metamorphosis (Baker and Tata, 1990; Yaoita and Brown, 1990; Banker et al., 1991; Kawahara et al., 1991). It has been hypothesized that the early expression of TRα establishes the hormone responsiveness of tadpole tissues (see Baker and Tata, 1990; Shi et al., 1996). TRβ mRNA is not detected until early prometamorphosis, but its expression increases during prometamorphosis in parallel with TH synthesis (Yaoita and Brown, 1990; Kawahara et al., 1991; Baker and Tata, 1992; Kanamori and Brown, 1992). Several studies have shown that the TR genes are up-regulated by T_3 in X. laevis and R. catesbeiana (Yaoita et al., 1990; Kawahara et al., 1991; Schneider and Galton, 1991; Helbing et al., 1992), a phenomenon termed autoinduction (see Tata et al., 1993; Davey et al., 1994; Rabelo and Tata, 1997). A thyroid response element (TRE), to which TRs can bind and regulate transcription, has been identified in the X. laevis TRβA gene (Ranjan et al., 1994; Machuca et al., 1995).

The specific functions for the different receptors in amphibia are unknown. The results of gene-targeting experiments in mice point to a network of specific and common TR pathways, but have failed to provide a clear picture of the roles for these different receptors (Forrest and Vennstrom, 2000). There is evidence in mammals that the TRs possess different functional characteristics (Zhu et al., 1999) and can mediate different cellular responses to T_3 (Lebel et al., 1993), presumably by regulating different sets of genes (Guissouma et al., 1998; Sandhofer et al., 1998; Denver et al., 1999). Studies addressing specific functions for the different TRs have not been done in amphibians.

TRs function as dimers; that is, the DNA consensus sequences that TRs bind to are six nucleotides in length and are referred to as half-sites. Two of these half-sites make up a TRE (Williams and Brent, 1995). These TREs can be located in the promoter, in the structural part of the gene, or upstream of the transcription start site. Homodimers of TRα or TRβ can form on most TREs, but the preferred configuration appears to be as a heterodimer with retinoid-X receptor (RXR) (see Wong and Shi, 1995; Puzianowska-Kuznicka et al., 1997). TR-RXR heterodimers bind DNA and transactivate TRE-containing genes much more effectively than TR homodimers. In the unliganded form, the TR-RXR complex functions as a transcriptional repressor (Wong and Shi, 1995). The TR-RXR heterocomplex recruits cofactor proteins that mediate the repressive or activational actions of the complex (Shi, 2000; Wu and Koenig, 2000). The TR and RXR genes exhibit more or less coordinated regulation during metamorphosis, and this coordination may be essential to the timing of tissue-specific changes (Wong and Shi, 1995).

Hormone binding to the TR-RXR complex induces gene expression in target tissues. A detailed discussion of the characteristics of the gene-regulation cascades and the functions of the gene products induced in different tissues during metamorphosis is beyond the scope of this chapter. The reader is referred to Shi (2000) for a thorough treatment of this topic.

C. Corticoids

Although TH is the primary morphogen controlling metamorphosis, corticoids may synergize with TH to accelerate metamorphosis (Kikuyama et al., 1993). Corticoids are the primary vertebrate stress hormones and are produced in response to a variety of environmental signals (Selye, 1976). The production of corticoids changes with development and probably reflects the functional maturation of the hypothalamic-hypophyseal-interrenal axis.

1. Roles of Corticoids in Amphibian Growth and Development

Corticoids (also referred to as corticosteroids) may influence growth and development in larval anurans, but their influence may be more complex than that of TH. Exogenous corticoids can either accelerate or decelerate metamorphosis, depending on the animal's developmental stage and TH status. Studies using relatively large doses of exogenous corticoids have shown that these hormones inhibit forelimb emergence when administered during premetamorphosis (Frieden and Naile, 1955; Kobayashi, 1958; Gray and Janssens, 1990; Hayes et al., 1993; Wright et al., 1994; Hayes, 1995). The effects of exogenous corticoids on tadpole growth are more straightforward than their developmental effects. The administration of various corticoid doses to both pre- and prometamorphic tadpoles inhibits growth (Hayes and Licht, 1993; Wright et al., 1994; Hayes, 1995; Glennemeier and Denver, 2002a).

Although exogenous corticoids when administered alone during premetamorphosis can inhibit growth and development, the hormones accelerate TH-induced metamorphosis in most species (Frieden and Naile, 1955; Kikuyama et al., 1983, 1993; Gray and Janssens, 1990; Hayes, 1995). In one study, prometamorphic *Bufo boreas* tadpoles exposed to exogenous corticosterone alone also showed accelerated metamorphosis, probably due to synergy of the corticosterone with rising endogenous TH levels (Hayes et al., 1993).

The studies in which tadpoles were treated with exogenous corticoids with or without TH suggest, but do not prove, a physiological role for endogenous corticoids in the regulation of tadpole development. Inhibitors of corticoid synthesis have been used to address the role of endogenous corticoids. Hayes and Wu (1995) found that a 33% reduction in corticosterone by treatment with metyrapone (an inhibitor of corticoid biosynthesis) slowed TH-induced acceleration of hind-limb development, but did not affect the rate of tail resorption (Hayes, 1995; Hayes and Wu, 1995). Glennemeier and Denver (2002a) found that a 50% reduction in whole-body corticosterone by treatment with metyrapone throughout prometamorphosis increased size at metamorphosis by more than 10%, but did not affect the rate of metamorphosis in *R. pipiens* tadpoles. More work is required to determine a potential role for endogenous corticoids in tadpole growth and development.

In summary, the dose of corticoid administered, the stage at which the hormone is given, and whether it is administered with TH determines the developmental effects of the steroid (Glennemeier and Denver, 2002a). Whether these effects represent physiological actions remains to be determined. If these actions turn out to be physiologically relevant, then we predict that increased corticoid biosynthesis (perhaps in response to a stressor) in premetamorphic tadpoles might retard growth and delay metamorphosis. Conversely, increased corticoids in prometamorphic tadpoles might retard growth but accelerate metamorphosis.

2. Hormones Produced by Amphibian Interrenal Glands

Corticosterone and aldosterone appear to be the major corticoids produced by the amphibian interrenal glands (Carstensen et al., 1961; Macchi and Phillips, 1966). In many species there is an elevation in plasma concentrations of these hormones during metamorphic climax that is more or less synchronous with plasma TH increases (see later).

The interrenal gland is generally less active in early premetamorphic developmental stages and more active during prometamorphosis and metamorphic climax (see Dodd and Dodd, 1976). The ultrastructural appearance of *X. laevis* interrenal cells indicates relative inactivity in mid-prometamorphs, increasing to peak activity at metamorphic climax (reviewed in Dodd and Dodd, 1976; however, see later for contradictory evidence). Activity of the interrenal enzyme Δ^5-3β-hydroxysteroid dehydrogenase (HSD) is present throughout development in *R. catesbeiana* and *X. laevis*, but increases at metamorphic climax in *R. catesbeiana* (Hsu et al., 1980; Kang et al., 1995). Carr and Norris (1988) found a similar pattern for plasma corticosterone and interrenal HSD activity in the tiger salamander, *Ambystoma tigrinum*.

Radioimmunoassays for corticoids have been done on plasma samples collected throughout the metamorphic period for a number of amphibian species—*R. catesbeiana* (Jaffe, 1981; Krug et al., 1983; Kikuyama et al., 1986), *B. japonicus* (Niinuma et al., 1989), *X. laevis* (Jolivet-Jaudet and Leloup-Hatey, 1984), and *A. tigrinum* (Carr and Norris, 1988). Whole-body measures of corticoid content have also been determined throughout development (*S. hammondii*: Denver, 1998)—*X. laevis* (Kloas et al., 1997; Glennemeier and Denver, 2002b), and *R. pipiens* (Glennemeier and Denver, 2002b). The majority of these studies show a marked increase in corticoid production at metamorphic climax, more or less in parallel with the rise in THs. The only exception to this rule is whole-body corticoid content in *X. laevis*. Kloas and colleagues (1997) reported that whole-body corticosterone content in *X. laevis* increases during premetamorphosis to reach a peak at NF stage 48, then declines during prometamorphosis, and is low at metamorphic climax; we have obtained similar results although we did observe a small but significant increase at metamorphic climax (Glennemeier and Denver, 2002b). Kloas and colleagues (1997) also measured whole-body aldosterone and found a similar increase during premetamorphosis, but the peak production was during early prometamorphosis (NF stage 54) and it declined thereafter. Whether these findings in *X. laevis* represent species differences or whether changes in whole-body corticoid content are not representative of changes in plasma concentrations is unknown.

Few have analyzed the activity of the hypothalamic-pituitary-interrenal axis throughout metamorphosis at levels other than the interrenal gland. Carr and Norris (1990) reported low immunoreactive corticotropin-releasing hormone (CRH) in the median eminence and arginine vasotocin (AVT) in the preoptic nucleus of premetamorphic *R. catesbeiana* tadpoles, which increased dramatically by late prometamorphosis. Both CRH and arginine vasopressin (AVP)—AVT is the amphibian hormone—are potent stimulators of adrenocorticotropic hormone (ACTH) secretion by cultured adult frog pituitaries (Tonon et al., 1986). Note also that CRH is a potent and potentially important regulator of TSH secretion in tadpoles (discussed later). To our knowledge, no direct measures of ACTH production over development have been reported in amphibia. However, the expression of the messenger RNA for the precursor of ACTH, proopiomelanocortin (POMC) in the anterior pituitary of bullfrog tadpoles is low during premetamorphosis, increases during prometamorphosis, and remains high during metamorphic climax (Aida et al., 1999). Whether this mRNA expression pattern reflects the production and secretion of ACTH peptide is unknown.

The tadpole hypothalamic-hypophyseal-interrenal axis becomes functional during premetamorphosis. For example, the interrenal glands of premetamorphic tadpoles of *R. pipiens* and *X. laevis* respond to ACTH injections *in vivo* by increasing whole-body corticosterone content (Glennemeier and Denver, 2002b). These experiments show that functional ACTH receptors are expressed before metamorphosis. The functionality of higher levels of the hypothalamic-hypophyseal-interrenal axis in premetamorphic animals is shown by their ability to mount a corticosterone response (increased whole-body corticosterone content) following exposure to an artificial stressor (handling and shaking stress in the laboratory; Glennemeier and Denver, 2002b). Thus, there is the potential for environmental stressors to cause elevations in endogenous corticoid biosynthesis during premetamorphosis. Such early activation of the hypothalamic-hypophyseal-interrenal axis could result in growth retardation and metamorphic inhibition (see previous discussion).

3. Control of Corticoid Production and Transport

The major regulator of interrenal corticoid production is the pituitary hormone ACTH (Kikuyama et al., 1993). Injections of ACTH increased serum corticoids and accelerated T_4-induced metamorphosis in several amphibian species (see White and Nicoll, 1981; Kikuyama et al., 1993). The secretion of ACTH may be controlled by the neurohormones CRH and AVT (see previous discussion).

Corticoids, being lipophilic, are transported in blood bound to plasma proteins. Corticoid-binding globulin (CBG) is the primary plasma protein to which corticoids bind in mammals, although albumin also plays a transport role (Hammond, 1990; Rosner, 1990). The binding properties of a putative CBG present in amphibian serum (*A. tigrinum*) were reported by Orchinik *et al.* (2000). However, the expression of CBG has not been studied in amphibians nor is there anything known of the role that this protein might play in maintaining corticoid balance in frogs or tadpoles.

4. Mechanisms of Corticoid Action

Corticoids, like all steroid hormones, act primarily through binding to receptors that function as ligand-dependent transcription factors. These receptors are members of the same superfamily of receptor proteins that include the TRs (see previous discussion). Corticoid receptors are found primarily in the cytosol in the absence of ligand, where they are complexed with a series of heat-shock proteins and immunophilins (a foldosome) that serve to maintain the receptors in a conformation that favors ligand binding (Pratt and Toft, 1997). The binding of the hormone results in the dissociation of the foldosome complex and translocation of the receptor to the nucleus (Pratt and Toft, 1997). Vertebrates possess two distinct corticoid receptors (designated glucocorticoid and mineralocorticoid) and both types have been isolated in *X. laevis* (Gao *et al.*, 1994a,b; Csikos *et al.*, 1995).

How might corticoids act to inhibit growth and development? In mammals, corticoids are known to produce growth inhibition through actions at multiple levels. At the organismal physiological level, corticoids mobilize stored fuels during increased metabolic demand—for example, fight-or-flight response, exercise, or fasting (see Sapolsky *et al.*, 2000). The chronic elevation of plasma corticoid concentrations promotes protein catabolism and muscle wasting. Corticoids are known to down-regulate growth hormone (GH) biosynthesis in the anterior pituitary gland of mammals (see Harvey *et al.*, 1995).

Corticoids may enhance the developmental actions of TH by several mechanisms. Corticoids have been shown to increase maximal nuclear binding capacity for T_3 in a dose-dependent manner and thus alter tissue responsiveness (Niki *et al.*, 1981; Suzuki and Kikuyama, 1983; Kikuyama *et al.*, 1993). Our studies (R. J. Denver and E. D. Hoopfer, unpublished results) have found that corticosterone up-regulates TRα and TRβ mRNAs in *X. laevis* tail cultures. Corticosterone may also increase 5'-deiodinase activity, thereby increasing the availability of T_3 at peripheral tissues (Galton, 1990).

D. Prolactin and Growth Hormone

The pituitary hormones GH (also called somatotropin) and prolactin (PRL; also called lactotropin) are simple polypeptides approximately 200 amino acids in length and are paralogous members of a multigene family. A key component of Etkin's (1968) model was that the stimulatory actions of TH on metamorphosis were counterbalanced by the inhibitory effects of the pituitary hormone PRL. Etkin proposed that PRL production would be high during larval life and then decline at metamorphic climax. This prediction was based largely on the inhibitory effects that preparations of mammalian PRLs had on metamorphosis when injected into tadpoles (see White and Nicoll, 1981). Based on the antimetamorphic actions of these mammalian PRL preparations, several investigators suggested that PRL exerted a juvenilizing action in amphibian larvae akin to that of juvenile hormone in insects (Bern *et al.*, 1967; Etkin and Gona, 1967).

The early studies that led to the development of the Etkin model have been extensively reviewed (see Dodd and Dodd, 1976; White and Nicoll, 1981; Kikuyama *et al.*, 1993; Denver, 1996; Kaltenbach, 1996). Studies using primarily mammalian preparations of GH or PRL suggested different roles for these hormones, with PRL enhancing larval growth and blocking the actions of TH on metamorphosis, and GH primarily stimulating postmetamorphic growth as it does in other vertebrates (see Denver, 1996). A role for GH in regulating body growth in amphibia as it does in other vertebrates (see Harvey *et al.*, 1995) has been borne out by numerous studies in which GH was injected into tadpoles or frogs (see White and Nicoll, 1981; Kikuyama *et al.*, 1993; Denver, 1996) and through the use of transgenic techniques in *X. laevis* (Huang and Brown, 2000a). A role for PRL in the stimulation of tadpole growth and the inhibition of metamorphosis has been questioned (see Huang and Brown, 2000b).

The early studies supported the view that treatment of tadpoles with PRL inhibits metamorphosis and stimulates larval growth. Most of these studies, done with mammalian PRL (and GH) preparations, showed that tadpole tissues have the capacity to respond to PRL-like or GH-like molecules; functional receptors are expressed in amphibian tissues that can transmit a signal that can both promote tadpole growth and block T_3-induced metamorphosis, probably by preventing the autoinduction of the TRs (see Tata et al., 1993). Furthermore, studies with amphibian PRL preparations show that the homologous PRL has effects similar to the mammalian hormones (see Kikuyama et al., 1993). Passive immunization studies with PRL antisera suggested a physiological role for endogenous PRL (see Kikuyama et al., 1993; Denver, 1996).

But do these effects represent pharmacological actions of the exogenous hormones? The strongest argument against a role for PRL as a juvenilizing hormone in amphibians comes from expression analyses. Recall that Etkin (1968) proposed that larval growth and metamorphosis are controlled by a balance between TH and PRL and that the two should show an inverse relationship in their blood concentrations at metamorphic climax. The rise in circulating concentrations of TH during prometamorphosis and climax have been confirmed (see previous discussion). However, circulating concentrations of PRL and levels of pituitary PRL mRNA are low during premetamorphosis and also rise, more or less in parallel with TH, during late prometamorphosis and climax (Clemons and Nicoll, 1977; Yamamoto and Kikuyama, 1982; Takahashi et al., 1990; Niinuma et al., 1991a; Buckbinder and Brown, 1993), thus contradicting the earlier hypothesis of an inverse relationship of the two hormones (Etkin, 1968). The rise in PRL production tends to occur slightly later than the rise in TSH expression and circulating TH (see Buckbinder and Brown, 1993). Similarly, [^{125}I]-PRL binding to kidney membrane fractions was low in premetamorphic bullfrog tadpoles and increased during metamorphic climax (White and Nicoll, 1979). Huang and Brown (2000b) measured PRL receptor (PRL-R) mRNA by northern blotting in whole X. laevis tadpole and tail tissue and found increased expression at metamorphic climax. Taken together, these PRL and PRL-R expression analyses argue against the hypothesis that PRL plays a juvenilizing role in amphibian metamorphosis (see Buckbinder and Brown, 1993; Huang and Brown, 2000b). However, Kikuyama and colleagues (1993) have argued, based on their experiments with passive immunization with antiserum to bullfrog PRL, that low levels of PRL during the premetamorphic to early prometamorphic period might be sufficient to support larval growth and inhibit TH action.

Huang and Brown (2000a,b) used a transgenesis approach to address the question of the roles of GH and PRL in amphibian development. They created transgenic tadpoles of X. laevis that overexpressed X. laevis GH, X. laevis PRL, or ovine PRL. The expression of the transgenes was driven by the simian cytomegalovirus (sCMV) promoter; thus, all tissues expressed the transgenes (i.e., expression was not restricted to the pituitary gland where the hormones are normally expressed). They found that overexpression of GH had no effect on the timing of metamorphosis, but resulted in larger tadpoles and larger juvenile frogs, a finding that confirms earlier studies in frogs and other vertebrates that GH promotes growth (see Harvey et al., 1995). The overexpression of X. laevis PRL (xPRL) or ovine PRL (oPRL) did not alter the timing of metamorphosis, but blocked tail resorption in some tadpoles. The overexpression of the mRNAs was confirmed by northern blotting; however, they were unable to detect the xPRL in serum of transgenic frogs by western blotting, but apparently were able to detect the oPRL. The authors concluded that their results disprove the hypothesis that PRL is a juvenile hormone in X. laevis. One caution in this interpretation is that the PRL was overexpressed in all tissues throughout the entire developmental period. Such stage-inappropriate overexpression of a hormone might result in compensatory changes in physiological systems; alternatively, the PRL-responsive cells could become desensitized by receptor internalization following chronic exposure to very high concentrations of the hormone, which is a common phenomenon in endocrine systems.

Whether or not PRL plays any role in larval growth or development, the rise in PRL biosynthesis at metamorphic climax suggests that the hormone might either modulate the rapid tissue transformations that occur at climax (e.g., provide a brake on TH action in concert with the up-regulation of the 5-monodeiodinase; see Denver, 1996) or perhaps play an important physiological role in the postmetamorphic frog (see Huang and Brown, 2000b).

E. Neuroendocrine Control of Amphibian Development

The vertebrate neuroendocrine system comprises the hypothalamus and the pituitary gland. The major pituitary hormones and their roles in amphibian development have already been described. The secretion of these pituitary hormones and thus the production of hormones by peripheral endocrine glands (e.g., the thyroid and interrenals) are controlled by hypothalamic neurohormones. These neurohormones (termed releasing and release-inhibiting factors) are released from modified nerve terminals in the median eminence into capillaries that drain into the hypophyseal portal vessels that deliver blood to the anterior pituitary gland (Fig. 3). The importance of hypothalamic control of metamorphosis has long been recognized (reviewed by Kikuyama et al., 1993; Denver, 1996). The anterior pituitary gland controls both the thyroid gland and the interrenals by the production of TSH and ACTH, respectively.

Although environmental influences on the timing of metamorphosis can occur at the level of peripheral tissues (e.g., direct thermal effects and osmotic effects), much environmental information is gathered by neural sensory systems and integrated in the hypothalamus to alter the secretion of pituitary hormones and, consequently, the activity of peripheral endocrine glands. The neuroendocrine system serves as an interface between the central nervous system and the endocrine system, and transduces signals obtained through a variety of sensory inputs into appropriate physiological responses.

1. Neurohormones and the Control of Pituitary Secretion

Early studies suggested that the pituitary hormones TSH and ACTH are primarily under stimulatory hypothalamic control in amphibians (reviewed by Denver, 1996). There have been far fewer studies done on the hypothalamic control of ACTH in amphibia than on TSH. The available data show that ACTH can be stimulated by CRH and AVT *in vitro* (Tonon *et al.*, 1986). However, whether CRH or AVT play important roles in controlling ACTH secretion *in vivo* in amphibia, as they do in mammals, has not been established.

2. Thyrotropin-Releasing Hormone (Pyro-glutamyl-histidyl-proline-amide)

The tripeptide pyro-glutamyl-histidyl-proline-amide was the first hypophysiotropic peptide to be isolated and have its structure determined (Reichlin, 1989). It was named thyrotropin-releasing hormone (TRH) for its ability to stimulate the release of TSH in mammals, where it appears to be the principal stimulator of TSH secretion (see Morley, 1981). However, its role as a TSH-releasing factor (TRF) in nonmammalian vertebrates is less certain. Although TRH is expressed in the brain of larval and adult amphibia, injections of TRH are without effect on the thyroid axis or in altering the timing of tadpole metamorphosis (see Norris and Dent, 1989; Kikuyama *et al.*, 1993; Denver, 1996). However, TRH can elevate plasma TH concentrations when injected into adult frogs (Darras and Kuhn, 1982) and can stimulate the release of thyrotropic bioactivity in cultured pituitaries from adults of several frog species (Denver, 1988; Jacobs and Kuhn, 1992). The possibility that TRH plays a hypophysiotropic role in larval amphibians is uncertain. It appears that pituitary TSH cell responsiveness to TRH is regulated in a developmental-stage-specific manner (see Denver, 1988; Denver and Licht, 1989a). Future studies should address the regulation of TRH receptor expression in the amphibian pituitary to explain changes in the responsiveness of the gland to the tripeptide.

3. Corticotropin-Releasing Hormone Is a Thyrotropin-Releasing Factor

Studies have shown that the stress neurohormone CRH is a potent stimulator of the thyroid axis in larval amphibians and other nonmammalian vertebrates (reviewed by Denver, 1999). CRH is a 41-amino-acid polypeptide that was first isolated based on its ability to stimulate ACTH secretion in mammals (Vale *et al.*, 1981; Turnbull and Rivier, 1997). The regulation of ACTH secretion by CRH in mammals is considered to be its primary hypophysiotropic role (Vale *et al.*, 1997). In mammals, the actions of CRH peptides, in addition to their hypophysiotropic role, include control of appetite, behavioral responses to stress (arousal and escape), and modulation of immune responses, among others (Vale *et al.*, 1997).

In nonmammalian species, CRH (and related peptides, sauvagine and urotensin I) have been found to be potent releasers of TSH. CRH stimulates the thyroid axis in a fish (salmon; Larsen *et al.*, 1998), several amphibians, reptiles, and a bird (reviewed by Denver, 1999). For example, CRH injections result in elevations in circulating TH concentrations in the frog (*Rana ridibunda*), the chick embryo Meeuwis *et al.*, 1989), and adult turtle (*Trachemys scripta*; R. J. Denver and P. Licht, unpublished data; see Kuhn *et al.*, 1998). Injections of CRH peptides also elevate whole-body TH content in tadpoles of several species (Gancedo *et al.*, 1992; Denver, 1993, 1997a). A direct action of CRH on TSH secretion by the pituitary gland is supported by tissue culture studies using pituitaries from representatives of each nonmammalian vertebrate class. Specific radioimmunoassays for TSH in the salmon (Larsen *et al.*, 1998) and turtle (Denver and Licht, 1989b, 1991) have verified that secretion of TSH protein is stimulated by CRH. In species in which a specific TSH radioimmunoassay is not yet available, the release of TSH was demonstrated by bioassay—for example, amphibians (Denver, 1988; Denver and Licht, 1989a; Jacobs and Kuhn, 1992)—or by a subtractive method using specific RIAs for the gonadotropin β subunits and the α subunit (chicken: Geris *et al.*, 1996; Kuhn *et al.*, 1998). Interestingly, although CRH is stimulatory to TSH secretion by cultured salmon pituitaries, TRH lacks activity in this regard (Larsen *et al.*, 1998). Matz and Hofeldt (1999) demonstrated that CRH-immunoreactive fibers terminate in regions that contain TSH-positive pituitary cells in Chinook salmon. They proposed that the contiguous localization of CRH-positive fibers and TSH cells supports a physiological role for CRH in mediating TSH release, which supports the findings of Larsen and colleagues (1998), who showed that CRH is a potent TSH-releasing factor in salmon.

Taken together, the data point to an important and perhaps primitive role for CRH in the regulation of both the thyroid and the interrenal (adrenal) axes. A role for CRH in influencing thyroid activity in tadpoles and thus regulating metamorphosis comes from studies from several labs in different species, which showed that injections of CRH-like peptides can accelerate metamorphosis. Injections of CRH and related peptides accelerated metamorphosis in the anurans *Rana perezi* (Gancedo *et al.*, 1992), *R. catesbeiana*, *Spea* (*Scaphiopus*) *hammondii* (Denver, 1993, 1997a), and *Bufo arenarum* (Miranda *et al.*, 2000) and in the salamander *Ambystoma tigrinum* (Boorse and Denver, 2002). CRH injections elevated whole-body TH content of *R. perezi* and *S. hammondii* tadpoles (Gancedo *et al.*, 1992; Denver, 1993). In *S. hammondii*, injections of synthetic *X. laevis* CRH (which is identical in primary structure to *S. hammondii* CRH; G. C. Boorse and R. J. Denver, unpublished) produced a dose-dependent increase in whole-body T_3, T_4, and corticosterone when measured 4 hours after injection (Denver, 1997a).

Passive immunization with CRH antiserum slowed spontaneous metamorphosis in *R. catesbeiana* tadpoles (Denver, 1993). Also, injections of the CRH receptor antagonist α-helical CRH$_{(9-41)}$ blocked simulated pond drying-induced metamorphosis in *S. hammondii* (Denver, 1997a). Furthermore, hypothalamic CRH peptide content was increased in spadefoot toad tadpoles that accelerated metamorphosis in response to simulated pond drying (Denver, 1997a). Taken together, these findings support a physiological role for CRH in controlling metamorphosis. Because CRH is a stress neurohormone we hypothesized that endogenous CRH participates in environmentally induced (stress-induced) metamorphosis (Denver, 1997b; see Section V).

All vertebrates studied possess at least two CRH receptor (CRHR) subtypes and a secreted CRH binding protein (CRH-BP) (Fig. 5). There is nothing known of the tissue distribution, developmental expression, or hormonal regulation of the CRHRs in amphibians. The CRH-BP has a high-affinity binding for CRH peptides (in the range of the receptors) and may play an important role in the modulation of CRH bioavailability (see Behan *et al.*, 1996). Analyses of the primary structures of the vertebrate CRH-BPs reveal a protein with high evolutionary conservation, which suggests strong selective pressure to maintain its structure and function (see Valverde *et al.*, 2001, also unpublished data). In mammals, CRH-BP is expressed in multiple tissues, including the liver, brain, and pituitary gland. CRHBP circulates in the blood in humans but not in rats, which may be explained by the lack of expression in rat liver. The *X. laevis* CRH-BP was originally isolated from a subtractive-tadpole-tail cDNA library as a T_3-regulated gene (Brown *et al.*, 1996). We found that this gene is expressed in the frog brain, intestine, liver, and pituitary (Valverde *et al.*, 2001) and preliminary data suggest that it is expressed in several other tissues (e.g.,

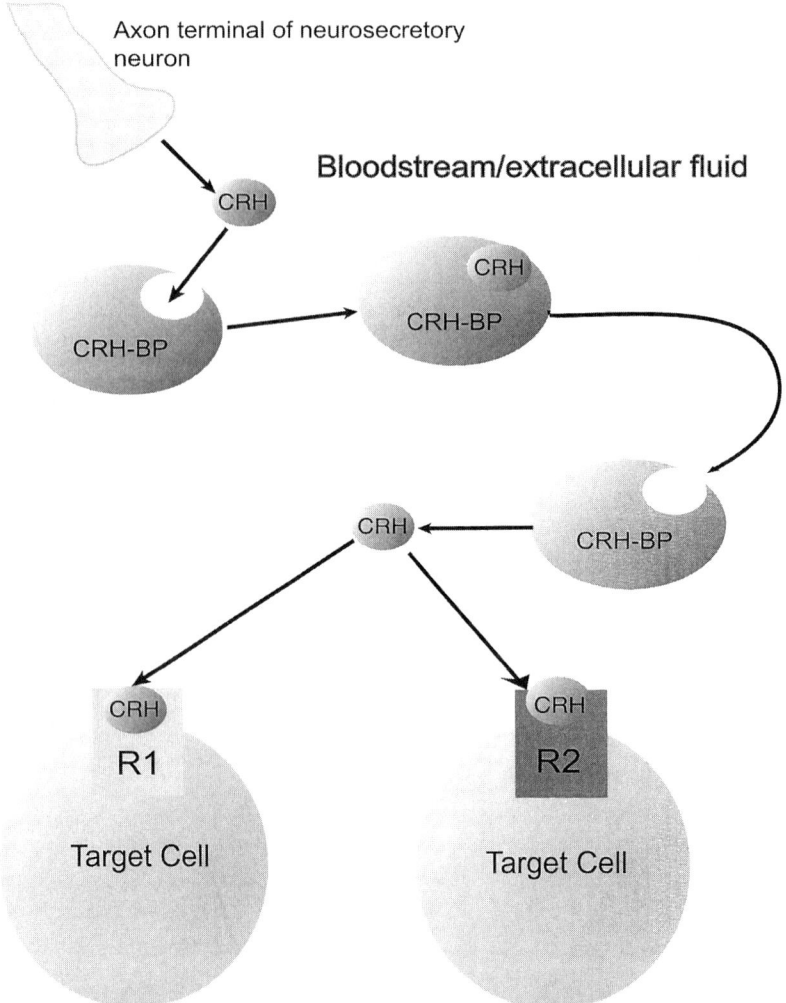

FIGURE 5 Regulation of CRH bioavailability by CRH binding protein (CRH-BP). Schematic representation of CRH interactions with its binding protein and two receptor subtypes.

the gonads and skin; R. A. Valverde and R. J. Denver, unpublished). The role that this protein plays in modulating CRH action in any species is poorly understood, and few comparative studies in nonmammalian species have been done (see Valverde et al., 2001). The protein could modulate CRH action by binding it, and thus blocking its availability to receptors, or by targeting the peptide for clearance, as has been proposed in humans (Behan et al., 1996). Alternatively, the CRH-BP might serve to maintain high concentrations of CRH in tissues or in tissue fluids, perhaps facilitating CRH action. Brown and colleagues (1996) suggested that the upregulation of this protein during metamorphic climax might serve a negative feedback function by sequestering CRH and thus modulating its bioavailability; this hypothesis has not been tested.

4. Other Neurohormones Regulating Thyroid-Stimulating Hormone

Although CRH is the only hypophysiotropic peptide known to stimulate TSH release in tadpoles, the possibility that other hypothalamic hormones regulate TSH must be considered. Gonadotropin-releasing hormone (GnRH) was found to stimulate the thyroid axis in axolotls and adult frogs (Jacobs et al., 1988b; Jacobs and Kuhn, 1988), acting directly on the pituitary gland

(Denver, 1988). The physiological significance of this finding is unknown, and it is also unknown whether GnRH is stimulatory to TSH during the larval stage.

IV. ENDOCRINOLOGY OF PAEDOMORPHOSIS

A. Overview

Paedomorphosis is common among salamanders. Four out of nine families of salamanders are entirely paedomorphic, and the five other urodele families contain at least one paedomorphic species (Duellman and Trueb, 1994). Although there is a high frequency of paedomorphosis among salamanders, its physiological basis remains poorly understood (but see Rosenkilde and Ussing, 1996). To understand the underlying physiological mechanisms controlling paedomorphosis, two separate endocrine pathways must be considered. As described in Section III, metamorphosis in anurans is driven by the activation of the thyroid axis. This also appears to be the case in facultative paedomorphic salamanders. Because paedomorphs become sexually mature while remaining in the larval habitat, we discuss here the endocrine pathways controlling gonadal development and maturation and their possible interaction with hormones controlling metamorphosis.

B. Thyroid Axis

1. Facultative Paedomorphs

In facultative paedomorphic salamanders, metamorphosis can be induced by exposure to exogenous T_3 or T_4 (Norris and Platt, 1974). The injection of mammalian TSH can also induce metamorphosis in paedomorphs (Norris *et al.*, 1973). Because both the peripheral tissues and the thyroid gland are competent to respond to hormonal stimulation, it has been suggested that the failure to metamorphose results from the lack of stimulation of the secretion of pituitary hormones by hypothalamic neurohormones. Norris and Gern (1976) provided evidence that the lack of metamorphosis in facultative paedomorphs results from insufficient hypothalamic development. They induced metamorphosis in paedomorphic *A. tigrinum* salamanders by intrahypothalamic administration of T_4; intraperitoneal injection of the same dose did not induce metamorphosis. Intrahypothalamic administration led to an activation of the thyroid axis not seen after systemic administration, apparently as a result of the differentiation of the hypothalamic neurosecretory system (Norris and Gern, 1976).

TRH injections did not accelerate metamorphosis when administered intrahypothalamically (Norris, 1978). However, similar to anurans (discussed in Section III), later studies suggested that TRH is not active in TSH secretion in larval salamanders (see Darras and Kuhn, 1983; Jacobs and Kuhn, 1987). We found that CRH injections in larval *A. tigrinum* (derived from a facultative paedomorphic population in Michigan) accelerated metamorphosis (see Fig. 7). Experiments with CRH in paedomorphic animals are necessary to determine whether this neurohormone can induce such animals to metamorphose.

2. Obligate Paedomorphs

Obligate paedomorphs can be further divided based on a species' response to TH treatment. Although all obligate paedomorphs do not metamorphose in the wild, inducible obligates do metamorphose when treated with TH. Permanent obligates, on the other hand, are insensitive to TH treatment (Wakahara, 1996).

The best-studied inducible obligate is the axolotl, *Ambystoma mexicanum*. It appears that low levels of circulating TH, low 5'-deiodinase activity, and low receptor number all contribute to the obligate paedomorphic lifestyle of the axolotl (Galton, 1992). The axolotl thyroid gland contains a large amount of thyroglobulin and is competent to respond to stimulation by TSH (Jacobs *et al.*, 1988a). The presence of an axolotl pituitary protein that has potent TSH-like activity has been demonstrated (Schultheiss, 1980). Thus, the paedomorphic state seems to be a result of the axolotl's lack of TSH release. Whether this is due to lack of hypothalamic stimulation, the presence of inhibitory factors, or an inability of the pituitary to respond to stimulatory neurohormones is uncertain.

Permanent obligates fail to respond to TH. This finding led to the hypothesis that TRs are not expressed or are somehow defective in these species. Partial TRα and TRβ sequences have been isolated from two members of the permanent obligate family Proteidae, Mudpuppy (*Necturus maculosus*) and *Proteus anguinus* (Safi *et al.*, 1997). Reverse transcriptase polymerase chain reaction (RT-PCR) analyses failed to demonstrate TRβ

expression in *N. maculosus* (Safi *et al.*, 1997). The authors suggested that failure to express this receptor may explain the insensitivity to TH in *Necturus*. Although both TRα and TRβ genes were found in *Proteus*, expression studies were not conducted on this species. The TR sequences of both *Necturus* and *Proteus* were found to contain nonconservative mutations that could potentially affect the hormone-binding domain (although, the binding affinities of these receptors for THs have not been examined).

C. Reproductive Development

Although sex determination and primary sexual differentiation occur during embryonic and larval development in amphibians (see Hayes, 1998, for review), many species do not reach sexual maturity until several years after metamorphosis (Duellman and Trueb, 1994). For most amphibians, the transition from the larval to the postmetamorphic form must occur before the initiation of maturation. Sexual maturation is arrested until a certain age when proper body size, body weight, or stage of nervous system development allows for the final stages of sexual maturation. Ryan and Semlitsch (1998) proposed that the decoupling of metamorphosis and sexual maturation has allowed paedomorphosis to evolve. The physiological mechanisms and environmental influences that contribute to the initiation of maturation in paedomorphic salamanders are probably very similar to those in amphibians that mature after metamorphosis.

The onset of sexual maturation is controlled by poorly understood central nervous system mechanisms that lead to the activation of GnRH neurons in the hypothalamus. GnRH acts on the anterior pituitary, which secretes GtHs (LH and FSH). The GtHs act on the gonads to bring about gonadal maturation and sex steroid secretion. In males, GtHs increase testosterone production, promote spermatogenesis, and increase testicular size by promoting the growth of interstitial cells and seminiferous tubules. In females, GtHs are responsible for promoting ovarian growth, sex steroid production, and oocyte maturation (Jorgensen, 1992). Circulating GtHs are also required for the ongoing maintenance of gametogenesis and reproductive structures. Hypophysectomy of sexually mature amphibians results in the degradation of vitellogenic oocytes (Lofts, 1974), arrested spermatogenesis, and degeneration of seminiferous tubules (Guha and Jorgensen, 1978a). Replacement of GtHs in hypophysectomized animals restores gonadal function in both males and females (Jorgensen, 1975; Guha and Jorgensen, 1978b).

Although the central mechanisms controlling the onset of maturation in amphibians are incompletely understood, nutritional status and growth rates are important factors. These relationships have been studied both in nature and in the laboratory. The high-altitude plethodontid salamander, *Bolitoglossa subpalmata*, grows in its native habitat at a rate of <0.5 mm/month. In the laboratory at their preferred temperature (10°C) and fed *ad libitum,* salamanders grew 1.3 mm/month. The growth rates of wild and lab-reared animals were positively correlated with the timing of sexual maturation. Laboratory-reared males matured at 1.5 years of age and females at 3 years of age, compared to 6 and 12 years for wild males and females, respectively (Houck, 1982).

Sexual maturation is typically correlated with an abrupt decline in somatic growth in anurans (Hemelaar, 1988) and in urodeles (Tiley, 1980). This is especially apparent in females, in which somatic growth may approach zero concurrent with the initiation of the first bout of reproduction (Jorgensen, 1986a). Vitellogenesis represents a large maternal investment; in gravid females, the ovaries may constitute 20–30% of body mass. Thus, during vitellogenesis energy is reallocated from somatic growth to reproduction (Jorgensen, 1986a). In males, sexual maturation and somatic growth are less tightly coupled because of the significantly lower investment that males must make in testicular development (Jorgensen, 1986a). Mature gonads in males contribute less than 1% to total body mass.

There may be a functional linkage between fat stores (which are dependant on nutritional status) and gonadal development in amphibia. Fat bodies are located in close proximity to the gonads in amphibians and an inverse relationship has been demonstrated between the size of the fat body and the size and stage of development of testes or ovaries in both anurans and urodeles (Fitzpatrick, 1976). Fat bodies are greatly reduced in size in sexually mature amphibians, whereas the fat bodies of immature amphibians are comparatively larger in size (Fitzpatrick, 1976).

Investigations into a possible linkage between fat bodies and gonads involved excising fat bodies and examining the effects on the gonads. In the newt *Notophthalmus viridescens,* fat-body removal caused the degeneration of gametes in both males and females (Adams and Rae, 1929). In the salamander *Amphiuma means,* fat-body removal prevented vitellogenic growth of the oocytes (Rose, 1968). Removal of fat bodies in anurans had a similar effect on gonads in males (Kobayashi and Iwasawa, 1984) and females (Pierantoni *et al.,* 1983). Unilateral excision of the fat body affected gametogenesis only in the gonad located on same side from which the fat body was removed; gametogenesis proceeded normally in the contralateral gonad, where the fat body remained intact (Adams and Rae, 1929). These findings prompted the hypothesis that a local mechanism mediated the fat–gonadal interaction. However, careful investigation of the vascularization revealed that there are independent blood supplies for the fat bodies and gonads and that fat bodies of some species spread along blood vessels near the ovary (Jorgensen, 1986b). Thus, there is the possibility that impaired gonadal development in these experiments was due to an experimental artifact, related to the disruption of blood supply to the gonad, rather than the removal of signals originating in the fat body.

Although the relationship between the amphibian fat bodies and the gonads is unclear, the fact remains that fat bodies tend to be large in immature animals and smaller in mature animals. This correlation could reflect the importance of fat stores for sexual maturation. Similarly, plenthodontid salamanders, who store fat in their tails, show a correlation between tail size and oocyte size, possibly reflecting the size of nutrient stores (Fraser, 1980). Removal of the tail prevented sexual maturation in these animals (Maiorana, 1977).

Although nutritional status is important for determining the onset of maturation, the physiological signal that communicates that there is ample energy for sexual maturation is unknown. A polypeptide called leptin, secreted by fat tissue in mammals, has received considerable interest (for review, see Houseknecht *et al.,* 1998; Wauters *et al.,* 2000). Leptin injections into female mice reduced food intake by 20 percent, but accelerated all measured indices of maturation (e.g., age at first estrus, ovarian weight, and ovulatory index) compared to pair-fed control animals. Animals fed *ad libitum* exhibited the same timing of events as leptin-injected animals (Cheung *et al.,* 1997). These findings and others have led to the hypothesis that leptin, which is released in greater amounts as fat stores increase (Houseknecht *et al.,* 1998; Wauters *et al.,* 2000), signals positive energy balance and thus brings about the onset of sexual maturation (i.e., puberty). However, it is unclear whether leptin serves as a trigger for the onset of sexual maturation or acts in a permissive manner. The presence or absence of such a hormone in amphibians has not, to our knowledge, been studied. Studies in lizards (*Sceloporus undulatus*) show that injections of mammalian leptin can increase metabolic rates, lower food intake, and increase body temperature (Niewiarowski *et al.,* 2000).

Hormones involved in regulating growth may also be important for the onset of maturation. As discussed in Section III, GH is important for growth of adult structures, but probably does not play a significant role in larval amphibians. Based on expression analyses and functional studies (see Section III), it is unclear whether PRL plays a role in controlling growth in larval amphibians. To our knowledge, PRL expression in paedomorphs has not been analyzed. It is uncertain which hormones play important roles in controlling larval growth in amphibians.

V. INTEGRATING EVOLUTION, ECOLOGY, AND ENDOCRINOLOGY

A. Metamorphosis

The activity of the thyroid axis in tadpoles can be regulated at multiple levels (see Section III; Fig. 6) and this activity ultimately determines when larvae enter metamorphosis and the rate at which metamorphosis progresses. Because the stress hormonal axis is closely linked to the thyroid axis, central nervous stress pathways may play a critical role in transducing environmental information and regulating metamorphic timing. From a developmental and physiological perspective, the upper and lower limits to the larval period in different species is established genetically through programming the developmental schedules for each of the components of the endocrine system (the establishment of functional endocrine cells and tissue competence to respond to thyroid and steroid

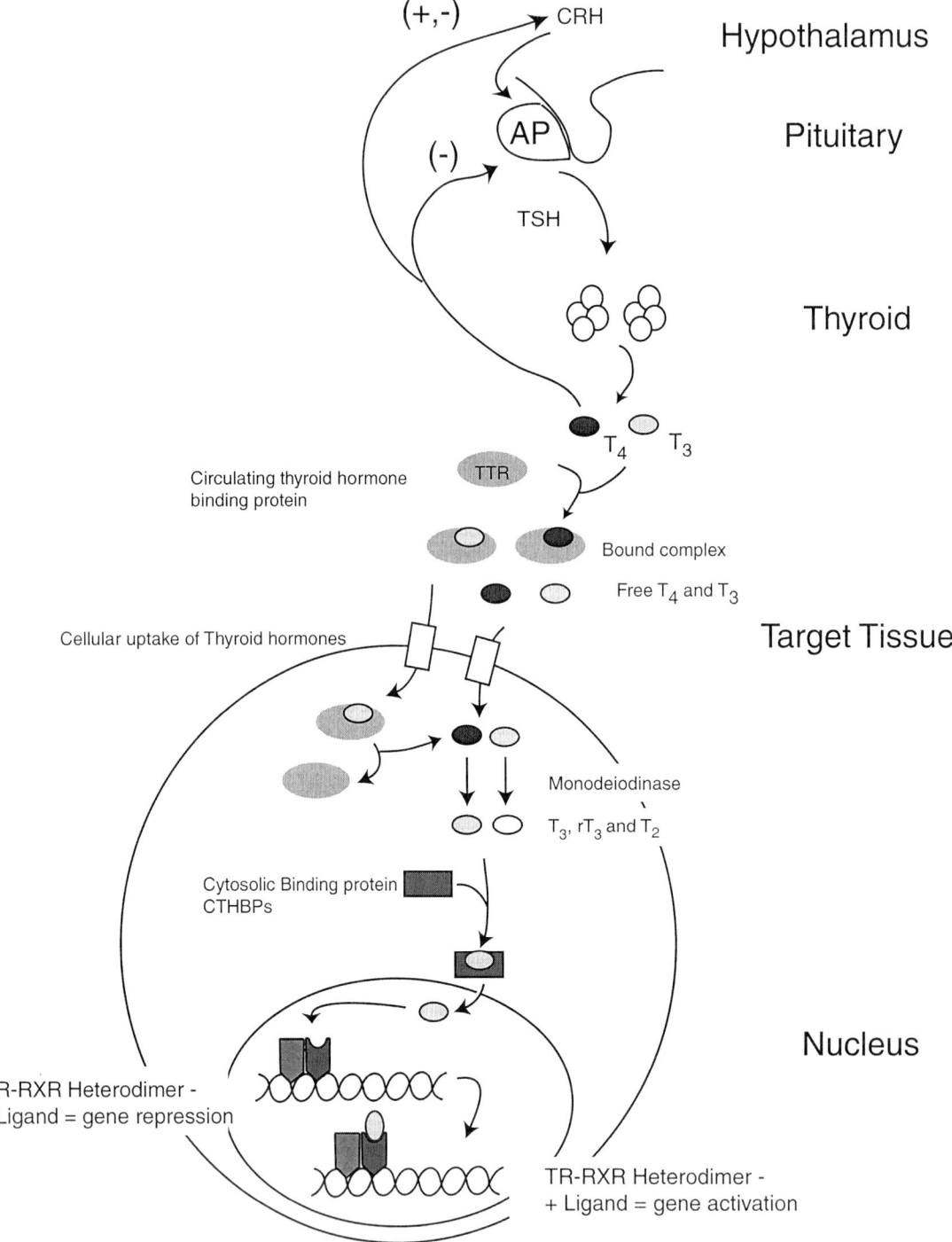

FIGURE 6 The integrated thyroid axis. Environmental regulation of the thyroid axis occurs at multiple levels. AP, anterior pituitary; CRH, corticotropin-releasing factor; RXR, retinoid-X receptor; T_3, 3,5,3'-triiodothyronine; T_4, thyroxine; TR, thyroid hormone receptor; TSH, thyroid-stimulating hormone; TTR, transthyretin. Minuses indicate a negative feedback. In the case of T_4 and T_3 effects on the brain, (+/−) indicates that these hormones promote differentiation of neurosecretory centers (and other brain regions) in addition to their negative feedback effects on neurohormone and pituitary hormone secretion.

hormones) and epigenetically through the regulated secretion, metabolism, and action of hormones. The environment could impact the developmental schedules and most certainly impacts the production and perhaps the actions of the hormones. Also, antagonism between growth-promoting hormones and morphogenic hormones might underlie the trade-offs between growth rate and development rate.

Few studies have addressed these issues from an integrative perspective (physiology and ecology). Here we discuss these issues and develop several hypotheses to explain how the limits to the larval period are established (in a physiological and developmental sense) and how plasticity in metamorphic timing within those limits is controlled.

1. Limits to the Length of the Larval Period

Why do amphibians differ in the lower and upper limits to the lengths of their larval periods and what determines tadpole growth and development rates and size at transformation? How does the timing of metamorphosis evolve? Few studies have attempted to address natural selection for the timing of metamorphosis; however, there is strong correlative evidence for the hypothesis that the length of the larval period is a reflection of the characteristics of the ancestral habitat (permanence and predictability, resource availability and competition, thermal environment, predation, etc.). The most important variable in this equation is likely to be habitat permanence because amphibian larvae depend on an aquatic environment for growth and development. It is also important to consider how factors operating in both life history stages (larval and adult) influence selection for the timing of metamorphosis (see Werner, 1986). Such questions have been addressed by ecologists (see Section II). Here we consider the question: What specific physiological regulatory systems in amphibian larvae might be targets for selection?

a) Lower Limit The earliest time at which tadpoles initiate metamorphosis in nature is probably influenced by the animal's size and the environmental conditions. But what determines the earliest possible time that a tadpole can enter metamorphosis and why does this timing differ among species? As discussed in Section II, the Wilbur-Collins model (Wilbur and Collins, 1973) proposes that tadpoles must reach a minimum body size before metamorphosis is possible. Thus, there must be a lower size limit, below which metamorphosis is impossible. This lower limit results from morphological and physiological constraints; for example, prey-catching ability and the size of prey, susceptibility to desiccation (higher surface-to-volume ratio of smaller animals) and susceptibility to predation, among others. Clearly, amphibians show considerable variation in the lower size limits for metamorphosis. For example, some species such as *Pseudacris* and *Bufo* grow very little during the larval phase and thus metamorphose at a very small size (7–9 mm snout to vent length), whereas others exhibit considerable growth and metamorphose at a large size (e.g., *Rana catesbeiana*, 20–60 mm snout to vent length; reviewed by Werner, 1986).

Is the minimum taxon-specific size for metamorphosis correlated with the establishment of competence to respond to metamorphic hormones? In *X. laevis* the capacity to respond to TH (i.e., increased RNA and protein synthesis) is established early, just after hatching (see Tata, 1968). Thus, competence to respond to TH is established well before the minimum size for normal metamorphosis is reached. Is the minimum size correlated with the establishment of competence to produce metamorphic hormones in sufficient quantities to drive morphogenesis? The capacity to up-regulate hormone production takes longer to develop and depends on the maturation of the neuroendocrine system (reviewed by Denver, 1996).

There is considerable variation among species in the time it takes to proceed from hatching to the first appearance of limb buds (premetamorphosis), and then from limb bud appearance to late prometamorphosis. These two periods are likely to be independent targets for selection. During the premetamorphic period, selection for growth rate may be most important. Plasticity in the length of the premetamorphic period depends primarily on growth opportunities, and tadpoles have no choice but to make a living in the larval habitat and attain the minimum size for metamorphosis. During the prometamorphic period, selection for development of the endocrine system is probably the more important factor. During this period, a tadpole's endocrine system is sufficiently developed to allow it to make developmental decisions. That is, if conditions are favorable, the rate of TH production remains low and tadpoles continues to capitalize on favorable growth conditions. If conditions deteriorate, tadpoles have the capacity to activate endocrine systems and transition from the aquatic to the terrestrial habitat.

Where is the metamorphic clock located? Etkin (1970) argued that the clock is located in the hypothalamus. For example, autotransplantation of the pituitary primordium to the tail of the frog embryo (separation from stimulatory control by the hypothalamus) results in more rapid growth compared with controls and a failure to metamorphose (see Etkin, 1970). Destruction of the preoptic nucleus or surgical removal of the primordium of the posterior hypothalamus (and thus isolation of the pituitary from the brain) prevents metamorphosis (reviewed by Denver, 1996). Studies of the normal development of the neurosecretory centers of the hypothalamus and the median eminence further support this hypothesis (see Etkin, 1970).

Although the neuroendocrine system is likely to be central to the control of metamorphic timing, this timing may be influenced at other levels. Other sites of regulation might involve the production of hormone transport proteins such as TTR, tissue monodeiodinases, membrane TH transporters, and CTH-BPs (see Fig. 5; discussion in Section III). We know so little about the roles of these proteins (with the exception of the monodeiodinases) in metamorphosis and the regulation of their biosynthesis that it is difficult to predict whether their regulation is an important site for the control of metamorphic timing.

A potentially important site for the regulation of metamorphic timing is at the level of hormone receptor synthesis. The timing of the expression of receptors for neurohormones in the pituitary gland may be regulated, but this has not been studied in any amphibian. We know that TH receptor expression, primarily TRβ, is up-regulated during prometamorphosis and that this up-regulation depends on TH. The hormone must be present for the receptors to be expressed and to function, and the finding of TR autoinduction supports the view that the clock is in the hypothalamus where hormone production is controlled. Other possible points of regulation of TR action include the expression of RXRs, and coactivator and corepressor proteins.

In conclusion, although several sites for regulation are possible, evidence suggests that the primary clock that determines when a tadpole can enter metamorphosis is related to the degree of development of the neuroendocrine system.

b) Upper Limit An environment with good growth conditions and low predation favors a longer larval period in most species; under such circumstances tadpoles would be expected to push the upper limit. But even if we maintain tadpoles in the laboratory under constant favorable conditions they do ultimately metamorphose; they won't grow indefinitely. What physiological or developmental mechanism is responsible for the spontaneous activation of the endocrine system controlling metamorphosis? Perhaps the slow increase in thyroid activity eventually reaches a threshold such that the system is pushed into metamorphic climax. The better the conditions, the lower the thyroid activity, but it eventually reaches a level where positive feedback is initiated. Or perhaps the activation follows from the animal reaching some upper size limit, and the subsequent decline in growth-promoting hormones removes antagonism on the thyroid system. Because anurans are not paedomorphic, the costs of remaining in the larval habitat longer should eventually outweigh the benefits of larger size at metamorphosis.

2. Plasticity in the Timing of Metamorphosis

Within the lower and upper limits to the larval period, tadpoles exhibit considerable plasticity in their timing of metamorphosis. This phenotypic plasticity depends on environmental factors, that is, the quality and suitability of the larval habitat for growth and survival. The majority of amphibians that have been studied exhibit phenotypic plasticity within the limits of the length of the larval period, rather than exhibiting a fixed rate of development. Here we address the question: What physiological systems enable plasticity in the timing of development and are thus targets for selection?

a) Integrated Endocrine System Controlling Metamorphosis and Potential Loci for Environmental Modification of Endocrine Activity Points of regulation by the environment might include the neuroendocrine system, peripheral endocrine organs, hormone transport and metabolism, and hormone action. But how are environmental factors sensed? Thermal, osmotic, and effects related to the gaseous environment could be sensed directly by most or all tissues. The influence of other factors, such as photoperiod, resource availability, predator presence, and crowding are likely integrated by the neuroendocrine system and transduced by the hypothalamus into changes in peripheral endocrine gland activity.

The availability of biologically active hormone is regulated in tissues by the monodeiodinases and the expression of these enzymes could be modified either directly or indirectly by environmental factors. An example of indirect regulation of monodeiodinases by environmental factors is by corticoids, which have been shown to increase 5′-deiondinase activity with the result that more of the active hormone T_3 is generated. This regulatory relationship might indicate that stress and stress hormones can accelerate metamorphosis by upregulating 5′-deiodinase (see Section III). Similarly, TR synthesis might be regulated directly or indirectly by environmental factors, which would then influence metamorphic timing. There is little known about which factors, physiological or environmental, regulate nuclear receptor expression in any species. As for monodeiodinase, evidence suggests that the corticoids can enhance TH action by up-regulating TR expression, and so TR biosynthesis is an additional site where stress and stress hormones may modulate timing (see Section III).

b) Plasticity Mediated by the Neuroendocrine System As described, the neuroendocrine system is likely to be the clock regulating spontaneous metamorphic timing. Furthermore, the external and internal environments can modify the activity of the neuroendocrine system. Many biotic and abiotic environmental factors are detected by animal sensory systems, integrated in higher brain centers, and then transduced via the neuroendocrine system.

The most important environmental variable for a tadpole is water availability, and duration of the aquatic habitat can profoundly influence the rate of metamorphosis in many species (see Section II; Table 1). This is especially true for desert amphibians that tend to breed in ephemeral habitats. We have studied the phenotypic and physiological responses of tadpoles of the western spadefoot toad (*S. hammondii*) to pond drying in the laboratory (see Section II).

As described in Section III, injections of CRH-like peptides accelerated metamorphosis in tadpoles of several amphibian species including the western spadefoot toad. Conversely, we found that the developmental acceleration induced by water-volume reduction could be attenuated by the treatment of tadpoles with the CRH receptor antagonist α-helical CRH$_{(9-41)}$ or by passive immunization with anti-CRH serum. Furthermore, spadefoot toad tadpoles had elevated hypothalamic CRH content at the time that they first responded (morphologically and endocrinologically) to the water-volume reduction in the laboratory (Denver, 1997a); these tadpoles also exhibited a precocious elevation in whole-body TH and corticosterone contents (Denver, 1998). Because the secretion of CRH is activated by stress, we hypothesized that CRH may play a central role in mediating a tadpole's developmental response to a deteriorating larval habitat. We also proposed that CRH may represent a phylogenetically ancient developmental cue that vertebrates use to assess changes in their habitat and to mount an appropriate developmental and physiological response. We based this hypothesis on data from mammals that show that CRH of fetal or placental origin controls the timing of the length of gestation and may shorten the gestational period under conditions of fetal stress (Smith, 1998).

But do other environmental factors that are known to alter the timing of metamorphosis also act through the neuroendocrine stress axis? We have observed elevated whole-body corticosterone content in *R. pipiens* tadpoles fed limited resources or subjected to high conspecific density, compared to their high-resource low-density counterparts (Glennemeier and Denver, 2002c). Both low food and increased density resulted in slowed growth and development in premetamorphic tadpoles, which agrees with other studies showing growth- and development-inhibiting effects of these factors in premetamorphs (but contrast this with prometamorphic animals, which accelerate development in response to food restriction or crowding; see Section II). This slowed growth caused by crowding stress was reversed in tadpoles by treatment with the corticosterone-synthesis inhibitor metyrapone, again suggesting a functional role for the hypothalamic-hypophyseal-interrenal axis in mediating the larval developmental response to environmental conditions (Glennemeier and Denver, 2002c). Hayes (1997) also reported an elevation in whole-body corticosterone content in *B. boreas* tadpoles caused by crowding. Predation, temperature, photoperiod, or other environmental factors could conceivably work through similar neuroendocrine pathways to exert their effects on larval development. If larvae have a means of detecting the state of environmental conditions, through visual, chemical, or other sensory systems, then the neuroendocrine system is a likely pathway through which developmental responses to the environment can operate.

B. Facultative Paedomorphosis

How (in an ultimate sense) are different life history trajectories selected (paedomorphosis vs metamorphosis)? Why (in a proximate sense) do some animals become paedomorphic, whereas others become metamorphic? The life history trajectory is influenced by the environment, but ultimately expressed via a change in hormone production and action. The components of the endocrine system are likely to be targets for selection.

As already discussed, the neuroendocrine system serves to transduce many environmental factors into changes in development and physiology. To understand the physiological processes involved in the determination, development, and maintenance of each morphology, two separate antagonistic developmental pathways must be considered. Metamorphs activate their thyroid axis, which results in the morphological changes necessary for adaptation to the terrestrial habitat. Paedomorphs have increased activity of the hypothalamic-pituitary-gonadal axis, which results in precocious sexual maturation. In the discussion that follows we address the possibility that interactions between the thyroid and gonadal axes may underlie the mechanism of the selection of the life history trajectory of a facultative paedomorphic salamander.

1. Integrated Organismal Responses to the Environment—Metamorphosis vs Paedomorphosis

Metamorphosis allows developing larvae to escape a deteriorating aquatic habitat and move into the terrestrial habitat. The environmental conditions that trigger metamorphosis (discussed in Section II) in facultative paedomorphic salamanders probably do so by activating neuroendocrine pathways, as discussed previously for anurans. In support of this hypothesis, we observed that injections of the stress neuropeptide CRH accelerated metamorphosis in larvae of the tiger salamander (*A. tigrinum*; Fig. 7; Boorse and Denver, 2002). We also observed that captured tiger salamander larvae metamorphose within 2 days of transfer to the laboratory (R. J. Denver, unpublished observations). Earl Werner (personal communication) found that several paedomorphic *A. tigrinum* brought into the laboratory from experimental ponds (at the E. S. George Reserve, Pinckney, MI) quickly metamorphosed. That they were indeed paedomorphs was verified by dissection, which showed scars on the ovaries, indicating that reproduction in the larval stage had occurred. We interpret these anecdotal observations as evidence for capture-stress-induced activation of the endocrine system controlling metamorphosis.

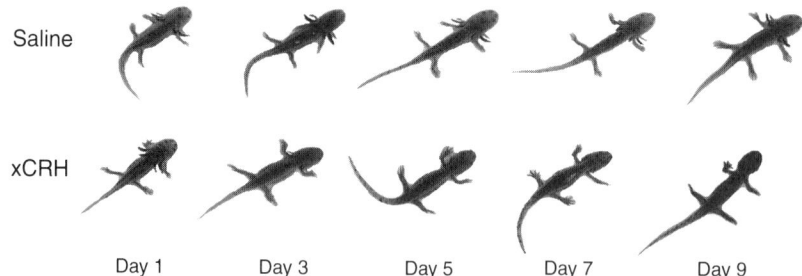

FIGURE 7 Effects of CRH on metamorphosis in *Ambystoma tigrinum*. Injections of ovine CRH (oCRH, 1 μg, i.p.) or saline (0.6%) were administered daily ($n = 6$). Digital images were captured every other day to access metamorphic progression. Note the gill resorption in larvae receiving oCRH injections. **See insert for a color version of this figure.**

Limitations in food availability result in trade-offs among allocation of energy to maintenance, growth, reproduction, and storage. We hypothesize that a favorable nutritional state of facultatively paedomorphic salamanders allows for early age at maturity. Adequate nutritional status appears to be a major factor in determining the onset of sexual maturation (see Section IV). The environmental conditions that produce paedomorphs presumably have higher per capita resources and less competition among larvae (Scott, 1993; Ryan and Semlitsch, 1998), as low larval density corresponds to lower interference rates or less crowding of larvae; constant water level provides stable larval density and stable resources. Considerable time and energy must be invested in the extensive morphological and biochemical restructuring that takes place during metamorphosis. Because paedomorphs do not undergo metamorphosis, they do not have this additional energetic cost.

The effects of differential resource allocation during larval development have not been studied in paedomorphic salamanders, but studies in metamorphic species have demonstrated that larvae allocate resources differently depending on environmental conditions, which then affects both growth and reproduction. Marbled salamander (*Ambystoma opacum*) larvae maintained at low densities had higher lipid stores at metamorphosis and exhibited longer survival in captivity. Lower larval densities also translated into benefits for the terrestrial adult as demonstrated by their larger size at first reproduction, earlier age at first reproduction, and greater clutch size (Scott, 1994). Juvenile *A. opacum* females exposed to high food levels exhibited larger size, higher lipid levels, larger clutch size, and earlier age at first reproduction than juveniles exposed to medium or low food levels (Scott and Fore, 1995). Each of these traits can contribute to an individual's overall lifetime reproductive success.

2. Physiological and Ecological Trade-offs between Metamorphosis and Paedomorphosis

The environment determines the life history trajectory by influencing the activity of endocrine glands. We hypothesize that there are antagonistic interactions among the endocrine pathways controlling growth, metamorphosis, and sexual maturation, and the strength of these interactions underlies the choice of developmental pathway taken.

a) *Thyroid Axis Inhibition of Gonadal Development*

The cost of morphological and biochemical restructuring during metamorphosis decreases the amount of resources available for gonadal development in metamorphs. The thyroid and interrenal hormones that drive metamorphosis may also directly inhibit gonadal development. Both stress hormones and THs have been demonstrated to inhibit gonadal function in vertebrates.

Stress is well known to inhibit reproduction in all vertebrate taxa. Stress hormones can influence sexual function at all levels of the hypothalamic-pituitary-gonadal axis: the hypothalamus to inhibit GnRH release, the pituitary to interfere with GnRH-induced LH and FSH release, and the gonads to alter the stimulatory effect of GtHs on sex steroid secretion (Rivier and Rivest, 1991) (Fig. 8). Both CRH and glucocorticoids are known to inhibit gonadal activity. Intracerebroventricular injections of CRH inhibited GnRH secretion in rodents and primates, whereas administration of CRHR antagonists reversed the inhibitory effects of stress on GnRH (Rivier *et al.*, 1986). Elevated plasma glucocorticoid concentrations also reduced GnRH secretion (Suter and Schwartz, 1985). Corticoid receptors and, surprisingly, CRH mRNA are expressed in rodent gonads, and CRH has been shown to directly inhibit steroidogenesis (Saez *et al.*, 1977; Ulisse *et al.*, 1989; Fabbri *et al.*, 1990). The stress hormones may directly inhibit sex steroidogenesis by reducing sensitivity to GtH stimulation (Charpenet *et al.*, 1981, 1982).

The activation of the stress hormonal axis in metamorphic salamanders may result in the inhibition of sexual maturation. Examples of such actions in amphibia include studies in adult *X. laevis* in which crowding and underfeeding reduced ovarian growth (Alexander and Bellerby, 1938); such effects could be reversed by injections of human chorionic gonadotropin (hCG), even in toads that were emaciated from starvation (Jorgensen, 1982). The stress to the frogs of being captured and brought into the lab caused a threefold increase in atresia of vitellogenic oocytes, which was attributed to a decrease in circulating GtHs (Pancharatna and Saidapur, 1992). These findings lead to the hypothesis that elevated stress hormones in metamorphs delays gonadal development.

Increasing plasma TH concentrations during metamorphosis may also play an important role in inhibiting

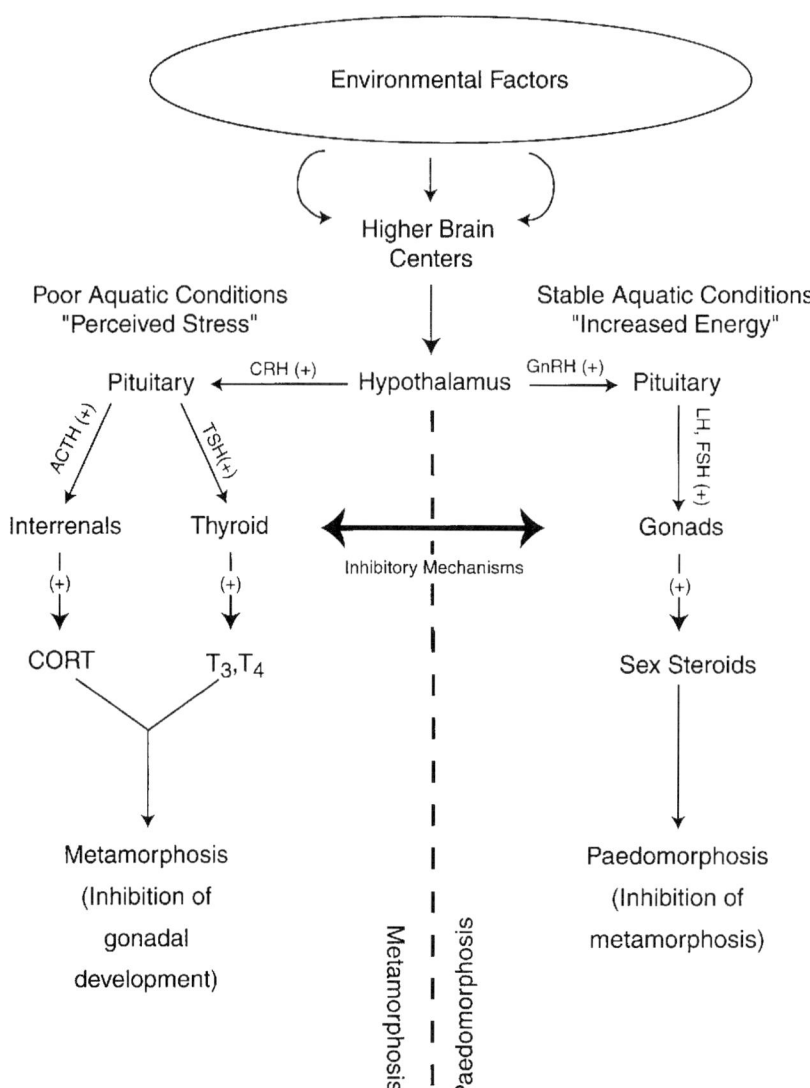

FIGURE 8 Environmental regulation of hormonal axes controlling metamorphosis and paedomorphosis in facultatively paedomorphic salamanders. Pluses indicate a stimulatory effect. Components of a given pathway (metamorphosis vs paedomorphosis) may inhibit the development of the alternative morphology. ACTH, adrenocorticotropin; CORT, corticosterone; CRH, corticotropin-releasing factor; FSH, follicle-stimulating hormone; GnRH, gonadotropin-releasing hormone; LH, luteinizing hormone; T_3, 3,5,3′-triiodothyronine; T_4, thyroxine; TSH, thyroid-stimulating hormone.

gonadal development. Wakahara (1994) treated larvae of the facultative paedomorphic salamander *Hynobius retardatus* with a goitrogen (antithyroid compound) and this both inhibited metamorphosis (as expected) and caused accelerated spermatogenesis and increased testicular growth (Wakahara, 1994). These findings suggest that TH exerts an inhibitory action on gonadal development in these animals. The mechanism by which TH inhibits gonadal development is unknown. However, it may be conserved across vertebrate taxa because goitrogen treatment of neonatal rats resulted in an increase in adult testis size (Cooke and Meisami, 1991).

Thus, both TH and stress hormones have been shown to inhibit gonadal development. Elevation in the production of these hormones at metamorphosis may explain why gonadal development is delayed in metamorphs compared with paedomorphs.

b) Sex Steroid Inhibition of the Thyroid Axis Facultative paedomorphs retain the ability to metamorphose, which is important for escaping mortality in a deteriorating aquatic habitat. However, if an individual matures early and then undergoes metamorphosis, the benefits of increased survival and higher quality offspring are lost because the age at first reproduction is the same as other metamorphs. Early maturation may then carry significant costs such as reduced body size or reduced parental investment at time of reproduction (Stearns, 1991).

We hypothesize that because paedomorphs carry an added cost associated with metamorphosis, especially if metamorphosis occurs before first reproduction, paedomorphs may not metamorphose as readily as sexually immature larvae. Paedomorphs are expected to delay metamorphosis and remain in a deteriorating habitat until the cost of remaining in the aquatic habitat is greater than the cost of metamorphosis. Paedomorphs may be less sensitive to metamorphic hormones; for example, sexually mature larvae of *A. tigrinum* required higher doses of exogenous TH to induce metamorphosis than immature larvae (Norris and Platt, 1974). We predict that elevated plasma concentrations of sex steroids in the paedomorph reduce its likelihood of metamorphosing by decreasing sensitivity to metamorphic hormones. Although sex steroids have not been quantified in paedomorphs, sex steroid production is presumably higher than in sexually immature larvae or metamorphic juveniles. Paedomorphs exhibit well-developed mature gonads in both males and females that require circulating gonadotropins for their maintenance (Jorgensen, 1975; Guha and Jorgensen, 1978b). Male paedomorphs exhibit secondary sexual characteristics (i.e., enlarged cloaca) that are dependent on elevated plasma testosterone concentrations (Norris *et al.*, 1989).

Both testosterone and estradiol inhibit TH-induced metamorphosis in *X. laevis* (Gray and Janssens, 1990). The inhibitory effects were only seen *in vivo* and not *in vitro*. This suggests the inhibitory action of sex steroids is not at the peripheral tissues but at a higher level in the thyroid axis (Fig. 8). Sex steroids also inhibit metamorphosis in Japanese flounder (*Paralichthys olivaceus*; Dejesus *et al.*, 1992); metamorphosis in flounder is endocrinologically similar to amphibian metamorphosis (Dejesus *et al.*, 1993).

The initiation of sexual maturation in larvae is tightly coupled to nutritional status, a good indicator of environmental quality. Paedomorphosis in stable aquatic conditions allows for the continued exploitation of resources. Facultative paedomorphs (or immature larvae) may respond to a deteriorating habitat by activating neuroendocrine stress pathways (see previous discussion). Although sex steroids may suppress the metamorphic pathways, we predict that the effects of thyroid and interrenal hormones dominate the sex steroid effects. The neuroendocrine stress pathway may be an evolutionary-conserved mechanism that allows animals to monitor their environment and to respond to deleterious changes in habitat quality by metamorphosing.

The decision to metamorphose or to become paedomorphic and remain in the larval habitat can have critical fitness-related consequences. Understanding the relationship between fitness and the phenotypes produced by different environments will be necessary to evaluate such consequences. Approaches that attempt to place the mechanistic bases of development in an ecologically relevant context are essential for understanding the potential physiological constraints on the evolution of paedomorphosis and metamorphosis.

Acknowledgments

G.C.B. was supported by a predoctoral fellowship from the NSF, and K.A.G. received support from the Michigan Department of Environmental Quality. This work was supported by NSF grant IBN9974672 to R.J.D.

References

Abe, T., Kakyo, M., Sakagami, H., Tokui, T., Nishio, T., Tanemoto, M., Nomura, H., Hebert, S. C., Matsuno, S., Kondo, H., and Yawo, H. (1998). Molecular characterization and tissue distribution of a new organic anion transporter subtype (Oatp3) that transports thyroid hormones and taurocholate and comparison with Oatp2. *J. Biol. Chem.* **273**, 22395–22401.

Adams, A., and Rae, E. (1929). An experimental study of the fat bodies in *Triturus (diemyctylus) viridescens. Anat. Rec.* **41**, 181–204.

Aida, T., Iwamuro, S., Miura, S., and Kikuyama, S. (1999). Changes of pituitary proopiomelanocortin mRNA levels during metamorphosis of the bullfrog larvae. *Zool. Sci.* **16**, 255–260.

Alexander, S., and Bellerby, C. (1938). Experimental studies on the sexual cycle of the South African clawed toad (*Xenopus laevis*). *J. Exp. Biol.* **15**, 74–81.

Ashizawa, K., and Cheng, S. Y. (1992). Regulation of thyroid-hormone receptor-mediated transcription by a cytosol protein. *Proc. Natl. Acad. Sci. U.S.A.* **89**, 9277–9281.

Baker, B. S., and Tata, J. R. (1990). Accumulation of proto-oncogene c-erb-a related transcripts during *Xenopus* development: Association with early acquistition of response to thyroid hormone and estrogen. *EMBO J.* **9**, 879–885.

Baker, B. S., and Tata, J. R. (1992). Prolactin prevents the autoinduction of thyroid-hormone receptor messenger-RNAs during amphibian metamorphosis. *Dev. Biol.* **149**, 463–467.

Banker, D. E., Bigler, J., and Eisenman, R. N. (1991). The thyroid-hormone receptor gene (c-erba-alpha) is expressed in advance of thyroid gland maturation during the early embryonic development of *Xenopus laevis*. *Mol. Cell. Biol.* **11**, 5079–5089.

Beachy, C. K. (1995). Effects of larval growth history on metamorphosis in a stream dwelling salamander (*Desmognathus ochrophaeus*). *J. Herpetol.* **29**, 375–382.

Becker, K. B., Stephens, K. C., Davey, J. C., Schneider, M. J., and Galton, V. A. (1997). The type 2 and type 3 iodothyronine deiodinases play important roles in coordinating development in *Rana catesbeiana* tadpoles. *Endocrinology (Baltimore)* **138**, 2989–2997.

Behan, D. P., DeSouza, E. B., Potter, E., Sawchenko, P., Lowry, P. J., and Vale, W. W. (1996). Modulatory actions of corticotropin-releasing factor-binding protein. *Ann. N.Y. Acad. Sci.* **780**, 81–95.

Bern, H. A., Nicoll, C. S., and Strohman, R. C. (1967). Prolactin and tadpole growth. *Proc. Soc. Exp. Biol. Med.* **126**, 518–520.

Berven, K. A., and Chadra, B. G. (1988). The relationship among egg size, density and food level on larval development in the wood frog (*Rana sylvatica*). *Oecologia* **75**, 67–72.

Berven, K. A., and Gill, D. E. (1983). Interpreting geographic variation in life-history traits. *Am. Zool.* **23**, 85–97.

Blair, W. F. (1972). "Evolution of the Genus *Bufo*." University of Texas Press, Austin.

Boorse, G. C., and Denver, R. J. (2002). Acceleration of *Ambystoma tigrinum* metamorphosis by corticotropin-eleasing hormone. In press.

Brady, L. D., and Griffiths, R. A. (2000). Developmental responses to pond desiccation in tadpoles of the British anuran amphibians (*Bufo bufo, B. Calamita* and *Rana temporaria*). *J. Zool.* **252**, 61–69.

Brockelman, W. Y. (1969). An analysis of density effects and predation in *Bufo americanus* tadpoles. *Ecology* **50**, 632–644.

Brooks, A. R., Sweeney, G., and Old, R. W. (1989). Structure and functional expression of a cloned *Xenopus* thyroid hormone receptor. *Nucleic Acids Res.* **17**, 9395–9405.

Brown, D. D., Wang, Z., Furlow, J. D., Kanamori, A., Schwartzman, R. A., Remo, B. F., and Pinder, A. (1996). The thyroid hormone-induced tail resorption program during *Xenopus laevis* metamorphosis. *Proc. Natl. Acad. Sci. U.S.A.* **93**, 1924–1929.

Bruneau, M., and Magnin, E. (1980). Larval life of bullfrogs *Rana catesbeiana* shaw (Amphibia:Anura) from Laurentides, Quebec. *Can. J. Zool.* **58**, 169–174.

Buckbinder, L., and Brown, D. D. (1993). Expression of the *Xenopus laevis* prolactin and thyrotropin genes during metamorphosis. *Proc. Natl. Acad. Sci. U.S.A.* **90**, 3820–3824.

Burns, J. T., Patyna, R., and Ryland, S. (1987). A circadian rhythm in the effect of thyroxine in the stimulation of metamorphosis in the African clawed frog, *Xenopus laevis. J. Interdiscip. Cycle Res.* **18**, 293–296.

Buscaglia, M., Leloup, J., and De Luze, A. (1985). The role and regulation of monodeiodination of thyroxine to 3,5,3′-triiodothyronine during amphibian metamorphosis. In "Metamorphosis" (M. Balls and M. Bownes, eds.), pp. 273–293. Clarendon Press, Oxford.

Carr, J. A., and Norris, D. O. (1988). Interrenal activity during metamorphosis of the tiger salamander, *Ambystoma tigrinum. Gen. Comp. Endocrinol.* **71**, 63–69.

Carr, J. A., and Norris, D. O. (1990). Immunohistochemical localization of corticotropin-releasing factor-like and arginine vasotocin-like immunoreactivities in the brain and pituitary of the American Bullfrog (*Rana catesbeiana*) during development and metamorphosis. *Gen. Comp. Endocrinol.* **78**, 180–188.

Carstensen, H., Burgers, A. C. J., and Li, C. H. (1961). Demonstration of aldosterone and corticosterone as the principal steroids formed in incubates of adrenals of the american bullfrog *Rana catesbeiana* and stimulation of their production by mammalian adrenocorticotropin. *Gen. Comp. Endocrinol.* **1**, 37–50.

Charpenet, G., Tache, Y., Forest, M. G., Haour, F., Saez, J. M., Bernier, M., Ducharme, J. R., and Collu, R. (1981). Effects of chronic intermittent immobilization stress on rat testicular androgenic function. *Endocrinology (Baltimore)* **109**, 1254–1258.

Charpenet, G., Tachey, B. M., Ducharme, J. R., and Collu, R. (1982). Stress-induced testicular hyposensitivity to gonadotropin in rats. Role of the pituitary gland. *Biol. Reprod.* **27**, 616–623.

Cheng, S. Y., Maxfield, F. R., Robbins, J., Willingham, M. C., and Pastan, I. H. (1980). Receptor mediated uptake of 3,3′,5-triiodo-L-thyronine by cultured fibroblasts. *Proc. Natl. Acad. Sci. U.S.A.* **77**, 3425–3429.

Cheng, S. Y., Gong, Q. H., Parkison, C., Robinson, E. A., Appella, E., Merlino, G. T., and Pastan, I. (1987). The nucleotide sequence of a human cellular thyroid-hormone binding protein present in endoplasmic reticulum. *J. Biol. Chem.* **262**, 11221–11227.

Cheung, C. C., Thornton, J. E., Kuijper, J. L., Weigle, D. S., Clifton, D. K., and Steiner, R. A. (1997). Leptin is a metabolic gate for the onset of puberty in the female rat. *Endocrinology (Baltimore)* **138**, 855–858.

Clemons, G. K., and Nicoll, C. S. (1977). Effects of antisera to bullfrog prolactin and growth hormone on metamorphosis of *Rana catesbeiana* tadpoles. *Gen. Comp. Endocrinol.* **31**, 495–497.

Cooke, P., and Meisami, E. (1991). Early hypothyroidism in rats causes increased adult testis and reproductive organ size but does not change testosterone levels. *Endocrinology (Baltimore)* **129**, 237–243.

Crump, M. L. (1989a). Effect of habitat drying on developmental time and size at metamorphosis in *Hyla pseudopuma*. *Copeia*, pp. 794–797.

Crump, M. L. (1989b). Life-history consequences of feeding versus non-feeding in a facultatively non-feeding toad larva. *Oecologia* **78**, 486–489.

Csikos, T., Tay, J., and Danielsen, M. (1995). Expression of the *Xenopus laevis* mineralocorticoid receptor during metamorphosis. *Recent Prog. Horm. Res.* **50**, 393–396.

D'Angelo, S. A., Gordon, A. S., and Charipper, H. A. (1941). The role of the thyroid and pituitary glands in the anomalous effect of inanition on amphibian metamorphosis. *J. Exp. Zool.* **87**, 259–277.

Darras, V. M., and Kuhn, E. R. (1982). Increased plasma levels of thyroid hormones in a frog *Rana ridibunda* following intravenous administration of TRH. *Gen. Comp. Endocrinol.* **48**, 469–475.

Darras, V. M., and Kuhn, E. R. (1983). Effects of TRH, bovine TSH, and pituitary extracts on thyroidal T_4 release in *Ambystoma mexicanum*. *Gen. Comp. Endocrinol.* **51**, 286–291.

Davey, J. C., Schneider, M. J., and Galton, V. A. (1994). Cloning of a thyroid hormone responsive *Rana catesbeiana* c-erba-beta gene. *Dev. Genet.* **15**, 339–346.

Dejesus, E. G., Hirano, T., and Inui, Y. (1992). Gonadal-steroids delay spontaneous flounder metamorphosis and inhibit T3-induced fin ray shortening in vitro. *Zool. Sci.* **9**, 633–638.

Dejesus, E. G., Hirano, T., and Inui, Y. (1993). Flounder metamorphosis—its regulation by various hormones. *Fish. Physiol. Biochem.* **11**, 323–328.

Denoel, M., and Joly, P. (2000). Neoteny and progenesis as two heterochronic processes involved in paedomorphosis in *Triturus alpestris* (Amphibia: Caudata). *Proc. R. Soc. London or Ser* **267**, 1481–1485.

Denver, R. J. (1988). Several hypothalamic peptides stimulate in vitro thyrotropin secretion by pituitaries of anuran amphibians. *Gen. Comp. Endocrinol.* **72**, 383–393.

Denver, R. J. (1993). Acceleration of anuran amphibian metamorphosis by corticotropin-releasing hormone like peptides. *Gen. Comp. Endocrinol.* **91**, 38–51.

Denver, R. J. (1996). Neuroendocrine control of amphibian metamorphosis. In "Metamorphosis: Postembryonic Reprogramming of Gene Expression in Amphibian and Insect Cells" (L. I. Gilbert, J. R. Tata, and B. G. Atkinson, eds.), pp. 434–464. Academic Press, San Diego, CA.

Denver, R. J. (1997a). Environmental stress as a developmental cue: Corticotropin-releasing hormone is a proximate mediator of adaptive plasticity in amphibian metamorphosis. *Horm. Behav.* **31**, 169–179.

Denver, R. J. (1997b). Proximate mechanisms of phenotypic plasticity in amphibian metamorphosis. *Am. Zool.* **37**, 172–184.

Denver, R. J. (1998). Hormonal correlates of environmentally induced metamorphosis in the western spadefoot toad, *Scaphiopus hammondii*. *Gen. Comp. Endocrinol.* **110**, 326–336.

Denver, R. J. (1999). Evolution of the corticotropin-releasing hormone signaling system and its role in stress-induced phenotypic plasticity. *Ann. N.Y. Acad. Sci.* **897**, 46–53.

Denver, R. J., and Licht, P. (1989a). Neuropeptide stimulation of thyrotropin secretion in the larval bullfrog—evidence for a common neuroregulator of thyroid and interrenal activity in metamorphosis. *J. Exp. Zool.* **252**, 101–104.

Denver, R. J., and Licht, P. (1989b). Synthetic neuropeptide antagonists stimulate in vitro thyrotropin and growth hormone secretion by hatchling turtle pituitaries. *J. Exp. Zool.* **252**, 169–173.

Denver, R. J., and Licht, P. (1991). Several hypothalamic peptides stimulate thyrotropin and growth hormone secretion by adult turtle pituitary glands. *Comp. Biochem. Physiol. A* **100**, 603–606.

Denver, R. J., Pavgi, S., and Shi, Y. B. (1997). Thyroid hormone-dependent gene expression program for *Xenopus* neural development. *J. Biol. Chem.* **272**, 8179–8188.

Denver, R. J., Mirhadi, N., and Phillips, M. (1998). Adaptive plasticity in amphibian metamorphosis: Response of *Scaphiopus hammondii* tadpoles to habitat desiccation. *Ecology* **79**, 1859.

Denver, R. J., Ouellet, L., Furling, D., Kobayashi, A., Fujii-Kuriyama, Y., and Puymirat, J. (1999). Basic transcription element-binding protein (BTEB) is a thyroid hormone-regulated gene in the developing central nervous system. Evidence for a role in neurite outgrowth. *J. Biol. Chem.* **274**, 23128–23134.

Denver, R. J., Krain, L. P., Hoopfer, E. D., and Farley, B. F. (2002). Auto- and cross-regulation of nuclear hormone receptors during *Xenopus* metamorphosis. *(Submitted.)*

Divino, C. M., and Schussler, G. C. (1990). Receptor mediated uptake and internalization of transthyretin. *J. Biol. Chem.* **265**, 1425–1429.

Docter, R., Krenning, E. P., Bos, G., Fekkes, D. F., and Hennemann, G. (1982). Evidence that the uptake of tri-iodo-L-thyronine by human erythrocytes is carrier mediated but not energy dependent. *Biochem. J.* **208**, 27–34.

Dodd, M. H. I., and Dodd, J. M. (1976). The biology of metamorphosis. *In* "Physiology of the Amphibia" (B. Lofts, ed.), Vol. 3, pp. 467–599. Academic Press, New York.

Duellman, W. E., and Trueb, L. (1994). "Biology of Amphibians." Johns Hopkins University Press, Baltimore, MD.

Edwards, M. L. O., and Pivorun, E. B. (1991). The effects of photoperiod and different dosages of melatonin on metamorphic mate and weight gain in *Xenopus laevis* tadpoles. *Gen. Comp. Endocrinol.* **81**, 28–38.

Ekins, R. (1990). Measurement of free hormones in blood. *Endocr. Rev.* **11**, 5–46.

Etkin, W. (1968). Hormonal control of amphibian metamorphosis. *In* "Metamorphosis: A Problem in Developmental Biology" (W. Etkin and L. I. Gilbert, eds.), pp. 313–348. Appleton-Century-Crofts, New York.

Etkin, W. (1970). The endocrine mechanism of amphibian metamorphosis, an evolutionary achievement. *Mem. Soc. Endocrinol.* **18**, 137–155.

Etkin, W., and Gona, A. G. (1967). Antagonism between prolactin and thyroid hormone in amphibian development. *J. Exp. Zool.* **165**, 249–258.

Fabbri, A., Tinajero, J. C., and DuFau, M. I. (1990). Corticotropin-releasing factor is produced by rat leydig cells and has a major local anti-reproductive role in the testes. *Endocrinology (Baltimore)* **127**, 1541–1543.

Feder, M. E., and Moran, C. M. (1985). Effect of water depth on costs of aerial respiration and its alternatives in tadpoles of *Rana pipiens. Can. J. Zool.—Rev. Can. Zool.* **63**, 643–648.

Fitzpatrick, L. (1976). Life history patterns of storage and utilization of lipids for energy in amphibians. *Am. Zool.* **16**, 725–732.

Forrest, D., and Vennstrom, B. (2000). Functions of thyroid hormone receptors in mice. *Thyroid* **10**, 41–52.

Fraser, D. (1980). On the environmental control of oocyte maturation in a plethodontid salamander. *Oecologia* **46**, 302–307.

Frieden, E. (1981). The dual role of thyroid hormones in vertebrate development and calorigenesis. *In* "Metamorphosis: A Problem in Developmental Biology" (L. Gilbert and E. Frieden, eds.), pp. 545–564. Plenum Press, New York.

Frieden, E., and Naile, B. (1955). Biochemistry of amphibian metamorphosis .1. Enhancement of induced metamorphosis by glucocorticoids. *Science* **121**, 37–38.

Friesema, E. C. H., Docter, R., Moerings, E., Stieger, B., Hagenbuch, B., Meier, P. J., Krenning, E. P., Hennemann, G., and Visser, T. J. (1999). Identification of thyroid hormone transporters. *Biochem. Biophys. Res. Commun.* **254**, 497–501.

Funkenstein, B., Perrot, V., and Brown, C. L. (1999). Cloning of putative piscine *(Sparus aurata)* transthyretin: Developmental expression and tissue distribution. *Mol. Cell. Endocrinol.* **157**, 67–73.

Galton, V. A. (1988). Iodothyronine 5′-deiodinase activity in the amphibian *Rana catesbeiana* at different stages of the life cycle. *Endocrinology (Baltimore)* **122**, 1746–1750.

Galton, V. A. (1989). The role of 3,5,3′-triiodothyronine in the physiological action of thyroxine in the premetamorphic tadpole. *Endocrinology (Baltimore)* **124**, 2427–2433.

Galton, V. A. (1990). Mechanisms underlying the acceleration of thyroid hormone induced tadpole metamorphosis by corticosterone. *Endocrinology (Baltimore)* **127**, 2997–3002.

Galton, V. A. (1991). Iodothyronine 5′-deiodinase activity in the amphibian *Rana catesbeiana* at different stages of the life cycle. *Endocrinology (Baltimore)* **122**, 1746–1750.

Galton, V. A. (1992). Thyroid hormone receptors and iodothyronine deiodinases in the developing Mexican axolotl, *Ambystoma mexicanum. Gen. Comp. Endocrinol.* **85**, 62–70.

Galton, V. A., and Hiebert, A. (1988). The ontogeny of iodothyronine 5′-monodeiodinase activity in *Rana catesbeiana* tadpoles. *Endocrinology (Baltimore)* **122**, 640–645.

Galton, V. A., St. Germain, D. L., and Whittemore, S. (1986). Cellular uptake of 3,5,3′-triiodothyronine and thyroxine by red blood and thymus cells. *Endocrinology (Baltimore)* **118**, 1918–1923.

Gancedo, B., Corpas, I., Alonso-Gomez, A. L., Delgado, M. J., Morreale de Escobar, G., and Alonso-Bedate, M. (1992). Corticotropin-releasing factor stimulates metamorphosis and increases thyroid hormone concentration in prometamorphic *Rana perezi* larvae. *Gen. Comp. Endocrinol.* **87**, 6–13.

Gao, X. M., Kalkhoven, E., Petersonmaduro, J., Vanderburg, B., and Destree, O. H. J. (1994a). Expression of the glucocorticoid receptor gene is regulated during early embryogenesis of *Xenopus laevis. Biochim. Biophys. Acta* **1218**, 194–198.

Gao, X. M., Stegeman, B. I., Lanser, P., Koster, J. G., and Destree, O. H. J. (1994b). GR transcripts are localized during early *Xenopus laevis* embryogenesis and overexpression of GR inhibits differentiation after dexamethasone treatment. *Biochem. Biophys. Res. Commun.* **199**, 734–741.

Geris, K. L., Kotanen, S. P., Berghman, L. R., Kuhn, E. R., and Darras, V. M. (1996). Evidence of a thyrotropin-releasing activity of ovine corticotropin-releasing factor in the domestic fowl (*Gallus domesticus*). *Gen. Comp. Endocrinol.* **104,** 139–146.

Glennemeier, K. A., and Denver, R. J. (2002a). Moderate elevation of corticosterone content affects fitness components in northern leopard frog (*Rana pipiens*) tadpoles. In press.

Glennemeier, K. A., and Denver, R. J. (2002b). Developmental changes in interrenal responsiveness in anuran amphibians. In press.

Glennemeier, K. A., and Denver, R. J. (2002c). A role for corticoids in mediating the response of *Rana pipiens* tadpoles to intraspecific competition. *J. Exp. Zool.* **292,** 32–40.

Gosner, K. L. (1960). A simplified table for staging anuran embryos and larvae with notes on indentification. *Herpetologica* **16,** 183–190.

Gould, S. (1977). "Ontogeny and Phylogeny." Harvard University Press, Cambrige, MA.

Gracia-Navarro, F., Lamacz, M., Tonon, M. C., and Vaudry, H. (1992). Pituitary adenylate cyclase-activating polypeptide stimulates calcium mobilization in amphibian pituitary-cells. *Endocrinology (Baltimore)* **131,** 1069–1074.

Gray, K. M., and Janssens, P. A. (1990). Gonadal hormones inhibit the induction of metamorphosis by thyroid hormones in *Xenopus laevis* tadpoles *in vivo*, but not *in vitro*. *Gen. Comp. Endocrinol.* **77,** 202–211.

Gudernatsch, J. F. (1912). Feeding experiments on tadpoles. I. The influence of specific organs given as food on growth and differentiation. A contribution to the knowledge of organs with internal secretion. *Wilhelm Roux' Arch. Entwicklungsmech. Org.* **35,** 457–483.

Guha, K., and Jorgensen, C. (1978a). Effects of hypophysectomy on structure and function of testis in adult toads, *Bufo bufo bufo* (l.). *Gen. Comp. Endocrinol.* **36,** 201–210.

Guha, K., and Jorgensen, C. (1978b). Effects of human chorionic gonadotropin and salmon gonadotropin on testis in hypsphysectomized toads (*Bufo bufo bufo* l.). *Gen. Comp. Endocrinol.* **36,** 371–379.

Guissouma, H., Ghorbel, M. T., Seugnet, I., Ouatas, T., and Demeneix, B. A. (1998). Physiological regulation of hypothalamic TRH transcription in vivo is T3 receptor isoform specific. *FASEB J.* **12,** 1755–1764.

Gutierrez, P., Delgado, M. J., and Alonsobedate, M. (1984). Influence of photoperiod and melatonin administration on growth and metamorphosis in *Discoglossus pictus* larvae. *Comp. Biochem. Physiol. A* **79,** 255–260.

Hammond, G. L. (1990). Molecular properties of corticosteroid binding globulin and the sex-steroid binding-proteins. *Endocr. Rev.* **11,** 65–79.

Harrington, C. R. (1926). Chemistry of thyroxine. II. Constitution and synthesis of desiodo-thyroxine. *Biochem. J.* **20,** 300.

Harrington, C. R., and Barger, G. (1927). Chemistry of thyroxine. III. Constitution and synthesis of thyroxine. *Biochem. J.* **21,** 169.

Harris, R. N. (1987). Density-dependent paedomorphosis in the salamander *Notophthalmus viridescens dorsalis*. *Ecology* **68,** 705–712.

Harvey, S., Scanes, C. G., and Daughaday, W. H. (1995). "Growth Hormone." CRC Press, Boca Raton, FL.

Hayes, T. B. (1995). Interdependence of corticosterone hormones and thyroid-hormones in larval toads (*Bufo boreas*) .1. Thyroid hormone-dependent and hormone-independent effects of corticosterone on growth and development. *J. Exp. Zool.* **271,** 95–102.

Hayes, T. B. (1997). Steroids as potential modulators of thyroid hormone activity in anuran metamorphosis. *Am. Zool.* **37,** 185–194.

Hayes, T. B. (1998). Sex determination and primary sex differentiation in amphibians: Genetic and developmental mechanisms. *J. Exp. Zool.* **287,** 373–399.

Hayes, T. B., and Licht, P. (1993). Metabolism of exogenous steroids by anuran larvae. *Gen. Comp. Endocrinol.* **91,** 250–258.

Hayes, T. B., and Wu, T. H. (1995). Role of corticosterone in anuran metamorphosis and potential role in stress-induced metamorphosis. *Neth. J. Zool.* **45,** 107–109.

Hayes, T. B., Chan, R., and Licht, P. (1993). Interactions of temperature and steroids on larval growth, development, and metamorphosis in a toad (*Bufo boreas*). *J. Exp. Zool.* **266,** 206–215.

Helbing, C., Gergely, G., and Atkinson, B. G. (1992). Sequential up-regulation of thyroid-hormone beta-receptor, ornithine transcarbamylase, and carbamyl-phosphate synthetase messenger-RNAs in the liver of *Rana catesbeiana* tadpoles during spontaneous and thyroid hormone-induced metamorphosis. *Dev. Genet.* **13,** 289–301.

Hemelaar, A. (1988). Age, growth, and other population characteristics of *Bufo bufo* from different latitudes and altitudes. *J. Herpetol.* **22,** 369–388.

Hennemann, G., Everts, M. E., de Jong, M., Lim, C. F., Krenning, E. P., and Docter, R. (1998). The significance of plasma membrane transport in the bioavailability of thyroid hormone. *Clin. Endocrinol. (Oxford)* **48,** 1–8.

Houck, L. (1982). Growth rates and age at maturity for the plethodontid salamander *Bolitoglossa subpalmata*. *Copeia*, pp. 474–478.

Houseknecht, K. L., Baile, C. A., Matteri, R. L., and Spurlock, M. E. (1998). The biology of leptin: A review. *J. Anim. Sci.* **76,** 1405–1420.

Hsu, C. Y., Yu, N. W., and Chen, S. J. (1980). Development of delta-5-3-beta-hydroxysteroid dehydrogenase activity in the interrenal gland of *Rana catesbeiana*. *Gen. Comp. Endocrinol.* **42**, 167–170.

Huang, H., Marsh-Armstrong, N., and Brown, D. D. (1999). Metamorphosis is inhibited in transgenic *Xenopus laevis* tadpoles that overexpress type III deiodinase. *Proc. Natl. Acad. Sci. U.S.A.* **96**, 962–967.

Huang, H. C., and Brown, D. D. (2000a). Overexpression of *Xenopus laevis* growth hormone stimulates growth of tadpoles and frogs. *Proc. Natl. Acad. Sci. U.S.A.* **97**, 190–194.

Huang, H. C., and Brown, D. D. (2000b). Prolactin is not a juvenile hormone in *Xenopus laevis* metamorphosis. *Proc. Natl. Acad. Sci. U.S.A.* **97**, 195–199.

Jackson, M. E., and Semlitsch, R. D. (1993). Paedomorphosis in the salamander *Ambystoma talpoideum*—effects of a fish predator. *Ecology* **74**, 342.

Jacobs, G. F. M., and Kuhn, E. R. (1987). TRH injection induces thyroxine release in the metamorphosed but not in the neotenic axolotl *Ambystoma mexicanum*. *Gen. Comp. Endocrinol.* **66**, 40.

Jacobs, G. F. M., and Kuhn, E. R. (1988). Luteinizing hormone-releasing hormone induces thyroxine release together with testosterone in the neotenic axolotl *Ambystoma mexicanum*. *Gen. Comp. Endocrinol.* **71**, 502–505.

Jacobs, G. F. M., and Kuhn, E. R. (1992). Thyroid-hormone feedback-regulation of the secretion of bioactive thyrotropin in the frog. *Gen. Comp. Endocrinol.* **88**, 415–423.

Jacobs, G. F. M., Michielsen, R. P., and Kuhn, E. R. (1988a). Thyroxine and triiodothyronine in plasma and thyroids of the neotenic and metamorphosed axolotl *Ambystoma mexicanum*: Influence of TRH injections. *Gen. Comp. Endocrinol.* **70**, 145–151.

Jacobs, G. F. M., Goyvaerts, M. P., Vandorpe, G., Quaghebeur, A. M., and Kuhn, E. R. (1988b). Luteinizing hormone-releasing hormone as a potent stimulator of the thyroidal axis in ranid frogs. *Gen. Comp. Endocrinol.* **70**, 274–283.

Jaffe, R. C. (1981). Plasma concentration of corticosterone during *Rana catesbeiana* tadpole metamorphosis. *Gen. Comp. Endocrinol.* **44**, 314–318.

Jolivet-Jaudet, G., and Leloup-Hatey, J. (1984). Interrenal function during amphibian metamorphosis—in vitro biosynthesis of radioactive corticosteroids from (4c-14) progesterone by interrenal in *Xenopus laevis* tadpoles. *Comp. Biochem. Physiol. B* **79**, 239–244.

Jorgensen, C. B. (1975). Factors controlling the annual ovarian cycle in the toad *Bufo bufo bufo* (l.). *Gen. Comp. Endocrinol.* **25**, 264–273.

Jorgensen, C. B. (1982). Factors controlling the ovarian cycle in a temperate zone anuran, the toad *Bufo bufo*: Food uptake, nutritional state, and gonadotropin. *J Exp. Zool.* **224**, 437–443.

Jorgensen, C. B. (1986a). External and internal control of patterns of feeding, growth and gonadal function in a temperate zone anuran, the toad *Bufo bufo*. *J. Zool.* **210A**, 211–241.

Jorgensen, C. B. (1986b). Effect of fat body excision in female *Bufo bufo* on the ipsilateral ovary, with a discussion of fat body-gonad relationships. *Acta Zool. (Stockholm)* **67**, 5–10.

Jorgensen, C. B. (1992). Growth and reproduction. In "Environmental Physiology of the Amphibians" (M. Feder and W. Burggren, eds.), pp. 439–466. University of Chicago Press, Chicago.

Just, J. J. (1972). Protein-bound iodine and protein concentration in plasma and pericardial fluid of metamorphosing anuran tadpoles. *Physiol. Zool.* **45**, 143–152.

Kaltenbach, J. C. (1996). Endocrinology of amphibian metamorphosis. In "Metamorphosis: Postembryonic Reprogramming of Gene Expression in Amphibian and Insect Cells" (L. I. Gilbert, J. R. Tata, and B. G. Atkinson, eds.), pp. 403–431. Academic Press, San Diego, CA.

Kanamori, A., and Brown, D. D. (1992). The regulation of thyroid hormone receptor beta genes by thyroid hormone in *Xenopus laevis*. *J. Biol. Chem.* **267**, 739–745.

Kang, L., Marin, M., and Kelley, D. (1995). Androgen biosynthesis and secretion in developing *Xenopus laevis*. *Gen. Comp. Endocrinol.* **100**, 293–307.

Kanki, K., and Wakahara, M. (2000). Spatio-temporal expression of TSH beta and FSH beta genes in normally metamorphosing, metamorphosed, and metamorphosis-arrested *Hynobius retardatus*. *Gen. Comp. Endocrinol.* **119**, 276–286.

Kawahara, A., Baker, B. S., and Tata, J. R. (1991). Developmental and regional expression of thyroid-hormone receptor genes during *Xenopus* metamorphosis. *Development (Cambridge, UK)* **112**, 933–943.

Kawahara, A., Gohda, Y., and Hikosaka, A. (1999). Role of type III iodothyronine 5-deiodinase gene expression in temporal regulation of *Xenopus* metamorphosis. *Dev., Growth Differ.* **41**, 365–373.

Kaye, N. W. (1960). The pituitary-thyroid axis in the premetamorphic tadpole. *Anat. Rec.* **137**, 370.

Kaye, N. W. (1961). Interrelationships of the thyroid and pituitary in embryonic and premetamorphic stages of the frog, *Rana pipiens*. *Gen. Comp. Endocrinol.* **1**, 1–19.

Kendall, E. C. (1915). The isolation in crystalline form of the compound which occurs in the thyroid: Its chemical nature and physiologic activity. *JAMA J. Am. Med. Assoc.* **64**, 2042.

Kikuyama, S., Niki, K., Mayumi, M., Shibayama, R., Nishikawa, M., and Shintake, N. (1983). Studies on corticoid action on the toad tadpole tail in vitro. *Gen. Comp. Endocrinol.* **52**, 395–399.

Kikuyama, S., Suzuki, M. R., and Iwamuro, S. (1986). Elevation of plasma aldosterone levels of tadpoles at metamorphic climax. *Gen. Comp. Endocrinol.* **63**, 186–190.

Kikuyama, S., Kawamura, K., Tanaka, S., and Yamamoto, K. (1993). Aspects of amphibian metamorphosis—hormonal control. *Int. Rev. Cytol.* **145**, 105–148.

Kloas, W., Reinecke, M., and Hanke, W. (1997). Stage-dependent changes in adrenal steroids and catecholamines during development in *Xenopus laevis*. *Gen. Comp. Endocrinol.* **108**, 416–426.

Kobayashi, H. (1958). Effect of desoxycorticosterone acetate on metamorphosis induced by thyroxine in anuran tadpoles. *Endocrinology (Baltimore)* **62**, 371–377.

Kobayashi, M., and Iwasawa, H. (1984). Effects of fat body excision on testicular ultrastucture in young frogs of *Rana nigromaculata*. *Zool. Sci.* **1**, 972.

Krenning, E., Docter, R., Bernard, B., Visser, T., and Hennemann, G. (1981). Characteristics of active-transport of thyroid-hormone into rat hepatocytes. *Biochim. Biophys. Acta* **676**, 314–320.

Krenz, J., and Sever, D. (1995). Mating and oviposition in paedomorphic *Ambystoma talpoideum* precedes the arrival of terrestrial males. *Herpetologica* **51**, 387–393.

Krug, E. C., Honn, K. V., Battista, J., and Nicoll, C. S. (1983). Corticosteroids in serum of *Rana catesbeiana* during development and metamorphosis. *Gen. Comp. Endocrinol.* **52**, 232–241.

Kuhn, E. R., Geris, K. L., van der Geyten, S., Mol, K. A., and Darras, V. M. (1998). Inhibition and activation of the thyroidal axis by the adrenal axis in vertebrates. *Comp. Biochem. Physiol. A* **120**, 169–174.

Larras-Regard, E., Taurog, A., and Dorris, M. (1981). Plasma-T4 and plasma-T3 levels in *Ambystoma tigrinum* at various stages of metamorphosis. *Gen. Comp. Endocrinol.* **43**, 443–450.

Larsen, D. A., Swanson, P., Dickey, J. T., Rivier, J., and Dickhoff, W. W. (1998). In vitro thyrotropin-releasing activity of corticotropin-releasing hormone-family peptides in coho salmon, *Oncorhynchus kisutch*. *Gen. Comp. Endocrinol.* **109**, 276–285.

Laurila, A., and Kujasalo, J. (1999). Habitat duration, predation risk and phenotypic plasticity in common frog (*Rana temporaria*) tadpoles. *J. Anim. Ecol.* **68**, 1123–1132.

Lazar, M. A. (1993). Thyroid hormone receptors: Multiple forms, multiple possibilities. *Endocr. Rev.* **14**, 184–193.

Lebel, J. M., L'Herault, S., Dussault, J. H., and Puymirat, J. (1993). Thyroid hormone up-regulates thyroid hormone receptor beta gene expression in rat cerebral hemisphere astrocyte cultures. *Glia* **9**, 105–112.

Leloup, J., and Buscaglia, M. (1977). Triiodothyronine, hormone of amphibian metamorphosis. *C.R. Hebd. Seances Acad. Sci., Ser. D* **284**, 2261–2263.

Leonard, J. L., and Visser, T. J. (1986). Biochemistry of deiodination. *In* "Thyroid Hormone Metabolism" (G. Hennemann, ed.), pp. 189–229. Dekker, New York.

Liang, V. C., Sedgwick, T., and Shi, Y. B. (1997). Characterization of the *Xenopus* homolog of an immediate early gene associated with cell activation: Sequence analysis and regulation of its expression by thyroid hormone during amphibian metamorphosis. *Cell Res.* **7**, 179–193.

Licht, L. E. (1992). The effect of food level on growth rate and frequency of metamorphosis and paedomorphosis in *Ambystoma gracile*. *Can. J. Zool.* **70**, 87–93.

Lindsay, R. H., Buettner, L., Wimberly, N., and Pittman, J. A. (1967). Effects of thyroxine analogs on isolated tadpole tail-tips. *Gen. Comp. Endocrinol.* **9**, 416–421.

Lofts, B. (1974). Reproduction. *In* "Physiology of Amphibia" (B. Lofts, ed.), Vol. 2, pp. 107–218. Academic Press, New York.

Loman, J. (1999). Early metamorphosis in common frog *Rana temporaria* tadpoles at risk of drying: An experimental demonstration. *Amphibia-Reptilia* **20**, 421–430.

Low, B. S. (1976). The evolution of amphibian life histories in the desert. *In* "Evolution of Desert Biota" (D. W. Goodall, ed.), pp. 149–195. University of Texas Press, Austin.

Macchi, I. A., and Phillips, J. G. (1966). In vitro effect of adrenocorticotropin on corticoid secretion in the turtle, snake, and bullfrog. *Gen. Comp. Endocrinol.* **6**, 170–182.

Machuca, I., Esslemont, G., Fairclough, L., and Tata, J. R. (1995). Analysis of structure and expression of the *Xenopus* thyroid-hormone receptor-beta gene to explain its autoinduction. *Mol. Endocrinol.* **9**, 96–107.

Maiorana, V. (1977). Tail autotomy: Functional conflicts and their resolution by a salamander. *Nature (London)* **265**, 533–535.

Mangelsdorf, D. J., and Evans, R. M. (1995). The RXR heterodimers and orphan receptors. *Cell (Cambridge, Mass.)* **83**, 841–850.

Marian, M. P., and Pandian, T. J. (1985). Effect of temperature on development, growth and bioenergetics of the bullfrog tadpole *Rana tigrina*. *J. Therm. Biol.* **10**, 157–161.

Marsh-Armstrong, N., Huang, H. C., Remo, B. F., Liu, T. T., and Brown, D. D. (1999). Asymmetric growth and development of the *Xenopus laevis* retina during metamorphosis is controlled by type III deiodinase. *Neuron* **24**, 871–878.

Matz, S. P., and Hofeldt, G. T. (1999). Immunohistochemical localization of corticotropin-releasing factor in the brain and corticotropin-releasing factor and thyrotropin-stimulating hormone in the pituitary of chinook salmon (*Oncorhynchus tshawytscha*). *Gen. Comp. Endocrinol.* **114**, 151–160.

Mayhew, W. W. (1968). Biology of desert amphibians and reptiles. *In* "Desert Biology" (G. W. Brown, ed.), Vol. 1, pp. 195–356. Academic Press, New York.

McKinney, M. L., and MacNamara, K. J. (1991). "Heterochrony. The Evolution of Neoteny." Plenum Press, New York.

Meeuwis, R., Michielsen, R., Decuypere, E., and Kuhn, E. R. (1989). Thyrotropic activity of the ovine corticotropin-releasing factor in the chick embryo. *Gen. Comp. Endocrinol.* **76**, 357–363.

Mendel, C. M. (1989). The free hormone hypothesis: A physiologically based mathematical model. *Endocr. Rev.* **10**, 232–274.

Merila, J., Laurila, A., Pahkala, M., Rasanen, K., and Laugen, A. T. (2000). Adaptive phenotypic plasticity in timing of metamorphosis in the common frog *Rana temporaria*. *Ecoscience* **7**, 18–24.

Miaud, C., Guyetant, R., and Elmberg, J. (1999). Variations in life-history traits in the common frog *Rana temporaria* (Amphibia: Anura): A literature review and new data from the French Alps. *J. Zool.* **249**, 61–73.

Miaud, C., Guyetant, R., and Faber, H. (2000). Age, size, and growth of the alpine newt, *Triturus alpestris* (Urodela: Salamandridae), at high altitude and a review of life-history trait variation throughout its range. *Herpetologica* **56**, 135–144.

Miranda, L. A., Affanni, J. M., and Paz, D. A. (2000). Corticotropin-releasing factor accelerates metamorphosis in *Bufo arenarum*: Effect on pituitary ACTH and TSH cells. *J. Exp. Zool.* **286**, 473–480.

Miyauchi, H., Larochelle, F. T., Suzuki, M., Freeman, M., and Frieden, E. (1977). Studies on thyroid-hormones and their binding in bullfrog tadpole plasma during metamorphosis. *Gen. Comp. Endocrinol.* **33**, 254–266.

Mondou, P. M., and Kaltenbach, J. C. (1979). Thyroxine concentrations in blood-serum and pericardial fluid of metamorphosing tadpoles and of adult frogs. *Gen. Comp. Endocrinol.* **39**, 343–349.

Morey, S. R., and Janes, D. N. (1994). Variation in larval habitat duration influences metamorphosis in *Scaphiopus couchii*. *In* "Proceedings of the Symposium on Herpetology of the North American Deserts," Spec. Publ. No. 5. Serpent's Tale Books, Excelsior, M.

Morey, S. R., and Reznick, D. (2000). A comparative analysis of plasticity in larval development in three species of spadefoot toads. *Ecology* **81**, 1736–1749.

Moriceau-Hay, D., Doerrschott, J., and Dubois, M. P. (1982). Immunohistochemical demonstration of TSH-cell, LH-cell and ACTH-cell in the hypophysis of tadpoles of *Xenopus laevis* d. *Cell Tissue Res.* **225**, 57–64.

Morley, J. E. (1981). Neuroendocrine control of thyrotropin secretion. *Endocr. Rev.* **2**, 396–436.

Newman, R. A. (1988). Adaptive plasticity in development of *Scaphiopus couchii* tadpoles in desert ponds. *Evolution (Lawrence, Kans.)* **42**, 774–783.

Newman, R. A. (1989). Developmental plasticity of *Scaphiopus couchii* tadpoles in an unpredictable environment. *Ecology* **70**, 1775–1787.

Newman, R. A. (1992). Adaptive plasticity in amphibian metamorphosis. *BioScience* **42**, 671–678.

Newman, R. A. (1994). Effects of changing density and food level on metamorphosis of a desert amphibian, *Scaphiopus couchii*. *Ecology* **75**, 1085–1096.

Newman, R. A. (1998). Ecological constraints on amphibian metamorphosis: Interactions of temperature and larval density with responses to changing food level. *Oecologia* **115**, 9–16.

Nieuwkoop, P. D., and Faber, J. (1956). "Normal Table of *Xenopus laevis* Daudin." North-Holland Publ. Amsterdam.

Niewiarowski, P. H., Balk, M. L., and Londraville, R. L. (2000). Phenotypic effects of leptin in an ectotherm: A new tool to study the evolution of life-histories and endothermy. *J. Exp. Biol.* **203**, 295–300.

Niinuma, K., Mamiya, N., Yamamoto, K., Iwamuro, S., Vaudry, H., and Kikuyama, S. (1989). Plasma concentrations of aldosterone and prolactin in *Bufo japonicus* tadpoles during metamorphosis. *Bull. Sci. Eng. Res. Lab., Waseda Univ.* **122**, 17–21.

Niinuma, K., Yamamoto, K., and Kikuyama, S. (1991a). Changes in plasma and pituitary prolactin levels in toad (*Bufo japonicus*) larvae during metamorphosis. *Zool. Sci.* **8**, 97–101.

Niinuma, K., Tagawa, M., Hirano, T., and Kikuyama, S. (1991b). Changes in tissue concentrations of thyroid-hormones in metamorphosing toad larvae. *Zool. Sci.* **8**, 345–350.

Niki, K., Yoshizato, K., and Kikuyama, S. (1981). Augmentation of nuclear-binding capacity for triiodothyronine by aldosterone in tadpole tail. *Proc. Jpn. Acad., Ser. B* **57**, 271–275.

Noble, C. K., and Putnam, P. G. (1931). Observations on the life history of *Ascaphus truei* stejneger. *Copeia*, pp. 97–101.

Norris, D. O. (1978). Hormonal and environmental factors involved in the determination of neoteny in urodeles. *In* "Comparative Endocrinology" (P. Gallard and H. Boer, eds.), pp. 109–112. Elsevier/North-Holland Biomedical Press, Amsterdam.

Norris, D. O., and Dent, J. N. (1989). Neuroendocrine aspects of amphibian metamorphosis. *In* "Development, Maturation and Senescence of Neuroendocrine Systems: A Comparative Approach" (C. G. Scanes and M. P. Schreibman, eds.), pp. 63–90. Academic Press, San Diego, CA.

Norris, D. O., and Gern, W. A. (1976). Thyroxine-induced activation of hypothalamo-hypophysial axis in neotenic salamander larvae. *Science* **194**, 525–527.

Norris, D. O., and Platt, J. E. (1974). T3- and T4-induced rates of metamorphosis in immature and sexually mature larvae of *Ambystoma tigrinum* (Amphibia: Caudata). *J. Exp. Zool.* **189**, 303–310.

Norris, D. O., Jones, R. E., and Cohen, D. C. (1973). Effects of mammalian gonadotropins (LH, FSH, hCG) and gonadal steroids on TSH-induced metamorphosis of *Ambystoma tigrinum* (Amphibia: Caudata). *Gen. Comp. Endocrinol.* **20**, 467–473.

Norris, D. O., Austin, H. B., and Hijazi, A. S. (1989). Induction of cloacal and dermal skin glands of tiger salamander larvae (*Ambystoma tigrinum*): Effects of testosterone and prolactin. *Gen. Comp. Endocrinol.* **73**, 194–204.

Okada, R., Iwata, T., Kato, T., Kikuchi, M., Yamamoto, K., and Kikuyama, S. (2000). Cloning of bullfrog thyroid-stimulating hormone (TSH) beta subunit cDNA: Expression of TSH beta mRNA during metamorphosis. *Gen. Comp. Endocrinol.* **119**, 224–231.

Oppenheimer, J. H., Schwartz, H. L., and Strait, K. A. (1995). An integrated view of thyroid hormone actions *in vivo*. In "Molecular Endocrinology: Basic Concepts and Clinical Correlations" (B. D. Weintraub, ed.), pp. 249–268. Raven Press, New York.

Orchinik, M., Matthews, L., and Gasser, P. J. (2000). Distinct specificity for corticosteroid binding sites in amphibian cytosol, neuronal membranes, and plasma. *Gen. Comp. Endocrinol.* **118**, 284–301.

Pancharatna, K., and Saidapur, S. (1992). A study of ovarian follicular kinetics, oviduct, fat-body, and liver mass cycles in laboratory-maintained *Rana cyanophlyctis* in comparison with wild-caught frogs. *J. Morphol.* **214**, 123.

Parris, M. J. (2000). Experimental analysis of hybridization in leopard frogs (Anura: Ranidae): Larval performance in desiccating environments. *Copeia* **2000**, 11–19.

Pierantoni, R., Varriale, B., Simeoli, C., Di Matteo, L., Milone, M., Rastogi, R., and Chieffi, G. (1983). Fat body and autumn recrudescence of the ovary in *Rana esculenta*. *Comp. Biochem. Physiol. A* **76A**, 31–35.

Pierce, J. G., and Parsons, T. F. (1981). Glycoprotein hormones—structure and function. *Annu. Rev. Biochem.* **50**, 465–495.

Power, D. M., Elias, N. P., Richardson, S. J., Mendes, J., Soares, C. M., and Santos, C. R. A. (2000). Evolution of the thyroid hormone-binding protein, transthyretin. *Gen. Comp. Endocrinol.* **119**, 241–255.

Pratt, W. B., and Toft, D. O. (1997). Steroid receptor interactions with heat shock protein and immunophilin chaperones. *Endocr. Rev.* **18**, 306–360.

Puzianowska-Kuznicka, M., Damjanovski, S., and Shi, Y. B. (1997). Both thyroid hormone and 9-cis retinoic acid receptors are required to efficiently mediate the effects of thyroid hormone on embryonic development and specific gene regulation in *Xenopus laevis*. *Mol. Cell. Biol.* **17**, 4738–4749.

Rabelo, E. M. L., and Tata, J. R. (1997). Prolactin inhibits auto- and cross-induction of thyroid hormone and estrogen receptor and vitellogenin genes in adult *Xenopus* (Amphibia) hepatocytes. *Braz. J. Genet.* **20**, 619–624.

Ranjan, M., Wong, J., and Shi, Y. B. (1994). Transcriptional repression of *Xenopus* TR beta gene is mediated by a thyroid hormone response element located near the start site. *J. Biol. Chem.* **269**, 24699–24705.

Rao, G. S., Eckel, J., Rao, M. L., and Breuer, H. (1976). Uptake of thyroid-hormone by isolated rat-liver cells. *Biochem. Biophys. Res. Commun.* **73**, 98–104.

Regard, E., and Mauchamp, J. (1971). Ultrastructure of thyroid gland of normal and hypophysectomized larval *Xenopus*—correlation with biosynthesis of thyroglobulin. *J. Ultrastruct. Res.* **37**, 664–678.

Regard, E., and Mauchamp, J. (1973). Peroxidase activity in *Xenopus* thyroid gland through larval development—correlation with iodide organification and thyrotropic control. *J. Microsc. (Oxford)* **18**, 291–306.

Regard, E., Taurog, A., and Nakashima, T. (1978). Plasma thyroxine and triiodothyronine levels in spontaneously metamorphosing *Rana catesbeiana* tadpoles and in adult anuran amphibia. *Endocrinology (Baltimore)* **102**, 674–684.

Reichlin, S. (1989). TRH—historical aspects. *Ann. N.Y. Acad. Sci.* **553**, 1–6.

Reilly, S. M., Wiley, E. O., and Meinhardt, D. J. (1997). An integrative approach to heterochrony: The distinction between interspecific and intraspecific phenomena. *Biol. J. Linn. Soc.* **60**, 119–143.

Ritchie, J. W. A., Peter, G. J., Shi, Y. B., and Taylor, P. M. (1999). Thyroid hormone transport by 4f2hc-iu12 heterodimers express in *Xenopus* oocytes. *J. Endocrinol.* **163**, R5–R9.

Rivier, C., and Rivest, S. (1991). Effect of stress on the activity of the hypothalamic-pituitary-gonadal axis: Peripheral and central mechanisms. *Biol. Reprod.* **45**, 523–532.

Rivier, C., Rivier, J., and Vale, W. (1986). Stress-induced inhibition of reproductive functions: Role of endogenous corticotropin-releasing factor. *Science* **231**, 607–609.

Roff, D. A. (1992). "The Evolution of Life Histories." Chapman & Hall, New York.

Rose, F. (1968). Seasonal changes in lipid levels of the salamander *Amphiuma means*. *Copeia* **1967**, 662–666.

Rosenkilde, P. (1978). Thyroid-hormone synthesis in metamorphosing and adult *Xenopus laevis*. *Gen. Comp. Endocrinol.* **34**, 95–96.

Rosenkilde, P., and Ussing, A. P. (1996). What mechanisms control neoteny and regulate induced metamorphosis in urodeles? *Int. J. Dev. Biol.* **40**, 665–673.

Rosner, W. (1990). The functions of corticosteroid-binding globulin and sex hormone-binding globulin—recent advances. *Endocr. Rev.* **11**, 80–91.

Rowe, C. L., and Dunson, W. A. (1995). Impacts of hydroperiod on growth and survival of larval amphibians in temporary ponds of central Pennsylvania, USA. *Oecologia* **102**, 397–403.

Ryan, T., and Semlitsch, R. (1998). Intraspecific heterochrony and life history evolution: Decoupling somatic and sexual development in a facultatively paedomorphic salamander. *Proc. Natl. Acad. Sci. U.S.A* **95**, 5643–5648.

Saez, J. M., Morera, A. M., Haour, F., and Evain, D. (1977). Effects of *in vivo* administration of dexamethasone, corticotropin and human chorionic gonadotropin on steroidogenesis and protein and DNA synthesis of testicular interstitial cells in prepuberal rats. *Endocrinology (Baltimore)* **101**, 1256–1263.

Safi, R., Begue, A., Hanni, C., Stehelin, D., Tata, J. R., and Laudet, V. (1997). Thyroid hormone receptor genes of neotenic amphibians. *J. Mol. Evol.* **44**, 595–604.

Sandhofer, C., Schwartz, H. L., Mariash, C. N., Forrest, D., and Oppenheimer, J. H. (1998). Beta receptor isoforms are not essential for thyroid hormone dependent acceleration of pcp-2 and myelin basic protein gene expression in the developing brains of neonatal mice. *Mol. Cell. Endocrinol.* **137**, 109–115.

Sapolsky, R. M., Romero, L. M., and Munck, A. U. (2000). How do glucocorticoids influence stress responses? Integrating permissive, suppressive, stimulatory, and preparative actions. *Endocr. Rev.* **21**, 55–89.

Saxén, L., Saxén, E., Toivonen, S., and Salimaki, K. (1957a). The anterior pituitary and the thyroid function during normal and abnormal development of the frog. *Ann. Zool. Soc. Zool. Bot. Fenn. Vanamo* **18**, 1–44.

Saxén, L., Saxén, E., Toivonen, S., and Salimaki, K. (1957b). Quantitative investigation on the anterior pituitary-thyroid mechanism during frog metamorphosis. *Endocrinology (Baltimore)* **61**, 35–44.

Schneider, M. J., and Galton, V. A. (1991). Regulation of c-erba-alpha messenger-RNA species in tadpole erythrocytes by thyroid-hormone. *Mol. Endocrinol.* **5**, 201–208.

Schultheiss, H. (1980). Isolation of pituitary proteins from Mexican axolotls, *Ambystoma mexicanum*, by polyacrylamide gel electrophoresis. 1. Assay for thyrotropic activity. *J. Exp. Zool.* **213**, 351–358.

Schussler, G. C. (2000). The thyroxine-binding proteins. *Thyroid* **10**, 141–149.

Scott, D. E., and Fore, M. (1995). The effect of food limitation on lipid levels, growth, and reproduction in the marbled salamander, *Ambystoma opacum*. *Herpetologica* **51**, 462.

Scott, D. E. (1990). Effects of larval density in *Ambystoma opacum*—an experiment in large scale field enclosures. *Ecology* **71**, 296–306.

Scott, D. E. (1993). Timing of reproduction of paedomorphic and metamorphic *Ambystoma talpoideum*. *Am. Midl. Nat.* **129**, 397–402.

Scott, D. E. (1994). The effect of larval density on adult demographic traits in *Ambystoma opacum*. *Ecology* **75**, 1383–1396.

Selye, H. (1976). "The Stress of Life." Mcgraw-Hill, New York.

Semlitsch, R. D., Scott, D. G., and Pechmann, J. H. K. (1988). Time and size at metamorphosis related to adult fitness in *Ambystoma talpoideum*. *Ecology* **69**, 184–192.

Semlitsch, R. D. (1985). Reproductive strategy of a facultatively paedomorphic salamander *Ambystoma talpoideum*. *Oecologia* **65**, 305–313.

Semlitsch, R. D. (1987a). Paedomorphosis in *Ambystoma talpoideum*: Effects of density, food, and pond drying. *Ecology* **68**, 994–1002.

Semlitsch, R. D. (1987b). Density-dependent growth and fecundity in the paedomorphic salamander *Ambystoma talpoideum*. *Ecology* **68**, 1003–1008.

Semlitsch, R. D., and Gibbons, J. W. (1985). Phenotypic variation in metamorphosis and paedomorphosis in the salamander *Ambystoma talpoideum*. *Ecology* **66**, 1123–1130.

Semlitsch, R. D., and Wilbur, H. M. (1998). Effects of pond drying time on metamorphosis and survival in the salamander. *Copeia* **1988**, 978–983.

Shi, Y. B. (1996). Thyroid hormone-regulated early and late genes during amphibian metamorphosis. *In* "Metamorphosis: Postembryonic Reprogramming of Gene Expression in Amphibian and Insect Cells" (L. I. Gilbert, J. R. Tata, and B. G. Atkinson, eds.), pp. 505–538. Academic Press, San Diego, CA.

Shi, Y. B. (2000). "Amphibian Metamorphosis. From Morphology to Molecular Biology." Wiley-Liss, New York.

Shi, Y. B., and Brown, D. D. (1993). The earliest changes in gene expression in tadpole intestine induced by thyroid hormone. *J. Biol. Chem.* **268**, 20312–20317.

Shi, Y. B., Liang, V. C., Parkison, C., and Cheng, S. Y. (1994). Tissue-dependent developmental expression of a cytosolic thyroid hormone protein gene in *Xenopus*: Its role in the regulation of amphibian metamorphosis. *FEBS Lett.* **355**, 61–64.

Shi, Y. B., Wong, J., Puzianowska-Kuznicka, M., and Stolow, M. A. (1996). Tadpole competence and tissue-specific temporal regulation of amphibian metamorphosis: Roles of thyroid hormone and its receptors. *BioEssays* **18**, 391–399.

Shumway, W. (1940). Stages in the normal development of *Rana pipiens*. *Anat. Rec.* **78**, 139–144.

Smith, D. C. (1983). Factors controlling tadpole populations of the chorus frog (*Pseudacris triseriata*) on Isle Royale, Michigan. *Ecology* **64**, 501–510.

Smith, D. C. (1987). Adult recruitment in chorus frogs: Effects of size and date at metamorphosis. *Ecology* **68**, 344–350.

Smith, R. (1998). Alterations in the hypothalamic pituitary adrenal axis during pregnancy and the placental clock that determines the length of parturition. *J. Reprod. Immunol.* **39,** 215–220.

Spieler, M. (2000). Developmental plasticity and behavioural adaptations of two West African anurans living in an unpredictable environment (Amphibia, Anura). *Bonn. Zool. Monogr.* **46,** 109–120.

Sredl, M., and Collins, J. (1992). The interaction of predation, competition, and habitat complexity in structuring an amphibian community. *Copeia,* pp. 607–614.

Stearns, S. C. (1989). The evolutionary significance of phenotypic plasticity. *BioScience* **39,** 436–445.

Stearns, S. C. (1991). "The Evolution of Life Histories." Oxford University Press, New York.

Stebbins, R. C. (1951). "Amphibians in Western North America." University of California Press, Berkeley.

Stewart, M. M. (1967). "Amphibians of Malawi." State University of New York Press, Albany.

St. Germain, D. L. (1994). Iodothyronine deiodinases. *Trends Endocrinol. Metab.* **5,** 36–42.

St. Germain, D. L., and Galton, V. A. (1997). The deiodinase family of selenoproteins. *Thyroid* **7,** 655–668.

St. Germain, D. L., Schwartzman, R. A., Croteau, W., Kanamori, A., Wang, Z., Brown, D. D., and Galton, V. A. (1994). A thyroid hormone-regulated gene in *Xenopus laevis* encodes a type III iodothyronine 5-deiodinase. *Proc. Natl. Acad. Sci. U.S.A.* **91,** 7767–7771.

Suter, D. E., and Schwartz, M. (1985). Effects of glucocorticoids on responsiveness of luteinizing hormone and follicle-stimulating hormone to gonadotropin-releasing hormone by male rat pituitary cells *in vitro. Endocrinology (Baltimore)* **117,** 855–859.

Suzuki, M. R., and Kikuyama, S. (1983). Corticoids augment nuclear-binding capacity for triiodothyronine in bullfrog tadpole tail fins. *Gen. Comp. Endocrinol.* **52,** 272–278.

Suzuki, S., and Suzuki, M. (1981). Changes in thyroidal and plasma iodine compounds during and after metamorphosis of the bullfrog, *Rana catesbeiana. Gen. Comp. Endocrinol.* **45,** 74–81.

Takahashi, N., Yoshihama, K., Kikuyama, S., Yamamoto, K., Wakabayashi, K., and Kato, Y. (1990). Molecular cloning and nucleotide sequence analysis of complementary DNA for bullfrog prolactin. *J. Mol. Endocrinol.* **5,** 281–287.

Tanaka, S., Sakai, M., Park, M. K., and Kurosumi, K. (1991). Differential appearance of the subunits of glycoprotein hormones (LH, FSH, and TSH) in the pituitary of bullfrog (*Rana catesbeiana*) larvae during metamorphosis. *Gen. Comp. Endocrinol.* **84,** 318–327.

Tata, J. R. (1968). Early metamorphic competence of *Xenopus* larvae. *Dev. Biol.* **18,** 415–440.

Tata, J. R., Baker, B. S., Machuca, I., Rabelo, E. M. L., and Yamauchi, K. (1993). Autoinduction of nuclear receptor genes and its significance. *J. Steroid Biochem. Mol. Biol.* **46,** 105–119.

Taylor, A. C., and Kollros, J. J. (1946). Stages in the normal development of *Rana pipiens* larvae. *Anat. Rec.* **94,** 7–23.

Taylor, B., and Scott, D. (1997). Effects of larval density dependence on population dynamics of *Ambystoma opacum. Herpetologica* **53,** 132–145.

Tiley, S. G. (1980). Life histories and comparative demography of two salamander populations. *Copeia,* pp. 806–821.

Tonon, M. C., Cuet, P., Lamacz, M., Jegou, S., Cote, J., Gouteaux, L., Ling, N., Pelletier, G., and Vaudry, H. (1986). Comparative effects of corticotropin-releasing factor, arginine vasopressin, and related neuropeptides on the secretion of ACTH and alpha-MSH by frog anterior pituitary cells and neurointermediate lobes in vitro. *Gen. Comp. Endocrinol.* **61,** 438–445.

Torrents, D., Estevez, R., Pineda, M., Fernandez, E., Lloberas, J., Shi, Y. B., Zorzano, A., and Palacin, M. (1998). Identification and characterization of a membrane protein (y(+)L amino acid transporter-1) that associates with 4f2hc to encode the amino acid transport activity y(+)L-A candidate gene for lysinuric protein intolerance. *J. Biol. Chem.* **273,** 32437–32445.

Turnbull, A. V., and Rivier, C. (1997). Corticotropin-releasing factor (CRF) and endocrine responses to stress: CRF receptors, binding protein, and related peptides. *Proc. Soc. Exp. Biol. Med.* **215,** 1–10.

Ulisse, S., Fabbri, A., and Dufau, M. L. (1989). Corticotropin-releasing factor receptors and action in rat Leydig cells. *J. Biol. Chem.* **264,** 2156–2163.

Vale, W., Speiss, J., Rivier, C., and Rivier, J. (1981). Characterization of a 41-amino acid residue ovine hypothalamic peptide that stimulates the secretion of corticotropin and b-endorphin. *Science* **213,** 1394–1397.

Vale, W., Vaughan, J., and Perrin, M. (1997). Corticotropin-releasing factor (CRF) family of ligands and their receptors. *Endocrinologist* **7,** S3–S9.

Valverde, R. A., Seasholtz, A. F., Cortright, D. N., and Denver, R. J. (2001). Biochemical characterization and expression analysis of the Xenopus laevis corticotropin-releasing hormone binding protein. *Mol. Cell. Endocrinol.* **173,** 29–40.

Wager, V. A. (1965). "The Frogs of South Africa." Purnell & Sons, Capetown.

Wahlborg, A., Bright, C., and Frieden, E. (1964). Activity of some new triiodothyronine analogs in tadpole. *Endocrinology (Baltimore)* **75,** 561–566.

Wakahara, M. (1994). Spermatogenesis is extraordinarily accelerated in metamorphosis-arrested larvae of a salamander, *Hynobius retardatus. Experientia* **50,** 94–98.

Wakahara, M. (1996). Heterochrony and neotenic salamanders: Possible clues for understanding the animal development and evolution. *Zool. Sci.* **13**, 765–776.

Wang, Z., and Brown, D. D. (1993). Thyroid hormone-induced gene expression program for amphibian tail resorption. *J. Biol. Chem.* **268**, 16270–16278.

Wassersug, R. J., and Seibert, E. A. (1975). Behavioral-responses of amphibian larvae to variation in dissolved-oxygen. *Copeia*, pp. 87–103.

Wauters, M., Considine, R. V., and Van Gaal, L. F. (2000). Human leptin: From an adipocyte hormone to an endocrine mediator. *Eur. J. Endocrinol.* **143**, 293–311.

Weber, G. M., Farrar, E. S., Tom, C. K. F., and Grau, E. G. (1994). Changes in whole-body thyroxine and triiodothyronine concentrations and total content during early development and metamorphosis of the toad *Bufo marinus*. *Gen. Comp. Endocrinol.* **94**, 62–71.

Weil, M. R. (1986). Changes in plasma thyroxine levels during and after spontaneous metamorphosis in a natural population of the green frog, *Rana clamitans*. *Gen. Comp. Endocrinol.* **62**, 8–12.

Werner, E. E. (1986). Amphibian metamorphosis—growth-rate, predation risk, and the optimal size at transformation. *Am. Nat.* **128**, 319–341.

White, B. A., and Nicoll, C. S. (1979). Prolactin receptors in *Rana catesbeiana* during development and metamorphosis. *Science* **204**, 851–853.

White, B. A., and Nicoll, C. S. (1981). Hormonal control of amphibian metamorphosis. *In* "Metamorphosis: A Problem in Developmental Biology" (L. I. Gilbert and E. Frieden, eds.), pp. 363–396. Plenum Press, New York.

Whiteman, H. H. (1994). Evolution of facultative paedomorphosis in salamanders. *Q. Rev. Biol.* **69**, 205–221.

Whiteman, H. H., Wissinger, S. A., and Brown, W. (1996). Growth and foraging consequences of facultative paedomorphosis in the tiger salamander, *Ambystoma tigrinum nebulosum*. *Evol. Ecol.* **10**, 433–446.

Wilbur, H. M. (1976). Density dependent aspects of metamorphosis in *Ambystoma* and *Rana sylvatica*. *Ecology* **57**, 1289–1296.

Wilbur, H. M. (1977). Density dependent aspects of growth and metamorphosis in *Bufo americanus*. *Ecology* **58**, 196–200.

Wilbur, H. M. (1980). Complex life-cycles. *Annu. Rev. Ecol. Syst.* **11**, 67–93.

Wilbur, H. M. (1987). Regulation of structure in complex-systems—experimental temporary pond communities. *Ecology* **68**, 1437–1452.

Wilbur, H. M., and Collins, J. P. (1973). Ecological aspects of amphibian metamorphosis. *Science* **182**, 1305–1314.

Williams, G. R., and Brent, G. A. (1995). Thyroid hormone response elements. *In* "Molecular Endocrinology: Basic Concepts and Clinical Correlations" (B. D. Weintraub, ed.), pp. 217–239. Raven Press, Bethesda, MD.

Wong, J. M., and Shi, Y. B. (1995). Coordinated regulation of and transcriptional activation by *Xenopus* thyroid-hormone and retinoid-X-receptors. *J. Biol. Chem.* **270**, 18479–18483.

Wright, M. L., Frim, E. K., Bonak, V. A., and Baril, C. (1986). Metamorphic rate in *Rana pipiens* larvae treated with thyroxine or prolactin at different times in the light/dark cycle. *Gen. Comp. Endocrinol.* **63**, 51–61.

Wright, M. L., Cykowski, L. J., Lundrigan, L., Hemond, K. L., Kochan, D. M., Faszewski, E. E., and Anuszewski, C. M. (1994). Anterior-pituitary and adrenal-cortical hormones accelerate or inhibit tadpole hindlimb growth and development depending on stage of spontaneous development or thyroxine concentration in induced metamorphosis. *J. Exp. Zool.* **270**, 175–188.

Wu, Y. F., and Koenig, R. J. (2000). Gene regulation by thyroid hormone. *Trends Endocrinol. Metab.* **11**, 207–211.

Yamamoto, K., and Kikuyama, S. (1982). Radioimmunoassay of prolactin in plasma of bullfrog tadpoles. *Endocrinol. Jpn.* **29**, 159–167.

Yamauchi, K., and Tata, J. R. (1994). Purification and characterization of a cytosolic thyroid-hormone-binding protein (ctbp) in *Xenopus* liver. *Eur. J. Biochem.* **225**, 1105–1112.

Yamauchi, K., Yamamoto, T., Hayashi, H., Koya, S., Takikawa, H., Toyoshima, K., and Horiuchi, R. (1987). Sequence of membrane-associated thyroid-hormone binding-protein from bovine liver—its identity with protein disulfide isomerase. *Biochem. Biophys. Res. Commun.* **146**, 1485–1492.

Yamauchi, K., Horiuchi, R., Koya, S., and Takikawa, H. (1989). Uptake of 3,5,3′-L-triiodothyronine into bullfrog red blood cells mediated by plasma membrane binding sites. *Zool. Sci.* **6**, 749–755.

Yamauchi, K., Kasahara, T., Hayashi, H., and Horiuchi, R. (1993). Purification and characterization of a 3,5,3′-L-triiodothyronine-specific binding-protein from bullfrog tadpole plasma—a homolog of mammalian transthyretin. *Endocrinology (Baltimore)* **132**, 2254–2261.

Yamauchi, K., Takeuchi, H., Overall, M., Dziadek, M., Munro, S. L. A., and Schreiber, G. (1998). Structural characteristics of bullfrog (*Rana catesbeiana*) transthyretin and its cDNA—comparison of its pattern of expression during metamorphosis with that of lipocalin. *Eur. J. Biochem.* **256**, 287–296.

Yamauchi, K., Nakajima, J., Hayashi, H., and Hara, A. (1999). Purification and characterization of thyroid-hormone-binding protein from masu salmon serum—a homolog of higher-vertebrate transthyretin. *Eur. J. Biochem.* **265**, 944–949.

Yamauchi, K., Prapunpoj, P., and Richardson, S. J. (2000). Effect of diethylstilbestrol on thyroid hormone binding to amphibian transthyretins. *Gen. Comp. Endocrinol.* **119**, 329–339.

Yaoita, Y., and Brown, D. D. (1990). A correlation of thyroid hormone receptor gene expression with amphibian metamorphosis. *Genes Dev.* **4**, 1917–1924.

Yaoita, Y., Shi, Y. B., and Brown, D. D. (1990). *Xenopus laevis* alpha and beta thyroid hormone receptors. *Proc. Natl. Acad. Sci. U.S.A.* **87**, 7090–7094.

Zhou, Y., Samson, M., Francon, J., and Blondeau, J. P. (1992). Thyroid hormone concentrative uptake in rat erythrocytes. *Biochem. J.* **281**, 81–86.

Zhu, X. G., Kaneshige, M., Parlow, A. F., Chen, E., Hunziker, R. D., McDonald, M. P., and Cheng, S. Y. (1999). Expression of the mutant thyroid hormone receptor PV in the pituitary of transgenic mice leads to weight reduction. *Thyroid* **9**, 1137–1145.

29

Sensorimotor Processing Model: How Vasotocin and Corticosterone Interact and Control Reproductive Behaviors in an Amphibian

Frank L. Moore
Department of Zoology
Oregon State University
Corvallis, Oregon 97331-2914

James D. Rose
Departments of Psychology and Zoology-Physiology
University of Wyoming
Laramie, Wyoming 82071

This chapter reviews research on amphibians, focusing on questions about the hormonal mechanisms that regulate reproductive behaviors. In the roughskin newt (*Taricha granulosa*) and other amphibians, reproductive behaviors are activated and maintained by the usual set of sex steroid hormones—testosterone, 5α-dihydrotestosterone, and 17β-estradiol. Sex steroids appear to act on the brain and activate reproductive behaviors, at least in part by stimulating the synthesis of arginine vasotocin (AVT) in specific neurons. AVT is a behaviorally active peptide that can enhance specific behaviors in amphibians (female sexual receptivity and egg-laying behaviors; male frog calling and courtship behaviors). Behavioral and neurophysiological studies reveal that AVT modulates behaviors in *Taricha* by acting on neuronal pathways associated with sensorimotor processing, not by acting on the animal's general state of arousal. When animals perceive harsh or life-threatening conditions, hormones in the stress axis typically suppress reproductive behaviors. In *Taricha*, corticosterone (CORT) rapidly inhibits male courtship by nongenomic mechanisms that use a membrane-associated corticosteroid receptor (mCR). This mCR appears to be a member of the G-protein-coupled receptor superfamily and has similarities to kappa opioid-like receptors. Neurophysiological recordings in medullary neurons show that CORT rapidly depresses spontaneous and stimulus-coupled neuronal activity and provide strong evidence that the behavioral effects of CORT involve the modulation of sensorimotor processing. Other studies in *Taricha* reveal that the propensity to exhibit courtship is affected by context-dependent interactions between AVT and CORT. We conclude that the hormonal control of amphibian reproductive behavior operates in diverse ways that depend on the specific neural subsystem affected (e.g., tectal, reticulospinal, or intraspinal), as well as concurrent interactions between steroids and neuropeptides in a subsystem.

I. INTRODUCTION

In the wild, animals usually perform courtship and mating behaviors during specific seasons and in species-specific contexts, typically when conspecific males and females are in breeding condition and when environmental conditions are favorable and appropriate. There is considerable complexity in the external and internal cues affecting courtship and mating behaviors and, as a result, considerable complexity in the hormonal regulation of these behaviors. Hormones control the development of sex- and species-specific neural circuitry and sexual structures bring the animals into breeding condition at the appropriate season and regulate the animals' behavioral state in response to the immediate environmental conditions. These hormonal mechanisms include stimulatory and inhibitory pathways that control when animals are ready and able to initiate courtship with prospective partners and to mate successfully.

Steroid hormones secreted by the gonads regulate the developmental and seasonal changes in the animals' breeding condition. In addition, there are short-term changes in behavioral state that influence whether an animal courts and mates in a particular time and place. These short-term changes are enhanced by certain hormones such as arginine vasotocin (AVT) and gonadotropin-releasing hormone (GnRH) and suppressed by other hormones such as corticosterone (CORT), corticotropin-releasing hormone (CRH), and the opioid peptides. The various hormones interact to enhance or suppress the longer-term development of the animals' reproductive state and the shorter-term modulation of the animals' behavioral responses to specific sexual stimuli.

These complex regulatory mechanisms have been studied using a wide variety of vertebrates, but this chapter focuses on research into the control of male reproductive behaviors in amphibians and emphasizes our research on the roughskin newt (*Taricha granulosa*, Family Salamandridae, Superfamily Salamandroidea, Order Caudata, Class Amphibia). Although the chapter emphasizes amphibians, these findings pertain to other vertebrates because many of the endocrine mechanisms, neural pathways, and hormonal interactions are similar. In fact, it has become increasing clear that, despite the diversity in reproductive behaviors and mating systems among species, the hormonal mechanisms that control reproductive behaviors are evolutionarily conserved.

Because of the following features, the roughskin newt is a particularly useful model for investigating the hormonal control of behaviors. Unlike many field-collected amphibians, *T. granulosa* reliably performs reproductive behaviors in the laboratory and under experimental conditions. These reproductive behaviors are highly stereotyped and are expressed readily during daylight hours and over an extended breeding season. The distinct seasonal cycles of reproduction in *Taricha* provide opportunities to run natural experiments. There also are a large number of individuals in the breeding ponds in the vicinity of the laboratory and collecting a sufficient number of animals for the experiments is not difficult and does not appear to affect the natural populations. Unlike other tetrapods, amphibians have no cortical structures in the brain (cerebral cortex or neocortex), which means that higher-brain processes are absent and probably explains why its behavioral responses are so sensitive to hormonal manipulations. Last, the same repertoire of chemical messengers act on homologous neuroanatomical pathways to modulate reproductive behaviors and stress responses in this amphibian and other vertebrates.

II. NEWT REPRODUCTIVE BEHAVIORS

The term "newt" refers to salamanders that are members of the family Salamandridae. The types of newts that have been most studied by comparative endocrinologists are *Cynops pyrrhogaster* and *C. ensicauda* (Japan), *Taricha granulosa* and *Notophthalmus viridescens* (North America), and *Triturus carnifex* and *T. alpestris* (Europe). These four genera have been geographically isolated for many thousands of years, probably dating back to when newts crossed an early Bering land bridge into North America. Despite this isolation, these genera have many similarities in their reproductive behaviors and hormonal control mechanisms, as described later.

Newts conduct courtship and mating behaviors in the water. The most pronounced behaviors that mark the onset of the breeding season occur when the newts migrate into breeding ponds. The migratory behaviors and the preference to stay in the water, rather than on land, are controlled by prolactin (PRL). In fact, an early bioassay for PRL was the red eft water drive (Grant and Grant, 1956). Subsequent studies confirmed that injecting newts with purified PRL enhances their preference to remain in water (Moore et al., 1978; Moriya and Dent, 1986) and administering antiserum against PRL to newts during the breeding season reduces their preference for the water (Toyoda et al., 1996). In most wild populations, males typically enter the breeding ponds first and wait for females to arrive. Breeding males develop species-specific secondary sexual structures, such as enlarged tail fins, cornified epithelium on the underside of the limbs and toes (nuptial pads), enlarged abdominal and lateral glands in the cloaca, and mental or hedonic glands on the chin and head. These secondary sexual structures in male newts apparently are regulated by elevated levels of circulating androgens and PRL (Moore et al., 1978; Mazzi and Vellano, 1987; Iwata et al., 2000).

Reproductive behaviors in newts can be divided into three distinct behavioral stages—preinsemination, insemination, and postinsemination (Salthe, 1967; Halliday, 1977; Verrell, 1982; Propper, 1991). There are, of course, species-specific differences in the behaviors among the newts, but there are many similarities as well.

A. Preinsemination Behaviors and Sexual Stimuli

Preinsemination behaviors include the preparatory courtship behaviors that lead up to the behaviors associated with sperm transfer and actual mating. Courtship in newts is initiated after a male is attracted to and recognizes another salamander as a prospective mate. The initial attraction of males to female newts involves visual cues such as the size, shape, color, and movements of the females (Roth, 1987; Thompson and Moore, 2000). After the initial sexual recognition, males use olfactory cues that are released by females. Male newts respond behaviorally to this pheromone and appear to use it to identify prospective mates and assess the female's reproductive state and sexual attractivity. In *Taricha*, the pheromone is relatively insoluble and seems to be detected by male olfactory investigation of the female's skin near the cloaca. Male *Taricha* respond to the pheromone by capturing the female with a highly stereotyped dorsal amplectic clasp (Thompson et al., 1999). Other newts also appear to use chemical cues to signal female sexual attractivity. In *Cynops*, combined treatment of females with 17β-estradiol (E_2) and PRL enhances the attractivity of females to male newts (Iwata et al., 2000).

In *Taricha*, amplexus persists on average for 7 hours, during which time the male firmly embraces the female with fore and hind limbs, rubs his submandibular mental glands against the female's nares (chin-rubbing behavior), and sharply contracts both hind limbs in unison against the female's abdomen. During amplexus, female behaviors change from sexually unreceptive to sexually receptive (Propper, 1991). The chin-rubbing behavior seems to transfer chemical signals from the male's mental glands to the female's olfactory epithelium and facilitate female sexual receptivity. In Plethodontid salamanders, males produce a peptide pheromone that induces female receptivity (Rollmann et al., 1999).

In contrast to *Taricha*, *Cynops* and *Triturus* do not use amplexus during courtship. (These salamanders apparently secondarily lost amplexus during evolution; Salthe, 1967). Instead, the males respond to sexually attractive females with blocking behaviors and tail vibrations (Salthe, 1967; Halliday, 1977; Iwata et al., 2000).

B. Neural Control of Clasping in *Taricha*

The essential element of clasping is bilateral, synchronized adduction of all four legs by limb flexor muscles. Thus, the inhibition of walking is required, but *Taricha* often swim with undulating trunk and tail muscle contractions during clasping. Head movements are also common during clasping, as exemplified by the male's rubbing of his lower jaw on the female's snout. In addition to sustained flexion of the legs, the clasping male periodically shows repetitive bilateral extension and flexion of the hind legs in a manner that stimulates the female's trunk and pulls her tightly against his ventrum. Consequently, the male retains a great deal of mobility while clasping, but alternate stepping movements are selectively absent. The tonic contraction of leg flexors in the absence of alternate stepping movements implies the operation of a central clasping generator that does not interfere with swimming or head movements but acts in opposition to the central pattern generator (CPG) for stepping.

Clasping in *Taricha* is triggered by ventral body stimulation, especially pressure on the cloaca. Our behavioral tests of newts (Rose et al., 1998) showed that clasping is often stimulus-bound to the duration of cloacal trigger stimuli, but that it sometimes persists after stimulus termination. Clasping can be blocked or overridden by the stimulation of the head or immobilization of the male. In addition, it is difficult to elicit reflexive clasping if the male is concurrently walking, again suggesting an antagonistic interaction between the CPG for stepping and the neural generator of clasping. Finally, the clasping male can make adjustments in the ongoing clasp depending on diverse sensory information, such as movements by the female or encroachment by competing males.

The neural control of amplexus has been more extensively studied in anurans than in urodelele amphibians. In both taxa, the medulla and spinal cord are principally involved. In anurans, amplexus is often performed mainly or solely by the forelimbs, which show anatomical specializations, including sexually dimorphic flexor muscles innervated by motor neurons that bind testosterone (Erulkar et al., 1981). In addition, the motor neurons innervating homonymous as well as functionally related forelimb and hind limb muscles are electrically coupled (Westerfield and Frank, 1982). Corresponding information is lacking for urodeles, but male *Taricha* show highly visible hypertrophy of several body regions during the breeding season (Deviche et al., 1990). It would seem reasonable to expect similar types of functional specializations, including the hind limbs, in this urodele.

In anurans, high spinal transection or decapitation (to remove brain influences) results in strong sustained clasping (Smith, 1938), indicating that the termination of episodes of clasping requires an influence from the brain. Brain-stem transection studies suggest that the upper medulla probably facilitates clasping, whereas the forebrain and upper-brain-stem regions transmit a combination of inhibitory and facilitatory influences to medullary-spinal clasp-control mechanisms (Aronson and Noble, 1945). In *Taricha,* premedullary brain-stem transections lead to a decline in clasp probability or strength (J. D. Rose, unpublished observations). This pattern differs from results with anurans, which show strong amplexus after high medullary transections (Aronson and Noble, 1945; Hutchison and Poynton, 1963; Smith, 1938). However, severing the connection between the medulla and cervical spinal cord in *Taricha,* as in anurans, results in strong sustained clasp responses to ventral body stimulation (Lewis and Rose, 2000). The clasp-inhibiting system may be more caudal in *Taricha* because it shows strong hind-limb clasping.

Knowledge that the medulla is a critical structure regulating amplectic clasping led us to examine medullary neurons for properties likely to be involved in the control of clasping. For the medulla to regulate the onset, strength, and duration of clasp responses, we expected that many medullary neurons, including reticulospinal neurons, would show sensory responses to cloacal stimuli. We used two experimental approaches for recording responses to cloacal pressure stimuli from single medullary neurons: (1) newts that were unanesthetized and immobilized with a myoneural blocking agent (Rose et al., 1993, 1995a) and (2) newts that were chronically implanted with microwire electrodes and were freely moving (Rose et al., 1995b, 1998). Recording from freely moving newts conveys a powerful strategic advantage because it is possible to identify in real time the patterns of neuronal activity that control the clasping response and to observe hormone-induced changes in this neuronal activity as the hormone effects on clasping responses appear. An additional strategic refinement of these studies contributing to their analytic power was the use of antidromic invasion (Fig. 1) to identify reticulospinal neurons. In this way, we were able to examine clasping-related activity in those neurons that transmit the brain's influence to spinal neural networks controlling clasping.

In recordings from unanesthetized, paralyzed newts (Rose et al., 1993, 1995a), we found that the majority of reticulospinal and surrounding nonreticulospinal neurons showed strong responses to cloacal pressure that closely paralleled the onset, duration, and offset of the cloacal stimulus. These neurons were located in an extensive paramedian reticular zone of the rostral medulla that overlaps the location of reticulospinal neurons in *Taricha* (G. S. Marrs and J. D. Rose, unpublished observations) and other urodeles (Naujoks-Manteuffel and Mantueffel, 1988). The sensory responsiveness of these neurons was relatively broad in that they typically responded, in varying degrees, to stimulation of the head or limbs. But cloacal pressure had extremely potent effects, frequently producing greater changes in firing than could be elicited by the stimulation of other body locations.

Recordings from single medullary neurons in freely behaving newts have led to a better understanding of

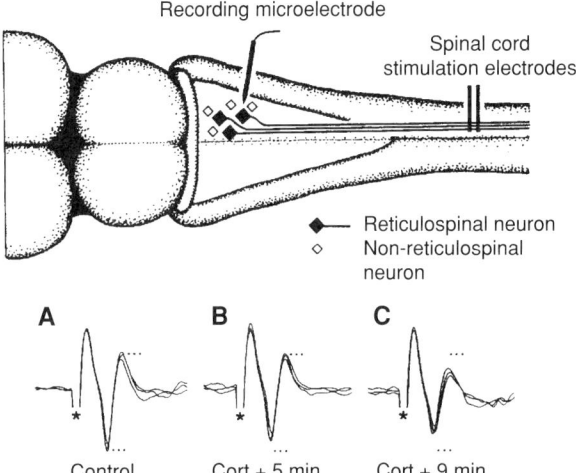

FIGURE 1 Upper figure: Dorsal surface of the newt brain stem showing the recording and stimulating electrode configuration used for identification and testing of reticulospinal and nonreticulospinal neurons. Neurons that were tested for a role in courtship clasping and for effects of CORT were in the rostromedial medulla. Reticulospinal neurons (filled symbols) were identified by recording an antidromically conducted (backfired) action potential elicited by electrical stimulation of the descending spinal cord axons of these neurons. These antidromic action potentials are sensitive indicators of the state of neural excitability and the antidromic testing method was used to assess CORT effects on the spike-generating capability of reticulospinal neurons. Nonreticulospinal neurons (unfilled symbols) did not have axons descending in the spinal cord. These neurons tended to show more spontaneous and sensory-stimulus-elicited firing than reticulospinal neurons. Lower figure: Antidromic action potentials recorded from a reticulospinal neuron in an unanesthetized newt immobilized with a myoneural blocking agent. Each set of traces (A–C) shows a series of three sequential superimposed antidromic action potentials. The asterisk by the break in the recording designates the electrical artifact due to stimulation of the spinal cord. In this neuron, as in most reticulospinal neurons tested with CORT injection, the peak-to-peak amplitude of the antidromic action potential in (A), designated by the dashed lines, was rapidly reduced after CORT injection. At (B) 5 min and (C) 9 min after CORT, the amplitude of the spike was reduced by 14% and 38%, respectively. The magnitude of this amplitude decline increased with time. Each set of traces is 8 msec in duration. Reproduced with permission from Rose (2000).

the critical role of this brain-stem region in the control of clasping (Rose *et al.*, 1995b, 1998). Most neurons in the rostral medulla, including identified reticulospinal neurons and nonreticulospinal neurons, showed activity that closely reflected the occurrence of cloacal stimulation as well as the expression and quality of reflexive hind-limb clasping. The onset of cloacal stimulation and the concurrent occurrence of clasping was usually associated with a burst of firing, as was the offset of cloacal pressure and termination of clasping (Fig. 2). During sustained cloacal pressure and concurrently maintained clasping, most medullary neurons showed a decline or cessation in firing but a few neurons showed continuously elevated discharge during cloacal pressure and sustained clasping. In addition, reticulospinal neurons showed fluctuations in antidromic excitability closely time-locked with or even predictive of the specific motor events of clasping. Thus, as a population, both the reticulospinal and nonreticulospinal medullary neurons show sensorimotor properties that are compatible with control of clasping.

In addition to the propensity to exhibit clasping-related activity, most medullary reticular neurons in behaving newts showed firing that was closely related to other motor events, especially locomotion, head movements, and breathing. Thus, the activity of these neurons was broadly associated with movements, although sustained clasping, a largely immobile state, was usually associated with decreased firing, whereas overt movements such as walking were associated with increased firing. The properties of reticulospinal neurons were tied to movements to a greater degree than was activity of nonreticulospinal neurons. This observation is consistent with the major role of reticulospinal neurons as the controllers of spinal-cord locomotor pattern generators (Grillner *et al.*, 1998a,b).

The clasp-related activity of both reticulospinal and nonreticulospinal neurons typically operates in a manner opposite to that shown by the same neurons during walking. Specifically, these neurons show mainly enhanced activity or antidromic excitability during waking, but a depression of activity or excitability during clasping. This pattern could represent the opposing effects of these neurons on a CPG for locomotion. Less commonly, medullary neurons showed tonically increased activity or excitability during clasping, a pattern that might reflect facilitation of a central clasping generator. The onset and offset of clasping involves a switching of motor states, typically a switching from clasping to walking. A large proportion of the reticulospinal and unidentified neurons show stimulus-driven or motor

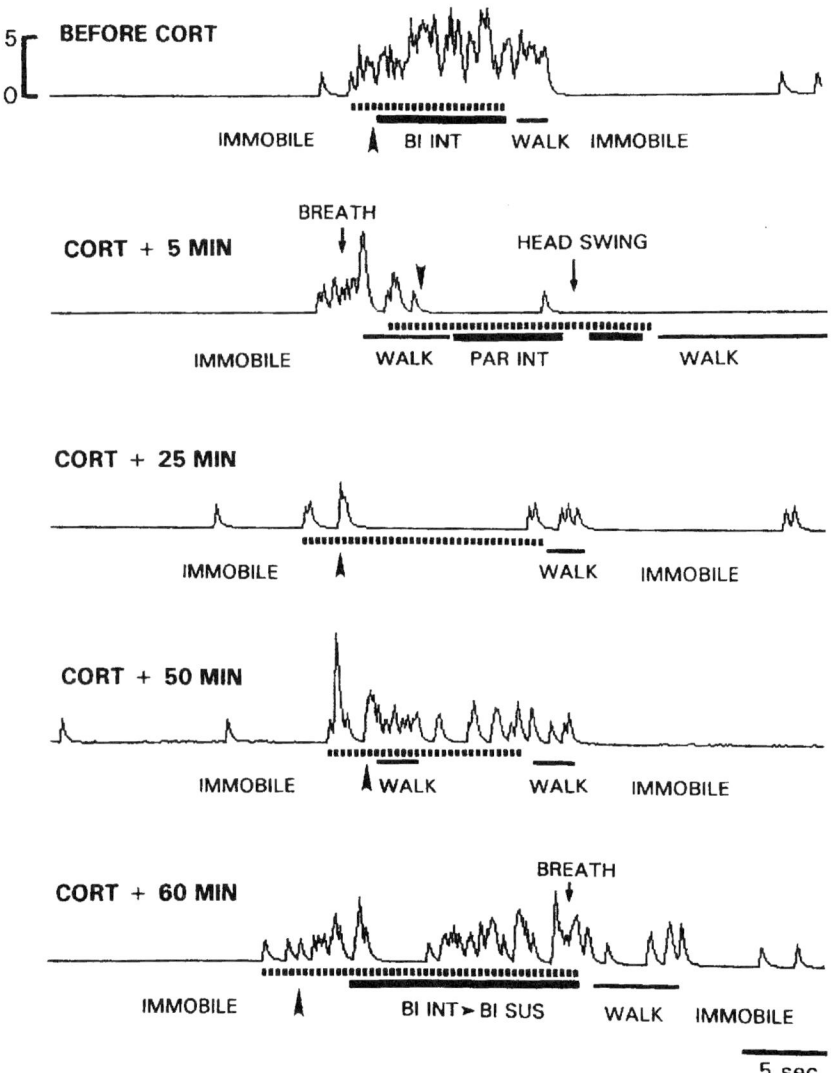

FIGURE 2 Illustration of the loss of clasping-related firing in a reticulospinal neuron and simultaneously impaired reflexive clasping due to CORT in a freely moving roughskin newt. Each of the traces shows a 45-s segment of neuronal activity recorded during a test of clasping in response to cloacal stimulation. The vertical deflection on each trace is an integrator record showing the firing rate of the neuron. The broken line beneath the record of integrated single neuron activity indicates the duration of stimulating probe contact with the cloaca. This initial contact was light and insufficient to evoke clasping. The arrowhead shows the onset of increased cloacal pressure, adequate for triggering clasping, which continued until the end of the broken line. The thicker solid line indicates the occurrence of clasping and the thinner line the occurrence of walking. Each record begins with the newt immobile, as indicated by the label beneath the traces. Before CORT injection, the neuron showed a strong sustained increase in firing that began with pressure on the cloaca reached its maximum during full bilateral, intermittent clasping (BI INT) and continued during a brief episode of walking at the end of the clasp test. At 5 min after CORT injection, this neuron showed acceleration of firing during movements associated with the newt taking a breath, a pattern present prior to CORT injection. Now, cloacal stimulation failed to elicit sustained firing during clasping, which had deteriorated to just a partial intermittent closure of the legs (PART INT). In this neuron, firing

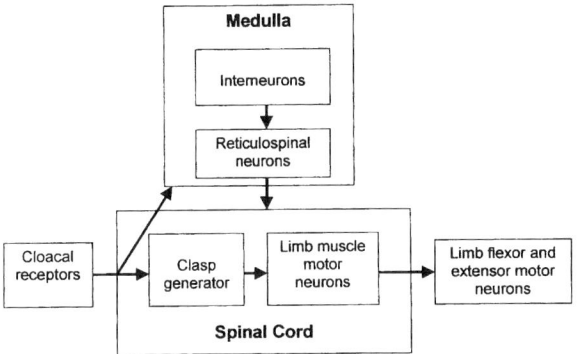

FIGURE 3 A diagram illustrating the principal neural systems controlling clasping in *Taricha*. For simplicity in this depiction, the sensory control of clasping is limited to stimulation of the cloaca. Pressure on the cloaca activates receptors that trigger a clasp-generating neural process in the spinal cord. This clasp generator acts on limb muscle motor neurons to excite limb flexor motor neurons and, presumably, inhibit extensor motor neurons. The spinal clasp generator also receives descending influences from the brain, principally from reticulospinal neurons that control clasp onset, clasp termination, and adjustments of clasp quality. Activity elicited by cloacal stimulation also ascends to the medulla, producing mainly an increase in the firing of non-reticulospinal neurons (designated interneurons in the diagram) and a mixture of increases and decreases in reticulospinal neuron firing. These responses of medullary neurons, collectively, are closely associated with the onset, maintenance, and offset of clasping. The roles of reticulospinal neurons in clasping appear to be similar to their role in locomotion control. Thus, reticulospinal neurons through their action on the spinal clasp generator, regulate the onset, strength, and offset of clasping. Exact details of the neuroanatomical connections between neuron types represented in the diagram have not been elucidated, but are inferred from our neurophysiological data from *Taricha* and neuroanatomical studies on other amphibian species.

state transition-related activity that could be a controlling event for this switching. A model summarizing the neural control of clasping in *Taricha* is presented in Fig. 3.

C. Insemination Behaviors

In species that use amplexus during courtship, such as *Taricha*, the mating sequence starts when the male releases the female from amplexus and moves forward to a position in front of the female. At this stage, male *Taricha* stop in front of the female and exhibit tail vibration behaviors. While the male vibrates his tail and deposits a spermatophore, the female keeps her nares close to the male's cloaca. The behaviors that follow amplexus in *Taricha* are similar to the blocking and tail vibration behaviors exhibited by species of *Cynops* and *Triturus*. When males are exhibiting tail vibration behaviors, female newts are attracted to secretions from the males. Female *Taricha* are probably attracted to a pheromone secreted from the male's cloaca, as has been shown in *Cynops* and *Triturus* (Cedrini and Fasolo, 1970; Toyoda *et al.*, 1994; Kikuyama *et al.*, 1995; Yamamoto *et al.*, 2000).

The female-attracting pheromone in *Cynops* is called sodefin (Toyoda *et al.*, 1994; Kikuyama *et al.*, 1995). Sodefin is produced in the abdominal gland of the male and, when secreted into the water, functions to attract sexually receptive females. Molecular studies discovered that sodefin is a unique decapeptide (Kikuyama *et al.*, 1995) that is synthesized from a larger precursor protein consisting of 189 amino acid residues (Iwata *et al.*, 1999). The synthesis of sodefin appears to be controlled by the elevated levels of androgen and PRL in breeding males; treating male *Cynops* with androgen plus PRL maximally stimulates the synthesis of sodefin (Yamamoto *et al.*, 1996). AVT injections into courting male *Cynops* stimulate sodefin secretion, suggesting AVT involvement (Iwata *et al.*, 2000).

Successful mating in newts occurs when the female moves over the spermatophore and the sperm cap adheres to her cloaca. Spermatozoa in the sperm cap then move from the cloacal orifice into the lumen and enter

---

(*Continued*) was not reliably present during walking as it had been before CORT. At CORT + 25 min, only a few spikes were fired at the onset and offset of cloacal pressure and clasping was absent. At CORT + 50 min, cloacal contact by the stimulating probe and application of pressure elicited a transiently high, and then reduced level of firing, but no clasping. A low level of firing continued during the brief episode of walking after the end of stimulation. At CORT + 60 min, the rate of firing had increased during cloacal pressure and during the subsequent, long-latency intermittent then sustained (SUS) clasping. Firing during walking was still depressed relative to the pre-CORT level. In most reticulospinal neurons, CORT did not affect walking-related firing. Reproduced from Rose *et al.* (1998).

the sperm-storage organ (spermatotheca) in the female (Propper, 1991).

D. Postinsemination Behaviors

In *Taricha,* males recapture the females with the amplectic clasp approximately 30 seconds after depositing a spermatophore. The pair remains quiescent for a period of time. Some pairs regress to preinsemination behaviors, but more often sperm transfer is accomplished with one spermatophore deposited. Postinsemination clasping persists for many hours (ranging from 4 hr to 4 days) and, when terminated, the female is not sexually attractive to other males (Propper, 1991).

Female *Taricha* begin to ovulate starting approximately 11 days after mating and continuing for several weeks thereafter. In *Taricha* and presumably other newts, fertilization occurs when freshly ovulated eggs move through the oviducts and are deposited on substrates (e.g., aquatic vegetation, stones, or sticks) in the pond (Moore *et al.,* 1979). Ovulation in female *Taricha* apparently is induced by sensory cues received with the spermatozoa because female newts do not ovulate when mated with vasectomized males (S. P. Spielvogel and F. L. Moore, unpublished data).

E. Modifying Factors in Reproductive Behaviors

As in other animals, numerous external factors modulate the timing and occurrence of reproduction in newts. The dominant environmental cues are photoperiod and average ambient temperature. Research with European newts indicates that the combined effects of photoperiod and average ambient temperature modify the time when newts becomes fully developed sexually (Paniagua *et al.,* 1990; Zerani *et al.,* 1991a,b). In *Taricha,* the breeding season starts earlier and lasts longer for populations living near the Pacific coast where it is mild and moist, compared to the higher-elevation populations living further inland in the mountains. As in other vertebrates, annual reproductive cycles are controlled predominantly by GnRH, which stimulates secretion of the gonadotropins luteinizing hormone (LH) and follicle-stimulating hormone (FSH) which in turn stimulate gametogenesis and steroid synthesis in the gonads.

There also are short-term effects of external factors and hormones on the animals' behavioral state. For example, newts usually migrate into the breeding ponds during periods of rainy weather and moderate temperatures. Perhaps the rainy weather stimulates the secretion of hormones, such as PRL (Toyoda *et al.,* 1996), that control migratory behaviors.

When a newt or other animal in the wild is exposed to a threatening stimulus, the most common response is to switch from nonessential behaviors, such as courtship, to behaviors essential to survival, such as fleeing or hiding. Thus it is not surprising that stress hormones exert rapid inhibitory effects on reproductive behaviors. Studies in *Taricha* reveal that reproductive behaviors are suppressed when the animal is exposed to mild short-term stress and that this change in behavioral state is controlled by the classic stress hormones that include CRH, adrenocorticotropin hormone (ACTH), CORT, and dynorphin (Deviche and Moore, 1987; Moore *et al.,* 1995).

III. ACTIVATION OF MALE REPRODUCTIVE BEHAVIORS: STEROIDS

A. Testicular Steroids in Amphibians

Much of what researchers have learned from mammals about the actions of testicular steroids on reproductive behaviors seems to apply to amphibians as well. But many unanswered questions remain for amphibians. Early developmental and organizational effects of androgens on sexual differentiation and development in amphibians have been studied most extensively in *Xenopus*. Those studies are reviewed in Kelley (Chap. 27 in this volume).

In general, adult amphibians have high plasma testosterone (T) concentrations in males and high plasma 17β-estradiol (E_2) concentrations in females. But the picture is more complex and interesting than this. Plasma samples from male and female amphibians frequently have measurable amounts of T, E_2, 5α-dihydrotestosterone (DHT), and progesterone (P4) (Lecouteux *et al.,* 1985; Moore *et al.,* 2000; Gobbetti and Zerani, 1999; Zerani *et al.,* 1991b). In *Triturus,* for example, although plasma E_2 concentrations are higher in females than males, E_2 concentrations peak during the breeding season in both males and females (Zerani et al., 1991b). In *Taricha*, significant amounts of T and DHT occur in the plasma of both males and females (Moore et al., 2000). Plasma DHT concentrations are similar in males and females, but plasma T concentrations are higher in males than females (Moore et al., 2000). To add further complexity, research in frogs reveals that not only are T and DHT synthesized and secreted into the plasma by the gonads, but these androgens also are synthesized by glial cells in the telencephalon of males and females (Mensah-Nyagan et al., 1996a,b). As in other vertebrates, responses to androgens and estrogens by target cells in the brain and peripheral tissues depend on the concentrations of androgens and estrogens in blood, the types and availability of steroid-binding proteins in the blood, the types and activities of steroid-synthesizing enzymes in and around the target cells, and the prevalence and activity of specific subtypes of estrogen receptors (ERs) and androgen receptors (ARs) in the targets cells.

B. Seasonal Cycles in Sex Steroids

Seasonal changes in circulating sex steroids have been studied in a variety of amphibians from temperate climates. In male newts (*Cynops*, *Taricha*, and *Triturus*), seasonal studies reveal consistent temporal patterns of change in the testes, secondary sexual characteristics, reproductive hormones, and reproductive behaviors. Testicular changes reflect the annual cycle of regression and recrudescence typical of seasonally breeding animals. Testis weights reach maximum values with the completion of spermatogenesis and spermiogenesis in late summer and early autumn (4–6 months before the breeding season for most males). The testis weights diminish gradually starting in October or November and continuing into the breeding season, and they reach minimum values in March or April with the completion of spermiation (Tanaka and Iwasawa, 1979; Specker and Moore, 1980; Deviche et al., 1990). This testicular cycle results in males' having mature sperm in the duct system during the period when they are most likely to encounter sexually developed females.

Testicular cycles in amphibians are associated with annual variations in the amount of T, DHT, and E_2 secreted from the testes (D'Istria et al., 1974; Specker and Moore, 1980; Imai et al., 1985; Harvey et al., 1997; Norris et al., 1985; Gobbetti et al., 1991a,b; Garnier, 1985). In newts, androgen (T plus DHT) concentrations typically are lowest during the later stages of the spring breeding season (before males become completely inactive sexually) and remain low into the summer. Androgen concentrations rise rapidly in August and September, when spermatogenesis is nearly complete and spermiogenesis is underway, and they reach peak levels in late fall and early spring (Tanaka and Takikawa, 1983; Specker and Moore, 1980; Garnier, 1985; Imai et al., 1985; Deviche et al., 1990; Gobbetti et al., 1991a). In *Taricha*, this seasonal pattern of change in androgenic steroids can be attributed to seasonal changes in plasma T concentrations (Moore et al., 2000). In male *Taricha*, T concentrations reach peak values by the onset of the breeding season; whereas, DHT concentrations only increase slightly in August and remain at modest and stable levels during other seasons. Interestingly, whereas T concentrations are significantly higher in breeding males than females, DHT concentrations are similar in breeding males and females (Moore et al., 2000).

Nearing the end of the breeding season, T concentrations diminish precipitously and in parallel with the decline in the percentage of sexually active males (Deviche et al., 1990). By the end of the breeding season, which occurs in early June for *Taricha*, T concentrations are at seasonal lows in males and at similar levels in males and females (Moore et al., 2000).

In male newts, the annual increase in circulating androgens plays important roles in the development of secondary sexual characteristics. In newts, androgens and PRL work in conjunction to stimulate the growth and development of the tail fin, abdominal glands, and other secondary sexual characteristics in males (Kikuyama et al., 1980; Vellano et al., 1967; Mosconi et al., 1994), preparing them for the breeding season. In *Cynops* and *Triturus*, plasma PRL concentrations change seasonally and reach peak concentrations by the onset of the breeding season (Matsuda et al., 1990; Mosconi et al., 1994). These elevated levels of PRL are thought to contribute to controlling the migratory behaviors into the breeding ponds and enhancing male reproductive behaviors (see later).

Male newts have measurable amounts of circulating E_2 (Lecouteux et al., 1985; Moore et al., 2000; Gobbetti and Zerani, 1999; Zerani et al., 1991b). In *Taricha*, males have lower E_2 concentrations than females throughout the year (Moore et al., 2000). Therefore, there are sex differences in circulating sex steroids in newts—males have higher T concentrations than females, and females have higher E_2 concentrations than males. These two steroids, in our judgement, play important roles in the seasonal development of sex-specific behaviors. Specifically, the elevated concentrations of T in the plasma of males prior to the onset of the breeding season induce the development of male-like behaviors, whereas the elevated concentrations of E_2 in the plasma of females prior to the breeding season induce female-like reproductive behaviors. Additional support for this conclusion comes from studies showing that, in ovariectomized newts, E_2-implanted animals showed female-like behaviors and T-implanted females showed male-like behaviors (Moore et al., 1992).

Steroid concentrations in newts change in response to the performance of reproductive behaviors. In *Triturus*, when males perform courtship behaviors, T concentrations decrease and E_2 concentrations increase (Zerrani et al., 1991b). Furthermore, aromatase enzyme activity in the brain increases, which is consistent with the observed drop in T and rise in E_2. Other studies in *Triturus* (Gobbetti and Zerani, 1995) provide evidence that when males perform courtship, circulating levels of prostaglandin $F_{2\alpha}$ increase; the increase in $PGF_{2\alpha}$ enhances aromatase activity in the brain to control the conversion of T to E_2. Gobbetti and Zerani (1995) hypothesize that short-term changes in aromatase activity and increased conversion of T to E_2 might trigger courtship behaviors in male *Triturus*. This hypothesis seems to suggest that E_2 exerts rapid effects on male courtship behaviors and that these effects of E_2 pertain to the performance of male reproductive behaviors rather than to the hormonal control of the male's propensity to exhibit the behaviors.

C. Castration and Steroid-Replacement Studies in Amphibians

In amphibians, as in most other vertebrates, castration eliminates male reproductive behaviors (Palka and Gorbman, 1973; Wada and Gorbman, 1977; Andreoletti et al., 1983; Moore, 1978; Kelley and Pfaff, 1976). But despite the studies showing a postcastration decline in male reproductive behaviors, studies with steroid-replacement threatment in castrated amphibians have produced mixed results. In some cases, the administration of androgens to castrated males has maintained or restored male reproductive behaviors (Andreoletti et al., 1983; Kelley and Pfaff, 1976; Moore, 1978; Deviche and Moore, 1988). However, other studies found that androgen treatment to castrated or sexually inactive males had no effect on either restoring or inducing male behaviors (Malacarne and Giacoma, 1980; Moore et al., 1978; Palka and Gorbman, 1973; Wada and Gorbman, 1977). It seems that testicular androgens (and perhaps estrogens) are necessary, but not sufficient, for activating male reproductive behaviors (Moore, 1978).

Castration and steroid-replacement studies in *Taricha* found that androgen implants (T, DHT, or T plus DHT) maintain male reproductive behaviors if the males are sexually activate when castrated. But if males are sexually inactive when castrated, androgen implants do not affect male behaviors (Moore, 1978). Furthermore, when males are castrated and implanted with steroids (T, DHT, or T plus DHT) several months prior to the breeding season, T-implanted males exhibit reproductive behaviors during the normal breeding season, but not before that time of year (Deviche and Moore, 1988). Thus the season of the year affected the effectiveness of T to induce male behaviors. These observations support the hypothesis that nontesticular hormones become elevated during the breeding season and function in combination with testicular steroids to enhance male reproductive behaviors in newts. The primary candidates for behaviorally important nontesticular hormones are GnRH (Moore et al., 1982, 1987; Propper and Dixon, 1997), PRL (Toyoda et al., 1996; Mosconi et al., 1994), and AVT (reviewed next).

IV. ACTIVATION OF MALE REPRODUCTIVE BEHAVIORS: VASOTOCIN

A. Behavioral Responses to Vasotocin Injections in Amphibians

The first evidence that AVT modulates reproductive behaviors was published in a paper by Wilhelmi, Pickford, and Sawyer (1955) reporting that neurohypophysial extracts induce spawning behaviors in killifish (*Fundulus heteroclitus*). Since then, many other papers have reported that injecting AVT alters specific social behaviors in fish, amphibians, reptiles, birds, and mammals (for a review of early comparative literature, see Moore, 1992). In amphibians, AVT administration has been found to enhance sexual receptivity in female frogs (Diakow, 1978), advertisement and territorial calls in male frogs (Boyd, 1994a; Marler *et al.*, 1995; Propper and Dixon, 1997; Semsar *et al.*, 1998; Chu *et al.*, 1998; Tito *et al.*, 1999), egg-laying behaviors in female *Taricha* (Moore *et al.*, 1992), and courtship behaviors in male *Taricha*.

The actions of AVT on courtship behaviors have been studied in considerable detail in *Taricha* (for earlier reviews, see Moore, 1983, 1992). Early experiments in *Taricha* revealed that exogenous AVT administration increases the incidence of amplectic clasping (courtship) behaviors in male newts (Moore and Zoeller, 1979; Moore and Miller, 1983). Evidence that AVT is acting on target cells in the brain comes from studies showing that the potency of AVT to induce male courtship behaviors in *Taricha* is over 1000 times more potent when AVT is administered intracerebroventricularly (ICV) compared to intraperitoneal (IP) injections (Moore and Miller, 1983). During the peak breeding season, when essentially all male *Taricha* are sexually active, ICV injections of AVT antagonists or anti-AVT antiserum suppress courtship behaviors. Similar experiments with *C. pyrrhogaster* found that AVT administration enhances the incidence and frequency of courtship behaviors and that an injection of AVT antagonists suppresses courtship behaviors (Iwata *et al.*, 2000). It is noteworthy that AVT enhances courtship in both species even though their courtship behaviors are different—*Taricha* capturing the females with an amplectic clasp to initiate courtship and *Cynops* never exhibiting amplectic clasping behaviors. These observations suggest that AVT enhances the expression of species-typical motor patterns, perhaps by enhancing the animals' motivational state. But as we describe later, AVT also appears to control reproductive behaviors by modulating the processing of sensory stimuli that normally elicit sexual responses.

In *Taricha* we have observed that AVT enhances neuronal responses to clasp-triggering stimuli (Rose *et al.*, 1995a). AVT was applied to the medulla in unanesthetized immobilized newts and the activity of single neurons was recorded. In seconds or a small number of minutes, AVT application increased the spontaneous firing and the enhanced magnitude of sensory responses to cloacal stimulation in 93% of these neurons.

An enhancement of neuronal responses to noncloacal stimuli was also produced by AVT, but in a smaller proportion of the neurons. Thus, the previously documented facilitation of clasping by AVT (Moore and Zoeller, 1979) might be due partly to an enhancement of caudal-brain-stem neuronal responses to clasp-triggering stimuli.

B. Sex and Seasonal Variations in Vasotocin

Immunocytochemical studies reveal that the neuroanatomical distribution of AVT immunoreactive (ir) neurons in *Taricha* is complex, containing at least 19 distinct populations of AVT-synthesizing neurons and many AVT-containing fibers and terminal fields in the brain (Lowry *et al.*, 1997; Moore and Lowry, 1998). Seven of the 19 AVT-ir populations are sexually dimorphic (Moore *et al.*, 2000). Three populations are masculinized, with a greater number of AVT-ir neurons in males than in females. The masculinized AVT-ir populations are located in three brains areas—the bed nucleus of the stria terminalis (BNST), amygdala, and anterior preoptic area—that have been linked to the control of male sexual behaviors in diverse vertebrates. Four of the 19 AVT-ir populations are feminized, with a greater number of AVT-ir neurons in females than males. One feminized AVT-ir cell group is located in the pars dorsalis hypothalami and ventromedial hypothalamus, brain regions frequently associated with stress responses and female mating behaviors (Moore *et al.*, 2000). In *Rana catesbeiana*, specific brain sites have a greater amount of AVT-ir and a greater number of AVT-ir-labeled neurons in males than females (Boyd *et al.*, 1992; Boyd and Moore, 1992). It seems likely that the masculinized AVT neurons are involved in regulating male-specific behaviors and the feminized AVT neurons are involved in regulating female-specific behaviors.

Other studies confirm that the AVT content in specific sites in the brain correlates with the amphibians' reproductive and behavioral status. In *Taricha*, the AVT-ir concentrations in the optic tectum of males change seasonally, with highest levels during the breeding season (Zoeller and Moore, 1986). AVT-ir concentrations were higher in sexually responsive than in unresponsive males in specific brain sites (dorsal preoptic area, optic tectum, ventral infundibulum, and cerebrospinal fluid) (Zoeller and Moore, 1988). In the cricket frog (*Acris crepitans*), a greater number of cells and fibers show AVT-ir labeling in the medial amygdala and nucleus accumbens of satellite males than in calling males (Marler *et al.*, 1999). In bullfrogs (*R. catesbeiana*), AVT-ir distribution and abundance are highest in neural areas associated with vocalizations (Boyd, 1997; Boyd *et al.*, 1992; Boyd and Moore, 1992). As in amphibians, studies in fish and birds show that there are behavioral and sexual differences in AVT in specific brain sites linked to reproductive behaviors (Godwin *et al.*, 2000; Goodson and Bass, 2000; Grober and Sunobe, 1996; Foran and Bass, 1998; Ota *et al.*, 1999; Viglietti-Panzica *et al.*, 1992; Panzica *et al.*, 1999; Jurkevich *et al.*, 1997).

C. Effects of Sex Steroids on the Vasotocin System

Steroid hormones exert organizational and activational effects on reproductive behaviors in amphibians, as in other vertebrates. Various types of evidence support the hypothesis that some of the sex steroid effects on reproductive behaviors involve site-specific regulation of AVT synthesis and AVT release by neurons in the brain. Some of this evidence comes from the observations that there are sex differences in the predominant type of sex steroid in the plasma (androgen in males; estrogen in females) and sex differences in the AVT system in behaviorally important brain areas (see previous discussion). Sex steroids must have localized effects, targeting specific neurons, to produce site-specific sex differences in AVT. Localized effects of steroids are well documented (Boyd *et al.*, 1992; Boyd and Moore, 1992; Moore *et al.*, 2000) and are explained by localized differences in the activity of steroidogenic enzymes (e.g., aromatase and 5α-reductase) and differences in intracellular ARs and ERs.

The neuroanatomical distribution of ARs and ERs has been studied in amphibians using immunocytochemistry (Davis and Moore, 1996) and *in vivo* autoradiography (Di Meglio *et al.*, 1987; Morrell *et al.*, 1975; Kelley *et al.*, 1975, 1978). These studies indicate that there is some overlap, but not complete concordance, between steroid receptor localization and AVT sexual dimorphism. Thus AVT sexual dimorphism in the brain cannot be explained completely by the distribution of the steroid receptors.

Gonadectomy and steroid-replacement experiments in *R. catesbeiana* investigated the question of steroid control of AVT sex differences (Boyd, 1994b, 1997). Following gonadectomy, AVT concentrations decrease in certain brain areas (amygdala, septal area, and habenula) in both sexes and in several other areas (optic tectum, torus semicircularis, and pretrigeminal nucelus) in males only. In gonadectomized frogs, DHT treatment maintained AVT content in all six brain areas; whereas, E_2 treatment restored AVT content in the septal area, habenula, and amygdala. These results indicate that sex steroids can control AVT synthesis and release in specific brain areas, and that these effects of steroids are influenced by the sex of the animal.

Sex steroids also appear to control the abundance of AVT receptors in specific brain areas, perhaps indirectly. In male and female *Taricha*, gonadectomy reduces the number of AVT binding sites in the amygdala, but not in other brain areas (Boyd and Moore, 1991). In *R. catesbeiana*, AVT receptor concentrations are sexually dimorphic in specific brain areas (amygdala, hypothalamus, pretrigeminal nucleus, and dorsolateral nucleus), and the concentrations decrease following the removal of gonads (Boyd, 1997). In male and female bullfrogs, gonadectomy reduces and E_2 treatment restores the number of AVT binding sites in the amygdala. On the other hand, DHT treatment increases AVT binding sites in the pretrigeminal nucleus of males, but not females (Boyd, 1997). These studies indicate that sex steroids exert site-specific effects on AVT receptors.

These studies of AVT receptors relate to behavioral responses. Castration and steroid-replacement studies in *Taricha* show that the induction of courtship behavior by AVT is androgen-dependent and that there is a slow postcastration decline in AVT responses (Zoeller and Moore, 1982).

D. Effects of Castration and Steroid Replacement on Heterotypical Reproductive Behavior

Female newts were found to exhibit male-like courtship behaviors (i.e., clasp other females in amplexus) when gonadectomized, implanted with DHT, and then after 30 days injected with AVT (Moore *et al.*, 1992). In contrast, AVT administration did not elicit clasping behaviors in gonadectomized females that had no steroid implants. In *Taricha*, AVT administration to intact females induces egg-laying behaviors, where the female clasps an inanimate object and deposits an egg. Female egg-laying behavior and male amplectic clasping behavior use similar motor patterns and, in both behaviors, the animals clasp an object. When gonadectomized, AVT-injected females are given a choice between clasping aquatic vegetation or a conspecific female, the E_2-implanted females did not preferentially clasp aquatic vegetation over other females. In contrast, gonadectomized AVT-injected females implanted with DHT preferentially clasped other females (Moore et al., 1992). Therefore, in *Taricha*, exposure to estrogens or androgens appears to control the orientation of the AVT-induced clasping such that estrogen maintains egg-laying behavior and androgen maintains amplectic clasping. This research on newt male courtship and female egg-laying behaviors suggests that sex steroids might control reproductive behaviors by acting directly or indirectly on the AVT system and, by some unknown mechanism, modify behavioral responses to specific releasing stimuli.

E. Vasotocin as a Regulator of Sensorimotor Processing

The preceding sections support the conclusion that AVT acts centrally and, working through steroid-dependent pathways, regulates specific behaviors in amphibians. Research in fish, birds, and mammals adds further support to this conclusion and establishes that the regulation of social behaviors by AVT-like peptides is evolutionarily conserved (Moore, 1992).

But many unanswered questions remain about the mechanisms through which AVT (and other AVT-like peptides) modulates reproductive behaviors. Four distinct mechanisms might be involved:

1. AVT could influence reproductive behaviors as a secondary consequence of its effects on the general processes of sensory orientation or arousal (Ebner et al., 1999; Landgraf et al., 1995; Born et al., 1986).
2. AVT could enhance the animals' probability of engaging in sexual behavior (Bohus, 1977).
3. AVT could influence reproductive behaviors by modulating specific sensory pathways, for example, by affecting the processing of species-specific social-releasing stimuli. A sensory processing mechanism seems to be supported in studies of auditory responses in frogs (Boyd, 1994a) and olfactory responses in voles (Young et al., 1999).
4. AVT could influence reproductive behaviors by acting on motor pathways to modulate species-specific stereotypical motor output patterns (Pickford and Strecker, 1977; Goodson and Bass, 2000).

Generalizing from known mechanisms of hormonal action on the neural control of sexual behavior (Rose, 1990a), it appears likely that AVT could exert multiple actions on sensorimotor mechanisms controlling sexual behaviors in *Taricha*.

1. Vasotocin Effects on Sensory Orientation and Responses to Sex Pheromones

A series of experiments investigated the effects of AVT on general arousal and sensory orientation in male newts by determining the effects of AVT on locomotor activity and behavioral responses to functionally unrelated sensory cues (Thompson and Moore, 2000). AVT administration in *Taricha* was found to decrease general locomotor activity, which is contrary to what is expected if AVT increases general arousal.

Other experiments investigated the effects of AVT on behavioral responses to sex-related and food-related stimuli. These two types of stimuli were used because they are functionally different from one another and because in *Taricha* AVT administration enhances male sexual behaviors, but not feeding behaviors (Moore and Zoeller, 1979; Thompson and Moore, 2000). One set of experiments tested the effects of AVT administration on behavioral responses to sex-related olfactory information (female sex pheromones) and to food-related olfactory information (earthworm odors). AVT injections enhanced appetitive responses to sex pheromones and not to worm odors, providing evidence that AVT does not cause general increases in the animals' responses to functionally significant stimuli. These results suggest that AVT influences reproductive behaviors by increasing the animal's central motivational state or that AVT modulates the processing of species-specific social-releasing stimuli (Thompson and Moore, 2000).

2. Vasotocin Effects on Visual Sexual Cues

Other experiments with *Taricha* tested the effects of AVT administration on behavioral responses to sex-related visual information (sexually mature female newts viewed through clear glass) and food-related visual information (earthworms viewed through clear glass). These studies found that AVT administration increases appetitive responses to both types of visual information. These results leave open the possibility that AVT might influence the male's orientation or attraction to a visual feature common to females and worms, such as movement. As described earlier, our experiments with medullary AVT application demonstrated enhanced neuronal responses to somatic stimuli (Rose et al., 1995a). Some of these same medullary neurons also developed pronounced responses to moving visual stimuli. The functional significance of this AVT effect is uncertain because only large, moving, overhead stimuli were tested. Nonetheless, this effect demonstrates an AVT modulation of sensory influences converging on a neuron population involved in regulating clasping.

Studies using microdissection and radioimmunoassay found seasonal changes in AVT-ir concentrations in the optic tectum of male *Taricha* that are coincident with seasonal changes in male sexual behaviors (Zoeller and Moore, 1986). Electrophysiological studies revealed that the direct application of AVT to the optic tectum produces a rapid reversible decline in the amplitude of field potentials evoked by flashes of light (Rose et al., 1997). This attenuation of tectal response is opposite to other neurophysiological effects of AVT that we have documented in *Taricha* and shows that the peptide does not always enhance sensory activity. This AVT effect could be a mechanism regulating a newt's reactivity to intense light. During spring breeding season, which begins in late February and ends in early June, a period when day length and solar radiation increases markedly, male *Taricha* occupy sites in shallow water at the margins of breeding ponds where they intercept females moving into the ponds. The progressive increase in tectal AVT could provide a means for attenuating the somewhat photophobic male newt's reactivity. In this way, males are more likely to maintain their highly exposed positions in shallow water rather than retreating from the intense light into the depths of the ponds.

3. Conclusions about Vasotocin and Sensorimotor Processing Controlling Reproductive Behavior

In the foregoing review, there are many examples cited implicating AVT in sensorimotor processing. These examples include the presence of AVT systems in proximity to brain structures with known roles in sensory processing, motor control, or integrative sensorimotor functions. We have described numerous behavioral and neurophysiological examples from our research with *Taricha* in which AVT has exerted specific actions on types of sensory processing critical for sexual behavior, including olfactory, visual, and somatic sensory modalities. In some cases, as exemplified by AVT effects on medullary reticular neurons, the neuropeptide's action has occurred at a level best regarded as integrative, that is, between specifically sensory input and motor output levels. Thus, the AVT effects consitute an array of highly specific, yet diverse actions on multiple facets of sensorimotor processing. The neural systems controlling sexual behavior are highly species-specific (Rose, 1990a,b), and the steroid and neuropeptide hormones regulating these behaviors are few in number and common to vertebrates generally. Furthermore, the behavioral actions of AVT and the neuroanatomical sites of AVT synthesis are evolutionarily conserved (Moore, 1992; Moore and Lowry, 1998). By selectively modulating sensorimotor responsiveness to specific sensory stimuli, AVT in nonmammals and vasopressin in mammals can modulate species-typical social behaviors.

V. SUPPRESSION OF MALE REPRODUCTIVE BEHAVIORS: CORTICOSTERONE

Hormonal activation of male reproductive behaviors is only one side of the control mechanism. An animal's behavioral state also depends on hormones and neurotransmitters that suppress or inhibit specific behavioral responses. These positive and negative regulators of behavioral state are analogous to the endocrine mechanisms that control essential physiological functions. For example, the counteracting actions of insulin and glucagon control plasma glucose concentrations and the counteracting actions of calcitonin and parathyroid hormone control plasma calcium concentrations. In much the same way, the counteracting actions of stimulatory and inhibitory hormones control reproductive behaviors.

When wild animals confront harsh or threatening conditions (such as an approaching predator or the freezing temperatures of a severe ice storm), their behaviors usually switch from nonessential behaviors such as courtship or territorial defense to more essential survival behaviors, such as fleeing from the predator or seeking shelter (see Wingfield, 1994). Animals in the wild sometimes survive because neuroendocrine mechanisms can rapidly suppress courtship and mating behaviors.

From fishes to mammals, adaptive behavioral and physiological responses to harsh or threatening conditions are regulated by a common repertoire of hormones, the stress hormones. Three hormones are typically included in the stress axis: stressor → CRH → ACTH → glucocorticoid hormones (CORT or cortisol) → adaptive responses. However, a more complete picture includes additional hormones such as epinephrine, AVT and vasopressin, β-endorphin, dynorphin, and orphanin FQ (nociceptin). These stress hormones control multiple functions, not just the hypothalamic-pituitary-adrenal (HPA) axis and not just stress responses. For example, CRH not only controls ACTH secretion, but it also binds to receptors in the brain and modifies the animals' locomotor activity (Dunn and Berridge, 1990; Lowry and Moore, 1991). Vasopressin and AVT (in nonmammals) not only function as antidiuretic hormones, but also stimulate ACTH secretion in response to specific stressors (Kovacs, 1998). Similarly, the endogenous opioid peptides (dynorphin, β-endorphin, and orphanin FQ) frequently are secreted in response to physiological and social challenges and are involved in the control of many behavioral and physiological responses to specific stressors (Pfaus and Gorzalka, 1987; Reinscheid et al., 1995).

Unfortunately, animal models for studying how stress hormones inhibit reproductive behaviors are rare. Laboratory and domesticated animals generally are insensitive to the effects of stress on reproductive behaviors, whereas many species of wild animals are so sensitive to stress that stress responses are difficult to study in the laboratory. *Taricha* falls between these extremes and has contributed to understanding the hormonal control of stress-induced inhibition of reproductive behaviors.

A. Corticosterone Inhibits Courtship Behaviors in *Taricha*

In *Taricha*, courtship behaviors are suppressed in males that have been injected with specific types of stress hormones—namely CORT, CRH, or κ-opioid-like agonists (Moore and Miller, 1984; Deviche and Moore, 1987). Other studies found that injections of male newts with agonist drugs for γ-aminobutyric acid (GABA) and dopamine receptors also can inhibit male reproductive behaviors (Boyd and Moore, 1990; P. Deviche, unpublished data, with ergocryptine). Although many unanswered questions remain about which of these hormones actually control the newt reproductive behaviors, it is clear that CORT plays an important role.

Follow-up experiments in *Taricha* showed that endogenous CORT rapidly inhibits male reproductive behaviors during acute stress (Moore and Miller, 1984). Male *Taricha* exhibit a typical vertebrate stress response—within a few minutes of exposure to harsh stimuli, plasma corticosterone concentration increases (Moore and Miller, 1984; Moore and Zoeller, 1985). Correlated with the stress-induced increase in plasma corticosterone, male newts show a marked decrease in the propensity to exhibit courtship behaviors. When CORT concentrations are elevated experimentally, such as by exposure to confinement stress or by injecting either CRH or CORT, courtship clasping in male *Taricha* is potently and rapidly suppressed (Moore and Miller, 1984). Treating stressed newts or CRH-injected ones with metyrapone (a competitive inhibitor of 11β-hydroxylation and CORT synthesis) not only blocks the increase in plasma CORT, but also blocks the decrease in courtship behaviors. These studies support the conclusion that, during acute stress, elevated CORT levels act to inhibit newt courtship behaviors.

An interesting fact about this inhibitory effect of CORT on courtship is that it occurs rapidly, within a time frame of a few minutes. For example, in one set of studies (Orchinik et al., 1991) in which sexually active males were tested during the breeding season, a significant number of control males (untreated or saline-injected) initiated courtship by capturing a female in amplexus within 8 minutes of starting the behavior tests. In contrast, none of the CORT-injected males exhibited amplexus at any time during the test (Orchinik et al., 1991). Because of the rapidity of this response, it seems unlikely that CORT works through traditional genomic mechanisms. The search for an explanation led to the discovery of a novel membrane-associated receptor for CORT in *Taricha* brains.

B. Membrane Receptor for Corticosterone

The possibility that the potent inhibitory effects of CORT on courtship in *Taricha* might involve nongenomic receptor mechanisms was supported by two observations. The first has been mentioned: the response is too fast to be explained easily by genomic steroid action, which in the traditional model requires the steroid to enter the cell, bind to a nuclear steroid receptor (a ligand-dependent transcription factor), induce changes in mRNA, and synthesize a protein to produce a response. This series of steps takes at least many minutes and usually several hours to produce physiological responses. The second observation came from a paper by Majewska and colleagues (1986) reporting that metabolites of progesterone and deoxycorticosterone can act on and modulate the $GABA_A$ receptor/chloride channel. Based on this discovery, it seemed reasonable to hypothesize that in *Taricha* the CORT (or its metabolite) binds to the $GABA_A$ receptor and inhibits courtship. This hypothesis was initially attractive because behavioral studies with *Taricha* showed that GABA agonists inhibited amplectic clasping (Boyd and Moore, 1990). Considerable effort went into testing this hypothesis and provided fairly conclusive evidence that the hypothesis is false (Orchinik *et al.*, 1994). CORT probably does not inhibit newt courtship by acting on the $GABA_A$ receptor. Incidentally, those studies found that the pharmacological responses of the $GABA_A$ receptor to steroids in *Taricha* closely match those in mammals (Orchinik *et al.*, 1994).

Using the same assay conditions that he developed to study the $GABA_A$ receptor in *Taricha*, Orchinik discovered a high-affinity binding site for radiolabeled CORT (^{3}H-CORT) in neuronal membranes (Orchinik *et al.*, 1991). This high-affinity binding site has been characterized pharmacologically, biochemically, and behaviorally (described later) and has been shown to meet all the criteria of a legitimate receptor. Henceforth, it is referred to as mCR.

Pharmacological characterization of mCR in *Taricha* was accomplished using ligand-binding assays in kinetic and equilibrium saturation binding studies. This mCR has a binding site that is saturable and binds ^{3}H-CORT with specificity and high-affinity ($K_d = 0.5$ nM) (Orchinik *et al.*, 1991). Estimates of receptor density with respect to ^{3}H-CORT specific binding ($B_{max} = 130$–150 fmol/mg protein) are comparable to the density of neuropeptide receptors, but lower than the densities for the major neurotransmitters. Competition binding studies compared the effectiveness of various steroids to inhibit ^{3}H-CORT specific binding and found that the binding site is highly specific for CORT and cortisol. The ^{3}H-CORT binding site in *Taricha* does not recognize most steroids and has modest to extremely low affinity for dexamethasone, T, progesterone, RU28362, and RU38486 (Orchinik *et al.*, 1991). Data from competition binding studies in *Taricha* were used to calculate inhibition constants (K_i values) and revealed the following rank-order potency of steroids to inhibit ^{3}H-CORT specific binding: CORT > cortisol > aldosterone > RU28362 > dexamethasone. This same rank-order potency for these five steroids holds for the high-affinity binding site for ^{3}H-CORT in neuronal membranes from *Xenopus laevis* (Moore *et al.*, 1995). Because this binding site only has modest affinity for aldosterone ($K_i = 293$ nM) and very low affinity for dexamethasone ($K_i > 5000$ nM), the pharmacological signature for mCR clearly distinguishes it from the intracellular glucocorticoid receptor (iGR). Studies in *Ambystoma tigrinum* confirm that the high-affinity binding sites for ^{3}H-CORT in the neuronal membranes (e.g., mCR) and cytosolic fractions (e.g., iGR) are pharmacologically distinguishable (Orchinik *et al.*, 2000; also see Orchinik *et al.*, Chap. 51 in this volume).

1. Behavioral Function for the Membrane Corticosterone Receptor

Given the initial findings, the critical question became, Does the mCR control the rapid behavioral responses to corticosterone? To address this question, dose–response studies were run to determine the relative potency of specific steroids to rapidly inhibit courtship behaviors in *Taricha* (Orchinik *et al.*, 1991). Unstressed male *Taricha* received an IP injection (saline, CORT, cortisol, aldosterone, RU28362, or dexamethasone) and then were tested for courtship clasping behavior in a standardized 20-minute behavioral test. Data from the dose–response studies, when converted to ED_{50} values (half-maximal effective dose), revealed the following rank-order potency to rapidly inhibit sex behavior:

CORT > cortisol > aldosterone > RU28362 > dexamethasone. Comparisons of ED_{50} values from the behavioral tests with the K_i values from competition binding studies show a strong correlation ($r = 0.98$). It is important to note that, the concordance between ligand-binding assays and the dose–response behavioral studies support the conclusion that mCR is a functional receptor (Orchinik et al., 1991). These results are unique to the literature and provide strong evidence that rapid responses to steroid hormones involve membrane-associated receptor mechanisms (for reviews of steroid membrane receptors, see Wehling, 1997; Moore and Evans, 1999; Kelly and Wagner, 1999). In this amphibian, there is good reason to believe that CORT controls the rapid inhibition of reproductive behaviors by binding to and activating the mCR in neuronal membranes.

2. Evidence That the Membrane Corticosterone Receptor Is a G-Protein-Coupled Receptor

Of the three major types of membrane receptors—the ligand-gated ion channels, enzyme-linked receptors, and G-protein-coupled receptors (GPCR)—the most prevalent in the brain are the GPCRs. Ligand-binding studies in *Taricha* indicate that the mCR has similar pharmacological characteristics to known receptors in the GPCR superfamily. These studies found that ^{3}H-CORT specific binding in neuronal membranes is negatively modulated by nonhydrolyzable guanine nucleotide analogs, especially GTP-γ-S (guanosine 5'-[γ-thio]triphosphate). Furthermore, ^{3}H-CORT specific binding is enhanced in a concentration-dependent manner by adding Mg^{2+} to the assay buffer. Together, these data suggest that the mCR is a GPCR (Orchinik et al., 1992).

3. Biochemical Studies of the Membrane Corticosterone Receptor

Studies have attempted to determine the molecular identity of the mCR (i.e., identify its amino acid sequence) by isolating the receptor protein from *Taricha* neuronal membranes. As a first step, conditions were optimized for solubilizing neuronal membranes with nonionic detergents and maintaining binding activity (Evans et al., 1998). Ligand-binding assays with the solubilized mCR confirmed that it binds ^{3}H-CORT with high affinity and specificity. Competition binding studies revealed that solubilization does not change the mCR pharmacological signature and maintains the same rank-order potency of steroids to inhibit ^{3}H-CORT binding (CORT > cortisol > aldosterone > dexamethasone).

The second step in the search for the mCR's molecular identity involved evaluating different chromatographic schemes for purifying the receptor protein. Partial purification of solubilized mCR was accomplished with sequential enrichment using ammonium sulfate fractionation, then wheat germ agglutinin (WGA) agarose chromatography, then hydroxylapatite chromatography, then immobilized ligand affinity resin (affinity chromatography with CORT-Sepharose), and finally SDS-PAGE gel electrophoresis (Evans et al., 2000a). Ligand binding assays confirmed that each chromatographic step enriched the active mCR. Because WGA chromatography was found to greatly enrich the mCR, it seems likely that this receptor protein is glycosylated (as are all known GPCRs). After four purification steps, SDS-PAGE gels revealed a single putative receptor protein with an apparent mass of 63 kDa (Evans et al., 2000b).

Two independent approaches confirm that the estimated mass of *Taricha*'s mCR is 63 kDa (Evans et al., 2000a). First, differential-display chromatography visualized the putative receptor protein on 2-D SDS-PAGE gels that contained proteins eluted from parallel CORT-Sepharose affinity columns. One column contained active mCR, and the other column contained occupied mCR (excess CORT in buffer). Second, the putative receptor protein was identified with a photoreactive form of CORT (azido-CORT) by visualizing the photoaffinity-labeled proteins on 2-D SDS-PAGE gels with western blot methodology and anticorticosterone antiserum (Evans et al., 2000a; Evans and Moore, 2001). Both of these techniques identified the putative receptor protein as having an estimated mass of 63 kDa. This mass matches the mass of many known GPCRs, including the opioid-like receptors.

These studies have identified the biochemical strategies for purifying and sequencing the mCR protein from brain tissue. In addition, these studies provide further evidence that the mCR is not a membrane-associated iGR, because it is glycosylated and has a mass that is too small for known intracellular glucocorticoid receptors ($\sim$92 kDa).

4. κ-Selective Ligand Binding to the Membrane Corticosterone Receptor

Grazzini et al. (1998) presented evidence that progesterone binds to and inhibits the oxytocin receptor, a member of the GPCR superfamily. That paper prompted us to investigate whether an analogous phenomenon might explain the high-affinity binding site for ^{3}H-CORT in *Taricha*, testing the possibility that the mCR might be a functional binding site on a known GPCR. The initial screening studies evaluated the effects of 21 ligands (at 10 μM) on inhibiting ^{3}H-CORT specific binding (Evans et al., 2000b). Many of these competitors had been shown in behavioral tests to enhance or suppress courtship behaviors in *Taricha*. Three of the 21 competitors inhibited ^{3}H-CORT binding. Naloxone (a nonselective opioid antagonist) and U50,488 (a κ-selective opioid agonist) inhibited about 70% of ^{3}H-CORT specific binding, whereas, dynorphin, the endogenous κ-selective opioid peptide, inhibited about 25% of ^{3}H-CORT binding in *Taricha* membrane preparations. Therefore, the initial screening showed that two κ-selective agonists and one nonselective antagonist are recognized by the ^{3}H-CORT binding site (Evans et al., 2000b).

In follow-up studies, various opioid ligands were tested in equilibrium competition studies with ^{3}H-CORT and membrane preparations from *Taricha*. The ligand with the highest affinity for the ^{3}H-CORT binding site is dynorphin ($K_i < 1$ nM). The rank-order potency of the various opioids to inhibit ^{3}H-CORT binding is: dynorphin > U50,488 > naloxone > bremazocine > EKC (ethylketocyclazocine) (Evans et al., 2000b). All of these compounds are κ-selective agonists, except for naloxone, the nonselective opioid antagonist (Raynor et al., 1994). Kinetic studies provided evidence that U50,488 and corticosterone interact directly (not allosteroically) by competing for the same binding pocket (Evans et al., 2000b). Four ligands that normally have high-affinity binding to the κ-opioid receptor in mammals and amphibians (U69,593, diprenorphine, nor-BNI [nor-binaltorphimine], and etorphin) did not inhibit ^{3}H-CORT binding.

The pharmacology of the ^{3}H-CORT binding site in *Taricha* is interesting because the site recognizes several κ-selective agonists. But this site differs from known kappa opioid binding sites because of the modest to low affinities for bremazocine, EKC, and naloxone and the failure to recognize several other opioid ligands. Another important observation is that the κ-selective ligands only inhibited a maximum of 70% of ^{3}H-CORT binding, suggesting that there are opioid-sensitive and opioid-insensitive binding sites for ^{3}H-CORT. In conclusion, these studies suggest that ^{3}H-CORT might be binding to several high-affinity sites and that the predominant site recognizes specific κ-selective opioids.

5. Membrane Corticosteroid Receptor and Opioid Receptors

The overlap in binding-site selectivity between the mCR and κ-opioid-like receptors could be misleading or it could reveal that the mCR is structurally related to the opioid receptor family. A generalization in endocrinology is that the more related receptors are structurally, the more closely related they are pharmacologically, meaning that their binding sites recognize similar subsets of ligands. There are, of course, exceptions to this generalization, namely the cases in which the same ligands bind to structurally unrelated receptors (e.g., many of the same ligands bind to the structurally unrelated GABA$_A$ and GABA$_B$ receptors).

Opioid receptors—the δ-, μ-, κ-, and orphanin FQ receptors—are structurally related members of the GPCR superfamily. The basic biochemical properties of these opioid receptors and many other GPCRs match those of the mCR in *Taricha* in that they are glycosylated proteins with a mass of 58–64 kDa. Also as already mentioned, ligand-binding assays show that the mCR in *Taricha* responds to quanine nucleotide analogs and Mg^{2+} in the same ways as known GPCRs (Orchinik et al., 1992). Finally, the subset of κ-selective ligands that have been shown to inhibit ^{3}H-CORT binding partially matches the binding site selectivity of the κ-opioid receptor and the orphanin FQ receptor, not matching either exactly, but overlapping with both. Because of these considerations, it seems reasonable to entertain the hypothesis that the mCR in *Taricha* is a κ-opioid-like receptor (Evans et al., 2000b).

Behavioral studies in *Taricha* reveal that CORT and κ-selective agonists have similar effects. Specifically, amplectic clasping responses in males are suppressed by injections of CORT (Moore and Miller, 1984) or injections of the κ-agonists bremazocine or EKC (Deviche and Moore, 1987). The inhibitory effects of stress on amplectic clasping are ameliorated by pretreating males with metyrapone (Moore and Miller, 1984) or naloxone (nonselective opioid antagonist that binds to the mCR) (Deviche and Moore, 1987).

C. Neural Mechanisms of mCR-Mediated Corticosterone Effects on Clasping

We have identified rapid neural effects of CORT at multiple levels of the brain in *Taricha*, but most of our research has focused on neurons in the medulla, an important brain area for controlling amplectic clasping. These neurophysiological studies have identified many rapid actions of CORT that are likely to be critical to the hormone's effect on clasping.

1. Corticosterone Rapidly Blocks Neuronal Responses to Clasp Trigger Stimuli

In unanesthetized, immobilized newts (Rose *et al.*, 1993), CORT injection in a dose producing circulating levels similar to those produced by a moderate stress (32 nmol, IP), eliminated or greatly attenuated neuronal responses to cloacal pressure (Fig. 2). This effect was very rapid, appearing within 3–7.5 min and occurring in the great majority of the neurons tested. However, in a substantial portion of these same neurons, robust responses to stimulation of the face or limbs remained. Another pervasive effect of CORT, with a similar onset latency, was a depression or elimination of spontaneous neuronal activity. This effect even occurred in neurons in which responsiveness to noncloacal stimuli persisted after CORT. Of particular importance is the fact that injections of dexamethasone (DEX), a synthetic glucocorticoid that has low affinity for mCR (Orchinik *et al.*, 1991), failed to alter sensory responsiveness or spontaneous activity of any medullary neurons. DEX injections were not completely without effect, however. A DEX injection 30 min prior to CORT blocked the usual CORT effects on sensory responsiveness and spontaneous activity in medullary neurons. The mechanism through which DEX exerts this effect is unknown.

The examination of CORT effects on the excitability properties of reticulospinal neurons by means of antidromic invasion revealed multiple changes in excitability of these neurons. These effects included a slowing of the generation of the antidromic action potential, attenuated action potential amplitude (Fig. 1.), increased current threshold for antidromic spike elicitation, and prolonged recovery cycle for responsiveness to paired-pulse stimuli. All of these effects represented depressed excitability of a type that could have been produced by a membrane hyperpolarization (Lipski, 1981). These changes in excitability began to occur with a short latency, usually in 4–8 min, intensified with time, and also involved progressively more neurons with time. DEX injections usually produced no effects.

Although reticulospinal neurons in the immobilized newts tended not to show firing in response to sensory stimuli, the application of cloacal pressure often altered the probability of antidromic firing or modified the waveform of the antidromic spike, reflecting the action of a sensory input to the reticulospinal neuron. This sensory influence on reticulospinal neurons was rapidly blocked by CORT. These CORT effects were also present in newts with a premedullary brain-stem transection, indicating a hormone action on the caudal neuraxis that was independent of the rostral regions of the brain.

CORT effects on medullary neurons are closely associated with the suppression of clasping. In freely behaving newts, we examined medullary neuronal activity during CORT-induced impairment or elimination of reflexive clasping (Rose *et al.*, 1995b, 1998). CORT injection rapidly depressed the probability and quality of reflexive clasping. This effect was apparent in some newts as soon as 5 min after injection and persisted for most of the subsequent hour. In some newts, clasping began to recover 1 hour after CORT injection. In contrast to the pronounced impairment of clasping, locomotion and other behaviors appeared to be quite normal.

Neurophysiological observations in the behaving newts replicated the principal CORT effects in immobilized newts already described. But in the behaving animals the functional properties of medullary neurons were very closely tied to clasping and other behaviors displayed by the newts. Consequently, the association between CORT-induced changes in the properties of these neurons and CORT-induced impairment of clasping was clearly apparent. The nature of CORT effects on medullary neurons was consistent with the selective effect of CORT on clasping. Of the reticulospinal and other medullary neurons that initially showed clasping-related activity, more than three-quarters of these neurons lost this activity after CORT injection. This CORT effect appeared within 5 min of injection in many of these neurons and involved progressively more neurons with increasing time. The principal aspects of neuronal activity that were associated with clasping, such as the burst of firing at the onset and offset of cloacal pressure, were reduced or eliminated by CORT (Fig. 2). For most of these neurons the CORT effect was behaviorally specific, showing a trial-by-trial association with clasp quality. For example, the degree that a neuron responded (or failed to respond) to the onset of cloacal pressure could predict the quality or failure of clasping in response to that particular stimulus. Neuronal activity that was associated with nonclasping motor events such as locomotion usually persisted with little or no change (Fig. 2). Only approximately one-third of the neurons that initially showed such nonclasping activity exhibited a loss of movement-associated firing. In these cases, the affected neurons showed very global changes in function, in which all observable dimensions of activity, such as spontaneous firing rates, were profoundly altered by the hormone. Antidromic spikes from neurons showing the more global, steady-state effects of CORT typically showed indications of reduced excitability or total loss of responsiveness to spinal stimuli.

We believe that these CORT-induced changes in medullary neuronal activity are causally linked with the depression of reflexive clasping for the following reasons: (1) they occurred in a brain region of known importance for clasping control, (2) the trial-by-trial properties of neuronal activity had a predictable association with individual episodes of clasping or clasp impairment, (3) the types of functional alterations in these neurons that were produced by CORT (e.g., loss of response to cloacal stimuli) are of a form that could underlie impaired clasping, (4) the time course of changes in neuronal activity following CORT corresponded well with the time course of CORT effects on clasping, (5) the magnitude of the CORT effect on individual neurons and number of neurons affected is consistent with concurrent impairment of clasping, and (6) there was a dissociation between impaired clasping and related neuronal activity, on one hand, and the relative lack of impairment of other sensorimotor functions and their associated neuronal activity, on the other.

2. Spinal Corticosterone Effect on Clasping

As explained previously, the basic display of amplexus in *Taricha*, as in other amphibians, is spinally controlled, but subject to regulation by descending reticulospinal influences. It is clear that these types of CORT effects on medullary neurons could account for the hormone's rapid effect on clasping. However, the possibility of a direct spinal action remains. In a study in newts with a high cervical spinal transection (Lewis and Rose, 2000), CORT rapidly depressed the maintenance but not elicitation of clasping by cloacal stimulation. These results indicate that mCR is probably present in spinal neurons. But the selective CORT effect on clasp maintenance suggests a lack of action on primary afferent neurons or on neuromuscular components of clasping, including spinal motor neurons and the motor units they innervate. It appears more likely that CORT affected the hypothesized spinal clasp-generating mechanism that regulates the sustained expression of clasping.

D. Rapid Corticosterone Effects on Forebrain Neurons

Single neuron and multiunit activity were recorded in various forebrain regions including the dorsal pallium and hippocampal primordium in behaving newts (Rose and Moore, 1992). Before CORT injection, the neural activity in these regions was broadly correlated with diverse types of movements displayed by the newt as well as sensory stimuli such as cloacal pressure. Within 10 minutes of CORT injection, the activity of these forebrain regions became dissociated from sensory and motor events (such as locomotion and head movements in response to sensory stimuli), suggesting that the forebrain was no longer receiving or responding to sensory inputs or signals related to the generation of motor events by brain-stem-spinal motor networks. This dissociation in the continued presence of sensorimotor function in these newts indicates that the forebrain contributes relatively little to the control of these behaviors. It is clear from the investigation of medullary neurons in freely behaving newts that the effects of CORT can be much more selective and functionally specific than a simple depression of neuronal function. However, the results from these forebrain recordings, together with our findings from other brain systems make it clear that a rapid depression of neural function, especially sensory processing, is a widespread CORT effect on the brain.

E. General Conclusions Concerning the Rapid Neural Actions of Corticosterone

In addition to the foregoing conclusions, some additional interpretations can be presented about the mCR-mediated actions of CORT in *Taricha*.

1. The widespread effects of CORT in the brain and spinal cord imply that the mCRs are present in most neurons or that neurons with such receptors have widespread influences on other neurons.

2. The neuronal effects of CORT on medullary neuronal activity take two forms: a functionally specific effect in which clasping-related neuronal activity is selectively lost and a global effect consisting of a steady-state depression of neuronal sensory responsiveness, spike-generating capability, and spontaneous firing. Both types of effects can be occurring in different neurons at the same time.

3. The functionally specific CORT effects are so closely tied to clasping-related neural processes that these effects are observable only when neuronal activity and hormone-sensitive behaviors are monitored concurrently.

4. The different properties of the functionally specific and global CORT effects suggest that the hormone's neuronal actions are diverse. The character of the global effect suggests a general depression of neuronal excitability. In contrast, the functionally specific effect seems more likely to result from a change in the way neurons operate within a particular functional network (e.g., clasping) apart from the operations of the same neurons in different functional networks (e.g., locomotion).

VI. NEUROPHYSIOLOGICAL INTERACTIONS BETWEEN CORTICOSTERONE AND THE NEUROPEPTIDES CRH AND VASOTOCIN

The rapid nongenomic actions of CORT on the brain in *Taricha* have been found to interact potently with rapid neural actions of CRH and AVT. As explained previously, AVT causes an enhancement of spontaneous firing and responsiveness to somatic stimuli, especially cloacal pressure, by medullary neurons. CORT injection 10–17 min after AVT application caused an unexpected effect—the rapid potentiation of neuronal spontaneous activity and response to cloacal and other somatic stimuli (Rose et al., 1996). Thus, prior exposure of the medulla to AVT reversed the usual effect of CORT. In contrast, CORT injection 30 min before AVT application to the medulla caused the neuropeptide's effect to be reversed, resulting in a rapid decrease in the number of medullary reticular neurons responsive to cloacal and other somatic stimuli. The basic patterns of these interactive AVT–CORT effects on medullary neurons are shown in Fig. 4. These interactive effects of CORT and AVT could produce finely tuned behavioral responses to stressful conditions in the context of reproduction in the following ways. Among breeding *Taricha*, if an unpaired male were attacked by a predator but escaped, the subsequently elevated plasma CORT would suppress courtship behavior by making the male less responsive to female sexual stimuli. This effect could protect the male from further imminent risk of predation that would be associated with the conspicuous nature of courtship behaviors. But suppose a male that was under the neural influence of AVT action had already initiated clasping and subsequently, as mating newts frequently do, numerous other males surrounded this clasping male, competing for access to the clasped female. Being at the center of this aggregation of competing males would probably cause CORT secretion by this clasping male, but subsequent to the on-going AVT action, this CORT would rapidly act on the medullary neurons to increase their response to cloacal stimuli generated by clasping, thereby intensifying the clasp. In this particular case, given the competitive nature of courtship in *Taricha*, it would probably be the most successful reproductive strategy for a male that is already clasping a female to continue clasping rather than respond to stressful stimuli with the interruption of courtship behavior.

We have also identified interactions between CORT and AVT in the optic tectum (Rose et al., 1997), but the pattern of these interactions is different from those that we observed in the medulla. CORT effects on visual system functioning were assessed in waking immobilized newts by recording field potentials evoked from the midbrain optic tectum in response to flashes of light. Consistent with other effects of CORT, the injection of the steroid caused a depression in magnitude of the optic tectum evoked response within 5–10 min. Thus,

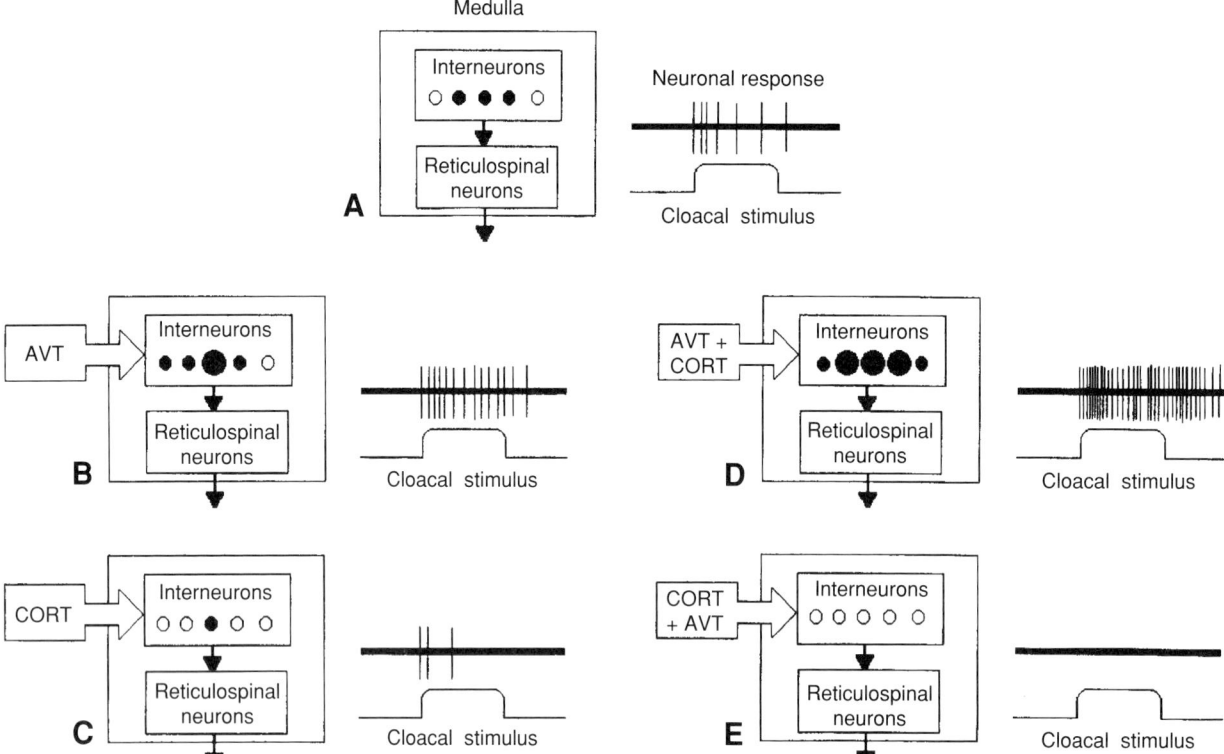

FIGURE 4 Schematic illustration of the actions and interactions of CORT and AVT in a medullary neuronal population. The figure is a simulation illustrating results of experiments (Rose *et al.*, 1993, 1995a) showing that (1) the response of medullary reticular neurons to cloacal pressure, a clasp-triggering stimulus, is strongly and rapidly affected by AVT as well as CORT; concurrent action of these two hormones has an even stronger effect either hormone alone; and the direction of this joint effect depends on the order of administration of AVT and CORT. Each insert A–E shows the medullary level of the newt brain stem with two classes of neurons, reticulospinal neurons, which provide the chief output of the brain to the spinal cord, and interneurons, which represent medullary reticular neurons that do not project to the spinal cord, but may have connections in the brain, including reticulospinal neurons. In the rectangle representing interneurons, the symbols depict neurons that in a given state respond (filled circles) or do not respond (open circles) to pressure on the cloaca. The larger filled circles represent stronger responses. At the right of each medullary diagram is a hypothetical depiction of a single interneuron's response to an application of cloacal pressure of several second's duration, under the hormonal conditions in A–E. (A) Under conditions of relatively low prevailing CORT or AVT action on the medulla, a majority of the neurons respond to cloacal pressure and their response is of an intermediate magnitude. (B) During the action of AVT on the medullary interneurons, a greater proportion of the neurons respond to cloacal pressure and the responses are enhanced in magnitude. (C) During the action of CORT at the mGR, very few neurons respond and response magnitude is very small. (D) AVT action on the medulla followed within a few minutes by CORT action at the mGR causes the great majority of the neurons to respond and their individual responses to be very pronounced in magnitude. (E) CORT action on the medulla at the mGR followed within minutes by AVT action leads to an extreme depression of the number of neurons responding and great reduction of response magnitude or complete elimination of responses.

the effects of CORT and AVT, acting separately on tectal responses to light flashes, were similar. However, CORT injected within 20 min after tectal AVT application produced an increase rather than a decrease in tectal-evoked responses to light flashes. So, although the hormone effects were somewhat different in medullary and tectal recording studies, the reversal of a CORT effect by prior AVT action was seen in both. In the case of the tectum, we have interpreted the tectal action of AVT as a mechanism through which the peptide could decrease reactivity to bright light and enable newts to maintain exposed positions in the shallow margins of mating ponds. The CORT interaction with AVT could, in contrast, provide a rapid means of reversing this tolerance of bright light, such that a newt in mating condition (presumably with an AVT-influenced brain) that was exposed to a stressor and subsequently secreted CORT would become rapidly more photophobic and inclined to retreat to a safer location in the darker depths of the pond rather than maintain its position in shallow water. The mechanisms through which these CORT–AVT interactions occur in the medulla and midbrain are not known.

Similar patterns of interaction occur between CRH and CORT (Rose *et al.*, 1996). We have reported that intraventricular CRH infusion potentiates the firing levels of single medullary neurons that have locomotion-related properties (Lowry *et al.*, 1996). This increase in neuron activity is closely associated with the stimulation of locomotion by CRH. In subsequent recordings from immobilized unanesthetized newts (Rose *et al.*, 1996), we found that CRH application to the medulla in Taricha causes a rapidly appearing increase in neuronal spontaneous activity in both reticulospinal and nonreticulospinal neurons and responsiveness to somatic stimuli, including cloacal pressure. CORT injection 5–10 min after CRH was followed by further enhancement of activity and excitability of these medullary neurons instead of the usual depression of activity and sensory responsiveness.

Collectively, the evidence for interactions between CORT and these neuropeptides reveals that the rapid neural actions of CORT are potentially quite diverse and likely to depend on the neuroendocrine milieu of the brain when CORT effects ensue. In contrast to the high-stress situation in which CORT effects might predominate, a condition in which AVT action in the brain was occurring prior to stress-induced CORT release (as in ongoing clasping) could lead to an intensification of clasping.

A. Rapid Stress Hormone Actions on the Neural Control of Clasping: A Summary Model

The following presents a synthesis of the neural actions of CORT, AVT, and CRH on reflexive clasping. The basic components of this neural system and known levels of hormone action are shown in Fig. 5. Circulating CORT binds with mCR in neurons in widespread brain and spinal cord locations to produce rapidly appearing changes in multiple aspects of neuronal function. CORT effects in the medulla and spinal cord are sufficient by themselves to account for the disruption of clasping that occurs within a small number of minutes after the first changes in neuronal function appear. Clasping deteriorates with a sequence of changes that includes a decline in clasp quality, in which partial, poorly sustained, and sometimes unilateral clasps appear, after which cloacal stimulation fails to trigger a clasp at all.

The changes in medullary reticular neuronal function that are most closely associated with CORT's reduction of clasping are a loss of cloacal stimulus-related changes in firing and concurrently a loss of firing specifically associated with clasping movements. These changes occur in most reticulospinal and nonreticulospinal neurons. For most medullary neurons, the loss of response to cloacal stimulation is selective, with responses to stimulation of other body regions being retained.

The CORT-induced loss of clasping-related activity is also selective in that neuronal activity related to other kinds of motor events usually persists. The selective loss of response to cloacal stimulation probably involves a CORT effect presynaptic to medullary neurons but is probably not due to a change in primary afferent function. The CORT-induced changes in clasping-related reticulospinal-neuron firing patterns are highly specific and precisely associated on a second-by-second basis with the appearance of impaired clasping. These functional changes, such as a loss of the usual suppression of firing during clasping, appear to be due to a loss of the brief changes in reticulospinal neuron excitability that underlie the normal clasp-associated activity. These same neurons continue to show dynamic excitability changes during other behaviors, such as walking or head movements. This observation suggests that CORT produces an impairment in a clasp-controlling mechanism in the medulla because afferent input from cloacal mechanoreceptors can no longer trigger a switch in motor control from an ongoing nonclasping motor state to a state of clasping. The fact that these specific clasping-related changes in reticulospinal neuron function are evident only in the dynamic expression of a functional operation implies a type of CORT effect that operates specifically on dynamic aspects of neuronal function. A minority of reticulospinal and nonreticulospinal neurons undergo a rapidly developing, global, steady-state depression of activity level and excitability.

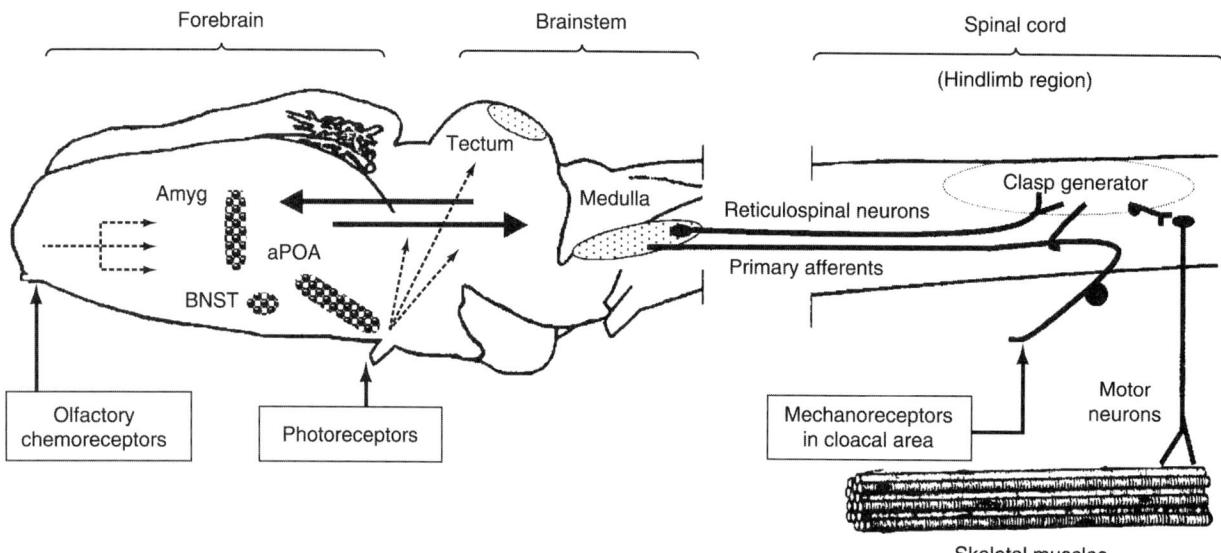

FIGURE 5 This schematic illustrates the sites where vasotocin and corticosterone could interact and control male courtship behaviors. Sexually active males initiate courtship behaviors in response to species-specific olfactory and visual sensory stimuli. The sensorimotor processing of these sexual stimuli appears to be modulated by antagonistic and synergistic interactions between vasotocin and corticosterone. In the forebrain, vasotocin has been shown to enhance behavioral responses to sex pheromones and to be sexually dimorphic in the amygdala (Amyg), bed nucleus of stria terminalis (BNST), and anterior preoptic area (aPOA). In the brain stem, vasotocin and corticosterone modulate neuronal and behavioral responses at sites in the optic tectum and the medulla. Additional sites of interaction include neurons that respond to tactile sensory input from mechanoreceptors (primary afferent sensory neurons) and the reticulospinal neurons associated with the clasp-generating motor neurons.

The properties of this effect are consistent with a membrane hyperpolarization and imply a membrane effect of CORT on processes regulating action potential generation. Although fewer neurons show this global change in function, this type of CORT action is likely to contribute to the hormone's effect on clasping because of its magnitude and the types of neurons involved. The distinction between the two types of CORT effect suggests that the hormone alters some neuronal signaling mechanisms and network processes differently from others. CORT action at the spinal level is limited to an effect on the clasp-generating process, whereby the duration of a given clasp following the termination of the cloacal-eliciting stimulus is shortened. Due to the rather limited nature of the spinal CORT effects it appears that most of the effects of CORT on clasping are due to the hormone's effect on the brain, principally the medulla. The effects on this system of a single CORT injection typically undergo a reversal in less than 1 hour, which suggests that the nongenomic action of CORT is separate from a longer latency genomic action.

The CORT actions on medullary neurons are subject to modification by the prior actions of the neuropeptides AVT and CRH. AVT causes a rapidly appearing enhancement of spontaneous activity and responsiveness to cloacal stimulation of medullary neurons. This neuropeptide also reverses the usual effect of CORT, such that the steroid strongly enhances medullary on neuronal activity and responsiveness to cloacal stimuli if it is given within a few minutes of AVT. In contrast, the administration of CORT a few minutes before AVT reverses the effect of the neuropeptide. CRH, which like AVT increases activity and sensory response of medullary neurons to cloacal stimulation, also reverses the effect of subsequent CORT administration, causing a further enhancement of spontaneous activity and sensory responsiveness. The rapidity of these neuropeptide interactions with CORT indicates that they are tied to CORT action at the mCR. Functionally, these interactions allow for very rapid, adaptive adjustments in the probability and strength of clasping behavior as a consequence changing environmental factors, such as competition with other males or attack by predators.

References

Andreoletti, G. E., Malacarne, G., and Vellano, C. (1983). Androgen control of male sexual behavior in the crested newt (*Triturus cristatus carnifex* Laur.): Castration and sex steroid administration. *Horm. Behav.* **17**, 103–110.

Aronson, L. R., and Noble, G. K. (1945). The sexual behavior of anura—2. Neural mechanisms controlling mating in the male leopard frog, *Rana pipiens*. *Bull. Am. Mus. Nat. Hist.* **86**, 83–140.

Bohus, B. (1977). Effect of desglycinamide-lysine vasopressin (DG-LVP) on sexually motivated T-maze behavior of the male rat. *Horm. Behav.* **8**, 52–61.

Born, J., Fehm-Wolfsdorf, G., Lutzenberger, W., Voigt, K., and Fehm, H. (1986). Vasopressin and electrophysiological signs of attention in man. *Peptides (N.Y.)* **7**, 189–193.

Boyd, S. K. (1994a). Arginine vasotocin facilitation of advertisement calling and call phonotaxis in bullfrogs. *Horm. Behav.* **28**, 232–240.

Boyd, S. K. (1994b). Gonadal steroid modulation of vasotocin concentrations in the bullfrog brain. *Neuroendocrinology* **60**(2), 150–156.

Boyd, S. K. (1997). Brain vasotocin pathways and the control of sexual behaviors in the bullfrog. *Brain Res. Bull.* **44**, 345–350.

Boyd, S. K., and Moore, F. L. (1990). Autoradiographic localization of putative arginine vasotocin receptors in the kidney of a urodele amphibian. *Gen. Comp. Endocrinol.* **78**, 344–350.

Boyd, S. K., and Moore, F. L. (1991). Gonadectomy reduces the concentrations of putative receptors for arginine vasotocin in the brain of an amphibian. *Brain Res.* **541**, 193–197.

Boyd, S. K., and Moore, F. L. (1992). Sexually dimorphic concentrations of arginine vasotocin in sensory regions of the amphibian brain. *Brain Res.* **588**, 304–306.

Boyd, S. K., Tyler, C. J., and De Vries, G. J. (1992). Sexual dimorphism in the vasotocin system of the bullfrog (*Rana catesbeiana*). *J. Comp. Neurol.* **325**, 313–325.

Cedrini, L., and Fasolo, A. (1970). Olfactory attractants in sex recognition of the crested newt: An electrophysiological research. *Monit. Zool. Ital. [N.S.]* **5**, 223–229.

Chu, J., Marler, C. A., and Wilczynski, W. (1998). The effects of arginine vasotocin on the calling behavior of male cricket frogs in changing social contexts. *Horm. Behav.* **34**, 248–261.

Davis, G. A., and Moore, F. L. (1996). Neuroanatomical distribution of androgen and estrogen receptor-immunoreactive cells in the brain of the male roughskin newt. *J. Comp. Neurol.* **372**, 294–308.

Deviche, P., and Moore, F. L. (1987). Opioid Kappa-receptor agonists suppress sexual behaviors in male rough-skinned newts. *Horm. Behav.* **21**, 371–383.

Deviche, P., and Moore, F. L. (1988). Steroidal control of sexual behavior in the rough-skinned newt (*Taricha granulosa*): Effect of testosterone, estradiol, and dihydrotestosterone. *Horm. Behav.* **22**, 26–34.

Deviche, P., Propper, C. R., and Moore, F. L. (1990). Neuroendocrine, behavioral, and morphological changes associated with the termination of the reproductive period in a natural population of male rough-skinned newts (*Taricha granulosa*). *Horm. Behav.* **24**, 284–300.

Diakow, C. (1978). Hormonal basis for breeding behavior in female frogs: Vasotocin inhibits the release call of *Rana pipiens*. *Science* **199**, 1456–1457.

Di Meglio, M., Morrell, J. I., and Pfaff, D. W. (1987). Localization of steroid-concentrating cells in the central nervous system of the frog *Rana esculenta*. *Gen. Comp. Endocrinol.* **67**, 149–154.

D'Istria, M., Delrio, G., Botte, V., and Chieffi, G. (1974). Radioimmunoassay of testosterone, 17beta-oestradiol and oestrone in the male and female plasma of plasma of *Rana esculenta* during sexual cycle. *Steroids Lipids Res.* **5**, 42–48.

Dunn, A. J., and Berridge, C. W. (1990). Physiological and behavioral responses to corticotropin-releasing factor administration: Is CRF a mediator of anxiety or stress responses? *Brain Res. Rev.* **15**, 71–100.

Ebner, K., Wotjak, C. T., Holsboer, F., Landgraf, R., and Engelmann, M. (1999). Vasopressin released within the septal brain area during swim stress modulates the behavioral stress response in rats. *Eur. J. Neurosci.* **11**, 997–1002.

Erulkar, S. D., Kelly, D. B., Jurman, M. E., Zemlan, F. P., Schneider, G. T., and Krieger, N. R. (1981). Modulation of the neural control of the clasp reflex in male *Xenopus laevis* by androgens: A multidisciplinary study. *Proc. Natl. Acad. Sci. U.S.A.* **78**, 5876–5880.

Evans, J. E., Moore, F. L., and Murray, T. F. (1998). Solubilization and pharmacological characterization of a glucocorticoid membrane receptor from an amphibian brain. *J. Steroid Biochem. Mol. Biol.* **67**, 1–8.

Evans, S. J., and Moore, F. L. (2001). Non-radioactive photoaffinity labeling of steroid receptors using a western blot detection system. *Meth. Mol. Biol.* **176**, 261–272.

Evans, S. J., Murray, T. F., and Moore, F. L. (2000a). Partial purification and biochemical characterization of a membrane glucocorticoid receptor from an amphibian brain. *J. Steroid Biochem. Mol. Biol.* **72**, 209–221.

Evans, S. J., Searcy, B. T., and Moore, F. L. (2000b). A subset of kappa opioid ligands bind to the membrane glucocorticoid receptor in an amphibian brain. *Endocrinology (Baltimore)* **141**, 2294–2300.

Foran, C. M., and Bass, A. H. (1998). Preoptic AVT immunoreactive neurons of a teleost fish with alternative reproductive tactics. *Gen. Comp. Endocrinol.* **111**, 271–282.

Garnier, D. H. (1985). Androgen and estrogen levels in the plasma of *Pleurodeles waltl*, Michah., during the annual cycle. I. Male cycle. *Gen. Comp. Endocrinol.* **58**, 376–385.

Gobbetti, A., and Zerani, M. (1995). Prostaglandin E2-9-ketoreducatase and prostaglandin F 2a activate brain aromatase to induce courtship in the male crested newt, *Triturus carnifex*. *Horm. Behav.* **29**, 267–277.

Gobbetti, A., and Zerani, M. (1999). Hormonal and cellular brain mechanisms regulating the amplexus of male and female water frog (*Rana esculenta*). *J. Neuroendocrinol.* **11**, 589–596.

Gobbetti, A., Zerani, M., and Botte, V. (1991a). Plasma prostaglandin $F_{2\alpha}$ in the male *Triturus carnifex* (Laur.) during the reproductive annual cycle and effects of exogenous prostaglandin on sex hormones. *Prostaglandins* **41**, 67–74.

Gobbetti, A., Zerani, M., Bolelli, G. F., and Botte, V. (1991b). Seasonal changes in plasma prostaglandin F2 alpha and sex hormones in the male water frog, *Rana esculenta Gen. Comp. Endocrinol.* **82**, 331–336.

Godwin, J., Sawby, R., Warner, R. R., Crews, D., and Grober, M. S. (2000). Hypothalamic arginine vasotocin mRNA abundance variation across sexes and with sex change in a coral reef fish. *Brain, Behav. Evol.* **55**, 77–84.

Goodson, J. L., and Bass, A. H. (2000). Vasotocin innervation and modulation of vocal-acoustic circuitry in the teleost *Porichthys notatus*. *J. Comp. Neurol.* **422**, 363–379.

Grant, W. C. J., and Grant, J. A. (1956). The induction of water drive in the land stage of *Triturus viridescens* following hypophysectomy. *Anat. Rec.* **125**, 604.

Grazzini, E., Guillon, G., Mouillac, B., and Zingg, H. H. (1998). Inhibition of oxytocin receptor function by direct binding of progesterone. *Nature (London)* **392**, 509–512.

Grillner, S., Ekeberg, Ö., El Manira, A., Lasner, A., Parker, D., Tegnér, J., and Wallén, P. (1998a). Intrinsic function of a neuronal network a vertebrate central pattern generator. *Brain Res. Rev.* **26**, 184–197.

Grillner, S., Parker, D., and El Manira, A. (1998b). Vertebrate locomotion—a lamprey perspective. *Ann. N.Y. Acad. Sci.* **860**, 1–18.

Grober, M. S., and Sunobe, T. (1996). Serial adult sex change involves rapid and reversible changes in forebrain neurochemistry. *NeuroReport* **7**, 2945–2949.

Halliday, T. R. (1977). The courtship of European newts: An evolutionary perspective. *In* "The Reproductive Biology of Amphibians" (D. Taylor, S. I. Guttman, and K. Yamamoto, eds.), pp. 185–232. Plenum Press, New York.

Harvey, L. A., Propper, C. R., Woodley, S. K., and Moore, M. C. (1997). Reproductive endocrinology of the explosively breeding desert spadefoot toad, *Scaphiopus couchii*. *Gen. Comp. Endocrinol.* **105**, 102–113.

Hutchison, J. B., and Poynton, J. C. (1963). A neurological study of the clasp reflex in *Xenopus laevis* (daudin). *Behaviour* **22**, 41–63.

Imai, K., Tanaka, S., and Takikawa, H. (1985). Annual cycle of gonadotropin and testicular steroid hormones in the Japanese red-bellied newt. *In* "Current Trends in Comparative Endocrinology" (B. Lofts and W. N. Holmes, eds.), pp. 247–249. Hong Kong University Press, Hong Kong.

Iwata, T., Umezawa, K., Toyoda, F., Takahashi, N., Matsukawa, H., Yamamoto, K., Miura, S., Hayashi, H., and Kikuyama, S. (1999). Molecular cloning of newt sex pheromone precursor cDNAs: evidence for the existence of species-specific forms of pheromones. *FEBS Lett.* **457**, 400–404.

Iwata, T., Toyoda, F., Yamamoto, K., and Kikuyama, S. (2000). Hormonal control of urodele reproductive behavior. *Comp. Biochem. Physiol. B* **126**, 221–229.

Jurkevich, A., Barth, S. W., and Grossmann, R. (1997). Sexual dimorphism of arg-vasotocin gene expressing neurons in the telencephalon and dorsal diencephalon of the domestic fowl. An immunocytochemical and in situ hybridization study. *Cell Tissue Res.* **287**, 69–77.

Kelley, D. B., and Pfaff, D. W. (1976). Hormone effects on male sex behavior in adult South African clawed frogs, *Xenopus laevis*. *Horm. Behav.* **7**, 159–182.

Kelley, D. B., Morrell, J. I., and Pfaff, D. W. (1975). Autoradiographic localization of hormone-concentrating cells in the brain of an amphibian, *Xenopus laevis* I. Testosterone. *J. Comp. Neurol.* **164**, 47–62.

Kelley, D. B., Lieberburg, I., McEwen, B. S., and Pfaff, D. W. (1978). Autoradiographic and biochemical studies of steroid hormone-concentrating cells in the brain of *Rana pipiens*. *Brain Res.* **140**, 287–305.

Kelly, M. J., and Wagner, E. J. (1999). Estrogen modulation of G-protein-coupled receptors. *Trends Endocrinol. Metab.* **10**, 369–374.

Kikuyama, S., Yamamoto, K., and Seki, T. (1980). Prolactin and its role in growth, metamorphosis and reproduction in amphibians. *Gunma Symp. Endocrinol.* **17**, 3–13.

Kikuyama, S., Toyoda, F., Ohmiya, Y., Matsuda, K., Tanaka, S., and Hayashi, H. (1995). Sodefrin: A female-attracting peptide pheromone in newt cloacal glands. *Science* **267**, 1643–1645.

Kovacs, K. J. (1998). Functional neuroanatomy of the parvocellular vasopressinergic system: Transcriptional responses to stress and glucocorticoid feedback. *Prog. Brain Res.* **119**, 31–43.

Landgraf, R., Gerstberger, R., Montkowski, A., Probst, J. C., Wotjak, C. T., Holsboer, F., and Engelmann, M. (1995).

V1 vasopressin receptor antisense oligodeoxytnucleotide into septum reduces vasopressin binding, social discrimination abilities, and anxiety-related behavior in rats. *J. Neurosci.* **15**, 4250–4258.

Lecouteux, A., Garnier, D. H., Bassez, T., and Joly, J. (1985). Seasonal variations of androgens, estrogens, and progesterone in the different lobules of the testis and in the plasma of *Salamandra salamandra*. *Gen. Comp. Endocrinol.* **58**, 211–221.

Lewis, C. M., and Rose, J. D. (2000). A rapid spinal effect of corticosterone on a component of amphibian reproductive behavior. *Soc. Neurosci. Abstr.* **26**, 999.

Lipski, J. (1981). Antidromic invasion as a tool in the study of the central nervous system. *J. Neurosci. Methods* **4**, 1–32.

Lowry, C. A., and Moore, F. L. (1991). Corticotropin-releasing factor (CRF) antagonist suppresses stress-induced locomotor activity in an amphibian. *Horm. Behav.* **25**, 84–96.

Lowry, C. A., Rose, J. D., and Moore, F. L. (1996). Corticotropin-releasing factor enhances locomotion and medullary neuronal firing in an amphibian. *Horm. Behav.* **30**, 50–59.

Lowry, C. A., Richardson, C. F., Zoeller, R. T., Miller, L. J., Muske, L. E., and Moore, F. L. (1997). Neuroanatomical distribution of vasotocin in a urodele amphibian (*Taricha granulosa*) revealed by immunohistochemical and *in situ* hybridization techniques. *J. Comp. Neurol.* **385**, 43–70.

Majewska, M. D., Harrison, N. L., Schwartz, R. D., Barker, J. L., and Paul, S. M. (1986). Steroid hormone metabolites are barbiturate-like modulators of the GABA receptor. *Science* **232**, 1004–1007.

Malacarne, G., and Giacoma, C. (1980). Influence of testosterone on mating behavior in the male crested newt (*Triturus cristatus carnifex* Laur.). *Boll. Zool.* **47**, 107–111.

Marler, C. A., Chu, J., and Wilczynski, W. (1995). Arginine vasotocin injection increases probability of calling in cricket frogs, but causes call changes characteristic of less aggressive males. *Horm. Behav.* **29**, 554–570.

Marler, C. A., Boyd, S. K., and Wilczynski, W. (1999). Forebrain arginine vasotocin correlates of alternative mating strategies in cricket frogs. *Horm. Behav.* **36**, 53–61.

Matsuda, K., Yamamoto, K., and Kikuyama, S. (1990). Development and application of homologous radioimmunoassay for newt prolactin. *Gen. Comp. Endocrinol.* **79**, 83–88.

Mazzi, V., and Vellano, C. (1987). Prolactin and reproduction. *In* "Hormones and Reproduction in Fishes, Amphibians, and Reptiles" (D. O. Norris and R. E. Jones, eds.), pp. 87–115. Plenum Press, New York.

Mensah-Nyagan, A. G., Do-Rego, J. L., Feuilloley, M., Marcual, A., Lange, C., Pelletier, G., and Vaudry, H. (1996a). In vivo and in vitro evidence for the biosynthesis of testosterone in the telencephalon of the female frog. *J. Neurochem.* **67**, 413–422.

Mensah-Nyagan, A. M., Feuilloley, M., Do-Rego, J. L., Marcual, A., Lange, C., Tonon, M. C., Pelletier, G., and Vaudry, H. (1996b). Localization of 17beta-hydroxysteroid dehydrogenase and characterization of testosterone in the brain of the male frog. *Proc. Natl. Acad. Sci. U.S.A.* **93**, 1423–1428.

Moore, F. L. (1978). Differential effects of testosterone plus dihydrotestosterone on male courtship of castrated newts, *Taricha granulosa*. *Horm. Behav.* **11**, 202–208.

Moore, F. L. (1983). Behavioral endocrinology of amphibian reproduction. *BioScience* **33**, 557–561.

Moore, F. L. (1992). Evolutionary precedents for behavioral actions of oxytocin and vasopressin. *Ann. N.Y. Acad. Sci.* **652**, 156–165.

Moore, F. L., and Evans, S. J. (1999). Steroid hormones use non-genomic mechanisms to control brain functions and behaviors: A review of evidence. *Brain, Behav. Evol.* **54**, 41–50.

Moore, F. L., and Lowry, C. A. (1998). Comparative neuroanatomy of vasotocin and vasopressin in amphibians and other vertebrates. *Comp. Biochem. Physiol. C* **119**, 251–260.

Moore, F. L., and Miller, L. J. (1983). Arginine vasotocin induces sexual behavior of newts by acting on cells in the brain. *Peptides (N.Y.)* **4**, 97–102.

Moore, F. L., and Miller, L. J. (1984). Stress-induced inhibition of sexual behavior: Corticosterone inhibits courtship behaviors of a male amphibian (*Taricha granulosa*). *Horm. Behav.* **18**, 400–410.

Moore, F. L., and Zoeller, R. T. (1979). Endocrine control of amphibian sexual behavior: Evidence for a neurohormone-androgen interaction. *Horm. Behav.* **13**, 207–213.

Moore, F. L., and Zoeller, R. T. (1985). Stress-induced inhibition of reproduction: Evidence of suppressed secretion of LHRH in an amphibian. *Gen. Comp. Endocrinol.* **60**, 252–258.

Moore, F. L., Seide, R. L., Specker, J. L., and Swanson, L. W. (1978). Effects of prolactin and methallibure on second metamorphosis and plasma androgens in male newts, *Taricha granulosa*. *Comp. Biochem. Physiol.* **61**, 419–422.

Moore, F. L., McCormack, C., and Swanson, L. (1979). Induced ovulation: Effects of sexual behavior and insemination on ovulation and progesterone levels in *Taricha granulosa*. *Gen. Comp. Endocrinol.* **39**, 262–269.

Moore, F. L., Miller, L. J., Spielvogel, S. P., Kubiak, T., and Folkers, K. (1982). Luteinizing hormone-releasing hormone involvement in the reproductive behavior of a male amphibian. *Neuroendocrinology* **35**, 212–216.

Moore, F. L., Muske, L., and Propper, C. R. (1987). Regulation of reproductive behaviors in amphibians by LHRH. *Ann. N.Y. Acad. Sci.* **519**, 108–116.

Moore, F. L., Wood, R. E., and Boyd, S. K. (1992). Sex steroids and vasotocin interact in a female amphibian (*Taricha granulosa*) to elicit female-like egg-laying behavior or male-like courtship. *Horm. Behav.* **26**, 156–166.

Moore, F. L., Orchinik, M., and Lowry, C. (1995). Functional studies of corticosterone receptors in neuronal membranes. *Receptor* **5**, 21–28.

Moore, F. L., Richardson, C., and Lowry, C. A. (2000). Sexual dimorphism in numbers of vasotocin-immunoreactive neurons in brain areas associated with reproductive behaviors in the roughskin newt. *Gen. Comp. Endocrinol.* **117**, 281–298.

Moriya, T., and Dent, J. N. (1986). Hormonal interaction in the mechanism of migratory movement in the newt, *Notophthalmus viridescens*. *Zool. Sci.* **3**, 669–676.

Morrell, J. I., Kelley, D. B., and Pfaff, D. W. (1975). Autoradiographic localization of hormone-concentrating cells in the brain of an amphibian, *Xenopus laevis*. *J. Comp. Neurol.* **164**, 63–77.

Mosconi, G., Yamamoto, K., Kikuyama, S., Carnevali, O., Mancuso, A., and Vellano, C. (1994). Seasonal changes of plasma prolactin concentration in the reproduction of the crested newt (*Triturus carnifex* Laur.). *Gen. Comp. Endocrinol.* **95**, 342–349.

Naujoks-Manteuffel, C., and Manteuffel, G. (1988). Origins of descending projections to the medulla oblongata and rostral medulla spinalis in the urodele *Salamandra salamandra* (Amphibia). *J. Comp. Neurol.* **273**, 187–206.

Norris, D. O., Norman, M. F., Pancak, M. K., and Duvall, D. (1985). Seasonal variations in spermatogenesis, testicular weights, vasa deferentia, and androgen levels in neotenic male tiger salamanders, *Ambystoma tigrinum*. *Gen. Comp. Endocrinol.* **60**, 51–57.

Orchinik, M., Murray, T. F., and Moore, F. L. (1991). A corticosteroid receptor in neuronal membranes. *Science* **252**, 1848–1851.

Orchinik, M., Murray, T. F., Franklin, P. H., and Moore, F. L. (1992). Guanyl nucleotides modulate binding to steroid receptors in neuronal membranes. *Proc. Natl. Acad. Sci. U.S.A.* **89**, 3830–3834.

Orchinik, M., Murray, T. F., and Moore, F. L. (1994). Steroid modulation of $GABA_A$ receptors in an amphibian brain. *Brain Res.* **646**, 258–266.

Orchinik, M., Matthews, L., and Gasser, P. J. (2000). Distinct specificity for corticosteroid binding sites in amphibian cytosol, neuronal membranes, and plasma. *Gen. Comp. Endocrinol.* **118**, 284–301.

Ota, Y., Ando, H., Ueda, H., and Urano, A. (1999). Seasonal changes in expression of neurohypophysial hormone genes in the preoptic nucleus of immature female masu salmon. *Gen. Comp. Endocrinol.* **116**, 31–39.

Palka, Y. S., and Gorbman, A. (1973). Pituitary and testicular influenced sexual behavior in male frogs, *Rana pipiens*. *Gen. Comp. Endocrinol.* **59**, 308–315.

Paniagua, R., Fraile, B., and Saez, F. J. (1990). Effects of photoperiod and temperature on testicular function in amphibians. *Histol. Histopathol.* **5**, 365–378.

Panzica, G. C., Plumari, L., Garcia-Ojeda, E., and Deviche, P. (1999). Central vasotocin-immunoreactive system in a male passerine bird (*Junco hyemalis*). *J. Comp. Neurol.* **409**, 105–117.

Pfaus, J. G., and Gorzalka, B. B. (1987). Opioids and sexual behavior. *Neurosci. Biobehav. Rev.* **11**, 1–34.

Pickford, G. E., and Strecker, E. L. (1997). The spawning reflex response of the killifish, *Fundulus heteroclitus*: Isotocin is relatively inactive in comparison with arginine vasotocin. *Gen. Comp. Endocrinol.* **32**, 132–137.

Propper, C. R. (1991). Courtship in the rough-skinned newt *Taricha granulosa*. *Anim. Behav.* **41**, 547–554.

Propper, C. R., and Dixon, T. B. (1997). Differential effects of arginine vasotocin and gonadotropin-releasing hormone on sexual behaviors in an anuran amphibian. *Horm. Behav.* **32**, 99–104.

Raynor, K., Kong, H., Chen, Y., Yasuda, K., Yu, L., Bell, G. I., and Reisine, T. (1994). Pharmacological characterization of the cloned kappa-, delta-, and mu-opioid receptors. *Mol. Pharmacol.* **45**, 330–334.

Reinscheid, R. K., Nothacker, H. P., Bourson, A., Ardati, A., Henningsen, R. A., Bunzow, J. R., Grandy, D. K., Langen, H., Monsma, F. J., Jr., and Civelli, O. (1995). Orphanin FQ: A neuropeptide that activates an opioid like G protein-coupled receptor. *Science* **270**, 92–94.

Rollmann, S. M., Houck, L. D., and Feldoff, R. C. (1999). Proteinaceous pheromone affecting female receptivity in a terrestrial salamander. *Science* **285**, 1907–1909.

Rose, J. D. (1990a). Brainstem influences on sexual behavior. In "Brainstem Mechanisms of Behavior" (W. R. Klemm and R. P. Vertes, eds.), pp. 407–463. Wiley, New York.

Rose, J. D. (1990b). Forebrain influences on brainstem and spinal mechanisms of copulatory behavior: A current perspective on Frank Beach's contribution. *Neurosci. Biobehav. Rev.* **14**, 207–215.

Rose, J. D. (2000). Corticosteroid actions from neuronal membrane to behavior: Neurophysiological mechanisms underlying rapid behavioral effects of corticosterone. *Biochem. Cell. Biol.* **78**, 307–315.

Rose, J. D., and Moore, F. L. (1992). Neurophysiological effects of corticosterone related to behavior and reproduction in an amphibian. *Soc. Neurosci. Abstr.* **19**, 895.

Rose, J. D., Moore, F. L., and Orchinik, M. (1993). Rapid neurophysiological effects of corticosterone on medullary neurons:

Relationship to stress-induced suppression of courtship clasping in an amphibian. *Neuroendocrinology* **57**, 815–824.

Rose, J. D., Kinnaird, J. R., and Moore, F. L. (1995a). Neurophysiological effects of vasotocin and corticosterone on medullary neurons: Implications for hormonal control of amphibian courtship behavior. *Neuroendocrinology* **62**, 406–417.

Rose, J. D., Marrs, G., and Moore, F. L. (1995b). Rapid corticosterone effects on reticulospinal neurons and behavior. *Soc. Neurosci. Abstr.* **21**, 699.

Rose, J. D., Marrs, G., and Moore, F. L. (1996). CRF alters corticosterone effects on medullary sensorimotor integration and neural excitability. *Soc. Neurosci. Abstr.* **22**, 1149.

Rose, J. D., Marrs, G., and Moore, F. L. (1997). Vasotocin and corticosterone modulate neurophysiological responsiveness of optic tectum to photic stimuli. *Soc. Neurosci. Abstr.* **23**, 895.

Rose, J. D., Marrs, G. S., and Moore, F. L. (1998). Rapid, corticosterone-induced disruption of medullary sensorimotor integration related to suppression of amplectic clasping in behaving roughskin newts *(Taricha granulosa)*. *Horm. Behav.* **34**, 268–282.

Roth, G. (1987). "Visual Behavior in Salamanders." Springer-Verlag, Berlin.

Salthe, S. N. (1967). Courtship patterns and the phylogeny of the urodeles. *Copeia*, pp. 100–117.

Semsar, K., Klomberg, K. F., and Marler, C. (1998). Arginine vasotocin increases calling-site acquisition by nonresident male grey treefrogs. *Anim. Behav.* **56**, 983–987.

Smith, C. L. (1938). The clasping reflex in frogs and toads and the seasonal variation in the development of the brachial musculature. *J. Exp. Biol.* **15**, 1–9.

Specker, J. L., and Moore, F. L. (1980). Annual cycle of plasma androgens and testicular composition in the rough-skinned newt, *Taricha granulosa*. *Gen. Comp. Endocrinol.* **42**, 297–303.

Tanaka, S., and Iwasawa, H. (1979). Annual change in testicular structure and sexual character of the Japanese red-bellied newt, *Cynops pyrrhogaster pyrrhogaster*. *Zool. Mag.* **88**, 295–305.

Tanaka, S., and Takikawa, H. (1983). Seasonal changes in plasma testosterone and 5 alpha-dihydrotestosterone levels in the adult male newt, *Cynops pyrrhogaster pyrrhogaster*. *Endocrinol. Jpn.* **30**, 1–6.

Thompson, R. R., and Moore, F. L. (2000). Vasotocin stimulates appetitive responses to the visual and pheromonal stimuli used by male roughskin newts during courtship. *Horm. Behav.* **38**, 75–85.

Thompson, R. R., Tokar, Z., Pistohl, D., and Moore, F. L. (1999). Behavioral evidence of chemosensory signaling in roughskin newts, *Taricha granulosa*. In "Chemical Signals in Vertebrates" (R. E. Johnston, D. Müller-Schwarze, and P. Sorenson, eds.), pp. 421–429. Plenum Press, New York.

Tito, M. B., Hoover, M. A., Mingo, A. M., and Boyd, S. K. (1999). Vasotocin maintains multiple call types in the gray treefrog, *Hyla versicolor*. *Horm. Behav.* **36**, 166–175.

Toyoda, E., Tanaka, S., Matsuda, K., and Kikuyama, S. (1994). Hormonal control of response to and secretionn of sex attractants in Japanese newts. *Physiol. Behav.* **55**, 569–576.

Toyoda, E., Masuda, K., Yarnamoto, K., and Kikuyama, S. (1996). Involvement of endogenous prolactin in the expression of courtship behavior in the newt, *Cynops pyrrhogaster*. *Gen. Comp. Endocrinol.* **102**, 191–196.

Vellano, C., Peyrot, A., and Mazzi, V. (1967). Effects of prolactin on the pituitary-thyroid axis, integument and behavior of the adult male crested newt. *Monit. Zool. Ital.* **1**, 207–227.

Verrell, P. (1982). The sexual behavior of the red-spotted newt, *Notophthalmus viridescens* (Amphibia: Urodela: Salamandridae). *Anim. Behav.* **30**, 1224–1236.

Viglietti-Panzica, C., Anselmetti, G. C., Balthazart, J., Aste, N., and Panzica, G. (1992). Vasotocinergic innervation of the septal region in the Japanese quail: sexual differences and the influence of testosterone. *Cell Tissue Res.* **267**, 261–263.

Wada, M., and Gorbman, A. (1977). Relation of mode of administration of testosterone to evocation of male sex behavior in frogs. *Horm. Behav.* **8**, 310–319.

Wehling, M. (1997). Specific, nongenomic actions of steroid hormones. *Annu. Rev. Physiol* **59**, 365–393.

Westerfield, M., and Frank, E. (1982). Specificity of electrical coupling among neurons innervating forelimb muscles of the adult bullfrog. *J. Neurophysiol.* **48**, 904–913.

Wilhelmi, A. E., Pickford, G. E., and Sawyer, W. H. (1955). Initiation of the spawning reflex response in *Fundulus* by the administration of fish and mammalian neurohypophysial preparations and synthetic oxytocin. *Endocrinology (Baltimore)* **57**, 243–252.

Wingfield, J. C. (1994). Control of territorial aggression in a changing environment. *Psychoneuroendocrinology* **19**, 709–721.

Yamamoto, K., Toyoda, F., Tanaka, S., Hayashi, H., and Kikuyama, S. (1996). Radioimmunoassay of a newt sex pheromone, sodefrin, and influence of hormones on its level in the abdominal gland. *Gen. Comp. Endocrinol.* **104**, 356–363.

Yamamoto, K., Kawai, Y., Hayashi, T., Ohe, Y., Hayashi, H., Toyoda, F., Kawahara, G., Iwata, T., and Kikuyama, S. (2000). Selefrin, a sodefrin-like pheromone in the abdominal gland of the sword-tailed newt, *Cynops ensicauda*. *FEBS Lett.* **472**, 267–270.

Young, L. J., Nilsen, R., Waymire, K. G., MacGregor, G. R., and Insel, T. R. (1999). Increased affiliative response to vasopressin in mice expressing the V1a receptor from a monogamous vole. *Nature (London)* **400**, 766–768.

Zerani, M., Amabili, F., and Gobbetti, A. (1991a). Plasma testosterone and 17 beta-estradiol concentrations, and aromatase activity, during courtship in male *Triturus carnifex*. *Horm. Behav.* **26**, 56–61.

Zerani, M., Vellano, C., Amabili, F., Carnevali, O., Andreoletti, G. E., and Polzonetti-Magni, A. (1991b). Sex steroid profile and plasma vitellogenin during the annual reproductive cycle of the crested newt (*Triturus carnifex* Laur.). *Gen. Comp. Endocrinol.* **82**, 337–344.

Zoeller, R. T., and Moore, F. L. (1982). Duration of androgen treatment modifies behavioral response to arginine vasotocin in *Taricha granulosa*. *Horm. Behav.* **16**, 23–30.

Zoeller, R. T., and Moore, F. L. (1986). Correlation between immunoreactive vasotocin in optic tectum and seasonal changes in reproductive behaviors of male rough-skinned newts. *Horm. Behav.* **20**, 148–154.

Zoeller, R. T., and Moore, F. L. (1988). Brain arginine vasotocin concentrations related to sexual behaviors and hydromineral balance in an amphibian. *Horm. Behav.* **22**, 66–75.

30

Hormones, Brain, and Behavior in Reptiles

John Godwin
Department of Zoology
North Carolina State University
Raleigh, North Carolina 27695-7617

David Crews
Institute for Cellular and Molecular Biology
University of Texas at Austin
Austin, Texas 78712

I. INTRODUCTION

The living group of animals we refer to as reptiles consists of at least three evolutionary lineages that encompass one of the major amniote vertebrate radiations (Fig. 1). In addition to familiar forms, such as lizards, snakes, turtles, and crocodilians, the reptiles also encompass the approximately 10,000 species of birds (Padian and Chiappe, 1998). From a general standpoint, the key value of studies of reptiles lies in two features. The first of these is the enormous diversity of patterns of sexual differentiation observed across species. The second is the presence of many primitive (in the phylogenetic sense) characters in reptiles. Among the diverse patterns represented are temperature-dependent sex determination, parthenogenesis in all-female species, and other species that exhibit distinct alternate male phenotypes.

This chapter focuses on variation in the neural substrates of sexual behavior in reptiles. We begin with a short review of diversity in sex determination, sexual differentiation, and hormone-behavior relationships observed in reptiles. This is followed by a discussion of anatomical differences, including intersexual variation in the size of neuron soma and brain nuclei and the within vs between sex differences in the function of neurons as revealed by the 2-deoxyglucose utilization and cytochrome oxidase techniques. Next, we consider within and between sex differences in the neurochemistry of brain areas subserving sexual behavior in reptiles. Reptiles show some differences in steroid receptor regulation that are similar to those described for mammals, whereas the diversity of reproductive patterns enables some comparisons not possible with mammals or birds and so extends these findings. Finally, we summarize some research directions that are likely to prove especially promising.

A. Advantages as Models

Modern reptiles exhibit phenotypes that are in many ways similar to what we assume the ancestral amniote vertebrate must have been like. These characteristics include ectothermy, oviparity, and the lack of a well-developed cerebral cortex. The presence of structures homologous to those found in mammals and birds coupled with the lack of complex cortical development characteristic of birds and mammals makes modern reptiles useful systems for examining basic behavioral controlling mechanisms in vertebrates. Such comparative research has revealed that the areas in the limbic forebrain involved in the regulation of social and sexual behaviors are ancient and conserved among vertebrates. This research has also demonstrated that differences in the distribution of sex-steroid-concentrating neurons are rare, but differences in the distribution of steroid hormone receptors and differences in the regulation of steroid hormone receptors are common. Further,

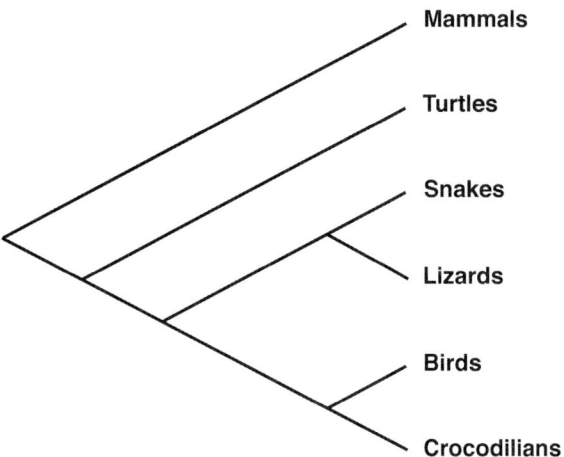

FIGURE 1 Phylogeny of amniote vertebrates. Mammals are believed to have arisen from turtle-like therapsid reptiles approximately 350 mya and modern birds from crocodilian-like archosaurs approximately 250 mya.

species differences in plasma levels of sex hormones are paralleled by differences in behavioral sensitivity to these hormones as well as by differences in the regulation of genes coding for steroid hormone receptors. Other features modern reptiles probably share with the first amniote vertebrates are mechanisms of sex determination that are variable in terms of the important cues (genotype vs environment) and in the type of genotypic sex determination that is displayed in groups (male vs female heterogamety).

This combination of diversity and conserved characters provides a variety of natural experiments with which to ask questions about basic principles of sex determination and sexual differentiation (cf. Crews and Gans, 1992). This has two consequences. First, phenomena heretofore unrecognized in other amniote groups are evident in reptiles, leading to renewed study in mammals that increases our understanding of the neuroendocrine control of sexual behavior. For example, the discovery that progesterone is important in the control of male-like pseudocopulatory behavior in parthenogenetic whiptail lizards led to studies with rats and transgenic mice that, together, revealed the importance of progesterone and its receptor in the control of male sexual behavior. Second, this diversity also allows for a variety of comparisons between species exhibiting differing patterns and for many processes, there are a sufficient of number of species, including outgroups, to generate an adequate sample size for comparisons. For example, viviparity has evolved independently from oviparity perhaps 100 or more times in reptiles (Blackburn, 1999; Guillette, 1991).

B. Pivotal Place in Amniote Evolutionary History

Reptiles as a group gave rise to two major lineages, the birds and the mammals, approximately 250 and 300 million years ago, respectively. The closest living relatives of birds are the crocodilians and their closest extinct relatives are the dinosaurs. Indeed, the skull of ratites (the ancient birds including the ostrich, emu, rhea, and kiwi) resembles that of a crocodilian in many respects. This has led to the suggestion that modern birds fall within the phylogenetic classification of reptiles. Early reptiles gave rise to today's turtles and mammals. Thus, research on the neural and endocrine control of behavior in extant reptiles help us better understand the patterns we see in birds and mammals and how these patterns may have originated.

C. Reptilian Brain as an Experimentally Tractable Model

The lack of a well-developed cortex in reptiles is experimentally advantageous in many ways. Greenberg refers to reptiles as "walking limbic systems" and notes the value of interpretations not being subject to the complications presented by a well-developed cortex (Greenberg *et al.*, 1979). Modern reptiles are probably also primitive in the neural circuitry that mediates intromission behavior and sexual receptivity. Sexual behaviors have been important for our understanding of behavioral neuroendocrinology generally and an understanding of the ancestral state of neuroendocrine mechanisms controlling these behaviors should help us better understand how they have evolved and function in birds and mammals.

II. DIVERSITY IN SEX DETERMINATION, SEXUAL DIFFERENTIATION, AND HORMONE–BEHAVIOR RELATIONSHIPS

Reptiles show an extraordinary diversity of sex determination and differentiation patterns. In addition to genotypic sex-determining mechanisms, many reptiles possess primitive traits (e.g., temperature-dependent sex determination, TSD) or specialized traits (e.g., obligate parthenogenesis and alternative mating tactics) that have added new dimensions to our understanding of reproductive neuroendocrine mechanisms underlying reproduction in mammals. One important benefit deriving from the diversity seen in reptiles relates to studying variation in sexual behavior. Sexual behaviors and aggressive behaviors often show discontinuous variation between the sexes in birds and mammals, although there is typically considerable individual variation within the sexes (Crews, 1998). In contrast, many reptiles show more continuous variation in these behaviors. Examples include all-female species in which individuals alternate between the display of female- and male-like pseudosexual behavior during the course of the ovarian cycle, species with TSD that show substantial behavioral variation within sexes across incubation temperatures, and species that exhibit distinct alternate male phenotypes. Viewing sexuality as a continuous variable should facilitate thinking about how modern states of sexuality in birds and mammals arose. This section highlights diversity in reptilian sex determination and differentiation patterns and the research opportunities that this diversity presents.

A. Sex Determination and Sexual Differentiation in Reptiles Lacking Sex Chromosomes

Many reptiles exhibit genotypic sex determination similar to that of mammals (XX:XY) and birds (ZZ:ZW); some reptiles exhibit male heterogamety similar to mammals, whereas others exhibit female heterogamety similar to birds. However, in all crocodilians (alligators, crocodile, caiman, etc.), most turtles (all marine turtles and tortoises and many freshwater turtles), and some lizards (various Geckkonid and Agamid species), gonadal sex is established by the temperature experienced by the incubating egg (Viets *et al.*, 1994).

1. Molecular Genetics of Temperature-Dependent Sex Determination

Three basic patterns of TSD have been documented (Fig. 2). First, relatively high temperatures produce males, whereas relatively low temperatures produce females. The inverse pattern also exists in some species, as well as a sex-determining pattern in which inter-

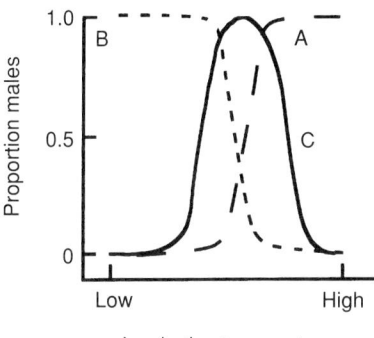

FIGURE 2 Response of hatchling sex ratio to incubation temperature in various egg-laying reptiles. These graphs represent only the approximate pattern of the response and are not drawn according to any single species. The three patterns recognized are (A) only females produced from low incubation temperatures, males at high temperatures; (B) only males produced from low incubation temperatures, females at high temperatures; and (C) only females produced at the temperature extremes, with male production at the intermediate incubation temperatures. Genotypic sex determination also occurs in reptiles with the result that the hatchling sex ratio is fixed at 1:1 despite incubation conditions.

mediate temperatures produce males and high and low temperatures produce males. The sensitivity to temperature is restricted to the mid-trimester of development, the temperature-sensitive period (TSP) (Crews, 1994, 1996a). TSD is believed to be ancestral to the genotypic sex-determining pattern characteristic of birds and mammals (Crews, 1994).

Sex steroid hormones are implicated in the process of TSD, and estrogen, in particular, appears essential in female sex determination (Crews *et al.*, 1994, 1996a; Lance, 1997; Wibbels *et al.*, 1998). Estrogens applied exogenously to red-eared slider turtle (*Trachemys scripta*) eggs incubating at a male-producing temperature override the temperature effect and female hatchlings result (Crews *et al.*, 1991; Wibbels and Crews 1992). Exogenously applied inhibitors of aromatase override a female-producing incubation temperature, and male hatchlings result (Crews and Bergeron, 1994; Wibbels and Crews, 1994).

Research with a variety of turtle species such as the European pond turtle (*Emys orbicularis*) has shown a correlation between female incubation temperatures and increased levels of endogenous aromatase mRNA and enzyme activity in the putative ovary during the TSP (cf. Desvages and Pieau, 1992; Jeyasuria and Place,

1997, 1998). Other researchers have found that aromatase activity increases in the turtle brain prior to the time it increases in the gonad at a female-producing temperature, suggesting that the brain, rather than the gonad, is the sex-determining source of estrogen (Jeyasuria and Place, 1998; Merchant-Larios, 1998). Whatever the endogenous source of estrogen, the gonads of putative females and males are receptive to its effect because both express estrogen receptors (ERs), albeit differentially, throughout the TSP (Bergeron et al., 1998).

Male sex determination can be manipulated by exogenously applied dihydrotestosterone (DHT), a non-aromatizable androgen, its derivatives, and reductase inhibitors (Wibbels et al., 1992; Wibbels and Crews, 1992, 1995, Crews and Bergeron, 1994). This effect is less striking than that of estrogen in female sex determination and is only seen at intermediate, or less potent, incubation temperatures. Nevertheless, steroid hormones are undoubtedly a part of TSD in both males and females.

It is evident that the downstream events in the differentiation of the gonad in TSD reptiles and mammals and birds are similar and that both an ovary-determining cascade and a testis-determining cascade coexist in the embryo (Fig. 3). With the exception of *Sry* (in mammals) or the sex-determining gene associated with the W chromosome (in birds), the genetic cascade thus far described in the gonadal development of mammals has been identified in birds and in reptiles with TSD. For example, steroidogenic factor 1 (SF-1) is a transactivator of most enzymes involved in the biosynthesis of steroid hormones, including sex steroids (Morohashi et al., 1999). SF-1 is encoded by the *ftz-f1* gene, a homolog of the *Drosophila ftz-f1* gene, and study of mice with a targeted disruption of *ftz-f1* reveals the abnormal function of pituitary gonadotropes (Morohashi et al., 1999) as well as a malformed ventromedial hypothalamus (VMH) (Shinoda et al., 1995; Luo et al., 1994). Analysis indicates that SF-1 is expressed at the earliest stages of urogenital ridge development; in mice the disruption of the gene encoding SF-1 results in newborns that lack adrenal glands and gonads (Ikeda et al., 1994; Luo et al., 1994; Shen et al., 1994). Both male and female embryos express SF-1; shortly after differentiation of the Sertoli cells and formation of testicular cords, SF-1 expression persists in males but diminishes in females (Luo et al., 1994). In addition to being critical to sex steroid biosynthesis, SF-1, along with SOX9, up-regulates the expression of Müllerian inhibiting substance (MIS) in the Sertoli cells of developing testes and the MIS receptor in testes and Müllerian ducts (Arango et al., 1999). MIS in turn appears to down-regulate aromatase gene expression (DiClemente et al., 1992; Rouiller-Fabre et al., 1998). A brain-specific transcript of aromatase has been detected in rats, and the gene encoding it contains a consensus SF-1 binding site (Honda et al., 1994). In reptiles and birds, it is thought that SF-1 might regulate aromatase, and hence the synthesis of ovary-determining estrogen, in developing ovaries (Fleming et al., 1999; Western et al., 2000; Smith et al., 1999).

The pattern of SF-1 expression in the chicken and alligator following histological distinction of gonadal sex differs from that in mammals. As gonadal sex becomes distinct, SF-1 levels become less abundant in the genetically or temperature-determined male than in the female chicken (Smith et al., 1999) and alligator (Western et al., 2000), respectively. In the chicken, SF-1 message expression falls to an almost negligible level in males but remains high in females, correlating with the pattern of aromatase expression in chickens (Andrews et al., 1997; Smith et al., 1999). Aromatase is up-regulated by SF-1 in mammalian granulosa cells (Carlone and Richards, 1997), where it converts testosterone (T) to estradiol (E_2).

Studies of the expression of SF-1 mRNA in the red-eared slider turtle, a species with TSD, reveals that SF-1 is equivalent at male- and female-producing temperatures in the early gonadal ridge (Fleming et al., 1999). At this stage, gonads from the two incubation temperatures are bipotential and histologically indistinguishable. As the gonads become histologically distinct, the pattern of SF-1 expression changes, continuing to increase at the male-producing incubation temperature but declining at the female-producing incubation temperature. SF-1 mRNA is also evident in the brain. Shifting eggs from a male- to a female-producing incubation temperature—or vice versa—at the middle of the TSP results in the down-regulation of SF-1 message levels to a female level (Fleming and Crews, 2000). The opposite pattern is observed when eggs are shifted from a female- to a male-producing incubation temperature; that is, there is an up-regulation of SF-1 mRNA levels.

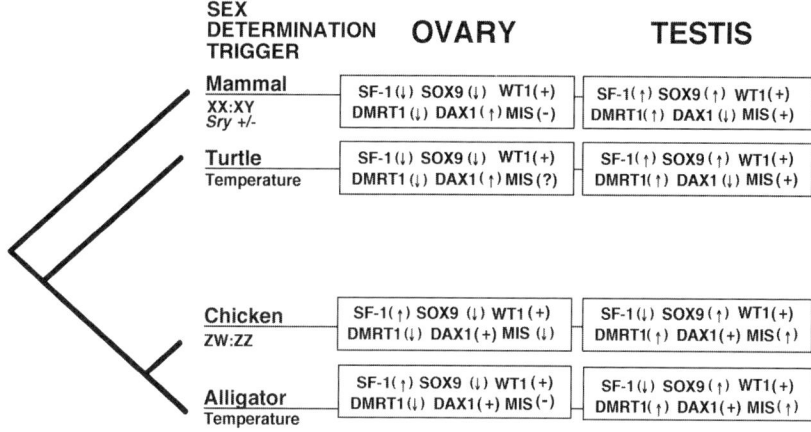

FIGURE 3 Selected genes underlying differentiation of the genital ridge into an ovary (upper panel) or testis (lower panel) in amniote vertebrates. Phylogenetic relationship of different groups is indicated at the left. In mammals and birds, gonadal sex is established by the genetic composition inherited at fertilization, a process known as genotypic sex determination (GSD). In some reptiles, gonadal sex depends ultimately on the temperature of the incubating egg, a process known as temperature- dependent sex determination (TSD). The trigger for gonad determination in mammals is the presence (or absence) of *Sry*; in birds the trigger is unknown but appears to be the ratio of the Z chromosome and autosomes. Note that many of the same genes appear to be involved in gonadal differentiation for species exhibiting GSD (mammals and birds) and TSD (turtles and crocodilians). Note also that for these selected genes the patterns of expression appear to reflect phylogenetic relationships, with mammals being similar to turtles, and birds more similar to crocodilians. The regulatory mechanisms behind the expression patterns for most of these selected genes are being investigated, but timing of SOX9 and MIS expression during testis development appears to fall along phylogenetic lines; in mammals and turtles SOX9 expression precedes MIS expression, whereas in alligator and bird the reverse pattern is seen. Finally, by manipulating the genetic, physical, or chemical environment in the various amniote vertebrates it is possible to modify gonadal sex in both GSD and TSD amniote vertebrates. DAX1, dosage-sensitive sex-reversal adrenal hypoplasia congenital critical region on the X chromosome; DMRT1, DM-related transcription factor one; MIS, Müllerian inhibiting substance; SF-1, steroidogenic factor one; SOX9, SRY-related HMG box nine; SRY, Sex-determining region on the Y chromosome; WT1, Wilm's tumor one. Plus (+) indicates presence and minus (−) indicates absence. Up arrow (↑) indicates up-regulation and down arrow (↓) indicates down-regulation.

Gonadal sex in the red-eared slider turtle and other reptiles with TSP can also be manipulated during the TSP by treating eggs incubating at a male-producing temperature with E_2 or by treating eggs incubating at a female-producing temperature with an aromatase inhibitor. Such manipulations produce female and male offspring, respectively. Following E_2 treatment of eggs incubating at a male-producing temperature, gonadal SF-1 expression is down-regulated and becomes statistically and histologically indistinguishable from temperature-derived females. The treatment of eggs incubating at a female-biased temperature with aromatase inhibitor has the opposite effect.

2. Organizing Influence of Incubation Temperature

There are two levels in the organization of sexuality (Crews, 1998b). Primary organization refers to the process of differentiation of the primary and secondary structures (gonads and associated duct systems) and accessory sex characters (various glands and morphological features). Here is where most studies in behavioral neuroendocrinology concentrate, focusing on group mean differences in sexually dimorphic traits. Secondary organization follows primary organization and is manifest as the unique morphological, physiological, and behavioral aspects of an individual's sexual phenotype. Studies in this realm focus on individual variation in sexually dimorphic traits. Individual variation is the substance of evolutionary change. If we are to understand how the neuroendocrine mechanisms underlying an individual's behavior or physiology evolved, we must concentrate our efforts on understanding the prenatal and postnatal experiences, as well as on how stimuli arising from the abiotic and biotic environment influence the development of the individual (Crews, 1999). This requires both new paradigms and animal model systems that allow the separation of the effects of genes and hormones from environmental and experiential stimuli. For example, the great majority of the research on the proximate mechanisms underlying sexually dimorphic traits has emphasized the role of gonadal sex hormones. Further, this work almost invariably has used species in which gonadal sex is determined by sex chromosomes. In such species, genetic sex and gonadal sex, and hence the nature and pattern of hormones produced, are linked, making it difficult to distinguish environmental from genetic and hormonal contributions to individual differences.

Animals with environmental sex determination, such as lizards with TSD, are particularly suitable for this type of work. The leopard gecko, in particular, has proven to be an excellent model system for several reasons. First, the investigator has precise control of the critical environmental variables (in this case, incubation temperature) that determine gonadal sex and, hence, its products. Thus, by comparing males and females at certain incubation temperatures it is possible to determine the effect of gonadal sex steroids on sexually dimorphic aspects of the nervous system. Comparing same-sex individuals across a range of incubation temperatures, on the other hand, can assess individual differences among males and females. This is analogous to comparing males and females from different intrauterine positions in rodents (see Chapter 68 in Volume 4) and alternative sexual phenotypes in genotypic sex determination (GSD) reptiles (see later). Finally, these animals eliminate possible sex-specific genetic effects (see Chapter 63) because they lack sex chromosomes. What we have discovered is that the temperature experienced during embryogenesis has organizational effects on the morphology, physiology, and behavior of adults that are independent of the hormones produced by gonads. By incubating eggs at various temperatures and then following individuals as they age, we have found that incubation temperature accounts for much of the phenotypic variation seen among adults both between (sexual dimorphisms) and within (individual differences) the sexes (Crews et al., 1998).

For example, in the leopard gecko (Eublepharis macularius) the incubation of eggs at 26°C produces only female hatchlings, incubation at 30°C produces a female-biased sex ratio, and incubation at 32.5°C produces a male-biased sex ratio; incubation of 34–35°C again produces virtually all females (Fig. 4). Hence, females from eggs incubated at 26°C are referred to

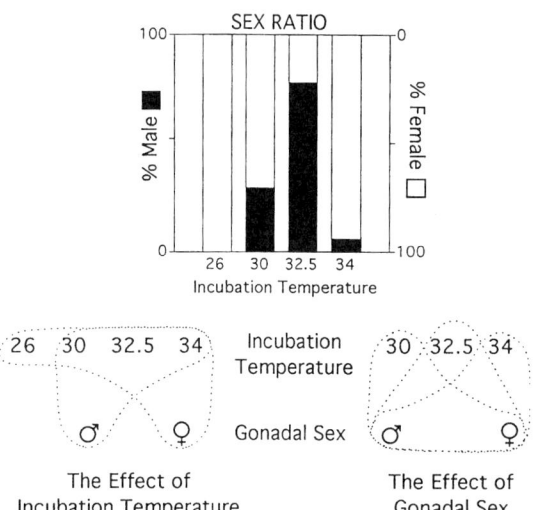

FIGURE 4 Pattern of temperature-dependent sex determination in the leopard gecko. (A) Effect of incubation temperature on sex ratio. Extreme temperatures produce females, whereas intermediate temperatures produce different ratios. Because the effects of incubation temperature and gonadal sex covary, any difference between individuals could be due to the incubation temperature of the egg, the gonadal sex of the individual, or both factors combined. To assess the contribution of each, they must be dissociated. (B) Studying same-sex animals that differ only in the incubation temperature experienced reveals the effects of temperature. (C) Comparing males and females from the same incubation temperature reveals the effects of gonadal sex. Dotted lines group comparisons made in each condition.

as low-temperature females and females from eggs incubated at 34°C are referred to as high-temperature females; the two intermediate incubation temperatures are referred to as female-biased (30°C) and male-biased (32.5°C) temperatures. Adult leopard geckos are sexually dimorphic, with males having open secretory pores anterior to the cloaca. In low-temperature females these pores are closed, whereas in females from a male-biased temperature they are open (Gutzke and Crews, 1988). Head size is also sexually dimorphic, with males having wider heads than females; yet in females, those from a male-biased temperature have wider heads than do those from a low temperature (Gutzke and Crews, 1988). Similarly, although males are the larger sex, incubation temperature has a marked effect on growth within a sex. Females from a male-biased temperature grow faster and larger than do females from female-biased temperatures and become as large as males from female-biased temperatures (Tousignant and Crews, 1995). Indeed, female geckos from estrogen-treated eggs incubated at a male-biased temperature (which overcomes the male-determining temperature effect and produces females) do not differ in growth rates from unmanipulated females from the same temperature.

Circulating concentrations of T in both newborn and adult males are approximately 100 times higher than in adult females (Table 1) (Gutzke and Crews, 1988; Tousignant and Crews, 1995). However, the en-

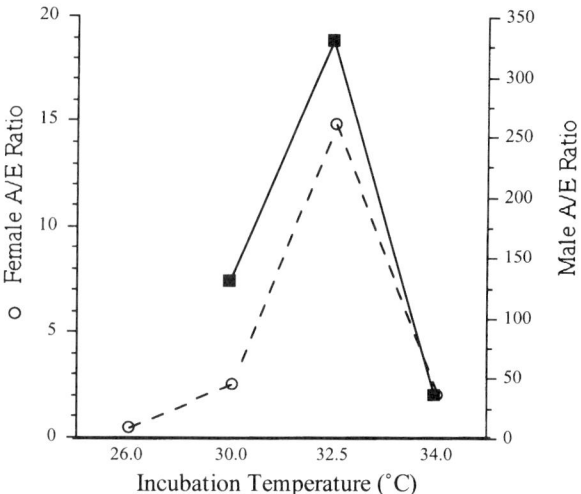

FIGURE 5 Ratio of the plasma levels of total androgens (A) and estrogens (E) in adult female (dashed line) and male (solid line) leopard geckos *(Eublepharis macularius)* from different incubation temperatures. Data from Coomber *et al.* (1997); Gutzke and Crews (1988).

docrine physiology of the adult varies in part due to the temperature experienced during incubation (Fig. 5) (Coomber *et al.*, 1997; Tousignant *et al.*, 1995). For example, plasma estrogen levels are significantly higher in males from female-biased temperatures than in males from a male-biased temperature. Circulating estrogen levels are significantly higher and androgen levels are significantly lower in low-temperature females than in females from a male-biased temperature. Although circulating concentrations of sex hormones do differ between male and female hatchlings (Table 1), whether this also is the case in hatchlings from different incubation temperatures is not known.

Incubation temperature also has a major influence on the nature and frequency of the behavior displayed by the adult leopard gecko. Females usually respond aggressively only if attacked, whereas males posture and then attack other males, but rarely females (Gutzke and Crews, 1988; Flores *et al.*, 1994). However, males from a female-biased temperature are less aggressive than males from the higher male-biased temperature and, although not as aggressive as males from that same incubation temperature, females from a male-biased temperature are significantly more aggressive toward males than are females from a low or female-biased temperature. These same females show the male-typical pattern

TABLE 1
Circulating Concentrations of Steroid Hormones in Hatchling and Adult Leopard Geckos, Female-Biased Incubation Temperature (30°C)

Sex	Number	Testosterone	Estradiol-17β
Hatchlings			
Male	5	1.43 (.70)	0.14 (.03)
Female	6	0.20 (.02)	0.12 (.02)
Adults			
Male	6	77.92 (26.40)	0.48 (.06)
Female	7	1.23 (.45)	0.49 (.05)

[a]Mean concentration (ng/ml) is presented; standard error in parentheses. For hatchlings, due to the small blood volumes of hatchlings, samples were pooled (n = 2–6 hatchlings/pool) and number indicates number of pooled samples. For adults, number indicates individual animals.

of offensive aggression and, as is the case for body growth, females from estrogen-treated eggs incubated at the male-biased temperature are as aggressive as their unmanipulated counterparts.

Incubation temperature also influences the ability of exogenous T to restore aggression. Following ovariectomy and T treatment, low-temperature females do not exhibit increased levels of aggression toward male stimulus animals, whereas females from male-biased temperatures return to the high levels exhibited while gonadally intact (Flores and Crews, 1995). Similarly, males from the male-biased embryonic temperature scent mark more than males from the female-biased embryonic temperature when treated with DHT or T; treatment with E_2, decreases submissive behavior in males from a male-biased embryonic temperature compared to males from a female-biased embryonic temperature (Rhen and Crews, 1999). Such data suggest that incubation temperature influences how the individual responds to steroid hormones in adulthood.

Courtship is a male-typical behavior. In a sexual encounter, the male slowly approaches the female, touching the substrate or licking the air with his tongue. Males also have a characteristic tail vibration, creating a buzzing sound, when they detect a female. Intact females have never been observed to exhibit this tail-vibration behavior, regardless of their incubation temperature. However, if ovariectomized females from low and male-biased temperatures are treated with T, they begin to tail-vibrate toward female, but not male, stimulus animals; males appear to regard such females as male because they are attacked (Flores and Crews, 1995).

Attractiveness is a female-typical trait and is measured by the intensity of a sexually active male's courtship behavior toward the female. Females from a male-biased temperature are less attractive than are females from lower incubation temperatures (Flores *et al.*, 1994). Interestingly, attractiveness in high-temperature females is greater than that of females from male-biased temperatures and not different from that of low-temperature females. Long-term castrated males are attractive and initially courted by intact males, but on olfactory inspection they are attacked. This suggests that both sexes can produce both a female-typical attractiveness pheromone and a male-typical recognition pheromone, as does the red-sided garter snake (Mason *et al.*, 1989). As is the case in females, incubation temperature influences sensitivity to exogenous hormones in males. Estrogen treatment induces receptive behavior in castrated males if they were incubated at a female-biased temperature, but not if they were incubated at a male-biased temperature.

As might be predicted, these behavioral differences among and between male and female leopard geckos from different incubation temperatures also reflect differences in the neural substrates regulating these behaviors, including the size and metabolic activity of different limbic areas (see later).

3. Parthenogenesis

Another variation in sex determination found in reptiles is obligate parthenogenesis. In three families of lizard (teiid, agamid, and lacertid lizards) there are species that consist only of females that reproduce by cloning. Among the whiptail lizards (*Cnemidophorus* spp.) fully one-third of the species reproduce by obligate parthenogenesis. The best studied to date is the triploid *Cnemidophorus uniparens*. This particular species arose from the hybrid mating between two sexual species, and restriction analysis of mitochondrial DNA indicates that two-thirds of its genome comes from *C. inornatus* (Densmore *et al.*, 1989) (Fig. 6).

Parthenogenesis in *C. uniparens* is accompanied by a fascinating reproductive adaptation—females display male-like pseudocopulatory behavior that is indistinguishable from the male-typical courtship and mounting behavior seen in males of their direct sexual ancestor, *C. inornatus* (Crews and Fitzgerald, 1980) (Fig. 7). This behavior functions to facilitate reproduction among the females, much like male courtship serves to stimulate and synchronize reproductive activity in conspecific females (Crews *et al.*, 1980). Indeed, the process is fundamental to reproduction in all living organisms, including various forms in which males do not exist (Crews, 1996b, 1998a). The display of pseudosexual behavior is associated predominantly with the postovulatory phase of the ovarian cycle when progesterone (P) levels are elevated (Moore *et al.*, 1985a,b). The P sensitivity of male-like pseudosexual behavior in *C. uniparens* has an evolutionary antecedent in *C. inornatus*, in which P acting alone and in synergism with androgens stimulates male-typical mounting and intromission behavior (Lindzey and Crews, 1992).

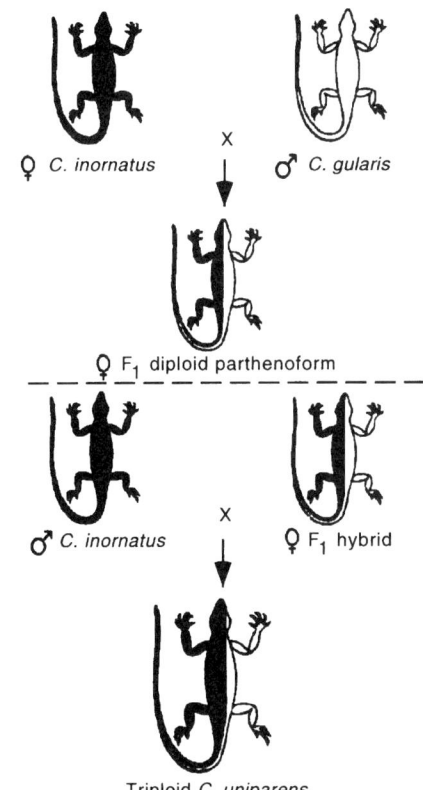

FIGURE 6 Most whiptail lizard species (genus *Cnemidophorus*) are gonochoristic, having both male and female individuals that reproduce sexually. However, one-third of the 45 species of whiptail lizards are unisexual, consisting only of individuals that reproduce by true parthenogenesis. The parthenogenetic species arose fully formed from the hybrid mating of two sexual whiptail species. Indeed, in many instances, we know which species were involved. The best-studied parthenogen is *C. uniparens*. The maternal ancestor of *C. uniparens* is the Little Striped Whiptail, *C. inornatus*. The paternal ancestor is still under dispute, with some favoring *C. gularis* and others favoring *C. burti*. Whatever the paternal species, it is known that *C. uniparens* arose from the F1 hybrid mating in a backcross with *C. inornatus*.

This discovery of P sensitivity in male lizards led to a revisitation of the question and the demonstration of similar sensitivity in male rats (Witt *et al.*, 1995).

B. Functional Associations in Hormones, Gamete Production, and Mating Behavior

Species that evolved under different constraints presumably exhibit different patterns of reproduction and therefore are likely to have fundamentally different neuroendocrine mechanisms controlling their reproduction and associated behaviors. The display of reproductive behavior in reptiles and other vertebrate groups shows one of three basic temporal relationships to gamete production (Fig. 8). The most common relationship is an associated reproductive pattern. Animals displaying this pattern exhibit sexual behavior when their gonads are actively producing gametes and steroid hormone levels are elevated. Reptilian examples of this pattern are the green anole lizard (*Anolis carolinensis*), the sea turtles discussed in the next part of this section, and many of the other species discussed in this chapter. The display of mating behavior may also be temporally uncoupled from gamete production. This is a dissociated reproductive pattern. The most thoroughly reptilian example of this pattern remains the red-sided garter snake, *Thamnophis sirtalis parietalis* (Crews, 1983). This species is discussed at length later. The third possible temporal relationship between gametogenic activity and reproductive behavior is a constant reproductive pattern. This pattern is characterized by the maintenance of reproductive readiness (mature sperm and ovarian follicles), but with actual reproduction and the display of associated behaviors limited to typically short and unpredictable periods when environmental conditions are such that reproduction can be successful. Although this pattern has not been documented in any reptile, it does characterize wild populations of zebra finches in unpredictable desert environments (Sossinka, 1980; Allen and Hume, 1997) and remains a possibility for reptiles facing similar challenges.

This prediction that the wide variety of neuroendocrine mechanisms that subserve sexual behavior observed among vertebrate animals arose as adaptations to various ecological, phylogenetic, developmental, and physiological constraints has been borne out. Carefully chosen comparisons have led to some unexpected outcomes and insights. For example, there is a tendency to assume that there is a fundamental functional association among the three basic components of vertebrate reproduction—gametes, steroid hormones, and behavior (Fig. 9). Beginning with studies of reptiles (Crews *et al.*, 1984) and extending to other vertebrates (Crews, 1987), it has become clear that there is no intrinsic linkage between the production of gametes, the secretion of gonadal steroid hormones, and the expression

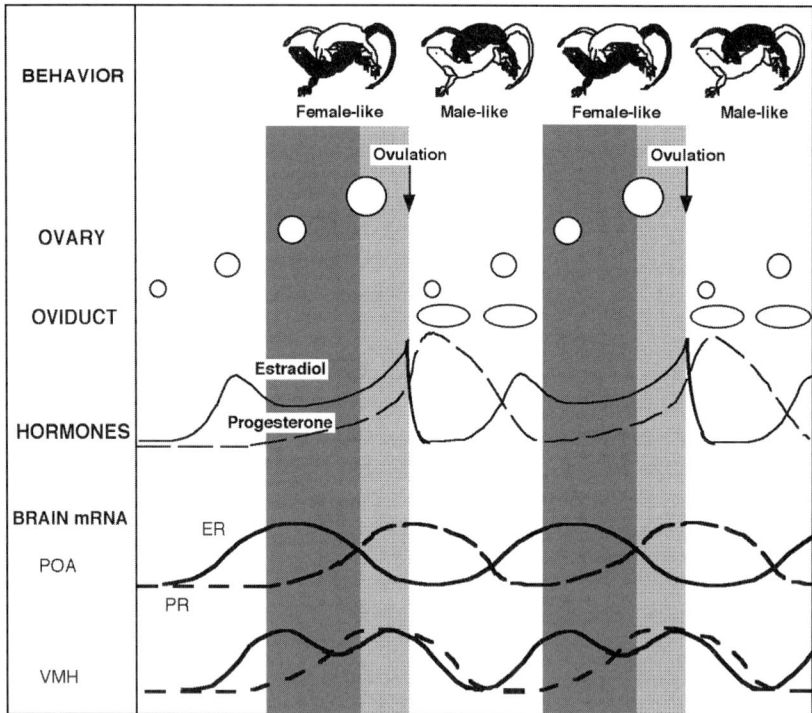

FIGURE 7 Relation among male-like and female-like pseudosexual behavior, ovarian state, and circulating levels of E_2 and progesterone (P) during various stages of the reproductive cycle of the parthenogenetic whiptail lizard. The transition from receptive to mounting behavior occurs at the time of ovulation (arrow). Also shown are the relative changes in abundance of the gene transcripts coding for ERs and progesterone receptors (PR) in the preoptic area (POA) and the VMH, brain areas that are involved in the regulation of male- and female-typical sexual behaviors. Redrawn from Crews et al., 1998a.

of sexual behavior. Indeed, of the six relationships possible among these three elements, only one can be regarded as fundamental, namely that gametes cannot be produced independent of steroid hormone secretion (Crews et al., 1984; Crews, 1987). A number of studies now have shown that sexual behavior need not depend on increased levels of sex steroid hormones and, further, that males and females of a particular species may regulate similar reproductive (behavioral) events by using different proximate cues and mechanisms.

C. Alternative Mating Strategies

Many species of reptiles show discrete alternate male phenotypes that exhibit discontinuous variation in male morphology, physiology, and behavior. Alternative male phenotypes are also found in other vertebrate groups, including fishes, amphibians, birds, and mammals, as well as in many invertebrates. Often one male phenotype in these systems is similar to females and the other shows exaggerated male characters. These systems have the advantage of allowing comparisons of differing behavioral phenotypes without the confound of a difference in gonadal sex (Moore, 1991). For this reason, it has been suggested that alternate reproductive phenotypes present a valuable opportunity to explore the physiological and neural mechanisms underlying individual variation in behavior and morphology. Males and females also represent alternate reproductive phenotypes, but sex comparisons face an important confounding factor—the groups being compared differ in both behavior and the type of gonad they possess. Moore (1991) proposed that alternate reproductive phenotypes within a sex avoid this complication (because the groups being compared do not differ in

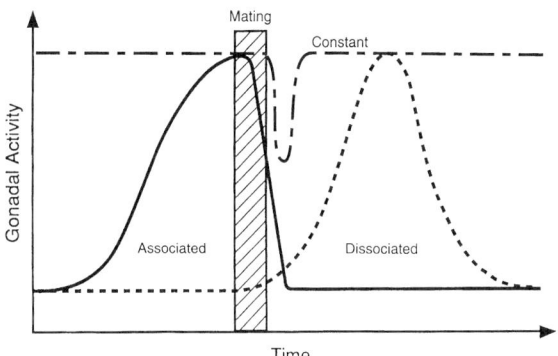

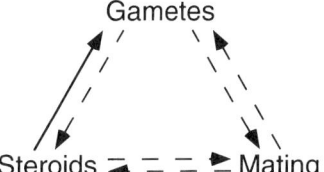

FIGURE 8 Vertebrates display a variety of reproductive patterns. Here gonadal activity is defined as the development of eggs and sperm or increased sex-steroid-hormone secretion. Individuals exhibiting the associated reproductive pattern (solid line) live in temperate regions where seasonal cycles are regular and prolonged; in such species, the gonads are fully developed at the time of mating and circulating levels of sex hormones are maximal. Individuals exhibiting the dissociated reproductive pattern (dashed line) live in extreme environments in which seasonal changes are regular, but the length of time available for breeding is limited; in such species, the gonads are small and sex-steroid-hormone levels are low at the time of mating. Individuals exhibiting a constant reproductive pattern (hatched line) live in harsh environments where breeding conditions are completely unpredictable; in such species, the gonads are maintained at nearly maximal development so that when breeding conditions do arise, breeding can occur immediately. Just as the reproductive cycles have adapted to the environment, so too have the neuroendocrine mechanisms subserving breeding behavior. The temporal uncoupling of sexual behavior and gonadal recrudescence in vertebrates exhibiting these different reproductive patterns is reflected in the dynamics of their hormone–brain–behavior relationship. The dimension of reproductive pattern is depicted here as mutually exclusive extremes only for the sake of argument; intermediate forms are known to exist.

FIGURE 9 The three major components of the reproductive process in vertebrates. In species in which the pattern of gonadal activity is associated temporally with mating, as occurs in many mammals and birds, these elements are functionally associated. This has led to the paradigm that mating behavior is activated by increasing levels of gonadal steroid hormones in the circulation. However, there is no intrinsic functional association among these elements. Indeed, studies indicate that the dependence of mating behavior on sex hormones depends on the reproductive pattern exhibited, which in turn depends on various ecological, phylogenetc, developmental, and physiological constraints. The solid line indicates the only functional association shared by all living vertebrates, indicating that it is the primitive or ancient characteristic. The dashed lines represent the various functional associations observed in vertebrates. Whether these are derived associations that evolved independently in the different genera, and therefore are analogous, or they were present in the common ancestor of each Class (e.g., mammals) and therefore are homologous can only be determined through comparative analysis.

type of gonad) and are therefore valuable models for exploring the bases of ubiquitous individual variation within the sexes.

In order for this approach to be a useful one conceptually and operationally, the physiological mechanisms operating to generate differences in behavior and morphology between alternate within-sex phenotypes should be similar to those documented to produce between-sex differences. The organizational concept proposed by Phoenix and coworkers (1959) has provided the most valuable framework for understanding

sex differences and has been applied to understanding the endocrine bases of alternate male phenotypes (reviewed in Moore *et al.*, 1998; see later), although the applicability of this model to other variations in vertebrate sexual determination and differentiation has been questioned (Crews, 1993).

The behavioral and ecological correlates of alternative reproductive phenotypes in reptiles are better explored than their endocrine bases so far. The hormonal bases of these alternate phenotypes have been addressed in only a few species of reptiles and the neural correlates of behavioral differences in these species have received little detailed study. However, studies in fishes that display alternate male phenotypes suggest that this will be a productive area of research in reptiles (see Grober and Bass, Chapter 23). Moore (1991) proposed the relative plasticity hypothesis as a basis for understanding the diversity of behavioral and morphological expression observed with alternate male phenotypes. Briefly, this hypothesis proposes that fixed differences between alternate phenotypes are due to organizational actions of steroid hormones, whereas more plastic differences are due to activational influences of these hormones. Moore, Hews, and Knapp (1998) refined this hypothesis to account for cases in which permanent phenotypic effects might require the actions of the relevant hormones only during critical developmental windows.

We briefly review two cases here for which physiological information is available regarding alternative reproductive phenotypes in reptiles. We also consider a genus of iguanid lizards (*Sceloporus* spp.) in which variation in male phenotypes is common both in and across closely related species. The best-characterized models of alternate reproductive phenotype variation from a physiological perspective include the red-sided garter snake *(Thamnophis sirtalis parietalis)* and the tree lizard *(Urosaurus ornatus)* (reviewed later). There are a number of other reptiles displaying alternate reproductive phenotypes whose behavior and ecology are becoming well understood, but for which the endocrinology and neurobiology of behavioral variation have not been studied. These promising models include the side-blotched lizard *(Uta stansburiana)* (e.g., Sinervo and Lively, 1996) and a variety of *Sceloporus* species (see later).

The first physiological studies exploring alternate male phenotypes focused on the red-sided garter snake. As previously described, this species exhibits a reproductive pattern in which peak levels of gonadal hormones are temporally dissociated from the display of reproductive behavior (Crews, 1991). Males emerge from winter hibernacula before females and vigorously court and attempt copulations in multimale mating balls as females emerge (Crews, 1983). Two pheromones underlie male courtship behavior (Mason *et al.*, 1989). The first is an estrogen-dependent attractivity pheromone produced by females that elicits vigorous courtship from males. The second pheromone, which most males produce, identifies them as males and hence not the object of courtship. However, a small proportion of males (termed she-males) actually produces the attractivity pheromone that characterizes females (Mason and Crews, 1985). This female mimicry serves to confuse other males in mating aggregations and appears to increase the chances of successful mating by the she-males. She-males have higher circulating concentrations of T (Mason and Crews, 1985) and a greater abundance of aromatase in the skin (Krohmer, 1989), which presumably converts the endogenous T to estrogen, thereby stimulating production of the female attractiveness pheromone.

The most thoroughly studied reptile exhibiting alternative mating strategies is the tree lizard. In this species, the males possess colored dewlaps that are extended during both aggressive and sexual interactions (Thompson and Moore, 1991a; reviewed in Moore *et al.*, 1998). The color of this dewlap varies among males and shows at least nine geographic variants with one to five variants occurring in any given location (Thompson and Moore, 1991b). Experiments in which males are raised in a common laboratory environment indicate that the basis of this dewlap color variation is either genetic or maternal in origin because the orange and orange-blue phenotypes develop in approximately the same proportions as are observed in the wild source populations (Thompson *et al.*, 1993; Hews *et al.*, 1997). Most attention has focused on one Arizona location in which two male morphs exist—one with orange-blue dewlaps (orange-blue males) that is site attached and holds territories encompassing the territories of three to four females and one with orange dewlaps (orange males) that is more nomadic under poor habitat conditions (i.e., in drought years) and sedentary with small home ranges under good habitat conditions. Orange-blue males are more aggressive both in the laboratory and in nature (Thompson and Moore, 1991a, 1992).

The effects of gonadal steroid and glucocorticoid hormones in male tree lizards support the predictions of Moore's relative plasticity hypothesis. Adult T and corticosterone levels do not differ between orange-blue and orange males, and neither castration nor androgen manipulations alter dewlap color expression in adult males (Moore *et al.*, 1998). In contrast, the castration of neonatal male tree lizards increases the proportion developing into orange males, whereas T implants given on hatching or 30 days thereafter increase the proportion developing into orange-blue males (Hews *et al.*, 1994) (Fig. 10). By 60 days posthatching, T implants are ineffective in altering dewlap color, indicating a defined early critical period for the development of this trait, as has been shown for behavioral organization by steroid hormones in mammals. Patterns of plasma androgens in developing male tree lizards do suggest a possible bimodality in male androgen levels during the period in which dewlap color develops (Moore *et al.*,

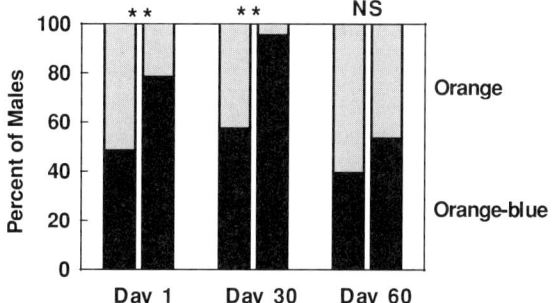

FIGURE 10 Testosterone manipulations of hatchlings alter adult dewlap coloration (day 90) in male tree lizards. This figure shows the results of T manipulation experiments begun at different times following hatching. The left bar of each pair represents morph frequency in control males who did not receive T, and the right bar depicts the frequency of different morphs for males receiving T implants. Significant differences are indicated by asterisks; NS indicates no significant difference was found between the groups. Redrawn from Moore et al. (1998).

1998), but much more striking is a clear bimodality in P levels on the day of hatching. This possible role for P in determining morph type has experimental support. Single injections of P on the day of hatching significantly increased the proportion of males developing as orange-blue males (Moore et al., 1998). This organizational role for P may point to an unrecognized developmental role for this steroid in other vertebrate systems. It is also reminiscent of the important role played by P in stimulating male-typical sexual behavior and male-like pseudosexual behaviors in whiptail lizards, as already discussed.

Corticosteroids play important roles in short-term behavioral responses in male tree lizards, supporting the relative plasticity hypothesis and adding to a growing body of information indicating these steroids are important mediators of behavioral plasticity. Corticosterone levels vary in both orange and orange-blue males depending on habitat conditions, being higher in dry years (Moore et al., 1998). In the aggressive orange-blue males, corticosterone levels are temporarily higher in losers of long-term laboratory dominance interactions, but show the opposite pattern in winners of short-duration encounters (Knapp and Moore, 1995). In the field, the less aggressive orange males show both less intense aggressive behavior and greater corticosterone elevations in response to an aggressive encounter than do orange-blue males (Knapp and Moore, 1996). Males of the two morphs also differ in their response to exogenous corticosterone. Both morphs show decreases in circulating T, but this decrease is greater in the subordinate orange males. Knapp and Moore (1997) hypothesize that the greater sensitivity of T levels to elevations in corticosterone in subordinate orange males accounts for the fact that these males switch between roving and sedentary satellite patterns of space use depending on habitat conditions, whereas changes in space use are not seen in the more aggressive orange-blue males (Fig. 11).

The work on the tree lizard is supported by studies in the side-blotched lizard (U. stansburiana). This species has three male morphs that are distinct in both morphological characteristics and behavior (Sinervo and Lively, 1996). Unlike tree lizards, there is some plasticity in male morph type in side-blotched lizards, in that the female-mimic yellow-throated males can become mate-guarding blue-throated males, but not the ultradominant orange-throated morph. The orange-throated morph has higher plasma levels of T, lower year-to-year survivorship, greater endurance, higher activity generally, and a larger home range that overlaps the areas used by more females than either the yellow- or blue-throated males (Sinervo et al., 2000). A series of studies have shown that corticosterone decreases aggression by adult males in aquaria (Denardo and Licht, 1993) and both home-range size and activity levels in the field (Denardo and Sinervo, 1994a), even when corticosterone is given in combination with T. This effect of corticosterone on male home range appears to depend on interactions with neighboring males (Denardo and Sinervo, 1994b). Corticosterone-implanted males decreased home-range size if some neighboring males were saline-implanted, but not if all neighboring males received corticosterone implants. Testosterone implants can increase home-range size in male side-blotched lizards if not given with corticosterone (Denardo and Sinervo, 1994b). Experimentally elevating T levels in yellow- and blue-throated males to those found in orange-throated males also increases both endurance and access to females in nature (Sinervo et al., 2000).

Although not as well studied from the standpoint of endocrine physiology, other groups of reptiles present opportunities for exploring the mechanisms underlying behavioral variation in and across species. One particularly promising group is the speciose lizard

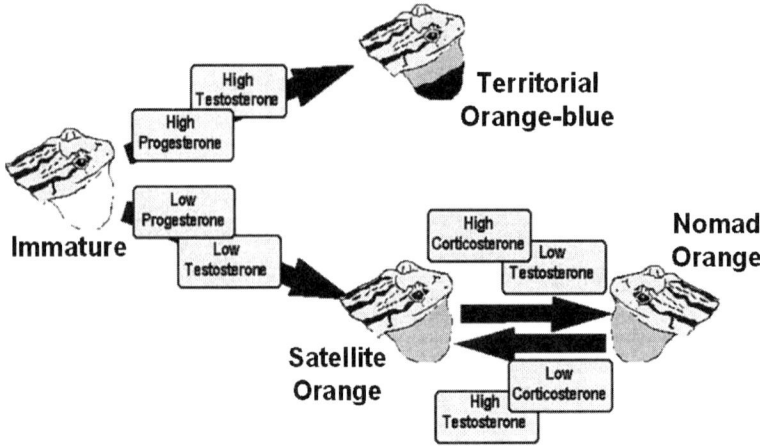

FIGURE 11 Moore and coworkers' model for organizational and activational influences on male phenotype development in tree lizards. Both testosterone and progesterone act during early development to affect adult dewlap coloration. Plastic switches between satellite and nomadic tactics in adult males of the less-aggressive orange morph are hypothesized to be due to an interplay of testosterone and corticosterone. Redrawn from Moore et al. (1998).

genus *Sceloporus*. There is a large body of behavioral and ecological information for *Sceloporus* species and both phylogenetic relationships in the genus as a whole (Wiens, 1993), and the evolution of dimorphic coloration and behavior in and across species have received attention (Wiens et al., 1999; Wiens, 2000). Finally, there is a growing body of information on the endocrine bases of sexual phenotype development and the hormonal consequences of social interactions in this genus.

As with alternate male types in the tree lizard, various *Sceloporus* species show geographic variation in male coloration (Rand, 1990; Wiens et al., 1999). There are also effects of steroid hormones on coloration in *Sceloporus*. Both orange facial color and a blue ventral coloration are influenced by T implants in adult red-lipped western fence lizards (*Sceloporus undulatus erythrocheilus*), with effects on ventral coloration being greater in males than females (Rand, 1992). In contrast, no effects were seen on the final size or intensity of blue throat or ventral patches in striped plateau lizards (*Sceloporus virgatus*) when T implants were put in hatchling males and females (Abell, 1998).

Androgens affect aggressive behavior in both male and female *Sceloporus*. Moore (1986) found elevated T associated with territorial behavior during the nonbreeding season in male mountain spiny lizards (*Sceloporus jarrovi*). This territorial aggression is affected by both castration and T replacement (Moore, 1987a,b; Moore and Marler, 1987). It is possible that aromatization is important for aggression in mountain spiny lizards, at least in females because aggressiveness in females is correlated with seasonal elevations in both T and estradiol (Woodley and Moore, 1999a), but ovariectomized T-implanted females lacked some elements of aggressive behavior observed in sham-operated controls (Woodley and Moore, 1999b). Elevated T and the associated territorial behavior have substantial energetic and survival costs in male *S. jarrovi* that appear to result from increases in energy expenditure without compensating increases in energy intake (Marler and Moore, 1989, 1991; Marler et al., 1995). Comparable energetic and growth costs of experimentally elevated T levels are seen in male northern fence lizards (*Sceloporus undulatus hyacinthus*) (Klukowski et al., 1998).

Sceloporus males can also show the short-term steroid hormone responses to encounters described for tree lizard and *U. stansburiana* males. Male *S. undulatus* show T elevations in response to a series of staged laboratory encounters with other males during the breeding season, but not in response to similar staged encounters with females or other males outside the breeding season (Smith and John-Alder, 1999). Corticosterone levels in males are increased by both male and female encounters, whereas females do not show hormonal responses to either male or female encounters.

D. Sex Steroids and Behavior: Other Reptiles

Reptiles display a diversity of relationships between circulating steroid hormones and reproductive behavior. These relationships were comprehensively reviewed by Whittier and Tokarz (1992) for female reptiles and by Moore and Lindzey (1992) for male reptiles. Findings related to this topic also appear elsewhere in this chapter as they relate to TSD, parthenogenesis, and alternate reproductive phenotypes. We briefly review information presented in these earlier contributions by taxon and along with information that has been presented since these reviews were published.

As with other aspects of brain–behavior relationships in reptiles, steroid hormone effects on behavior are best understood in lizards and snakes. This is primarily due to the ease of husbandry and adaptability of many of these species to laboratory conditions. Many lizards are also very amenable to studies in the natural habitat. Exceptions to this focus on lizards and snakes are studies on sea turtles and tuataras. Both are of interest in part because of their endangered status. The hope is that better information on their reproductive biology may be applied to aiding in their conservation.

1. Turtles

This group has been the subject of a great deal of research related to TSD, but relatively little work has addressed hormone–behavior relationships in turtles. It is known that both luteinizing hormone (LH) and folliale-stimulating hormone (FSH) rise during the breeding period in female green sea turtles (*Chelonia mydas;* Licht *et al.*, 1979, 1980). P and T also rise during this period, although E_2 does not rise significantly. Patterns in the loggerhead sea turtle (*Caretta caretta*) show similarities—P, T, and corticosterone all decline over the course of the mating season through repeated nesting episodes (Wibbels *et al.*, 1990; Whittier *et al.*, 1997). Sea turtles are most easily sampled during the nesting period when they emerge onto beaches. Less information is available on steroid levels during other seasons. Rostal and coworkers (1998) approached this problem by sampling from captive Kemp's Ridley sea turtles (*Lepidochelys kempi*) under seminatural conditions. Male Kemp's Ridley turtles show T peaks several months prior to mating and these levels decline slightly by the mating season in March; they decline sharply following the cessation of breeding. Females exhibit peak levels of T, E_2, and P at the time of mating. Both T and E_2 decline sharply after mating, whereas P declines more slowly.

Social interactions also influence circulating steroid levels in green sea turtles during the mating period. Jessop and coworkers (1999a) found that female green sea turtles have higher levels of plasma corticosterone at nesting beaches (rookeries) with a high density of other nesting females than at comparable low-density nesting beaches. A combined measure of plasma androgens showed no difference with nesting-female density in this study. In contrast, male green sea turtles do show effects on plasma androgens related to social interactions (Jessop *et al.*, 1999b). Males near, or actually mounting, females have elevated androgen levels, whereas males that are the recipients of aggression from rival males or males that exhibit courtship damage resulting from this male–male aggression have lower circulating levels of androgen.

Although there are data on seasonal cycles in gonadal steroid hormones for other turtles and tortoises (e.g., Callard *et al.*, 1978; Lewis *et al.*, 1979; Sarkar *et al.*, 1996; Mahmoud and Licht, 1997; Schramm *et al.*, 1999; Shelby *et al.*, 2000), no studies have addressed the behavioral correlates of this variation. The single exception is work in musk turtles (*Sternotherus odoratus*) in which there is some evidence of both photoperiod and androgen control of sexual behavior (Mendonca, 1987a,b).

2. Crocodilians, Tuatara, and Amphisbaenians

The 21 species of crocodilians represent the most primitive extant members of the archosauromorph lineage that includes modern birds and the extinct dinosaurs. As with turtles, considerable information is available regarding steroid hormones and the process of TSD for crocodilians (represented by the American alligator, *Alligator missipiensis*). Some information is also available regarding gametogenic cycles and circulating steroid hormones in the group (Guillette et al., 1997). However, no experimental work has addressed the relationship of steroid hormones in crocodilians to behavior, and there are relatively few studies on the mating behavior of the group generally (e.g., Compton, 1981; Webb et al., 1983; Thorbjarnason and Hernandez, 1993; Tucker et al., 1998).

Data on tuataras, limited to a single extant species representing the order Sphenodontida, are similarly limited. Female tuatara exhibit a prolonged reproductive cycle, carrying eggs in the oviduct for 6–8 months and nesting only once every 4 years on average (Cree et al., 1992). Tuataras appear to exhibit an associated reproductive pattern. Gametogenesis and testosterone levels in males follow an annual cycle—low during the winter, rising in the spring, and peaking in mid-summer to early autumn during the mating period. Female tuatara show elevated levels of E_2, and T during vitellogenesis, which fall at ovulation when P levels rise. Females also show elevations in plasma AVT during oviposition relative to during the nest digging and guarding stages that are probably associated with oviducal contractions (Guillette et al., 1991).

As when this topic was last comprehensively reviewed (Whittier and Tokarz, 1992; Moore and Lindzey, 1992), no information is available regarding the relationship of steroid hormones to either reproduction or behavior in Amphisbaenians.

III. NEUROANATOMICAL SUBSTRATES OF SEXUAL BEHAVIOR IN REPTILES

Most work on the neural substrates of behavior in reptiles has focused on the squamate reptiles, lizards and snakes. This is the most speciose group and their typically small body sizes and ease of husbandry facilitates experimental studies in the laboratory as well as in the field. Research to date has focused primarily on the limbic system. The first studies established the role of limbic nuclei as critical integrative areas in the control of sexual behavior. Another area of research has been the metabolic and neurochemical differences between the sexes and within sexes across seasons and incubation conditions. The metabolic work has used 2-deoxyglucose (2DG) and cytochrome oxidase (CO) histochemistry. The neurochemistry work has focused on neurotransmitters, neuropeptides, and the expression and regulation of steroid receptor mRNAs.

A. Integrative Centers for Sexual Behaviors

The primary integrative centers for sexual behavior in reptiles are in the hypothalamus, as in other vertebrates (Sachs and Meisel, 1994; Pfaff et al., 1994). The final common pathway for male-typical mounting and intromission behavior appears to be the preoptic area–anterior hypothalamus (POAH), whereas that of female-typical receptive behavior is the ventromedial portion of the hypothalamus (VMH; comparable to the ventromedial nucleus of the hypothalamus of rodents). Both of these areas are rich in steroid hormone receptors and their activity and neurochemistry responds to both steroid hormones and environmental signals. Experimental support for the critical importance of the POAH in regulating male-typical and VMH in regulating female-typical suites of reproductive behaviors comes mainly from two types of experiments.

Electrolytic lesion experiments involve creating localized damage in candidate regions followed by behavioral assays to assess disruptions of function. Lesions of the POAH impair courtship and copulatory behavior in male green anole lizards (Anolis carolinensis; Wheeler and Crews, 1978) and little striped whiptail lizards (Cnemidophorus inornatus; Kingston and Crews, 1994), whereas lesions of the VMH in the parthenogenetic whiptail lizard C. uniparens abolish receptive behavior; it is significant that only those lesions that encompassed the area containing ERs were effective (Kendrick et al., 1995) (Fig. 12). Interestingly, POAH lesions also impair male-like pseudocopulatory behavior in the unisexual C. uniparens. This suggests that pseudosexual behavior in the descendant species of this pair is mediated by the same neural circuits responsible for copulatory and receptive behaviors in males and females of its ancestral species.

The second type of experiment providing critical support for the roles of the POAH and VMH in mediating sexual behaviors in reptiles involves intracranial implantation of minute amounts of steroid hormones directly into candidate brain regions of animals lacking gonads. This approach has been shown to effectively restore male-typical sexual behaviors in rats

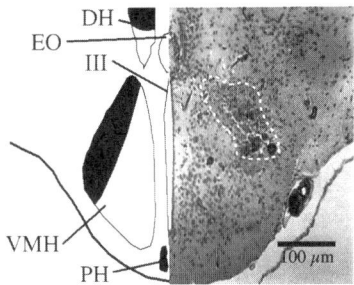

FIGURE 12 Composite illustration of the ventral portion of the hypothalamus of *Cnemidophorus uniparens* at the level of the ventromedial hypothalamus (VMH). Left: The outlines of the VMH, dorsal hypothalamus (DH), the ependymal organ (EO), the third ventricle (III), and the periventricular hypothalamus (PH). The black regions represent the location of estrogen receptor mRNA. Right: Photomicrograph of brain tissue stained with cresyl violet. The dashed white line demarks the tissue damage caused by an electrolytic lesion. Only those lesions of the dorsolateral VMH effectively prevented estrogen induction of sexual receptivity. From Kendrick et al. (1995).

and other mammals (reviewed in Sachs and Meisel, 1994). The implantation of androgens directly into the POAH reinstates courtship and copulatory behaviors in castrated male green anoles (Morgentaler and Crews, 1978). Likewise, intracranial implantation of androgen into the POAH induces copulatory behaviors in both castrated male whiptails (*C. inornatus*; Rozendaal and Crews, 1989) and the parthenogenetic *C. uniparens* (Mayo and Crews, 1987) (Fig. 13). Intracranial implantation of P rather than androgen is also effective in restoring courtship and copulatory behavior in a subset of *C. inornatus* males that are sensitive to intraperitoneal P implants (Crews et al., 1996b).

As with male-typical sexual behavior, the implantation of estrogen directly into the VMH of ovariectomized female and unisexual whiptail lizards reinstates receptive behavior (Wade and Crews, 1991) (Fig. 13). This finding agrees well with the characterized distribution and regulation of both ERs and PRs in this brain region (see later).

B. Variation in Brain Nuclei and Neuron Soma Sizes

Several sex differences in reptilian brain nuclei or soma sizes are best characterized in the whiptail lizards and green anoles. In the sexual species of whiptail lizard, *C. inornatus*, males have larger POAH than do females, whereas females have a larger VMH (Crews et al., 1990). These sexual dimorphisms in size are under the control of gonadal androgens in the male (Fig. 14). That is, castration of breeding animals results in a reduction in the area of the preoptic area (POA) and an enlargement in the area of the VMH, whereas androgen replacement therapy reverses these effects of castration. It is significant that only the male shows these responses to hormonal manipulation. These overall differences in nucleus size are correlated with differences in soma size in these areas. Male *C. inornatus* have larger soma sizes in the POA, whereas females have larger soma sizes in the VMH (Wade and Crews, 1992). Interestingly, the brains of the all-female *C. uniparens* show patterns similar to those of females of the sexual species, despite the fact that these females regularly show male-like pseudosexual behavior. This finding is also true when the parthenogenetic females are sex-reversed using fadrozole, an inhibitor of aromatase that effectively induces male development in *C. uniparens* (Wennstrom and Crews, 1995; Wennstrom et al., 1999). This result indicates that, although useful, measurements of brain nucleus volume and soma size probably do not reflect many important differences in function. We return to this topic later when considering metabolic capacity, neurotransmitter function, and regulation of steroid-hormone-receptor expression.

Seasonal variation in the size of brain areas has been documented in a variety of vertebrate species, particularly in the song system of many birds (see Ball and Balthazart, Chap. 32 in this volume; Schlinger and Brenowitz, Chap. 33 in this volume). Many reptiles also show seasonal reproduction, but the neural correlates of this seasonality are less well documented. In the Canadian red-sided garter snake (*Thamnophis sirtalis parietalis*) the volume of the POA varies seasonally in females, but not in males (Crews et al., 1993). The POA of female snakes is smaller than that of males during the hibernation period. The lack of variation in males may be related to the fact that, unlike the songbirds that are the focus of most studies, these garter snakes exhibit a dissociated reproductive pattern in which seasonal mating behavior and gonadal steroid hormone peaks are temporally offset (Crews, 1991).

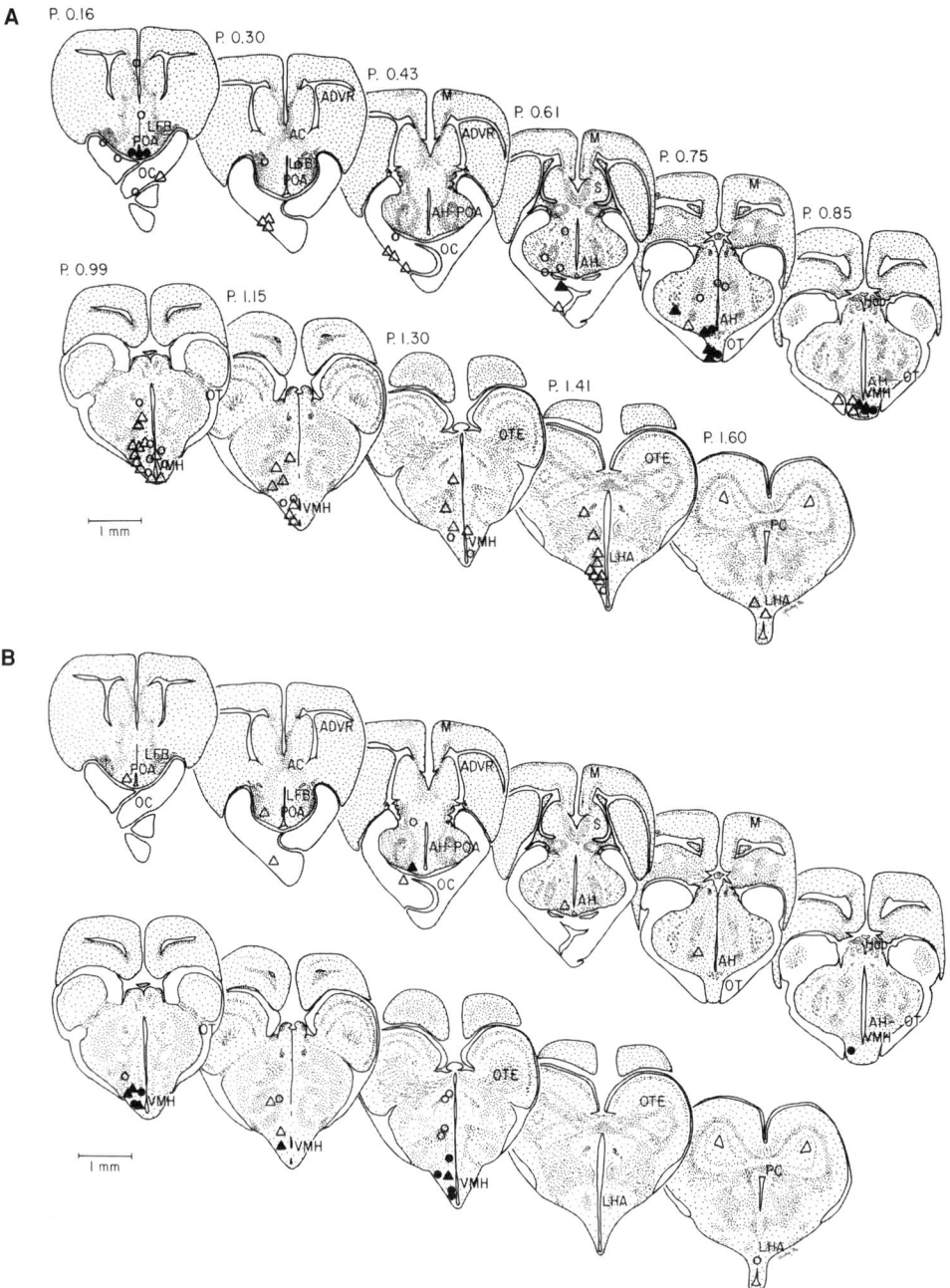

FIGURE 13 Frontal sections through the brain of a representative whiptail lizard, showing locations of the approximate center of hormone implants that elicited (A) mounting and copulatory behavior or (B) sexual receptivity in whiptail lizards. Numerals indicate distance posterior to zero point. (A) Solid triangles indicate locations of dihydrotestosterone implants that resulted in male-like pseudocopulatory behavior in ovariectomized parthenogenetic whiptails (*Cnemidophorus uniparens*), whereas solid circles indicate implants that result in male-typical copulatory behavior in castrated male whiptails (*C. inornatus*). Open symbols represent placement of implants that failed to respond. (B) Solid triangles indicate locations of estrogen implants that resulted in female-like sexual receptivity in ovariectomized parthenogenetic whiptails (*Cnemidophorus uniparens*), whereas solid circles indicate implants that result in female-typical sexual receptivity in ovariectomized female whiptails (*C. inornatus*). Open symbols represent placement of implants that failed respond. AC, anterior commissure; ADVR, anterodorsal ventricular ridge; AH, anterior hypothalamus; LFB, lateral forebrain bundle; LHA, lateral hypothalamic area; OC, optic chiasm; OT, optic tract; OTE, optic tectum; PC, posterior commissure; POA, preoptic area; VMH, ventromedial hypothalamus.

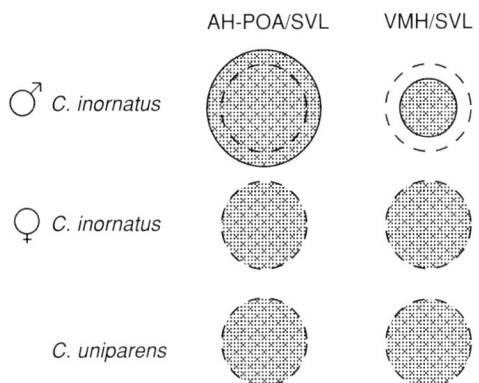

FIGURE 14 Schematic representations of the volumes of the sexually dimorphic areas in the brain relative to body size in sexual and parthenogenetic whiptails. To aid in comparison, the volume of the POAH and the VMH of female *C. inornatus* is represented as a solid outline in other figures to indicate significant differences (SVL refers to snout-vent length, a standard measure of body size in reptiles).

Information has become available on sexual dimorphisms in both the brain stem and limbic system of green anoles. Sexual and aggressive behaviors in green anoles are well characterized (Crews, 1975b; Crews *et al.*, 1978; Andrews and Summers, 1996; Propper *et al.*, 1991). The control of these behaviors by gonadal steroid hormones in green anoles has also received a good deal of attention (Valenstein and Crews, 1977; Crews *et al.*, 1978; Crews and Morgentaler, 1979; Tokarz and Crews, 1979, 1980, 1981; Jones *et al.*, 1983). Males perform push ups, as in many male lizards, and are also able to greatly extend a red-pigmented portion of skin on the ventral side of the neck (termed the dewlap) through flexion of the hyoid apparatus (Crews, 1975a); although female green anoles have similar pigmentation in the gular region and use this as an aggressive signal, neither the skin nor the hyoid is as well developed as in males (Crews, 1975b). Both of these signals are used in social contexts, with dewlap extension being shown only in males. The muscle primarily responsible for dewlap extension, the ceratohyoideus muscle, is innervated from the nucleus ambiguus (AmbX) as well as the glossopharyngeal portion of the AmbX and the ventral portion of the motor nucleus of the facial nerve (AmbIX/VIImv). Neurons in both brain regions are larger in males than in females (Wade 1998). The motor neuron number does not vary by sex or across the breeding and nonbreeding seasons, but nerve cross-sectional area and both muscle fiber size and number are greater in males than females (O'Bryant and Wade, 2000a). However, there is no consistent relationship between either the breeding and nonbreeding season or androgen treatment (T propionate) and these characteristics. Another study found that, unlike some other vertebrate systems in which the sexes differ in their display behavior (Gurney, 1981; Devoogd and Nottebohm, 1981; Kelley *et al.*, 1988; Bass and Baker, 1990), green anoles show no sex difference in the dendritic arborization of motoneurons in AmbX or AmbIX/VIImv (O'Bryant and Wade, 2000b). These findings suggest that changes in this system during adulthood do not underlie sex or seasonal differences in the dewlap-extension behavior. O'Bryant and Wade propose that this may be due to the fact that, although the extension of the dewlap is associated with male courtship, females also lower the hyoid, thereby exposing the patch of red.

The described research with whiptail and green anole lizards focused on species with the familiar pattern of GSD. The other end of the genotype–environment spectrum is represented by species that exhibit TSD. In the leopard gecko (*Eublepharis macularius*), both low and high incubation temperatures produce females, whereas intermediate temperatures result in male determination and differentiation (Fig. 4). Interestingly, sexuality covaries with incubation temperature somewhat independently of gonadal sex, such that females produced at higher temperatures are masculinized compared to females incubated at low temperatures. This variation is reminiscent of the intrauterine position effect in mammals and may provide a powerful experimental system for addressing the causes and consequences of prenatal hormonal effects as well as maternal effects on offspring phenotypes.

Coomber, Crews, and Gonzalez-Lima (1997) found that females from male-biased incubation temperatures had larger POA volumes than those from female-biased incubation temperatures (Fig. 15). There are parallel differences in the VMH, but this varies with age; for example, old females have a larger POA and VMH than do young females. Differences are also seen in males with age, but these contrast with those found in females (Crews *et al.*, 1997). Young males show larger volumes for the POA and VMH than do older males. Sociosexual experience does not have strong effects on brain nucleus

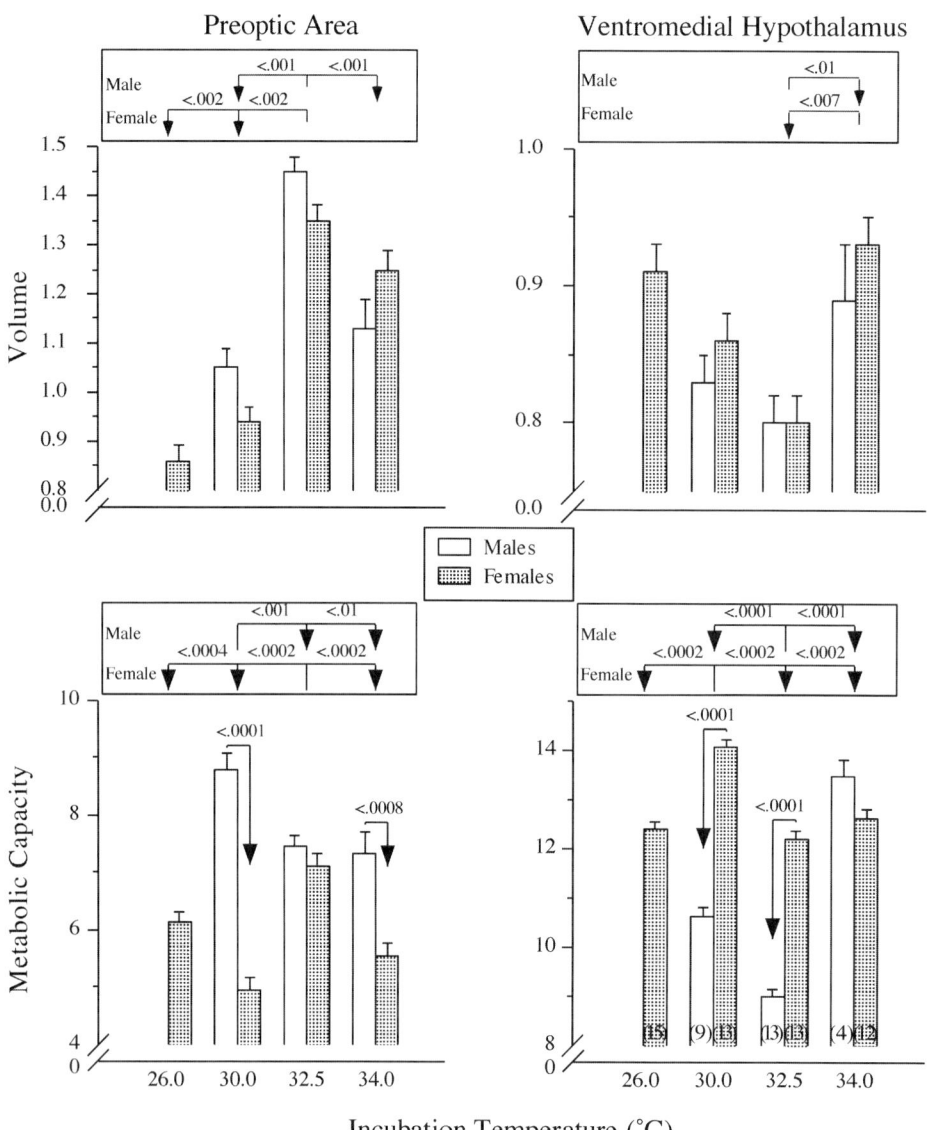

FIGURE 15 Effect of incubation temperature and gonadal sex on the volume (top panels) and cytochrome oxidase (CO) activity (μmol/min/g tissue wet weight) (bottom panels) of the preoptic area (POA) (left panels) and ventromedial hypothalamus (VMH) (right panels) in the leopard gecko (*Eublepharis macularius*). Volumes are normalized by entire forebrain volume. Significant differences (entries are p values) within each sex are illustrated in boxes above each panel, indicating the effect of incubation temperature. Significant differences between the sexes are illustrated above bars, indicating the effect of gonadal sex. Sample sizes are in parentheses. Means are depicted with vertical bars representing standard error. Data from Coomber et al. (1997).

volume (possibly an increase in POA volume in female geckos from female-determining temperatures), but experience does strongly affect the metabolic capacity of brain areas functionally linked to sexual and aggressive behavior (see later).

IV. METABOLIC INDICATORS OF NEURAL ACTIVITY

Although informative, measurements of brain nucleus volume and soma size represent only an indirect assessment of function. One exciting development in our ability to assess sex differences in the neural substrates of sexual behavior has been the introduction and implementation of measurements of acute metabolic activity and sustained metabolic capacity in the brains of reptiles and other vertebrates. The 2-DG technique utilizes the dependence of neurons on glucose as a source of energy and an analog of glucose that can be taken up by cells, but not metabolized. This allows ^{14}C-labeled 2-DG to accumulate in cells and this accumulation can be assessed by the relative amounts of radioactivity present in tissue sections (Cada et al., 1995). CO catalyzes the rate-limiting step in oxidative respiration in brain tissue and levels of this enzyme provide a useful indicator of the total metabolic capacity (Wong-Riley, 1989).

A. Acute Metabolic Activity Associated with Behavioral State: 2-Deoxyglucose Utilization

Even when no morphometric differences are apparent across behavioral phenotypes, indicators of metabolic activity can demonstrate differences in function. Rand and Crews (1994) found that the acute metabolic activity of the parthenogenetic *C. uniparens* depended on whether they were displaying male-like or female-like pseudosexual behavior (Table 2). Specifically, animals displaying male-like pseudocopulatory behavior showed a sixfold greater accumulation of 2-fluoro-2-DG in the medial POA than did animals showing female-like behavior. Conversely, individuals showing female-like receptive pseudosexual behavior exhibited a greater accumulation of 2-DG in the VMH.

The results from *C. uniparens* are paralleled across seasons in red-sided garter snakes. Male red-sided garter snakes that actively court females show a significantly higher 2-DG accumulation in the POAH than males who either are exposed to females but fail to court or males that are not exposed to females (Allen and Crews, 1992). Interestingly, simply being exposed to females increases the overall 2-DG accumulation in garter snake males. These results suggest both a generalized arousal effect as well as a more specific effect of active courting that is restricted to the brain region very directly involved in mediating this behavior.

Radiolabeled 2-DG has also been used to study patterns of neural activity associated with the change from a receptive to an unreceptive state in female red-sided garter snakes (Mendonça and Crews, 2001). On emergence from hibernation, females initially are receptive to male courtship behavior but become unreceptive immediately following mating. Females that are courted and then mate have significantly higher activity in the POA and significantly lower activity in the VMH compared to females who are courted but do not mate (Fig. 16). Because intromission during mating is responsible for the loss of sexual receptivity in the female (Mendonça and Crews, 1990, 2001; Ross and Crews, 1977; Whittier and Crews, 1989; Whittier et al., 1985, 1987), the injection of a local anesthetic (tetracaine or lidocaine) into the cloacal region desensitizes the female to mating stimuli (Mendonça and Crews, 1990, 2001). Not only does this treatment prevent the mating-induced surge in estrogen levels in the plasma and subsequent ovarian recrudescence, but the pattern of 2-DG accumulation in tetracaine-treated females is similar to courted but unmated females and to females exposed only to other females. These results suggest that in the female red-sided garter snake sensory input from the cloaca during mating alters patterns of metabolism in those brain areas most often associated with sexual receptivity. The increased activity in the POA accompanied by a decrease in activity in the VMH after mating supports the hypothesis that mating initiates a neuroendocrine reflex that results in a loss of receptivity in female red-sided garter snakes.

TABLE 2
Optical Density Scores of the Medial Preoptic Area and Ventromedial Hypothalamus in *Cnemidophorus uniparens*

Behavior	(N)	mPOA score	VMH score
Courtship	(6)	−5.86 ± 0.79 ⎤ +	+4.58 ± 1.03 ⎤ *
Receptive	(5)	+0.12 ± 1.70 ⎦	+0.66 ± 0.63 ⎦

^{a}Subjects exhibit either male-like pseudocopulatory (courtship) or female-like (receptive) behavior. Lower scores indicate higher 2DG accumulations; + indicates significance at $P = 0.008$; * indicates significance at $P = 0.006$.

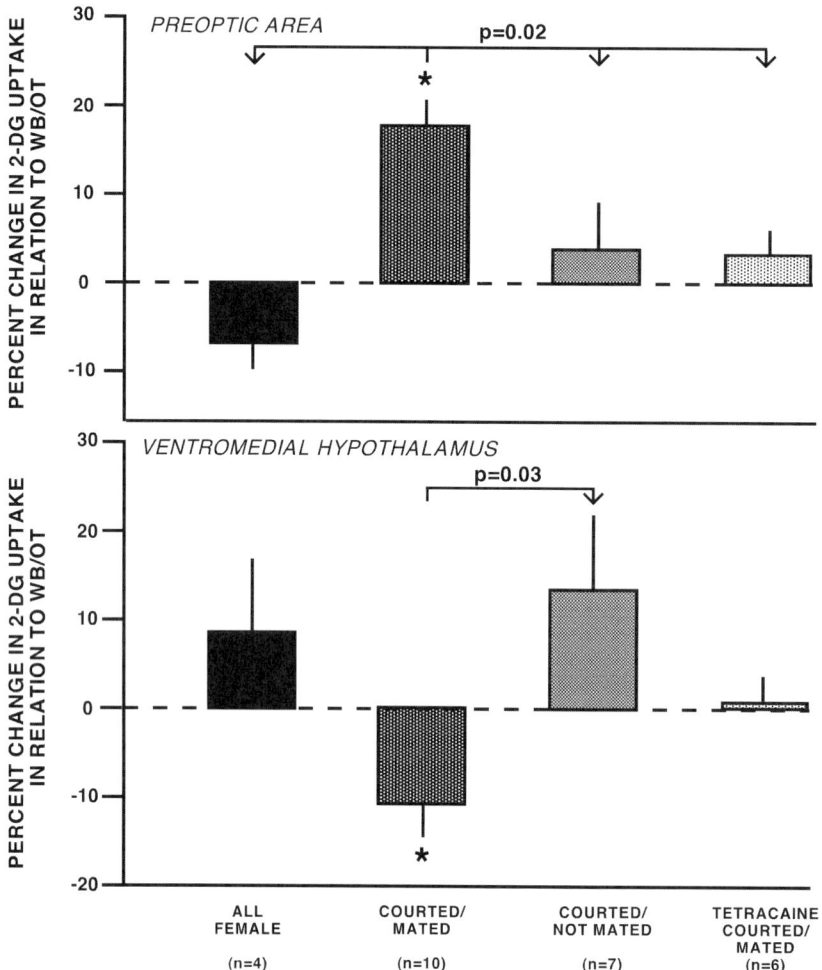

FIGURE 16 Mean relative change in 2-deoxyglucose (2-DG) uptake in the red-sided garter snake (*Thamnophis sirtalis parietalis*). Values for different treatment groups relative to whole brain/optic tract (WB/OT). The dashed line indicates background brain levels (e.g., zero difference from background). A positive change represents higher accumulation; a negative change represents lower accumulation than background. The vertical lines represent 1 standard error. The asterisk represents significant differences. The p level of the difference is indicated. A. Uptake of 2-DG in the preoptic area–optic tract. B. Uptake of 2-DG in the ventromedial hypothalamus–optic tract.

B. Metabolic Capacity Associated with Behavioral Phenotype: Cytochrome Oxidase Histochemistry

As with brain nucleus volume, a variety of factors influence metabolic capacity in the brain of leopard geckos. These include incubation temperature, age, and sexual experience. Incubation temperature affects CO activity in both females and males, although the effect varies depending on the brain nucleus being considered. Females from a male-biased incubation temperature have increased metabolic capacity of the anterior hypothalamus (AH), external amygdala, dorsolateral hypothalamus, dorsoventricular ridge, nucleus sphericus, lateral septum, and striatum, but do not increase capacity in the posterior hypothalamus or periventricular POA (Fig. 17). Of particular interest is the finding that young females from a male-biased incubation temperature show greater CO levels in the medial POA than young females from a female-biased

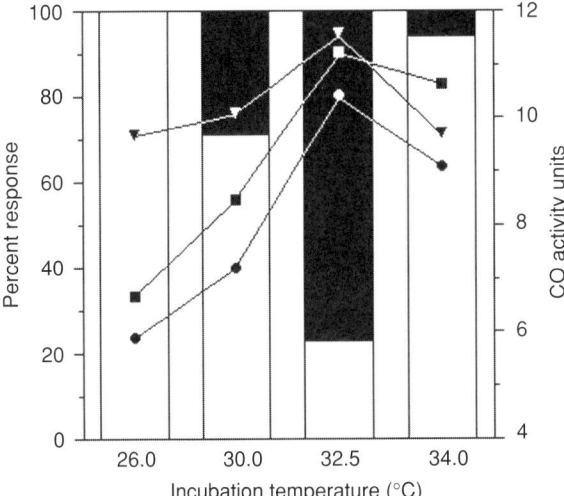

FIGURE 17 Relationship between sex ratio, aggressive behavior, and cytochrome oxidase activity in the amygdala in female leopard geckos. Sex in the leopard gecko is determined by the incubation temperature of the egg; the sex ratio produced at the temperatures indicated is reflected in the bar graph (proportion male is indicated by darkened areas of bars). The proportion of females responding aggressively toward a courting male indicated by squares. Cytochrome oxidase activity in the nucleus sphericus and external amygdala of females from these same incubation temperatures are shown by inverted triangles and circles, respectively. In reptiles, the nucleus sphericus and external amygdala are homologous to the medial and basolateral amygdala of mammals, respectively; as in mammals, both areas are involved in the control of aggression. Thus, embryonic experience with temperature affects the level of aggressive behavior and brain metabolism in the amygdala of adult females.

incubation temperature. Females from a male-biased incubation temperature are more aggressive and less sexually attractive than females from a female-biased incubation temperature. CO levels in male leopard geckos are also influenced by incubation temperature, with males from a female-biased incubation temperature having greater levels of CO in the POA and VMH than males from a male-biased incubation temperature. Such findings are reminiscent of the finding that in mice males positioned between two females *in utero* are more sexually active than their male siblings positioned between two males (cf. Clark and Galef, 1995).

Age and sexual experience are also important factors determining metabolic activity in limbic nuclei in both male and female geckos. For example, age is associated with a decrease in the size of the POA and VMH in males, but not in females. CO activity increases in the POA, nucleus sphericus, and external amygdala (reptilian counterparts to the mammalian amygdala) with age in males, but the precise effects of age on CO levels in different brain nuclei in female leopard geckos vary with incubation temperature, indicating a complex interaction of these factors (Coomber *et al.*, 1997).

Sexual experience also influences the metabolic capacity of limbic nuclei in leopard geckos, again in complex ways (Crews *et al.*, 1997). Several nuclei, including the VMH and AH, have higher metabolic capacities in sexually experienced males than in sexually inexperienced males. In contrast, there is no difference with experience in the POA or several other limbic nuclei in males. On the other hand, sexually experienced female leopard geckos show a higher CO abundance in the POA than sexually inexperienced females regardless of incubation temperature history; the results were mixed for other nuclei.

Sakata and coworkers (2000) assessed functional connectivity among limbic nuclei in the leopard gecko by analyzing covariance patterns in metabolic capacity, as revealed by quantitative CO histochemistry. As previously indicated, incubation temperature during embryonic development influences an individual's aggressive and sexual behaviors in adulthood. For example, an increase in incubation temperature results in an increase in adult aggressivity in both males and females. Correlated with this are increased amounts of CO in the AH and both the septum and POA. Similarly, female-typical sexual behaviors decline with increasing incubation temperature, and the correlations between the VMH and both the dorsoventricular ridge and septum were significant only in females. Correlations among preoptic, hypothalamic, and amygdalar areas tend to be distributed across both sexes, suggesting that there may exist shared pathways underlying the expression of male-typical and female-typical behaviors.

Thus, a variety of factors including gonadal sex, age, sexual experience, and incubation temperature history influence the volume and metabolic capacity of brain nuclei and the connectivity among these nuclei in leopard geckos. The dominant influence, however, is incubation temperature. This work provided the first unequivocal demonstration that factors other than gonadal sex and gonadal hormones can influence the sexual differentiation of the brain in vertebrates.

V. NEUROCHEMICAL BASES OF SEXUAL AND AGGRESSIVE BEHAVIOR IN REPTILES

The relationship of neurotransmitters and neuropeptides to sexual and other behaviors in reptiles has received relatively little attention. Propper and coworkers (1992a) examined the distribution of AVT in the green anole and found labeling in the cortex, around the olfactory ventricle, in the diagonal band of Broca, and in the amygdala area, dorsal ventricular ridge, striatum, nucleus accumbens, septum, VMH, lateral hypothalamus, medial forebrain bundle, median eminence, pars nervosa, nucleus of the solitary tract, locus coeruleus, cerebellar cortex (granular layer), dorsal part of the nucleus of the lateral lemniscus, substantia nigra, and myelencephalon. There is generally greater intensity of staining in males than females. The distribution of AVT immunoreactivity has also been examined in a turtle (*Pseudemys scripta*) and a python (*Python regius*) (Smeets *et al.*, 1990). No sex differences were described in vasopressin-like or oxytocin-like (presumably AVT and mesotocin) immunoreactivity in the brain of the chameleon, although differences were found for females across the ovarian cycle (Bennis *et al.*, 1995). This variation in AVT also occurs in female green anoles, in which females with large preovulatory follicles have higher AVT concentrations in the supraoptic area than do females with small preovulatory follicles (Propper *et al.*, 1992b).

Dominance interactions influence monoamine metabolism in male lizards. For example, aggressive interactions increase plasma epinephrine and norepinephrine in male green anoles and these levels are higher in males winning encounters than in males that lose (Summers and Greenberg, 1994). This response and the speed of the correlated eyespot darkening are reduced by castration, suggesting an influence of testosterone. Both dominant and subordinate male anoles show changes in central monoamine metabolism following aggressive encounters, but these changes are more pronounced in subordinates. Subordinate male green anoles show elevated ratios of 5-hydroxyindoleacetic acid (5-HIAA) to 5-hydroxytryptamine (5-HT) and the substrate for 5-HT, 5-hydroxytryptophan (5-HTP), indicating enhancement of both serotonin turnover and production, 1 hour after an encounter with a dominant individual (Summers and Greenberg, 1995). The difference between subordinate and both dominant and control males diminishes thereafter. Dominant males show broadly similar patterns, but return to baseline turnover levels more rapidly. Neither the dopaminergic nor adrenergic systems showed similar patterns, indicating this response is specific to the serotonergic system. This serotonergic response is also regionally specific. The nucleus accumbens and hippocampal cortex show the most dramatic changes 1 hour following an aggressive interaction, but the medial and lateral amygdala show a more delayed response with serotonergic activity, peaking at 1 week postinteraction in subordinate males (Summers *et al.*, 1998). The amygdalar region is important in regulating sexual and aggressive behaviors in green anoles (Greenberg *et al.*, 1984).

Both plasma and brain-region-specific alterations in monoamine metabolism can also be induced in male anoles by manipulating a key aggressive signal and exposing males to a mirror (Korzan *et al.*, 2000a,b). Masking a male's eyespot with green paint suggests a less aggressive or subordinate opponent when the animal observes this opponent (itself) in a mirror. Males whose eyespots were painted green showed the highest frequency of biting behavior. These males also showed elevated plasma levels of dopamine, epinephrine, and norepinephrine compared to isolated controls and males whose eyespots were painted black. In the brain, males with green-painted eyespots showed increased serotonergic and adrenergic activity (but lower dopaminergic activity) in the subiculum (dorsal cortex), hippocampus, nucleus accumbens, and medial amygdala compared to males whose eyespots were darkened (suggesting an aggressive or dominant opponent) (Fig. 18).

The patterns of monoamine metabolism in mountain spiny lizards (*Sceloporus jarrovi*) are similar to those in anoles—higher serotonergic activity is seen in non-territorial satellite (subordinate) males than in territorial males (Matter *et al.*, 1998). As with anoles, aggressive defense of territory in *S. jarrovi* males results in increases both in 5-HTP and in 5-HIAA/5-HT ratios. These interactions also increase the activity of the

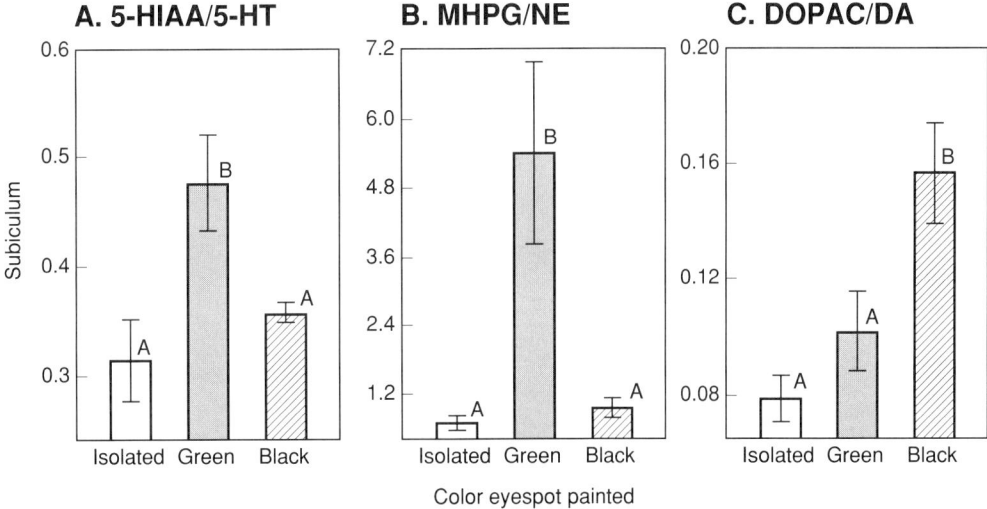

FIGURE 18 Monoaminergic profiles in the dorsal cortex (subiculum) of male green anoles following 10 minutes exposure to mirror presentations in one of two conditions (gray bars, subject male's eyespot was painted green; black bars, subject's eyespot was painted black; white bars, isolated controls). Neurotransmitter activity is depicted as ratios of important catabolite levels to levels of the neurotransmitter itself for (a) serotonin (5-HIAA/5-HT), (b) norepinephrine (MHPG/NE), and (c) dopamine (DOPAC/DA). Bars are mean ± S.E.M.; means with a different letter labels are significantly different. 5-HIAA, 5-hyddroxyindoleacetic acid; 5-HT, 5-hydroxytryptophan; DA, dopamine; DOPAC, 3,4-dihydroxyphenylacetic acid; MHPG, 4-hydroxy-3-methoxyphenylglycol; NE, norepinephrine. Reprinted from Korzan *et al.* (2000a) with permission from Elsevier Science.

central dopamine and epinephrine systems. Plasma levels of norepinephrine and epinephrine also rise rapidly during restraint stress or following territorial interactions in *S. jarrovi* (Matt *et al.*, 1997).

The rapid alterations in serotonergic metabolism during aggressive interactions in male green anoles may be modulated by alterations in circulating steroid hormones. In green anoles, serotonin turnover (5-HIAA/5-HT) was enhanced in the hippocampus and medial amygdala 20 minutes after males received low-dose systemic injections of corticosterone (1.6–2.0 mg/kg), but not following 10-fold-higher corticosterone doses (16–20 mg/kg) (Summers *et al.*, 2000) (Fig. 19). Testosterone injections (1.6–2.0 mg/kg) enhanced serotonin turnover in the hippocampus, but not the medial amygdala. There were no changes found in several other brain regions or in the activity of other monoaminergic systems. The authors note the possibility that the injected testosterone could have been converted before having this effect. The brain of green anoles does show both aromatase and 5α-reductase activity (Wade, 1997) and at least aromatase activity is important in some behavioral contexts (Winkler and Wade, 1998). Aggressive interactions influence plasma steroid levels in green anoles and other male lizards (Greenberg and Crews, 1990; Knapp and Moore, 1995, 1996). Testosterone levels are also typically elevated during the breeding season and influence aggression (Moore and Crews, 1986; Moore, 1986, 1988), although plasma T levels do not necessarily change following an aggressive encounter (e.g., Moore, 1987b). The steroid hormone mediation of serotonergic metabolism demonstrated in green anole males was suggested as part of a mechanism enabling an individual to respond to changing social situations.

Differences are also found with social status in female anoles (Summers *et al.*, 1997). Females housed with males singly did not differ from isolated females. However, there were differences among females housed in groups of five with a male. In contrast to results obtained with green anole males, dominant females in this experiment showed higher 5-HT and dopamine (DA) activity in the telencephalon than did subordinate females, whereas subordinate females showed higher serotonergic activity in the brain stem. It was suggested that the heightened serotonergic activity in dominant

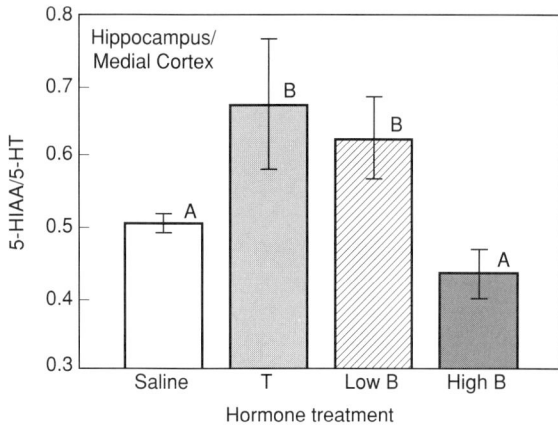

FIGURE 19 Serotonergic activity in the hippocampus and medial cortex of male green anoles 20 minutes following an intraperitoneal injection of a saline control solution, 10 μg T, 10 μg corticosterone (low B), or 100 μg corticosterone (high B). Serotonergic activity is assessed as the ratio of the primary metabolite 5-hydroxyindoleacetic acid (5-HIAA) to serotonin (5-HT). Bars are mean ± S.E.M.; Means with a different letter label are significantly different. Redrawn from Summers et al. (2000).

females is more directly related to interactions with males than to those with other females.

DA also is integral to the display of copulatory behaviors in male mammals and birds. Woolley and colleagues (2001) determined that a DA D1 receptor agonist facilitates the display of courtship and copulatory behaviors in both castrated sexual (C. inornatus) and ovariectomized parthenogenetic (C. uniparens) whiptail lizards. In both species, the D1 agonist SKF 81297 increases the proportion of individuals mounting and decreases the latency to mount (Fig. 20). Moreover, there is a difference in sensitivity to the agonist between the species—mounting is elicited at a lower dose in C. uniparens than in C. inornatus. This suggests that, as is the case for sensitivity to exogenous estrogen (see previous discussion), the heightened sensitivity in the triploid parthenogen is due to the increased ploidy, indicating that the parthenogen may have elevated levels of D1 receptor in limbic brain areas that modulate courtship behavior. Not only does this work extend to reptiles the central role of DA in the modulation of copulatory behavior, it also indicates that DA can elicit male-typical mounting behavior from both a "male" (C. inornatus) and a "female" (C. uniparens) brain.

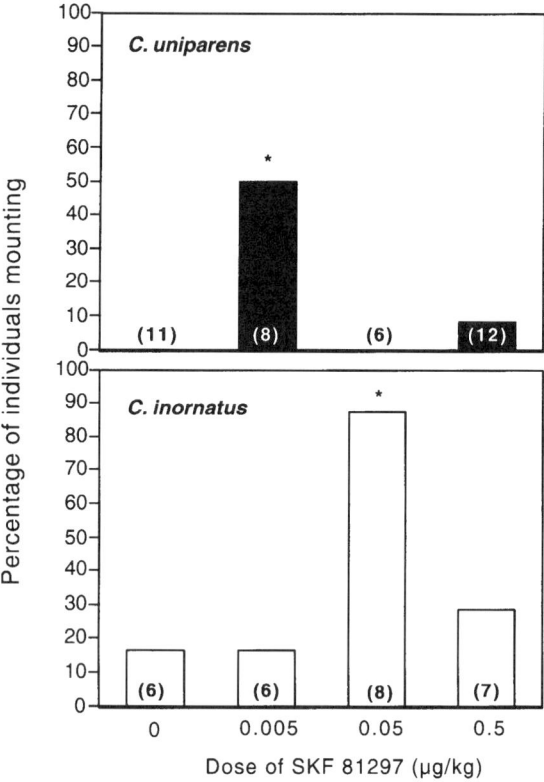

FIGURE 20 The percentage of individuals of each species mounting across all treatment groups (in Cnemidophorus uniparens (black bars) and C. inornatus (white bars)). In each species, an asterisk indicates a dose that is significantly different than vehicle treatment ($P < 0.05$). Redrawn from Woolley et al. (2001).

VI. DISTRIBUTION AND REGULATION OF SEX STEROID HORMONE RECEPTORS

Studies of sex steroid receptors in the brain of reptiles have focused exclusively on lizards and snakes. These studies have taken one of three approaches. Early studies examined the accumulation of radiolabeled sex steroid hormones T, DHT, or E_2 in specific brain nuclei. Later, steroid hormone receptors have been cloned from reptiles, allowing cellular-level localization of their mRNAs and studies of the factors influencing their abundance. Immunocytochemistry has also been used to map androgen receptor distribution.

A. Distribution

The accumulation of tritium-labeled E_2, T, and DHT is found at a variety of sites in the brain of green anole lizards (Morrell et al., 1979). Halpern and coworkers (1982) performed a similar study with labeled E_2 and T in the brain of red-sided garter snakes. These studies, similar to those in mammals and other vertebrates (see Morrell and Pfaff, 1978), reveal substantial E_2 binding in the POA, AH, amygdaloid nuclei, VMH, and posterior hypothalamic nuclei, with lighter labeling in several areas including the septum, torus semicircularis, central gray, and some brain-stem areas. In the green anole, the binding of tritiated T and DHT is very similar to patterns for tritiated E_2, but there are some differences in the pallial and the mesencephalic tegmental area.

A series of studies have explored the location and hormonal and social regulation of the mRNAs encoding the estrogen receptor-α (ERα), androgen receptor (AR), and progesterone receptor (PR) in whiptail lizards. These studies have elucidated the brain regions where each of these receptor mRNAs is expressed, variation in receptor mRNA abundances over the course of the ovarian cycle, species differences in expression levels and behavioral correlates of this expression, sex and species differences in the hormonal regulation of this expression, developmental influences on the sexual differentiation of hormonal responsiveness in receptor mRNA expression, and documented social influences on ER and PR mRNA abundance in the hypothalamic nuclei.

The mapping of the distribution of steroid receptor mRNA expression has relied on cloning portions of genes coding for sex steroid hormone receptors using reverse transcription–polymerase chain reactions (Young et al., 1994). The resulting clones were used to generate riboprobes for use in *in situ* hybridization. The partial ER clone generated is homologous to ERα, although an isoform of the ER lacking exon 4 has been identified in whiptail lizards; a homolog of this ER isoform has also been found in rats (Skipper et al., 1993). In general, *in situ* hybridization studies have documented the expression of ERs and ARs in the same regions as previous work using tritiated label to identify neurons concentrating sex steroid hormones, although some additional regions not found using steroid autoradiography have been described (see later).

Strong ER mRNA expression is found in the periventricular and medial POA, AH, periventricular nuclei of the hypothalamus, septal nuclei, the optic tectum, and the dorso-, postero-, and ventromedial hypothalamus

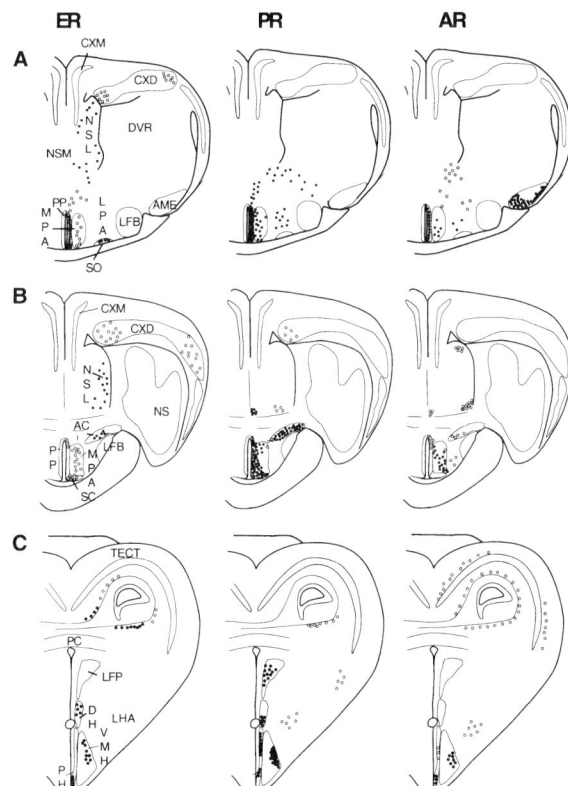

FIGURE 21 Distribution of cells expressing steroid receptor mRNA in selected sections of the brain of whiptail lizards. Shown are the positions of cells expressing mRNA for estrogen receptor (ER column), progesterone receptor (PR column), and androgen receptor (AR column) in the right half of brain sections. Solid circles indicate heavily labeled cells and open circles indicate lightly labeled cells. AC, anterior commissure; AME, nucleus externus amygdalae; CXD, cortex dorsalis; CXM, cortex medialis; DH, nucleus dorsalis hypothalami; DVR, dorsoventricular ridge; LFB, lateral forebrain bundle; LHA, lateral hypothalamic area; LPA, lateral preoptic area; LTP, lentiformis thalami pars plicta; MPA, medial preoptic area; NS, nucleus sphericus; NSL, nucleus septalis lateralis; NSM, nucleus septalis medialis; PC, posterior commissure; PH, nucleus periventricularis hypothalami; PP, nucleus periventricularis preopticus; SC, nucleus suprachiasmaticus; SO, nucleus supraopticus; TECT, optic tectum; VMH, nucleus ventromedialis hypothalami. Redrawn from Young et al., *J. Comp. Neurol.* **347**, 288–300, copyright © 1994, Wiley-Liss, Inc., a subsidiary of John Wiley & Sons, Inc.

(Fig. 21). Weaker labeling is found in the dorsal cortex, near the nucleus accumbens, the lateral and medial septal areas, and the supraoptic nucleus. Previous work with green anole lizards suggested little difference in androgen- and estrogen-concentrating neurons in the brain (Morrell *et al.*, 1979). However, this previous study used tritiated E_2 and T, respectively, and it is possible that some of the T label was aromatized to E_2 (see Wade, 1997) and then bound to the ER. This is discussed at greater length later.

PR mRNA expression is also widely distributed through the brain of whiptail lizards. An especially strong expression is seen in the VMH and both the periventricular and medial POA. Strong labeling is also found in the medial septum, lateral POA, central amygdala, AH, the postero-, dorso- and ventromedial hypothalamus, the lentiformis thalamis pars plicta, and the torus semicircularis. Lower levels of PR mRNA are evident in the lateral hypothalamic area, near the premammilary nucleus, and in parts of the optic tectum.

In both the whiptail lizard and the leopard gecko, AR mRNA expression occurs in the dorsoventricular ridge, external nucleus of the amygdala, medial POA, AH, lateral septum, dorsolateral anterior nucleus, VMH, periventricular nuclei of the hypothalamus, and especially the premammilary nucleus (Young *et al.*, 1994; Rhen and Crews, 2000). This distribution reveals differences from previously documented distributions in the brains of green anole lizards and garter snakes based on steroid autoradiography. Specifically, AR mRNA is more abundant than ER mRNA in the lateral septum, and ER mRNA does not occur in the external amygdala of whiptail lizards. Of particular interest from a comparative perspective is the expression of AR mRNA in the dorsoventricular ridge (DVR) of the lizard. The DVR appears homologous to the AR expressing magnocellular nucleus of the anterior neostriatum (MAN) in songbirds (Balthazart *et al.*, 1992). There are also some strong similarities between the patterns of AR expression in whiptail lizards and those in mammals.

Mapping AR gene expression by using *in situ* hybridization has also been employed in green anole lizards to examine the distribution of AR mRNA expression (Rosen *et al.*, 2000). These workers found AR mRNA in many of the same areas that express this message in the brain of whiptail lizards, with some differences. The regions of similarity include the POA, septum, amygdala, striatum, premammilary nucleus, VMH, torus semicircularis and brain-stem motor nuclei. In contrast to the patterns observed in whiptail lizards, AR mRNA expression was not localized to the DVR of green anole lizards in this study.

Moga and coworkers (2000) used an antibody directed at a conserved sequence in the N-terminal domain of the AR protein (residues 1–21 of the rat AR) to map AR immunoreactivity (AR-ir) in the fence lizard, *S. undulatus*. This method allows them to distinguish between staining in the nucleus and cytoplasm and also reveals AR-ir in axons and dendrites with a high anatomical specificity. AR-ir in the brain of *S. undulatus* showed good, but not complete, agreement with the distribution of AR determined in other species and by other methods previously described. AR staining was found in males in the medial and dorsal cortices, medial septum, and several cell groups in the amygdala as well as the adjacent bed nucleus of the stria terminalis. These investigators also found nuclear staining in the medial POA, periventricular hypothalamus, and ventromedial, premammillary, and arcuate nuclei. AR-ir fiber staining occurred throughout the AH and POA and in a variety of other diencephalic areas. Females showed nuclear AR-ir in fewer areas than males, with nuclear staining only in the ventroposterior amygdala and VMH (the ventroposterior amygdala appears homologous to the external amygdala of whiptail lizards based on anatomy and AR expression; Moga *et al.*, 2000). Fiber staining in male and female fence lizards was broadly similar. The sex difference in distribution found here for *S. undulatus* could represent a species difference or a difference in the sensitivity of the immunocytochemical method employed relative to the *in situ* hybridization approach used in other studies. Male whiptail lizards do show higher levels of AR mRNA in the medial POA (MPOA) than females (Godwin *et al.*, 2000). The results reported for fence lizards could be very similar if females do express AR mRNA in the MPOA, but they express AR protein at levels too low to be detected by immunocytochemistry. A difference in the sensitivity of the technique could also account for the lack of AR-ir observed in the dorsolateral thalamic nucleus and anterodorsal ventricular ridge, a result that also contrasts with the described distribution of AR mRNA in whiptail lizards (Young *et al.*, 1994).

As in other groups of vertebrates, reptiles show what Pfaff and coauthors termed a lawfulness of steroid receptor distribution in the brain (Pfaff *et al.*, 1994). Indeed, this conservation in distribution provides evidence of neural homologies, as with the expression of AR in the lizard DVR and the avian MAN. Sex steroid receptors are widely distributed in areas of the brain that play critical integrative roles in sociosexual behavior, including the POAH and VMH. The identification of sites outside these areas expressing steroid receptors has been facilitated by the development of *in situ* hybridization techniques and antibodies directed at conserved regions of the receptor proteins. In contrast to what is known about mammals and fishes (Kuiper *et al.*, 1996; Hawkins *et al.*, 2000), there is no information available on different forms of the sex steroid receptors in reptiles. The *in situ* hybridization data presented for ER in lizard brain are for ERα (Young *et al.*, 1994). It is also not known whether the alternatively spliced form of the ER, Δ-4, identified in turtles, lizards, and rats shows a distribution in the brain that differs from the full-length form (Skipper *et al.*, 1993). *In situ* hybridization has proven very useful for determining sites of steroid receptor synthesis, but immunocytochemical work further exploring regions of steroid responsiveness has been limited due to the lack of immunoreactivity of most antibodies available (M. Gahr and D. Crews, unpublished). Studies in this area and immunocytochemical work exploring colocalization of different receptor types in cells will be particularly useful.

B. Regulation

The ability to localize and compare relative levels of abundance of the three main gonadal steroid hormone receptors in whiptail lizards has allowed a variety of questions related to sex and species differences in their regulation to be addressed. A key species difference in whiptail lizards is unisexuality and the display of male-like pseudocopulatory behavior by the parthenogenetic *C. uniparens*, but not by females of its sexual ancestor *C. inornatus* (Crews and Fitzgerald, 1980).

E_2 increases ER mRNA abundance in discrete brain regions in the whiptail lizards. Young and coworkers documented this using a 0.5-μg injection of estradiol benzoate (EB) and measuring ER mRNA abundance 24 hours after administration. The EB effectively stimulates female-typical receptive behavior in parthenogenetic whiptail lizards (Young *et al.*, 1995a), and it increases ER mRNA in some regions (torus semicircularis and VMH), decreases it in others (lateral septum), and causes no change in still other nuclei (periventricular nuclei of the hypothalamus, periventricular nucleus of the POA, and the dorsal hypothalamus). The increase seen in ER mRNA in the VMH is particularly interesting for three reasons. First, as previously mentioned, this nucleus critically regulates female-typical sexual behavior in both the sexual and unisexual parthenogenetic whiptail lizards. Second, the pattern of increased ER mRNA in the mediobasal hypothalamus is opposite that seen in rats, in which estrogen down-regulates its receptor. This difference between whiptail lizards and rats may relate to differences in the nature of their ovarian cycles. Whiptail lizards have elevated E_2 levels for a relatively long period prior to ovulation and display receptive behavior for the duration of this period, whereas female rats are receptive for only a short window following ovulation. Young and Crews (1995) suggest that prolongation of the time span E_2 levels are elevated and of sexual receptivity may be quite common in mammals (e.g., cats and rabbits). Last, species comparisons indicate that parthenogenetic whiptails have higher concentrations of ER mRNA expression in the POA than do sexually reproducing female whiptails (Young *et al.*, 1995b). This observation led in turn to the sensitivity compensation hypothesis (Fig. 22), which proposes that an inverse relationship exists between the expression of the genes coding for sex steroid hormone receptors in the POA and circulating concentrations of sex steroid hormone. The increased level of ER gene expression in the POA results in a greater sensitivity to the circulating concentrations of E_2 that, in turn, results in lower levels of circulating E_2 through feedback effects.

E_2 also stimulates increases in PR mRNA abundance in lizard brains, but again typically in a manner specific to species, sex, and region. Female green anoles show increases in progestin binding sites with estrogen treatment (Tokarz *et al.*, 1981) as well as induction of sexual receptivity (Tokarz and Crews, 1980). EB treatment strongly induces PR mRNA in the VMH of whiptail lizard females. The degree of this induction is tightly correlated with the display of female-typical receptive behavior in *C. inornatus* and female-like pseudosexual behavior in the parthenogenetic *C. uniparens* (Fig. 23) (Young *et al.*, 1995b), with EB being more effective in the parthenogenetic *C. uniparens*. EB also effectively stimulates increases in PR mRNA in the POA of female *Cnemidophorus* again with similar dosages being more effective in the parthenogen *C. uniparens* than

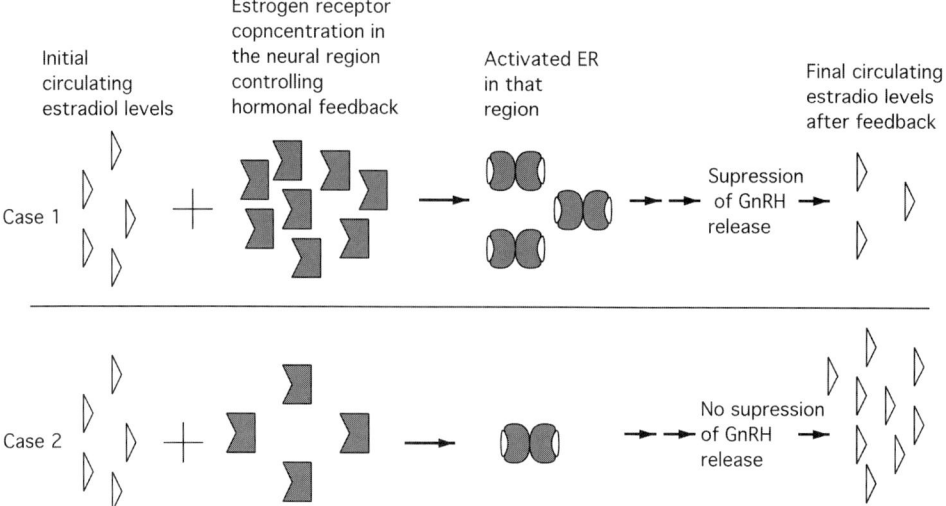

FIGURE 22 Schematic illustrating the sensitivity compensation model for species differences in the circulating concentrations of sex steroid hormones. Two cases (species) are illustrated that differ in the abundance of estrogen receptor (ER) in the neurons involved in the negative feedback loop. Under the initial conditions illustrated, both systems are presented with identical hormone concentrations. However, due to differences in the number of receptor molecules, the neurons in case 1 have more activated estrogen receptors, which results in an inhibition of gonadotropin-releasing-hormone (GnRH) release and ultimately a lower circulating concentration of hormone. In case 2, less activated receptors are formed, GnRH release is not inhibited significantly, and hormone levels remain the same or rise.

in females of the sexual ancestor *C. inornatus* (Godwin and Crews, 1999). This greater estrogen stimulation of PR mRNA in the brain region mediating male-like pseudosexual behavior in *C. uniparens* may be related to the display of male-like pseudosexual behavior by *C. uniparens*, but not by *C. inornatus* females.

Although E_2 increases PR mRNA in both the VMH and POA of female and parthenogenetic whiptail lizards, exogenous P inhibits both female-typical receptive behavior and decreases estrogen-stimulated ER and PR mRNA in the VMH (Godwin et al., 1996). This effect of P on both receptivity and on ER and PR mRNA abundance is similar to patterns in well-studied rodent models (Blaustein and Turcotte, 1990; Blaustein et al., 1994; Brown and Maclusky, 1994). In contrast, exogenous P has no effect on PR mRNA abundance in the periventricular POA in this experiment.

Neither the effective induction of female-typical receptive behavior nor increases in ER and PR mRNA in the VMH seen in female and parthenogenetic whiptail lizards occur in short-term castrate males (1 week) (Godwin and Crews, 1995). This lack of responsiveness to estrogen in the VMH of male whiptail lizards parallels patterns in rats (Lauber et al., 1991a,b). In contrast, male *C. inornatus* castrated for longer periods (6 weeks) showed PR mRNA responses to estrogen that were not different from females (Wennstrom and Crews, 1998). Females implanted with T, however, did not show an attenuation of the female pattern of responsiveness. These results indicate that the maintenance of the male-typical pattern of nonresponsiveness requires the activational effects of T, whereas the female-typical pattern is less plastic.

The abundance of PR mRNA is also correlated to the display of male-typical sexual behavior in male *C. inornatus* (Crews et al., 1996b). Male *C. inornatus* can be classified as either P-sensitive or P-insensitive based on the effectiveness of exogenous P delivered in Silastic capsules implanted intraperitoneally in reinstating sexual behavior following castration (Lindzey and Crews, 1992). Males classified as P-sensitive are also significantly more likely to respond to intracranial implants of P (directed at the POA) than are P-insensitive males (Crews et al., 1996b). Interestingly, there are also

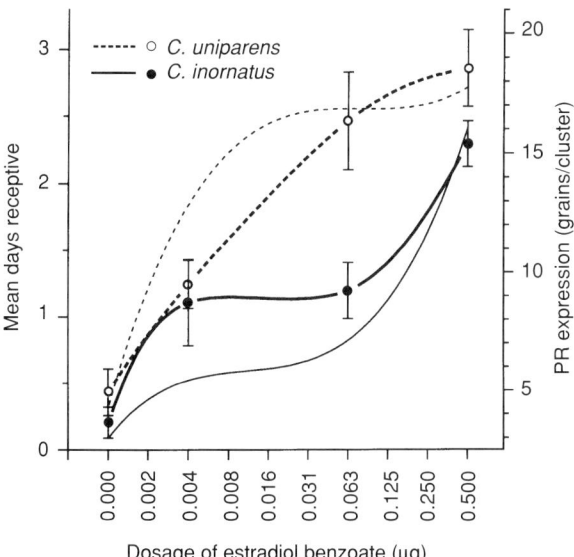

FIGURE 23 Species differences in the induction of sexual receptivity (thin lines) and progesterone receptor mRNA expression (bold lines) by estradiol benzoate (EB) in ovariectomized whiptail lizards. Ovariectomized animals were given a single injection of EB and either were tested daily for receptivity for 4 days following the injection or had their brains removed 24 hours after treatment and analyzed using *in situ* hybridization. Vertical error bars represent standard errors of the mean.

differences in both PR and AR mRNA abundance between the two groups following intracranial implantation of P. Progesterone-sensitive males display lower abundances of PR mRNA in both the medial and periventricular portions of the POA, but higher abundances of AR mRNA in the medial POA, external amygdala, and lateral septum. No differences are seen between P-sensitive and P-insensitive males without an intracranial implant.

Sex and species differences are also found in the androgenic regulation of ER, PR, and AR mRNA. The implantation of gonadectomized male and female *C. inornatus* and parthenogen female *C. uniparens* with either T or DHT reveals a diversity of effects, suggesting that gonadal sex, aromatization, and gene dosage (ploidy) all influence steroid receptor mRNA response (Godwin *et al.*, 2000; see also Young *et al.*, 1995a, for PR mRNA). For example, males have higher AR mRNA in the MPOA than females of either species and these levels decrease with T treatment in males, but not in females. In contrast, ER and PR mRNA levels in the VMH are higher with androgen treatment, but these effects do not differ by sex. There also are species effects in that the triploid parthenogen shows higher steroid receptor mRNA abundances overall than the diploid sexual females. Finally, aromatization of T to estrogen is probably important in some regions. PR mRNA in the periventricular POA is increased in both males and females by T, but not by nonaromatizable DHT.

Last, individual experiences might influence gene expression in the brain directly rather than via the modulation of the endocrine physiology of the partner. For example, in the hamster and the rat, exposure to the sexual behavior of the opposite sex induces expression of the immediate to early gene c-*fos* in those brain regions that mediate sexual behavior (see Chapters 1, 2, and 15). Using ovariectomized, hormone-primed, parthenogenetic whiptail lizards, Hartman and Crews (1996) demonstrated that participating either as a male or as a female during a pseudosexual encounter significantly alters the abundance of ER and PR mRNA in the hypothalamus of whiptail lizards.

In contrast to the conservation of steroid receptor distribution in the brain in reptiles and other vertebrates, the patterns of steroid receptor regulation vary greatly. Studies in lizards show that steroid receptors in the brain are regulated by both their own ligands and other steroid hormones. This regulation shows variation across brain nuclei, both within and between the sexes, between closely related species, and with social interactions. Some of the patterns found are strikingly similar to those seen in well-studied rodent models, but there are also differences that appear to be related to differences in the nature of the reproductive cycles. It is important to note that most of the studies examining steroid receptor regulation have either shown behavioral effects or used behaviorally relevant dosages of hormone, supporting a role for this regulation in behavioral display. Remaining challenges in this area include determining the degree of colocalization of receptor types in neurons and cross talk between signalling systems, exploring the influences of other mediators (e.g., corticosteroids, thyroid hormones, and neurotransmitters) on receptor regulation, and characterizing the downstream effects of steroid receptor activation.

VII. CONCLUSION AND FUTURE DIRECTIONS

Reptiles enable the study of the neuroendocrine mechanisms underlying sociosexual behaviors in ways not possible with conventional animal model systems. This work has had two important impacts on our understanding of sociosexual behavior. First, it has revealed the great diversity that exists among vertebrates in reproductive behaviors and the neuroendocrine mechanisms underlying these behaviors. For example, the study of species with dissociated reproductive tactics and unisexual species has suggested three factors that may explain species differences in endocrine physiology and behavior: (1) sensitivity to sex steroid hormones, (2) hormone-dependent regulation of sex-steroid-hormone-receptor gene expression, and (3) neuroanatomical distribution of steroid receptor gene expression, especially in nonlimbic structures.

The second major impact arises from explorations of this diversity within and across major taxa. These explorations allow us to begin defining which mechanisms show strong conservation and which are evolutionarily more labile. Reptiles and mammals diverged approximately 300 million years ago, yet research in reptiles has revealed the apparent conservation of many behavior-controlling mechanisms between these groups. For example, research in reptiles has led us to reexamine certain assumptions in behavioral neuroendocrinology—for example, that progesterone is a female-specific hormone with no function in males. Experiments with four lizard species demonstrated that progesterone is vital to the display of male copulatory behavior in lizards and, further, that androgen and progesterone synergize in males much like estrogen and progesterone synergize in females to facilitate sexual receptivity; subsequent studies with mice and rats have revealed similar roles for progesterone and its receptor in male sexual behavior in male mammals. Continuing to identify those mechanisms that are fundamentally important in all vertebrates and those that represent axes along which evolutionary change may take place will lead to a more complete understanding of the diversity we see and how this diversity arose.

Research in reptiles has also contributed and continues to contribute to our understanding of animal sexuality and the nature of individual variation. For example, the study of animals that lack sex-linked sex-determining genes has reinforced the conclusion that the same genes are involved in the development of testes (in males) and ovaries (in females) and are contained in each individual. That is, the species may differ in their patterns of regulation, but the genes associated with sex determination are conserved. What differs is the trigger; in some it is sex chromosomes at fertilization, in others it is environmental factors during embryogenesis, and in still others it is the social context in which the adult might find itself. This understanding is changing the classic paradigm idea of an organized and a default sex; rather, we now regard both sexes as organized and pose the question, Why does the activation of one cascade (e.g., the ovary-determining cascade) actively suppress the complementary sex-determining cascade? This in turn has led to a new paradigm to take the place of the organized–default paradigm, namely that the female is the ancestral sex and the male the derived sex. A logical extension of this paradigm is the question, Why might males be more like females (rather than females being like males)?

The mechanisms that generate individual variation are an important focus across modern biology. Understanding these mechanisms is of fundamental importance for addressing basic issues, such as how evolutionary change takes place, and applied problems in human health. Research in reptile behavioral neuroendocrinology has contributed to our understanding of behavioral variation, particularly as it relates to sexually dimorphic behaviors. For example, it has been proposed that some behavioral sex differences in mammals may be mediated directly by expression of *Sry* in the brain (see Chapter 63). Evidence of direct genetic influences on the organization of behavior was first proposed in studies of nonmammalian vertebrates that completely lack sex chromosomes—the neural organization underlying sex-typical behaviors may depend on behavioral or physical stimuli in the environment (Crews, 1994). Sex-changing fish typify the first, the social environment effectively switching the brain and behavior, and ultimately the gonad, from one sex to the other (Godwin *et al.*, 2000). Dependence on the second stimulus is characteristic of reptiles that exhibit TSD in with the temperature of the incubating egg in the mid-trimester of embryonic development determining gonadal sex. Another example of this idea comes from studies of parthenogenetic, or all-female, whiptail lizards. These unique animals arose from the hybridization of sexually reproducing species and sex chromosomes appear to exist in the ancestral sexual species with male heterogamety (XY). The expected sexual dimorphisms are present in morphology, physiology, brain anatomy, and behavior, all of which are under testicular hormone control. In the descendant unisexual species, however, no males exist and all individuals have a female phenotype. Remarkably, these parthenogens reliably and regularly exhibit both male-like and female-like pseudosexual behaviors during the course of their reproductive cycle. Although males do not exist, the gene(s) for male development have not been lost but, instead, appear to be repressed. Although the genetic trigger for male development (Y) is absent, the male-determining cascade can be activated by treating embryos with aromatase inhibitor, thereby producing fully functional males. Such animals exhibit only male-like copulatory behavior and are insensitive to exogenous estrogen. However, their brain anatomy remains similar to that of normal parthenogens who, despite the bisexual nature of their behavior, have strictly female-like brain morphology. Thus, the expression of Y chromosome gene products in whiptail lizards not only influences brain anatomy, but suppresses the display of female-like behavior and sensitivity to exogenous estrogen.

Many challenges remain in the study of hormones, brain, and behavior in reptiles. Nearly all the information available regarding the hormonal and neural bases of behavior in reptiles comes from studies of lizards and snakes. Although this gives insight into these mechanisms in the most speciose group of reptiles, little is known about hormone–brain–behavior relationships in the other major lineages of reptiles, the turtles and crocodilians. Modern birds represent the most derived forms in the archosauromorph lineage, with crocodilians being the most primitive and the extinct dinosaurs falling in between. Our understanding of behavioral mechanisms in birds would benefit from a more thorough understanding of these mechanisms in the primitive members of the lineage, the crocodilians.

The lack of correspondence between structure of the nervous system and behavioral phenotype highlights the need for more comparisons of a functional nature. Insights from measurements of neural metabolic activity and capacity, neurotransmitter metabolism and influences, and the regulation and actions of steroid hormone receptors all show the value of these approaches.

The diversity of patterns in sex determination and differentiation seen in reptiles has provided important evidence that factors other than gonadal steroid hormones can have critical influences on the differentiation of the neural substrates of behavior. Elucidating these influences and the interplay of factors such as temperature and social interactions with gonadal steroids in shaping the function of the adult nervous system is an important research direction.

References

Abell, A. J. (1998). The effect of exogenous testosterone on growth and secondary sexual character development in juveniles of *Sceloporus virgatus*. *Herpetologica* **54**(4), 533–543.

Allen, E. E., and Crews, D. (1992). Sexual-behavior and 2-deoxyglucose uptake in male red-sided garter snakes (*Thamnophis sirtalis parietalis*). *Brain, Behav. Evol.* **40**(1), 17–24.

Allen, L. R., and Hume, I. D. (1997). The importance of green seed in the nitrogen nutrition of the zebra finch *Taeniopygia guttata*. *Aust. J. Ecol.* **22**(4), 412–418.

Andrews, J. E., Smith, C. A., and Sinclair, A. H. (1997). Sites of estrogen receptor and aromatase expression in the chicken embryo. *Gen. Comp. Endocrinol.* **108**, 182–190.

Andrews, T. J., and Summers, C. H. (1996). Aggression, and the acquisition and function of social dominance in female *Anolis carolinensis*. *Behaviour* **133**, 1265–1279.

Arango, N. A., Lovell-Badge, R., and Behringer, R. R. (1999). Targeted mutagenesis of the endogenous mouse mis gene promoter: In vivo definition of genetic pathways of vertebrate sexual development. *Cell (Cambridge, Mass.)* **99**(4), 409–419.

Balthazart, J., Foidart, A., Wilson, E. M., and Ball, G. F. (1992). Immunocytochemical localization of androgen receptors in the male songbird and quail brain. *J. Comp. Neurol.* **317**(4), 407–420.

Bass, A. H., and Baker, R. (1990). Sexual dimorphisms in the vocal control-system of a teleost fish—morphology of physiologically identified neurons. *J. Neurobiol.* **21**(8), 1155–1168.

Bennis, M., Tramu, A. M., and Reperant, J. (1995). Vasopressin-like and oxytocin-like systems in the chameleon brain. *J. Brain Res.* **36**(4), 445–450.

Bergeron, J. M., Gahr, M., Horan, K., Wibbels, T., and Crews, D. (1998). Cloning and in situ hybridization analysis of estrogen receptor in the developing gonad of the red-eared slider turtle, a species with temperature-dependent sex determination. *Dev. Growth Differ.* **40**(2), 243–254.

Blackburn, D. G. (1999). Are viviparity and egg-guarding evolutionarily labile in squamates? *Herpetologica* **55**(4), 556–573.

Blaustein, J. D., and Turcotte, J. C. (1990). Down-regulation of progestin receptors in guinea-pig brain—new findings using an immunocytochemical technique. *J. Neurobiol.* **21**(5), 675–685.

Blaustein, J. D., Tetel, M. J., Ricciardi, K. H. N., Delville, Y., and Turcotte, J. C. (1994). Hypothalamic ovarian-steroid hormone-sensitive neurons involved in female sexual-behavior. *Psychoneuroendocrinology* **19**(5–7), 505–516.

Brown, T. J., and Maclusky, N. J. (1994). Progesterone modulation of estrogen-receptors in microdissected regions of the rat hypothalamus. *Mol. Cell. Neurosci.* **5**(3), 283–290.

Cada, A., Gonzalez-Lima, F., Rose, G. M., and Bennett, M. C. (1995). Regional brain effects of sodium azide treatment on cytochrome oxidase activity: A quantitative histochemical study. *Metab. Brain Dis.* **10**, 303–320.

Callard, I. P., Lance, V., Salhanick, A. R., and Barad, D. (1978). Annual ovarian cycle of *Chrysemys picta*-correlated changes in plasma steroids and parameters of vitellogenesis. *Gen. Comp. Endocrinol.* **35**(3), 245–257.

Carlone, D. L., and Richards, J. S. (1997). Functional interactions, phosphorylation, and levels of 3′,5′-cyclic adenosine monophosphate-regulatory element binding protein and steroidogenic factor-1 mediate hormone-regulated and constitutive expression of aromatase in gonadal cells. *Mol. Endocrinol.* **11**, 292–304.

Clark, M. M., and Galef, B. G. (1995). Prenatal influences on reproductive life-history strategies. *Trends Ecol. Evol.* **10**(4), 151–153.

Compton, A. W. (1981). Courtship and nesting-behavior of the freshwater crocodile, *Crocodylus johnstoni,* under controlled conditions. *Aust. Wildl. Res.* **8**(2), 443–450.

Coomber, P., Crews, D., and Gonzalez-Lima, F. (1997). Independent effects of incubation temperature and gonadal sex on the volume and metabolic capacity of brain nuclei in the leopard gecko *(Eublepharis macularius),* a lizard with temperature-dependent sex determination. *J. Comp. Neurol.* **380**(3), 409–421.

Cree, A., Cockrem, J. F., and Guillette, L. J. (1992). Reproductive-cycles of male and female tuatara *(Sphenodon punctatus)* on Stephens Island, New Zealand. *J. Zool.* **226**, 199–217.

Crews, D. (1975a). Effects of different components of male courtship behaviour on environmentally induced ovarian recrudescence and mating preferences in the lizard, *Anolis carolinensis. Anim. Behav.* **23**, 349–356.

Crews, D. (1975b). Inter- and intraindividual variation in display patterns in the lizard, *Anolis carolinensis. Herpetologica* **31**, 37–47.

Crews, D. (1983). Control of male sexual behavior in the Canadian red-sided garter snake. In "Hormones and Behavior in Higher Vertebrates" (J. Balthazart, E. Pröve, and R. Gilles, eds.), pp. 398–406. Plenum Press, London.

Crews, D. (1987). Diversity and evolution of behavioral controlling mechanisms. In "The Psychobiology of Reproductive Behavior: An Evolutionary Perspective" (D. Crews, ed.), pp. 88–119. Prentice-Hall, Englewood Cliffs, NJ.

Crews, D. (1991). Trans-seasonal action of androgen in the control of spring courtship behavior in male red-sided garter snakes. *Proc. Natl. Acad. Sci. U.S.A.* **88**(9), 3545–3548.

Crews, D. (1993). The organizational concept and vertebrates without sex-chromosomes. *Brain, Behav. Evol.* **42**(4–5), 202–214.

Crews, D. (1994). Temperature, steroids, and sex determination. *J. Endocrinol.* **142**, 1–8.

Crews, D. (1996a). Temperature-dependent sex determination: The interplay of steroid hormones and temperature. *Zool. Sci.* **13**, 1–13.

Crews, D. (1996b). Species diversity and the evolution of behavioral controlling mechanisms. In "The Integrative Neurobiology of Affiliation" (C. S. Carter, I. Izja Lederhendler, and B. Kirkpatrick, eds.), pp. 1–21. N. Y. Acad. Sci., New York.

Crews, D. (1998a). The evolutionary antecedents of love. *Psychoneuroendocrinology* **23**, 751–764.

Crews, D. (1998b). On the organization of individual differences in sexual behavior. *Am. Zool.* **38**(1), 118–132.

Crews, D. (1999). Sexuality: The environmental organization of phenotypic plasticity. In "Reproduction in Context" (K. Wallen and J. Schneider, eds.), pp. 473–499. MIT Press, Cambridge, MA.

Crews, D., and Bergeron, J. M. (1994). Role of reductase and aromatase in sex determination in the red-eared slider *(Trachemys scripta),* a turtle with temperature-dependent sex determination. *J. Endocrinol.* **143**(2), 279–289.

Crews, D., and Fitzgerald, K. T. (1980). Sexual-behavior in parthenogenetic lizards *(Cnemidophorus). Proc. Natl. Acad. Sci. U.S.A.* **77**(1), 499–502.

Crews, D., and Gans, C. (1992). The interaction of hormones, brain, and behavior: An emerging discipline in herpetology. In "Biology of the Reptilia" (C. Gans and D. Crews, eds.), Vol. 18, pp. 1–23. University of Chicago Press, Chicago.

Crews, D., and Morgentaler, A. (1979). Effects of intracranial implantation of estradiol and dihydrotestosterone on the sexual-behavior of the lizard *Anolis carolinensis. J. Endocrinol.* **82**(3), 373–381.

Crews, D., Traina, V., Wetzel, F. T., and Muller, C. (1978). Hormonal-control of male reproductive-behavior in lizard, *Anolis carolinensis*—role of testosterone, dihydrotestosterone, and estradiol. *Endocrinology (Baltimore)* **103**(5), 1814–1821.

Crews, D., Camazine, B., Diamond, M., Mason, R., Tokarz, R. R., Garstka, W. R. (1984). Hormonal independence of courtship behavior in the male garter snake. *Horm. Behav.* **18**, 29–41.

Crews, D., Grassman, M., and Lindzey, J. (1986). Behavioral facilitation of reproduction in sexual and unisexual whiptail lizards. *Proc. Natl. Acad. Sci. U.S.A.* **83**, 9547–9550.

Crews, D., Wade, J., and Wilczynski, W. (1990). Sexually dimorphic areas in the brain of whiptail lizards. *Brain, Behav. Evol.* **36**, 262–270.

Crews, D., Bull, J. J., and Wibbels, T. (1991). Estrogen and sex reversal in turtles—a dose-dependent phenomenon. *Gen. Comp. Endocrinol.* **81**(3), 357–364.

Crews, D., Robker, R., and Mendonca, M. (1993). Seasonal fluctuations in brain nuclei in the red-sided garter snake and their hormonal control. *J. Neurosci.* **13**(12), 5356–5364.

Crews, D., Bergeron, J. M., Bull, J. J., Flores, D., Tousignant, A., Skipper, J. K., and Wibbels, T. (1994). Temperature-dependent sex determination in reptiles—proximate mechanisms, ultimate outcomes, and practical applications. *Dev. Genet.* **15**(3), 297–312.

Crews, D., Cantu, A. R., and Bergeron, J. M. (1996a). Temperature and non-aromatizable androgens: A common pathway in male sex determination in a turtle with temperature-dependent sex determination? *J. Endocrinol.* **149**(3), 457–463.

Crews, D., Godwin, J., Hartman, V., Grammer, M., Prediger, E. A., and Sheppherd, R. (1996b). Intrahypothalamic implantation of progesterone in castrated male whiptail lizards (*Cnemidophorus inornatus*) elicits courtship and copulatory behavior and affects androgen receptor- and progesterone receptor-mRNA expression in the brain. *J. Neurosci.* **16**(22), 7347–7352.

Crews, D., Coomber, P., and Gonzalez-Lima, F. (1997). Effects of age and sociosexual experience on the morphology and metabolic capacity of brain nuclei in the leopard gecko (*Eublepharis macularius*), a lizard with temperature-dependent sex determination. *Brain Res.* **758**(1–2), 169–179.

Crews, D., Sakata, J., and Rhen, T. (1998). Developmental effects on intersexual and intrasexual variation in growth and reproduction in a lizard with temperature-dependent sex determination. *Comp. Biochem. Physiol. C* **119**, 229–241.

Denardo, D. F., and Licht, P. (1993). Effects of corticosterone on social-behavior of male lizards. *Horm. Behav.* **27**(2), 184–199.

Denardo, D. F., and Sinervo, B. (1994a). Effects of corticosterone on activity and home-range size of free-ranging male lizards. *Horm. Behav.* **28**(1), 53–65.

Denardo, D. F., and Sinervo, B. (1994b). Effects of steroid-hormone interaction on activity and home-range size of male lizards. *Horm. Behav.* **28**(3), 273–287.

Densmore, L. D., Moritz, C., Wright, J. W., and Brown, W. M. (1989). Mitochondrial-DNA analysis and the origin and relative age of parthenogenetic lizards (Genus *Cnemidophorus*). IV. Nine *sexlineatus*-group unisexuals. *Evolution (Lawrence, Kans.)* **43**, 969–983.

Desvages, G., and Pieau, C. (1992). Aromatase-activity in gonads of turtle embryos as a function of the incubation-temperature of eggs. *J. Steroid Biochem. Mol. Biol.* **41**(3–8), 851–853.

Devoogd, T. J., and Nottebohm, F. (1981). Sex-differences in dendritic morphology of a song control nucleus in the canary—a quantitative golgi-study. *J. Comp. Neurol.* **196**(2), 309–316.

DiClemente, N., Ghaffari, S., Pepinsky, R. B., Pieau, C., Josso, N., Cate, R. L., and Vigier, B. (1992). A quantitative and interspecific test for biological-activity of anti-mullerian hormone—the fetal ovary aromatase assay. *Development (Cambridge, UK)* **114**(3), 721–727.

Fleming, A., and Crews, D. (2000). Estradiol and incubation temperature modulate regulation of steroidogenic factor 1 in the developing gonad of the red-eared slider turtle. *Endocrinology (Baltimore)* **142**, 1403–1411.

Fleming, A., Wibbels, T., Skipper, J. K., and Crews, D. (1999). Developmental expression of steroidogenic factor 1 in a turtle with temperature-dependent sex determination. *Gen. Comp. Endocrinol.* **116**(3), 336–346.

Flores, D. L., and Crews, D. (1995). Effect of hormonal manipulation on sociosexual behavior in adult female leopard geckos (*Eublepharis macularius*), a species with temperature-dependent sex determination. *Horm. Behav.* **29**, 458–473.

Flores, D. L., Tousignant, A., and Crews, D. (1994). Incubation temperature affects the behavior of adult leopard geckos (*Eublepharis macularius*). *Physiol. Behav.* **55**, 1067–1072.

Godwin, J., and Crews, D. (1995). Sex-differences in estrogen and progesterone-receptor messenger-ribonucleic-acid regulation in the brain of little striped whiptail lizards. *Neuroendocrinology* **62**(3), 293–300.

Godwin, J., and Crews, D. (1999). Hormonal regulation of progesterone receptor mRNA expression in the hypothalamus of whiptail lizards: Regional and species differences. *J. Neurobiol.* **39**(2), 287–293.

Godwin, J., Hartman, V., Grammer, M., and Crews, D. (1996). Progesterone inhibits female-typical receptive behavior and decreases hypothalamic estrogen and progesterone receptor messenger ribonucleic acid levels in whiptail lizards (genus *Cnemidophorus*). *Horm. Behav.* **30**(2), 138–144.

Godwin, J., Hartman, V., Nag, P., and Crews, D. (2000). Androgenic regulation of steroid hormone receptor mRNAs in the brain of whiptail lizards. *J. Neuroendocrinol.* **12**(7), 599–606.

Greenberg, N., and Crews, D. (1990). Endocrine and behavioral-responses to aggression and social dominance in the green anole lizard, *Anolis carolinensis*. *Gen. Comp. Endocrinol.* **77**(2), 246–255.

Greenberg, N., MacLean, P. D., and Ferguson, J. L. (1979). Role of the paleostriatum in species-typical display behavior of the lizard *(Anolis carolinensis)*. *Brain Res.* **172**, 229–241.

Greenberg, N., Scott, M., and Crews, D. (1984). Role of the amygdala in the reproductive and aggressive behavior of the lizard, *Anolis carolinensis*. *Physiol. Behav.* **32**(1), 147–151.

Guillette, L. J. (1991). The evolution of viviparity in amniote vertebrates—new insights, new questions. *J. Zool.* **223**, 521–526.

Guillette, L. J., Propper, C. R., Cree, A., and Dores, R. M. (1991). Endocrinology of oviposition in the tuatara *(Sphenodon punctatus)*. 2. Plasma arginine vasotocin concentrations during natural nesting. *Comp. Biochem. Physiol. A* **100**(4), 819–822.

Guillette, L. J., Woodward, A. R., Crain, D. A., Masson, G. R., Palmer, B. D., Cox, M. C., Qui, Y. X., and Orlando, E. F. (1997). The reproductive cycle of the female american alligator *(Alligator mississippiensis)*. *Gen. Comp. Endocrinol.* **108**(1), 87–101.

Gurney, M. E. (1981). Hormonal-control of cell form and number in the zebra finch song system. *J. Neurosci.* **1**(6), 658–673.

Gutzke, W. H. N., and Crews, D. (1988). Embryonic temperature determines adult sexuality in a reptile. *Nature (London)* **332**, 832–834.

Halpern, M., Morrell, J. I., and Pfaff, D. W. (1982). Cellular [H^3]-labeled estradiol and [H^3]-labeled testosterone localization in the brains of garter snakes—an autoradiographic study. *Gen. Comp. Endocrinol.* **46**(2), 211–224.

Hartman, V., and Crews, D. (1996). Sociosexual stimuli affect ER- and PR-mRNA abundance in the hypothalamus of all-female whiptail lizards. *Brain Res.* **741**(1–2), 344–347.

Hawkins, M. B., Thornton, J. W., Crews, D., Skipper, J. K., Dotte, A., and Thomas, P. (2000). Identification of a third distinct estrogen receptor and reclassification of estrogen receptors in teleosts. *Proc. Natl. Acad. Sci. U.S.A.* **97**, 10751–10756.

Hews, D. K., Knapp, R., and Moore, M. C. (1994). Early exposure to androgens affects adult expression of alternative male types in tree lizards. *Horm. Behav.* **28**(1), 96–115.

Hews, D. K., Thompson, C. W., Moore, I. T., and Moore, M. C. (1997). Population frequencies of alternative male phenotypes in tree lizards: Geographic variation and common-garden rearing studies. *Behav. Ecol. Sociobiol.* **41**(6), 371–380.

Honda, S., Harada, N., and Takagi, Y. (1994). Novel exon-1 of the aromatase gene-specific for aromatase transcripts in human brain. *Biochem. Biophys. Res. Commun.* **198**(3), 1153–1160.

Ikeda, Y., Shen, W. H., Ingraham, H. A., and Parker, K. L. (1994). Developmental expression of mouse steroidogenic factor-1, an essential regulator of the steroid hydroxylases. *Mol. Endocrinol.* **8**(5), 654–662.

Jessop, T. S., Limpus, C. J., and Whittier, J. M. (1999a). Plasma steroid interactions during high-density green turtle nesting and associated disturbance. *Gen. Comp. Endocrinol.* **115**(1), 90–100.

Jessop, T. S., FitzSimmons, N. N., Limpus, C. J., and Whittier, J. M. (1999b). Interactions between behavior and plasma steroids within the scramble mating system of the promiscuous green turtle, *Chelonia mydas*. *Horm. Behav.* **36**(2), 86–97.

Jeyasuria, P., and Place, A. R. (1997). Temperature-dependent aromatase expression in developing diamondback terrapin *(Malaclemys terrapin)* embryos. *J. Steroid Biochem. Mol. Biol.* **61**(3–6), 415–425.

Jeyasuria, P., and Place, A. R. (1998). Embryonic brain-gonadal axis in temperature-dependent sex determination of reptiles: A role for p450 aromatase (cyp19). *J. Exp. Zool.* **281**(5), 428–449.

Jones, R. E., Guillette, L. J., Summers, C. H., Tokarz, R. R., and Crews, D. (1983). The relationship among ovarian condition, steroid-hormones, and estrous behavior in *Anolis carolinensis*. *J. Exp. Zool.* **227**(1), 145–154.

Kelley, D. B., Fenstemaker, S., Hannigan, P., and Shih, S. (1988). Sex-differences in the motor nucleus of cranial nerve-IX-X in *Xenopus laevis*—a quantitative golgi-study. *J. Neurobiol.* **19**(5), 413–429.

Kendrick, A. M., Rand, M. S., and Crews, D. (1995). Electrolytic lesions to the ventromedial hypothalamus abolish receptivity in female whiptail lizards, *Cnemidophorus uniparens*. *Brain Res.* **680**(1–2), 226–228.

Kingston, P. A., and Crews, D. (1994). Effects of hypothalamic lesions on courtship and copulatory-behavior in sexual and unisexual whiptail lizards. *Brain Res.* **643**(1–2), 349–351.

Klukowski, M., Jenkinson, N. M., and Nelson, C. E. (1998). Effects of testosterone on locomotor performance and growth in field-active northern fence lizards, *Sceloporus undulatus hyacinthinus*. *Physiol. Zool.* **71**(5), 506–514.

Knapp, R., and Moore, M. C. (1995). Hormonal responses to aggression vary in different types of agonistic encounters in male tree lizards, *Urosaurus ornatus*. *Horm. Behav.* **29**(1), 85–105.

Knapp, R., and Moore, M. C. (1996). Male morphs in tree lizards, *Urosaurus ornatus*, have different delayed hormonal responses to aggressive encounters. *Anim. Behav.* **52**, 1045–1055.

Knapp, R., and Moore, M. C. (1997). Male morphs in tree lizards have different testosterone responses to elevated levels of corticosterone. *Gen. Comp. Endocrinol.* **107**(2), 273–279.

Korzan, W. J., Summers, T. R., Ronan, P. J., and Summers, C. H. (2000a). Visible sympathetic activity as a social signal in *Anolis carolinensis*: Changes in aggression and plasma catecholamines. *Horm. Behav.* **38**(3), 193–199.

Korzan, W. J., Summers, T. R., and Summers, C. H. (2000b). Monoaminergic activities of limbic regions are elevated during aggression: Influence of sympathetic social signaling. *Brain Res.* **870**(1–2), 170–178.

Krohmer, R. W. (1989). Reproductive physiology and behavior of a gynandromorph redsided garter snake, *Thamnophis sirtalis parietalis*, from central Manitoba, Canada. *Copeia*, 1064–1068.

Kuiper, G. G. J. M., Enmark, E., Pelto-Huikko, M., Nilsson, S., and Gustafsson, J.-A. (1996). Cloning of a novel estrogen receptor expressed in rat prostate and ovary. *Proc. Natl. Acad. Sci. U.S.A.* **93**, 5925–5930.

Lance, V. A. (1997). Sex determination in reptiles: An update. *Am. Zool.* **37**(6), 504–513.

Lauber, A. H., Mobbs, C. V., Muramatsu, M., and Pfaff, D. W. (1991a). Estrogen-receptor messenger-RNA expression in rat hypothalamus as a function of genetic sex and estrogen dose. *Endocrinology (Baltimore)* **129**(6), 3180–3186.

Lauber, A. H., Romano, G. J., and Pfaff, D. W. (1991b). Sex difference in estradiol regulation of progestin receptor messenger-rna in rat mediobasal hypothalamus as demonstrated by *in situ* hybridization. *Neuroendocrinology* **53**(6), 608–613.

Lewis, J., Mahmoud, I. Y., and Klicka, J. (1979). Seasonal fluctuations in the plasma concentrations of progesterone and oestradiol-17-beta in the female snapping turtle (*Chelydra serpentina*). *J. Endocrinol.* **80**(1), 127–131.

Licht, P., Wood, J., Owens, D. W., and Wood, F. (1979). Serum gonadotropins and steroids associated with breeding activities in the green sea turtle *Chelonia mydas*. 1. Captive animals. *Gen. Comp. Endocrinol.* **39**(3), 274–289.

Licht, P., Rainey, W., and Cliffton, K. (1980). Serum gonadotropin and steroids associated with breeding activities in the green sea turtle, *Chelonia mydas*. 2. Mating and nesting in natural-populations. *Gen. Comp. Endocrinol.* **40**, 116–122.

Lindzey, J., and Crews, D. (1992). Interactions between progesterone and androgens in the stimulation of sex behaviors in male little striped whiptail lizards, *Cnemidophorus inornatus*. *Gen. Comp. Endocrinol.* **86**(1), 52–58.

Luo, X. R., Ikeda, Y. Y., and Parker, K. L. (1994). A cell-specific nuclear receptor is essential for adrenal and gonadal development and sexual differentiation. *Cell (Cambridge, Mass.)* **77**(4), 481–490.

Mahmoud, I. Y., and Licht, P. (1997). Seasonal changes in gonadal activity and the effects of stress on reproductive hormones in the common snapping turtle, *Chelydra serpentina*. *Gen. Comp. Endocrinol.* **107**(3), 359–372.

Marler, C. A., and Moore, M. C. (1989). Time and energy costs of aggression in testosterone-implanted free-living male mountain spiny lizards (*Sceloporus jarrovi*). *Physiol. Zool.* **62**(6), 1334–1350.

Marler, C. A., and Moore, M. C. (1991). Supplementary feeding compensates for testosterone-induced costs of aggression in male mountain spiny lizards, *Sceloporus jarrovi*. *Anim. Behav.* **42**, 209–219.

Marler, C. A., Walsberg, G., White, M. L., and Moore, M. (1995). Increased energy expenditure due to increased territorial defense in male lizards after phenotypic manipulation. *Behav. Ecol. Sociobiol.* **37**(4), 225–231.

Mason, R. T., and Crews, D. (1985). Female mimicry in garter snakes. *Nature (London)* **316**, 59–60.

Mason, R. T., Fales, H. M., Jones, T. H., Pannell, L. K., Chinn, J. W., and Crews, D. (1989). Sex pheromones in snakes. *Science* **245**, 290–293.

Matt, K. S., Moore, M. C., Knapp, R., and Moore, I. T. (1997). Sympathetic mediation of stress and aggressive competition: Plasma catecholamines in free-living male tree lizards. *Physiol. Behav.* **61**(5), 639–647.

Matter, J. M., Ronan, P. J., and Summers, C. H. (1998). Central monoamines in free-ranging lizards: Differences associated with social roles and territoriality. *Brain, Behav. Evol.* **51**(1), 23–32.

Mayo, M., and Crews, D. (1987). Neural control of male-like pseudocopulatory behavior in the all-female lizard, *Cnemidophorus uniparens*: Effects of intracranial implantation of dihydrotestosterone. *Horm. Behav.* **21**, 181–192.

Mendonca, M. T. (1987a). Photothermal effects on the ovarian cycle of the musk turtle, *Sternotherus odoratus*. *Herpetologica* **43**(1), 82–90.

Mendonca, M. T. (1987b). Timing of reproductive-behavior in male musk turtles, *Sternotherus odoratus*—effects of photoperiod, temperature and testosterone. *Anim. Behav.* **35**, 1002–1014.

Mendonça, M. T., and Crews, D. (1990). Mating-induced ovarian recrudescence in the red-sided garter snake. *J. Comp. Physiol. A* **166**, 629–632.

Mendonça, M. T., and Crews, D. (2000). Control of attractivity and receptivity in female red-sided garter snakes, *Thamnophis sirtalis parietalis*: *Horm. Behav.* **40**, 43–50.

Mendonça, M. T., Daniels, D., Faro, C., and Crews, D. (2000). Receptivity and 2-deoxyglucose uptake in female red-sided garter snakes. (In preparation.)

Merchant-Larios, H. (1998). Brain as a sensor of temperature during sex determination in the sea turtle *Lepidochelys olivacea*. *J. Exp. Zool.* **281**, 510–518.

Moga, M. M., Geib, B. M., Zhou, D., and Prins, G. S. (2000). Androgen receptor-immunoreactivity in the forebrain of the eastern fence lizard (*Sceloporus undulatus*). *Brain Res.* **879**(1–2), 174–182.

Moore, M. C. (1986). Elevated testosterone levels during nonbreeding-season territoriality in a fall-breeding lizard, *Sceloporus jarrovi*. *J. Comp. Physiol. A* **158**(2), 159–163.

Moore, M. C. (1987a). Castration affects territorial and sexual behavior of free-living male lizards, *Sceloporus jarrovi*. *Anim. Behav.* **35**, 1193–1199.

Moore, M. C. (1987b). Circulating steroid hormones during rapid aggressive responses of territorial male mountain spiny lizards, *Sceloporus jarrovi*. *Horm. Behav.* **21**(4), 511–521.

Moore, M. C. (1988). Testosterone control of territorial behavior—tonic-release implants fully restore seasonal and short-term aggressive responses in free-living castrated lizards. *Gen. Comp. Endocrinol.* **70**(3), 450–459.

Moore, M. C. (1991). Application of organization activation theory to alternative male reproductive strategies—a review. *Horm. Behav.* **25**(2), 154–179.

Moore, M. C., and Crews, D. (1986). Sex steroid-hormones in natural-populations of a sexual whiptail lizard *Cnemidophorus inornatus*, a direct evolutionary ancestor of a unisexual parthenogen. *Gen. Comp. Endocrinol.* **63**(3), 424–430.

Moore, M. C., and Lindzey, J. (1992). The physiological basis of sexual behavior in male reptiles. *In* "Hormones, Brain and Behavior" (C. Gans and D. Crews, eds.), Vol. 18, pp. 70–113. University of Chicago Press, Chicago.

Moore, M. C., and Marler, C. A. (1987). Effects of testosterone manipulations on nonbreeding season territorial aggression in free-living male lizards, *Sceloporus jarrovi*. *Gen. Comp. Endocrinol.* **65**(2), 225–232.

Moore, M. C., Whittier, J. M., and Crews, D. (1985a). Sex steroid-hormones during the ovarian cycle of an all-female, parthenogenetic lizard and their correlation with pseudosexual behavior. *Gen. Comp. Endocrinol.* **60**, 144–153.

Moore, M. C., Whittier, J. M., Billy, A. J., and Crews, D. (1985b). Male-like behavior in an all-female lizard—relationship to ovarian cycle. *Anim. Behav.* **33**, 284–289.

Moore, M. C., Hews, D. K., and Knapp, R. (1998). Hormonal control and evolution of alternative male phenotypes: Generalizations of models for sexual differentiation. *Am. Zool.* **38**(1), 133–151.

Morgentaler, A., and Crews, D. (1978). Role of the anterior hypothalamus-preoptic area in the regulation of reproductive behavior in the lizard, *Anolis carolinensis*: Implantation studies. *Horm. Behav.* **11**, 61–73.

Morohashi, K., Tsuboi-Asai, H., Matsushita, S., Suda, M., Nakashima, M., Sasano, H., Hataba, Y., Li, C. L., Fukata, J., Irie, J., Watanabe, T., Nagura, H., and Li, E. (1999). Structural and functional abnormalities in the spleen of an mftz-f1 gene-disrupted mouse. *Blood* **93**(5), 1586–1594.

Morrell, J. I., and Pfaff, D. W. (1978). A neuroendocrine approach to brain function: Localization of sex steroid concentrating cells in vertebrate brain. *Am. Zool.* **18**, 447–460.

Morrell, J. I., Crews, D., Ballin, A., Morgentaler, A., and Pfaff, D. W. (1979). Estradiol-h-3, h-3-testosterone and dihydrotestosterone-H^3 localization in the brain of the lizard *Anolis carolinensis*—autoradiographic study. *J. Comp. Neurol.* **188**(2), 201–223.

O'Bryant, E. L., and Wade, J. (2000a). Sexual and seasonal dimorphisms in the green anole forebrain. *Soc. Neurosci.*, New Orleans, LA, Abstr. 77.3.

O'Bryant, E. L., and Wade, J. (2000b). Arborization of dewlap motoneurons in the green anole lizard (*Anolis carolinensis*) is not sexually dimorphic. *Neurosci. Lett.* **281**(2–3), 115–118.

Padian, K., and Chiappe, L. M. (1998). The origin and early evolution of birds. *Biol. Rev. Cambridge Philos. Soc.* **73**(1), 1–42.

Pfaff, D. W., Schwartz-Giblin, S., McCarthy, M. M., and Kow, L.-M. (1994). Cellular and molecular mechanisms of female reproductive behaviors. *In* "The Physiology of Reproduction" (E. Knobil and J. D. Neill, eds.), pp. 107–220. Raven Press, New York.

Phoenix, C. H., Goy, R. W., Gerall, A. A., and Young, W. C. (1959). Organizing action of prenatally administered testosterone propionate on the tissues mediating mating behavior in the female guinea pig. *Endocrinology (Baltimore)* **65**(3), 369–382.

Propper, C. R., Jones, R. E., Rand, M. S., and Austin, H. (1991). Nesting-behavior of the lizard *Anolis carolinensis*. *J. Herpetol.* **25**(4), 484–486.

Propper, C. R., Jones, R. E., and Lopez, K. H. (1992a). Distribution of arginine vasotocin in the brain of the lizard *Anolis carolinensis*. *Cell Tissue Res.* **267**(2), 391–398.

Propper, C. R., Jones, R. E., Dores, R. M., and Lopez, K. H. (1992b). Arginine vasotocin concentrations in the supraoptic nucleus of the lizard *Anolis carolinensis* are associated with reproductive state but not oviposition. *J. Exp. Zool.* **264**(4), 461–467.

Rand, M. S. (1990). Polymorphic sexual coloration in the lizard *Sceloporus undulatus erythrocheilus*. *Am. Midl. Nat.* **124**(2), 352–359.

Rand, M. S. (1992). Hormonal control of polymorphic and sexually dimorphic coloration in the lizard *Sceloporus undulatus erythrocheilus*. *Gen. Comp. Endocrinol.* **88**(3), 461–468.

Rand, M. S., and Crews, D. (1994). The bisexual brain—sex behavior differences and sex differences in parthenogenetic and sexual lizards. *Brain Res.* **663**(1), 163–167.

Rhen, T., and Crews, D. (1999). Embryonic temperature and gonadal sex organize male-typical sexual and aggressive behavior in a lizard with temperature-dependent sex determination. *Endocrinology (Baltimore)* **140**, 4501–4508.

Rhen, T., and Crews, D. (2001). Distribution of androgen and estrogen receptor mRNA in the brain and reproductive tissue of the leopard gecko, *Eublepharis macularius. J. Comp. Neurol.* **437**(4), 385–397.

Rosen, G., Matthews, J., Zacharewski, T., and Wade, J. (2000). Distribution of androgen receptor mRNA in the green anole brain. *Soc. Neurosci.*, New Orleans, LA, Abstr. 77.4.

Ross, P., and Crews, D. (1977). Influence of the seminal plug on mating behavior in the garter snake. *Nature (London)* **267**, 344–345.

Rostal, D. C., Owens, D. W., Grumbles, J. S., MacKenzie, D. S., and Amoss, M. S. (1998). Seasonal reproductive cycle of the kemp's ridley sea turtle *(Lepidochelys kempi). Gen. Comp. Endocrinol.* **109**(2), 232–243.

Rouiller-Fabre, V., Carmona, S., Abou Merhi, R., Cate, R., Habert, R., and Vigier, B. (1998). Effect of anti-mullerian hormone on sertoli and leydig cell functions in fetal and immature rats. *Endocrinology (Baltimore)* **139**(3), 1213–1220.

Rozendaal, J. C., and Crews, D. (1989). Effects of intracranial implantation of dihydrotestosterone on sexual behavior in male *Cnemidophorus inornatus*, a direct sexual ancestor of a parthenogenetic lizard. *Horm. Behav.* **23**, 194–202.

Sachs, B., and Meisel, R. L. (1994). The physiology of male sexual behavior. *In* "The Physiology of Reproduction" (E. Knobil and J. Neill, eds.), Vol. 2, pp. 3–106. Raven Press, New York.

Sakata, J. T., Coomber, P., Gonzalez-Lima, F., and Crews, D. (2000). Functional connectivity among limbic brain areas: Differential effects of incubation temperature and gonadal sex in the leopard gecko, *Eublepharis macularius. Brain, Behav. Evol.* **55**(3), 139–151.

Sarkar, S., Sarkar, N. K., and Maiti, B. R. (1996). Seasonal pattern of ovarian growth and interrelated changes in plasma steroid levels, vitellogenesis, and oviductal function in the adult female soft-shelled turtle *Lissemys punctata punctata. Can. J. Zool.* **74**(2), 303–311.

Schramm, B. G., Casares, M., and Lance, V. A. (1999). Steroid levels and reproductive cycle of the galapagos tortoise, *Geochelone nigra*, living under seminatural conditions on Santa Cruz island (Galapagos). *Gen. Comp. Endocrinol.* **114**(1), 108–120.

Shelby, J. A., Mendonca, M. T., Horne, B. D., and Seigel, R. A. (2000). Seasonal variation in reproductive steroids of male and female yellow-blotched map turtles, *Graptemys flavimaculata. Gen. Comp. Endocrinol.* **119**(1), 43–51.

Shen, W. H., Moore, C. C. D., Ikeda, Y., Parker, K. L., and Ingraham, H. A. (1994). Nuclear receptor steroidogenic factor-1 regulates the mullerian-inhibiting substance gene—a link to the sex determination cascade. *Cell (Cambridge, Mass.)* **77**(5), 651–661.

Shinoda, K., Lei, H., Yoshii, H., Nomura, M., Nagano, M., Shiba, H., Sasaki, H., Osawa, Y., Ninomiya, Y., Niwa, O., Morohashi, K., and Li, E. (1995). Developmental defects of the ventromedial hypothalamic nucleus and pituitary gonadotroph in the ftz-f1 disrupted mice. *Dev. Dyn.* **204**(1), 22–29.

Sinervo, B., and Lively, C. M. (1996). The rock-paper-scissors game and the evolution of alternative male strategies. *Nature (London)* **380**, 240–243.

Sinervo, B., Miles, D. B. M., Frankino, W. A., Klukowski, M., and Denardo, D. F. (2000). Testosterone, endurance, and darwinian fitness: Natural and sexual selection on the physiological bases of alternative male behaviors in side-blotched lizards. *Horm. Behav.* **38**(4), 222–233.

Skipper, J. K., Young, L. J., Bergeron, J. M., Tetzlaff, M. T., Osborn, C. T., and Crews, D. (1993). Identification of an isoform of the estrogen-receptor messenger-RNA lacking exon 4 and present in the brain. *Proc. Natl. Acad. Sci. U.S.A* **90**(15), 7172–7175.

Smeets, W., Sevensma, J. J., and Jonker, A. J. (1990). Comparative analysis of vasotocin-like immunoreactivity in the brain of the turtle *Pseudemys scripta elegans* and the snake *Python regius. Brain, Behav. Evol.* **35**(2), 65–84.

Smith, C. A., Smith, M. J., and Sinclair, A. H. (1999). Expression of chicken steroidogenic factor-1 during gonadal sex differentiation. *Gen. Comp. Endocrinol.* **113**(2), 187–196.

Smith, L. C., and John-Alder, H. B. (1999). Seasonal specificity of hormonal, behavioral, and coloration responses to within- and between-sex encounters in male lizards *(Sceloporus undulatus). Horm. Behav.* **36**(1), 39–52.

Sossinka, R. (1980). Ovarian development in an opportunistic breeder, the zebra finch *Poephila guttata castanotis. J. Exp. Zool.* **211**(2), 225–230.

Summers, C. H., and Greenberg, N. (1994). Somatic correlates of adrenergic activity during aggression in the lizard, *Anolis carolinensis. Horm. Behav.* **28**(1), 29–40.

Summers, C. H., and Greenberg, N. (1995). Activation of central biogenic-amines following aggressive interaction in male lizards, *Anolis carolinensis. Brain, Behav. Evol.* **45**(6), 339–349.

Summers, C. H., Larson, E. T., Summers, T. R., Renner, K. J., and Greenberg, N. (1998). Regional and temporal separation of serotonergic activity mediating social stress. *Neuroscience* **87**(2), 489–496.

Summers, C. H., Larson, E. T., Ronan, P. J., Hofmann, P. M., Emerson, A. J., and Renner, K. J. (2000). Serotonergic responses to corticosterone and testosterone in the limbic system. *Gen. Comp. Endocrinol.* **117**(1), 151–159.

Summers, T. R., Hunter, A. L., and Summers, C. H. (1997). Female social reproductive roles affect central monoamines. *Brain Res.* **767**(2), 272–278.

Thompson, C. W., and Moore, M. C. (1991a). Throat color reliably signals status in male tree lizards, *Urosaurus ornatus*. *Anim. Behav.* **42**, 745–753.

Thompson, C. W., and Moore, M. C. (1991b). Syntopic occurrence of multiple dewlap color morphs in male tree lizards, *Urosaurus ornatus*. *Copeia* **2**, 493–503.

Thompson, C. W., and Moore, M. C. (1992). Behavioral and hormonal correlates of alternative reproductive strategies in a polygynous lizard—tests of the relative plasticity and challenge hypotheses. *Horm. Behav.* **26**(4), 568–585.

Thompson, C. W., Moore, I. T., and Moore, M. C. (1993). Social, environmental and genetic factors in the ontogeny of phenotypic differentiation in a lizard with alternative male reproductive strategies. *Behav. Ecol. Sociobiol.* **33**(3), 137–146.

Thorbjarnarson, J. B., and Hernandez, G. (1993). Reproductive ecology of the orinoco crocodile (*Crocodylus intermedius*) in Venezuela. 2. Reproductive and social-behavior. *J. Herpetol.* **27**(4), 371–379.

Tokarz, R. R., and Crews, D. (1979). Temporal pattern of estrogen-induction of female sexual receptivity in the lizard, *Anolis carolinensis. Am. Zool.* **19**(3), 966–966.

Tokarz, R. R., and Crews, D. (1980). Induction of sexual receptivity in the female lizard, *Anolis carolinensis*—effects of estrogen and the anti-estrogen CI-628. *Horm. Behav.* **14**(1), 33–45.

Tokarz, R. R., and Crews, D. (1981). Effects of prostaglandins on sexual receptivity in the female lizard, *Anolis carolinensis. Endocrinology (Baltimore)* **109**(2), 451–457.

Tokarz, R. R., Crews, D., and McEwen, B. S. (1981). Estrogen-sensitive progestin binding-sites in the brain of the lizard, *Anolis carolinensis. Brain Res.* **220**(1), 95–105.

Tousignant, A., and Crews, D. (1995). Incubation temperature and gonadal sex affect growth and physiology in the leopard gecko (*Eublepharis macularius*), a lizard with temperature-dependent sex determination. *J. Morphol.* **224**, 159–170.

Tousignant, A., Viets, B., Flores, D., and Crews, D. (1995). Ontogenetic and social factors affect the endocrinology and timing of reproduction in the female leopard gecko (*Eublepharis macularius*). *Horm. Behav.* **29**, 141–153.

Tucker, A. D., McCallum, H. I., Limpus, C. J., and McDonald, K. R. (1998). Sex-biased dispersal in a long-lived polygynous reptile (*Crocodylus johnstoni*). *Behav. Ecol. Sociobiol.* **44**(2), 85–90.

Valenstein, P., and Crews, D. (1977). Mating-induced termination of behavioral estrus in female lizard, *Anolis carolinensis. Horm. Behav.* **9**(3), 362–370.

Viets, B. E., Ewert, M. A., Talent, L. G., and Nelson, C. E. (1994). Sex-determining mechanisms in squamate reptiles. *J. Exp. Zool.* **270**, 45–56.

Wade, J. (1997). Androgen metabolism in the brain of the green anole lizard (*Anolis carolinensis*). *Gen. Comp. Endocrinol.* **106**(1), 127–137.

Wade, J. (1998). Sexual dimorphisms in the brainstem of the green anole lizard. *Brain, Behav. Evol.* **52**(1), 46–54.

Wade, J., and Crews, D. (1991). The effects of intracranial implantation of estrogen on receptivity in sexually and asexually reproducing female whiptail lizards, *Cnemidophorus inornatus* and *Cnemidophorus uniparens. Horm. Behav.* **25**(3), 342–353.

Wade, J., and Crews, D. (1992). Sexual dimorphisms in the soma size of neurons in the brain of whiptail lizards (*Cnemidophorus* species). *Brain Res.* **594**(2), 311–314.

Webb, G. J. W., Buckworth, R., and Manolis, S. C. (1983). *Crocodylus johnstoni* in the McKinlay River nt. 6. Nesting biology. *Aust. Wildl. Res.* **10**(3), 607–637.

Wennstrom, K. L., and Crews, D. (1995). Making males from females—the effects of aromatase inhibitors on a parthenogenetic species of whiptail lizard. *Gen. Comp. Endocrinol.* **99**(3), 316–322.

Wennstrom, K. L., and Crews, D. (1998). Effect of long-term castration and long-term androgen treatment on sexually dimorphic estrogen-inducible progesterone receptor mRNA levels in the ventromedial hypothalamus of whiptail lizards. *Horm. Behav.* **34**(1), 11–16.

Wennstrom, K. L., Blesius, F., and Crews, D. (1999). Volumetric analysis of sexually dimorphic limbic nuclei in normal and sex-reversed whiptail lizards. *Brain Res.* **838**(1–2), 104–109.

Western, P. S., Harry, J. L., Graves, J. A. M., and Sinclair, A. H. (2000). Temperature-dependent sex determination in the American alligator: Expression of SF-1, WT-1 and DAX1 during gonadogenesis. *Gene* **241**(2), 223–232.

Wheeler, J. M., and Crews, D. (1978). Role of the anterior hypothalamus-preoptic area in the regulation of male reproductive-behavior in the lizard, *Anolis carolinensis*—lesion studies. *Horm. Behav.* **11**(1), 42–60.

Whittier, J. M., and Crews, D. (1989). Mating increases plasma levels of prostaglandin F2 alpha in female garter snakes. *Prostaglandins* **37**, 359–366.

Whittier, J. M., and Tokarz, R. (1992). Physiological regulation of sexual behavior in female reptiles. In "Hormones, Brain and Behavior" (C. Gans and D. Crews, eds.), Vol. 18, pp. 24–69. University of Chicago Press, Chicago.

Whittier, J. M., Mason, R. T., and Crews, D. (1985). Mating in the red-sided garter snake, *Thamnophis sirtalis parietalis*. Differential effects on male and female sexual behavior. *Behav. Ecol. Sociobiol.* **16**, 257–261.

Whittier, J. M., Mason, R. T., and Crews, D. (1987). Plasma steroid hormone levels of female red-sided garter snakes, *Thamnophis sirtalis parietalis:* Relationship to mating and gestation. *Gen. Comp. Endocrinol.* **67**, 33–43.

Whittier, J. M., Corrie, F., and Limpus, C. (1997). Plasma steroid profiles in nesting loggerhead turtles *(Caretta caretta)* in Queensland, Australia: Relationship to nesting episode and season. *Gen. Comp. Endocrinol.* **106**(1), 39–47.

Wibbels, T., and Crews, D. (1992). Specificity of steroid hormone-induced sex determination in a turtle. *J. Endocrinol.* **133**(1), 121–129.

Wibbels, T., and Crews, D. (1994). Putative aromatase inhibitor induces male sex determination in a female unisexual lizard and in a turtle with temperature-dependent sex determination. *J. Endocrinol.* **141**(2), 295–299.

Wibbels, T., and Crews, D. (1995). Steroid-induced sex determination at incubation temperatures producing mixed-sex ratios in a turtle with TSD. *Gen. Comp. Endocrinol.* **100**(1), 53–60.

Wibbels, T., Owens, D. W., Limpus, C. J., Reed, P. C., and Amoss, M. S. (1990). Seasonal-changes in serum gonadal-steroids associated with migration, mating, and nesting in the loggerhead sea turtle *(Caretta caretta)*. *Gen. Comp. Endocrinol.* **79**(1), 154–164.

Wibbels, T., Bull, J. J., and Crews, D. (1992). Steroid hormone-induced male sex determination in an amniotic vertebrate. *J. Exp. Zool.* **262**(4): 454–457.

Wibbels, T., Cowan, J., and LeBoeuf, R. (1998). Temperature-dependent sex determination in the red-eared slider turtle, *Trachemys scripta*. *J. Exp. Zool.* **281**(5), 409–416.

Wiens, J. J. (1993). Phylogenetic relationships of phrynosomatid lizards and monophyly of the *Sceloporus* group. *Copeia* **2**, 287–299.

Wiens, J. J. (2000). Decoupled evolution of display morphology and display behavior in phrynosomatid lizards. *Biol. J. Linn. Soc.* **70**(4), 597–612.

Wiens, J. J., Reeder, T. W., and De Oca, A. N. M. (1999). Molecular phylogenetics and evolution of sexual dichromatism among populations of the Yarrow's spiny lizard *(Sceloporus jarrovi)*. *Evolution (Laurence, Kans.)* **53**(6), 1884–1897.

Winkler, S. M., and Wade, J. (1998). Aromatase activity and regulation of sexual behaviors in the green anole lizard. *Physiol. Behav.* **64**(5), 723–731.

Witt, D. M., Young, L. J., and Crews, D. (1995). Progesterone modulation of androgen-dependent sexual behavior in male rats. *Physiol. Behav.* **57**, 307–313.

Wong Riley, M. T. T. (1989). Cytochrome-oxidase—an endogenous metabolic marker for neuronal activity. *Trends Neurosci.* **12**(3), 94–101.

Woodley, S. K., and Moore, M. C. (1999a). Female territorial aggression and steroid hormones in mountain spiny lizards. *Anim. Behav.* **57**, 1083–1089.

Woodley, S. K., and Moore, M. C. (1999b). Ovarian hormones influence territorial aggression in free-living female mountain spiny lizards. *Horm. Behav.* **35**(3), 205–214.

Woolley, S. C., Sakata, J. T., Gupta, A., and Crews, D. (2001). Evolutionary conservation of dopaminergic modulation of sexual behavior in two related species of lizard. *Horm. Behav.* **40**, 483–489.

Young, L. J., and Crews, D. (1995). Comparative neuroendocrinology of steroid receptor gene expression and regulation: Relationship to physiology and behavior. *Trends Endocrinol. Metab.* **6**(9–10), 317–323.

Young, L. J., Lopreato, G. F., Horan, K., and Crews, D. (1994). Cloning and *in situ* hybridization analysis of estrogen-receptor, progesterone-receptor, and androgen receptor expression in the brain of whiptail lizards *(Cnemidophorus uniparens* and *C. inornatus)*. *J. Comp. Neurol.* **347**(2), 288–300.

Young, L. J., Nag, P. K., and Crews, D. (1995a). Regulation of estrogen-receptor and progesterone-receptor messenger-ribonucleic-acid by estrogen in the brain of the whiptail lizard *(Cnemidophorus uniparens)*. *J. Neuroendocrinol.* **7**(2), 119–125.

Young, L. J., Nag, P. K., and Crews, D. (1995b). Species-differences in behavioral and neural sensitivity to estrogen in whiptail lizards—correlation with hormone-receptor messenger ribonucleic acid expression. *Neuroendocrinology* **61**(6), 680–686.

31

Ecophysiological Studies of Hormone-Behavior Relations in Birds

John C. Wingfield
Department of Zoology
University of Washington
Seattle, Washington 98195

Bengt Silverin
Department of Zoology
University of Göteborg
S-405 30 Göteborg, Sweden

I. INTRODUCTION

Most, if not all, vertebrates live in changing environments in which morphology, physiology, and behavior are regulated to maximize fitness in any habitat configuration. Environmental fluctuations can be predictable (e.g., night and day, the seasons, and low tide and high tide) allowing organisms to respond to environmental signals that trigger appropriate changes in morphology, physiology, and behavior (Wingfield et al., 1992b, 1993). There is also a stochastic component to environmental fluctuations that require emergency responses to unpredictable, severe storms and other potentially catastrophic events (Wingfield, 1988; Silverin, 1998a; Wingfield et al., 1998). Environmental signals, usually transduced through hormone secretions, result in the activation or deactivation of appropriate behaviors (e.g., during the reproductive season). However, throughout an individual's life cycle, responses to environmental change are also influenced by social interactions—even in species that may spend much of their lives in isolation (e.g., Harding, 1981; Balthazart, 1983; Wingfield et al., 1994c, 2000).

Despite the complexity of social systems and responses to environmental change, there is a clear interaction of environmental signals and expression of behavior through neuroendocrine and endocrine functions. The mechanisms involved remain obscure partly because of a lack of integration of field studies and laboratory experimentation. On the one hand, experimental studies of neural pathways for environmental signals that regulate neuroendocrine function can only be done in the laboratory. On the other hand, the interpretation of laboratory data in the contexts of animals in their natural habitats must involve a field component at some stage in the investigation. The emergence of field endocrinology is one way by which laboratory and field investigations can be integrated effectively. It should be emphasized here that the integration of field and laboratory studies is a critical process. Either alone is ineffective in unraveling the mechanisms underlying interactions of hormones, behavior, and their ecological bases.

Some impediments to field endocrine investigations include the need to develop new techniques, including molecular approaches, for the study of wild species. Early investigations of wild species focused largely on histological studies of endocrine glands. Many experimental studies of, for example, photoperiodic control of gonadal function and comparative endocrinology were conducted under captive conditions (Wingfield and Farner, 1993). The endocrinology of wild species in their natural habitats was inferred, and the potential confounding effects of captivity on endocrine functions were largely ignored. The earliest investigations in the field involved the effects of testosterone implants on free-living California quail (*Callipepla californica*; Emlen and Lorenz, 1945), red grouse (*Lagopus lagopus scotticus*; Watson, 1970), and sharp-tailed grouse (*Tympanuchus phasianellus*; Trobec and Oring, 1972). Ecophysiological studies of hormone–behavior interactions in birds under natural conditions then gained momentum in all vertebrate classes from the mid-1970s on (see Wingfield and Kenagy, 1991; Wingfield and Farner, 1993). The result is several hundred published papers on field endocrinology, but it is only since the 1990s that attempts have been made to review these data in a framework that involves ecological bases of hormone–behavior interactions and provides testable hypotheses.

Here we review the ecophysiology of wild species with particular focus on the endocrine aspects of reproductive behavior and associated annual events such as migration, molt, and responses to stress. The history of avian endocrinology, particularly in wild species; the structure and function of endocrine glands in birds; and the isolation, identification, and assay of avian hormones have been reviewed extensively in Wingfield and Farner (1993). Other general publications providing useful background on avian endocrinology include Assenmacher (1973), Kobayashi and Wada (1973), Lofts and Murton (1973), Tixier-Vidal and Follett (1973), Murton and Westwood (1977), and Balthazart (1983). Symposium volumes providing valuable information are Epple and Stetson (1980), Mikami *et al.* (1983), Follett *et al.* (1985), Johnson et al. (1984), Wada *et al.* (1990), Silverin (1992), Sharp (1993), and Harvey and Etches (1997). We have adopted a theoretical framework that allows us to look for general principles that may have heuristic value in an attempt to identify the ecological bases of hormone systems. The hypotheses and predictions that result can then be taken to the cell and molecular levels. If nothing else, we hope this approach will promote further studies directed at drawing together the vast diversity of processes and their mechanisms in vertebrates in general.

A. Temporal Sequence of Life History Stages

Endocrine secretions regulate many aspects of homeostasis as well as transitions in morphology, physiology, and behavior in relation to predictable changes in the environment. Because most vertebrates live in fluctuating environments, they adjust their state to maximize survival at different times of year. These changes can be summarized as a finite-state machine (FSM) consisting of a temporal sequence of life history stages (LHSs) that maximizes lifetime fitness (Jacobs 1996; Jacobs and Wingfield, 2000). Hormone secretions have several roles in the regulation of LHSs. They are involved in developmental trajectories and transitions between LHSs, they activate and deactivate physiological and behavioral state in a LHS, and they orchestrate facultative responses to unpredictable events in the environment (e.g., Gorbman *et al.*, 1983; Nelson, 1999; Wingfield *et al.*, 1999; Jacobs and Wingfield, 2000). Most life history trajectories involve ontogenetic stages followed by a transition into cyclic adult LHSs. During ontogeny, hormones regulate growth and differentiation including the determination of sex. It is during this process that morphological, physiological, and behavioral phenotypes are developed. These characteristic are largely irreversible (Arnold and Breedlove, 1985) or can be expressed in a fixed number of ways regulated by hormone action in the adult (relative plasticity model of Thompson and Moore, 1992). Adult LHSs also involve growth and differentiation as the individual changes morphology, physiology, and behavior from one stage to the next. Unlike ontogeny, developmental changes associated with adult LHSs are reversible and usually cyclic. These are hormone dependent, but may be markedly different from ontogeny (Jacobs and Wingfield, 2000).

The LHSs in the life cycle of vertebrates are distinct stages and independent of one another, although they may overlap to varying degrees (Wingfield *et al.*, 1997b; Jacobs and Wingfield, 2000). Examples of LHSs in birds are given in Figs. 1 and 2. Each box represents a distinct LHS with several unique substages. In species with more than two LHSs the sequence cannot be reversed. For example, in the migratory Gambel's white-crowned sparrow (*Zonotrichia leucophrys gambelii*), it is not possible to revert to vernal migration after the breeding LHS. The sequence must move on to the next stage—prebasic molt (Fig. 1). All LHSs must be expressed in the correct sequence before vernal migration is again attained.

A number of substages exist in each LHS. Because different combinations of substages can be expressed depending on local environmental conditions, they define the state of the individual at that time (Wingfield

Gambel's White-crowned Sparrow

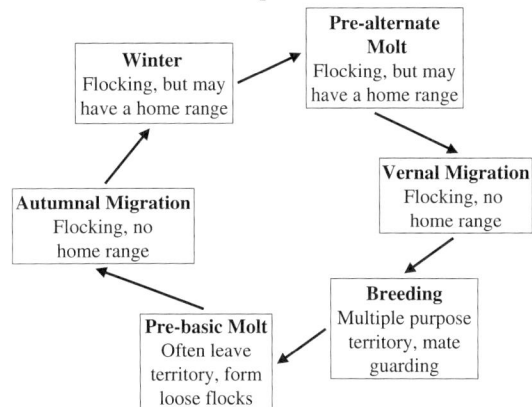

FIGURE 1 An example illustrating finite-state machine (FSM) theory of the cycle of life history stages (LHSs) in the Gambel's white-crowned sparrow, *Zonotrichia leucophrys gambelii*. Each box represents a LHS in which are indicated some substages (in relation of behavior). The LHSs progress in a one-way temporal sequence with each timed to occur at a time of year characteristic of that stage. For example, breeding LHS occurs in spring and summer, whereas the nonbreeding stage is typical of the winter months. The sequence cannot be reversed. Some LHSs cannot be expressed at the same time as others, whereas some can overlap to varying degrees. The timing, overlap, and diversity of LHSs have been discussed in detail by Wingfield and Jacobs (1999). Substages are characteristic of the LHS in which they are expressed. However, the sequences and overlap of substages in a LHS are far more flexible (Wingfield and Jacobs, 2000). The combination of substages expressed in a LHS in relation to environmental and social cues gives state of the organism at that moment. State can be highly changeable, especially in complex social situations. Note also that FSM theory predicts that apparently similar substages expressed in different LHSs will have different context of expression and there is no reason to assume that hormonal control mechanisms will be similar. From Jacobs and Wingfield (2000), courtesy of the Cooper Ornithological Society.

and Jacobs 1999; Wingfield *et al.*, 1997b). They may be altered further by, for example, changes in social status. Whereas most studies of life history strategies have focused on population differences or individual phenotypes in a population, it is important also to assess changes of physiology, behavior, and morphology in an individual in response to environmental signals. In other words, the progression of LHSs in individuals is analogous to the switching of phenotypes at the population level, except that the switch occurs within an individual. Differences in how the repertoires of LHSs and their substages vary and what the endocrine mechanisms underlying them are may provide extensive new insight into how individuals cope with a changing and sometimes capricious environment.

Substages (Figs. 1–2) are expressed in many sequences and combinations in LHSs (Jacobs, 1996; Wingfield and Jacobs, 1999; Jacobs and Wingfield, 2000). A number of potential states can thus be manifest in each LHS. These represent not only the actual LHS and the combination of substages, but also factors often included in the extended phenotype such as territory quality and presence of a mate (Dawkins, 1982). State varies with time, associated with changes in the extended phenotypic factors, as well as adjustments in the morphology, physiology, and behavior of the organism as it acclimates to fluctuations in its environment. Note again that these changes are triggered by environmental cues in a manner different from the transition between LHSs.

It is important to bear in mind that there are three phases in the expression of a LHS. Each has a development phase followed by a mature capability in which a number of substages can then be activated. The LHS is terminated at an appropriate time, although there may be varying degrees of overlap with other LHSs. Hormones play a major role in the development of each stage (and its termination) as well as the activation of substages (Jacobs and Wingfield, 2000). Some species may have more LHSs than others (Fig. 2), and in an individual some LHSs may have a more complex set of substages than others. The rock ptarmigan (*Lagopus mutus*) has as many as seven distinct LHSs (Wingfield and Jacobs, 1999; Jacobs and Wingfield, 2000). At the opposite end of the spectrum, rock doves (*Columba livia*) have only two adult LHSs (Fig. 2). Because the transitions between stages and activation of substages are regulated by hormones, it is possible that there are major species differences in mechanisms at cell and molecular levels. In addition, it is highly likely that some aspects of this FSM are genetic and others experiential.

The duration of each LHS can be measured by field observations. In birds (Figs. 1–2), individuals may be in breeding condition for 1–3 months, whereas prebasic molt may require only 1 month (Wingfield and Jacobs, 1999). The extent of overlap of LHSs varies too. Some LHSs (such as winter and molt) may be more compatible in terms of overlap, whereas others

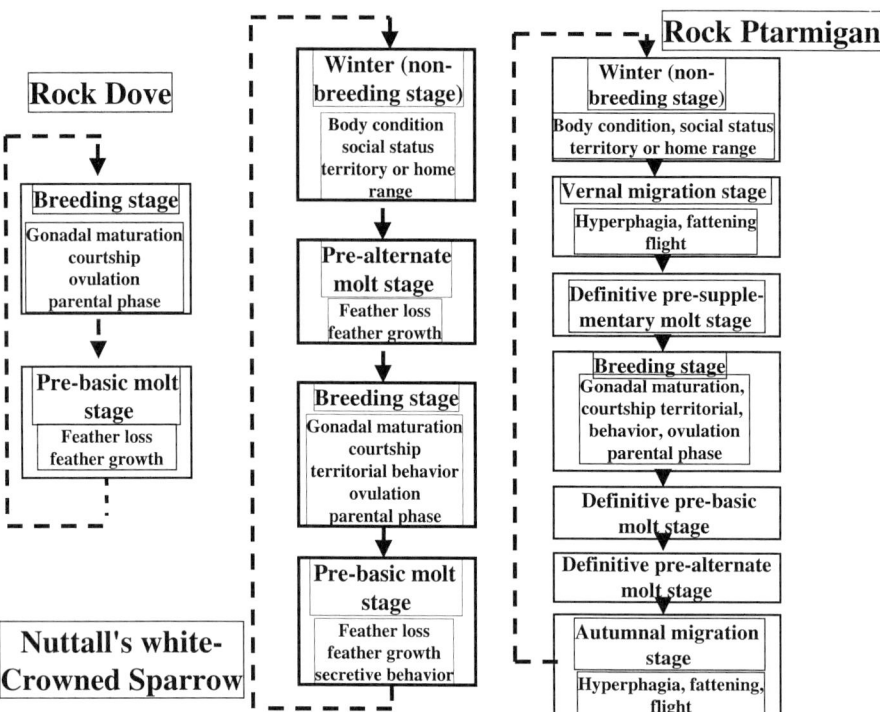

FIGURE 2 A comparison of life history stages (LHSs) in different avian taxa. The rock dove (*Columba livia*) has only two LHSs and these can show considerable overlap, thus imbuing a high degree of flexibility in the life cycle. Contrast this with the rock ptarmigan (*Lagopus mutus*), which has as many as seven LHSs. Given that each LHS has a development phase, mature capability, and a termination phase, there is a limit to the number of LHSs any organism can express in a year simply because of the time constraints. To change from one LHS to another requires the cell cycle be activated in some cells and deactivated in others. Cell growth and differentiation, and the reverse, require time. Onset of the actual LHS also has a time component. For example, the minimum time required to breed (nest, lay eggs, and raise young) is 5–6 weeks. The nonmigratory Nuttall's white-crowned sparrow (*Zonotrichia leucophrys nuttalli*) is intermediate in the number of LHSs and thus may show flexibility in timing in some LHS and less in others. From Wingfield and Jacobs (1999); Jacobs and Wingfield (2000), courtesy of the Cooper Ornithological Society.

such as migration and breeding are mutually exclusive. Obviously, it is not possible for a bird to build a nest and incubate eggs while covering long distances on migration.

B. Expression of Substages That Give State

The expressed set of substages at any point in a specific LHS is the overall morphological, physiological, and behavioral state of the organism. Complex states may exist if two LHSs overlap or during the transition from one LHS to another. State is dictated by a number of environmental and social factors that may vary in an individual from moment to moment or among individuals in a population according to microhabitats and experience. An illustration of variation in complexity of substages is given in Fig. 3 for the Gambel's white-crowned sparrow (Wingfield and Jacobs, 1999). The reproductive stage is complex with at least eight distinct substages. During the development phase, gonads recrudesce, resulting in mature capability, following which onset of actual breeding can begin. This involves the onset of yolk deposition, leading to ovulation and oviposition. Several substages may follow including the establishment of a breeding territory, courtship and pair-bonding, nest building, ovulation, copulation, and egg laying. Later, parental substages are expressed such as incubation, feeding

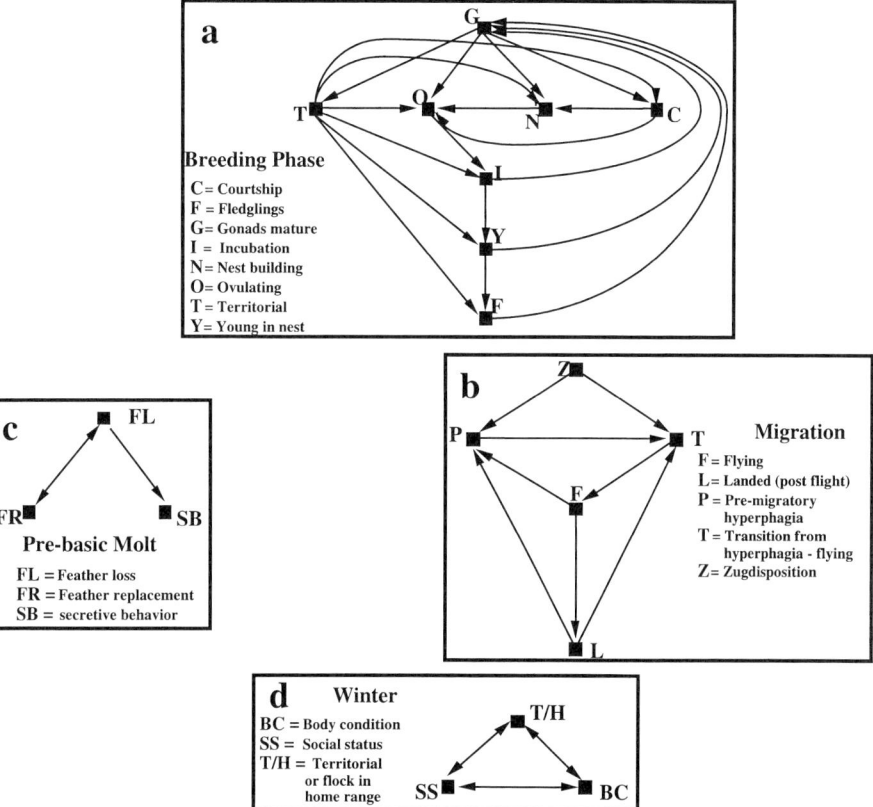

FIGURE 3 Schematic showing the connectivity of substages in some life history stages (LHSs) of Gambel's white-crowned sparrow (*Zonotrichia leucophrys gambelii*). The most complex LHS is breeding, with up to eight substages. However, these may not switch in all possible combinations. The arrows show how most transitions among substages occur. Some substages can overlap extensively (e.g., territorial behavior is expressed throughout breeding and thus overlaps with all other stages). Some sequences can be repeated. For example, the sexual and parental phases can be repeated in multiple-brooding species. Other LHSs are less complex. Note that during migration some sequences are repeatable—hyperphagia, fattening, flight, and landing can be repeated multiple times as the individual moves many thousands of kilometers between wintering grounds and breeding areas. From Wingfield and Jacobs (1999), courtesy of Bird Life International, Johannesburg, South Africa.

nestlings, and fledging. Note that despite the plasticity of the expression of substages, they are not expressed in random sequences. The arrows in Fig. 3 indicate the known transitions between substages or indicate when more than one substage can be expressed simultaneously (from Wingfield and Jacobs, 1999). The connections possible for the reproductive LHS have been identified in field studies of white-crowned sparrows (from Blanchard, 1941; Blanchard and Erickson, 1949; Mewaldt and King, 1977; Wingfield and Farner, 1978a,b). There is a time-dependent temporal sequence of these events in the breeding LHS, but it differs from the temporal sequence of LHSs because it can be interrupted and initiate a new breeding attempt if the nest or eggs are lost to a predator. Furthermore, if the breeding LHS is prolonged, the sexual and parental substages can be repeated (Wingfield and Moore, 1987; Jacobs and Wingfield, 2000).

C. Transitions between Life History Stages

The development phase of a LHS usually requires the stimulation of the cell cycle followed by cell differentiation and growth. An example is the recrudescence of gonads in seasonally breeding birds. In the development phase, hormones act either via genomic receptors (e.g., steroids and thyroid hormones) or by membrane receptors that influence the cell cycle (Hadley, 1999). The phase of mature capability must be attained before the LHS can be expressed fully, and the process is reversed as the LHS is terminated. At this time, the development of the next LHS begins.

D. Timing of Life History Stages

If a given population lives in a predictably fluctuating environment that requires several LHSs, then each must be timed to coincide with its appropriate habitat configuration. Social status may also require further adjustments, but the end result is selection for precise timing of LHSs that maximize fitness (Jacobs and Wingfield, 2000). It is well known that signals emanating from the environment can be used by individuals to time many aspects of the life cycle. Indeed, there is a vast literature on the responses of vertebrates to environmental signals (Immelmann, 1971, 1973). Although the complexity of these cues and responses is bewildering, the environmental information used by animals can be organized into five major types, based on the major effects of these signals (Wingfield, 1983; Wingfield and Kenagy, 1991; Jacobs and Wingfield, 2000).

1. Developmental cues. These include growth factors and morphogens, tissue interactions, intrinsic factors, and external factors. They most often originate from the internal environment of the embryo, such as growth factors, but extrinsic cues come directly from the external environment. An example is low environmental temperature that tends to slow down embryonic development.

2. Initial predictive information. This provides very reliable long-term predictive information so that an individual can begin preparing for a future event several weeks or even months in advance. For example, it is well known that the seasonal change in day length can act as a signal to promote gonadal development in anticipation of the breeding season.

3. Supplementary factors. These provide short-term predictive information. In most habitats, there is temporal variation in predictive events. For example, at mid-latitudes some springs are early and warm, whereas others are late and cool. Thus individuals need to fine-tune changes in the development phase, onset (mature capability), and termination of any LHS induced by initial predictive information to give maximum fitness. Note that the types of supplementary factors at each phase may or may not be similar, but the mechanisms by which they act in each phase are likely to be different. Examples of supplementary cues are local temperature, availability of food, and rainfall. The integration of changes in LHS in response to predictable fluctuations of the environment is coordinated precisely by type 2 and 3 signals.

4. Integrating and synchronizing information. This group comprises all the behavioral interactions, inter- and intrasexual, among groups and between adults and young. They serve to integrate changes in behavior with reproductive state and also synchronize the behavior of a breeding pair or group during nesting (Wingfield and Moore, 1987; Wingfield *et al.*, 1994c). A great deal of research over since the 1950s indicates that integrating and synchronizing information impinges on all aspects of an animal's life. However, the critical importance of social influences and the profound implications for an individual's physiology have not been appreciated fully.

5. Modifying information. These are also called labile perturbation factors (e.g., Wingfield *et al.*, 1998, 2000). These trigger the emergency LHS that redirects the individual away from its normal LHS and allows it to survive the perturbation in the best condition possible. The animal then returns to the normal LHS when the perturbation passes or if an alternate habitat is located.

E. Field Studies in Environmental Endocrinology: Why and How

FSM theory, the temporal sequence of LHSs and expression of their substages, allows us to develop a framework to compare the life cycles of vertebrates in diverse habitats. However, investigations of the hormone–behavior interactions that occur throughout an animal's life cycle require experimental approaches in both the laboratory and field. It is appropriate at this point to briefly discuss how field endocrine techniques have been developed and how they can provide essential context and guides for further experimentation in the laboratory. In this way it is possible to identify what the important questions are and what the best approaches may be to determine mechanisms.

To illustrate this point further, comparisons of LH (luteinizing hormone) and testosterone cycles in the plasma of captive and free-living populations of song sparrows (Melospiza melodia) show markedly different patterns (Figs. 4–5). In the laboratory, males exposed to long days complete spermatogenesis, develop all accessory organs, and express the full repertoire of sexual and aggressive behavior. Accompanying development of these traits is an increase in the plasma levels of LH and testosterone that remain high through much of the breeding period and then decline as photorefractoriness develops. In contrast, birds captured at intervals during a natural breeding cycle show much more complex patterns of LH and testosterone (Figs. 4–5). In addition, testosterone levels in birds sampled in the field may be almost an order of magnitude higher than those from captive birds (Fig. 5; Wingfield and Farner, 1980, 1993; Wingfield and Moore, 1987). These data clearly suggest that environmental cues in the field, but absent under captive conditions, have marked effects on reproductive function. Because mature capability of breeding develops under laboratory conditions, it is likely that the different patterns in free-living birds are a result of social interactions (Wingfield and Farner, 1993; Wingfield et al., 1990a). It should also be pointed out that the presence of such interactions and their impact on hormone patterns may have been overlooked in studies using only captive animals.

Experiments with domesticated and semidomesticated species have enhanced our knowledge of how the life cycle of birds is initiated, synchronized, and integrated (e.g., Hinde and Steel, 1978; Cheng, 1979; Silver, 1978; Murton and Westwood, 1977). However, domesticated species have lost, to varying degrees, the ability to respond to the environmental information used by their ancestors. They are ideal for investigations of fundamental endocrine mechanisms, but the application to diverse scenarios in the field should be made with caution. The investigation of the mechanisms involved in the temporal adjustment of LHSs rely on investigations of populations living in their natural habitat or recently removed from it.

Techniques are now well established whereby blood samples, including serial samples, can be collected from free-living birds immediately after capture in Japanese

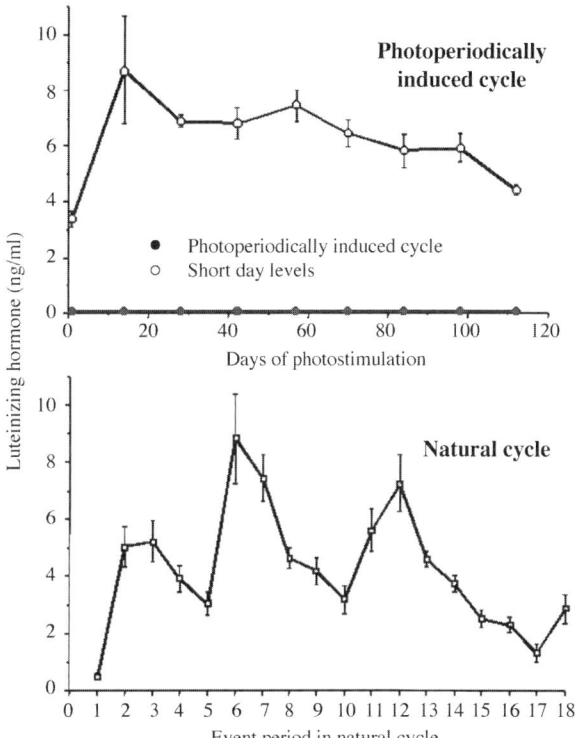

FIGURE 4 Upper panel: Plasma levels of luteinizing hormone (LH) in captive male song sparrows (Melospiza melodia) exposed to long days to simulate spring. Open circles are means ±SE for photostimulated males and solid circles are means ±SE for short-day controls. Note that LH levels in the blood rise rapidly, remain high for several weeks, and then decline slowly as photorefractoriness sets in to mark the termination of the breeding LHS. Lower panel: Changes in plasma levels of LH in free-living males going through a normal breeding cycle in spring. Each number of the event period in natural cycle represents a specific state (i.e., combination of substages expressed in a LHS such as breeding). These could include territory establishment, egg-laying, and feeding of young. Note that the pattern of LH secretion is markedly different from those of captive birds despite the fact that captive males showed full reproductive development and expressed the full repertoire of reproductive behavior. These comparisons indicate clearly that environmental and social cues in the field have a far more profound effect on hormone secretion than we would expect from laboratory studies only. From Wingfield (1984, 1994); Wingfield et al. (2000), courtesy of MIT Press.

mist nets or traps (Wingfield and Farner, 1976). After the withdrawal of blood, each bird is color-banded, following which data such as body mass, fat score, and mensural characters can be measured. It is also possible

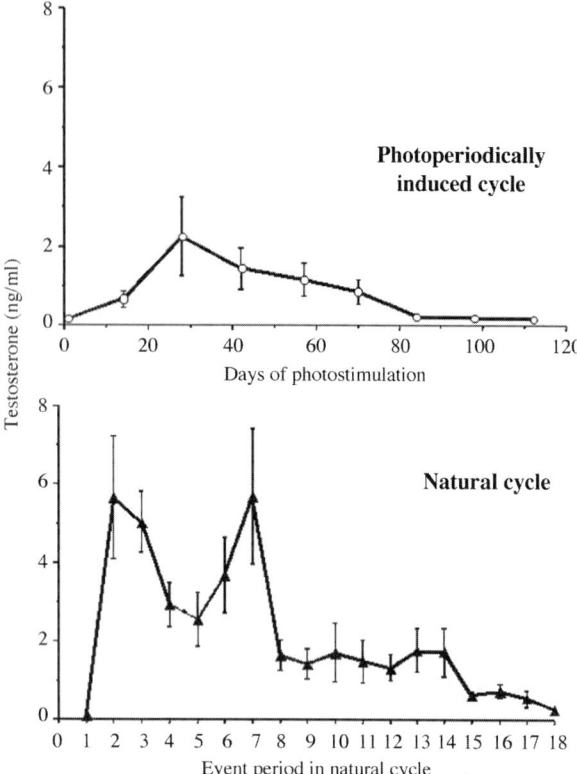

FIGURE 5 A comparison of the pattern of testosterone levels in the blood of male song sparrows (*Melospiza melodia*) (upper panel) exposed to long days in the laboratory (to simulate spring breeding conditions), and (lower panel) going through a natural breeding cycle in the field. See Fig. 4. Note the marked difference in patterns of testosterone secretion, indicating that field studies reveal far more information about the potential control of a reproductive cycle than we would expect from simple laboratory studies. From Wingfield (1984, 1994); Wingfield et al. (2000), courtesy of MIT Press.

to perform a laparotomy, give injections, or implant hormones and their blockers with appropriate controls in field experiments to manipulate the expression of substages in a LHS or to prolong one LHS and determine the effects on fitness (e.g., Ketterson et al., 1996). Birds are then released for subsequent observation—still under natural conditions. Recapture, reexamination, and collection of further blood samples are then possible. Analyses of hormone levels in blood samples can be related directly to stages of the annual cycle, behavior, weather, and other variables (Wingfield and Farner, 1976). Behavioral observations can be made directly or after experimental challenges such as a simulated territorial intrusion (e.g., Wingfield, 1985; Silverin, 1993). These types of approaches allow multiple options for collecting data or experimentally manipulating the system. Such information provides critical bases for designing appropriate laboratory or field experiments to investigate mechanisms. Most important, they provide a solid database for new research directions and concepts that could probably not be approached in the laboratory (e.g., Wingfield et al., 1990b).

F. Overview: Ecophysiological Studies of Hormone–Behavior Relations in Birds

Having reviewed the organization of life cycles in birds, the ways by which hormones might influence them, and how we go about studying the ecological bases of hormone–behavior interactions, it is important here to discuss how the extremely diverse, and sometimes conflicting, studies of birds are dealt with in the next sections. We have chosen to adhere to a FSM approach. Beginning with the prealternate molt stage, we discuss, in sequence, vernal migration, breeding, prebasic molt, autumnal migration, and winter stages. The emphasis is on hormone–behavior interactions and, where possible, attention to the development, mature capability, and termination phases are included. Obviously some stages are more complex than others, and we know a great deal about some and much less about others. Finally, we cover the responses to unpredictable events and the expression of the emergency LHS.

II. PREALTERNATE MOLT

A. A True Life History Stage?

Many, but not all, avian species molt at least part of their plumage in late winter and early spring. This has been termed a prealternate molt by Humphrey and Parkes (1959). Note this is distinct from the prebasic molt that usually occurs after breeding (see later). In prealternate molt, selected feathers such as contour feathers and a few rectrices, or in some species the entire plumage, may be replaced prior to the onset of the migration and breeding LHSs. In some species there is no change in color pattern during this molt, whereas others may develop a bright nuptial plumage influenced to varying degrees by reproductive hormones (Witschi, 1961; Owens and Short, 1995). There is still some confusion about whether prealternate molt is indeed a true LHS. In those species in which the molt does not involve any reproductive context, it may be a distinct LHS. For those that develop a nuptial plumage, prealternate molt could be included in the development phase of the breeding LHS along with other secondary sex characters. The intriguing possibility now arises that the prealternate molt that is independent of the breeding LHS may be an entirely different phenomenon from the prealternate molt that gives rise to a nuptial plumage. Further studies taking into account the FSM approach might resolve this issue and point toward possible mechanisms. Bearing this in mind, we discuss all types of prealternate molt in this section. It should also be pointed out that this molt and its control are very poorly understood (Wingfield and Farner, 1980). For example, we know nothing about the development phase and even the onset and termination of the molt itself remains enigmatic. Nevertheless, the literature available is very provocative, indicating a potentially rich area for research with the techniques available. Furthermore, it must be emphasized that the plumages developed in this molt are essential for behavioral traits expressed in later LHSs.

B. Prealternate Molt, Development of Nuptial Plumages, and Their Hormonal Control

Species differences in plumage patterns can be classified roughly into two types—those that show seasonal variation in plumage and other external appendages, and those that do not. The number of species that undergo a seasonal change is only approximately 25% of all those breeding at north temperate latitudes, and the plumages developed are very diverse. Often external secondary characters are restricted to males, although in some cases the female may develop a nuptial plumage that is duller than that of the male but brighter than the nonbreeding (or basic; Humphrey and Parkes, 1959) plumage (e.g., the ruff, *Philomachus pugnax*). In a few cases, both sexes may show a seasonal change, with the female attaining a brighter plumage than the male (e.g., in *Phalaropus* sp.). On the other hand, some species show a seasonal change in plumage and other external appendages that is of equal intensity in both sexes (i.e., a seasonal change but no dimorphism, as in many Charadriiformes, Gaviiformes, and Podicipediformes). Thus we can, for purposes of discussing hormonal control mechanisms, classify avian plumages including other external appendages into four categories:

1. No seasonal change and monomorphic
2. No seasonal change and dimorphic
3. Seasonal change and monomorphic
4. Seasonal change and dimorphic

The majority of avian species fall in categories 1 and 2, showing no seasonal change in plumage. In many instances, however, the juvenile plumage is distinct and adult plumage is attained during an ontogenetic molt. Plumage pattern does not change in further molts (Humphrey and Parkes, 1959). In cases 1 and 2 a prealternate molt, if it occurs, is a distinct LHS. Species that fall in categories 3 and 4 also have juvenile plumages that are different from both breeding and nonbreeding plumages of the adult. In these cases, the postjuvenile molt is ontogenetic and not repeated, whereas the molt into nuptial plumage may be part of the development phase of the breeding LHS and distinct from a true prealternate LHS in categories 1 and 2. It should also be noted that many avian taxa show changes in color and size of other components of the integument that include wattles, combs, and brightly colored patches of skin mostly on the head, eye rings, beak, and legs. These have long been known to be regulated by sex steroid hormones (Witschi, 1961; Owens and Short, 1995) and are clearly part of the development phase of the breeding LHS. Although the idea of different types of prealternate molt has not been tested, we next discuss the disparate and very sparse literature within this framework. This subject has also been reviewed by Owens and Short (1995), although their emphasis is more on the diversity of hormonal regulation of nuptial plumage and secondary sex characters rather than on prealternate molt itself.

1. Species Showing No Seasonal Change

In those species that show no seasonal change in plumages (categories 1 and 2), it appears that plumage color and pattern may be relatively independent of

TABLE 1
Effects of Castration and Testosterone on Secondary Sex Characters; Prealternate Molt; and Color of Beak, Legs, Eye Ring, and Iris in Adult Male White-Crowned Sparrows (*Zonotrichia leucophrys gambelii*)[a]

	T plasma level (ng/ml)	LH plasma level (ng/ml)	Length of cloacal protuberance (mm)	Diameter of vas deferens (mm)
Castrate + empty implant	0.23	10.0	2.8	0.1
	$\bar{n}$*** 0.09	$\bar{n}$*** 1.3	$\bar{n}$** 0.37	$\bar{n}$* 0.0
Castrate + T implant	7.83	0.75	6.8	0.52
	$\bar{n}$ 0.50	$\bar{n}$ 0.14	$\bar{n}$ 1.0	$\bar{n}$ 0.12

	Prealternate molt	Color of beak	Color of leg	Color of eye ring	Color of iris
Castrate + empty implant	Molt completed in 30 days	Orange, brown tip	Brown/orange	Gray	Brown
Castrate + T implant	No molt	Orange, brown tip	Orange	Gray	Brown

[a] N = 5 in all cases. * indicates $p < 0.05$; ** indicates $p = 0.005$; *** indicates $p < 0.001$ (Mann-Whitney U test, 2-tailed, castrate with empty implant vs castrate with T implant). LH, luteinizing hormone; $\bar{n}$, standard errors; T, Testosterone.
From J. C. Wingfield and D. S. Farner (unpublished).

hormonal control, at least in the adult, although the timing probably does involve endocrine regulation (see later). Lofts and Murton (1973) have suggested that in these cases plumage coloration develops on a purely genetic basis and cannot be altered further by hormonal treatment. For example, castration had no effect on the plumage color of monomorphic species such as the blue jay (*Cyanocitta cristata*; C. G. Danforth, cited in Witschi, 1961). Castration followed by testosterone treatment had no effect on the plumage or color of the legs, beak, and eye ring of white-crowned sparrows (see Table 1) or song sparrows (J. C. Wingfield, unpublished).

In the sexually dimorphic bullfinch (*Pyrrhula pyrrhula*) and chaffinch (*Fringilla coelebs*) males have much brighter plumage than females. Their plumage was also not affected by castration (Novikov, 1936, 1937). Furthermore, sex steroid hormone treatment had no effect even though estrogen resulted in the development of the oviduct in female bullfinches (Novikov, 1936). In the house sparrow (*Passer domesticus*) females always have drab brown and gray plumage, and the male, although variable, is always distinct with chestnut and gray plumage on the back and head and a prominent black chin and upper breast. This plumage difference cannot be altered by gonadectomy (Keck, 1934), although it should be noted that this species does show a marked seasonal change in beak color that is hormone dependent (see later). In the American robin (*Turdus migratorius*) the male is more brightly colored than the female, although both have varying degrees of red color on the breast feathers. When skin from a robin embryo was grafted onto the embryo of a chicken, colored feathers typical of the robin developed in the host (Rawles, 1939). Apparently melanoblasts migrated from the grafted tissue into the feather germs of the developing host (Ralph, 1969) and were unaffected by the host's hormonal milieu.

Further evidence for the genetic control of plumage color and patterns comes from Le Douarin *et al.* (1984), who transplanted neural primordia from quail embryos into chick embryos. The resulting chimeras had a chicken body but the pigmentation typical of the quail on the back and wings. Thus, whether dimorphic or not, the color and pattern of the plumage may be genetically determined and independent of hormonal control, although it is possible that hormones could have an effect during ontogeny in some cases (and in other vertebrates; Thompson and Moore, 1992). Such generalizations should be made with caution, however, because in at least one dimorphic species that shows no seasonal change, the house finch (*Carpodacus mexicanus*) castration did result in reversion to drab female plumage, whereas controls retained bright red feathers on the head, neck, and breast. In addition, injection of estradiol into intact males resulted in the regeneration of female plumage (Tewary and Farner, 1973). A similar situation exists in the domestic chicken, which generally shows no seasonal change in adult plumage and other external appendages. The castration of young cockerels completely suppresses development of the comb and wattles (Witschi, 1961). Curiously, gonadectomy can result in male-type plumage in the female, and hen plumage (shape and color pattern) is stimulated by estradiol (Witschi, 1961).

2. Species Showing a Seasonal Change

All species studied that display some seasonal change in plumage pattern reveal the hormonal dependence of the changing character. The mechanisms involved, however, are complex. For those species in which both sexes undergo the same change in plumage and other parts of the integument, it appears that testosterone is involved in males and females. For example, in the European starling (*Sturnus vulgaris*) the bills of both sexes are black in nonbreeding plumage and turn bright yellow when breeding, although females attain full color approximately 1 full month later than males. Gonadectomy in both sexes leads to permanently black bills, whereas testosterone administration results in a rapid transition to yellow, starting at the base of the bill and progressing to the tip. Testosterone is also effective in inducing the yellow color in females; progesterone, deoxycorticosterone, and estradiol are without effect (Witschi, 1961). Measurements of circulating levels of testosterone during the bill color change do not, however, always support the experimental evidence. In captive European starlings (Chase, 1982), plasma levels of testosterone are basal while the yellow color is being developed. However, in free-living males, development of the yellow beak is correlated with a slight elevation of testosterone, but the level is still only one-tenth to one-twentieth the maximal levels attained later in the spring (Ball and Wingfield, 1987; Dawson, 1983). Thus pigmentation of the beak is sensitive to very low levels of testosterone, in some cases below the sensitivity of the assay systems employed. In females, plasma levels of testosterone are basal during development of yellow pigment in the beak (Ball and Wingfield, 1987), although it is possible that a metabolite such as 5α-dihydrotestosterione (DHT) may fulfill such a role. Clearly this problem needs more investigation. It should also be noted that because the amount of testosterone required to induce a change in beak color is so low, the degree of yellow coloration should not be used as an indicator of circulating testosterone level.

In the black-headed gull (*Larus ridibundus*) and the laughing gull (*L. atricilla*) both sexes develop dark brown or black plumage on the head, and the eye ring, beak, and legs become bright red just prior to the breeding season. This transformation is abolished in gonadectomized males and females and can be induced by transplants of testicular fragments or by injection of testosterone (van Oordt and Junge, 1930, 1933; Noble and Wurm, 1940). At least in the laughing gull, estradiol is without effect (Noble and Wurm, 1940). In the herring gull, premature development of adult beak color and plumage were induced by androgen treatment; estradiol was without effect (Boss, 1943; Boss and Witschi, 1941). Similarly in the black-headed gull, implants of testosterone into chicks induced premature darkening of the head plumage and precocial development of long call vocalizations (Groothuis and Meeuwissen, 1992). In the American coot (*Fulica americana*) both males and females have a fleshy frontal shield on the forehead above the upper mandible that is white with a reddish-brown callus at the tip. This shield enlarges in both sexes during late winter and early spring and appears to be used in agonistic interactions over territory. The administration of testosterone accelerates development of this shield in both males and females. In males, development of the shield is correlated with the proliferation of Leydig cells in the testis, although no such correlation was noted with ovarian follicular development in females. Estradiol was generally without effect, but sample sizes were low (Gullion, 1951). This effect was confirmed in the closely related European coot (*F. atra*) by Eens *et al.* (2000). Many other examples are given in Witschi (1961).

As previously indicated, species that show pronounced sexual dimorphism and a seasonal transition in plumage, or other characters of the integument, also show the hormonal dependence of these changes. In the house sparrow, plumage is dimorphic, shows no great seasonal change, and is independent of hormonal control (Witschi, 1961), although the size of the black bib may be influenced by testosterone (Evans *et al.*, 2000). However, in males the beak is pale-buff- or ivory-colored in the nonbreeding season and becomes completely black before onset of breeding. Injections of testosterone induce rapid darkening of the bill to jet black (Keck, 1934; Haase, 1975). Females also show a testosterone-dependent darkening of the beak to varying degrees, although it is never as black as in the male (Keck, 1934). Lofts *et al.* (1973), on the other hand, could find no effect of testosterone alone on beak pigmentation in male house sparrows treated on short winter-like days. They found that a combination of testosterone and LH or LH and follicle-stimulating hormone (FSH) were required to induce an effect at this time. Although gonadotropins may be necessary for the full effect of testosterone on blackening of the beak, it is clear that testosterone is itself the major factor. This is supported by the findings of Donham *et al.* (1982), Evans *et al.* (2000), and Hegner and Wingfield (1990) that development of the black beak in photostimulated males correlates with increasing titers of testosterone in blood. Note that plasma levels are low at this time and similar to those in European starlings during development of the yellow color of the beak. These data again emphasize that changes in plumage patterns and other integumentary structures are sensitive to very low levels of testosterone, one-tenth to one-twentieth of peak breeding levels.

Changes in external secondary sex characters have been demonstrated to be dependent on gonadal hormones in several other species that show sexual dimorphism. In the ruff there is a dramatic seasonal change not only in color, but also elongation of pectoral feathers to form the ruff used in agonistic displays with other males at the lek (a natural arena in which males display and compete for matings with females). Castration in early winter abolishes these changes (van Oordt and Junge, 1936). Implants of testosterone into female ruffs (called reeves) not only resulted in male-like nuptial ruffs, but also activated two types of breeding behavior typical of males but not females (Lank *et al.*, 1999). In winter, the male plumage is similar to that of the reeve, although the male is considerably larger than the female. Testosterone implants in reeves also induced a prebreeding rise in body weight typical of males. Thus, the polymorphisms in male reproductive behavior, breeding plumage, and body-size dimorphism appear to be testosterone-dependent. Furthermore, the effects of testosterone on male-like behavior in reeves supports an autosomal model of inheritance (the traits occurred in testosterone-treated reeves in the same rates as in males) rather than a sex-linked model. The effects of testosterone were also reversible, and reeves bred normally in subsequent seasons (Lank *et al.*, 1998).

3. Polyandrous Species

It is pertinent here to consider the hormonal control of bright nuptial plumage in the polyandrous phalaropes, in which females are brighter than males. Injection of testosterone into male and female Wilson's phalaropes (*Steganopus tricolor*) and northern phalaropes (*Lobipes lobatus*) resulted in regeneration of bright nuptial plumage in plucked areas of both species. Estradiol and prolactin alone, or in combination, were without effect (Johns, 1964). The biosynthesis of testosterone by the ovary of the Wilson's phalarope is greater than that of the testis (Höhn, 1970; Höhn and Cheng, 1967), and this has led to the hypothesis that in polyandrous species there has been a sex reversal not only of behavior but also of endocrine physiology. However, a high rate of synthesis of testosterone in the ovary does not mean that this steroid is secreted into the peripheral circulation in greater amounts than in the male. Investigations of free-living Wilson's phalaropes indicate that females do not have higher plasma levels of testosterone than males (Fivizzani *et al.*, 1986). In females a vernal increase in plasma levels of testosterone does occur, but not more so than in females of other nonpolyandrous, species. Also, the literature indicates that it is not unusual for seasonal changes in plumage in females to be controlled by testosterone. Thus it appears that development of bright nuptial plumage in female phalaropes is similar to that in other species that are not polyandrous (see previous discussion) and a simple sex reversal hypothesis is not justified. Perhaps more interesting questions are why males do not develop as bright a nuptial plumage as females and what are the hormonal mechanisms involved? The androgen metabolizing enzyme, 5α-reductase has been shown to be absent in male skin, suggesting that conversion to DHT is important for the development of nuptial plumage and thus males do not respond (Fivizanni *et al.*, 1990).

The concept of patterns of testosterone in females of some species being identical to males has been the subject of debate. Because birds are relatively easy to observe under natural conditions and their natural history is very well known, it is not surprising that we have hormone data from males and females in over thirty species. Wingfield (1994a) formulated a dimorphism index that included differences in body size, plumage pattern, and territorial aggression. In those species in which males and females were similar, patterns of testosterone secretion were identical in males and females. As dimorphism increased, then patterns of testosterone secretion diverged (Wingfield, 1994a; Wingfield et al., 2000). These data suggest there is a rich source of potential research on sexual dimorphism here.

4. Species Undergoing More Than Two Plumage Changes per Year

One of the most complex series of plumages known is that shown by the willow ptarmigan (*Lagopus lagopus lagopus*). There may be as many as four distinct plumages in the male and three in the female (e.g., Stokkan, 1979). The winter plumage of both sexes is white, and in early spring males develop a nuptial plumage in which the head, neck, upper breast, and back become reddish-brown. A red wattle above the eye of the male also increases 100% in size. After mating, a summer plumage in which the body is yellow-brown with dark bars appears; this is very similar to the summer plumage of females. In the autumn, both sexes develop dark-brown and black feathers and finally molt into pure white winter plumage by the end of October. Thus, the male may be in molt almost continuously from March to October!

Photostimulation of captive male Norwegian willow ptarmigan results in rapid molt to the pigmented nuptial plumage. However, castrated males show a much slower molt directly into the summer plumage, similar to that of the female. An experiment in which males held on short day lengths had feathers plucked on the head, back, and breast revealed that intact controls regenerate pure white feathers. Testosterone-treated intact males develop pigmented feathers typical of the nuptial plumage and, curiously, castrated males also develop pigmented feathers, suggesting a possible role for LH. Intact testosterone-treated males showed a 100% increase in comb height, whereas no such development was noted in castrated males (Stokkan, 1979). It is possible that winter, summer, and autumnal plumages (possibly each a separate LHS) of both sexes are genetically based (as an antipredator mechanism) and independent of hormonal control, or at least of the influence of sex steroid hormones. Superimposed on this is the nuptial plumage of the male (possibly resulting from sexual selection) that does appear to be testosterone dependent.

There is evidence in this species that hormones other than androgens can influence plumage color. Experiments on willow ptarmigan in Canada indicated that α-MSH, LH, and FSH induced pigmented plumage in feathers regenerated after plucking (all birds were held on short day lengths). Cholesterol-treated birds (controls) regenerated only white feathers (Höhn and Braun, 1980). α-Melanocortin-stimulating hormone (MSH) was also effective in producing pigmented plumage in the white-tailed ptarmigan (*L. leucurus*), whereas controls grew only white feathers. Höhn and Braun (1980) also found that thyroid-stimulating hormone (TSH) and thyroxine (T_4) were effective in the induction of pigmented feathers, although they point out that sample sizes were small and this effect needs to be confirmed. Note also that thyroid hormones do not appear to influence feather color in the willow ptarmigan (K.-A. Stokkan, personal communication, cited in Höhn and Braun, 1980). Further investigation is required before the significance of control of plumage color by multiple hormones can be understood.

5. Effects of Estradiol on Plumage

Seasonal changes in plumage are not always controlled by androgens. In the mallard (*Anas platyrhynchos*) the male has a bright basic plumage that is attained after a molt in September. However, in mid-summer the body feathers of males molt to produce an eclipse plumage that is similar to the drab cryptic plumage of females. Gonadectomy results in the assumption of a permanent bright male plumage, even in females. Female-like plumage can be induced by injection of estradiol, but not testosterone (Witschi, 1961). Mueller (1976) showed that the skin of male embryos of the mallard can be permanently feminized by exposure to estradiol. However, this experiment is difficult to interpret because adult females develop male plumage if gonadectomized, suggesting no permanent feminization.

Color of the beak may also be affected by estradiol in some species. For example, male and female red-billed queleas (*Quelea quelea*) have blood-red beaks. Female bill color changes to light yellow during breeding, whereas males and castrates never show a change in beak color (Witschi, 1961). It is possible that estrogens may control this change in females, although the appropriate experiments in gonadectomized birds have not been performed.

6. Effects of Luteinizing Hormone on External Secondary Sex Characteristics

In yet other species the situation is even more complicated, and breeding plumage may be dependent on sex steroid hormones and LH. In the paradise whydah (*Vidua (Steganura) paradisea*) castrates show the same seasonal plumage change as intact males, and injections of preparations containing LH induced a darkening of the beak (Witschi, 1961). The reaction of females to this treatment is unknown. Weaver finches of the genus *Euplectes* develop a nuptial plumage that appears to be independent of stimulation by sex steroids (in contrast to beak color; Witschi, 1961). Castrated males develop a normal nuptial plumage and females that normally do not develop such a plumage do so after ovariectomy. Injections of estradiol or testosterone result in development of a female plumage in both males and females. In this case it appears that LH induces nuptial plumage and injection of sex steroids tends to reduce LH levels due to negative feedback, thus resulting in a female plumage. Testosterone, however, mobilizes carotenoids in the liver, and the feathers become suffused with red, but not in the same way as in the intact male (Witschi, 1961), suggesting a synergism of LH and testosterone. Similar indications of LH-dependent nuptial plumage have been demonstrated for the baya weaver (*Ploceus phillipinus*) and the lal munia (*Estrilda amandava*; Thapliyal and Saxena, 1961; Thapliyal and Tewary, 1961), although in the latter species the effect of LH can be blocked by treatment with T_4 (Thapliyal and Gupta, 1984). LH appears to stimulate the synthesis of melanin that then infiltrates the feather papillae (see also Ralph *et al.*, 1967a,b). This action has been used as a bioassay for LH. The breast feathers of weaver finches are plucked, and the finches are then treated with various doses of LH. As the feathers regenerate, the degree of black pigment is an indication of the amount of LH injected (Witschi, 1961). Similar effects can be shown for the yellow pigmentation of feathers in the baya weaver (Thapliyal and Saxena, 1961).

7. Is There a Relationship between Hormonal Control and Plumage Type?

From the diverse investigations summarized so far, it is clear that the control of plumage color pattern in birds is complex; although several species have been investigated, it is not possible to come to any firm generalizations (see also Owens and Short, 1995). However, it is perhaps of heuristic value to speculate that in those species that show no sexual dimorphism and no seasonal change plumage and other external characters are largely hormonally independent, at least in the adult. This may also be true of sexually dimorphic species in which there is also no seasonal change, although there is one notable exception, the house finch (Tewary and Farner, 1973). On the other hand, in all species that undergo a seasonal development of external secondary sex characters, whether dimorphic or not, these changes are hormone dependent, at least in all species studied. The control of such seasonal changes is, however, complex and may involve a testosterone-dependent male nuptial plumage with the female plumage being basic or an estradiol-dependent female plumage with the bright male plumage basic. In yet others, nuptial plumage is apparently dependent on LH, possibly in synergy with sex steroid hormones.

At least one investigation has suggested that the determination of adult plumage in sexually dimorphic species is partly genetic and partly hormonal. In the ring-necked pheasant (*Phasianus colchicus*) and the Reeve's pheasant (*Syrmaticus reevesi*) transplants of male skin to female and vice versa produce an intermediate plumage in the graft. Also, injections of both androgens and estrogens have a partially feminizing effect on feather pattern (Danforth, 1937) This array of possible hormonal mechanisms, intermingled with genetic effects, is bewildering in its diversity even though only a small fraction of the 9000 or so species have been studied. It should be noted, however, that many of these investigations were conducted in the 1970s and before, when hormone preparations were known to be less pure. Further research incorporating modern techniques would be highly desirable for this fascinating field.

C. Timing Mechanisms

Internal secondary sex characters and external appendages such as wattles and combs develop in parallel with gonadal recrudescence and are largely sex steroid dependent. In these cases, seasonal development is regulated by initial predictive information as part of the breeding LHS. Changes in plumage are usually only achieved during a molt in which the old feathers are shed and the nuptial plumage develop in their place (although in a few species the erosion of feathers can result in a color pattern change independent of molt). The prealternate molt involves a change in only the body (contour) feathers, although in some species the central tail feathers (rectrices) may also be replaced. The rest of the rectrices and also the primaries are not molted at this time (Stresemann and Stresemann, 1966), although one exception is the sharp-tailed sparrow (*Ammospiza caudacuta*) which undergoes a complete molt in spring (Humphrey and Parkes, 1959). It is also possible that prealternate molt in the absence of any seasonal change in plumage pattern may be a separate LHS, whereas molt to a nuptial plumage is part of the breeding LHS and controlled entirely differently (see previous discussion).

The prealternate molt is completed well before onset of the breeding season. Species in which an immature plumage is maintained during the nonbreeding period also undergo a prealternate type molt into adult plumage (e.g., sparrows of the genus *Zonotrichia*; Blanchard, 1941; Blanchard and Erickson, 1949; Michener and Michener, 1943). Generally this molt occurs well in advance of the breeding season and, in migratory species, before vernal migration because the energetic requirements of molt and migration are incompatible. Although in a few species the prealternate molt has been well described, its regulation has been less well studied. This may be due to difficulties in quantifying the progression of the molt because generally only the body feathers are replaced. However, despite the paucity of information, it does appear that mechanisms inducing the onset of prealternate molt include exposure to the lengthening days of spring in indigo buntings (*Passerina cyanea*; Emlen, 1969), white-crowned sparrows (Farner and Mewaldt, 1955), and white-throated sparrows (*Zonotrichia albicollis*; Lesher and Kendeigh, 1941).

The timing and duration of the molt can be variable. In Gambel's white-crowned sparrow, the prealternate molt begins earlier in the more southerly wintering populations, and moving north the molt begins later, is shorter in duration, and is more synchronized in timing among the members of the local population (Mewaldt and King, 1978). In the coastal populations of white-crowned sparrow (*Z. l. nuttalli* and *Z. l. pugetensis*) prealternate molt is also variable, with northern populations showing a heavy molt and more southerly birds showing only a moderate molt or, in some individuals, no molt at all (Mewaldt *et al.*, 1968). Thus, it appears that day length can also act as initial predictive information to time prealternate molt, but other factors such as temperature (changing with latitude) may provide supplementary information to slow down or accelerate the progression. Clearly, more experimental evidence is required before any conclusions on the regulation of prealternate molt in north temperate birds can be made.

Onset of prealternate molt is not affected by castration, although its duration may be lengthened (Morton and Mewaldt, 1962; Mattocks, 1976). Administration of testosterone can arrest the molt or even prevent it entirely (see Table 1). In immature *Z. l. gambelii* exposed to long days in the laboratory, gonadal development is so rapid that testosterone levels in the blood increase and block the prealternate molt (Mattocks, 1976; J. C. Wingfield, unpublished; Table 1). In these cases, it is possible to have birds that are sexually mature but in immature plumage. In other species, especially transequatorial migrants and those that winter in tropical regions, a role for endogenous circannual rhythms has been postulated (see Gwinner, 1977a, 1981b, 1986). In the yellow wagtail (*Motacilla flava*; Curry-Lindahl, 1958; Marshall and Williams, 1959) and old world warblers of the genera *Phylloscopus,* and *Sylvia* (e.g., Gwinner, 1977b) that winter in equatorial regions where day length is less useful as initial predictive information, prealternate molt occurs in mid-winter.

In these cases, endogenous rhythms play an important role in timing of the molt. However, day length may also play a role because in the willow warbler (*P. trochilus*) that winters deep in the tropics, the transfer of captive individuals held on winter-like day lengths to long days accelerates the prealternate molt (Gwinner, 1971, 1972).

Species that live at mid-latitudes may also have an endogenous component involved in the timing of prealternate molt. In the dark-eyed junco (*Junco hyemalis*) and the white-throated sparrow held on a short day of 9 hours light: 15 hours dark (9L:15D) for 18 months showed initiation of prealternate molt at the normal time in the first and second years of short-day treatment. However, this molt was greatly protracted and incomplete (Weise, 1962). Finally, it should be pointed out that development of a nuptial plumage does not always require a molt. In the house sparrow, prebasic molt (a LHS that occurs after breeding) (Humphrey and Parkes, 1959) results in a plumage in which the black feathers of the chin and upper breast of the male are tipped with gray and buff, thus reducing the intensity of the black nuptial gorget. However, as the winter progresses, the buff and gray tips are eroded, thus exposing the jet-black plumage underneath. So here we have a case of full nuptial plumage being attained by abrasion rather than by a molt (Newton, 1973; Palmer, 1972; Summers-Smith, 1963). Similar mechanisms occur in the snow bunting (*Plectrophenax nivalis*) in which the winter plumage is white with brown patches and flecks on the head, flanks, and rump. The normally black back is also streaked with brown. As the winter progresses, these brown tips to the contour feathers become abraded revealing the striking white and black nuptial plumage (Amadon, 1966). The iridescent breeding plumage of the starling also appears to be acquired by erosion of the duller distal portions of contour feathers (Amadon, 1966).

There is clearly enormous diversity in the control mechanisms for prealternate molt and the associated changes of the integument in spring. It is intriguing that the tissues involved appear to show almost limitless plasticity, and their sensitivity to reproductive hormones appears to have evolved multiple times. Despite this diversity, the class Aves may be a relatively monophyletic group. As such, birds provide many exciting possibilities for further studies of control mechanisms at the cell and molecular levels.

III. VERNAL MIGRATION

In a seasonally changing environment, temperature and food availability increase or decrease over time at a particular geographic location or habitat. In this situation, individuals in a population migrate to take advantage of seasonally abundant resources in environments that are hostile for much of the rest of the year (Gauthreux, 1982)—if an individual cannot withstand a period of unfavorable conditions during the seasonal changes in the environment, it must change localities to survive. The behavioral components involved in the changing of localities are termed migration, generally defined precisely (e.g., Farner, 1955) as the annual movement of the members of a species or a population between discrete breeding and wintering (or nonbreeding) areas. There are two distinct periods of migration, each a separate LHS. Vernal migration refers to the movement toward a breeding area; autumnal migration is the opposite. FSM theory suggests that although vernal and autumnal migrations may appear similar as far as behaviors go, the mechanisms may be different. That is, same distance may be covered but different strategies are used (O'Reilly and Wingfield, 1995; Wingfield and Jacobs, 1999).

In late winter and early spring, many populations of birds breeding at higher latitudes begin a migration from the wintering grounds to breeding areas. This phenomenon has fascinated humans for millennia, but the control mechanisms remain largely unknown. Some migrations are intercontinental, whereas others may be short distances and altitudinal. The whole process requires a development phase in which migratory capability is obtained. This includes muscle hypertrophy, deposition of fuel reserves (fat), and the modification of other organs such as the gut to minimize weight carried while in flight (Piersma, 1998). The vernal migration LHS can partially overlap the prealternate molt and breeding LHSs, but migration must be terminated before onset of breeding can occur (see Wingfield and Jacobs, 1999).

A. Migration Strategies Prebreeding

The mechanisms controlling migration probably evolved many times (see also Dorst, 1955; Schüz, 1971; Dolnik, 1975). In northern areas, as many as 61% of avian species that breed in temperate regions are migratory and about another 6% generally can disperse at irregular intervals in all directions, such as in the western Palaearctic. In North America, approximately 72% of the species are migrants and about 8% tend to disperse. Of all animal behaviors, the phenomenon of migration has probably received more attention over many hundreds of years than any other behavioral trait. Much has been written on the control of orientation and navigation as birds are migrating or homing, but this topic is beyond the scope of this review. In general, migration is thought to be under photoperiodic control. Almost all migrations observed among bird species are classical south–north movements or, in the southern hemisphere, north–south, with the breeding area being at the higher latitude and the wintering area at lower latitude. In some cases, there are longitudinal migrations east–west especially on the edge of continents where some species winter along the milder coasts and breed in the interior, but leave before the more severe climate inland gives way to winter. In other cases, altitudinal migrations exist in which species that breed above the timberline in high mountain ranges generally winter at lower altitudes. Thus, there is a full spectrum from short-distance migrations of just a few kilometers in the case of altitudinal migration to vast distances covered by some seabirds from the Arctic Ocean coast to the Antarctic and back again the following spring.

Migration has a high-energy requirement; there is an accumulation of fat in specific adipose tissue organs (see Farner, 1985; King, 1972; Berthold, 1977; Dolnik, 1975, 1976). There appears to be a programmed hyperphagia resulting in an increase in fat in most species studied. Fat is an ideal storage medium because of the high caloric yield and water produced by hydrolysis. For species that make long uninterrupted flights over ocean or deserts, the initial fat reserve may be as much as 50% body weight (Biebach, 1990). Migration over land or the ocean in some seabirds is often interrupted at intervals for the replenishment of stores. After migration is terminated, the hyperphagia seen in most species tends to be reduced to a lower level and fat stores are reduced. The development of fat in the adipose tissue sites and the accompanying hyperphagia are prerequisites for premigratory behavior (Ramenofsky, 1990). This state is called zugdisposition (Farner, 1955; Putzig, 1939).

B. Hormone Control Mechanisms in Vernal Migration

Vernal migration occurs prior to, and may also overlap the development phase of, the breeding LHS when gonadal development and increased secretion of reproductive hormones occur. In contrast, autumnal migratory behavior occurs after the reproductive season has been terminated and the gonads have regressed to a completely inactive state. Thus, autumnal migration occurs at a time when reproductive hormones are basal. It is possible that the factors timing and controlling the temporal sequence of events during the two migratory LHSs are distinct, even though both migrations require hyperphagic states, deposition of fat, and long-distance flights. The endocrine mechanisms by which these migrations may be regulated has been reviewed extensively by Wingfield et al. (1990a).

Circannual rhythms of migration and the application of internal periodic time-measuring processes were first postulated particularly for bird species that live at least part of the year in environments deficient in reliable seasonal variations (e.g., Gwinner, 1971, 1977a,b). Many permanent inhabitants of the tropics and migratory species that breed at high latitudes and winter close to the equator fall into this category. For example, the willow warbler (*Phylloscopus trochilus*) winters in equatorial areas where photoperiod is essentially constant and provides no cue when to start premigratory hyperphagia, fattening, and migration. However, each year these phenomena occur at exactly the same time. Willow warblers held in captivity on 12L:12D show strong evidence for rhythms and migratory fattening and restlessness. The free-running period of these migratory episodes is somewhat less than a year, and thus are termed circannual. Endogenous control mechanisms for the willow warbler appear to be more rigid than those for the chiffchaff (*P. collybita*), garden warbler (*Sylvia borin*), black-cap (*S. atricapilla*), and others that tend to overwinter at more northerly latitudes (Gwinner, 1971; Berthold et al., 1972). Circannual rhythms are synchronized by environmental cues called zeitgebers, such as the annual cycle and photoperiod. It is possible that changes in day length on the breeding ground are sufficient to entrain the circannual rhythm for a single year. Evidence shows that the different degrees of migratory distance and directions (including changes in direction en route) are genetically determined (Berthold, 1999).

In other species, especially those that winter at mid- to low latitudes, the increase in long days of spring induces vernal hyperphagia, migratory fattening, and migratory behavior itself (e.g., Farner and Lewis, 1971; Dolnik, 1975; Wingfield and Farner, 1980; Farner and Gwinner, 1980). In the white-crowned sparrow, soon after the completion of the prealternate molt, there begins a phase of photoperiodically induced hyperphagia that results in deposition of fat stores before and during migration (e.g., King et al., 1963). There is also an increase in the hematocrit at this time (see Wingfield and Farner, 1980). This phase requires the massive mobilization of energy reserves during prolonged flights and the increase in the oxygen-carrying capacity of the blood seems clearly adaptive.

A number of papers published in the 1940s implicated a role for thyroid hormones in the regulation of vernal migration (see Wingfield et al., 1990a). In white-crowned sparrows T_4 levels increase in April at the height of vernal migration, whereas there is no change in T_4 during spring in the sedentary house sparrow (*Passer domesticus*; Smith, 1982). In the migratory Canada goose (*Branta canadensis*) T_4 levels are lowest in postmigratory periods in autumn and highest in the vernal postmigratory period. Plasma levels of triiodothyronine (T_3), on the other hand, are maximal during spring migration (John and George, 1978). More detailed investigations of the red-headed bunting (*Emberiza bruniceps*) show an increase in the T_3 to T_4 ratio prior to vernal migration (Chandola and Pathak, 1980). Thyroidectomy decreased the migratory disposition (Pathak and Chandola, 1982a). Apparently T_3 may be the important hormone regulating migratory behavior in this species. In addition, there appears to be an increase in the activity of mondeiodinase that catalyzes the conversion of T_3 to T_4 during migration. The pharmacological blockade of this enzyme significantly decrease premigratory fattening (Pathak and Chandola, 1982b).

There is evidence that the role of thyroid hormones on migration may be associated with growth hormone. Thyrotrophin-releasing factor (TRF) increases the plasma levels of T_4 within 20 minutes of injection in the snow goose (*Chen caerulescens*) and TSH injections are effective within 15 minutes. Generally, increases in circulating T_3 lag behind those of T_4 (Campbell and Leatherland, 1979). However, TRF also results in an elevation of growth hormone (Pethes et al., 1979; Harvey et al., 1978).

It has been suggested that corticosterone and prolactin may synergize in the control of not only migratory distance, but also fattening and premigratory hyperphagia. The phase relationship of two circadian rhythms, plasma levels of corticosterone and prolactin vary as a function of day length or an endogenous circannual rhythm. The phase angle between these two rhythms, one usually associated with dawn, the other with dusk, determines the migratory direction and fattening vs no-fattening responses. Whether the temporal synergism of corticosterone or prolactin rhythms controls migration and other events in the annual cycle of a wide variety of species remains to be determined (Meier and Ferrell, 1978; Meier et al., 1980).

Although this hypothesis has been criticized (see Farner and Gwinner, 1980; Follett, 1984; Rankin, 1991), there is considerable evidence that adrenocortical secretions may influence migration. Péczely (1976) has presented extensive correlative evidence for a relationship between adrenocortical activity and migration. He measured corticosteroid production *in vitro* using adrenal glands collected from several species in the field. In nonmigrants such as the house sparrow, yellowhammer (*Fringilla citrinella*), linnet (*Carduelis cannabina*), and great tit (*Parus major*), corticosterone production is lowest in spring and highest during the summer, including the postbreeding period. In migratory species such as the stonechat (*Saxicola torquata rubicola*), white-throat (*Sylvia curruca*), redbacked shrike (*Lanius colurio*), and brambling (*Fringilla montifringilla*), corticosterone production is highest during the vernal migratory period. Evidence in migratory shore birds suggests that corticosterone levels in blood are high during flight and may be involved in the mobilization of energy, as opposed to the storage of fat during the hyperphagic period (O'Reilly and Wingfield, 1995; Ramenofsky *et al.*, 1995; Piersma and Ramenofsky, 1998; Piersma *et al.*, 2000). Given these correlations, it is of great interest to explore the seemingly complex relationship of corticosterone and other hormones such as T_3, T_4, and growth hormone with migration.

C. Substages of Fat Deposition, Fat Use, and Flight—Fluctuating Extremes of Migration

Hyperphagia increases with no change in energy expended, thus resulting in fat deposition. This state may persist so that fat reserves are replenished rapidly during stopover periods (King, 1961). Substages of the vernal migration LHS include hyperphagia and fat storage, followed by its mobilization for long flights—that is, fluctuating extremes of metabolism with dramatic switches from anabolism to catabolism (O'Reilly and Wingfield, 1995; Ramenofsky, 1990). There is great potential here for endocrine studies of control mechanisms but, the field is small and very little is known.

Migration has initial predictive and supplementary timing to initiate migration itself and to terminate the migratory period. For the immediate release or integration of migratory behavior, especially switches of substages involving hyperphagia and migratory flight, the birds must be in zugdisposition (mature capability phase of the vernal migration LHS). The increase in temperature in spring has been postulated as a major trigger of migratory activity (Schüz, 1952). The increase in temperature also enhances zugunruhe (migratory restlessness) in the white-crowned sparrow (Farner and Mewaldt, 1953). Bad weather may slow migration by decreasing food intake and zugunruhe. Evans (1970) emphasizes the role of initial predictive information in vernal migration; then supplementary factors that include food and weather advance or retard the onset of migratory activity. Also, temperature or wind velocity may affect short-term behavior en route.

It is well known that many hormones such as insulin, glucagon, epinephrine, and prolactin can affect energy balance and fat deposition, and these have been reviewed in relation to migration (Ramenofsky, 1990; Wingfield *et al.*, 1990a). Several experiments in which peptides were injected directly into the third ventricle of the white-crowned sparrow brain (Richardson and Boswell, 1993) showed marked effects on food intake. Neuropeptide Y and endorphin increased food intake in male white-crowned sparrows (Richardson *et al.*, 1995; Maney and Wingfield, 1998a), whereas cholecystokinin and corticotropin-releasing hormone (CRH) decreased it (Richardson *et al.*, 1993, 2000; Maney and Wingfield, 1998a). Food intake could also be altered by manipulating metabolic fuels, and responses to hormones also changed with day length (Boswell *et al.*, 1995; Richardson *et al.*, 1995). The relation this may have to migration in spring remains unclear.

D. Role of Testosterone in Control of Vernal Fattening and Zugunruhe

Both the premigratory hyperphagia and deposition of fat, as well as the increase in hematocrit, appear to be under the influence of gonadal hormones, at least during vernal migration (Weise, 1967; Wingfield *et al.*, 1990a). It was assumed that estradiol and androgens had identical functions in females and males, respectively (Farner, 1955; Berthold, 1977). However, ovariectomy abolishes vernal migratory behavior and can be reinstated by implants of small quantities of androgen (Schwabl and Farner, 1989a). Estradiol was without effect, although the blockade of the enzyme aromatase (that coverts androgen precursor to estradiol) did decrease migratory restlessness (Schwabl and Farner, 1989a). Furthermore, it is known that female white-crowned sparrow and other species have transient increases in testosterone and DHT just before or just at the onset of premigratory hyperphagia (see Wingfield and Farner, 1978a,b, 1980).

Castrated male white-crowned sparrows and bramblings show delayed or abolished onset of zugunruhe for at least 2 weeks. If it does occur, it is usually of shorter duration and less intense than in intact controls (Morton and Mewaldt, 1962; Weise, 1967; Lofts and Marshall, 1960; Wingfield *et al.*, 1990). Yokoyama (1976) was able to induce zugunruhe in male white-crowned sparrows with injections of prolactin and testosterone, suggesting that testosterone may be involved in the intensity of zugunruhe, but that its onset is triggered by other mechanisms. There has been much controversy as to whether castration affected vernal migration. Weise (1967) pointed out that in some studies using castrated migratory birds, the operations had all been performed in late winter or early spring. This is well before the normal migratory season, but after the onset of lengthening days. Therefore those birds had all been exposed to some photoperiodic stimulation before the experiments began. Over three seasons, Weise took white-throated sparrows from natural day lengths of approximately 9.5 hours light in mid-December into artificial daily photoperiods of 9L:15D and held the birds there for several weeks. Nine males were castrated and after 3–5 more weeks of short photoperiods they were exposed to stimulatory periods of 15L:9D. Twelve control birds and nine other attempted castrates with testicular regeneration were in adjacent cages. Throughout the 12 weeks of long-day photostimulation the castrates demonstrated only a slight trace of extensive zugunruhe shown by the intact and regenerated groups. Further, these castrates showed no rapid fat deposition in the manner of photostimulated birds or of spring migrants under outdoor conditions.

Stetson and Erickson (1971) confirmed and extended these results for white-crowned sparrows. This very strongly suggests that the gonads, presumably via sex hormones, must have an essential role in these functions. Mattocks (1976), in a detailed study on the effects of castration on migration and fattening in the white-crowned sparrow, showed that in birds castrated before the winter solstice the vernal migratory hyperphagia was completely eliminated and zugunruhe was greatly diminished in castrated males. Plasma levels of testosterone were undetectable and corticosterone was present only at a low level. However, implants of small quantities of testosterone for a limited time in February reinstated zugunruhe and fattening to varying degrees in the spring, at the same time as those of intact birds. Similar data have been obtained for female white-crowned sparrows by Schwabl and Farner (1989a). These fascinating data suggest that although testosterone is involved in the regulation of hyperphagia, fattening, and zugunruhe in spring, it acts early enough not to be part of the breeding LHS per se. Even a 2-week exposure to testosterone treatment in February was sufficient to reinstate full migratory capability 2.5 months later (Mattocks, 1976; Wingfield et al., 1990a).

Yokoyama (1976) showed that lesions of the posterior or entire median eminence decreased photoperiodically induced testicular growth, premigratory fattening, and zugunruhe. The destruction of the anterior median eminence alone had no appreciable effects on fattening or zugunruhe. Lesions in the basal infundibulum abolished zugunruhe, but allowed varying degrees of fattening. Systemic administration of prolactin, testosterone propionate, or a combination in birds with posterior-median-eminence lesions induced fattening but not zugunruhe. It is possible that testosterone may act by increasing the release of prolactin (see also Yokoyama, 1977). Subcutaneous implants of tesosterone propionate and daily injections of prolactin in birds with median eminence lesions increased food intake and body weight, but did not induce zugunruhe (Yokoyama, 1977). Furthermore, photostimulation through fiber optics inserted in the basal hypothalamus to stimulate encephalic photoreceptors increased zugunruhe even though the ambient photoperiod was only 8 hours (Yokoyama and Farner, 1978).

The factors terminating the vernal migration LHS are unknown (Weise, 1962). The control of the termination of the reproductive periods was thought to be related to increasing levels of sex steroids as spring progresses and as birds approach their breeding grounds. However, experiments on the white-crowned sparrow in captivity show that implants of testosterone do not reduce the duration of zugunruhe and may indirectly prolong it (Schwabl and Farner, 1989b). Thus, the control mechanisms for the termination of spring migration as birds arrive on their breeding grounds remains to be determined.

IV. BREEDING LIFE HISTORY STAGE

Reproductive function in vertebrates has been the subject of extensive research from evolutionary ecology to molecular biology. Nevertheless, we know little about the hormone mechanisms underlying reproductive function in free-living animals and even less about the neural pathways for environmental signals that influence neuroendocrine and endocrine secretions that regulate breeding. There is a vast literature that spans field and laboratory studies in birds, and the reader is referred to Murton and Wetswood (1977), Wingfield and

Kenagy (1991), and Wingfield and Farner (1993) for detailed reviews of the older literature. Here we again take a FSM approach and discuss hormonal mechanisms of development of the breeding LHS, mature capability and actual onset of nesting, and finally termination of breeding. The emphasis is on new promising areas of research and not on an exhaustive review of the literature.

A. Development of Reproductive Function in Ecological Contexts

How and why organisms breed at certain times and not others has fascinated biologists for centuries. What environmental signals do they use to time breeding, and why do some populations have very rigid breeding periods and others show great plasticity? Ecologists and evolutionary biologists have made significant headway at the ultimate (why) level (e.g., Lack, 1968; Perrins, 1970), but physiologists still have much to learn about proximate (how) mechanisms (Follett, 1984; Wingfield and Kenagy, 1991). Since the 1980s, there has been extensive investigation of how one environmental signal, the annual change in day length (photoperiod), regulates seasonal breeding (e.g., Follett, 1984; Gwinner, 1986; Nicholls et al., 1988). However, the degree to which other environmental signals are used to time reproductive development and the onset of breeding, and the neuroendocrine and endocrine mechanisms that orchestrate reproductive function, are by no means fully understood. This is especially true of species that show great plasticity in the timing of onset and duration of breeding seasons (e.g., in wild birds; Silverin, 1994; Silverin and Viebke, 1994; Jacobs, 1996; Hahn et al., 1997; Wingfield et al., 1997a; Jacobs and Wingfield, 2000).

The mathematical treatment of natural history data (Wingfield et al., 1992b, 1993) is useful as a template to investigate how reproductive processes are regulated by the interactions of environmental and social cues in birds. Techniques such as log-linear analysis and information theory can be used to model when, and if, individuals should integrate predictive environmental signals or rely more heavily on one or the other (Wingfield et al. 1992b, 1993). For example, if a future event is highly predictable and restricted in time, then only one reliable environmental cue is needed to trigger the appropriate preparation. Conversely, if a future event is much less predictable, the animal should monitor and respond to more environmental cues to coordinate the precise adjustment of reproductive state with changing environment. Using the predictability of a given habitat, we can calculate an environmental information factor (Ie) (Wingfield et al., 1992b, 1993). This factor reflects the degree to which a species in that habitat is predicted to use available environmental cues to regulate gonadal development and onset of breeding. If the Ie factor is low, individuals should focus on one or very few reliable cues (e.g., photoperiod), whereas a high Ie predicts that individuals should be sensitive to many environmental cues to make appropriate adjustments in their reproductive schedules (Wingfield et al., 1992b, 1993).

Research (e.g., Wingfield et al., 1996, 1997a) has shown this to be a powerful tool. Simple demographic data (e.g., the timing of breeding from egg-laying dates) and field endocrine data provide the bases from which to test these models further. Mechanisms by which the brain transduces such information can then be compared in populations that represent different extremes of responsiveness. The endocrine pathways by which this information is then passed on to specific tissues, and how those tissues respond, can also be investigated.

The photoperiodic control (initial predictive information) of the development phase has received many decades of attention (e.g., Farner and Follett, 1979; Nicholls et al., 1988; Silverin, 1995). However, the integration of supplementary information as well as variations in responsiveness to these specific cues seen among populations has not been well studied (see Wingfield et al., 1992b, 1993). How these cues may influence the phases of ovarian development and the termination of the breeding LHS are even less well known. Photoperiodic regulation of the development phase of reproduction involves increased secretion of chicken gonadotropin-releasing hormone 1 (cGnRH-1), the major GnRH in passerines (Sherwood et al., 1988). This then regulates release of the gonadotropins LH and FSH, which in turn orchestrate gonadal growth and the secretion of sex steroid hormones. The latter then trigger the development of secondary sex characters and reproductive behavior (see Wingfield and Farner,

1993, for a review of wild birds). Increased levels of gonadotropins in blood are accompanied by elevated LHβ-subunit mRNA titers in the anterior pituitary, and a rise in LH and FSH receptors in the testes of *Z. l. gambelii* (Ishii and Farner, 1976; Kubokawa *et al.*, 1994). In females, photoperiodic cues trigger the release of the same reproductive hormones and ovarian maturation follows, but only to the mature capability phase (e.g., King *et al.*, 1966; Wingfield and Farner, 1980). In *Zonotrichia* the development phase of ovarian growth culminates when follicles are about 2–3 mm in diameter and contain white yolk only. Females generally do not progress beyond this phase unless the environment is conducive to nesting (King *et al.*, 1966). A second set of supplementary factors (or inhibitors) regulates the mature capability phase and onset of nesting, rapid deposition of yellow yolk (under the control of estradiol secretion), and egg-laying (Wingfield and Farner, 1980). The interaction of initial predictive information (probably largely genetic) and supplementary information (probably largely experiential) provide varying degrees of plasticity in the timing and integration of the breeding LHS.

Temperature is one established supplementary factor that modulates gonadal maturation in both phases. Mathematical models of egg-laying dates in sparrows predict that species with a low Ie should be insensitive to supplementary environmental cues and be driven primarily by photoperiod. Experimental results are consistent with these predictions (Wingfield *et al.*, 1996, 1997a). *Z.l. pugetensis,* a species with a high Ie, showed effects of increasing temperature on testicular and ovarian maturation in the development phase. Furthermore, exposure to 30°C resulted in deposition of yellow yolk and rapid final maturation of the ovary, indicating onset of nesting in the mature capability phase. In contrast, *Z.l. gambelii*, a species with a low Ie, did not show these responses. Studies demonstrate that the effect of temperature is widespread in species with high Ie factors. Similarly, temperature may affect gonadal growth differently even in populations of the same species. For example, sedentary great tits breeding in the Mediterranean area have a high Ie, and their gonadal maturation, as well as LH secretion, is delayed by low temperatures. This is not the case in great tits from more northern populations (south Sweden and northern Norway) having much lower Ie (B. Silverin, unpublished data).

Although photoperiodically induced rises in gonadotropins are mediated through the stimulation of cGnRH-I from hypothalamic neurons (e.g., Follett, 1984; Nicholls *et al.*, 1988), the mechanisms by which temperature and other supplementary cues modulate this response remain unclear. In *Zontrichia* and *Melospiza*, there were no differences in patterns of plasma levels of LH or FSH in either sex, despite the profound effects of temperature on gonadal maturation in both phases (Wingfield *et al.*, 1997a). These data indicate that temperature effects may be signalized via pathways other than through control of GnRH secretion. Low temperature did not increase circulating levels of T_4 or T_3. Thus, it is unlikely that temperature effects on the first phase of gonadal maturation are mediated through the hypothalamic-pituitary-thyroid axis (Wingfield *et al.*, 1997a). Nor is it likely that low temperature is stressful because plasma levels of corticosterone (an indicator of stress; e.g., Wingfield, 1994c) were similar in all groups (Wingfield *et al.*, 1996, 1997a). It is possible that other hormonal pathways mediate the effect of temperature, including at the gonad level (e.g., gonadotropin receptors), because plasma levels of gonadotropins (and presumably GnRH) were unaffected.

There is a consistent correlation between circulating prolactin and temperature effects (Maney *et al.*, 1999b,c). Photostimulation resulted in an increase in prolactin levels in the blood of all avian species studied and is probably mediated through vasoactive intestinal peptide (VIP) of hypothalamic origin (e.g., Dawson and Sharp, 1998; Maney *et al.*, 1999a). In *Z. l. gambelii*, which shows no modulation of gonadal development by temperature, there was no correlation between circulating prolactin levels and temperature treatment. However, in *Z. l. pugetensis* and *Z. l. oriantha* there was a consistent tendency for elevated prolactin levels at higher temperatures in groups that showed acceleration of gonadal development and decreased levels at lower temperatures with retarded gonadal development (Maney *et al.*, 1999b,c). It is tempting to suggest that VIP neurons, via the secretion of prolactin, may mediate temperature effects—presumably by changing the responsiveness of the gonads to FSH. However, it is also possible that temperature-modulated prolactin levels are a result of changes in gonadal growth and not the cause of those effects. Further experiments are needed to resolve this issue.

1. Effects of Food

Availability of food, quality of nutrition, and endogenous reserves of fat and protein can have profound influences on reproductive function (see Follett, 1984; Knobil and Neill, 1988). However, the mechanisms by which the food supply acts as supplementary information remain equivocal (Wingfield and Kenagy, 1991). Many experiments have been done, but they may not be relevant to an individual in its natural environment because severe food restriction (i.e., nutritional stress) is often the experimental paradigm (Wingfield and Kenagy, 1991). Field information collected on the opportunistic breeder red crossbill (*Loxia curvirostra*) sheds new light on this problem. There appears to be a seasonal component to the crossbill reproductive cycle, probably regulated by photoperiod, that brings the birds into breeding condition in July. There is another potential reproductive period in winter that is entirely opportunistic (Hahn, 1997), controlled by factors other than day length and temperature (because the latter is at a seasonal low in January). A regulatory role of food supply is unlikely to be simply caloric intake because captive crossbills fed *ad libitum* failed to breed in winter. Photostimulated male crossbills fed a laboratory diet equal to what they normally would eat on short days, showed similar testicular growth to males fed *ad libitum* and much greater development than males held on short days (Hahn, 1995). After food-restricted males on long days were given food *ad libitum*, their testicular development was significantly greater than males that had continuous access to food. These exciting data suggest that the perception of food availability may affect gonadal development. Body mass and food intake were similar among groups regardless of availability of food.

2. Role of Social Interactions

All great tits in southern Sweden enter photorefractoriness at the same time (mid-July), but there is a huge variation between age and sex groups in the vernal FSH-secretion pattern (Silverin et al., 1997b), suggesting possible effects of experience and social status. Most experiments on the interaction of initial predictive and supplementary factors have been performed in environmental chambers in which males and females were housed together. Because it is well known that the presence of the opposite sex can enhance photoperiodically induced gonadal maturation in both phases (see Wingfield et al., 1994c, for review), experiments were conducted on *Z.l. pugetensis* in which sexes were isolated to remove intersexual social cues. The effects of temperature on testis growth persisted (Wingfield et al., 1997a). However, isolation from males resulted in retardation of the first phase of ovarian development at temperatures of 5° and 20°C (but not at 30°C). All temperature effects on the second phase of ovarian maturation were abolished in females isolated from males. These data clearly indicate that social cues and temperature interact to regulate both phases of gonadal maturation.

3. Pathways of Action of Environmental Signals

Exploration of the mechanisms underlying the transduction of environmental signals into neuroendocrine and endocrine secretions is still a largely unchartered area of biology (e.g., Ball, 1993). The use of a protein product of the immediate early gene (IEG) *c-fos*, as a marker of neuronal activation following stimulation by environmental cues has been applied to brain tissues of Japanese quail (*Coturnix japonica*), European starling (*Sturnus vulgaris*) and other avian species (Meddle and Follett, 1995; Sharp et al., 1995). An increase in Fos expression was detectable by immunocytochemistry (ICC) in the tuberal hypothalamus of Japanese quail during photostimulation (Meddle and Follett, 1995, 1997). Similarly, in *Z. l. gambelii* photostimulation caused Fos expression in the tuberoinfundibular complex. Evidence also strongly indicated that social cues in both sexes may result in the expression of IEGs. Exposure of adult male quail to a receptive female elicited an increase in Fos immunostaining in the preoptic region of the hypothalamus and the nucleus intercollicularis (Meddle et al., 1997). Females and males also showed increases of Fos expression following copulatory interactions, with prominent activation observed in the ventromedial hypothalamus (Meddle et al., 1997, 1999). The differential expression of Fos between the sexes provides valuable insights into the brain regions regulating hormonally sensitive stereotypic behavior.

4. Periodicity of Reproduction at Low Latitudes

The environmental control of reproductive function at mid- and high latitudes has received considerable attention especially in relation to photoperiodic controls (e.g., Follett, 1984; Wingfield and Farner, 1993). On the other hand, mechanisms by which breeding periodicity is regulated in tropical forest species are virtually unknown. In the spotted antbird *(Hylophylax naevioides)*, breeding in Soberania National Park, central Panama, nesting occurs seasonally or periodically over as many as 10 months of the year (e.g., Skutch, 1969; Leigh *et al.*, 1982). Food supply and predator avoidance are thought to be important ultimate factors determining these breeding seasons (Morton, 1980; Poulin *et al.*, 1992). However, it is unclear which proximate factors tropical species use to time breeding so that it coincides with favorable environmental conditions. Do tropical birds remain in breeding condition year round (i.e., with the development phase permanently complete)? If so, do they simply react to supplementary factors to trigger onset of breeding (i.e., mature capability phase and final development of ovarian function)? Alternately, do they prepare for reproduction by responding to initial predictive cues as do avian species at mid- and high latitudes (i.e., the breeding LHS occurs periodically)?

Field and laboratory experiments reveal that spotted antbirds are capable of responding to changes in day length as short as 20 minutes or less over the year (Hau *et al.*, 1998, 1999)—consistent with very small changes in annual photoperiod at 10°N latitude in Panama. Many tropical species may undergo marked seasonal changes in gonadal development (Wikelski *et al.*, 1999c, 2000). Furthermore, environmental cues asssociated with food had a dramatic stimulatory effect on gonadal development and singing behavior (Hau *et al.*, 2000a). Social interactions such as territorial challenges also resulted in increases in territorial aggression and testosterone secretion in both sexes (Wikelski *et al.*, 1999a; Hau *et al.*, 2000b).

B. Multiple Brooding

Avian species that breed at mid- to low latitudes have a breeding season that is long enough to allow them to raise more than one brood (Wingfield and Farner, 1978a, 1980). In female white-crowned sparrows (Z. l. *pugetensis*) and European blackbirds *(Turdus merula)* there were distinct cycles in plasma levels of LH and estrogens, with maxima at each egg-laying period. Males, however, show a more complex pattern of hormone secretion. Despite a second maximum in circulating LH during the second egg-laying period, there were no parallel increases in circulating testosterone (Wingfield and Farner, 1978a, 1980; Wingfield, 1984b; Schwabl *et al.*, 1980). High levels of testosterone associated with territory establishment and attraction of a mate were apparently unnecessary for the second brood (Wingfield and Moore, 1987). It has been shown that high levels of testosterone interfere with parental behavior (Fig. 6) (Silverin, 1980b; Hegner and Wingfield, 1987; Beletsky *et al.*, 1995; Ketterson *et al.*, 1992, 1996). In other species, (e.g. house sparrow), however, peaks of LH and testosterone occurred with each brood (Hegner and Wingfield, 1986a) because apparently males were susceptible to a nest-box takeover by other males at the time the young fledge. Parental behavior of males decreased, but females were able to compensate and fledge the young. The second brood was not initiated until the young of the first brood became independent (Hegner and Wingfield, 1986a,b). Similar results have been obtained in the European starling, although the second peak of testosterone was significantly less than the first (Ball and Wingfield, 1987). The second clutch was not initiated until the young of the first brood were independent.

In multibrooding great tits the LH secretion patterns are even more complex. Males show the same LH and testosterone patterns as male white-crowned sparrows—with LH and testosterone peaks during the period of territorial establishment, but only a peak in LH when laying a second clutch (Röhss and Silverin, 1983). However, female great tits show a much more complex pattern. After a persistent rise in LH levels at the beginning of winter (December), there is a photoperiodically induced rise in March to half the level induced by social and supplementary information when nest-building and egg-laying starts in early May (maximum levels of the year). At the onset of incubation, LH levels have decreased dramatically. Curiously enough, by the end of the incubation period LH levels peak again and have declined markedly by the end of the incubation period. While the birds are producing the second clutch, their LH again peaks at the same breeding

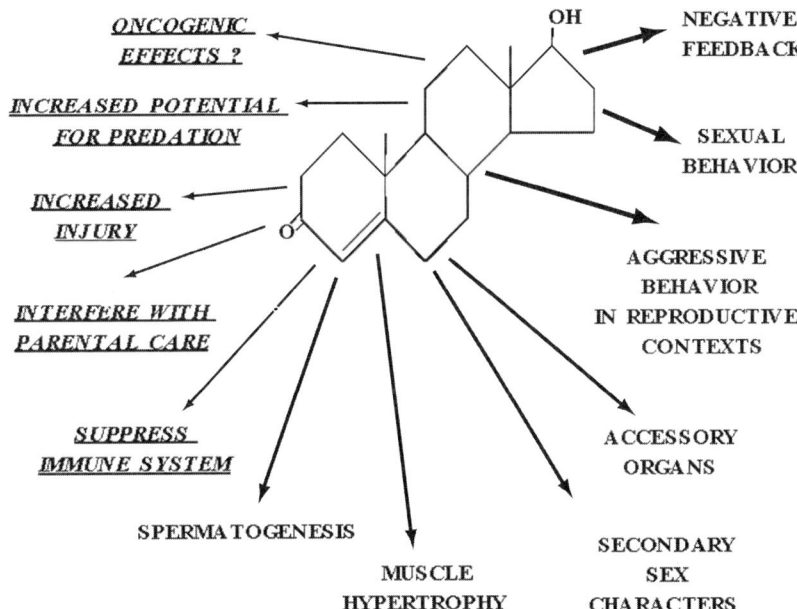

FIGURE 6 The benefits and costs of the steroid hormone testosterone. Beneficial effects of testosterone (physiological, morphological, and behavioral) are denoted on the right-hand side and lower part of the molecule in regular type. These are essential for normal reproductive function in the male. However, prolonged high levels of testosterone may incur costs that could actually reduce reproductive success and impair lifetime fitness (effects denoted in italics on left-hand side of the molecule). Experimental evidence suggests that there may be additional costs not shown here. Note also that if testosterone were secreted in a life history stage (LHS) other than breeding, the normal effects of this steroid may be inappropriate and incur further costs. Finite-state machine theory predicts that, for example, a behavior expressed in the breeding LHS that is testosterone dependent may be regulated by different means if that apparently same behavior is expressed in another LHS. The costs associated with prolonged high levels of secretion of a hormone such as testosterone or its secretion in an inappropriate LHS may have led to selection for many mechanisms that avoid these costs. Field endocrinology has made a major contribution in identifying such costs, and the mechanisms by which they may be avoided. From Wingfield et al. (1997, 2000), courtesy of MIT Press.

substages (i.e., nest-building and early egg-laying and late incubation), with a significant drop in between (Silverin, 1991a). A similar increase in LH during the second half of the incubation period has also been observed in some other species—European blackbirds (Schwabl et al., 1980) and pied flycatchers (Ficedula hypoleuca; Silverin and Wingfield, 1982). The cause and function of this incubation peak in LH is unclear.

The mechanisms by which testosterone levels remain low despite elevated LH during a second clutch in some species remain unknown. An antigonadal role for prolactin has been proposed (Moore, 1982, 1984; Wingfield and Moore, 1987) because during the parental substages blood levels of prolactin are elevated and, in turkeys and Japanese quail, have been shown to exert an antigonadal effect (Camper and Burke, 1977a,b). Stimuli from the young induce prolactin secretion in females (Lehrman, 1965; Goldsmith et al., 1981; Goldsmith, 1983, 1991), but this would be lost at fledging. Detailed studies on free-living pied flycatchers show that at least in the pied flycatcher the duration of the period with high prolactin secretion seems to be under endogenous control because the birds only have a limited capacity for an experimentally induced prolongation of the period with high prolactin secretion (Silverin and Goldsmith, 1984, 1990). Thus, the inhibition of prolactin on ovarian function (Camper and Burke, 1977a,b; El Halawani and Rozenboim, 1993) would be relieved and a second clutch initiated. In free-living dark-eyed juncos, removal of the male resulted in a decline in male prolactin levels, but had no effect on prolactin in females (Ketterson et al., 1990).

The antagonistic relationship of prolactin and reproductive hormones in the regulation of transitions between sexual and parental behavior may not be universal. In the song sparrow and white-crowned sparrow circulating prolactin was elevated in males and females during egg-laying, but showed no further major fluctuations until the breeding LHS was terminated. There were no correlations of prolactin titers with transitions between sexual and parental phases (Hiatt et al., 1987; Wingfield and Goldsmith, 1990). Removal of the nest to induce renesting did not result in a decline of prolactin in either male or female song sparrows despite significant second peaks of LH and sex steroid hormones (Wingfield and Goldsmith, 1990). Furthermore, implants of estradiol into females to maintain them in a sexual receptive state did not affect prolactin or the expression of parental care in females (Wingfield et al., 1989). In addition, male song sparrows mated to estrogen-treated females had higher levels of testosterone than did controls, but there was no difference in circulating concentrations of prolactin (Wingfield et al., 1989). Clearly there is no single mechanism underlying transitions between sexual and parental substages, but it should be pointed out that multiple brooding after successfully raising a first clutch is different from renesting after the loss of the nest to a predator or storm (see later; Wingfield and Moore, 1987; Wingfield and Farner, 1993).

C. Termination of Breeding

The development of refractory periods to long day length is the most intensively investigated environmentally induced function that terminates the breeding LHS (Nicholls et al., 1988). It is well established that the vernal increase in day length initiates gonadal growth in anticipation of the ensuing breeding season. If, for example, male great tits captured during winter are kept on short days for 2 years, they never grow testes (Silverin, 1994). Conversely, decreasing day length in late summer could act as predictive information for the termination of reproduction, as appears to be the case in pigeons of the genus *Columba* (Lofts et al., 1966; Lofts and Murton, 1968), and possibly also in the baya weaver (Thapliyal and Saxena, 1964). However, most passerine species and many others that breed in northern latitudes undergo spontaneous gonadal regression in mid-summer despite continuing long days that in spring were responsible for the stimulation of gonadal development. This absolute photorefractory condition (Nicholls et al., 1984) can also be induced by artificial long days, and when birds are in this state no known photoregime stimulates gonadal recrudescence. The number of long days required to induce photorefractoriness is a function of day length (Dolnik, 1976; Farner and Gwinner, 1980; Farner, 1985). In *Z. l. gambelii*, the gonads remain regressed for several years if the birds are maintained on permanently long days (Farner and Follett, 1979; D. S. Farner, R. A. Lewis, and R. S. Donham, unpublished).

The recovery of photosensitivity usually occurs only after birds have been exposed to short days for 40–60 days (Wolfson, 1966; Lofts and Murton, 1968; Turek, 1978; Dolnik, 1976; Farner and Follett, 1979; Farner, 1985; Silverin, 1994). Under natural conditions, photosensitivity is regained in late October and early November when day length is still decreasing. Gonadal recrudesence is thus prevented until days lengthen the following spring (Farner and Mewaldt, 1955). There is much evidence for an involvement of an endogenous circadian rhythm in the measurement of day length, although the underlying mechanisms remain somewhat obscure (for reviews, see Farner and Follett, 1979; Farner and Gwinner, 1980; Farner, 1985; Nicholls et al., 1984, 1988). Furthermore, it has also been demonstrated that *Zonotrichia* continue to measure day length in relation to the recovery of photosensitivity (Turek, 1978).

1. Nonphotoperiodic Regulation of Termination of Reproduction

There is evidence that the onset of photorefractoriness can be delayed by supplementary factors in relation to local conditions and to substages expressed in the breeding LHS. Investigations of captive and naturally breeding populations of *Z. l. gambelii* indicate that the timing of spontaneous gonadal regression is variable (Wingfield and Farner, 1979, 1993). The duration of maximum testicular size is only 10–12 days in captive conditions, whereas in the field unmated males undergo gonadal regression in the fourth week of June, breeding males and females in the first week of July, and renesting birds in the third week of July (Wingfield and Farner, 1978b, 1979, 1980). It obviously would not be advantageous for the parental phase to be terminated during the nestling substage because the young would not survive. However, the onset of photorefractoriness prevents initiation of clutches beyond a certain date, allowing the completion of a nesting phase that was initiated before this time. In the case of *Z. l. gambelii*, this period appears to be the third and fourth weeks of June (Wingfield and Farner, 1979). Studies on willow tits indicate that the time of testicular regression also is dependent on whether the male is mated, as well as the ambient temperature (Silverin and Viebke, 1994; Silverin and Westin, 1995).

Social interactions may also play a role. Runfeldt and Wingfield (1985) showed that free-living female song sparrows given subcutaneous implants of estradiol remained sexually receptive and delayed onset of the prebasic molt LHS until at least the beginning of October. Control females given empty implants became photorefractory and began molt by mid-August. Males mated to control females also were refractory by mid-August, but those mated to estradiol-implanted females delayed onset of refractoriness and began the prebasic molt LHS almost 1 month later than the controls. In contrast, untreated females mated to testosterone-implanted males became photorefractory and began the prebasic molt LHS at the same time as females mated to controls. The testosterone-implanted males remained on territory and delayed the onset of the prebasic molt LHS until the beginning of October (Runfedlt and Wingfield, 1985). Long-distance migrants such as the pied flycatcher, with a restricted time schedule of LHSs, showed a different response pattern. Experimental elevation of estradiol levels in females did not affect the time of gonadal regression in males, although their behavior during breeding was dramatically affected. Males paired to estradiol-treated females became more aggressive and spent more time mate-guarding than control males, indicating that cuckoldry is a potential problem for males of this species. In fact, males paired with estradiol-treated females were less successful than control males in attracting a second female to breed with (Silverin, 1991b).

These data indicate that males adjust termination of the breeding LHS to the reproductive state of their mates. Under natural conditions, we might expect that unmated males terminate breeding before mated males (Wingfield and Farner, 1979). However, apparently this is not always the case. Unmated male willow tits regress their testes much later than paired males, possibly to remain sexually active for a longer period of time to attract a female at all costs. Such males have no parental obligations and can maintain high plasma T levels, and sperm production for a longer period. After all, for many species of small birds there is a very little chance that they will live another year and breed again (Silverin *et al.*, 1986; Silverin and Westin, 1995). Reasons why males of some species terminate earlier in the breeding season than others remain to be determined. Females, on the other hand, do not adjust termination of the breeding LHS to the reproductive state of males.

D. Mating Systems and Breeding Strategies

There are now over 90 species of birds for which there are profiles of reproductive hormones under natural or near-natural conditions (see Wingfield and Farner, 1993; Wingfield, 1994c; Wingfield *et al.*, 2000). It is beyond the scope of this chapter to discuss all of these, but such a unique database has allowed us to begin assessing the hormonal bases of mating systems and breeding strategies. These analyses do have problems of phylogeny, but it is important to remember that the conclusions are not end points but generate hypotheses and predictions for further experimental testing. One of the central theses to come out of comparisons of avian taxa is that the profiles of testosterone appear to be roughly related to the mating system. Socially monogamous species, in which males provide significant parental care, have brief peaks of testosterone and a low breeding baseline. Implants of testosterone into these parental males tends to interfere with parental behavior (Wingfield *et al.*, 1990b, 1997b; Ketterson *et al.*, 1996). Polygynous species, on the other hand, have longer peaks of testosterone levels in the blood and breeding baselines tend to be higher (e.g., Wada et al., 1999). Most males of polygynous species provide little or no parental care and thus interference with paternal care is not a problem. This situation is especially clear in the pied flycatcher. Most males from this species are polyterritorial. The proportion, however, varies with the habitat (Silverin, 1990). Male pied flycatchers can be either strictly monogamous (a smaller proportion) or polyterritorial. The number of polyterritorial males succeeding in getting a second female to breed varies. In strictly monogamous males testosterone levels already reach basal levels at the end of the egg-laying period, whereas polyterritorial males maintain high testosterone levels until the end of the incubation period for the first female in the home territory (Silverin and Wingfield, 1982).

In socially monogamous males, there is now extensive evidence that male–male interactions over territory and mates can result in a marked increase in testosterone secretion—the challenge hypothesis (Wingfield et al., 1990b; 2000). However, parental care in males requires that testosterone levels be low. It has been suggested that the temporal patterns of testosterone in birds, and perhaps in vertebrates in general, is a trade-off between social interactions that tend to increase testosterone and paternal care that requires it to decrease (Wingfield et al., 1990b, 2000). Field endocrine techniques allowed experimental tests of this idea using implants of sex steroids and their blockers. The result was a series of papers that clearly indicate there may be many costs to high circulating levels of testosterone (Ketterson et al., 1996).

During the breeding LHS, testosterone has a number of morphological, physiological, and behavioral effects that are essential for normal reproductive function in males (Fig. 6). Experimental field studies show that elevated testosterone levels in parental males reduces parental care in pied flycatchers (Silverin 1980b), house sparrows (Hegner and Wingfield, 1987), dark-eyed juncos (Ketterson et al., 1996), yellow-headed blackbirds (*Xanthocephalus xanthocephalus*; Beletsky et al., 1995), and the barn swallow (*Hirundo rustica*; Saino and Møller, 1995). However, such an effect may not be universal because testosterone implants had a reduced (or no) effect on paternal care in Lapland longpurs (*Calcarius lapponicus*; Hunt et al., 1999) and great tits (van Duyse et al., 2000). Additional costs include wounding and increased mortality (Dufty, 1989), suppression of the immune system (Hillgarth and Wingfield, 1997), potential increased sensitivity to stress (Schoech et al., 1999), reduced overwinter survival, higher predation rates, and increased energetic costs (Fig. 6; Ketterson et al., 1996; Beletsky et al., 1995). On the other hand, testosterone implants may have some benefits, such as increased activity, successful territorial establishment, and larger territory size (Silverin, 1980b; Wingfield, 1984a; Chandler et al., 1994, 1997; Lynn et al., 2000). Raouf et al. (1997) showed that male dark-eyed juncos with testosterone implants actually gained more extrapair fertilizations (see also Enstrom et al., 1997). In addition, they may have higher sperm counts for longer periods (Kast et al., 1998), and energetic costs may not always be higher (Lynn et al., 2000).

There is a growing literature on the potential immunosuppressive actions of testosterone in male birds (see Hillgarth and Wingfield, 1997). This is a rapidly growing field, but much controversy remains (Hasselquist et al., 1999; Peters, 2000).

The concept that there are costs associated with high levels of testosterone for prolonged periods raises a number of issues that could be central for hormonal bases of many breeding strategies such as brood parasitism and cooperative breeding. In addition, it suggests that there may have been strong selection for mechanisms that avoid the costs of testosterone as well as for those that regulate increased secretion of this steroid hormone. It is highly unlikely that we would have become aware of this trade-off if field endocrine studies had not been conducted. Experimental investigations in the field and laboratory will explore endocrine mechanisms in a new light and hormone manipulations will also provide new insights into behavioral ecology and evolution of breeding strategies.

V. PREBASIC MOLT

Feathers are built by dead keratinzed epidermal cells that are constantly being worn. To maintain high flight maneuverability, it is therefore highly important for a bird to replace the worn-out feathers with new ones on a seasonal basis. When doing so, birds are especially vulnerable to predators. Some groups of birds (e.g., ducks and geese) even become flightless during molt. The prebasic molt is usually a complete molt (i.e., all feathers are replaced) and mostly occurs after breeding (as opposed to prealternate molt, which is partial and occurs generally before breeding). To grow new feathers is, however, energetically costly, and to maximize molting efficiency individuals must concentrate their behavior on foraging and predator avoidance. Anyone working with free-living birds is also aware that this is an extremely difficult period for capturing them. They are very shy, and consequently difficult to observe, and they do not respond to cues that at other times of the year would attract them to a capture place. For these reasons, very few studies have been performed on hormonal behavioral interactions in molting free-living birds.

To breed and molt at the same time is usually incompatible. Parents are not able to collect enough food for both the energy-requiring molting process and feeding of young. Natural selection therefore favors individuals that replace their feathers after breeding or start molt at the end of the nestling period, by which time the breeding LHS is being terminated and when circulating levels of reproductive hormones are low (Voitkevitch, 1966; Payne, 1972). Some degree of overlap occurs in some species (e.g., Stresemann and Stresemann, 1966; Payne, 1972; Jallageas and Assenmacher, 1985). Furthermore, migrating birds have a limited time available for molt. Ideally it should be finished before they leave their breeding grounds. However, because the molting process may take 6–8 weeks not all species finish molt before setting off for their wintering grounds. Some, such as many arctic shorebirds, may pause and molt somewhere along the migratory route south. It is therefore easy to understand that the molting process needs a very strict regulatory process and may be finely integrated with autumnal migration.

The molt itself consists of two processes—the shedding of the feathers, or ecdysis, and the growth of new plumage, or endysis. As with other LHSs, prebasic molt has a development phase, mature capability (when feathers are actually shed and then new ones begin to grow), and a termination phase. We do know that many species are very secretive during the molt, and some have a special migration to safe areas where food is plentiful and they are protected from predators (Payne, 1972). Very little is known about control mechanisms at any of these phases or the behavioral strategies involved.

A. Hormonal Bases of Prebasic Molt

It has long been known that the onset of prebasic molt is asynchronous among individuals in a population. Reproductive activities delay molt because brooding females start last and have an accelerated molt, whereas nonbreeding males tend to start first. The duration of molt in Pacific-seaboard white-crowned sparrows decreases by an average of 2.6 days per degree of latitude. In the south, it takes approximately 83 days, in the north, around the Puget Sound, 47 days. Males begin earlier than females by approximately 2 weeks, and molt onset is correlated not with exact date but with the end of the nesting season (Mewaldt and King, 1977). In the chaffinch (*Fringilla coelebs*) molt rate increases on short days and decreases on long days. This may be adaptive in synchronizing the end of the molt in individuals that start at different times (Dolnik and Gavrilov, 1980). In the white-crowned sparrow the onset of molt occurs sooner when exposed to 20 hours of light than 16 hours. There is generally no molt when birds are exposed only to 12 hours of light. Low air temperature (5°C) increases the rate and decreases the duration of molt, and the shedding interval of primaries is decreased. High temperatures of 25°C have no effect (Chilgren, 1978).

Voitkevich (1966) found in European starlings that the timing of thyroidectomy prior to the natural prebasic molt affected its progression, but effects were less deleterious when the interval between thyroidectomy and the onset of molt was decreased. This result suggests that thyroid secretions are involved in the metabolic preparation (development phase) for prebasic molt and that it occurs in advance of feather replacement (i.e., mature capability of the prebasic molt LHS). These data also indicate that thyroid hormones do not serve as sole causative agents for the loss and replacement of feathers because thyroidectomy at the onset of molt did not appear to have much effect on subsequent feather regeneration (Voitkevich, 1966).

B. Molt and the Incompatibility of High Thyroxine and Testosterone Secretion

Laboratory studies on American tree sparrows (*Spizella arborea*) indicate that the autumn molting process is already programmed early in spring (Wilson and Reinert, 1996). The process seems to be initiated by an elevation of thyroid hormones. Destruction of the thyroid suppresses molt (Haase and Paulke, 1980; Wilson and Reinert, 1993). Most seasonal studies on circulating levels of thyroid hormones also show dramatically elevated levels during molt (e.g., Haase and Paulke, 1980; Smith, 1982; Péczely and Pethes, 1982; Groscolas et al., 1986; Péczely, 1986; Cherel et al., 1988a). Other studies have shown T_4 levels to be very high immediately before molt and low during the actual molting process (Smith, 1982; Kern and Degraw, 1986). Whether it is T_4 or T_3 that is the active hormone in molt is unknown. Studies by Reinert and Wilson (1997), however, indicate that T_3 is not involved. The correlation between the time the thyroids increase secretion and the onset of molt is illustrated in two European tit species, willow tits (*Parus montanus*) and great tits (Silverin et al., 1989a). In Sweden, willow tits lay only one clutch, and the nestlings leave the nest in early to mid-June. At this time the parents start molting, and they also significantly increase their circulating levels of T_4, which remain elevated throughout molt and do not decrease to basal until late autumn when molt is terminated. The closely related great tit breeds in the same areas and similar habitats but, unlike willow tits, it frequently lays two clutches. It is therefore not surprising that great tits do not start their molting process until mid-July, approximately 1 month later than willow tits. In concordance with this difference, T_4 levels also start to increase 1 month later in great tits, and levels remain high only as long as the tits are molting. This time difference in the molting–T_4 pattern is also correlated with differences in times of gonadal regression and the time circulating levels of gonadal steroids and LH return to basal. Both of these events occur approximately 1 month earlier (mid-June) in willow tits than in great tits (mid-July; Viebke, 1991; Silverin, 1978).

There are, however, exceptions to this molting–T_4 pattern. Several studies did not find a correlation between high T_4 levels and molt. (e.g., Lincoln et al., 1980; Hissa et al., 1983; Dittami and Hall, 1983). In, for example, juvenile white-crowned sparrows only females have elevated T_4 levels during mid-molt, and T_3 levels remain unchanged throughout molt (Wingfield et al., 1980). Why these studies failed to find a correlation is unclear. That a causal relationship between a rise in T_4 levels and the onset of molt may exist was experimentally shown by Silverin (1980a). The administration of T_4 to male pied flycatchers (*Ficedula hypoleuca*) soon after their arrival on the breeding areas, before breeding had even started, induced an immediate molt. The intensity of the molt was also dependent on the dosage of T_4 given. Birds given higher dosages molted much more rapidly and vigorously.

In all studies on molting in free-living birds, the circulating levels of reproductive hormones have been found to be basal or even below the level of detectability (e.g., Wingfield and Farner, 1978a,b; Wingfield, 1984b; Dittami, 1987; Logan and Wingfield, 1990; Williams, 1992; Mauget et al., 1994). An experimental prolongation of a high testosterone level beyond breeding and beyond the time of gonadal regression delays or even prevents the onset of molt (Runfeldt and Wingfield, 1985; Dawson, 1994; Ketterson et al., 1996). In the starling (Schleussner and Gwinner, 1985) testosterone delayed the onset and rate of the molt, but it did not apparently affect its timing. In other words, molt ended at the normal time, so if the implants were removed molt did not renew or was not completed.

A late nesting attempt normally results in delayed peaks of reproductive hormones. A consequence of this is a delayed onset of molt (Wingfield and Farner, 1979; Dittami, 1987). A similar response occurs if the nest is depredated before the parents have become photorefractory. Such an event results in a resurgence of plasma levels of LH, testosterone, and estradiol, allowing the parents to produce a replacement clutch, thus delaying the onset of the prebasic molt. However, by some unknown system, the birds compensate for the delay by speeding up their molt so that it finishes at the normal time (Wingfield and Farner, 1979).

Experimental studies on white-crowned sparrows have clearly shown that environmental factors, such as low temperatures, that affect the onset of gonadal regression also affect the onset of molt (Wingfield *et al.*, 1997a). All these studies indicate that active gonads and molt are temporarily incompatible, at least in temperate-zone birds. The situation seems to be somewhat different in tropical birds. In some tropical starling species molt may extend over most of the year, resulting in extensive overlap between breeding and molt (Dittami, 1987). Likewise, molt in tropically breeding house sparrows *(Passer domesticus)* seems to be independent of the breeding LHS (Mathew and Naik, 1986).

In addition to low levels of gonadotrophins and gonadal hormones during molt, birds also generally have low circulating concentrations of corticosterone. Furthermore, many birds show a dramatically reduced sensitivity to stress during molt (Wingfield and Farner, 1979; Wingfield, 1984b; Astheimer *et al.*, 1995; Romero *et al.*, 1998a,b). The reasons for this are unknown, but might include avoidance of corticosterone-induced dispersal behavior (e.g., Heath, 1997), a behavior likely to be inconsistent with the costly molting process. Another possibility is that the reduced stress response evolved to avoid the risk of a detrimental corticosterone-induced protein mobilization during molt.

It is curious that the molting process has been neglected as a research topic. The great diversity of molt patterns, the dependence on photoperiod, the clear interaction of social cues and the onset of molt, and easy access to developing feather follicle tissue are potentially rich sources of experimental material. Future studies incorporating modern techniques would be very productive in this field.

VI. AUTUMNAL MIGRATION

A. Postbreeding Movements

Birds undergo several forms of movements during the postbreeding period. Some of these are very predictable—for example, postfledging dispersal and migration to wintering areas. Some species are also partial migrants. Within a population, the same individual is either consistently migratory or consistently sedentary across years, regardless of the prevailing environmental situation (obligate partial migration); this type of partial migration appears to be regulated by strict endogenous control. In other species, individuals may or may not migrate depending on the prevailing environmental conditions that particular year (facultative partial migration); the factors determining whether individuals migrate can be competition for a resource, establishment of a winter flock, age and dominance relationships, or date of hatching (Schwabl and Silverin, 1990). The distance partially migrating birds move is usually short (rarely more than a few hundred kilometers). Another type is irruptive migration that occurs on an unpredictable schedule; movements are in relation to food availability in a population's original breeding or wintering areas. During these irruptive movements, birds can move in enormous numbers. Most of these species are predators such as the snowy owl *(Nyctea scandiaca)*, but they also include seed-eating birds, such as crossbills *(Loxia spp.)* and nutcrackers *(Nucifraga caryocatactes)*.

Postbreeding movements are extremely complex and it is not surprising that experiments designed to explore hormone mechanisms are few and conflicting (Ramenofsky, 1990; Schwabl and Silverin, 1990; Wingfield *et al.*, 1990a). Applying FSM theory, we can suggest four LHSs that categorize these phenomena.

1. Juvenile dispersal that occurs as an ontogenetic LHS once in an individual's life cycle. Thus, the hormone mechanisms involved may be entirely distinct from those regulating other types of movements.

2. Regular autumnal migration LHS of the entire population—the mirror image of the vernal migration LHS.

3. Programmed partial migration in which certain individuals always show autumnal migration LHS (and, therefore, vernal migration also) and others never migrate. Presumably those that do migrate have control mechanisms similar to those in category 2. Experimental comparisons of individuals in the same population that do not migrate with those that do may be valuable (i.e., a natural experiment!).

4. Facultative migration or irruptive movements that occur in response to unpredictable perturbations of the environment. We include this type of movement in the emergency LHS with a completely different endocrine basis (see later).

B. Migration Strategies Postbreeding and Their Hormonal Bases

Given these categories of post-breeding movements of birds, we can explore what is known about endocrine mechanisms. Much more information is needed, but the diversity of strategies in very closely related species offers many exciting models for future experiments.

1. Postjuvenile Dispersal

Belthoff and Dufty (1998) suggest, based on a study of Western screech-owls (*Otus kennicotti*), that young birds in good body condition have high corticosterone levels, which would stimulate locomotor activity and thereby dispersal behavior. Lean birds are predicted to maintain low corticosterone levels, to keep gluconeogenesis low, and delay dispersal until their energy stores have improved. Once a set body condition is reached, corticosterone levels increase and induce dispersal. What factor causes elevated corticosterone levels in these birds? This hypothesis has not been tested on free-living birds.

2. Programmed Partial Migration

In 1954, Lack suggested that testosterone might suppress the migratory urge, thus avoiding the premature departure from the breeding grounds if breeding is delayed. This also seems to be true for regular migrants (Runfeldt and Wingfield, 1985; Schwabl and Silverin, 1990). Seasonal changes in testosterone levels have so far only been investigated in two partially migratory species—the European blackbird (*Turdus merula*; Schwabl *et al.*, 1984) and the willow tit (Silverin *et al.*, 1986). European blackbirds show no autumnal surge in testosterone plasma levels. In contrast, approximately 30% of juvenile female and male willow tits show a dramatic transitory autumnal peak in circulating testosterone. No adult willow tits show elevated testosterone levels during autumn. Furthermore, high testosterone levels are also found in some juveniles along the autumn migration route. In contrast, field experiments show that elevated testosterone levels during autumn do not affect the sedentary behavior of individuals that do not migrate (Silverin *et al.*, 1989b). Thus, the results from these two partially migratory species indicate that testosterone is not involved in the regulation of partial migration but may in some way be a result of it.

The scenario described for the willow tit differs from that postulated for dispersing nonterritorial sedentary birds. The latter birds may disperse from their natal areas even though there is plenty of food and an absence of parental aggression. The timing of their dispersal has been related to body condition, social status, or both. This is the situation for the nonterritorial marsh tit (*Parus palustris*; Nilsson and Smith, 1985). Birds in good condition disperse earlier than those in bad condition.

3. Regular Autumnal Migration

After the postnuptial molt and sometimes before the prebasic molt is complete, many birds of north temperate regions begin the autumnal migration (see Wingfield and Farner, 1980; Stresemann and Stresemann, 1966; Gavrilov and Dolnik, 1974). The mechanisms of autumn migration are even less well known than for vernal migration (Wingfield *et al.*, 1990a). It should also be noted that the autumnal migration occurs at a time when the gonads are completely regressed and plasma levels of sex steroid hormones are basal. This is in contrast to the control of vernal migration that occurs just prior to or during a period of gonadal recrudescence and ever-increasing levels of plasma sex steroids. Castration or ovariectomy of birds in mid-winter results in the complete abolishment of vernal fattening and migratory behavior but autumnal fattening and zugunruhe are unaffected (see Weise, 1967; Wingfield *et al.*, 1990a). There is also considerable evidence for circannual rhythms of migratory activity in some species (see Gwinner, 1986; Berthold, 1996). Berthold and Querner (1982) showed in studies of black caps (*Sylvia atricapilla*) that both migratory restlessness and the pattern of fat deposition can be under a genetic control. At least, migratory restlessness may include an endogenous circannual rhythm with a periodicity of approximately 10 months (Berthold, 1975). Initial predictive information results in the development of a migratory state (mature capability), and actual day-to-day migratory movements are controlled by supplementary factors that fine-tune the migratory process (Weise, 1962; Wingfield *et al.*, 1990a).

Migration probably evolved independently several times, and the physiological base for migration may therefore differ among species. Normally we may think of migratory birds as long-distance migrants, spending their breeding period at high latitudes and the winter period in tropical areas. Some species fly very long distances before stopping to refuel. A bird whose body weight is 50% fat or more can fly 3000–4000 km in 3–4 days without having to stop. Others make only shorter flights and make repeated stops to refuel. Many finches and sparrows, for example, only fly short distances and stop everyday to lay down new fat reserves. These differences most likely reflect the hormonal mechanisms regulating energy management between species with different migratory strategies (Biebach, 1990; Piersma, 1998).

Not only are there many different complex migratory patterns, but spring migrants and autumn migrants also experience different conditions during their flights. Spring migrants are normally in a big hurry, and early arrivers experience decreased food availability as they move north. Autumn migration is more protracted, and birds meet more favorable weather conditions and food situations as they fly south. In contrast to spring migrants, they do not have to arrive at their destination with maintained fat reserves. Thus, strategies for spring and autumn migration may differ (King et al., 1963; O'Reilly and Wingfield, 1995), and it is acknowledged that mechanisms regulating spring and autumn migration differ (e.g., Moore et al., 1982; Wingfield et al., 1990a; Romero et al., 1997).

The induction of migratory restlessness and fat deposition in autumn has only been studied in captive birds. The process is complex and a number of hormones seem to be involved in the activation of hyperphagia, the subsequent deposition of fat, and migratory restlessness—for example, growth hormone, thyroid hormones, corticosterone, catecholamines, insulin, glucagon, and prolactin (Wingfield et al., 1990a; Schwabl et al., 1991). In the green-winged teal (*Anas crecca*) there is a significant correlation of plasma T_4 and growth hormone, with the highest levels of both hormones occurring in August just before onset of autumnal migration (Scanes et al., 1980).

In an earlier review, Berthold (1984) concluded that corticosterone was not involved in the initiation of migratory behavior. Since then, results from several studies have changed this opinion. Corticosterone is thought to be one of the most important hormones in the control of events related to autumn migration. The adrenals of autumn migrants secrete more corticosterone than adrenals from nonmigratory birds, as shown in 1976 by Péczely. Corticosterone is involved in the induction of migratory restlessness, as demonstrated by Schwabl et al. (1991) in a study on captive garden warblers. These autumn migrants were found to have a diel corticosterone secretion pattern with high nocturnal levels and low diurnal levels. When the migratory state was experimentally interrupted, the diel pattern disappeared.

How do migrating birds meet the conflicting effects of corticosterone—such as induction of hypherphagia and lipogenesis on one hand, and catabolic effects on skeletal muscles on the other hand? Corticosterone secretion during migration and stopovers must be balanced between its stimulating effects on foraging and lipogenesis and the costs associated with its effects on muscle catabolism (not desirable for a migratory bird). In a study on gray catbirds (*Dumetella carolinensis*), Holberton et al. (1996) tested the hypotheses that migratory birds should have higher corticosterone levels during migration than during the period preceding migration and that birds should reduce their stress response during migration. In this study, they also tested migrating yellow-rumped warblers (*Dendroica coronata*) at stopover sites. In brief, they showed that migrating catbirds had higher baseline levels of corticosterone than did lean molting birds from the premigratory period. Furthermore, the fat migratory birds did not respond to stress during stopovers, whereas this was the case during molt. Nor did the warblers show a stress response at stopovers. Their conclusion was that corticosterone levels are maintained at only moderately high levels in migrating birds, enough to facilitate hyperphagia and lipogenesis, but low enough to avoid a detrimental effect on flight muscles. The reduced stress sensitivity is needed to avoid a further elevation of corticosterone. This has been called the migration modulation hypothesis. Contrary to the Holberton et al. (1996) study, Romero et al. (1997) could not find elevated baseline levels of corticosterone in autumn migrants of white-crowned sparrows. Although the stress response was not of the same magnitude as during breeding, migrating sparrows responded to stress by increasing circulating levels of corticosterone. Still another species, the western sandpiper (*Calidris mauri*), a long-distance migrant, showed a strong stress response during its autumn migration (O'Reilly and Wingfield,

1995). In addition, autumn-migrating garden warblers show low baseline levels of corticosterone and a pronounced stress response (Schwabl et al., 1991). Thus, it appears that different response patterns to stress exist not only between spring and autumn migrants, but also between autumn migrants with different migratory strategies.

Whether lean birds have higher corticosterone levels to facilitate fattening is a controversial question. Several studies of nonmigratory birds have shown this to be the case (e.g., Smith et al., 1994; Wingfield et al., 1994a), whereas other studies have failed to establish such a connection (e.g., Silverin et al., 1997a; Silverin and Wingfield, 1998). Wingfield et al. (1994a) also showed that the relationship between body condition and responsiveness to stress may change within a species over the year. Holberton et al. (1996) did not find any such correlation in either of the two species they studied during autumn migration. Instead, elevated corticosterone levels seemed to be maintained throughout migration regardless of short-term fluctuations in the birds' energetic condition. Romero et al. (1997) also did not find any correlation between body condition and corticosterone levels in their study of autumn-migrating white-crowned sparrows. On the other hand, in garden warblers during autumn migration across the Sahara Desert, corticosterone levels were negatively correlated with body conditions (Schwabl et al., 1991).

To determine if corticosterone levels were high or low during the actual autumn migratory flight, Gwinner et al. (1992) collected blood samples from several migrating bird species captured at a field station high up in the Alps. The results from this study clearly showed that endurance flights had not resulted in high corticosterone levels. They found high corticosterone levels only in one extremely lean pied flycatcher. From this they concluded that corticosterone levels may rise if energy depots decline during the flight. In a spring study on long-distance bar-tailed godwits (*Limosa limosa*) migrants, Ramenofsky et al. (1995) found lean godwits arriving at stopover sites in The Netherlands to have high corticosterone levels. During refeeding, while body mass increased, the corticosterone levels declined. This is in agreement with the observations on garden warblers, as well as with the results from the lean pied flycatcher captured by Gwinner et al. (1992). The actual role that corticosterone plays in regulating (managing) energy storage and mobilization in the fluctuating extremes of migratory substages remains to be determined.

VII. WINTER (NONBREEDING) LIFE HISTORY STAGE

Perhaps the most obvious change of behavior once the breeding season ends is that many birds stop singing and some gather in huge flocks. They no longer have to channel energy into reproduction, but must turn their efforts to survival. These changes are also reflected in the hormonal secretion patterns. While the nestlings from the last brood are preparing to leave the nest, the gonads of the adults are regressing very rapidly and circulating levels of gonadotropins and gonadal hormones are decreasing to basal levels (e.g., Silverin and Wingfield, 1982; Röhss and Silverin, 1983; Silverin et al., 1986, 1997b). In most species, prebasic molt follows (and then autumn migration) as they prepare for the winter LHS. In tropical species, for which there is no winter per se, there is a nonbreeding LHS (e.g., during the dry season). The ecology and behavior of birds in the nonbreeding LHS is very different from the rest of the year. In some species, this may entail changes in morphology and physiology too. For example, some species wintering in high latitudes turn white in winter, and their physiology is adjusted to allow the accumulation of fat for thermoregulation during long cold nights. Others may take advantage of shelters, even snow caves (e.g., Andreev, 1999). Even species wintering in the tropics may undergo marked adjustments in the morphology of the gastrointestinal tract as diet changes. For example, the Eastern kingbird (*Tyrannus tyrannus*) is territorial and insectivorous during the breeding LHS; in winter, in the neotropics, it flocks and eats primarily fruit (Baptista and Welty, 1987). Although there is a growing literature on wintering strategies in birds, most of the hormone mechanisms remain entirely unknown.

A. Wintering Strategies in Ecological Contexts

Once on their wintering or nonbreeding grounds, birds can follow several strategies. Some defend territories in small groups (4–5 individuals), but they also may have a strict social dominance hierarchy in the group. Others may form small flocks (5–40 individuals) with a home range that is not defended as a territory. They may or may not have a strict hierarchy in the flock. We have identified four major strategies.

A. Defend territories either alone, in pairs, or as a group (Ekman, 1989; Gwinner *et al.*, 1994; Wingfield, 1994d).

B. Form small flocks (up to 40 individuals) on a home range with a more or less rigid dominance hierarchy (Rohwer, 1977; Saitou, 1978, 1979).

C. Form enormous flocks that have extended home ranges or may be nomadic over many hundreds to thousands of kilometers. Although these flocks are too large for rigid dominance hierarchies, there are frequent dominance–subordinance interactions. In some cases, these interactions are reinforced by singing in both males and females (Baptista *et al.*, 1987).

D. Wander over a wintering area as individuals, associating in groups from time to time, but not forming discrete flocks or remaining associated with the same individuals over the winter. Many seabirds, especially large gulls (*Larus sp.*), follow this strategy.

Virtually all the endocrine studies of hormone–behavior interactions in the nonbreeding LHS have focused on strategies A and B. Field investigations of strategies C and D would be fascinating, but are intractable due to the large distances covered by individuals. However, as tracking devices become miniaturized, it may be possible to conduct experimental studies in the future.

B. Hormone–Behavior Interactions in Winter Territoriality (Strategy A)

Species forming territorial winter flocks (e.g., willow tits) normally have a social hierarchy in the flock. These flocks consist of just a few individuals, and those that survive the winter always establish their breeding territories within the borders of the winter territory. The function with the establishment of a social hierarchy in a territorial winter flock is to secure access to a resource (e.g., a future mate or good foraging). The willow tit winter flock normally consists of only 4–5 individuals—the two adults that previously bred in the area and 2–3 non-kin juveniles. The adult birds always dominate juveniles and, within each age group, males dominate females (Ekman, 1979, 1989). Dominance status is primarily associated with foraging sites in the tree canopy and not with food availability per se. Dominant birds forage in the upper, densely branched parts of the coniferous trees where they are less likely to be taken by predators. Subdominant individuals are forced to forage in the lower, more open parts of the canopy where they much more easily become the victims of attacking pygmy owls. There is no major difference in food availability between the two areas of the tree, but juveniles have to spend more time watching for predators than do the dominant birds (Ekman, 1979, 1989; Ekman *et al.*, 1981).

Because territorial behavior can also be expressed outside the breeding season, at these times hormones that are considered to be of importance for the expression of territorial behavior in spring are now basal (Wingfield, 1994a,b; Silverin *et al.*, 1986). Nonbreeding territories are defended and maintained by aggressive displays that are identical to those used during spring. It is therefore tempting to assume that testosterone in some way also plays a role in the regulation of territorial aggressiveness outside the breeding season. In the socially very stable willow tit flock in winter there are no differences among flock members in circulating levels of LH, and sex steroid titers are very low in all individuals (Silverin *et al.*, 1984). However, it is worth noting that the subdominant juvenile females have the highest testosterone and *DHT* levels, although these titers are much lower than in the breeding LHS. The hypothesis is also fostered by studies of some species that have a period of autumn sexuality, including male–male competition for different resources. One well-known example is the rook (*Corvus frugilegus*), which may even lay eggs after having returned to the rookery in autumn (Marshall and Coombs, 1957). These birds, of course, must have developed their gonads to maturity to produce and lay eggs, but as noted by Marshall and Coombs (1957) gonads in the population as a whole were not as developed as in spring. In a thorough study of rooks in England, Lincoln *et al.* (1980) could not, however, find any increase in testis size during autumn and winter. On the other hand, they found a pronounced LH peak, without an accompanying testosterone surge, during the sexually active period (courtship behavior) in autumn (October and November). There was even a FSH peak preceding the LH peak by approximately 1 month.

Similar transient autumn peaks in reproductive hormones have been found in other birds—herring gulls (*Larus argentatus;* Scanes *et al.,* 1974), red grouse (*Lagopus lagopus scoticus;* Sharp *et al.,* 1974), mallards (*Anas platyrhynchos;* Haase *et al.,* 1975), eider duck (*Somateria mollissima;* Gorman, 1974; Spurr and Milne, 1976), and different species of tits (*Parus* sp.; Röhss and Silverin, 1983; Silverin *et al.,* 1984). However, other species that also establish types of autumn territories do not show similar autumn peaks in testosterone or LH—sheathbills (*Chionis minor;* Burger and Millar, 1980) and European robins (Schwabl and Kriner, 1991), which establish feeding territories, and sedentary northern mockingbirds (*Mimus polyglottos;* Logan and Wingfield, 1990), whose autumn and winter territories are later used as breeding territories. Because those species showing an autumn peak of gonadal development and testosterone secretion all show some forms of reproductive behavior (forming pair bonds, establishing nest sites, etc.), it has been suggested that this marks the beginning of a potential breeding LHS (Wingfield *et al.,* 1997b). As winter ensues, further development and breeding is suppressed until spring. In these cases, then, the breeding and nonbreeding LHSs must overlap considerably.

Adrenal hormones may also be involved. For example, in normal-size willow tit winter flocks (4–5 flock members), subdominant birds of both sexes have significantly higher corticosterone levels than dominant birds, indicating that subdominants are exposed to more stress than dominants. However, this relationship depends on flock size. In small flocks (three flock members), there is no difference in corticosterone levels between subdominant and dominant individuals. Furthermore, the dominant birds have significantly higher corticosterone levels than dominant birds in normal-size groups, indicating that three is a suboptimal group size or that the occupied territory is of low quality (Silverin *et al.,* 1984).

1. Hormonal and Gonadal Activities during Winter

Other species also show a slight, but still pronounced, elevation of LH titers, but not FSH, during early winter. In both willow tits and great tits, LH secretion increases during early winter without a concomitant increase in the circulating levels of testosterone. Parallel with the rise in LH secretion, there is an increase in gonadal size (Silverin, 1978; Röhss and Silverin, 1983; Viebke, 1991; Silverin *et al.,* 1986, 1997b). The cause and functional significance of these winter increases are not known. These events occur at a time when tits start to sing (but only during days with sunny weather) and when willow tits stop storing food and instead start to live on cached food items. Crossbills are known to be opportunistic breeders in response to food availability. Like all other birds living in the northern hemisphere, the reproductive systems of red crossbills were found to terminate activities during autumn molt at a time when food availability was still high. However, after finishing molt, crossbills began gonadal growth if food availability was sufficient; these birds are known to breed during winter (Hahn, 1997). An important factor to bear in mind is that crossbills can become sexually mature at a few months of age (Hahn, 1997) and can also breed the following summer.

House sparrows in rural areas of New York differ from other temperate-zone birds in showing reproductive activities not only during spring and summer, but also during autumn and winter (Hegner and Wingfield, 1986c). Their gonads are regressed only during the brief period of molt (September–October). Later in autumn, when males compete for nest sites, gonads show a partial recrudescence followed by an increase, approximately 1 month later, in plasma levels of testosterone. This may be an adaptation to overlap the breeding and nonbreeding LHSs, so that if food is available in adequate quantities more broods can be produced per year. Studies in most other free-living species have failed to show changes in gonadal growth or secretion of gonadotropins at the beginning of winter (e.g., Dawson, 1983; Schwabl *et al.,* 1980; Wingfield and Farner, 1993).

2. Territoriality in the Nonbreeding Season

Migratory stonechats (*Saxicola torquata*) establish territories on their wintering grounds in Israel. These birds are very aggressive, but do not show any signs of elevated testosterone levels during this period (Gwinner *et al.,* 1994). If testosterone is involved in the expression of autumn sexuality, it must do so through a different mechanism than during spring. Furthermore, castrating a nonbreeding song sparrow does not influence its territorial behavior (Wingfield, 1994b). Despite the fact that male song sparrows holding autumn territories have basal levels of testosterone, they show the same aggressive response toward a simulated territorial intruder as does a male holding a breeding territory. A major difference between the two responses is that the intrusion results in a dramatic elevation of circulating levels of testosterone in spring, but not in autumn (Wingfield and Hahn, 1994), which is consistent with the observation that all free-living song sparrows show basal levels of testosterone during autumn. Nor does an experimental elevation of circulating levels of testosterone in male mockingbirds holding autumn and winter territories affect aggressive behavior. Singing behavior, mate acquisition, and other reproductive behaviors not normally occurring during autumn were increased (Logan and Carlin, 1991). Taken together, these results suggest that the expression of territorial aggression in autumn territories is independent of gonadal hormones.

This hypothesis is also supported by studies on subtropical and tropical species that show year-round territoriality and live in different types of habitats and have different social systems. Circulating levels of testosterone are very low year round with a small peak during breeding, and experimental field studies clearly have shown that aggression in these territorial species is uncoupled from testosterone. Although these birds respond to simulated territorial intrusions with extensive aggression year round and although subdominant males respond to the removal of a territorial male with an increase in aggressive interactions, plasma levels of testosterone are either unaffected (Dittami and Gwinner, 1985; Wingfield *et al.*, 1992a; Levin and Wingfield, 1992; Wingfield and Lewis, 1993; Levin, 1996) or increase only after prolonged interactions (Wikelski *et al.*, 1999a; Hau *et al.*, 2000b). In a study of tropical spotted antbirds, Wikelski *et al.* (1999a) found that individuals living in a socially unstable situation had high circulating levels of testosterone.

A similar situation is found among willow tits living in northern Europe, a species showing year-round territoriality. During late summer, before autumn territorial flocks are being established, all juvenile willow tits have basal levels of testosterone. However, by early autumn the social situation becomes very unstable as the young birds try to establish themselves as members of a territorial flock. At this time, a substantial proportion of the juveniles (males as well as females), but none of the adult birds, have very high circulating levels of testosterone (just as high as during the breeding season), most likely a result of intensive aggressive encounters (Silverin *et al.*, 1986). The social situation is not unstable for the adult birds. They do not have to fight for a place in a winter flock. The parents stay on their breeding territory, although they extend its borders dramatically, and by prior residence and age they are from the very beginning the dominant individuals of the future winter flock. Later, during autumn when flock composition is permanent but aggressive encounters still occur at territorial boundaries (Ekman, 1979, 1989), no free-living willow tits, juveniles or adults, are found with high testosterone levels. Willow tits in the socially stable winter flock are estimated to be involved in an aggressive encounter at least once every 2 hr. Thus, the hormonal situation and hormonal reaction patterns to aggressive encounters in willow tits during late autumn seem to agree very well with that in song sparrows and other species not showing high autumn levels of testosterone.

Thus, it is possible that behavior mediated via high testosterone levels may be important during periods of social instability in the breeding LHS, but not necessarily in other LHSs. Given that testosterone also has marked effects on sexual behavior as well as the morphology of reproductive accessory organs (see Fig. 6), the secretion of this hormone in an LHS other than breeding would lead to inappropriate results (Wingfield *et al.*, 1997b, 2000).

The hypothesis that nonbreeding territorial aggression is independent of gonadal steroids was, however, challenged by the observation that an experimental elevation of testosterone in male song sparrows holding autumn territories made them more aggressive (Wingfield, 1994b). To further examine a possible role of endogenous sex steroids on territorial behavior in nonbreeding song sparrows, field experiments were conducted using hormone receptor antagonists and hormone synthesis inhibitors. During the breeding period, the level of aggression displayed by individual males toward a territorial intruder is related to the rate with which the avian brain metabolizes testosterone to estradiol (Schlinger and Callard, 1990; Foidart *et al.*, 1998; Balthazart *et al.*, 1999; Silverin *et al.*, 1999). Thus, brain aromatase activity may be a key factor that limits the expression of aggressive behavior in breeding birds. The situation seems to be the same in territorial birds outside the breeding period. Treating free-living European robins, holding an autumn and winter territory, with just an antiandrogen does not affect territorial defense, suggesting that androgen receptors are not of primary importance for this behavior (Schwabl and Kriner, 1991). However, field experiments in nonbreeding territorial song sparrows combining the use of an androgen receptor antagonist with an aromatase inhibitor significantly reduced territorial behavior both during autumn and winter (Soma *et al.*, 1999a; Soma and Wingfield, 2000). The same result was obtained when just an aromatase inhibitor (Fadrozole) was used (Soma *et al.*, 2000a,b). By blocking the aromatase activity, but not by only blocking androgen receptors, autumn territorial aggressive behavior is reduced.

These results suggest that estrogens are involved in the regulation of territorial behavior outside the breeding season. An additional, very important experiment was one in which one group of birds was given an aromatase inhibitor in combination with estradiol implants. This replacement therapy completely restored the territorial aggressive behavior (Soma *et al.*, 2000a). These experiments very convincingly showed that the conversion of testosterone to estradiol is important for the expression of territorial aggression during autumn. If this is the case, why are circulating levels of gonadal hormones low during the nonbreeding period, and why doesn't castration affect territorial behavior?

During the breeding LHS, testosterone regulates a number of traits such as sexual displays, song, and aggressive behavior. It also regulates many morphological events such as the development of secondary sex characteristics and accessory organs. It affects spermatogenesis and muscle hypertrophy. Having high testosterone levels during breeding also implies costs such as increased risks for injuries or being killed by a predator (Fig. 6). High testosterone levels interfere with parental care (Silverin, 1980b; Hegner and Wingfield, 1987), and it may suppress the immune system (Hillgarth and Wingfield, 1997). If a bird has high testosterone levels also outside the breeding period, winter mortality increases (Dufty, 1989; Ketterson *et al.*, 1992). Ecological constraints and the costs associated with prolonged high levels of sex steroids, therefore, have an influence on the hormone–behavior mechanisms (Wingfield *et al.*, 1997b, 1999; Fig. 6). It is therefore important that testosterone secretion is turned off at the right time, so that, by having low circulating levels of testosterone outside the breeding season, a bird avoids the costly peripheral effects of high testosterone titers. Thus, it appears that the hormone-dependent cellular mechanisms controlling spring and autumn territoriality are the same, but that the mode by which hormones are delivered to the target cells in the brain differ. The expressions of the enzymes involved in the metabolism of testosterone may hold the key to the cellular and molecular mechanisms underlying strategies in behavioral ecology.

There are three ways that the potential costs of testosterone secreted into the blood in nonbreeding LHSs could be solved: (1) steroid production could occur in the brain *de novo* from cholesterol (the neurosteroid hypothesis); (2) a peripheral organ, such as the adrenals, could produce a biologically inactive precursor, such as dehydroepiandrosterone (DHEA), that can be converted to the active hormone in the brain (the precursor hypothesis); (3) the target organ could be sensitized to extremely low hormonal levels by regulation of the steroid receptors or changes in the aromatase activity (Soma and Wingfield, 2000).

There is evidence that the brain can synthesize sex steroids from cholesterol *de novo*, thereby creating high local concentrations of steroids, and that this is not reflected in circulating levels of the hormone (Robel and Baulieu, 1995; Tsutsui and Yamakazi, 1995; Baulieu, 1998; Nomura *et al.*, 1998). This is the neurosteroid hypothesis. The hypothesis is, however, controversial. Studies have given different results; some have shown the avian brain to have the capacity to produce steroids (e.g., Vanson *et al.*, 1996), whereas other studies have not (e.g., Lane *et al.*, 1996).

The precursor hypothesis attempts to explain how the endocrine signal gets to the brain to trigger the increase in territorial aggression. The hypothesis states that there is peripheral production of a biologically inert sex steroid and that this hormone is converted to an active hormone in the brain. There are several candidates, and DHEA is a possibility. Enzymatic activity in brain could convert this steroid to androstenedione, which in turn can be converted to testosterone or aromatized to estradiol (Lane et al., 1996; Labrie et al., 1995; Vanson et al., 1996; Schlinger et al., 1999; Ukena et al., 1999). The neurosteroid hypothesis and the precursor hypothesis need not be mutually exclusive.

The third alternative is the increased sensitivity of the brain to low levels of sex steroids during the nonbreeding period. Thus, sex steroids originating from nongonadal organs (e.g., the adrenals) could also be of importance for the maintenance of aggressive behavior during the autumn to winter period. This could occur through an up-regulation of steroid receptors and aromatase activity in the brain. This hypothesis does not seem likely because several studies indicate that birds may have a decreased sensitivity to testosterone outside the breeding season. Available data suggest that the number of androgen receptors is less and hypothalamic aromatase activity is reduced during the nonbreeding period (e.g., Hutchison et al., 1986; Nowicki and Ball, 1989; Schlinger and Callard, 1990; Silverin and Deviche, 1991; Soma et al., 1997, 1999b,c; Gahr and Metzdorf, 1997; Ball, 1999).

C. Hormone–Behavior Interactions in Social Hierarchies in Flocks (Strategy B)

Some species form huge autumn and winter flocks (bramblings), but normally they do not move large distances, they do not defend territories, and most likely there are no social hierarchies in such a flock. There are very few studies of free-living birds in winter flocks investigating the correlation between social dominance and circulating levels of hormones. Rohwer and Wingfield (1981) found no correlation between testosterone and social rank in winter flocks of Harris sparrows. It was speculated that one reason for this could be that social rank is indicated by individual differences in plumage. Nor did Wingfield and Farner (1978a,b) find elevated levels in migratory white-crowned sparrows in flocks in their wintering areas. Similar results were obtained in a study of caged dark-eyed juncos (*Junco hyemalis*; Holberton et al., 1989). Schwabl et al. (1988b) were unable to correlate plumage variations and social rank in white-throated sparrows (*Zonotrichia albicollis*) during autumn, although aggressiveness is related to morph variations during spring. Nor did the white-throated sparrows show any correlation between social rank and autumn testosterone levels.

Many studies have explored the relationship between social status and adrenocortical function in wintering birds. Morphological data point to a correlation between adrenal weight and an individual's status in the social hierarchy, with subdominant individuals having bigger adrenals—possibly indicating higher secretion activity (Fretwell, 1969; Murton et al., 1971). These early observations seem to be partly true also when using more sophisticated methods to assay adrenal activity. These results agree with those found in winter flocks of Harris sparrows. Under snow-free conditions, corticosterone levels are negatively correlated with social status. However, if conditions become severe, corticosterone levels in dominant birds are elevated and the difference between dominant and subdominant birds is abolished (Rohwer and Wingfield, 1981). These observations differ from those made in wintering European blackbirds (Schwabl et al., 1985). A change to a situation with intense food competition does not alter corticosterone levels in adult (dominant) blackbirds, but increases circulating levels of corticosterone in first-year subdominant birds. Similarly, Schwabl et al. (1988b) found that subordinate white-throated sparrows tended to have higher corticosterone levels, both baseline and stress-induced. Much more work remains to be done to determine the mechanisms, but fieldwork has identified several ideal models to pursue the cellular and molecular bases of wintering strategies. The work on adrenocortical function and stress also suggests an overlap with responses to unpredictable events in the environment.

VIII. EMERGENCY LIFE HISTORY STAGE

The development of LHSs, onset of mature capability, and termination follow roughly predictable schedules throughout an individual's life cycle, depending on the type of habitat. However, unpredictable perturbations of the environment can occur at any time in the life cycle (Fig. 7). Typically, reproduction is interrupted while the individual responds to the perturbation, but the reproductive system remains

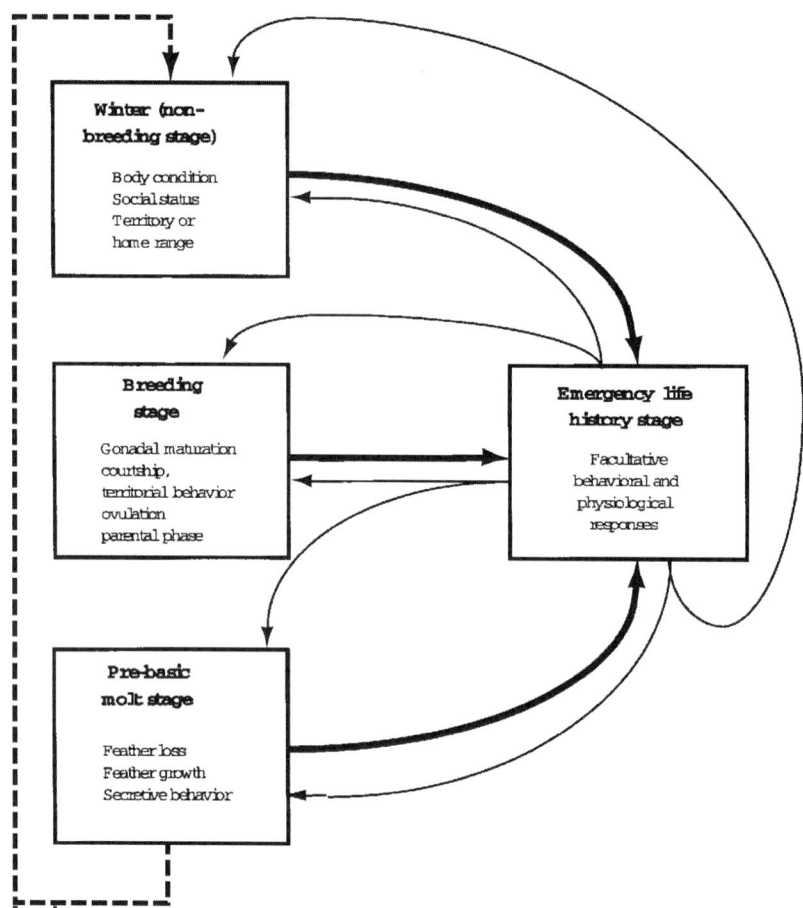

FIGURE 7 Schematic diagram showing the emergency life history stage (ELHS) that can be expressed from any normal life history stage (LHS) in the life cycle (the species here is the nonmigratory song sparrow, Melospiza melodia). The cycle of LHSs represents the predictable life cycle regulated according to the seasons and predictable changes in the environment. Superimposed on this predictable cycle are unpredictable events such as severe storms, failure of trophic resources, and influx of predators. These are called labile perturbation factors (LPFs) and have the potential to be stressful. The ELHS redirects an individual away from its normal LHS into a state that allows it to survive the perturbation in the best condition possible. Once the LPF passes, the individual can return to the same LHS. If the LPF is lasts longer, the next LHS may be the appropriate one to return to. No matter how long an LPF may be in effect, the cycle of normal LHSs continues, although they are not necessarily expressed while the individual is in an ELHS. The bold arrows indicate that the ELHS can be reached directly from any LHS. The finer arrows indicate potential LHSs that an individual can return to after the LPF passes. From Wingfield et al. (1998, 2000), courtesy of MIT Press.

in a near-functional state so that breeding can begin again once the perturbation passes (see Wingfield, 1988, 1994a). We use the term labile perturbation factors (LPFs) to classify these modifying factors because they are transitory, unpredictable, and always disruptive to the current LHS (Jacobs, 1996; Wingfield et al., 1998, 2000). LPFs trigger an emergency life history stage (ELHS), facultative behavioral and physiological responses that appear to be mediated by increases in corticosterone secretion (Wingfield et al.,

1998). There are several components to the ELHS (Wingfield Ramenofsky, 1997, 1999).

1. Deactivation of the current LHS (e.g., territorial behavior or current nesting effort).
2. Active response to the LPF: (a) movement away from the source of the LPF (leave-it strategy), (b) seeking refuge (take-it strategy), (c) seeking refuge first and then moving away if conditions do not improve (take-it first and then leave-it).
3. Mobilization of stored energy sources such as fat and perhaps protein to fuel movement or to provide energy while sheltering in a refuge.
4. Continued movement until a suitable habitat is discovered or the perturbation passes and settlement in the alternate habitat once an appropriate site is identified or return to the original site and resumption of the normal sequence of LHSs.

There have been numerous investigations of the hormonal bases of these facultative behavioral and physiological responses to LPFs, especially in relation to the ecology of animals in their natural environment (Silverin, 1997, 1998a,b,c; Wingfield et al., 1998, 2000). It is also clear that the hypothalamic-pituitary-adrenal (HPA) axis plays a major role in concert with the central actions of several peptides (Wingfield et al., 1998, 2000). The ELHS can be triggered at any time of year and from any LHS (Fig. 7), and the process may involve all times of year. Immediate-response LPFs (e.g., the fight or flight responses to predators) result in immediate avoidance behavior and possibly an increase in corticosterone within a few minutes. These responses are generally too short-lived to activate an ELHS (Wingfield and Ramenofsky, 1997).

Before discussing these endocrine components, it is important to first explore the types of LPFs than an organism may encounter in its habitat. These have been classified as indirect and direct LPFs (Wingfield, 1988). Indirect LPFs result in a change in habitat or social status that does not affect the individual directly (i.e., it is not stressed), but nonetheless results in a change in behavior and physiology. For example, the loss of the nest and young to a predator disrupts the reproductive process and renesting follows. This response to an indirect LPF is independent of the ELHS. In constrast, a LPF such as inclement weather or human disturbance may not affect the nest and young directly, but does decrease available food, temperature and so on. As a result, adults may become energetically stressed. This is a response to a direct LPF that triggers the ELHS via increased the secretion of corticosteroids from adrenocortical tissue (Wingfield and Ramenofsky, 1997; Wingfield et al., 1998). The ELHS is temporary (hours to days), and once the perturbation passes the individual returns to the same LHS or to the next if the ELHS was long in duration (Wingfield et al., 1998).

A. Nonstress Components of the Emergency Life History Stage

Breeding pairs of birds that have lost their nest and young to a storm or predator frequently renest. The loss of the nest is a considerable disruption to the normal temporal progression of the breeding LHS. A major reorganization of endocrine function and expression of substages is necessary to coordinate the renesting attempt. In *Z. l. gambelii*, LH, testosterone, and testis mass increased dramatically after loss of the nest. This was coincident with elevated LH and estrogens in females, leading to the production of a replacement clutch of eggs (Wingfield and Farner, 1979). Similarly, in female mallards after the experimental removal of the eggs (Donham et al., 1976) and in song sparrows that lost nests to extensive flooding (Wingfield and Farner, 1993), there are rapid increases in reproductive hormones just prior to renesting. It is important to note that in white-crowned sparrows there were also increased concentrations of testosterone when producing a replacement clutch. This is unlike multiple brooding after successfully raising young and suggests different mechanisms may initiate a second clutch in these two ecological contexts (see Section IV; Wingfield and Moore, 1987; Wingfield and Farner, 1993).

Why do circulating concentrations of testosterone rise when renesting, but not during the egg-laying period of a normal second brood? It is now well established that high levels of testosterone accompanied by increased territorial and mate-guarding aggression interfere with male parental behavior (see previous discussion; Silverin, 1980b; Hegner Wingfield, 1987) resulting in potential loss of reproductive success (Fig. 6; Beletsky et al., 1995; Ketterson et al., 1996). The fitness of the male has been shown to be greater if he feeds fledglings from the first brood to independence (their chances of survival are greater than for young from later broods; e.g., Perrins, 1970) and may outweigh neglecting current offspring to mate-guard the female and ensure the paternity of later clutches. However, if the eggs or young are lost, it would be advantageous to increase LH and testosterone secretion, enhancing aggression in relation to mate-guarding that in turn would lead to protection of the paternity of the replacement clutch (Wingfield and Moore, 1987). These explanations could be tested further in the field.

B. Behavioral and Physiological Responses to the Unpredictable Environment—Mechanisms to Avoid Chronic Stress

Corticosterone plays a major role in orchestrating physiological and behavioral response patterns to unpredictable environmental events (Wingfield and Ramenofsky, 1997, 1999; Silverin, 1998c). This has been shown both in controlled laboratory studies and field experiments. Free-living birds respond to stressful events such as food shortage, adverse weather, and the appearance of a predator by increasing their corticosterone secretion (Schwabl et al., 1985; Wingfield et al., 1983; Smith et al., 1994; Astheimer et al., 1995; Silverin, 1998a; Romero et al., 2000). In a laboratory experiment, Astheimer et al. (1992) showed how corticosterone may adapt birds to stressful situations. An experimental elevation of corticosterone levels in captive white-crowned sparrows resulted in a decreased activity (perch-hopping) if the birds at the same time had unlimited food availability. This is consistent with the behavior of a bird seeking a refuge while waiting for a stressful event to pass. However, if the food was removed from the corticosterone-treated white-crowned sparrows, they dramatically increased their perch-hoping activity. This resembles the escape behavior of a bird trying to get away from a LPF in the field. The first response is consistent with the take it response; the second is consistent with the leave it response (Wingfield and Ramenofsky, 1997, 1999). Experiments on white-crowned sparrows and some other species indicate that elevated corticosterone levels lower oxygen consumption in birds at rest (Buttemer et al., 1991), thereby saving energy.

There are corresponding observations on free-living birds. Breeding Lapland longspurs exposed to a prolonged snow storm did not abandon their nests until 2–3 days later. After abandoning their nests, longspurs had low baseline corticosterone levels but greatly increased sensitivity to stress (Astheimer et al., 1995). Experiments on breeding free-living pied flycatchers show that changes in parental behavior occur with increasing plasma levels of corticosterone. A slight increase enhances the parents feeding frequency with only minor effects on their body weights. Moderately high increases of corticosterone, however, lead to a decreasing feeding frequency of the nestlings. This results in a high mortality among the nestlings. The body weights of these adults remain constant during the nestling period. A further increase to high levels of corticosterone leads to territories and nests being abandonned. All the nestlings die, but the parents increase their body weight and possibly their survival rate. Thus, there is a clear change in strategy with increasing circulating levels of corticosterone. Behavior is redirected away from reproduction to survival (Silverin, 1986).

There is extensive experimental evidence to support the rapid effects of corticosterone, including suppressed reproductive and territorial behavior without inhibiting the reproductive system (in the chronic stressed state, sustained high levels of corticosteroids result in the marked atrophy of the gonads); increased gluconeogenesis; enhanced foraging behavior; promotion of escape-like behavior (consistent with moving away from the LPF), and conserved energy by reducing the standard metabolic rate at night (Wingfield, 1994b; Wingfield et al., 1998). The short-term effects of corticosterone correspond to many facets of the facultative behavioral and physiological responses typical of an ELHS. Neural peptides such as CRF and β-endorphin also appear to be involved (e.g., Maney and Wingfield, 1998a,b; Wingfield et al., 1998; Romero et al., 1998c). The sum of these is to redirect the individual away from the normal LHS for that time year to maximize survival.

1. Hormonal Changes after Exposure to a Direct Labile Perturbation Factor: The Emergency Life History Stage

A number of field investigations in birds have shown that plasma levels of corticosterone rise while responding to direct LPFs, such as storms, during the breeding season (see Wingfield, 1994b; Wingfield *et al.*, 1998). The behavioral and physiological responses were consistent with components of the ELHS already outlined. In breeding male *Z. l. pugetensis*, prolonged rain and windstorms in May and early June 1980 resulted in the abandonment of the nest and territory (i.e., an ELHS was triggered). Plasma levels of corticosterone were up to threefold higher than the normal levels expected at that time of year (Wingfield *et al.*, 1983), and behavioral and physiological changes characteristic of the ELHS were expressed (Wingfield, 1994b).

The importance of the HPA axis in regulating behaviors outside the breeding season was shown in a study of willow tits in southwest Sweden (Silverin, 1997). In winter, willow tits form stable winter flocks consisting of the two adults that had previously bred in the territory and two to four non-kin juveniles. In the flock there is a strict dominance hierarchy (Ekman, 1979, 1989; Hogstad, 1987, 1989). Because a forest area can host only a limited number of winter flocks, competition among juveniles for membership in a flock is severe during the period of flock establishment. It is crucial for a juvenile to become a flock member, even at the cost of being a subdominant individual. This is best illustrated by the fact that no willow tits survive the winter as solitary floaters, and juveniles showing irruptive movements are in a very poor condition. Juvenile floaters also quickly occupy vacancies in territorial flocks (Ekman *et al.*, 1981; Silverin *et al.*, 1989b). Furthermore, there is no immigration of willow tits to the forest in spring. Therefore, to have a chance to breed the following season, a juvenile must become a member of a winter flock. What allows one individual succeed in becoming a member while others fail and become floaters?

Only approximately 30% of juvenile tits succeed in becoming members of a winter flock. It is, therefore, not surprising that juvenile tits are very aggressive during early autumn (Hogstad, 1990). At this time of the year, approximately the same percentage of juveniles (males as well as females), but no adults, have very high circulating levels of testosterone in their blood (Silverin *et al.*, 1986), although an extensive field experiment could not confirm a role for testosterone in gaining territorial status (Silverin *et al.*, 1989b; see also Section VII).

In their study on flock establishment among juvenile willow tits, Thessing and Ekman (1994) showed that environmental conditions affect individuals in a cohort differently and that juveniles with a slow growth rate were less likely to succeed in becoming a permanent member of a flock. It is likely that these individuals where undernourished and were exposed to long-term nutritional stress—a situation known to increase corticosterone secretion in other species (Cherel *et al.*, 1988b). One of the more obvious results from studies on stress sensitivity in birds is the huge individual variation in the response. It has been suggested that at least part of this variation is caused by individual differences in body condition (Wingfield *et al.*, 1995b; Wingfield and Ramenofsky, 1999). Birds in better condition should be more resistant to an acute stressor. However, studies have not given uniform results— some studies show a relationship; others do not (Smith *et al.*, 1994; Wingfield *et al.*, 1994a,b, 1995a; Silverin *et al.*, 1997a; Silverin and Wingfield, 1998). Perhaps the results would be more uniform if researchers instead look at changes in body condition over time and compare that with the stress response.

It is possible that only a slight increase in corticosterone secretion triggers an ELHS, such as dispersal behavior. This would give floaters an opportunity to find a new area with better feeding conditions, and eventually places in winter flocks, or to create new flocks containing only juveniles. It is less likely that aggressive encounters between juveniles cause elevated corticosterone levels because this has never been found in juveniles defending their flock membership (Silverin *et al.*, 1989b). Because migrating juveniles also have higher plasma levels of corticosterone than territorial juveniles (Silverin *et al.*, 1989b), it is likely that the physiological mechanism regulating dispersal behavior involves the HPA axis. However, because corticosterone levels do not differ between migratory and sedentary European blackbirds prior to the onset of autumn migration (Schwabl *et al.*, 1984), it is also possible that the high corticosterone levels observed in migrating juvenile willow tits are due to energy demands during the actual migratory flight.

These issues were addressed in a field study in which willow tits were given either empty silastic implants or implants filled with corticosterone at a time when juveniles were fighting to become established as permanent flock members (Silverin, 1997). The results clearly showed that, at this time of the year, an experimental elevation of corticosterone levels caused a restlessness in the juvenile birds, but surprisingly not in the adult birds. Most of the juveniles implanted with corticosterone disappeared from the forest. Those remaining never settled in a territory, but kept wandering back and forth over the entire study area (several square kilometers). Adults given a corticosterone implant never left the territory in which they were originally captured. This may be a result of prior residency in the territory and, eventually, also a result of being the dominant individuals in the flock. The mechanisms by which juveniles show such a markedly different response to adults remain to be determined.

Because juveniles respond to elevated corticosterone levels by dispersing, normally a fatal behavior, sensitivity to stress should be selected against. This was investigated in an experiment in which juvenile and adult willow tits were exposed to a standardized stress situation (capture or handling stress) at different ecological stages during the autumn to winter period (Silverin, 1997). At the time that family flocks break up (July) and juveniles start to settle into the future winter flocks, neither juveniles nor adults show a strong adrenocortical response to capture stress. In September, a time when flock establishment is still going on, juveniles continue to respond very weakly to stress. Adults, on the other hand, have dramatically changed their reaction pattern and are now highly sensitive to stress. The significance of this change is unknown. This is a situation contrary to the one found in white-throated sparrows, in which dominant individuals in a flock normally show a lower stress response than subordinate individuals (Schwabl, 1995). Later in autumn (November) when there are no more willow tit floaters in the forest and flock composition has been permanently settled, juveniles (the subordinate individuals) and the dominant adults are equally highly sensitive to stress and baseline levels of corticosterone do not differ between the two groups.

Both of these situations are in contrast to cases of social groups of other birds. For example, in a wintering population of European blackbirds in southern Germany only the subdominant juveniles react to a LPF such as cold and snowy weather by increasing their corticosterone secretion; adult blackbirds do not. As a result, juvenile blackbirds migrate away from the area (Schwabl et al., 1985). However, willow tits differ from blackbirds in being strictly year-round territorial residents that live in flocks with a strict hierarchy. Subdominant and dominant individuals have access to the same amount of food, but are exposed to dramatically different predation pressure because they forage in different parts of the tree canopy.

2. Other Examples of Emergency Stages during Winter

Birds wintering in areas where the food resources may be covered with snow for a longer or shorter period are exposed to a risk of starvation. The only way to avoid this is to migrate away from certain severe snow conditions. This problem has been studied among ground-feeding species such as juncos and sparrows. However, tree-dwelling species face a similar problem when the winter weather rapidly changes from mild and wet to cold. A rapid drop in temperature covers tree branches with an icy snow cover that the birds cannot penetrate. Thus tree-dwelling species are exposed to the same risks of starvation as ground-feeding birds.

Ground-feeding birds in wintering flocks of dark-eyed juncos and white-throated sparrows use microhabitats, such a bare patches of ground under trees where the snow depth rarely exceeds 1–2 cm. These microhabitats are called qamaniq (Pruitt, 1970; Wingfield and Ramenofsky, 1999; Wingfield and Romero, 2000). A severe winter storm may, however, fill up the qamaniq, and, to acquire food, birds then have to dig through the snow cover. When the digging becomes too costly in relation to what is to be gained, flight away from the area is triggered. Juncos and the sparrows abandon their home range if the snow is more than 5 cm deep (Wingfield and Ramenofsky, 1997).

Dark-eyed juncos wintering in New York state had more fat stored in subcutaneous depots than juncos wintering much further south in Mississippi. Both populations had similar baseline plasma levels of corticosterone, but the birds wintering in New York showed a greater adrenocortical response to acute stress (Holberton and Able, 2000). These data suggest that birds wintering further north in potentially more severe and unpredictable winter environments have a higher responsiveness to stress that triggers movement out if conditions deteriorate. Furthermore, baseline plasma levels of corticosterone may also indicate habitat quality in wintering birds (Marra and Holberton, 1998).

Tree-foraging nonhoarding species, such as great tits, living in coniferous forests in southwest Sweden leave the forests if the winter weather deteriorates too far and foraging sites are covered with snow or ice. However, hoarding species, such as the willow tit, do not leave their winter territories (B. Silverin, unpublished data).

Dark-eyed juncos have higher plasma levels of corticosterone during an ongoing winter storm and while their home ranges are being abandoned than before or after the storm (when the birds again have found a refuge) (Rogers et al., 1993). Similar hormonal data have been obtained during severe winter weather for European blackbirds and Harris sparrows (Rohwer and Wingfield, 1981; Schwabl et al., 1985). In the case of the Harris sparrow, the birds did not leave their home range but, instead, became inactive and waited for the storm to pass. Common diving petrels (*Pelecanoides urinatrix*) that live and forage out on the open ocean, and thus in a completely different environment than the ground-feeding terrestrial species, also increase their corticosterone secretion in response to severe storms. As do the terrestrial birds, the petrels change their behavior and fly to islands where they can stay and seek shelter (Smith et al., 1994). Results from field studies such as these, coupled with data from controlled laboratory experiments, strongly suggest that corticosterone is directly involved in the induction of this ELHS.

C. Modulation of the Adrenocortical Response to Stress and Its Ecological Bases

We have already discussed that some populations appear to change sensitivity of the HPA axis to acute stress (due to LPFs). There are now many studies indicating the diverse ways in which the adrenocortical response to stress is modulated (Wingfield *et al.*, 1995b; Wingfield and Romero, 2000). Corticosterone levels increase within 5 minutes or so of capture, handling, and restraint and either continue to increase or plateau 30–60 minutes postcapture (Wingfield, 1994a). This standardized protocol can be used to compare the responses to acute stress across populations or in individuals within populations. The variation in the magnitude of adrenocortical responses to stress in birds resulted in three hypotheses concerning possible ecological bases (Wingfield *et al.*, 1995b).

1. *Body size and the modulation of adrenocortical responsiveness to acute stress.* Those species with greater body mass may have relatively greater reserves of fat and protein to combat LPFs such as inclement weather. They should be resistant to acute stress because stored energy (on fat) reserves are relatively greater than those for smaller species. Thus, they should be able to ride out the storm (take-it strategy). Smaller species have relatively limited reserves of fat and protein and may starve to death during a LPF. Therefore, smaller species should retain adrenocortical responsiveness to acute stress when breeding. However, there was no correlation of body mass with either maximum corticosterone level or the ratio of maximum to minimum levels, although there is the potential for a bias of phylogeny in the comparison of species (Wingfield *et al.*, 1995b).

2. *Age and the modulation of adrenocortical responsiveness to acute stress.* Species with a limited life span (one two breeding seasons) may be more resistant to LPFs when breeding so as to maximize reproductive success, even though the survival of the adults may be compromised. Long-lived species (5–10 or even more potential breeding seasons) may remain sensitive to LPFs and abandon the current breeding effort to survive in the best condition possible so as to attempt successful reproduction in a subsequent year. An analysis of several species according to age revealed no relationship of the adrenocortical response to the capture stress paradigm and age. There were no trends within groups of taxa, and it is unlikely that phylogeny was biasing the results (Wingfield *et al.*, 1995b).

3. *Degree of parental care and the modulation of adrenocortical responsiveness to acute stress.* The period of parental care is one of high energetic demands and there is a lot of evidence that the adrenocortical response to LPFs is reduced at this time (Wingfield *et al.*, 1995b; Wingfield and Romero, 2000). The sensitivity of the HPA axis may be a function of the degree of parental care provided by an individual. An analysis of several species showed clearly that those individuals expressing parental care had significantly lower stress levels of corticosterone. The baseline levels of

corticosterone were similar, however (Wingfield et al., 1995b).

Thus, it appears that the degree of parental care is one ecological correlate of modulation of the HPA axis to LPFs. Since that time, other possible ecological bases of stress modulation have been hypothesized, but much more fieldwork is required to test them. In general, it is thought that the modulation of the HPA axis response to LPFs at the population level occurs in species nesting in severe environments. Here the breeding LHS is short and birds are potentially exposed to inclement weather; shortages of food, especially early in the breeding season; and unpredictable numbers of predators (Wingfield and Romero, 2000). The onset of the parental phase in the breeding LHS also results in decreased sensitivity to LPFs regardless of severity of the breeding habitat. We also know that the modulation of the adrenocortical response to LPFs can occur at the individual level within a population. These responses are related to body condition and social status (Wingfield and Ramenofsky, 1999). Evidence in support of these hypotheses is provocative, but future field investigations will be critical to clarify these issues.

D. Mechanisms Modulating Responses to Stress

Although it is clear that the HPA axis changes sensitivity to LPFs, the mechanisms by which this is done appear to be complex and no clear trends are apparent (Wingfield and Romero, 2000). Male *Z. l. gambelii* actually increased their sensitivity to the capture stress protocol in the breeding LHS, possibly as a result of reduced sensitivity to glucocorticosteroid feedback (Astheimer et al., 1994). Investigations of several arctic-breeding passerines indicate that the mechanisms underlying the seasonal changes in the stress response may lie at the level of the adrenocortical cells, anterior pituitary or higher (Romero et al., 1998a,b,d; Romero and Wingfield, 1999). Also, we do not know what causes the seasonal change in the behavioral response to elevated corticosterone levels (Astheimer et al., 2000). Changes in the number and distribution of corticosterone receptors, the binding affinity and binding capacity of corticosterone-binding proteins (CBP), and the enzymes converting corticosterone to the biologically inactive 11-dehydrocorticosterone may be involved (Silverin, 1986; Wingfield and Romero, 2000).

Glucocorticosteroids act through classic intracellular receptors that bind to the genome and regulate gene expression (e.g., McEwen et al., 1993). Down-regulation of corticosteroid receptors in response to chronic high levels of corticosteroids may be a mechanism to reduce deleterious effects such as neuron loss (McEwen et al., 1993). However, genomic actions of steroid hormones require at least 30 min, and usually hours, whereas some actions appear to occur within minutes. For example, in white-crowned sparrows, noninvasive treatment with corticosterone induced an increase in locomotor activity within 15 minutes (Breuner et al., 1998), and this response appears to be modulated by season (Breuner and Wingfield, 2000). In amphibians there is evidence for a membrane receptor for corticosterone (Orchinik et al., 1991) that may transduce effects within minutes. An apparently similar membrane component that binds corticosterone has been identified in passerine birds (Breuner et al., unpublished). As cellular and molecular tools become modified and available for wild species, great advances in the mechanisms of stress modulation can be expected.

IX. CONCLUSION

It is encouraging, indeed surprising, that there are now several hundred published papers on field endocrinology of birds alone (and many more for vertebrates in general). However, most of these have little interconnection to each other except to explore how free-living animals cope with a changing environment. We now face the daunting challenge to move forward in a theoretical sense, to draw together this morass of information and mold it into a framework that predicts neuroendocrine and endocrine mechanisms underlying ecological processes. Such a framework will also allow a more meaningful approach at the evolutionary level. Although many theoretical approaches are possible, FSM theory has at least heuristic value insofar as it provides a common framework for all LHSs in an individual's life cycle and makes specific predictions that can be followed up in the field or in the laboratory. We also hope it will be a way to determine more sytematically how mechanisms at the cellular and molecular level underlie these responses to the environment. As the world of genomics progresses, it is hoped that molecular biology will flourish in wild species. The staggering biodiversity of species and populations in equally diverse habitats provides natural examples of any gene knockout or mutation that we could imagine. It should also be noted that they carry none of the problems of interpretation that engineered gene knockouts and mutations do. The possibilities are endless as we ponder the potential of an unprecedented new era of organismal biology.

Acknowledgments

The preparation of this manuscript and the formulation of ideas in it were facilitated by a John Simon Guggenheim Fellowship and a Bejamin Meaker Fellowship to J. C. W., and by financial support to B. S. from the Swedish National Research Council. J. C. W. is also grateful to the Division of Integrative Biology and Neurobiology and the Office of Polar Programs, National Science Foundation, for many years of generous grant support. He was also the recipient of a Shannon Award from the National Institutes of Health and the Russell F. Stark University Professorship from the University of Washington. Both awards had a major influence on the development of the ideas presented in this review.

References

Amadon, D. (1966). Avian plumages and molts. *Condor* **68**, 263–278.

Andreev, A. V. (1999). Energetics and survival of birds in extreme environments. *Ostrich* **70**, 13–22.

Arnold, A. P., and Breedlove, S. M. (1985). Organizational and activational effects of sex steroids on brain and behavior: A reanalysis. *Horm. Behav.* **19**, 469–498.

Assenmacher, I. (1973). The peripheral endocrine glands. *Avian Biol.* **3**, 183–286.

Astheimer, L. B., Buttemer, W. A., and Wingfield, J. C. (1992). Interactions of corticosterone with feeding, activity and metabolism in passerine birds. *Ornis Scand.* **23**, 355–365.

Astheimer, L. B., Buttemer, W. A., and Wingfield, J. C. (1994). Gender and seasonal differences in the adrenocortical response to ACTH challenge in an arctic passerine, *Zonotrichia leucophrys gambelii. Gen. Comp. Endocrinol.* **94**, 33–43.

Astheimer, L. B., Buttemer, W. A., and Wingfield, J. C. (1995). Seasonal and acute changes in adrenocortical responsiveness in an Arctic-breeding bird. *Horm. Behav.* **29**, 442–457.

Astheimer, L. B., Buttemer, W. A., and Wingfield, J. C. (2000). Corticosterone treatment has no effect on reproductive hormones or aggressive behavior in free-living male tree sparrows, *Spizella arborea. Horm. Behav.* **37**, 31–39.

Ball, G. F. (1993). The neurointegration of environmental information by seasonally breeding birds. *Am. Zool.* **33**, 185–199.

Ball, G. F. (1999). Neuroendocrine basis of seasonal changes in vocal behavior among songbirds. *In* "The Design of Communication" (M. Hauser and M. Konishi, eds.), pp. 213–254. MIT Press, Cambridge, MA.

Ball, G. F., and Wingfield, J. C. (1987). Changes in plasma levels of sex steroids in relation to multiple broodedness and nest site density in male starlings. *Physiol. Zool.* **60**, 191–199.

Balthazart, J. (1983). Hormonal correlates of behavior. *Avian Biol.* **7**, 221–365.

Balthazart, J., Foidart, A., Baillien, M., and Silverin, B. (1999). Brain aromatase in laboratory and free-living songbirds: Relationships with reproductive behaviour. *Proc. 22nd Int. Ornithol. Congr.*, Durban, pp. 1257–1289.

Baptista, L. F., and Welty, (1987). "The Life of Birds." Saunders Press, Philadelphia.

Baptista, L. F., DeWolfe, B. B., and Avery-Beausoleil, L. (1987). Testosterone, aggression, and dominance in Gambel's white-crowned sparrow. *Wilson Bull.* **99**, 86–91.

Baulieu, E. (1998). Neurosteroids: A novel function of the brain. *Psychoneuroendocrinology* **23**, 963–987.

Beletsky, L. D., Gori, D. F., Freeman, S., and Wingfield, J. C. (1995). Testosterone and polygyny in birds. *Curr. Ornithol.* **12**, 1–41.

Belthoff, J. R., and Dufty, A. M., Jr. (1998). Corticosterone, body condition and locomotor activity: A model for dispersal in screech owls. *Anim. Behav.* **55**, 405–415.

Berthold, P. (1977). Endogene Steuerung des Vogelzuges. *Vogelwarte* **29**, 4–15.

Berthold, P. (1996). "Control of Bird Migration." Chapman Hall Press, London.

Berthold, P. (1999). A comprehensive theory for the evolution, control and adaptability of bird migration. *Ostrich* **70**, 1–12.

Berthold, P., and Querner, U. (1982). Genetic basis of moult, wing-length and body weight in a migratory bird species *Sylvai atricapilla. Experientia* **38**, 801–802.

Berthold, P., Gwinner, E., and Klein, H. (1971). Circanuelle Periodik bei Grasmücken (*Sylvia*). *Experentia* **27**, 399.

Berthold, P., Gwinner, E., Klein, H., and Westrich, P. (1972a). Beziehungen zwischen Zugunruhe und Zugablauf bei Garten- und Mönchsgrasmücke (*Sylvia borin* und *S. atricapilla*). *Z. Tierpsychol.* **30**, 26–35.

Berthold, P., Gwinner, E., and Klein, H. (1972b). Circanuelle Periodik bei Grasmücken I. Periodik des Körpergewichtes, der Mauser und der Nachunruhe bei *Sylvia atricapilla* und *S. borin* unter verschiedenen konstanten Bedingungen. *J. Ornithol.* **113**, 170–190.

Biebach, H. (1990). Strategies of trans-sahara migrants. *In* "Bird Migration" (E. Gwinner, ed.), pp. 352–367. Springer-Verlag, Berlin.

Blanchard, B. D. (1941). The white-crowned sparrows (*Zonotrichia leucophrys*) of the Pacific seaboard: Environment and annual cycle. *Univ. Calif., Berkeley, Publ. Zool.* **46**, 1–178.

Blanchard, B. D., and Erickson, M. M. (1949). The cycle in the Gambel sparrow. *Univ. Calif., Berkeley, Publ. Zool.* **47**, 225–318.

Boss, W. R. (1943). Hormonal determination of adult characters and sex behavior in herring gulls (*Larus argentatus*). *J. Exp. Zool.* **94**, 181–209.

Boss, W. R., and Witschi, E. (1941). Male sex hormones inducing adult characters in juvenile herring gulls (*Larus argentatus*). *Anat. Rec.* **81**(Suppl.), 27–28.

Boswell, T., Richardson, R. D., Seeley, R. J., Ramenofsky, M., Wingfield, J. C., Friedman, M. I., and Woods, S. C. (1995). Regulation of food intake by metabolic fuels in white-crowned sparrows. *Am. J. Physiol.* **269**, R1462–R1468.

Breuner, C. W., and Wingfield, J. C. (2000). Rapid behavioral response to corticosterone varies with photoperiod and dose. *Horm. Behav.* **37**, 23–30.

Breuner, C. W., Greenberg, A. L., and Wingfield, J. C. (1998). Non-invasive corticosterone treatment rapidly increases activity in Gambel's white-crowned Sparrows (*Zonotrichia leucophrys gambelii*). *Gen. Comp. Endocrinol.* **111**, 386–394.

Burger, A. E., and Millar, R. P. (1980). Seasonal changes of sexual and territorial behavior and plasma testosterone levels in male lesser sheathbills (*Chionis minor*). *Z. Tierpsychol.* **52**, 397–406.

Buttemer, W. A., Astheimer, L. A., and Wingfield, J. C. (1991). The effect of corticosterone on standard metabolic rates of small passerines. *J. Comp. Physiol. B* **161**, 427–431.

Campbell, R. R., and Leatherland, J. F. (1979). Effect of TRH, TSH, and LHRH on plasma thyroxine and triiodothyronine in the lesser snow goose (*Anser caerulescens caerulescens*) and plasma thyroxine in the Rouen duck (*Anas platyrhynchos*). *Can. J. Zool.* **57**, 271–274.

Camper, P. M., and Burke, W. H. (1977a). The effects of prolactin on the gonadotropin induced rise in serum estradiol and progesterone of the laying turkey. *Gen. Comp. Endocrinol.* **32**, 72–77.

Camper, P. M., and Burke, W. H. (1977b). The effect of prolactin on reproductive function in female Japanese quail (*Coturnix coturnix japonica*). *Poul. Sci.* **56**, 1130–1134.

Chandler, C. R., Ketterson, E. D., Nolan, V., Jr., and Ziegenfus, C. (1994). Effects of testosterone on spatial activity in free-ranging male dark-eyed juncos, *Junco hyemalis*. *Anim. Behav.* **47**, 1445–1455.

Chandler, C. R., Ketterson, E. D., and Nolan, V., Jr. (1997). Effects of testosterone on use of space by male dark-eyed juncos when their mates are fertile. *Anim. Behav.* **54**, 543–549.

Chandola, A., and Pathak, V. (1980). Premigratory increase in circulating triiodothyronine/thyroxine ratio in the red-headed bunting (*Emberiza bruniceps*). *Gen. Comp. Endocrinol.* **42**, 39–46.

Chase, D. J. (1982). Gonadotropin specificity of acute testicular androgen secretion in birds. *Gen. Comp. Endocrinol.* **46**, 486–499.

Cheng, M.-F. (1979). Progress and prospectus in ring dove research: A personal view. *In* "Advances in the Study of Behavior" (J. S. Rosenblatt, R. A. Hinde, E. Shaw, and C. Beer, eds.), Vol. 9, pp. 97–129. Academic Press, New York.

Cherel, Y., Leloup, J., and Maho, Y. (1988a). Fasting in king penguin: II. Hormonal and metabolic changes during molt. *Am. J. Physiol.* **254**, R178–R184.

Cherel, Y., Robin, J.-P., and Maho, Y. (1988b). Physiology and biochemistry of long-term fasting in birds. *Can. J. Zool.* **66**, 159–166.

Chilgren, J. D. (1978). Effects of photoperiod and temperature on postnuptial molt in captive white-crowned sparrows. *Condor* **80**, 222–229.

Curry-Lindahl, K. (1958). Internal timer and spring migration in an equatorial migrant, the yellow wagtail (*Motacilla flava*). *Ark. Zool.* **11**, 541–557.

Danforth, C. H. (1937). An experimental study of plumage in Reeve's pheasants. *J. Exp. Zool.* **77**, 1–11.

Dawkins, R. (1982). "The Extended Phenotype. The Gene as the Unit of Selection." Freeman, Oxford.

Dawson, A. (1983). Plasma gonadal steroid levels in wild starlings (*Sturnus vulgaris*) during the annual cycle in relation to the stages of breeding. *Gen. Comp. Endocrinol.* **49**, 286–294.

Dawson, A. (1994). The effects of daylength and testosterone on the initiation and progress of moult in starlings *Sturnus vulgaris*. *Ibis* **136**, 335–340.

Dawson, A., and Sharp, P. J. (1998). The role of prolactin in the development of reproductive photorefractoriness and postnuptial molt in the European starling (*Sturnus vulgaris*). *Endocrinology (Baltimore)* **139**, 485–490.

Dittami, J. P. (1987). A comparison of breeding and molt cycles and life histories in two tropical starling species: The blue-eared glossy starling *Lamprotornis chalybaeus* and Rueppell's long-tailed glossy starling *Lamprotornis purpuropterus*. *Ibis* **129**, 69–85.

Dittami, J. P., and Gwinner, E. (1985). Annual cycles in the African stonechat *Saxicola torquata axillaris* and their relationship to environmental factors. *J. Zool.* **207**, 357–370.

Dittami, J. P., and Hall, M. R. (1983). Molt, thyroxine, and testosterone in adult male and female barheaded geese, *Anser indicus*. *Can. J. Zool.* **61**, 2695–2697.

Dolnik, V. R. (1975). Fotoperiodicheskii kontrol sezonnykh tsiklov beca tela linki i polovoi aktivnosti u zyablekov (*Fringilla coelebs*). *Zool. Zh.* **54**, 1048–1056.

Dolnik, V. R. (1976). Fotoperiodizm u ptits. *In* "Fotoperiodizm Zhivotnykhi Rastenii" (L. Zaslavsky, ed.), pp. 47–81. Akad. Nauk SSSR, Leningrad.

Dolnik, V. R., and Gavrilov, V. M. (1980). Photoperiodic control of the molt cycle in the chaffinch (*Fringilla coelebs*). *Auk* **97**, 50–62.

Donham, R. S., Dane, C. W., and Farner, D. S. (1976). Plasma luteinzing hormone and the development of ovarian follicles after loss of clutch in female mallards (*Anas platyrhynchos*). *Gen. Comp. Endocrinol.* **29**, 152–155.

Donham, R. S., Wingfield, J. C., Mattocks, P. W., Jr., and Farner, D. S. (1982). Changes in testicular and plasma androgens with photoperiodically induced increase in plasma LH in the house sparrow. *Gen. Comp. Endocrinol.* **48**, 342–347.

Dorst, J. (1955). Le déterminisme physiologique de l'impulsion migratoire. *Scientia* **49**, 1–5.

Dufty, A. M. (1989). Testosterone and survival. *Horm. Behav.* **23**, 185–193.

Eens, M., Van Duyse, E., Berghmann, L., and Pinxten, R. (2000). Shield characteristics are testosterone-dependent in both male and female moorhens. *Horm. Behav.* **37**, 126–134.

Ekman, J. (1979). Coherence, composition and territories of winter social groups of the willow tit *Parus montanus* and the crested tit *P. Cristatus*. *Ornis Scand.* **10**, 56–68.

Ekman, J. (1989). Ecology of non-breeding social systems of *Parus*. *Wilson Bull.* **101**, 263–288.

Ekman, J., Cederholm, G., and Askenmo, C. (1981). Spacing and survival in winter groups of willow tits *Parus montanus* and crested tits *P. Cristatus*: A removal study. *J. Anim. Ecol.* **50**, 1–9.

El Halawani, M. E., and Rozenboim, I. (1993). Incubation behavior in the turkey: Molecular and endocrinological implications. *In* "Avian Endocrinology" (P. J. Sharp, ed.), pp. 99–110. Soc. Endocrinol., Bristol, UK.

Emlen, J. T., and Lorenz, F. W. (1942). Pairing responses of free-living valley quail to sex hormone pellet implants. *Auk* **59**, 369–378.

Emlen, S. T. (1969). Bird migration: Influence of physiological state upon celestial orientation. *Science* **165**, 716–718.

Enstrom, D. A., Ketterson, E. D., and Nolan, V., Jr. (1997). Testosterone and mate choice in the dark-eyed junco. *Anim. Behav.* **54**, 1135–1146.

Epple, A., and Stetson, M. H. (1980). "Avian Endocrinology." Academic Press, New York.

Evans, M. R., Goldsmith, A. R., and Norris, S. R. A. (2000). The effects of testosterone on antibody production and plumage coloration in male house sparrows (*Passer domesticus*). *Behav. Ecol. Sociobiol.* **47**, 156–163.

Evans, P. R. (1970). Timing mechanisms and the physiology of bird migration. *Sci. Prog. (Oxford)* **58**, 263–275.

Farner, D. S. (1955). The annual stimulus for migration: Experimental and physiologic aspects. *In* "Recent Studies in Avian Biology" (A. Wolfson, ed.), University of Illinois Press, Urbana.

Farner, D. S. (1985). Annual rhythms. *Annu. Rev. Physiol.* **47**, 65–82.

Farner, D. S., and Follett, B. K. (1979). Reproductive periodicity in birds. *In* "Hormones and Evolution" (E. J. W. Barrington, ed.), pp. 829–872. Academic Press, New York.

Farner, D. S., and Gwinner, E. (1980). Photoperiodicity, circannual and reproductive cycles. *In* "Avian Endocrinology" (A. Epple and M. H. Stetson, eds.), pp. 331–366. Academic Press, New York.

Farner, D. S., and Lewis, R. A. (1971). Photoperiodism and reproductive cycles in birds. *In* "Photoperiodicity" (A. C. Giese, ed.), Vol. 6, pp. 325–370. Academic Press, New York.

Farner, D. S, and Mewaldt, L. R. (1953). The recording of diurnal activity patterns in caged birds. *Bird-Banding* **24**, 55–65.

Farner, D. S., and Mewaldt, L. R. (1955). The natural termination of the photorefractory period in the white-crowned sparrow. *Condor* **57**, 112–116.

Fivizzani, A. J., Colwell, M. A., and Oring, L. W. (1986). Plasma steroid hormone levels in free-living Wilson's phalaropes, *Phalaropus tricolor*. *Gen. Comp. Endocrinol.* **62**, 137–144.

Fivizzani, A. J., Oring, L. W., El Halawani, M. E., and Schlinger, B. A. (1990). Hormonal basis of male parental care and female intersexual competition in sex-role reversed birds. *In* "Endocrinology of Birds: Molecular to Behavioral" (S. Ishii, M. Wada, and C. G. Scanes, eds.), pp. 273–286. Jpn. Sci. Soc. Press, Tokyo/Springer-Verlag, Berlin.

Foidart, A., Silverin, B., Baillien, M., Harada, N., and Balthazart, J. (1998). Neuroanatomical distribution and variations across the reproductive cycle of aromatase activity and aromatase-immunoreactive cells in the pied flycatchers (*Ficedula hypoleuca*). *Horm. Behav.* **33**, 180–196.

Follett, B. K. (1984). Birds. *In* "Marshall's Physiology of Reproduction" (G. E. Lamming, ed.), Vol. 1, pp. 283–350. Churchill-Livingstone, Edinburgh.

Follett, B. K., Ishii, S., and Chandola, A. (1985). "The Endocrine System and the Environment." Jpn. Sci. Soc. Press, Tokyo/Springer-Verlag, Berlin.

Fretwell, S. D. (1969). Dominance behavior and winter habitat in juncos (*Junco hyemalis*). *Bird-Banding* **40**, 1–25.

Gahr, M., and Metzdorf, R. (1997). Distribution and dynamics in the expression of androgen and estrogen receptors in vocal control systems of songbirds. *Brain Res. Bull.* **44**, 509–517.

Gauthreaux, S. A., Jr. (1982). The ecology and evolution of avian migration systems. *Avian Biol.* **6**, 93–168.

Gavrilov, V. M., and Dolnik, V. R. (1974). Bioenergetics and regulations of the postnuptial and postjuvenile molt in chaffinches (*Fringilla coelebs coelebs*). *Dokl. Akad. Nauk SSSR* **60**, 14–62 (in Russian).

Goldsmith, A. R. (1983). Prolactin in avian reproductive cycles. *In* "Hormones and Behavior in Higher Vertebrates" (J. Balthazart, E. Pröve, and R. Gilles, eds.), pp. 375–387. Springer-Verlag, Berlin.

Goldsmith, A. R. (1991). Prolactin and avian reproductive strategies. *Acta 20th Congr. Int. Ornithol.*, pp. 2063–2071.

Goldsmith, A. R., Edwards, C., Koprucu, M., and Silver, R. (1981). Concentrations of prolactin and luteinizing hormone in plasma of doves in relation to incubation and development of the crop gland. *J. Endocrinol.* **90**, 437–443.

Gorbman, A., Dickhoff, W. W., Vigna, S. R., Clark, N. B., and Ralph, C. L. (1983). "Comparative Endocrinology." Wiley, New York.

Gorman, M. L. (1974). The endocrine basis of pair-formation behavior in the male eider *Somateria mollissima*. *Ibis* **116**, 451–465.

Groothuis, T., and Meeuwissen, G. (1992). The influence of testosterone on the development and fixation of the form of displays in two age classes of young black-headed gulls. *Anim. Behav.* **43**, 189–208.

Groscolas, R., Jallageas, M., Leloup, J., and Goldsmith, A. (1986). The endocrine control of reproduction in male and female emperor penguins (*Aptenodytes forsteri*). *Proc. 19th Int. Ornithol. Congr.*, pp. 1692–1701.

Gullion, G. W. (1951). The frontal shield of the American coot. *Wilson Bull.* **63**, 157–166.

Gwinner, E. (1971). Endogenous timing factors in bird migration. *In* "Animal Orientation and Navigation" (S. R. Galler, ed.), pp. 321–338. NASA, Washington, DC.

Gwinner, E. (1972). Adaptive functions of circannual rhythms in warblers. *Proc. 15th Int Ornithol. Congr.*, pp. 218–236.

Gwinner, E. (1977a). Circannual rhythms in bird migration. *Annu. Rev. Ecol. Syst.* **8**, 381–405.

Gwinner, E. (1977b). Über die Synchronization circannualer Rhythmen bei Vögeln. *Vogelwarte* **29**, 16–25.

Gwinner, E. (1981). Circannual systems: Perspective. *In* "Handbook of Behavioral Neurobiology" (J. Aschoff, ed.), Vol. 4, pp. 391–410. Plenum Press, New York.

Gwinner, E. (1986). "Circannual Rhythms." Springer-Verlag, Berlin.

Gwinner, E., Zeman, M., and Schwabl-Benzinger, I. (1992). Corticosterone levels of passerinebirds during migratory flight. *Naturwissenschaften* **79**, 276–278.

Gwinner, E., Rödl, T., and Schwabl, H. (1994). Pair territoriality of wintering stonechats: Behavior, function and hormones. *Behav. Ecol. Sociobiol.* **34**, 321–327.

Haase, E. (1975). The effects of testosterone propionate on secondary sexual characters and testes of the house sparrow, *Passer domesticus*. *Gen. Comp. Endocrinol.* **26**, 248–252.

Haase, E., and Paulke, E. (1980). Plasma concentrations of triiodothyronine, thyroxine and testosterone during the annual cycle of wild mallard drakes and the effects of thyroidectomy. *Zool. Anz.* **204**, 102–110.

Haase, E., Sharp, P. J., and Paulke, E. (1975). Annual cycle of plasma lueinizing hormone concentrations in wild mallard drakes. *J. Exp. Zool.* **194**, 553–558.

Hadley, M. E. (1999). "Endocrinology." Prentice Hall, Upper Saddle River, NJ.

Hahn, T. P. (1995). Integration of photoperiodic and food cues to time changes in reproductive physiology by an opportunistic breeder, the red crossbill, *Loxia curvirostra* (Aves: Carduelinae). *J. Exp. Zool.* **272**, 213–226.

Hahn, T. P. (1997). Reproductive seasonality in an opportunistic breeder, the red crossbill, *Loxia curvirostra*. *Ecology* **79**, 2365–2375.

Hahn, T. P., Boswell, T., Wingfield, J. C., and Ball, G. F. (1997). Temporal flexibility in avian reproduction: Patterns and mechanisms. *Curr. Ornithol.* **14**, 39–80.

Harding, C. F. (1981). Social modulation of circulating hormone levels in the male. *Am. Zool.* **21**, 223–232.

Harvey, S., and Etches, R. J., eds. (1997). "Perspectives in Avian Endocrinology." Journal of Endocrinology, Bristol.

Harvey, S., Scanes, C. G., Chadwick, A., and Bolton, N. J. (1978). The effect of thyrotropin-releasing hormone (TRH) and somatostatin (GHRIH) on growth hormone and prolactin secretion in vitro and in vivo in the domestic fowl (*Gallus domesticus*). *Neuroendocrinology* **26**, 249–260.

Hasselquist, D., Marsh, J. A., Sherman, P. W., and Wingfield, J. C. (1999). Is avian humoral immunocompetence suppressed by testosterone? *Behav. Ecol. Sociobiol.* **45**, 167–175.

Hau, M., Wikelski, M., and Wingfield, J. C. (1998). A neotropical bird can measure the slight changes in tropical photoperiod. *Proc. R. Soc. London, Ser. B* **265**, 1–7.

Hau, M., Wikelski, M., and Wingfield, J. C. (1999). Environmental control of reproduction in a neotropical rainforest bird. *Proc. 22nd Int. Ornithol. Congr.*, pp. 1720–1739.

Hau, M., Wikelski, M., and Wingfield, J. C. (2000a). Visual and nutritional food cues fine-tune timing of reproduction in a neotropical rainforest bird. *J. Exp. Zool.* **286**, 494–504.

Hau, M., Wikelski, M., Soma, K., and Wingfield, J. (2000b). Testosterone and year-round territorial aggression in a tropical bird. *Gen. Comp. Endocrinol.* **117**, 20–33.

Heath, J. (1997). Corticosterone levels during nest departure of juvenile American kestrels. *Condor* **99**, 806–811.

Hegner, R. E., and Wingfield, J. C. (1986a). Behavioral and endocrine correlates of multiple brooding in the semi-colonial house sparrow, *Passer domesticus*. I. Males. *Horm. Behav.* **20**, 294–312.

Hegner, R. E., and Wingfield, J. C. (1986b). Behavioral and endocrine correlates of multiple brooding in the semi-colonial house sparrow, *Passer domesticus*. II. Females. *Horm. Behav.* **20**, 313–326.

Henger, R. E., and Wingfiled, J. C. (1987). Effects of experimental manipulation of testosterone levels on parental investment and breeding success in male house sparrows. *Auk* **104**, 462–469.

Hegner, R. E., and Wingfield, J. C. (1990). Annual cycle of gonad size, reproductive hormones, and breeding activity of free-living house sparrows (*Passer domesticus* (L.) in rural New York. *In* "Granivorous Birds in the Agricultural Landscape" (J. Pinowski and J. D. Summers-Smith, eds.), pp. 123–135. Polish Academy of Sciences, Warsaw, Poland.

Hiatt, E. S., Goldsmith, A. R., and Farner, D. S. (1987). Plasma levels of prolactin and gonadotropins during the reproductive cycle of white-crowned sparrows (*Zonotrichia leucophrys*). *Auk* **104**, 208–217.

Hillgarth, N., and Wingfield, J. C. (1997). Parasite-mediated sexual selection: Endocrine aspects. *In* "Host-parasite Evolution" (D. H. Clayton and J. Moore, eds.), pp. 78–104. Oxford University Press, Oxford.

Hinde, R. A., and Steel, E. (1978). The influence of day length and male vocalizations on the oestrogen dependent behavior of female canaries and budgerigars, with discussion of data from other species. *In* "Advances in the Study of Behavior" (J. S. Rosenblatt, R. A. Hinde, C. Beer, and M.-C. Busnel, eds.), Vol. 8, pp. 39–73. Academic Press, New York.

Hissa, R., Saarela, S., Balthazart, J., and Etches, R. J. (1983). Annual variation in the concentrations of circulating hormones in capercaille (*Tetrao urogallus*). *Gen. Comp. Endocrinol.* **51**, 183–190.

Hogstad, O. (1987). Social rank in winter flocks of willow tits *Parus montanus*. *Ibis* **129**, 1–9.

Hogstad, O. (1989). Social organization and dominance behavior in some *Parus* species. *Wilson Bull.* **101**, 254–262.

Hogstad, O. (1990). Dispersal date and settlement of juvenile willow tits *Parus montanus* in winter flocks. *Fauna Norv., Ser. C* **13**, 49–55.

Höhn, E. O. (1970). Gonadal hormone concentration in northern phalaropes in relation to nuptial plumage. *Can. J. Zool.* **48**, 400–401.

Höhn, E. O., and Braun, C. E. (1980). Hormonal induction of feather pigmentation in ptarmigan. *Auk* **97**, 601–607.

Höhn, E. O., and Cheng, S. C. (1967). Gonadal hormones in Wilson's phalaropes (*Steganopus tricolor*) and other birds in relation to plumage and sex behavior. *Gen. Comp. Endocrinol.* **8**, 1–11.

Holberton, R. L., and Able, K. P. (2000). Differential migration and an endocrine response to stress in wintering dark-eyed juncos (*Junco hyemalis*). *Proc. R. Soc. London, Ser. B* **267**, 1889–1896.

Holberton, R. L., Able, K. P., and Wingfield, J. C. (1989). Status signalling in dark-eyed juncos, *Juncos hyemalis*: Plumage manipulations and hormonal correlates of dominance. *Anim. Behav.* **37**, 681–689.

Holberton, R. L., Parrish, J. D., and Wingfield, J. C. (1996). Modulation of the adrenocortical stress response in neotropical migrants during autumn migration. *Auk* **113**, 558–564.

Humphrey, P. S., and Parkes, K. C. (1959). An approach to the study of moults and plumages. *Auk* **76**, 1–31.

Hunt, K. E., Hahn, T. P., and Wingfield, J. C. (1999). Endocrine influences on parental care during a short breeding season: Testosterone and male parental care in Lapland longspurs (*Calcarius lapponicus*). *Behav. Ecol. Sociobiol.* **45**, 360–369.

Hutchison, J. B., Steimer, T., and Jaggard, D. (1986). Effects of photoperiod on formation of oestradiol-17β in the dove brain. *J. Endocrinol.* **109**, 371–377.

Immelmann, K. (1971). Ecological aspects of periodic reproduction. *Avian Biol.* **1**, 341–389.

Immelmann, K. (1973). Role of the environment in reproduction as a source of "predictive" information. *In* "Breeding Biology of Birds" (D. S. Farner, ed.), pp. 121–147. Natl. Acad. Sci., Washington, DC.

Ishii, S., and Farner, D. S. (1976). Binding of follicle-stimulating hormone by homogenates of testes of photostimulated white-crowned sparrows, *Zonotrichia leucophrys gambelii*. *Gen. Comp. Endocrinol.* **30**, 443–450.

Jacobs, J. D. 1996. Regulation of life history strategies within individuals in predictable and unpredictable environments. Ph.D. Dissertation, University of Washington, Seattle.

Jacobs, J. D., and Wingfield, J. C. (2000). Endocrine control of life-cycle stages: A constraint on response to the environment? *Condor* **102**, 35–51.

Jallageas, M., and Assenmacher, I. (1985). Endocrine correlates of molt and reproduction function in birds. *Acta 18th Congr., Int. Ornithol*, pp. 935–945.

John, T. M., and George, J. C. (1978). Circulating levels of thyroxine (T4) and triiodothyronine (T3) in the migratory Canada goose. *Physiol. Zool.* **51**, 361–370.

Johns, J. E. (1964). Testosterone-induced nuptial feathers in phalaropes. *Condor* **66**, 449–455.

Johnson, A. I., Pang, P., and Scanes, C. G. (1984). Third International Symposium on Avian Endocrinology. *J. Exp. Zool.* **232**, 385–745.

Kast, T. L., Ketterson, E. D., and Nolan, V., Jr. (1998). Variation in sperm reserves according to season, stage of reproduction, and testosterone treatment in the dark-eyed junco. *Auk* **115**, 684–693.

Keck, W. N. (1934). The control of secondary sex characters in the English sparrow, *Passer domesticus (Linnaeus)*. *J. Exp. Zool.* **67**, 315–347.

Kern, M. D., and DeGraw, W. A. (1986). Thyroid-molt relationships in Harris Sparrow (*Zonotrichia querula*). *Comp. Biochem. Physiol.* **85A**, 49–55.

Ketterson, E. D., Nolan, V., Jr., Wolf, L., and Goldsmith, A. R. (1990). Effect of sex, stage of reproduction, season and mate removal, on prolactin in dark-eyed juncos. *Condor* **92**, 922–930.

Ketterson, E. D., Nolan, V., Jr., Wolf, L., and Ziegenfus, C. (1992). Testosterone and avian life histories: Effects of experimentally elevated testosterone on behaviour and correlates of fitness in the dark-eyed junco (*Junco hyemalis*). *Am. Nat.* **140**, 980–999.

Ketterson, E. D., Nolan, V., Jr., Cawthorn, M. J., Parker, P. G., and Ziegenfus, C. (1996). Phenotypic engineering: Using hormones to explore the mechanistic and functional bases of phenotypic variation in nature. *Ibis* **138**, 70–86.

King, J. R. (1961). The bioenergetics of vernal premigratory fat deposition in the white-crowned sparrow. *Condor* **63**, 128–142.

King, J. R. (1972). Postnuptial and postjuvenal molt in rufous-collared sparrows in northwestern Argentina. *Condor* **74**, 5–16.

King, J. R., Barker, S., and Farner, D. S. (1963). A comparison of energy reserves during autumnal and vernal migratory periods in the white-crowned sparrow, *Zonotrichia leucophrys gambelii*. *Ecology* **44**, 513–521.

King, J. R., Follett, B. K., Farner, D. S., and Morton, M. L. (1966). Annual gonadal cycles and pituitary gonadotropin in *Zonotrichia leucophrys gambelii*. *Condor* **68**, 476–487.

Knobil, E., and Neill, J. D. (1988). "The Physiology of Reproduction." Raven Press, New York.

Kobayashi, H., and Wada, M. (1973). Neuroendocrinology in birds. *Avian Biol.* **3**, 287–347.

Kotschral, K., Hirschenhauser, K., and Möstl, E. (1998). Social stress and dominance: The relation is seasonal in greylag geese (*Anser anser*). *Anim. Behav.* **55**, 171–176.

Kubokawa, K., Ishii, S., and Wingfield, J. C. (1994). Effect of day length on luteinizing hormone α-subunit mRNA and subsequent gonadal growth in the white-crowned sparrow, *Zonotrichia leucophrys gambelii*. *Gen. Comp. Endocrinol.* **95**, 42–51.

Labrie, F., Bélanger, A., Simard, J., Luuthe, V., and Labrie, C. (1995). DHEA and peripheral androgen and estrogen formation: Intracrinology. *Ann. N.Y. Acad. Sci.* **774**, 16–28.

Lack, D. (1954). "The Natural Regulation of Animal Numbers." Oxford University Press, London.

Lack, D. (1968). "Ecological Adaptations for Breeding in Birds." Chapman & Hall, London.

Lane, N., Grisham, W., Brown, S., Thompson, L., Arnold, A., and Schlinger, B. (1996). Plasma testosterone and tissue 17alpha-hydroxylase activity in castrated and fadrozole-treated male zebra finches. *Soc. Neurosci. Abstr.* **22**, 156.

Lank, D. B., Coupe, M., and Wynne-Edwards, K. E. (1998). Testosterone-induced male traits in female ruffs (*Philomachus pugnax*): Autosomal inheritance and gender differentiation. *Proc. R. Soc. London, Ser. B* **266**, 2323–2330.

Le Douarin, N. M., Teillet, M. A., and Fontaine-Perus, J. (1984). Chimeras in the study of the peripheral nervous system of birds. *In* "Chimeras in Developmental Biology" (N. M. Le Douarin and A. McLaren, eds.), pp. 313–351. Academic Press, New York.

Lehrman, D. S. (1965). Interaction between internal and external environments in the regulation of the reproductive cycle of the ring dove. *In* "Sex and Behavior" (F. A. Beach, ed.), pp. 355–380. Wiley, New York.

Leigh, E. G., Rand, A. S., and Windsor, D. M., eds. (1982). "The Ecology of a Tropical Forest: Seasonal Rythms and Long-Term Changes." Smithsonian Inst. Press, Washington, DC.

Lesher, S. W., and Kendeigh, S. C. (1941). Effect of photoperiod on molting of feathers. *Wilson Bull.* **53**, 169–180.

Levin, R. N. (1996). Song behaviour and reproductive strategies in duetting wren, *Thryothorus nigricapillus*: I. Removal experiments. *Anim. Behav.* **52**, 1093–1106.

Levin, R. N., and Wingfield, J. C. (1992). The hormonal control of territorial aggression in tropical birds. *Ornis Scand.* **23**, 284–291.

Lincoln, G. A., Racey, P. A., Sharp, P. J., and Klandorf, H. (1980). Endocrine changes associated with spring and autumn sexuality of the rook *Corvus frugilegus*. *J. Zool.* **190**, 137–153.

Lofts, B., and Marshall, A. J. (1960). The experimental regulation of Zuguruhe and the sexual cycle in the brambling, *Fringilla montifringilla*. *Ibis* **102**, 209–214.

Lofts, B., and Murton, R. K. (1968). Photoperiodic and physiological adaptations regulating avian breeding cycles and their ecological significance. *J. Zool.* **155**, 327–394.

Lofts, B., and Murton, R. K. (1973). Reproduction in birds. *Avian Biol.* **3**, 1–107.

Lofts, B., Murton, R. K., and Westwood, N. J. (1966). Gonadal cycles and the evolution of breeding seasons in British Columbidae. *J. Zool.* **150**, 249–272.

Lofts, B., Murton, R. K., and Thearle, R. J. P. (1973). The effects of testosterone propionate and gonadotropins on the bill pigmentation and testes of the house sparrow *Passer domesticus*. *Gen. Comp. Endocrinol.* **21**, 202–209.

Logan, C. A., and Carlin, C. A. (1991). Testosterone stimulates reproductive behavior during autumn in mockingbirds (*Mimus polyglottos*). *Horm. Behav.* **25**, 229–241.

Logan, C. A., and Wingfield, J. C. (1990). Autumnal territorial aggression is independent of plasma testosterone in mockingbirds. *Horm. Behav.* **24**, 568–581.

Lynn, S. E., Houtman, A. M., Weathers, W. W., Ketterson, E. D., and Nolan, V., Jr. (2000). Testosterone increases activity but not daily energy expenditure in captive male dark-eyed juncos. *Anim. Behav.* **60**, 581–587.

Maney, D. L., and Wingfield, J. C. (1998a). Central opioid control of feeding behavior in the white-crowned sparrow, *Zonotrichia leucophrys gambelii*. *Horm. Behav.* **33**, 16–22.

Maney, D. L., and Wingfield, J. C. (1998b). Neuroendocrine suppression of female courtship in a wild passerine: Corticotropin-releasing factor and endogenous opioids. *J. Neuroendocrinol.* **10**, 593–599.

Maney, D. L., Schoech, S. J., Sharp, P. J., and Wingfield, J. C. (1999a). Effects of vasoactive intestinal peptide on plasma prolactin in passerines. *Gen. Comp. Endocrinol.* **113**, 323–330.

Maney, D. L., Hahn, T. P., Schoech, S. J., Sharp, P. J., Morton, M. L., and Wingfield, J. C. (1999b). Effects of ambient temperature on photo-induced prolactin secretion in three subspecies of white-crowned sparrow, *Zonotrichia leucophrys*. *Gen. Comp. Endocrinol.* **113**, 445–456.

Maney, D. L., Schoech, S. J., and Wingfield, J. C. (1999c). Environmental endocrinology and the timing of reproduction: Interaction of photoperiod and temperature. *Proc. 22nd Int. Ornithol. Congr.*, pp. 279–294.

Marra, P. P., and Holberton, R. L. (1998). Corticosterone levels as indicators of habitat quality: Effects of habitat segregation in a migratory bird during the non-breeding season. *Oecologia* **116**, 284–292.

Marshall, A. J., and Coombs, C. J. F. (1957). The interaction of environmental, internal and behavioural factors in the rook, *Corvus frugilegus* L. *Proc. Zool. Soc. London* **128**, 545–589.

Marshall, A. J., and Williams, M. C. (1959). The prenuptial migration of the yellow wagtail (*Motacilla flava*) from latitude 0ø04′ N. *Proc. Zool. Soc. London* **132**, 313–320.

Mathew, K. L., and Naik, R. M. (1986). Interrelation between molting and breeding in a tropical population of the house sparrow *Passer domesticus*. *Ibis* **128**, 260–265.

Mattocks, P. W., Jr. (1976). The role of gonadal hormones in regulation of the pre-migratory fat deposition in the white-crowned sparrow, *Zonotriochia leucophrys gambelii*. MS Thesis, University of Washington, Seattle.

Mauget, R., Jouventin, P., Lacroix, A., and Ishii, S (1994). Plasma LH and steroid hormones in king penguin (*Aptenodytes patagonicus*) during the onset of the breeding cycle. *Gen. Comp. Endocrinol.* **93**, 36–43.

McEwen, B. S., Sakai, R. R., and Spencer, R. L. (1993). Adrenal steroid effects on the brain: Versatile hormones with good and bad effects. In "Hormonally-Induced Changes in Mind and Brain" (J. Schulkin, ed.), pp. 157–189. Academic Press, San Diego, CA.

Meddle S. L., and Follett, B. K. (1995). Photoperiodic activation of fos-like immunoreactive protein in neurones within the tuberal hypothalamus of Japanese quail. *J. Comp. Physiol.* **176**, 79–89.

Meddle S. L., and Follett, B. K. (1997). Photoperiodic driven changes in Fos expression within the basal tuberal hypothalamus and median eminence of Japanese quail. *J. Neurosci.* **17**, 8909–8918.

Meddle, S. L., King, V. M., Follett, B. K., Wingfield, J. C., Ramenofsky, M., Foidart, A., and Balthazart, J. (1997). Copulation activates Fos-like immunoreactivity in the male quail forebrain. *Behav. Brain Res.* **85**, 143–159.

Meddle, S. L., Foidart, A., Wingfield, J. C., Ramenofsky, M., and Balthazart, J. (1999). Effects of sexual interactions with a male on fos-like immunoreactivity in the female quail brain. *J. Neuroendocrinol.* **11**, 771–784.

Meier, A. H., and Ferrell, B. R. (1978). Avian endocrinology. *Chem. Zool.* **10**, 213–271.

Meier, A. H., Ferrell, B. R., and Miller, L. J. (1980). Circadian components of the circannual mechanism in the white-throated sparrow. *Acta 17th Int. Ornithol. Congr.*, pp. 458–462.

Mewaldt, L. R., and King, J. R. (1977). The annual cycle of white-crowned sparrows (*Zonotrichia leucophrys nuttalli*) in coastal California. *Condor* **79**, 445–455.

Mewaldt, L. R., and King, J. R. (1978). Latitudinal variation in prenuptial molt in wintering Gambel's white-crowned sparrows. *North Am. Bird Bander* **3**, 138–144.

Mewaldt, L. R., Kibby, S. S., and Morton, M. L. (1968). Comparative biology of Pacific coastal white-crowned sparrows. *Condor* **70**, 14–30.

Michener, H., and Michener, J. R. (1943). The spring molt of the Gambel sparrow. *Condor* **45**, 113–116.

Mikami, S.-I., Homma, K., and Wada, M. (1983). "Avian Endocrinology: Environmental and Ecological Perspectives." Jpn. Sci. Soc. Press, Tokyo/Springer-Verlag, Berlin.

Moore, M. C. (1982). Hormonal responses of free-living male white-crowned sparrows to experimental manipulation of female sexual behavior. *Horm. Behav.* **16**, 323–329.

Moore, M. C. (1984). Changes in territorial defense produced by changes in circulating levels of testosterone. A possible hormonal basis for mate-guarding behavior in white-crowned sparrows. *Behaviour* **88**, 215–226.

Moore, M. C., Donham, R. S., and Farner, D. S. (1982). Physiological preparation for autumnal migration in white-crowned sparrows. *Condor* **84**, 410–419.

Morton, E. S. (1980). Adaptations to seasonal changes by migrant land birds in Panama Canal Zone. *In* "Migrant Birds in the Neotropics" (A. Keast and E. S. Morton, eds.), pp. 437–453. Smithsonian Inst. Press, Washington, DC.

Morton, M. L., and Mewaldt, L. R. (1962). Some effects of castration on a migratory sparrow (*Zonotrichia atricapilla*). *Physiol. Zool.* **35**, 237–247.

Mueller, N. S. (1976). Influence of embryonic estrogens on adult feather coloration in the duck *Anas platyrhynchos*. *J. Exp. Zool.* **195**, 207–214.

Murton, R. K., and Westwood, N. J. (1977). "Avian Breeding Cycles." Clarendon Press, Oxford.

Murton, R. K., Isaacson, A. J., and Westwood, N. J. (1971). The significance of gregarious feeding behavior and adrenal stress in a population of woodpigeons *Columba palumbus*. *J. Zool.* **165**, 53–84.

Nelson, R. (1999). "An Introduction to Behavioral Endocrinology." Sinauer Assoc., Sunderland, MA.

Newton, I. (1973). "Finches." Taplinger, New York.

Nicholls, T. J., Goldsmith, A. R., and Dawson, A. (1984). Photorefractoriness in European starlings: Associated hypothalamic changes and involvement of thyroid hormones and prolactin. *J. Exp. Zool.* **232**, 567–572.

Nicholls, T. J., Goldsmith, A. R., and Dawson, A. (1988). Photorefractoriness in birds and comparison with mammals. *Physiol. Rev.* **68**, 133–176.

Nilsson, J. Å., and Smith, H. G. (1985). Early fledgling mortality and the timing of juvenile dispersal in the marsh tit *Parus palustris*. *Ornis Scand.* **16**, 293–298.

Noble, G. K., and Wurm, M. (1940). The effect of hormones on the breeding of the laughing gull. *Anat. Rec.* **78** (Suppl.), 50.

Nomura, O., Nishimori, K., Nakabayashi, O., Yasue, H., and Mizuno, S. (1998). Determination by modified RT-PCR of transcript amounts from genes involved in sex-steroid synthesis in chicken organs including brain. *J. Steroid Biochem. Mol. Biol.* **67**, 143–148.

Novikov, B. G. (1936). Die Analyse des Geschlechtsdimorphismus bei den Sperlingsvogeln (Passeres). II. *Biol. Zentralbl.* **56**, 415–428.

Novikov, B. G. (1937). Die Analyse des Geschlechtsdimorphismus bei den Sperlingsvogeln (Passeres). IV. *Acta Zool.* **18**, 447–458.

Nowicki, S., and Ball, G. F. (1989). Testosterone induction of song in photosensitive and photorefractory male sparrows. *Horm. Behav.* **23**, 514–525.

Orchinik, M., Murray, T. F., and Moore, F. L. (1991). A corticosteroid receptor in neuronal membranes. *Science* **252**, 1848–1851.

O'Reilly, K. M., and Wingfield, J. C. (1995). Spring and autumn migration in Arctic shorebirds: Same distance, different strategies. *Am. Zool.* **35**, 222–233.

Owens, I. P. F., and Short, R. V. (1995). Hormonal basis of sexual dimorphism in birds: Implications for new theories of sexual selection. *Trends Ecol. Evol.* **10**, 44–47.

Palmer, R. S. (1972). Patterns of molting. *Avian Biol.* **2**, 65–103.

Pathak, V. K., and Chandola, A. (1982a). Thyroidal involvement in the development of migratory disposition in red-headed bunting (*Emberiza bruniceps*). *Horm. Behav.* **16**, 46–58.

Pathak, V. K., and Chandola, A. (1982b). Seasonal variations in extrathyroidal conversion of thyroxine to triiodothyronine and migratory disposition in red-headed bunting. *Gen. Comp. Endocrinol.* **47**, 433–439.

Payne, R. B. (1972). Mechanisms and control of molt. *Avian Biol.* **2**, 104–155.

Péczely, P. (1976). Etude circannuelle de la fonction corticosurrenalienne chez es spèces de passereaux migrants et non migrants. *Gen. Comp. Endocrinol.* **30**, 1–11.

Péczely, P. (1986). Hormonal regulation of moulting in blackheaded gull. *Proc. 19th Int. Ornithol. Congr.*, pp. 1710–1721.

Péczely, P., and Pethes, G. (1982). Seasonal cycle of gonadal thyroid and adrenocortical function in the rook (*Corvus frugilegus*). *Acta Physiol. Acad. Sci. Hung.* **59**, 59–74.

Perrins, C. M. (1970). The timing of birds' breeding seasons. *Ibis* **112**, 242–255.

Peters, A. (2000). Testosterone treatment is immunosuppressive in superb fairy-wrens, yet free-living males with high testosterone are more immunocompetent. *Proc. R. Soc. London, Ser. B* **267**, 883–889.

Pethes, G., Scanes, C. G., and Rudas, P. (1979). Effect of synthetic thyrotropin-releasing hormone on the circulating growth hormone concentration in cold and heat-stressed ducks. *Acta Vet. Acad. Sci. Hung.* **27**, 175–177.

Piersma, T. (1998). Phenotypic flexibiltiy during migration: Optimization of organ size contingent upon the risks and rewards of fueling and flight? *J. Avian Biol.* **29**, 511–520.

Piersma, T., and Ramenofsky, M. (1998). Long term decreases of corticosterone in captive migrant shorebirds that maintain seasonal mass and molt cycles. *J. Avian Biol.* **29**, 97–104.

Piersma, T., Reneerkens, J., and Ramenofsky, M. (2000). Baseline corticosterone peaks in shorebirds with maximal energy stores for migration: A general preparatory mechanism for rapid behavioral and metabolic transitions? *Gen. Comp. Endocrinol.* **120**, 118–126.

Poulin, B., Lefebvre, G., and McNeil, R. (1992). Tropical avian phenology in relation to abundance and exploitation of food resources. *Ecology* **73**, 2295–2309.

Pruitt, W. O., Jr. (1970). Some ecological aspects of snow. *In* "Ecology of the Subarctic Regions," pp. 83–99. United Nations Educational, Scientific and Cultural Organization, Paris.

Putzig, P. (1939). Beiträge zur Stoffwechsphysiologie des Zugvogels. *Vogelzug* **10**, 139–154.

Ralph, C. L. (1969). The control of color in birds. *Am. Zool.* **9**, 521–530.

Ralph, C. L., Grinwich, D. L., and Hall, P. F. (1967a). Studies of the melanogenic response of regenerating feathers in the weaver bird: Comparison of two species in response to two gonadotropins. *J. Exp. Zool.* **166**, 283–288.

Ralph, C. L., Grinwich, D. L., and Hall, P. F. (1967b). Hormonal regulation of feather pigmentation in African weaver birds: The exclusion of certain possible mechanisms. *J. Exp. Zool.* **166**, 289–294.

Ramenofsky, M. (1990). Fat storage and fat metabolism in relation to migration. *In* "Bird Migration" (E. Gwinner, ed.), pp. 214–231. Springer-Verlag, Berlin.

Ramenofsky, M., Piersma, T., and Jukema, J. (1995). Plasma corticosterone in bar-tailed godwits at a major stop-over site during spring migration. *Condor* **97**, 585–587.

Rankin, M. A. (1991). Endocrine effects on migration. *Am. Zool.* **31**, 217–230.

Raouf, S. A., Parker, P. G., Ketterson, E. D., Nolan, V., Jr., and Ziegenfus, C. (1997). Testosterone influences reproductive success by increasing extra-pair fertilizations in male dark-eyed juncos, *Junco hyemalis*. *Proc. R. Soc. London, Ser. B* **264**, 1599–1603.

Rawles, M. E. (1939). The production of robin pigment in white leghorn feathers by grafts of embryonic robin tissue. *J. Genet.* **38**, 517–532.

Reinert, B. D., and Wilson, F. E. (1997). Effects of thyroxine (T4) or triiodothyronine (T3) replacement therapy on the programming of seasonal reproduction and postnuptial molt in thyroidectomized male American tree sparrows (*Spizella arborea*) exposed to long days. *J. Exp. Zool.* **279**, 367–376.

Richardson, R. D., and Boswell, T. (1993). A method for third ventricular cannulation of small passerine birds. *Physiol. Behav.* **53**, 209–213.

Richardson, R. D., Boswell, T., Weatherford, S. C., Wingfield, J. C., and Woods, S. C. (1993). Cholescystokinin octapeptide decreases food intake in white-crowned sparrows. *Am. J. Physiol.* **264**, R852–R856.

Richardson, R. D., Boswell, T., Raffety, B. D., Seeley, R., Wingfield, J. C., and Woods, S. C. (1995). NPY increases food intake in white-crowned sparrows: Effect in short and long photoperiods. *Am. J. Physiol.* **268**, R1418–R1422.

Richardson, R. D., Boswell, T., Woods, S. C., and Wingfield, J. C. (2000). Intracerebroventricular corticotropin releasing factor decreases food intake in white-crowned sparrows. *Physiol. Behav.* **70**, 1–4.

Robel, P., and Baulieu, E. (1995). Dehydroepiandrosterone (DHEA) is a neuroactive neurosteroid. *Ann. N.Y. Acad. Sci.* **774**, 82–110.

Rogers, C. M., Ramenofsky, M., Ketterson, E. D., Nolan, V., Jr., and Wingfield, J. C. (1993). Plasma corticosterone, adrenal mass, winter weather, and season in non-breeding populations of dark-eyed juncos (*Junco hyemalis hyemalis*). *Auk* **110**, 279–285.

Röhss, M., and Silverin, B. (1983). Seasonal variation in the ultrastructure of the Leydig cells and plasma levels of luteinizing hormone and steroid hormones in juvenile and adult male great tits *Parus major*. *Ornis Scand.* **14**, 202–212.

Rohwer, S. (1977). Status signalling in Harris sparrows: Some experiments in deception behavior. *Behaviour* **61**, 107–129.

Rohwer, S., and Wingfield, J. C. (1981). A field study of social dominance; plasma levels of luteinizing hormone and steroid hormones in wintering Harris sparrows. *Z. Tierpsychol.* **47**, 173–183.

Romero, L. M., and Wingfield, J. C. (1999). Alterations in hypothalamic-pituitary-adrenal function associated with captivity in Gambel's white-crowned sparrows (*Zonotrichia leucophrys gambelii*). *Comp. Biochem. Physiol. B* **122**, 13–20.

Romero, L. M., Ramenofsky, M., and Wingfield, J. C. (1997). Season and migration alters the corticosterone response to capture and handling in an arctic migrant, the white-crowned sparrow (*Zonotrichia leucophrys gambelii*). *Comp. Biochem Physiol. C* **116**, 171–177.

Romero, L. M., Soma, K. K., and Wingfield, J. C. (1998a). Changes in pituitary and adrenal sensitivities allow the snow bunting (*Plectrophenax nivalis*), an Arctic-breeding song bird, to modulate corticosterone release seasonally. *J. Comp. Physiol. B* **168**, 353–358.

Romero, L. M., Soma, K. K., and Wingfield, J. C. (1998b). The hypothalamus and adrenal regulate modulation of corticosterone release in redpolls (*Carduelis flammea*). An arctic-breeding song bird). *Gen. Comp. Endocrinol.* **109**, 347–355.

Romero, L. M., Dean, S. C., and Wingfield, J.C. (1998c). Neurally active peptide inhibits territorial defense in wild birds. *Horm. Behav.* **34**, 239–247.

Romero, L. M., Soma, K. K., and Wingfield, J. C. (1998d). Hypothalamic-pituitary-adrenal axis changes allow seasonal modulation of corticosterone in a bird. *Am. J. Physiol.* **274**, 1338–1344.

Romero, L. M., Reed, J. M., and Wingfield, J. C. (2000). Effects of weather on corticosterone responses in wild free-living passerine birds. *Gen. Comp. Endocrinol.* **118**, 113–122.

Runfeldt, S., and Wingfield, J. C. (1985). Experimentally prolonged sexual activity in female sparrows delays termination of reproductive activity in their untreated mates. *Anim. Behav.* **33**, 403–410.

Saino, N., and Møller, A. P. (1995). Testosterone-induced depression of male parental behavior in the barn swallow: Female compensation and effects of seasonal fitness. *Behav. Ecol. Sociobiol.* **36**, 151–157.

Saitou, T. (1978). Ecological study of social organization in the great tit, *Parus major* L. I. Basic structure of the winter flocks. *Jpn. J. Ecol.* **28**, 199–214.

Saitou, T. (1979). Ecological study of social organisation in the great tit, *Parus major* L. III. Home range of the basic flock and dominance relationship of the members in a basic flock. *Misc. Rep., Yamashina Inst. Ornithol. Zool.* **11**, 149–171.

Scanes, C. G., Cheeseman, P., Phillips, J. G., and Follett, B. K. (1974). Seasonal and age variation of circulating immunoreactive luteinizing hormone in captive Herring gulls, *Larus argentatus*. *J. Zool.* **174**, 369–375.

Scanes, C. G., Jallageas, M., and Assenmacher, I. (1980). Seasonal variations in the circulating concentrations of growth hormone in male Pekin ducks (*Anas platyrhynchos*) and teal (*Anas crecca*); correlations with thyroidal function. *Gen. Comp. Endocrinol.* **41**, 76–89.

Schleussner, G., and Gwinner, E. (1988). Photoperidic time measurement during the termination of photoerfractoriness in the starling (*Sturnus vulgaris*). *Gen. Comp. Endocrinol.* **75**, 54–61.

Schlinger, B., Lane, N., Grisham, W., and Thompson, L. (1999). Androgen synthesis in a songbird: A study of Cyp17 (17α-hydroxylase/C17,20-lyase) activity in the zebra finch. *Gen. Comp. Endocrinol.* **113**, 46–58.

Schlinger, B. A., and Callard, G. V. (1990). Aromatization mediates aggressive behavior in quail. *Gen. Comp. Endocrinol.* **79**, 39–53.

Schoech, S., Ketterson, E. D., and Nolan, V., Jr. (1999). Exogenous testosterone and the adrenocortical response in the dark-eyed junco, *Junco hyemalis*. *Auk* **116**, 64–72.

Schüz, E. (1952). "Vom Vogelzug Grundiss der Vogelzugskunde." Schops, Frankfurt am Main.

Schüz, E. (1971). "Grundiss der Vogelsugkunde." Parey, Berlin.

Schwabl, H. (1995). Individual variation of the acute adrenocortical response to stress in the white-throated sparrow. *Zoology* **99**, 113–120.

Schwabl, H. (1999). Developmental changes and among sibling variation of corticosterone levels in an altricial avian species. *Gen. Comp. Endocrinol.* **116**, 403–408.

Schwabl, H., and Farner, D. S. (1989a). Dependency on testosterone of photoperiodically-induced vernal fat deposition in female white-crowned sparrows. *Condor* **91**, 108–112.

Schwabl, H., and Farner, D. S. (1989b). Endocrine and environmental control of vernal migration in male white-crowned sparrows, *Zonotrichia leucophrys gambelii*. *Physiol. Zool.* **62**, 1–10.

Schwabl, H., and Kriner, E. (1991). Territorial aggression and song of male European robins (*Erithacus rubecula*) in autumn and spring: Effects of antiandrogen treatment. *Horm. Behav.* **25**, 180–194.

Schwabl, H., and Silverin, B. (1990). Control of partial migration and autumnal behavior. In "Bird Migration" (E. Gwinner, ed.), pp. 144–155. Springer-Verlag, Berlin.

Schwabl, H., Wingfield, J. C., and Farner, D. S. (1980). Seasonal variation in plasma levels of luteinizing hormone and steroid hormones in the European blackbird *Turdus merula*. *Vogelwarte* **30**, 283–294.

Schwabl, H., Wingfield, J. C., and Farner, D. S. (1984). Endocrine correlates of autumnal behavior of sedentary and migratory individuals of a partially migratory population of the European blackbird *Turdus merula*. *Auk* **101**, 499–507.

Schwabl, H., Wingfield, J. C., and Farner, D. S. (1985). Influence of winter on endocrine state and behavior in European blackbirds *Turdus merula*. *Z. Tierpsychol.* **68**, 244–252.

Schwabl, H., Schwabl-Benzinger, I., Goldsmith, A. R., and Farner, D. S. (1988a). Effect of ovariectomy on long day-induced premigratory fat deposition, plasma levels of luteinizing hormone and prolactin, and molt in white-crowned sparrows, *Zonotrichia leuocphrys gambelii*. *Gen. Comp. Endocrinol.* **71**, 398–405.

Schwabl, H., Ramenofsky, M., Schwabl-Benzinger, I., Farner, D. S., and Wingfield, J. C. (1988b). Social status, circulating levels of hormones, and competition for food in winter flocks of the white-throated sparrow. *Behaviour* **107**, 107–121.

Schwabl, H., Bairlein, F., and Gwinner, E. (1991). Basal and stress-induced corticosterone levels of garden warblers, *Sylvia borin*, during migration. *J. Comp. Physiol. B* **161**, 576.

Sharp, P. J., ed. (1993). "Avian Endocrinology." Journal of Endocrinology, Bristol, UK.

Sharp, P. J., Moss, R., and Watson, A. (1974). Seasonal variation in plasma luteinizing hormone levelsin male red grouse, *Lagopus lagopus scoticus*. *J. Endocrinol* **64**, 1–44.

Sharp, P. J., Li, Q., Talbot, R. T., Barker, P., Huskisson, N., and Lea, R. W. (1995). Identification of hypothalamic nuclei involved in osmoregulation using fos immunocytochemistry in the domestic hen (*Gallus domesticus*), Ring dove (*Streptopelia* risoria), Japanese quail (*Coturnix japonica*) and Zebra finch (*Taenopygia guttata*). *Cell Tissue Res.* **282**, 351–361.

Sherwood, N. M., Wingfield, J. C., Ball, G. F., and Dufty, A. M. (1988). Identity of gonadotropin-releasing hormone in passerine birds: Comparison of GnRH in song sparrow (*Melospiza melodia*) and starling (*Sturnus vulgaris*) with five vertebrate GnRH's. *Gen. Comp. Endocrinol.* **69**, 341–351.

Silver, R. (1978). The parental behavior of ring doves. *Amer. Sci.* **66**, 209–215.

Silverin, B. (1978). Circannual rhythms in gonads and endocrine organs of the great tit *Parus major* in south-west Sweden. *Ornis. Scand.* **9**, 207–213.

Silverin, B. (1980a). Seasonal changes in the activity of the thyroid glands and its interaction with testicular function in the pied flycatcher *Ficedula hypoleuca*. *Gen. Comp. Endocrinol.* **41**, 122–129.

Silverin, B (1980b). Effects of long-acting testosterone treatment on free-living pied flycatchers, *Ficedula hypoleuca*, during the breeding period. *Anim. Behav.* **28**, 906–912.

Silverin, B. (1986). Corticosterone-binding proteins and behavioral effects of high plasma levels of corticosterone during the breeding period in the pied flycatcher. *Gen. Comp. Endocrinol.* **64**, 67–74.

Silverin, B. (1990). Testosterone and corticosterone and their relation to territorial and parental behavior in the pied flycatcher. In "Hormones, Brain and Behavior in Vertebrates" (J. Balthazart, ed.), Vol. 2, pp. 129–142. Karger, Basel.

Silverin, B. (1991a). Annual changes in plasma levels of LH, and prolactin in free-living female great tits (*Parus major*). *Gen. Comp. Endocrinol.* **83**, 425–431.

Silverin, B. (1991b). Behavioral, hormonal and morphological responses of free-living male pied flycatchers to estradiol treatment of their mates. *Horm. Behav.* **25**, 38–56.

Silverin, B., ed. (1992). "Endocrinology of the Non-breeding Season in Birds," Vol. 23. Ornis Scandinavica.

Silverin, B. (1993). Territorial aggressiveness and its relation to the endocrine system in the pied flycatycher. *Gen. Comp. Endocrinol.* **89**, 206–213.

Silverin, B. (1994). Photoperiodism in male great tits (*Parus major*). *Ethol. Ecol. Evol.* **6**, 131–157.

Silverin, B. (1995). Reproductive adaptations to breeding in the north. *Am. Zool.* **35**, 191–202.

Silverin, B. (1997). The stress response and autumn dispersal behaviour in willow tits. *Anim. Behav.* **53**, 451–459.

Silverin, B. (1998a). Behavioral and hormonal responses of pied flycatchers to environmental stressors. *Anim. Behav.* **55**, 1411–1420.

Silverin, B. (1998b). Territorial behavior and hormones of pied flycatchers in optimal and suboptimal habitats. *Anim. Behav.* **56**, 811–818.

Silverin, B. (1998c). Stress responses in birds. *Poult. Avian Rev.* **9**, 153–168.

Silverin, B., and Deviche, P. (1991). Biochemical characterization and seasonal changes in the concentration of testosterone-metabolizing enzymes in the European great tit (*Parus major*) brain. *Gen. Comp. Endocrinol.* **81**, 146–159.

Silverin, B., and Goldsmith, A. (1984). The effects of modifying incubation on prolactin secretion in free-living pied flycatchers. *Gen. Comp. Endocrinol.* **55**, 239–244.

Silverin, B., and Goldsmith, A. (1990). Plasma prolactin concentrations in breeding pied flycatchers (*Ficedula hypoleuca*) with an experimentally prolonged brooding period. *Horm. Behav.* **24**, 104–113.

Silverin, B., and Viebke, P. A. (1994). Low temperature affect the photoperiodically induced LH and testicular cycles differently in closely related species of tits (*Parus spp.*). *Horm. Behav.* **28**, 199–206.

Silverin, B., and Westin, J. (1995). Influence of the opposite sex on photoperiodically induced LH and gonadal cycles in the willow tit (*Parus montanus*). *Horm. Behav.* **29**, 207–215.

Silverin, B., and Wingfield, J. C. (1982). Patterns of breeding behaviour and plasma levels of hormones in a free-living population of pied flycatchers, *Ficedula hypoleuca*. *J. Zool.* **198**, 117–129.

Silverin, B., and Wingfield, J. C. (1998). Adrenocortical responses to stress in breeding pied flycatchers *Ficedula hypoleuca*: Relation to latitude, sex and mating status. *J. Avian Biol.* **29**, 228–234.

Silverin, B., Viebke, P. A., and Westin, J. (1984). Plasma levels of luteinizing hormones and steroid hormones in free-living winter groups of willow tits (*Parus montanus*). *Horm. Behav.* **18**, 367–379.

Silverin, B., Viebke, P. A., and Westin, J. (1986). Seasonal changes in plasma levels of LH and gonadal steroids in free-living willow tits *Parus montanus*. *Ornis Scand.* **17**, 230–236.

Silverin, B., Viebke, P. A., Westin, J., and Scanes, C. G. (1989a). Seasonal changes in body weight, fat depots, and plasma levels of thyroxine and growth hormone in free-living great tits (*Parus major*) and willow tits (*P. Montanus*). *Gen. Comp. Endocrinol.* **73**, 404–416.

Silverin, B., Viebke, P. A., and Westin, J. (1989b). Hormonal correlates of migration and territorial behavior in juvenile willow tits during autumn. *Gen. Comp. Endocrinol.* **75**, 148–156.

Silverin, B., Arvidsson, B., and Wingfield, J. C. (1997a). The adrenocortical responses to stress in breeding willow warblers *Phylloscopus trochilus* in Sweden: Effects of latitude and gender. *Func. Ecol.* **11**, 376–384.

Silverin, B., Kikuchi, M., and Ishii, S. (1997b). Seasonal changes in follicle-stimulating hormone in free-living great tits. *Gen. Comp. Endocrinol.* **108**, 366–373.

Silverin, B., Baillien, M., and Balthazart, J. (1999). Territorial aggression correlates with preoptic aromatase activity but not with plasma testosterone in free-living pied flycatchers. *Proc. Soc. Behav. Neuroendocrinol., Abstr.,* p. 64.

Skutch, A. F. (1969). Life histories of Central American birds. *Pac. Coast Avifauna* **35**, 172–179.

Smith, G. T., Wingfield, J. C., and Veit, R. R. (1994). Adrenocortical response to stress in the common diving petrel, *Pelecanoides urinatrix*. *Physiol. Zool.* **67**, 526–537.

Smith, J. (1982). Changes in blood levels of thyroid hormones in two species of passerine birds. *Condor* **84**, 160–167.

Soma, K. K., and Wingfield, J. C. (2000). Endocrinology of aggression in the nonbreeding season. *Proc. 22nd Int. Ornithol. Congr.,* Durban, pp. 1606–1620.

Soma, K. K., Hartman, V., Brenowitz, E. A., and Wingfield, J. C. (1997). Seasonal plasticity of the avian song nucleus HVc as indicated by androgen receptor immunocytochemistry in a wild songbird. *Soci. Neurosci. Abstr.* **23**, 1328.

Soma, K. K., Sullivan, K., and Wingfield, J. (1999a). Combined aromatase inhibitor and antiandrogen treatment decreases territorial aggression in a wild songbird during the nonbreeding season. *Gen. Comp. Endocrinol.* **115**, 442–453.

Soma, K., Hartman, V., Wingfield, J., and Brenowitz, E. (1999b). Seasonal changes in androgen receptor immunoreactivity in the song nucleus HVc of a wild bird. *J. Comp. Neurol.* **409**, 224–236.

Soma, K., Bindra, R., Gee, J., Wingfield, J., and Schlinger, B. (1999c). Androgen-metabolizing enzymes show region-specific changes across the breeding season in the brain of a wild songbird. *J. Neurobiol.* **41**, 176–188.

Soma, K. K., Tramontin, A. D., and Wingfield, J. C. (2000a). Oestrogen regulates male aggression in the nonbreeding season. *Proc. R. Soc. London, Ser. B* **267**, 1089–1096.

Soma, K. K., Sullivan, K. A., Tramontin, A. D., Saldanha, C. J., Schlinger, B. A., and Wingfield, J. C. (2000b). Acute and chronic effects of an aromatase inhibitor on territorial aggression in breeding and non-breeding male song sparrows. *J. Comp. Physiol. A* **186**, 759–769.

Spurr, E., and Milne, H. (1976). Adaptive significance of autumn pair formation in the common eider *Somateria mollissima* (L.). *Ornis Scand.* **7**, 85–89.

Stetson, M. H., and Erickson, J. E. (1971). Endocrine effects of castration in white-crowned sparrows. *Gen. Comp. Endocrinol.* **17**, 105–114.

Stokkan, K.-A. (1979). Testosterone and daylength dependent development of comb size and breeding plumage of male willow ptarmigan (*Lagopus lagopus lagopus*). *Auk* **96**, 106–115.

Stresemann, E., and Stresemann, V. (1966). Die Mauser der Vogel. *J. Ornithol.* **107**, 3–448.

Summers-Smith, D. (1963). "The House Sparrow." Collins, London.

Tewary, P. D., and Farner, D. S. (1973). Effect of castration and estrogen administration on te plumage pigment of the male house finch (*Carpodacus mexicanus*). *Am. Zool.* **13**, 1278.

Thapliyal, J. P., and Gupta, B. B. R. (1984). Thyroid and annual gonad development, body weight, plumage pigmentation, and bill color cycles of Lal munia, *Estrilda amandava*. *Gen. Comp. Endocrinol.* **55**, 20–28.

Thapliyal, J. P., and Saxena, R. N. (1961). Plumage control in Indian weaver bird, (*Ploceus phillipinus*). *Naturwissenschaften* **24**, 741–742.

Thapliyal, J. P., and Saxena, R. N. (1964). Abscence of refractory period in the common weaver bird. *Condor* **66**, 199–208.

Thapliyal, J. P., and Tewary, P. D. (1961). Plumage in Lal munia (*Amandava amandava*). *Science* **134**, 738–739.

Thessing, A., and Ekman, J. (1994). Selection on the genetical and environmental components of tarsal growth in juvenile willow tits (*Parus montanus*). *J. Evol. Biol.* **7**, 713–726.

Thompson, C. W., and Moore, M. C. (1992). Behavioral and hormonal correlates of alternative reproductive strategies in a polygynous lizard: Tests of the relative plasticity and challenge hypotheses. *Horm. Behav.* **26**, 568–585.

Tixier-Vidal, A., and Follett, B. K. (1973). The adenohypophysis. *Avian Biol.* **3**, 110–182.

Trobec, R. J., and Oring, L. W. (1972). Effects of testosterone propionate implantation on lek behavior of sharp-tailed grouse. *Am. Midl. Nat.* **87**, 531–536.

Tsutsui, K., and Yamakazi, T. (1995). Avian neurosteroids. I. Pregnenolone synthesis in the quail brain. *Brain Res.* **678**, 1–9.

Turek, F. W. (1978). Diurnal rhythms and the seasonal reproductive cycle in birds. *In* "Environmental Endocrinology" (D. S. Farner and I. Assenmacher, eds.), pp. 144–152. Springer-Verlag, Berlin.

Ukena, K., Honda, Y., Inai, Y., Kohchi, C., Lea, R., and Tsutsui, K. (1999). Expression and activity of 3β-hydroxysteroid dehydrogenase/Δ^5-Δ^4-isomerase in different regions of the avian brain. *Brain Res.* **818**, 536–542.

van Duyse, E., Pinxten, R., and Eens, M. (2000). Does testosterone affect the trade-off between investment in sexual/territorial behavior and parental care in male great tits? *Behaviour* **137**, 1503–1515.

van Oordt, G. J., and Junge, G. C. A. (1930). Die hormonale Wirking des Hodens auf Federkleid und Farbe des Schnabels und der Fusse bei der Lachmöwe (*Larus ridibundus* L.). *Zool. Anz.* **91**, 1–7.

van Oordt, G. J., and Junge, G. C. A. (1933). Die hormonale Wirkung der Gonaden auf Sommerund Prachtkleid. 1. Der Einfluss der Kastration bei mannlichen Lachmöwen (*Larus* ridibundus L.). *Wilhelm Roux' Arch. Entwicklungsmech. Org.* **128,** 166–180.

van Oordt, G. J., and Junge, G. C. A. (1936). Der Einfluss der Kastration auf mannliche Kampfleufer *(Philomachus pugnax)*. *Wilhelm Roux' Arch. Entwicklungsmech. Org.* **134,** 112–121.

Vanson, A., Arnold, A. P., and Schlinger, B. A. (1996). 3α-hydroxysteroid dehydrogenase/isomerase and aromatase activity in primary cultures of developing zebra finch telencephalon: Dehydroepiandrosterone as substrate for synthesis of androstendione and estrogens. *Gen. Comp. Endocrinol.* **102,** 342–350.

Viebke, P. A. (1991). Endocrine studies on the willow tit *Parus montanus*, with special emphasis on the male. Ph.D. Thesis, Göteborg University, Sweden.

Voitkevitch, A. A. (1966). "The Feathers and Plumage of Birds." Sidgwick & Jackson, London.

Wada, M., Ishii, S., and Scanes, C. G. (1990). "Endocrinology of Birds: Molecular to Behavioral." Jpn. Sci. Soc. Press, Tokyo/Springer-Verlag, Berlin.

Wada, M., Shimizu, T., Kobayshi, S., Yatani, A., Sandaiji, Y., Ishikawa, T., and Takemura, E. (1999). Behavioral and humoral basis of polygynous breeding in male bush warblers *(Cettia diphone)*. *Gen. Comp. Endocrinol.* **116,** 422–432.

Watson, A. (1970). Territorial and reproductive behavior of red grouse. *J. Reprod. Fertil., Suppl.* **11,** 3–14.

Weise, C. M. (1962). Migratory and gonadal responses of birds on long-continued short day-lengths. *Auk* **79,** 161–172.

Weise, C. M. (1967). Castration and spring migration in the white-throated sparrow. *Condor* **69,** 49–68.

Wikelski, M., Hau, M., and Wingfield, J. C. (1999a). Social instability increases plasma testosterone in a year-round territorial neotropical bird. *Proc. R. Soc. London, Ser. B* **266,** 551–556.

Wikelski, M., Lynn, S., Breuner, C., Wingfield, J. C., and Kenagy, G. J. (1999b). Energy metabolism, testosterone and corticosterone in white-crowned sparrows. *J. Comp. Physiol. A* **185,** 463–470.

Wikelski, M., Hau, M., Robinson, W. D., and Wingfield, J. C. (1999c). Seasonal endocrinology of tropical passerines—a comparative approach. *Proc. 22nd Int. Ornithol. Congr.,* Durban, pp. 1224–1241.

Wikelski, M., Hau, M., and Wingfield, J. C. (2000). Seasonality of reproduction in a neotropical rainforest bird. *Ecology* **81,** 2458–2472.

Williams, T. D. (1992). Reproductive endocrinology of macaroni *(Eudyptes chrysolophus)* and gentoo *(Pygoscelis papua)* penguins: I. Seasonal changes in plasma levels of gonadal steroids and LH in breeding adults. *Gen. Comp. Endocrinol.* **85,** 230–240.

Wilson, F. E., and Reinert, B. D. (1993). The thyroid and photoperiodic control of seasonal reproduction in American tree sparrows *(Spizella arbores)*. *J. Comp. Physiol. B* **163,** 563–573.

Wilson, F. E., and Reinert, B. D. (1996). The timing of thyroid-dependent programming in seasonally breeding male American tree sparrows *(Spizella arborea)*. *Gen. Comp. Endocrinol.* **103,** 82–92.

Wingfield, J. C. (1983). Environmental and endocrine control of reproduction: An ecological approach. *In* "Avian Endocrinology: Environmental and Ecological Aspects" (S.-I. Mikami and M. Wada, eds.), pp. 205–288. Japanese Scientific Societies Press, Tokyo, and Springer-Verlag, Berlin.

Wingfield, J. C. (1984a). Androgens and mating systems: Testosterone-induced polygyny in normally monogamous birds. *Auk* **101,** 665–671.

Wingfield, J. C. (1984b). Environmental and endocrine control of reproduction in the song sparrow, *Melospiza melodia*: I. Temporal organization of the breeding cycle. *Gen. Comp. Endocrinol.* **56,** 406–416.

Wingfield, J. C. (1985). Short-term changes in plasma levels of hormones during establishment and defense of a breeding territory in male song sparrows, *Melospiza melodia*. *Horm. Behav.* **19,** 174–187.

Wingfield, J. C. (1988). Changes in reproductive function of free-living birds in direct response to environmental perturbations. *In* "Processing of Environmental Information in Vertebrates" (M. H. Stetson, ed.), pp. 121–148. Springer-Verlag, Berlin.

Wingfield, J. C. (1994a). Hormone-behavior interactions and mating systems in male and female birds. *In* "The Difference Between the Sexes" (R. V. Short and E. Balaban, eds.), pp. 303–330. Cambridge University Press, London.

Wingfield, J. C. (1994b). Modulation of the adrenocortical response to stress in birds. *In* "Perspectives in Comparative Endocrinology" (K. G. Davey, R. E. Peter, and S. S. Tobe eds.), pp. 520–528. National Research Council, Ottawa, Canada.

Wingfield, J. C. (1994c). Control of territorial aggression in a changing environment. *Psychoneuroendocrinology* **19,** 709–721.

Wingfield, J. C. (1994d). Regulation of territorial behavior in the sedentary song sparrow, *Melospiza melodia morphna*. *Horm. Behav.* **28,** 1–15.

Wingfield, J. C., and Farner, D. S. (1976). Avian endocrinology—field investigations and methods. *Condor* **78,** 570–573.

Wingfield, J. C., and Farner, D. S. (1978a). The endocrinology of a naturally breeding population of the white-crowned sparrow *(Zonotrichia leucophrys pugetensis)*. *Physiol. Zool.* **51,** 188–205.

Wingfield, J. C., and Farner, D. S. (1978b). The annual cycle of plasma irLH and steroid hormones in feral populations of the white-crowned sparrow, *Zonotrichia leucophrys gambelii*. *Biol. Reprod.* **19,** 1046–1056.

Wingfield, J. C., and Farner, D. S. (1979). Some endocrine correlates of renesting after loss of clutch or brood in the white-crowned sparrow, *Zonotrichia leucophrys gambelii*. *Gen. Comp. Endocrinol.* **38**, 322–331.

Wingfield, J. C., and Farner, D. S. (1980). Environmental and endocrine control of seasonal reproduction in temperate zone birds. *Prog. Rep. Biol.* **5**, 62–101.

Wingfield, J. C., and Farner, D. S. (1993). The endocrinology of wild species. *Avian Biol.* **9**, 163–327.

Wingfield, J. C., and Goldsmith, A. R. (1990). Plasma levels of prolactin and gonadal steroids in relation to multiple brooding and renesting in free-living populations of the song sparrow, *Melospiza melodia*. *Horm. Behav.* **24**, 89–103.

Wingfield, J. C., and Hahn, T. P. (1994). Testosterone and territorial behaviour in sedentary and migratory sparrows. *Anim. Behav.* **47**, 77–89.

Wingfield, J. C., and Jacobs, J. D. (1999). The interplay of innate and experiential factors regulating the life history cycle of birds. *Proc. 22nd. Int. Ornithol. Congr.*, pp. 2417–2443.

Wingfield, J. C., and Kenagy, G. J. (1991). Natural regulation of reproductive cycles. *In* "Vertebrate Endocrinology: Fundamentals and Biomedical Implications" (M. Schreibman and R. E. Jones, eds.), Vol. 4, Part B, pp. 181–241. Academic Press, San Diego, CA.

Wingfield, J. C., and Lewis, D. M. (1993). Hormonal and behavioural responses to simulated territorial intrusion in the cooperatively breeding white-browed sparrow weaver, *Plocepasser mahali*. *Anim. Behav.* **45**, 1–11.

Wingfield, J. C., and Moore, M. C. (1987). Hormonal, social, and environmental factors in the reproductive biology of free-living male birds. *In* "Psychobiology of Reproductive Behavior: An Evolutionary Perspective" (D. Crews, ed.), pp. 149–175. Prentice-Hall, Englewood Cliffs, NJ.

Wingfield, J.C., and Ramenofsky, M. (1997). Corticosterone and facultative dispersal in response to unpredictable events. *Ardea* **85**, 155–166.

Wingfield, J. C., and Ramenofsky, M. (1999). Hormones and the behavioral ecology of stress. *In* "Stress Physiology in Animals" (P. H. M. Balm, ed.), pp. 1–51. Sheffield Academic Press, Sheffield, UK.

Wingfield, J. C., and Romero, L. M. (2000). Adrenocortical responses to stress and their modulation in free-living vertebrates. *In* "Handbook of Physiology" (B. S. McEwen, ed.), Sect. 7, Vol. 4, pp. 211–236. Oxford University Press, Oxford.

Wingfield, J. C., Smith, J. P., and Farner, D. S. (1980). Changes in plasma levels of luteinizing hormone, steroid and thyroid hormones during the postfledgling development of white-crowned sparrows, *Zonotrichia leucophrys*. *Gen. Comp. Endocrinol.* **41**, 372–377.

Wingfield, J. C., Moore, M. C., and Farner, D. S. (1983). Endocrine responses to inclement weather in naturally breeding populations of white-crowned sparrows. *Auk* **100**, 56–62.

Wingfield, J. C., Ronchi, E., Marler, C., and Goldsmith, A. R. (1989). Interactions of steroids and prolactin during the reproductive cycle of the song sparrow (*Melospiza melodia*). *Physiol. Zool.* **62**, 11–24.

Wingfield, J. C., Schwabl, H., and Mattocks, P. W., Jr. (1990a). Endocrine mechanisms of migration. *In* "Bird Migration: Physiology and Eco-physiology" (E. Gwinner, ed.), pp. 232–256. Springer-Verlag, New York.

Wingfield, J. C., Hegner, R. E., Dufty, A. M., Jr., and Ball, G. F. (1990b). The "Challenge Hypothesis": Theoretical implications for patterns of testosterone secretion, mating systems, and breeding strategies. *Am. Nat.* **136**, 829–846.

Wingfield, J. C., Hegner, R. E., and Lewis, D. M. (1991). Circulating levels of luteinizing hormone and steroid hormones in relation to social status in the cooperatively breeding white-browned sparrow weaver, *Plocepasser mahali*. *J. Zool.* **225**, 43–58.

Wingfield, J. C., Hegner, R. E., and Lewis, D. M. (1992a). Hormonal responses to removal of a breeding male in the cooperatively breeding white-browed weaver, *Plocepasser mahali*. *Horm. Behav.* **26**, 145–155.

Wingfield, J. C., Hahn, T. P., Levin, R., and Honey, P. (1992b). Environmental predictability and control of gonadal cycles in birds. *J. Exp. Zool.* **261**, 214–231.

Wingfield, J. C., Doak, D., and Hahn, T. P. (1993). Integration of environmental cues regulating transitions of physiological state, morphology and behavior. *In* "Avian Endocrinology" (P. J. Sharp, ed.), pp. 111–122. Journal of Endocrinology, Bristol, UK.

Wingfield, J. C., Deviche, P., Sharbaugh, S., Astheimer, L. B., Holberton, R., Suydam, R., and Hunt, K. (1994a). Seasonal changes of the adrenocortical responses to stress in redpolls, *Acanthis flammea*, in Alaska. *J. Exp. Zool.* **270**, 372–380.

Wingfield, J. C., Suydam, R., and Hunt, K. (1994b). Adrenocortical responses to stress in snow buntings and Lapland longspurs at Barrow, Alaska. *Comp. Biochem. Physiol.* **108**, 299–306.

Wingfield, J. C., Whaling, C. S., and Marler, P. R. (1994c). Communication in vertebrate aggression and reproduction: The role of hormones. *In* "Physiology of Reproduction" (E. Knobil and J. D. Neill, eds.), 2nd ed., pp. 303–342. Raven Press, New York.

Wingfield, J. C., Kubokawa, K., Ishida, K., Ishii, S., and Wada, M. (1995a). The adrenocortical response to stress in male bush warblers, *Cettia diphone*: A comparison of breeding populations in Honshu and Hokkaido, Japan. *Zool. Sci.* **12**, 615–621.

Wingfield, J. C., O'Reilly, K. M., and Astheimer, L. B. (1995b). Ecological bases of the modulation of adrenocortical responses to stress in Arctic birds. *Am. Zool.* **35**, 285–294.

Wingfield, J. C., Hahn, T. P., Wada, M., Astheimer, L. B., and Schoech, S. (1996). Interrelationship of day length and temperature on the control of gonadal development, body mass and fat depots in white-crowned sparrows, *Zonotrichia leucophrys gambelii*. *Gen. Comp. Endocrinol.* **101**, 242–255.

Wingfield, J. C., Hahn, T. P., Wada, M., and Schoech, S. J. (1997a). Effects of day length and temperature on gonadal development, body mass, and fat depots in white-crowned sparrows, *Zonotrichia leucophrys pugetensis*. *Gen. Comp. Endocrinol.* **107**, 44–62.

Wingfield, J., Jacobs, J., and Hillgarth, N. (1997b). Ecological constraints and the evolution of hormone-behavior interrelationships. *Ann. N. Y. Acad. Sci.* **807**, 22–41.

Wingfield, J. C., Breuner, C., Jacobs, J., Lynn, S., Maney, D., Ramenofsky, M., and Richardson, R. (1998). Ecological bases of hormone-behavior Interactions: The "Emergency Life History Stage." *Am. Zool.* **38**, 191–206.

Wingfield, J. C., Jacobs, J. D., Soma, K., Maney, D. L., Hunt, K., Wisti-Peterson, D., Meddle, S., Ramenofsky, M., and Sullivan, K. (1999). Testosterone, aggression, and communication: Ecological bases of endocrine phenomena. *In* "The Design of Animal Communication" (M. Hauser and M. Konishi, eds.), pp. 255–284. MIT Press, Cambridge, MA.

Wingfield, J. C., Jacobs, J. D., Tramontin, A. D., Perfito, N., Meddle, S., Maney, D. L., and Soma, K. (2000). Toward and ecological basis of hormone-behavior interactions in reproduction of birds. *In* "Reproduction in Context" (K. Wallen and J. Schneider, eds.), pp. 85–128. MIT Press, Cambridge, MA.

Witschi, E. (1961). Sex and secondary sexual characters. *In* "Biology and Comparative Physiology of Birds" (A. J. Marshall, ed.), Vol. 2, pp. 115–168. Academic Press, New York.

Wolfson, A. (1966). Environmental and neuroendocrine regulation of the annual gonadal cycles and migratory behavior in birds. *Recent Prog. Horm. Res.* **12**, 177–244.

Yokoyama, K. (1976). Hypothalamic and hormonal control of photoperiodically-induced vernal functions in the white-crowned sparrow, *Zonotrichia leucophrys gambelii*. 1. The effects of hypothalamic lesions and exogenous hormones. *Cell Tissue Res.* **174**, 391–416.

Yokoyama, K. (1977). Hypothalamic and hormonal control of photoperiodically-induced vernal functions in the white-crowned sparrow, *Zonotrichia leucophrys gambelii*. II. The effect of hypothalamic implantation of testosterone propionate. *Cell Tissue Res.* **176**, 91–108.

Yokoyama, K., and Farner, D. S. (1978). The induction of Zugunruhe by photostimulation of encephalic photoreceptors in white-crowned sparrows. *Science* **201**, 76–79.

32

Neuroendocrine Mechanisms Regulating Reproductive Cycles and Reproductive Behavior in Birds

Gregory F. Ball
Department of Psychological and Brain Sciences
Johns Hopkins University
Baltimore, Maryland 21218

Jacques Balthazart
Center for Cellular and Molecular Neurobiology
Research Group in Behavioral Neuroendocrinology
University of Liège
B-4020 Liège, Belgique

I. INTRODUCTION: DIVERSITY IN REPRODUCTIVE STRATEGIES IN BIRDS

This chapter concerns the interrelationships among hormones, brain, and behavior that mediate the occurrence of reproductive cycles and reproductive behavior among adults in avian species. The scope of the chapter is therefore quite broad, ranging from a consideration of the neuroendocrine basis of seasonal reproduction to a description of the neural and endocrine mechanisms that regulate male and female sexual behavior and parental behavior. Many of the individual sections of this chapter correspond to entire chapters in this multivolume work on hormones, brain, and behavior. What brings focus to our chapter is the fact that we limit our discussion to birds. It might be argued that it is somewhat archaic, and perhaps even a mistake, to organize a chapter concerning the neuroendocrine mechanisms mediating reproduction based on the consideration of a particular taxon. It is true that it has become clear that many neuroendocrine mechanisms relating behavior and other related complex processes are quite similar among vertebrates, especially at the cellular and molecular levels of analysis. It is also true that summarizing hormone action in relation to behavior among all taxa in relation to a given behavior could be quite informative. However, since the 1980s the field of neuroendocrinology has become highly specialized, with rapid progress being made based in studies of a relatively small number of rodent species that are generally thought to serve as model systems for our understanding of these processes in primates, especially humans. This trend, which has been apparent at least since the end of the Second World War, has become accelerated given the obvious utility of using mice for sophisticated genetic manipulations. Therefore integrating in a comprehensive and scholarly way all the information available on a given topic such as male sexual behavior for all vertebrate species (to say nothing of the rich literature on invertebrates) has become a daunting task. However, in addition to considering for one behavioral system the wealth of data available from highly studied mammalian species, useful insights can also be gained by considering in an integrative manner a variety of aspects of the neuroendocrinology of reproduction in a single taxon. We argue that the gap in research progress at the mechanistic level of analysis is not so extreme as to make a consideration of nonmammalian taxa without value to all workers in the field, including those interested in the comparative perspective. Indeed in some cases, even for questions posed at the cellular or molecular levels of analysis, studies of nonmammalian vertebrates remain vital.

A consideration of the neuroendocrine basis of reproductive cycles and reproductive behavior in bird species, (i.e., species that are members of the class Aves) is potentially particularly beneficial. Many of the pioneering studies concerning different aspects of the interrelations among hormones, brain, and behavior were conducted on birds (e.g., Berthold, 1849; Leinhart, 1927; Rowan, 1929; Riddle et al., 1935; Lehrman, 1959, 1964). Therefore, the history of avian studies in this field is as old as the field itself. Because of the tireless efforts of many field ethologists and field ecologists, there exists an extensive knowledge base of information on reproductive cycles and reproductive behavior in nature among avian species (Murton and Westwood, 1977; Perrins and Birkhead, 1983; Wingfield and Farner, 1993). This base of knowledge is arguably more extensive than for any other vertebrate class. Therefore the neuroendocrinology of reproductive behavior in birds can be considered in a natural context more easily than in many other taxa. Birds also exhibit some unusual attributes such as a well-defined neural substrate mediating the activation of many behaviors, a high level of adult neuroplasticity that includes adult neurogenesis (Nottebohm, 1989), and robust and well-characterized endocrine responses to environmental and social stimuli (Gwinner, 1986; Nicholls et al., 1988b, Ball and Bentley, 2000). These attributes make avian species a valuable resource for the elucidation of basic cellular and molecular mechanisms, independent of their ability to inform us about mechanisms regulating reproduction in a natural context. The literature on the neuroendocrinology of reproduction in birds is smaller than for mammalian species and therefore a large number of topics can be considered at once while still being reasonably comprehensive. Birds have long been a source of interesting insights into biological processes (Konishi et al., 1989); our goal in this chapter is to illustrate that they continue to provide valuable data from which general lessons can be gleaned. Our hope is that this chapter will be a resource for the future generations of behavioral biologists who will continue this tradition of investigating avian species.

A. Basic Aspects of Avian Reproduction

Birds are traditionally defined as any species that possesses feathers. Feathers may well represent a key adaptation that led to the evolution of the volant lifestyle (Feduccia, 1996; Chatterjee, 1997) that is widespread among birds, but by no means universal. A number of other traits generally relevant to all aspects of avian biology, including reproduction, appear to have evolved in association or as a result of their commitment to flight. Consequently, the natural history of reproduction in birds is unique in many respects. First and foremost, birds are obligately oviparous. They are the only vertebrate class in which there is not a single species exhibiting viviparity (Blackburn and Evans, 1986). In most species, as an adaptation to reduce overall body mass to promote flight, only the sinistral ovary is active (ground-dwelling species such as kiwis, Apterygiformes, are exceptions to this rule; Feduccia, 1996). The dextral ovary often, but not in all species, maintains the ability to recrudesce should the left ovary stop functioning or be removed experimentally. Males of most species also lack an intromittent organ of any sort, perhaps another adaptation for weight reduction. However, many are skeptical about this explanation for the widespread lack of an intromittent organ in birds and suggest that the loss of such organs occurred because it minimizes the acquisition of sexually transmitted diseases (Briskie and Montgomerie, 1997). In any case, a penis-like intromittent organ has been reacquired by large flightless birds such as ostriches and tinamous. An intromittent organ is also present in many waterfowl species and in storks and curassows (Birkhead and Moller, 1992; Briske and Montgomerie, 1997). Because of the lack of external genitalia, copulation in most birds involves brief cloacal contact movements in which the sperm is transferred from males to females. Another example of an adaptation designed to reduce body mass is the fluctuating pattern of breeding activity and gonadal recrudescence that is timed so that breeding is strictly limited to a relatively short window of time in the annual cycle (Baker, 1938; Murton and Westwood, 1977). Among male birds, there is remarkable seasonal variation in the size of the testis, with increases as large as

1000-fold in breeding males compared to nonbreeding males (Follett, 1984).

Avian species are also endothermic with a basal body temperature higher even than mammals (40°C ± 2°). This combination of universal oviparity and endothermy makes it essential that all eggs receive some sort of attention after oviposition, although it is not necessarily the case that the newly hatched young require any attention from their parents (Oring, 1982). Parental care, therefore, is a fundamental component of the life history of nearly all avian species. It appears to be a primitive life history characteristic that is a part of the group of morphological and behavioral adaptations that almost defines birds and differentiates them from their reptilian ancestors. The diversification of the class Aves has included patterns of parental behavior. Biparental care of some sort may be the primitive pattern and remains the most common (Lack, 1968; Silver et al., 1985). But the roles adopted by the sexes and the types of care provided to the offspring vary greatly among taxa. All birds lay eggs that require attendance of some sort for successful hatching. The type of posthatching care provided has coevolved with the mode of development of the young. Altricial development is most common in the class Aves, although it appears to be the derived condition, precocial development being the primitive condition (Ricklefs, 1983). Altricial young are generally helpless at hatching and therefore must be brooded and fed by their parents. Precocial young are somewhat independent at hatching and may only require supervision by the parents and no additional feeding.

Obligate parental care sets the stage for certain peculiarities of the life history strategies adopted by birds that influence the timing of reproduction. For example, in most avian species, food for the young at the time of hatching is particularly important because the successful survival of the progeny is closely tied to the types of food ingested during development (Baker, 1938; Perrins, 1970; Perrins and Birkhead, 1983). In altricial species food is provided by the parents to the young, whereas in precocial species the young are guided to food sources where they feed themselves (Ricklefs, 1983). In general, avian parents are unable to store energy as body fat and then provide it to their young at a later time. This is in contrast to certain mammalian species, in which the mother overeats and stores excess calories in the form of fat during a time of abundant food availability, and then converts her fat to milk during lactation and feeds her young on this milk at a later time when food availability is low (Bronson, 1989). For example, this pattern is very common among Pinnepeds. As we expect, there are of course exceptions among the living species of birds. Some species (especially in the corvid and parid families) store food so that they can initiate breeding before appropriate quantities and types of food are available (e.g., Sherry, 1989).

B. Avian Species That Have Been Studied in Detail

There are between 9000 and 10,000 living avian species on the planet (Bock and Farrand, 1980; del Hoyo et al., 1992). The estimate of the total living number of individuals ranges as high as 300 billion (del Hoyo et al., 1992). As we expect, endocrine and neuroendocrine mechanisms have been investigated in detail in only a relatively small subset of living species. However, there are some relevant data available in a rather large number of species, at least compared to other vertebrate taxa. The selection of species that have been investigated has not been based on a logical overall plan for the comprehensive investigation of birds but is, rather, influenced by the goals and intellectual traditions that have brought various scientists to study these questions in birds. Studies have been conducted on the neuroendocrinology of reproductive cycles and reproductive behavior in birds by several different types of investigators for several different reasons (Farner, 1981).

One group of investigators comes from the tradition of animal science and has focused on the neuroendocrinology of species of economic importance to humans, such as the domestic chickens and domestic turkeys. Studies of reproductive behavior in these species have the ultimate goal of improving the efficiency of breeding. Another group of scientists investigating neuroendocrine questions in birds comes from the tradition of ethology and physiological psychology and is interested in behavioral endocrinology. This group has studied semidomesticated species such as ring doves (*Streptopelia risoria*), canaries (*Serinus canaria*), and Japanese quail (*Coturnix japonica*) that breed in captivity or exhibit a wide range of reproductive behaviors under captive conditions. The neuroendocrine control of courtship behaviors, especially song in the case of canaries, has been the main focus of this group. Finally, there is the tradition of comparative endocrinology among zoologists. Scientists in this tradition have usually focused on wild species, most often members of the order Passeriformes (songbirds). This group initially was interested in the photoperiodic and environmental regulation of seasonal reproduction in species such as the white-crowned sparrow (*Zonotrichia leucophyrs;* Farner, 1986) or European starling (*Sturnus vulgaris;* Nicholls *et al.,* 1988b). With the advent of field endocrinology methods pioneered by Wingfield and Farner (1976), studies of wild birds in their natural habitat have expanded and have attracted physiological and behavioral ecologists.

These three different research traditions represent the historical roots of the field and investigators today ask questions and use methods that cut across the traditions that gave rise to the initial studies of these different groups of birds. In this chapter, our goal is to capture some of the most interesting work relevant to neuroendocrine mechanisms of reproductive behavior in birds. Therefore, we do not concentrate on the rich literature that has emerged from field studies (Wingfield and Silverin, Chapter 31) nor do we focus on the neuroendocrine basis of vocal behavior in songbirds, a field that has grown greatly in the 1990s (Schlinger and Brenowitz, Chapter 33).

C. Diversity in Breeding Cycles: Temperate vs Tropical Breeding Cycles

Birds originated in tropical climes and the majority of avian species living today are tropical. However, most studies of birds have been conducted by temperate-zone biologists on temperate-zone species. The organization of the avian breeding cycle appears to be quite different in the temperate zone than in the tropics. It is common for nontropical avian species to exhibit a clear pattern of seasonal reproduction. This means that reproductive activity is limited to the time of year when temperatures are relatively mild and the necessary food resources are present. Temperate-zone species often use specific cues in the environment, such as changes in photoperiod (the length of the daylight period) to coordinate gonadal recrudescence and the associated increases in endocrine activity with the appropriate season. Factors that limit reproductive success, such as food availability are usually referred to as ultimate causes (or factors) because their presence or absence directly affects the survival of the young. Factors that initiate reproductive processes in time for the breeding season, such as photoperiod, are usually referred to as the proximate causes (or cues) for successful breeding (Baker, 1938). Proximate cues can then be usefully subdivided into different categories (Wingfield, 1980, 1983; Wingfield and Kenagy, 1991). For example, photoperiod is a powerful initial predictive cue that initiates or terminates the period of reproduction in many nontropical species. Other cues provide essential supplementary information, synchronizing and integrating information (this category includes social interactions), or modifying information (this category includes storms and other natural stressors; Wingfield and Kenagy, 1991).

Species that seem to breed in response to the experience of a specific environmental cue other than photoperiod (such as rainfall) are often referred to as opportunistic breeders (Hahn *et al.,* 1997). It is sometimes thought that most tropical species are of this type because photoperiodic changes are minimal in the tropics and the pattern of breeding seems to be much less seasonal. Nonetheless, avian populations in the tropics still exhibit some form of periodic breeding. There is evidence that some species can measure the very small changes in photoperiod that occur in the tropics (e.g., Hau *et al.,* 1998) and it is also possible that periodic breeding is in response to some other cue such as rainfall (see Murton and Westwood, 1977). Seasonal cycles in hormone secretion are also more muted in tropical species than in temperate-zone species (e.g., Levin and Wingfield, 1992; Dittami and Gwinner, 1990). Thus, it seems highly likely that there are no qualitative differences between temperate and tropical breeding cycles and that the neuroendocrine mechanisms regulating these different cycles are also not qualitatively different (Hahn *et al.,* 1997).

D. Diversity in Mating Systems and Parental Care Patterns

Mating system refers to the breeding pattern adopted by males and females in sexually breeding species. The three most well-recognized types are monogamy (the association of a single male with a single female during the breeding period), polygyny (the association of a single male with multiple females), and polyandry (the association of a single female with multiple males). There are other less well-known variants such as polygynandry (the simultaneous association of multiple males and multiple females), as well as variations on the theme of promiscuity. One of the most interesting aspects of avian reproduction concerns the distribution of mating systems; for this reason, birds remain one of the most popular taxa for the study of the causes of variation in mating systems (e.g., Ligon, 1998). The first unusual aspect of the relative occurrence of mating systems in birds concerns the high rate of monogamy among avian species. Most estimates indicate that roughly 90% of living bird species (Lack, 1968; Silver et al., 1985; Ligon, 1998) exhibit at least a pattern of social monogamy in which a single female and a single male pair and tend a nest together. With the development of sophisticated methods for establishing paternity, such as DNA fingerprinting techniques, it has become apparent that many males in these socially monogamous species engage in mixed reproductive strategies (e.g., Westneat, 1990; Moller and Birkhead, 1993; Stuchbury et al., 1994). This means that, although they pair and associate with a single female, they attempt to copulate with neighboring females, as first predicted by Trivers (1972). This sets up a process of sperm competition. Field estimates have found that the percentage of eggs fathered by a male who is not tending a particular nest can vary from essentially 0% to nearly 60% (Westneat et al., 1990; Ligon, 1998). It has also become clear that females are active participants in this competitive process, based both on the active behavioral choices they make and on the influence they exert on the fertilization process once sperm is present in their reproductive tract (Gowaty, 1994).

Although birds are unique in that monogamy is quite widespread, they also stand out because of the diversity of mating systems. Polygyny, the most common mating system among mammalian species, is known to occur in approximately 8% of avian species. Polyandry, a very rare mating system among vertebrates, has been observed in approximately 2% of extant avian species, and other systems such as the complex polygynandry, described in acorn woodpeckers in California; (Koenig and Mumme, 1987) have been described in less than 1% of living bird species. This diversity in mating systems provides a tremendous opportunity for reproductive neuroendocrinologists. Most research of mating systems has been conducted by behavioral ecologists who have focused on the adaptive significance of this variation. Mechanistic studies have largely been limited to endocrine studies in which interesting correlates between variation in patterns of plasma hormone concentrations and variation in mating pattern have been identified (Wingfield and Farner, 1993; see Wingfield and Silverin, Chapter 31). However, this diversity in reproductive behavior cannot be explained only by variation in peripheral hormone secretion, as studies of polyandrous avian species have illustrated (e.g., Fivizzani and Oring, 1986). The diversity in neuroendocrine mechanisms have also evolved in concert with this variation in mating systems (Fivizzani and Oring, 1986).

The widespread occurrence of monogamy is thought to be related to the high rate of biparental care in birds. The argument has been that males and females can maximize their reproductive success by helping one another care for the eggs and the young (Lack, 1968; Oring, 1982). It is indeed the case that uniparental care provided by the female is much more common among polygynous species and similarly uniparental care provided by the male is most common among polyandrous species. However, parental care patterns do not simply covary with variation in mating systems. There are also some unique variants in parental care patterns among avian species that are not appreciated by merely considering variation in mating systems. For example, an interesting but relatively rare phenomenon is the reproductive strategy known as brood parasitism, which has been described in one or more species in five families of birds (Ligon, 1998). Birds engaging in this behavior lay their eggs in the nests of another species and allow the parents of the host species to incubate the egg and feed the nestling. In this way, these brood-parasitic species avoid the substantial energetic costs associated with parental care and can continue laying eggs throughout the breeding season. It has been estimated that a single female brown-headed cowbird (a North American brood parasite) can lay 40 eggs in a single breeding season (Scott and Ankney, 1980). Another unusual variant of parental care is observed in bird species that live in groups that are larger than a single breeding pair during the breeding season. In these group-living species, members of the group who are not the parents assist in some cases with incubation duties or parental feeding (see Brown, 1987, for a review). Brood parasitism and cooperative breeding also raise many interesting issues concerning the neuroendocrine regulation of reproductive behavior. Both of these problems have been addressed to varying degrees at the endocrine level, but neuroendocrine analyses have just started.

E. Species Diversity and Sexual Dimorphism in Behavior and Morphology

Variability in mating systems and parental care patterns are associated with extensive variability in behavior, morphology, and physiology among males and females. The variability among different species in the degree to which the sexes differ is striking. Some avian species are so monomorphic in appearance and even in most aspects of their behavior that determining the sex of an individual based on external characteristics is nearly impossible. In other species, sex differences in plumage or behavior or both are dimorphic to such a large degree that early naturalists classified males and females of a single species as being members of different species (Mayr, 1963). The ultimate reason for the occurrence of sex differences involves the differential action of sexual selection (Andersson, 1994). This question is not addressed in this review, but these sex differences and dimorphisms raise important issues for behavioral neuroendocrinologists interested in both the development of sex-typical systems and their activation in adulthood.

Although there is extensive variability among species, this variability is lawful. Monomorphism in plumage is associated with monogamous mating systems and extensive biparental care. There are some well-known exceptions, such as among raptors (accipiters), which breed monogamously but in which the females are larger than the males and in which there are plumage differences. Another exception involves members of the cardueline finch family (grosbeaks, cardinals, chaffinches, etc.), which are socially monogamous, but exhibit marked dimorphisms in plumage. Males in these species are typically much brighter in plumage than females. This pattern of male-biased differences in plumage is generally associated with polygynous mating patterns, in which males are typically larger and more brightly colored than females. The exact reverse is observed among polyandrous species, in which females are larger and more brightly colored than males.

Among mammalian species, one of the most obvious and well-documented dimorphisms in morphology associated with reproduction involves the genitals. In birds, such patterns are quite different. The cloaca serves both the function of elimination and the transfer of gametes. It is not obviously different in many avian species, although quantitative differences are often apparent during the breeding season. This means that sex differences in reproductive behavior can be directly related to sex differences in mechanisms of the central nervous system rather than influenced by prominent sex differences in peripheral effector systems. The more prominent sex differences in the genitals are observed in the few species that do exhibit intromittent organs in the males. This intromittent organ is a modification of the wall of the cloaca. It can be quite large in some cases, such as in the blue-billed duck in Australia in which it has been reported to be at least 10 cm in length and to trail after the male after copulation (see Birkhead and Moller, 1992). Perhaps the largest avian penis on record has been reported in the Argentine lake duck (*Oxyura vittata*), which has a 20-cm penis with spines (McCracken, 2000). As discussed previously, the occurrence of the intromittent organ is rarer than in other vertebrate groups and exhibits an unusual taxonomic distribution in avian species. There is no obvious single principle that easily explains why this organ appears in some taxa but not others (Birkhead and Moller, 1992). However, this organ does appear to facilitate sperm transfer and competition. Consistent with this notion is the trend for males in species that exhibit relatively high amounts of paternal care to possess such organs. This pattern suggests that these organs have been selected to facilitate sperm transfer and enhance a male's reproductive success, especially in species in which the fitness cost of failing to fertilize the mate's eggs is quite high due to the expenditure of parental effort (Briske and Montgomerie, 1997). There is also evidence that intromittent organs have appeared in species in which females produce relatively large eggs and may therefore have difficulty aborting them (Briske and Montgomerie, 1997). Females with such large investments in their eggs are thought to exert strong choice on their mates and male intromittent organs have appeared in these species due to males' attempts to exploit these large investments (Briske and Montgomerie, 1997).

F. Overall Organization of Reproductive Behavior

The study of reproductive behaviors in birds has been greatly influenced by the ethological concept of appetitive vs consummatory behaviors first articulated by pioneer ethologists such as Tinbergen (1951), Lorenz (1950), and Baerends (1988). The basic idea is that some stereotypic behaviors result in a functional outcome that is associated with a reduction in motivation, whereas other more variable behaviors allow an individual to converge on this functional outcome (Timberlake and Silva, 1995). This sort of dichotomy is potentially problematic when we try to apply it to complex sequences of behavior. For example, is the entire copulatory sequence the consummatory response or just the cloacal contact movements and associated sperm transfer? Therefore, the concept should be used cautiously, although the distinction continues to be useful to both ethologists and experimental psychologists in the elucidation of neuroendocrine mechanisms mediating a range of behaviors (Timberlake and Silva, 1995). The study of sexual behavior is an area in which this distinction has been particularly useful in guiding mechanistic studies. Beach (1956) formally introduced this idea to the field of behavioral endocrinology by pointing out its usefulness to the analysis of male sexual behavior based on his studies of rodents. This same paradigm has been applied usefully to studies of sexual behavior in females (e.g., Pfaus et al., 1999). Male- and female-typical avian reproductive behaviors are described separately and concisely in this section, although the behavior of the females needs to be discussed to understand male behaviors and vice versa.

1. Male Behavior

In males, appetitive sexual behavior consists in searching for and approaching a potential mate, whereas the consummatory component includes the actual contact between the sexes culminating in copulation (Beach, 1956). Appetitive male sexual behaviors include most courtship behaviors that function to attract females and stimulate them to bring them into a sexually receptive condition. In birds, males are known to exhibit a wide diversity of visual and vocal displays that function in this manner (Armstrong, 1947). As expected, there is a large amount of species variability. In some cases, stereotyped movements involving elaborate plumage displays are used to attract and stimulate females. In other cases, vocal behavior is paramount and in many cases there is a combination of these two sorts of displays. What is clear is that communication involving other sensory modalities such as olfaction or touch is not particularly important. Experimental paradigms for the investigation of appetitive male sexual behavior have been developed in domesticated species such as the Japanese quail (*Coturnix japonica*). It was discovered that when a male copulates with a female for a single time in an area there is a marked change in his behavior. After copulating with a female, the male stands in front of a window that provides him with visual access to the female for most of the day (Domjan and Hall, 1986a,b). This is a robust response that is easily quantifiable and provides a useful way to investigate the neuroendocrine mechanisms regulating male appetitive sexual behavior (Balthazart and Ball, 1998b).

Consummatory male sexual behavior consists of the copulatory act itself. This requires that males mount females so that gamete transfer can be facilitated. In most species, gamete transfer involves what is sometimes referred to as the cloacal kiss. These are cloacal contact movements that facilitate the deposition of sperm in the female. There are often other stereotyped motor patterns that precede cloacal contact movements per se. For example, in Japanese quail copulation consists of a sequence of stereotyped movements progressing from neck grab to mounts and cloacal contact movements (Adkins and Adler, 1972; R. E. Hutchison, 1978). In species with a penis-like intromittent organ, the copulatory act involves intromission as well. Most copulations between members of a pair are solicited by either the male or the female member of the pair (Birkhead and Moller, 1992). In a comparative study of 213 Palearctic bird species, it was found that females were more apt to solicit copulations than males, indicating that in most of these species females control pair copulations (Birkhead and Moller, 1992). However, males also play an important role in initiating copulations in many species, as was previously described for Japanese quail. In species in which female copulation solicitation is common, male neck-grabbing behavior prior to copulation is uncommon (Birkhead and Moller, 1992). Precopulatory and copulatory behavior is also often associated with the production of specific calls that again can be uttered by either the male or the female.

The timing and number of copulations engaged in by a pair varies widely among species and has been the target of a great deal of research due to a renewed interest in the study of sexual selection and sperm competition in birds (Birkhead and Moller, 1992). Often only a single mount and cloacal contact movement is observed, but in some species such as house sparrows multiple mounts and cloacal contact movements (up to 30 in quick succession) have been observed (Birkhead and Moller, 1992). In songbird species the duration of mounting and cloacal contact movements together last only 1–2 seconds (Birkhead et al., 1987). However, in larger species the duration can be much greater. In a comparative study of 69 species, a bimodal distribution in copulation duration was observed with most species either exhibiting a duration of less than 5 seconds or more than 30 seconds (Birkhead et al., 1987). The longest duration of mounting and cloacal contact movements was found to be 3.5 min in black terns (Birkhead et al., 1987). The variability in copulation duration was not explained by predation risk as we might assume. Rather, it appears to be related to mechanical constraints. Smaller birds are more agile and appear to require less time to transfer sperm (Birkhead et al., 1987). Pair copulations are usually clustered around the female's fertile period. Although it is clear that a relatively small number of copulatory acts are sufficient for fertilization (Cheng et al., 1981; Birkhead et al., 1987), the total number of copulations engaged in by a pair in a given species does vary widely. As was the case for copulation duration, comparative studies of copulation frequency reveal a bimodal distribution (Birkhead and Moller, 1992). In one group of species, copulations tend to be limited to 20 or less, whereas in other groups it is greater than 20; in some raptor species the number exceeds 500 copulations per clutch of eggs laid (Birkhead and Moller, 1992)! The frequency of copulatory behavior is correlated with the male's ability to guard the female during her fertile period and prevent her from copulating with other males (Birkhead and Moller, 1992). For example, in raptor species with high copulation rates males feed females during the egg-laying period and therefore frequently leave the females on the nest unattended while they forage for food. In species with low copulation rates, males guard and escort females during their entire fertile period and prevent other males from copulating with them (Birkhead and Moller, 1992). Relative gonad size is positively correlated with copulation frequency in male birds (Birkhead and Moller, 1992).

2. Female Behavior

The appetitive–consummatory dichotomy has also been applied to the study of female sexual behavior (Pfaus et al., 1999). Beach (1976) has argued that a distinction among the concepts of attractivity, receptivity, and proceptivity is useful when considering the mechanisms regulating female sexual behavior. Attractivity involves features of the female that influence the probability that the male initiates appetitive responses to the female. Proceptivity refers to the probability that the female exhibits appetitive behavior toward a male (which is influenced, in turn, by his attractivity). In mammals proceptivity is greatly enhanced in females during the period of behavioral estrus. Ovarian cycles in birds are not organized into periods of behavioral estrus as they are in mammals. However, females solicit male copulation with specialized displays that occur only during the breeding season when gonadal steroid hormone levels are high. Finally, receptivity involves the behaviors exhibited just prior and during copulation that are stimulated in response to the appropriate behavior by the male.

Field studies of female reproductive behavior have stressed the active role the female plays in soliciting male sexual behaviors and managing mating behavior in a way that is advantageous to the female's reproductive success (Gowaty, 1996). For example, it is clear in some species such as the dunnock (Prunella modularis), with a very complex mating system, that females actively solicit extrapair copulations in an apparently deceptive fashion (Davies, 1992). As mentioned previously, females in many species produce calls just prior to and during copulation (Birkhead and Moller, 1992). These calls are louder than would be expected if they were just communicating with their partner. It has been hypothesized that these calls signal to other males that the female is fertile and may also function as a solicitation of sorts for later extrapair copulations that might be beneficial to the female's reproductive success.

Although it is clear that female birds engage in complex appetitive sexual behaviors, the neural and hormonal basis of this repertoire has largely been neglected. No laboratory procedures have been developed for the experimental investigation of proceptive behaviors in females and, as is the case for male sexual behavior, most neuroendocrine work has concentrated on consummatory aspects of female sexual behavior.

II. ENVIRONMENTAL CONTROL OF THE REPRODUCTIVE CYCLE

As discussed in Section I, reproductive behavior in birds is embedded in an annual cycle that involves periods of breeding and of nonbreeding. In the temperate zone and boreal regions where bird populations breed in a highly seasonal manner, the timing of reproduction usually coincides with the late spring to early summer. In the tropics, breeding is still periodic for a given individual or pair, although populations may not breed as synchronously at particular times of the year as is common in the temperate zone. In this section, we review some basic facts about the different sorts of environmental stimuli that regulate the timing of reproduction in birds. Later in the chapter, we consider the neuroendocrine mechanisms mediating the effects of these stimuli on the environment. A complex configuration of environmental stimuli can influence the timing of avian reproduction, including geophysical cues such as variation in photoperiod, other aspects of the physical and biotic environment such as ambient temperature, nest-site access, food availability, and finally social interactions of various types. The theoretical orientation we adopt toward the environmental effects on seasonal reproduction is greatly influenced by Lehrman (1965) and Wingfield (1980, 1983). Lehrman made the crucial observation that the perception of a behaviorally active conspecific may have a profound effect on endocrine physiology, just as endocrine physiology has an important effect on the expression of various reproductive behaviors. He was the person who first made it clear that social interactions should be considered an environmental stimulus regulating endocrine physiology, just like other physical stimuli such as photoperiod. Wingfield provided a very valuable framework for organizing the various types of environmental stimuli that regulate seasonal reproduction, discussed in detail in this section. For more detailed reviews of the environmental regulation of seasonal reproduction in birds, the reader can consult a variety of reviews, such as those by Nicholls *et al.*, (1988b), Ball and Bentley (2000), and Dawson *et al.*, (2001).

A. Photoperiodic Regulation of Breeding

1. Photoperiodic and Extraphotoperiodic Cues

Changes in day length (or photoperiod) provide a valuable cue in the environment that allows animals to assess the time of year. If an individual is able to measure the current photoperiod and ascertain whether the photoperiod is decreasing or increasing, the individual can in theory determine with precision any date of the year. A wide range of avian species that live either in the tropics or in the temperate zone have evolved the ability to measure and respond to seasonal fluctuations in photoperiod (Murton and Westwood, 1977; Nicholls *et al.*, 1988b; Wilson and Donham, 1988). The photoperiodic response in birds can be characterized based on the physiological responses a given avian population exhibits as it experiences seasonal fluctuations in photoperiod. These responses are mediated by a complex system that includes both a neural component and an endocrine component (Follett, 1984). Variation in photoperiod is referred to as an initial predictive cue (Wingfield and Kenagy, 1991) because photoperiod regulates the onset and offset of breeding independent of any year-to-year variation in weather, food, or social conditions or any local geographic variation in the quality of such factors that a bird might encounter. For successful breeding to occur, photoperiodic responses must be fine-tuned by other cues in the environment that allow egg-laying to be timed optimally in response to variation in local conditions (Wingfield, 1980, 1983). In our consideration of avian photoperiodism, we focus on the photoperiodic regulation of reproduction. However, it should be noted that many other traits change seasonally and are regulated by photoperiod (such as plumage or body mass), whereas other traits may be impervious to photoperiodic changes. Some authors therefore argue that it is more accurate to refer to photoperiodic traits rather than photoperiodic individuals or populations.

2. Brief Description of the Photoperiodic Response

Birds are traditionally viewed as being long-day breeders (e.g., Murton and Westwood, 1977). By this, most authors mean that the hypothalamic-pituitary-gonadal axis responds to increasing day lengths after the winter solstice with a marked increase in gonadotropin secretion, gonadal growth, and a wide range of steroid-hormone-dependent processes, including changes in reproductive behaviors. Such a view of the photoperiodic regulation of reproduction leads logically to the simple hypothesis that photoperiods greater than 12 hours light:12 hours dark (12L:12D) stimulate the reproductive axis and day lengths shorter than 12:12 inhibit it (see Fig. 1). We would then predict a symmetrical function of gonadal activity centered on the summer solstice. It turns out that such breeding patterns are exceedingly rare. Perhaps the closest approximation of these symmetrical cycles is the annual cycle of certain gallinaceous birds such as the California quail (see Murton and Westwood, 1977) or columbiformes such as the wood pigeon (*Columba palumbus*) in the United Kingdom (Lofts *et al.*, 1966). It is more common that the photoperiodic response of birds exhibits physiological responses asymmetrical to seasonal changes in day length (Fig. 1). The effects on reproductive physiology of the lengthening periods of day light that are normally experienced by temperate-zone birds in the spring are twofold. One effect is to stimulate the hypothalamic-pituitary-gonadal axis to prepare and maintain the bird for reproduction. Birds that are reproductively active due to the stimulating effects of long days are said to be photostimulated (Follett, 1984; Nicholls *et al.*, 1988b). A second effect of long days is to initiate an inhibitory process that results in the regression of the hypothalamic-pituitary-gonadal axis. This inhibitory process has been well documented in many temperate-zone songbird species such as the European starling, tree sparrow, and white-crowned

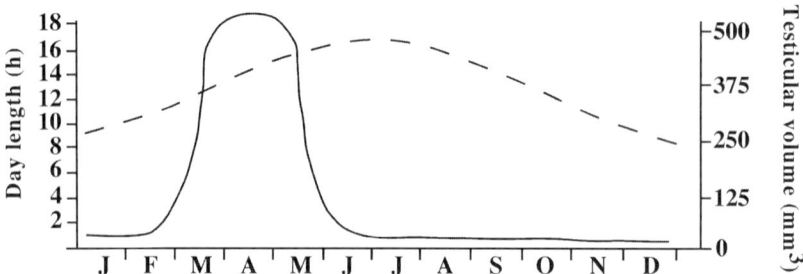

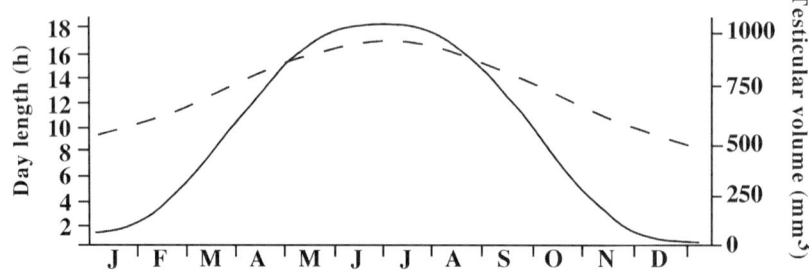

FIGURE 1 (A) Changes in testicular volume in European starlings throughout the annual cycle (solid line) and change in day length (dashed line) at 52°N. Note that in this species gonadal regression occurs while day lengths are still increasing, leading to an asymmetry in the breeding cycle relative to the changing photoperiod. (B) Changes in testicular volume characteristic of Japanese quail or wood pigeons at 52°N. Unlike starlings, the cycle is symmetrical and the gonads change in size in proportion to the ambient day length all year round.

he photoperiodic response in birds involves an
ogenous component (Gwinner, 1986). In many
ies, when maintained under conditions of con-
t photoperiod (e.g., 12L:12D) and temperature,
es of gonadal maturation and regression followed
eather molt can be observed for years (Gwinner,
, 1996). This phenomenon seems to be especially
alent in tropical species, but has also been ob-
d in temperate-zone species (e.g., Gwinner and
uerlein, 1999). For this reason, it has been hy-
esized that one mechanism by which photoperiod
ates seasonal breeding is through the entrainment
endogenous circannual rhythm (Gwinner, 1986,
). The exact nature of these endogenous seasonal
ms regulating seasonal reproduction remains to
icidated. In one particularly good test of the ex-
e of a circannual rhythm, dark-eyed juncos were
ained in conditions of constant dim light (rather
a constant photoperiod of some sort) and a per-
t rhythmicity of gonadal growth, regression, and
vas observed (Holberton and Able, 1992). How-
he period of this rhythm varied widely from 6 to
nths. Therefore this endogenous regulation of re-
ction may not involve a true circannual rhythm
analogous to circadian rhythms but rather a long-
ndogenous mechanism of a different sort.

v Is Variation in Day Length Measured?

length is measured in birds (as well as in mam-
vith the use of a circadian clock. For many years,
hypothesized that birds employed an hourglass
measure day length (see Farner, 1964, for a dis-
). The notion was that some sort of physiologi-
ess accumulated as a function of day length and
s was the way in which day length was encoded.
d by experiments completed on plants and other
ms (Bünning, 1960), Hamner (1963), based on
of house finches, demonstrated definitively that
ploy a circadian rhythm to complete this mea-
nt. The time of light onset entrains a circadian
of photoinducibility that in general occurs early
bjective night, and if a second period of light
dent with the photoinducible phase in the cir-
ycle the bird responds as if it has experienced a
Several types of experiments demonstrate that
hanism mediates the measurement of photope-
seasonal context (Follett, 1984). One of the

most convincing demonstrations was made by Ha[r]
and Enright (1967), who presented 6 hours of light
were either in phase or out of phase with the circa
cycle of photoinducibility in house finches. It was
from these studies that the amount of light experie[nced]
by the bird does not predict whether it exhibits a [long]
day-like response. Rather, the timing of the light p[ulse]
during the circadian phase is the critical factor pre[dict]
ing how the birds respond to the light.

B. Influence of Nonphotoperiodic Cu[es] on the Timing of Breeding

As discussed previously, in order to successfully
breeding birds must integrate an initial predictiv[e cue]
such as photoperiod with other types of cues tha[t pro]
vide them with information about local variations
environment that results from year-to-year fluctu[ations]
in weather conditions or in the geography, such a[s food]
availability and social interactions. The extent to
a given species or population integrates supplem[entary]
cues with an initial predictive cue such as photo[period]
is related to the predictability of the environmen[t in re]
lation to breeding. If a future event such as the o[nset of]
breeding is highly predictable, then only a selec[t num]
ber of reliable cues are required to time breedi[ng, and]
many other cues can be ignored (Cohen, 1967).
timing of the onset of the breeding season is le[ss pre]
dictable, then many cues are integrated to optim[ize the]
timing of breeding (Wingfield et al., 1992). Thi[s theo]
retical orientation has proven to be very useful
interpretation of species variability in the imp[ortance]
of nonphotoperiodic cues.

The critical physiological decision made by a [breed]
ing pair of birds is the decision to oviposit, m[ade by]
the female. Therefore the importance of the inte[gration]
of initial predictive cues with supplementary
synchronizing cues from the physical and soci[al envi]
ronment is most apparent in females. Initial pr[edictive]
cues such as photoperiod can stimulate ovaria[n devel]
opment to a prebreeding stage (Wingfield and
1980). This stage is followed by an exponentia[l growth]
stage that includes the synthesis and depos[ition of]
yolk that only occurs if the local conditions are
(e.g., Farner et al., 1966; Cheng, 1974; Johnson
Wild-caught females who are brought into cap[tivity of]
ten do not develop beyond the prebreeding sta[ge]

temperature in great tits on the photoinduction of gonadal growth, but a facilitating effect of warm temperatures in willow tits. There were, however, positive effects of warm temperatures on LH secretion (Silverin and Viebke, 1994) in great tits. In certain populations of Japanese quail (*Coturnix japonica*), decreases in temperature as well as decreases in photoperiod are required for the regression of various measures of reproductive physiology to be observed (e.g., Wada, 1993). In any case, temperature variation is clearly an important supplementary factor influencing the timing of laying under natural conditions in many species. In European starlings, a 10-year study of a naturally breeding population in southern Germany found a clear correlation between the initiation of breeding and the minimum temperature just prior to the initiation of egg-laying (Meijer et al., 1999). Furthermore, the manipulation of temperature in nest boxes during the night when females were sleeping in the boxes just prior to the egg-laying period could advance or retard the day of oviposition by 7–10 days.

As discussed previously, food is an important ultimate factor influencing the timing of reproduction, but generally is not thought to be a proximate cue. Stimuli such as photoperiod allow birds to predict the future amelioration of the environment and the concomitant increase in food. It has been hypothesized, after the initial observation about birds being long-day breeders, that gonadal growth ensued because the birds had more opportunities to feed in the presence of long photoperiods. However, careful experiments such as those conducted on starlings by Dawson (1986), which have restricted food intake to only a few hours per day, have clearly demonstrated that this hypothesis is false. Therefore, food itself is not generally thought to be a cue that directly stimulates reproductive development. This is not to say that food intake is irrelevant. The nutritional condition of the female can influence the timing of egg-laying, as supplementary feeding studies clearly indicate (Meijer et al., 1988). However, in these cases the presence of food per se does not seem to stimulate endocrine development but rather the energetic consequences of food intake are important. There are some interesting exceptions to this generalization. The neotropical spotted antbird is insectivorous and its insect prey increases in association with the onset of the rainy season. There is extensive year-to-year variation in the timing of the rainy season, making variation in photoperiod a poor predictor of the availability of food abundance. In these antbirds, the presentation of live crickets directly stimulates gonadal growth and singing behavior (Hau et al., 2000). This was not a nutritional effect because control animals received sufficient nutrients for gonadal growth. Song stimulation occurred even when the birds could see the crickets but not capture and handle them. Thus, in some species the actual perception of food can stimulate the reproductive neuroendocrine system (Hau et al., 2000).

C. Effects of Social Interactions on Reproductive Physiology

1. Effects of Male Behavior on Female Reproductive Physiology

One of the most important aspects of local conditions that needs to be met is for the female to have a mate and a nest site. Therefore, it is not surprising that the courtship behavior of males can exert a strong effect on the endocrine physiology of females. The investigation of the effects of male courtship behaviors on reproductive development in female birds has a relatively long history in the field of behavioral endocrinology. Pioneering studies were conducted by Polikarpova (1940) on house sparrows (*Passer domesticus*) and Burger (1942) on European starlings, both indicating that the presence of a male enhanced the seasonal development of the female reproductive system. In the 1960s, experimental programs investigating the social enhancement of female reproductive physiology were conducted by Brockway in female budgerigars (Brockway, 1969a), Hinde in canaries (Hinde, 1965), and by Lehrman and colleagues in female ring doves (Lehrman, 1960). In budgerigars, playbacks of the warbling vocalizations to females stimulates ovarian growth. Furthermore, certain components of the warble are more effective than others in stimulating this growth (Brockway, 1969a). Similarly, Lehrman and colleagues demonstrated that the presence of a female and other stimuli related to reproduction can enhance egg-laying in female ring doves (Lehrman et al., 1961). A series of experiments conducted over a 30-year period since this initial observation have dissected the stimulus conditions that facilitate this effect of male doves on female doves. It is worth covering these in some detail because of their experimental rigor. First, it was shown that the male had to engage in specific behaviors to stimulate ovulation. The castration of males eliminated male-typical displays such as the bow-coo, and females paired with such males had significantly smaller oviducts (a structure whose size is dependent on estrogen action) and were much less apt to lay eggs than females housed with an intact normally behaving male dove (Erickson and Lehrman, 1964). This response is dependent primarily on both auditory and visual cues emanating from the displaying male. Providing females with some combination of visual and auditory access to conspecifics works the best in enhancing endocrine activity (Lott and Brody, 1966), although providing or depriving female doves of information from only one modality can also influence various aspects of endocrine physiology (Lehrman and Friedman, 1969; Nottebohm and Nottebohm, 1971). The complexity of the social interaction between a male and a female that can influence endocrine activity was illustrated in an experiment that allowed six females to observe a single courting male simultaneously (Friedman, 1977). The cage was arranged so that in one case the male and female could see one another and in another case the female could see and hear the male but he could not see her. Two other variants were that the female could hear the male but see only reflections of the male in a direction perpendicular to the origin of the sound or that she could just hear the male but was visually isolated from conspecifics. A female dove exposed to a courting male, who is directing his behavior toward her, exhibits an enhanced endocrine response as measured by ovulation and follicle size compared to a female who sees the same male but from a view that indicates that he is not directing his courtship toward that specific female. Females who could see their own reflection and hear the male had the next highest level of stimulation and finally the females who heard the sound only had the lowest level of ovarian development (Friedman, 1977). These studies demonstrate that the neuroendocrine response to social stimuli is not a simple gating mechanism mediated by a simple stimulus–response relationship. Rather, females are making complex interpretations of male stimuli that then form the basis for the modification of the reproductive endocrine physiology. This is a complex interplay in which the female actively assesses the male but the male's response to the female also influences her behavior. Male doves respond aggressively to females whose behavior shows that they are advanced toward ovulation and slow them down, presumably to insure that they father the young (Erickson and Zenone, 1976; Zenone et al., 1979; Erickson, 1985).

Cheng (1986, 1992) has shown that in female ring doves the endocrine response to male courtship is the result of the female behaviorally stimulating herself by nest-cooing. If the female is devocalized and unable to nest-coo, her ovarian growth is attenuated relative to intact females that are able to coo. Playbacks of the female's vocalizations reinstates this ovarian growth. There is a direct relationship between this acoustic stimulation and LH release (Cheng et al., 1998). Interestingly, Cheng et al. (1998) hypothesize that this increase in LH secretion results from the release of an inhibition of hypothalamic gonadotropin-releasing-hormone neurons that regulate the pituitary gland rather than a direct stimulation of these cells. In any case, a further complication in our understanding of the behavioral effects on reproductive physiology is that females can fine-tune their physiological responses to males by modifying their own behavior.

In addition to the experimental work on ring doves and budgerigars, there is a large literature based both on laboratory studies and on field studies concerning the effects of male behavior on reproductive physiology in female songbirds. Much of the literature concerning field studies of behavioral interactions and female physiology are reviewed by Wingfield and Silverin (Chapt. 31 of this volume). We therefore focus on laboratory studies and some field experiments that elucidate the features of male behavior that stimulate female reproductive physiology. As mentioned previously, some of the earliest studies of the effects of males on females were conducted in songbirds (Polikarpova, 1940; Burger, 1942; Warren and Hinde, 1961). Because of the obvious salience of male courtship song in songbirds and the general interest in the function of these vocalizations, studies of the effects of male behavior on female songbirds often focused on the role played by male song. In several songbird species, most notably canaries and white-crowned sparrows (*Zonotrichia leucophrys gambelii*), male song has been shown to stimulate various aspects of endocrine development in conspecific females (Kroodsma, 1976; Hinde and Steel, 1978;

Morton *et al.*, 1985). Such specific effects of vocalizations are not limited to songbirds; in quail, Guyomarc'h and Guyomarc'h (1982) have also demonstrated that ovarian development in females can be stimulated by exposure to male vocalizations. One of the challenges of assessing the effects of song on reproductive development is establishing the stimulus specificity of conspecific song as opposed to heterospecific song or other organized sounds (Kroodsma and Byers, 1991). A comparison of the stimulatory effects on follicle growth, LH secretion and egg-laying in female canaries of the playback of male canary song, zebra finch song, and no song found that canary song was the most effective, but that zebra finch song also significantly enhanced follicle size and oviposition more than hearing no song at all (Fig. 2). Thus, females hearing heterospecific song had a state of ovarian development intermediate between females hearing conspecific song and no song at all (Bentley *et al.*, 2000). This suggests that the stimulus filter necessary to exhibit an endocrine response to song is not as tight as the one necessary to exhibit behavioral responses to song. This is consistent with some previous studies in canaries that found that certain parts of canary song were particularly important for females to exhibit copulation solicitation displays (Kreutzer and Vallet, 1991), but these same aspects of song did not enhance measures of endocrine activity such as egg-laying and nest-building (Leboucher *et al.*, 1998a). It is also possible that the playback of songs to isolated females presents the stimuli so out of context that females have a much lower threshold to respond to male-typical song. In zebra finches, male song enhances endocrine physiology and stimulates egg-laying in females if it is coupled with artificial models of the male (Tchernichovski *et al.*, 1998). Song playback in the absence of visual cues is not effective in finches. Even the placement of the male model from which song emanated could influence female responses. These data along with the study on doves by Friedman (1977) point to the complex processing that is made by females when responding to the various behavioral stimuli produced by the male.

2. Interaction between Photoperiod and the Effects of Social Stimuli from Male Birds on Female Reproductive Development

Sparrows and canaries exhibit tighter breeding seasons than ring doves, and their endocrine physiology is highly regulated by photoperiod. Therefore, the effects of males on females has been tested more in the context of the photoperiodically regulated reproductive cycle. For example, both Morton *et al.* (1985) and Hinde and Steel (1978) observed that song was not effective in enhancing reproductive development under all photoperiodic conditions. In the case of Gambel's white-crowned sparrows, there seems to be a photoperiodic threshold effect. Song played back to females in photoperiods of 11L:13D or 6L:18D did not enhance ovarian growth, but it did enhance ovarian growth in females in photoperiods of 12.5L:11.5D and 14L:10D (Morton *et al.*, 1985). In the case of canaries, playing back tape-recorded male song to female canaries in a photoperiod of 11L:13D significantly increased follicular growth and circulating levels of LH compared to females in 11L:13D who did not hear male song (Hinde and Steel, 1978). Females in photoperiods of 14L:10D did not exhibit enhanced reproductive development by exposure to song. Hinde and Steel (1978) suggested that this happened because a photoperiod of 14L:10D stimulated the reproductive system to a maximal extent and supplementary cues such as song could not stimulate it further.

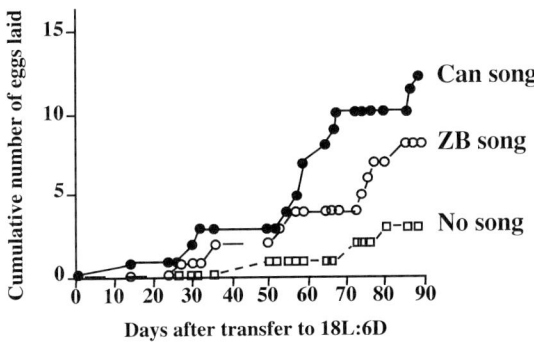

FIGURE 2 Graph of the total number of eggs laid by female canaries over time by three experimental groups that were housed individually and heard three different song types: male canary song (Can song), male zebra finch song (ZB song), or no song (No song), while maintained in a photoperiod of 11L:13D. They were then transferred to 18L:6D and the egg-laying rate was assessed. Each day marked with a data point denotes that at least one egg was laid in at least one of the groups. Note that the group exposed to conspecific song laid more eggs and began laying sooner than the group exposed to heterospecific song, which in turn laid more eggs and began laying sooner than the group exposed to no song. From Bentley *et al.* (2000).

Such interactions between photoperiod and male stimulation are also apparent in doves and quail, which exhibit annual cycles symmetrical around the summer solstice, as illustrated in Fig. 1. In most studies of ring doves, photoperiod was usually held constant at 14L:10D. All the effects of behavioral interactions were superimposed on this photoperiodic stimulation. Lehrman (1965) was well aware of this fact. Indeed, it is clear in doves that females can be stimulated to ovulate in 20 weeks when transferred to long days, but ovulation occurred after approximately 2 weeks in the same period when the females were paired with males (Cheng, 1976).

3. Effects of Female Behavior on Male Physiology

Just as males can clearly have important influences on female physiology, the reverse is also true. Pioneering studies were conducted on European starlings (Burger, 1953), in which it was shown that gonadal recrudescence in male starlings was greatly enhanced if they were placed with a female. Subsequently, it was demonstrated that several aspects of the photoperiodic response in males could be modified by females. Male starlings maintained in a photoperiod of 12L:12D exhibit annual rhythms in the growth and regression of their gonads (Gwinner, 1986). When such males are housed with females, there are differences in the timing of these cycles compared to males housed alone (Gwinner, 1975). Similarly, the timing of gonadal regression in starlings being held in long photoperiods is delayed in males housed with females compared to males housed alone (Schwab and Lott, 1969). Similar findings have been described in Gambel's white-crowned sparrows. Males photostimulated in the laboratory with long days in the presence of sexually active females (treated with exogenous estradiol, E_2) exhibited higher levels of testosterone and LH than males housed in the same photoperiod alone (Moore, 1983; Wingfield and Moore, 1987). Similarly, when the mates of free-living male sparrows received exogenous E_2 via implants that maintained high levels of female-typical behaviors, male testosterone and LH levels, which declined at the onset of female incubation in control pairs, were maintained. This is despite the fact that the females treated with E_2 did initiate incubation—they just continued to engage in sexual displays and stimulated the male. This finding suggests that the decline in male hormone levels at the onset of female incubation is a function of the decline in female sexual displays rather than a response to the onset of female incubation behavior. Maintaining high levels of female sexual displays by exogenous estrogen treatment also delays the termination of breeding in male song sparrows (Runfeldt and Wingfield, 1985). Female song sparrows were administered E_2 at the beginning of the period when they start feeding their young. This maintained high levels of sexual behavior for an additional 1–2 months compared to control females. Their untreated mates also maintained high levels of testosterone and continued defending territory compared to their counterparts mated to control females. These males had gone photorefractory and stopped breeding. Thus, maintaining the female in a high reproductive state modifies the onset of refractoriness in male sparrows. The converse experiment of manipulating male sexual activity to maintain the female reproductive system had no effect (Runfeldt and Wingfield, 1985).

Experimental analysis of the sensory bases of the effects of females on male endocrine physiology have been conducted in ring doves. Male doves exhibit a rise in testosterone within 4 hours when paired with a female (O'Connell et al., 1981a). This rise is attenuated if the male is paired with an ovariectomized female who does not exhibit sexual displays (O'Connell et al., 1981a). Also, if the male is deafened he does not exhibit a rise in testosterone and his hormonal levels are close to those of isolated males. Finally, males separated from females by a clear panel so that they could see and hear the female but could not have tactile interactions with her had hormone levels similar to those of males who could interact with the female (O'Connell et al., 1981a). Similar to the pattern described for sparrows, in male doves testosterone declines at the onset of incubation. This was also found to be a response to behavioral changes by the female. If the nests were experimentally destroyed and this inhibited the females from making the transition to incubation, male androgen levels failed to decline (O'Connell et al., 1981b). If males paired with sexually active females are switched to mates who incubate, their testosterone levels decline; but if they are switched to mates who are still courting, their testosterone levels are maintained at high levels. These results are quite consistent with the scenario proposed for sparrows—when female doves stop displaying to male doves testosterone levels decline.

Photoperiodic stimuli also can influence the effects of females on male endocrine physiology. In male doves that are hemicastrated, the presence of the female can influence compensatory hypertrophy. However, this was only apparent when males were housed in a 8L:16D photoperiod. Males housed in longer period exhibited no effects of the female (Cheng, 1974, 1976). In quail, exposing mature males in long days to females did not increase their tesotsterone levels (Delville et al., 1984b). However, exposing male during development to females did enhance reproductive maturation, but this effect was more pronounced in male housed in 12L:12D than in males housed in 16L:8D (Delville et al., 1984b).

III. ANATOMY OF THE REPRODUCTIVE NEUROENDOCRINE SYSTEM IN BIRDS

In this section, we review the basics of the chemical neuroanatomy that are relevant to the avian neuroendocrine system. We focus on a key neuropeptide, gonadotropin-releasing hormone (GnRH), which plays an important role in mediating the transduction of environmental information into changes in endocrine physiology and on the brain sites where receptors for sex steroid hormones and their associated metabolizing enzymes are present. These hormones are important regulators of reproductive behaviors. A special emphasis is placed on aspects of these systems that are unique to birds.

A. Gonadotropin-Releasing Hormone I and II Neuronal Systems

1. Structure

GnRH, the neuropeptide regulating gonadotropin secretion, was first isolated and characterized in mammalian species in the early 1970s (Amoss et al., 1971; Schally et al., 1971). The mammalian form of this releasing hormone was found to consist of a 10-residue amino acid sequence (this form is often referred to as mGnRH). Subsequent to this discovery, immunohistochemical studies in several avian species employing antibodies directed against the mammalian peptide sequence localized groups of immunoreactive cells in the diencephalon that project to the median eminence (Calas et al., 1973; Sharp et al., 1975; McNeil et al., 1976; Bons et al., 1978; Jozsa and Mess, 1982; Sterling and Sharp, 1982; Weindl and Sofroniew, 1982; Mikami et al., 1988). Peripheral injections of the mammalian peptide sequence confirmed that it was a potent releaser of both LH and follicle-stimulating hormone (FSH) in avian species (Bonney et al., 1974; Balthazart et al., 1980c; Godden et al., 1977; Wingfield et al., 1979; Storey and Nicholls, 1983). In the early 1980s GnRH was purified from chicken (*Gallus domesticus*) pituitaries and the structure characterized as varying from the mammalian form at residue 8, where glutamine is substituted for arginine (see Millar and King, 1984, for a review of these initial studies). At this time, a second form of GnRH was found in the chicken brain by Miyamoto and colleagues (1984). This form differed from the mammalian form by three amino acid substitutions. These two forms were then named chicken GnRH-I (cGnRH-I) and chicken GnRH-II (cGnRH-II). The primary structure cGnRH-I is thus $[Gln^8]mGnRH$ and the primary structure of cGnRH-II is $[His^5, Trp^7, Tyr^8]mGnRH$. Both these forms of GnRH have been found to be effective releasers of the gonadotropins LH and FSH *in vivo* (Hattori et al., 1986; Millar et al., 1986; Sharp et al., 1990a,b; Wingfield and Farner, 1993).

The presence of these two forms in the avian brain is not restricted to gallinaceous birds. For example, both forms of GnRH are apparently present in European starlings (*Sturnus vulgaris*), a species that is a member of the most recently evolved avian taxon, the Order Passeriformes (Sherwood et al., 1988). Extracts containing GnRH from the starling brain exhibited molecular heterogeneity and appeared to contain equal amounts of peptides similar in form to both cGnRH-I and cGnRH-II based on the high-performance liquid chromatography (HPLC) elution pattern and cross-reactivity with four different antisera (Sherwood et al., 1988). There was no evidence that the starling brain contains a form of GnRH that could be identified as mammalian, salmon, or lamprey. There may be species variability in the relative distribution of these peptides. Sherwood et al. (1988) found evidence for the presence of a peptide similar to cGnRH-I in the brain of another passerine species, the song sparrow (*Melospiza melodia melodia*), but they did not find evidence for cGnRH-II or any other form of GnRH in the brains of this species. The primary structure of these two peptides has yet to be determined in any avian species outside the order galliformes, so it is not known definitively if the exact forms of cGnRH-I and cGnRH-II are conserved throughout the avian class.

2. Distribution

The initial immunohistochemical studies of the distribution of GnRH immunoreactive cells and fibers in avian species completed in the 1970s and early 1980s used antisera raised against mGnRH and identified immunoreactive fibers in the median eminence and perikarya in the preoptic region, septum, and anterior hypothalamus (see Mikami, 1986, for a review). This septo-preoptic-infundibular GnRH pathway is characteristic of essentially all vertebrate species studied (Silverman et al., 1994) and has been described in all subsequent immunohistochemical studies of GnRH in birds (R. Foster et al., 1987; R. G. Foster et al., 1988; Mikami et al., 1988; Kuenzel and Blähser, 1991; Silver et al., 1992; Millam et al., 1993; Van Gils et al., 1993). The general distribution of these cells in birds is as follows. Cells extend from the preoptic area caudodorsally to the lateral septum. These perikarya send fibers to all zones of the anterior and posterior median eminence. The median eminence is supplied principally by two fiber bundles. The first bundle seems to originate from the more anterior perikarya, primarily in the preoptic area, and runs between the supraoptic decussation and the wall of the ventricle before entering the median eminence. The second bundle projects caudoventrally from the more dorsal GnRH cells in a relatively loose network throughout the infundibular regions before entering the median eminence. Some of the early avian studies of GnRH also suggested that there were GnRH-positive cells in the dorsal infundibular nucleus of certain species, such as mallard ducks *Anas platyrhynchos* (McNeil et al., 1976) and chickens (Hoffman et al., 1978; see Mikami, 1986, for a review). However, subsequent studies in ducks (Bons et al., 1978) and chickens have not detected immunoreactive perikarya in the dorsal infundibulum (Sterling and Sharp, 1982; Kuenzel and Blähser, 1991). There do seem to be genuine species differences, however, because a study of great tits reported immunoreactive cells in this region also (Silver et al., 1992).

In addition to the well-described septo-preoptic-infundibular GnRH pathway, cells and fibers immunoreactive for GnRH have been described in other parts of the brain. For example, perikarya have been found in the olfactory bulb, olfactory tubercle, parolfactory lobe (the anatomical homolog of the mammalian caudate nucleus), and the nucleus accumbens in the telencephalon and in the oculomotor complex in the mesencephalon—for example, European starlings (Foster et al., 1987), chicks (Hoffman et al., 1978), ring doves, (Silver et al., 1992), and great tits (Silver et al., 1992). Fibers have been described that terminate on the wall of the ventricle or in the capillary zone of the organum vasculosum of the lamina terminalis. Fibers have also been observed that terminate in the pituitary stalk (Blähser et al., 1986; Foster et al., 1987). Birds possess a terminal nerve (cranial nerve 0) and studies of pigeons (*Columba livia*) have revealed that this nerve contains GnRH immunoreactivity, as has been reported in other vertebrate species (Norgren et al., 1991). It has been hypothesized that both the terminal nerve and GnRH neurons are derived from the same embryological source, the olfactory placode (Muske and Moore, 1988). Studies of the development of the GnRH system are consistent with the notion that the GnRH immunoreactive neurons in the forebrain develop from the olfactory placode (Norgren and Lehman, 1991). Thus, perikarya containing GnRH in the terminal nerve may represent cells that originated in the olfactory epithelium and failed to finish their migration into the brain (Norgren et al., 1991).

Only a few studies have used antisera specific to cGnRH-I or cGnRH-II (Mikami et al., 1988; Millam et al., 1993; Van Gils et al., 1993). Immunohistochemical studies by Mikami et al. (1988) on chickens and quail revealed that terminals in the median eminence were strongly immunoreactive with antisera raised against cGnRH-I but not cGnRH-II. The primary group of perikarya that exhibits immunoreactivity for cGnRH-II is located in the mesencephalon in the oculomotor region, an area not known to project to the median eminence (Mikami et al., 1988). Studies in turkey hens (*Meleagris gallopavo*) revealed a large group of cells immunoreactive for cGnRH II in the midbrain in the oculomotor region (Millam et al., 1993). These authors also detected cells expressing cGnRH-II immunoreactivity in the lateral hypothalamus. Although they found a complex distribution of fibers immunoreactive for cGnRH-II in the telencephalon and diencephalon, they did not observe cGnRH-II immunoreactivity in the median eminence. The mRNA for the precursor protein of cGnRH-I, prepro-GnRH, has been localized in the turkey hen brain by *in situ* hybridization (Ball *et al.*, 1995). The distribution of cells expressing this mRNA is in excellent agreement with the cells identified as containing immunoreactive cGnRH-I but not cGnRH-II. Van Gils *et al.* (1993) designed antisera that recognize synthetic peptides derived from parts of the cGnRH-I and cGnRH-II sequence that demonstrate complete dissimilarity from each other. With these antisera, they also found cells expressing cGnRH-II immunoreactivity only in the midbrain in the oculomotor region of chickens and quail. Unlike the other studies mentioned, however, immunoreactive cGnRH-II fibers were detected in the median eminence, primarily in the external layer. This immunoreactivity was less prominent than that detected for cGnRH-I, but it nonetheless was significant. The GnRH-II in the median eminence was shown to be located in fibers that are different from the GnRH-I immunoreactive fibers. The presence of detectable levels of GnRH-I and -II in the median eminence was confirmed by HPLC combined with radioimmunoassays of separate chromatography fractions (D'Hondt, 2000). To exclude definitively possible artefacts that could be due to cross-reactions with GnRH-I of the antibody used to recognize GnRH-II, further confirmation of the presence of GnRH-II in the median eminence was obtained by mass spectrometry. The GnRH-II contained in the peptides extracted from the median eminence of 50 quail was first purified by affinity chromatography with the anti-GnRH-II antibody that had itself been first purified by affinity chromatography on a column containing immobilized synthetic GnRH-II. The purified fraction was then deposited into a glass capillary that was fitted to the nano-electrospray source of a Q-Tof mass spectrometer and a mass-spectrometry survey spectrum was acquired. This revealed the presence of a single peptide in the extract, and sequence analysis confirmed that this peptide is GnRH-II (D'Hondt, 2000). The presence of GnRH-II in the quail median eminence is therefore firmly established by these experiments, even if the origin of the discrepancies between the results of these and other studies remains unclear. In addition to these studies in gallinaceous birds, one study of cGnRH-II immunoreactivity in European starlings (Ball *et al.*, 1992) and another study in turkeys (Millam *et al.*, 1993) failed to find immunoreactive fibers in the median eminence.

An additional small group of cells immunoreactive for the serum against GnRH-II was detected in the infundibular region of chicken (D'Hondt, 2000). Lesions of this cell groups resulted in the disappearance of the GnRH-II immunoreactivity in the median eminence and, in addition, tract-tracing studies with dioctadecyl-tetramethyl-indocarbocyanine (DiI) indicated that neurons located at the same position as these GnRH-II neurons send projections to the median eminence (D'Hondt, 2000). This strongly suggests that the GnRH-II immunoreactive fibers identified in the median eminence originate in this new group of GnRH-II neurons located in the tuberal hypothalamus. This would explain why no projection from the mesencephalic GnRH-II cell group to the median eminence could be detected in previous tract-tracing studies.

The role of GnRH-II in the median eminence remains, however, unclear. Based on the anatomical studies reviewed, it seems most likely that the primary form of GnRH regulating reproduction is cGnRH-I. Several other lines of evidence also suggest that only cGnRH-I normally regulates pituitary function, even though cGnRH-II and cGnRH-I are potent in releasing LH and FSH from the pituitary when administered exogenously (Sharp *et al.*, 1990a,b; Wingfield and Farner, 1993). As discussed by Sharp *et al.* (1990a,b) in chickens, the brain content of cGnRH-I correlates well with reproductive status, but the brain content of cGnRH-II does not. This research group also found that active immunization against cGnRH-I, but not cGnRH-II, results in a loss of reproductive function, further suggesting that cGnRH-II is not released from the brain into the portal blood to control anterior pituitary activity. From these data it seems probable that the active form of GnRH in birds for the regulation of anterior pituitary function is cGnRH-I. In contrast to these studies, in turkey hens it was found that cGnRH-I and cGnRH-II content in the preoptic region and the hypothalamus as measured by radioimmunoassay increases after photostimulation and decreases during incubation and the subsequent onset of refractoriness (Rozenboim *et al.*, 1993). These changes in cGnRH-II over the reproductive cycle are consistent with a possible role of this peptide in the regulation of seasonal breeding. Another study in turkey hens also found that the brain levels of cGnRH-II change over the reproductive cycle, but that the highest levels in the hypothalamus were during the incubation period when the ovaries are regressed and plasma levels of LH are low (Millam et al., 1989). Overall, the function of cGnRH-II in birds remains unknown, but the studies by Van Gils et al. (1993) and Rozenboim et al. (1993) have reopened the possibility that cGnRH II may play some role in the regulation of reproductive events.

It must also be mentioned that in addition of the hypophyseal tract of GnRH-I fibers already discussed, a broad distribution of fibers immunoreactive for GnRH-I and, more important, for GnRH-II can be observed in wide areas of the avian brain including large parts of the telencephalon. This widespread distribution of GnRH-II was taken an indication of its role as a neurotransmitter (Katz et al., 1990), and it has been suggested that GnRH-I could be the prime regulator of gonadotropin release from the pituitary, whereas GnRH-II might have a neurotransmitter or neuromodulator role in brain areas outside the median eminence. The specific function of this widespread innervation is, however, not entirely clear; it appears likely that some of these fibers may be related to the behavioral effects of GnRH that are described later in this chapter.

B. Distribution of Sex Steroid Hormone Receptors

1. Androgen Receptors

The distribution of androgen receptors (AR) was originally studied in the avian brain by *in vivo* autoradiography with the use of tritiated testosterone as a ligand. However, because this steroid is readily converted in many parts of the brain to a variety of other steroids including estrogens (Balthazart, 1989), the binding sites described in these studies are likely to include estrogen receptors (ER) as well as AR. In a few selected cases, autoradiography was also carried out with tritiated 5α-dihydrotestosterone. Given that this compound cannot be aromatized into an estrogen, its localization provides in theory a more specific visualization of the AR. Unfortunately, 5α-dihydrotestosterone is rapidly metabolized in birds (Deviche et al., 1987), and this markedly limits its use as a ligand for *in vivo* autoradiography. Immunocytochemistry and *in situ* hybridization have also been used in a selected number of cases to confirm that the binding sites identified by autoradiography correspond to true receptors as identified by their protein or the corresponding mRNA.

In general, it appears that the distribution of AR in birds is restricted to the septal-preoptic area and to various nuclei in the hypothalamus and in the midbrain (Balthazart, 1983; Ball, 1990; Brenowitz, 1991). This corresponds to the common pattern that has been previously described in all vertebrate classes (Morrell et al., 1975; Pfaff, 1976; Stumpf and Sar, 1978).

In addition to the receptors located in these brain areas that seem to be present in all bird (and vertebrate) species, members of the suborder passeres (songbirds) possess androgen-sensitive brain areas that are part of the telencephalic network of sexually dimorphic nuclei that mediate the production and acquisition of male song (Arnold et al., 1976; Nottebohm and Arnold, 1976; Nottebohm, 1980; Konishi, 1985; Nottebohm et al., 1990). The high vocal center (HVc; previously misnamed caudal part of the ventral hyperstriatum), the robust nucleus of the archistriatum (RA), and the magnocelluar nucleus of the anterior neostriatum (MAN) appear to contain AR, based on both autoradiographic (Zigmond et al., 1973; Arnold et al., 1976; Lücke and Haase, 1980; Gahr, 1990; Ball, 1990; Brenowitz, 1991) and binding-assay (Harding et al., 1984) methods. Most of these autoradiographic studies used [^{3}H]-testosterone ([^{3}H]-T) as the ligand and therefore potentially confounded the identification of AR and ER. A few studies have employed a nonaromatizable androgen such [^{3}H]-dihydrotestosterone ([^{3}H]-DHT) and have in this way confirmed that these telencephalic binding sites identified by testosterone autoradiography are specific for androgens (Arnold, 1979; Arnold and Saltiel, 1979; E. J. Nordeen et al., 1987; Watson and Adkins-Regan, 1989b; Sohrabji et al., 1989).

Antibodies to the AR have become available (Tan et al., 1988; Lubahn et al., 1988; Van Laar et al., 1989; Demura et al., 1989; Marivoet et al., 1990; Chang et al., 1988; Husmann et al., 1990). They have been used to identify, in mammals, by immunocytochemistry (ICC) the AR in peripheral androgen target structures (Tan et al., 1988; Lubahn et al., 1988; Van Laar et al., 1989; Demura et al., 1989; Chang et al., 1989; Takeda et al., 1990; Husmann and McPhaul, 1991) and in the rat brain (e.g., Sar et al., 1990). These antibodies have also been used in a few species of birds to describe the distribution of AR in the brain—quail (Balthazart et al., 1992d, 1998c) and songbirds (Balthazart et al., 1992d; Smith et al., 1996; Soma et al., 1999b).

Finally, the AR has also been cloned and sequenced in canaries (Nastiuk and Clayton, 1994; Gahr and Metzdorf, 1997) and starlings (Bernard et al., 1999). This information was then used to prepare specific probes that could be used for visualizing the distribution of the AR mRNA in the canary brain (Nastiuk and Clayton, 1995; Fusani et al., 2000; Metzdorf et al., 1999) and starling brain (Bernard et al., 1999).

Studies using these complementary methods have described a concordant pattern of distribution for androgen receptors (see Fig. 3). In all species that were investigated, the most intense uptake of tritiated androgens or immunoreactivity for the AR was observed in the mesencephalic nucleus intercollicularis (ICo). Many nuclei of the preoptic-area (POA)-hypothalamic-limbic system also contain a large number of labeled cells. These nuclei include the medial preoptic nucleus (POM), the paraventricular nucleus (PVN), the ventromedial nucleus (VMN), and the tuberal hypothalamus, especially in the region of the nucleus infundibuli (IN) and the nucleus inferior hypothalami (IH).

These descriptions of the AR distribution generally apply to all species that were investigated in detail and include the domestic chicken (Barfield et al., 1978), Japanese quail (Watson and Adkins-Regan, 1989b; Balthazart et al., 1992d, 1998c), ring dove (Martinez-Vargas et al., 1975, 1976; Kim et al., 1978), and several species of songbirds (Zigmond et al., 1973; Arnold et al., 1976; Lücke and Haase, 1980; Gahr, 1990; Balthazart et al., 1992d; Smith et al., 1996; Soma et al., 1999b; Ball, 1990; Brenowitz, 1991).

In the quail brain, Watson and Adkins-Regan (1989b) used autoradiography to compare the uptake of [^{3}H]-T and [^{3}H]-DHT in males and females. They observed labeled cells for [^{3}H]-T in all the areas we have listed where AR immunoreactive cells were later observed by immunocytochemistry (Balthazart et al., 1992d, 1998c). However, they did not detect labeled cells in all these areas after injection with [^{3}H]-DHT. The highest intensity of labeling for [^{3}H]-DHT was observed in ICo. A few labeled cells were also present in the PVN and lateral hypothalamus, but no labeled

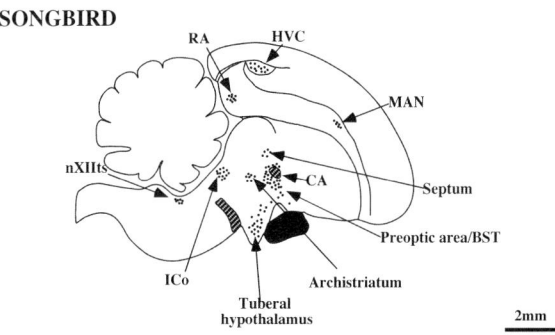

FIGURE 3 Schematic representation of the distribution of androgen receptors as observed by immunocytochemistry in the brain of the Japanese quail (nonsongbird) and of the zebra finch (songbird). Similar distributions have been observed by immunocytochemistry or in situ hybridization in a number of songbird and nonsongbird species. To permit immediate comparisons, all groups of cells expressing androgen receptors have been plotted on a slightly parasagittal section even if they are located more laterally. BST, nucleus striae terminalis; CA, commissura anterior; HVC, high vocal center (formely hyperstriatum ventralis, pars caudale); ICo, nucleus intercollicularis; MAN, nucleus anterioris magnocellularis; nXIIts, nucleus nervi hypoglossi, tracheosyringeal division; RA, nucleus robustus archistriatalis.

cells were observed in the POM, IH, or IN (which contain testosterone-binding sites and immunoreactive AR). Watson and Adkins-Regan (1989b) also saw a few cells accumulating [^{3}H]-DHT in the nucleus taeniae (Tn) and substantia grisea centralis (GCt).

The discrepancy between autoradiographic results obtained with tritiated T and DHT may relate in part to a difference in the specificity of the two methods—T autoradiography may also reveal estrogen-binding sites. However, the difference in sensitivity related to the high peripheral metabolism of DHT (Deviche et al., 1987) is likely to play a more important role in explaining the different results obtained by the two methods. This is the case because AR have been detected by immunocytochemistry in most brain areas that were binding tritiated T in autoradiographic studies and the discrepancies between T and DHT autoradiography occur mostly in areas where the signal for AR is low based either autoradiography or immunocytochemistry (see Balthazart et al., 1992d, for a more detailed discussion of these technical issues).

A limited number of additional discrepancies have been identified between studies that analyzed the distribution of AR in a given species by different methods. For example, Watson and Adkins-Regan (1989b) identified cells accumulating tritiated T and/or DHT in Tn and GCt, areas where no specific immunoreactivity for the AR could subsequently be detected with one antibody (Balthazart et al., 1992d), but were observed with another antibody raised against a different antigen (Balthazart et al., 1998b). AR immunoreactive (AR-ir) cells were observed by immunocytochemistry in the POA of zebra finches and canaries, but [^{3}H]-DHT uptake was never reported in the POA of any songbird species. [^{3}H]-T uptake was, however, reported in the POA of zebra finches (Arnold et al., 1976), bramblings (Lücke and Haase, 1980), and chaffinches (Zigmond et al., 1980), and high levels of AR were measured in the POA, PVN, and infundibulum of the zebra finch using the in vitro binding assay method (Harding et al., 1984). However as previously discussed, these limited discrepancies always occur in areas where AR appear to be relatively rare, and they are therefore likely to be explained by differences in the sensitivity (or sometimes specificity) of the detection methods.

The pattern of AR distribution in the POA-hypothalamic-limbic system (and ICo) of songbird species is similar to that described for the nonoscines, but major differences are observed in the telencephalon. Three nuclei, HVc, MAN, and RA, that are sexually dimorphic (Nottebohm and Arnold, 1976) and involved in the acquisition and production of birdsong (Nottebohm et al., 1976; Nottebohm, 1980) were found to either accumulate radioactive androgens based on autoradiographic studies (e.g., Arnold et al., 1976; Lücke and Haase, 1980; Zigmond et al., 1980) or contain AR-ir cells (e.g., Balthazart et al., 1992d; Smith et al., 1996; Soma et al., 1999b). The confirmation of the androgenic nature of these binding sites has been obtained by DHT autoradiography (Arnold and Saltiel, 1979; K. W. Nordeen et al., 1986; E. J. Nordeen et al., 1987; Sohrabji et al., 1989) and by in vitro binding assays with a nonaromatizable androgen (methyltrienolone) serving as the ligand (Harding et al., 1984) in the zebra finch. In these autoradiographic studies employing [^{3}H]-DHT as the ligand, AR were identified in three telencephalic song-control nuclei MAN, HVc, and RA (Arnold and Saltiel, 1979; K. W. Nordeen et al., 1986; E. J. Nordeen et al., 1987; Sohrabji et al., 1989). Similarly, the in vitro binding-assay method (Harding et al., 1984) found AR in HVc and RA (MAN was not investigated). Thus, these studies agree well with the previous finding based on testosterone autoradiography and with the immunocytochemical studies.

In the canary, HVc and MAN were also found to contain AR-ir cells. Weakly labeled cells containing AR-ir were, in addition, observed in canary RA and in a hook-like structure that is adjacent to RA and runs laterally and then ventrally (Balthazart et al., 1992d). This pattern has been previously described for RA when other neurochemical markers were used to define this nucleus. For example, Bottjer et al. (1989) observed a similar complex in and around RA in zebra finches when they defined the lateral MAN projection to RA by injecting the anterograde tracer horseradish peroxidase conjugated to wheat germ agglutinin. Similarly, Ball (1990, 1994) found that when RA is defined by autoradiographic procedures labeling α_2 adrenergic receptors, RA and the lateral structure both show a high receptor density for this receptor subtype. The precise relationship, either anatomical or functional, between this hook-like adjacent structure and RA is not understood.

RA provides inputs to medulary nuclei, the nucleus hypoglossus pars tracheosyringealis (syringeal motonucleus, nXIIts), the nucleus retroambigualis (RAm), and the rostroventral respiratory group (rVRG), which are thought to be present in all avian species (Mori and Striedter, 1992; Wild, 1997; Reinke and Wild, 1998). Interestingly, in songbirds these nuclei are also defined by the presence of AR (Gahr and Wild, 1997). No report has, however, to our knowldege mentioned the presence of AR in these nuclei in nonsongbirds, and there is actually evidence indicating that these receptors are not present in a diversity of species (Gahr, 2000). One exception to this rule has been reported—males of certain hummingbird species such as Anna's hummingbirds *(Calypte anna)* learn their song during postnatal development. Interestingly, these birds also possess a neural circuitry controling the learned vocalization that is largely similar (presumably analogous but not homologous because singing is supposed to have emerged independently in oscines and hummingbirds) to the song-control system of oscines. Several of these vocal nuclei in the Anna's hummingbird including nXIIts and the equivalents of the lateral MAN (lMAN) and HVc also express dense populations of AR-ir (Gahr, 2000).

As previously indicated, the results of *in situ* hybridization studies largely confirmed the distribution of the AR that had been identified by *in vivo* autoradiography or immunocytochemistry. The use of molecular biology has brought further support to the specificity of the previously identified signals. Northern blot analysis of mRNA extracted from the canary forebrain indicated the presence of a single low-abundance band between 8 and 10 kb in length, corresponding to the rat or human AR (Nastiuk and Clayton, 1994). Sequencing of the canary AR also confirmed the high degree of homology between this protein in birds and mammals.

In situ hybridization was also used to analyze the distribution of AR in the canary brain stem (Maney *et al.*, 2001). This study demonstrated the presence of significant levels of AR mRNA in several catecholaminergic nuclei, including the locus ceruleus, the substantia nigra, and the area ventralis of Tsai (homologous to the ventral tegmental area). AR mRNA had already been previously identified in the area ventralis of Tsai of canaries (Gahr and Metzdorf, 1997). The presence of AR both in the telencephalic song-control nuclei and in the catecholaminergic cell groups that are known to project to the song-control nuclei (Lewis *et al.*, 1981; Burd *et al.*, 1986; Appeltants *et al.*, 2000a) suggests that androgens could affect song learning and production both in a direct and in an indirect manner through the modulation of catecholaminergic inputs.

In summary, there is a large agreement among data obtained by binding assay, autoradiography, immunocytochemistry, and *in situ* hybridization even if limited discrepancies are observed in specific parts of the brain. These discrepancies presumably reflect differences in the sensitivity or specificity of the methods. A preferential identification of free vs occupied receptors by some methods could also contribute to the generation of these few differences (see Balthazart *et al.*, 1992d, for discussion). AR are localized in an anatomically discrete manner in the POA, hypothalamus, various parts of the limbic system, and ICo of all avian species that have been studied, that is, in areas that are homologous to brain regions where AR have been observed throughout vertebrates. In addition, a neurochemical specialization is detected in songbirds in which a few telencephalic nuclei involved in song learning and production also contain dense populations of AR-containing cells. The functional implications of this specialization are considered later.

2. Estrogen Receptors, α Subtype

A significant part of the behavioral effects of testosterone, in birds as in mammals, are produced at the cellular level by the action of estrogens produced by local aromatization of androgens. Estrogens play a critical role in the sexual differentiation and in the activation in adulthood of reproductive behavior. Estrogens also circulate in substantial amounts in the blood of females in most avian species and even in the blood of males in some species. Estrogens, act as transcription control factors after binding to specific receptors that have been shown to be distinct from AR in a number of model species. The distribution of ER has been investigated in a few avian species. As is the case for AR, several methods have been used for the studies—*in vivo* autoradiography, *in vitro* binding, immunocytochemistry, and, in a few cases, *in situ* hybridization.

At one time, a single ER was known to occur. However, in 1996, a new ER was cloned in rats (Kuiper *et al.*, 1996) and was rapidly shown to also occur in a variety of mammalian species (Mosselman *et al.*, 1996; Tremblay *et al.*, 1997). This second form of ER was called estrogen receptor β (ERβ) to distinguish it from the classic receptor that was then renamed ERα. ERβ has now been cloned in a few avian species and its distribution in the brain has been studied by *in situ* hybridization (Foidart *et al.*, 1999a; Bernard *et al.*, 1999; Ball *et al.*, 1999). These studies are summarized in a separate section. This section is specifically devoted to a review of studies that were performed before the second receptor was known and therefore concern the first identified form of receptor, ERα.

In vivo autroradiograhic studies originally identified the presence of estrogen-binding sites in a large number of limbic structures of the avian brain (e.g., Martinez-Vargas *et al.*, 1975, 1976; Kim *et al.*, 1978; Watson and Adkins-Regan, 1989b). The distribution of these regions is largely reminiscent of the distribution of AR. Similar to what has been observed for AR, ERα appear to be restricted to the hypothalamic and limbic structures, and to the mesencephalic ICo in non-songbirds; additional binding sites are found in telencephalic song-control nuclei of oscines (true songbirds; e.g., K. W. Nordeen *et al.*, 1987; Brenowitz and Arnold, 1989).

Immunocytochemical studies have confirmed and refined these general conclusions. Immunocytochemistry was first used to study the distribution of ERα in the brain of two songbird species, zebra finch and canary (Gahr *et al.*, 1987). This study used the monoclonal antibody H222SPγ raised against ERα purified from a human mammary tumor. As expected based on previous autoradiography data, in both species ERα-ir were observed in hypothalamic and limbic structures such as the PVM, nucleus medialis hypothalami posterioris (PMH), and Tn in the ICo, but also in the HVc of the canary and in adjacent telencephalic areas in both canaries and zebra finches.

The distribution of ERα was also analyzed in a nonsongbird brain, the Japanese quail, with the use of the same antibody (Balthazart *et al.*, 1989), and similar results were obtained except that in this species no label was detected in the telencephalon, with the exception of Tn. In particular, a high percentage of labeled cells was observed in the lateral septum, nucleus accumbens, preoptic medial nucleus, supraoptic nuclei, anterior medial hypothalamus, paraventricular magnocellular nucleus, caudal parts of the lateral hypothalamus, and whole tuberal and infundibular area. A small number of weakly labeled cells were also observed in the VMN. Although most of the positive cells were observed in the hypothalamus and POA, a few areas were also labeled in other parts of the brain. This was particularly the case for the Tn, ICo, and central gray. The distribution of labeled cells in this study closely matched the distribution of cells that accumulated radioactivity following the injection of tritiated E_2 in a previous study (Watson and Adkins-Regan, 1989b). The pattern of cells labeled by immunocytochemistry was also similar in males and females, and no evidence for a quantitative dimorphism in the percentage of labeled cells could be obtained. All nuclei containing cells labeled for ERα also contain significant levels of aromatase (with the exception of the ICo). The physiological significance of this coexistence is discussed later.

Similar studies have subsequently been carried out with the same antibody in many species ($n = 26$) belonging to a large number of avian orders, namely Anseriformes, Galliformes, Columbiformes, Psittaciformes, Apodiformes, and Passeriformes (17 species) (Gahr *et al.*, 1993). These data demonstrate that the distribution of ERα-ir cells in the diencephalic and limbic structures is very similar across all species that have been studied and resembles the distribution already described for the quail and canary. A total of 20 brain areas containing ERα-ir are considered in this study. A high degree of similarity is observed in general among species. All songbirds, however, display a telencephalic specialization in that they contain a significant number of cells that are intensely labeled by the antibody raised against ERα in three structures of the nonlimbic forebrain—the caudal neostriatum, including in some species the HVc; the dorsorostral area surrounding the RA; and an area in the rostral forebrain, dorsal to the lamina hyperstriatica and rostral to the nucleus magnocellularis anterioris. A fourth forebrain area, the hyperstriatum accessorium, also contained many ERα-ir cells in songbirds, but a few positive cells were also found in this location in the budgerigar (Gahr *et al.*, 1993) (see Fig. 4). In some species, changes in the microdistribution of ERα were observed in areas such as the hippocampus and anterior hypothalamus of suboscine species and in the POA of the Japanese quail. During the second half of the 1990s, molecular biology techniques were also used to clone the ERα in a few selected avian species, and the sequence information derived from theses studies was used to design probes that allowed a detailed analysis of the distribution of the mRNA encoding this receptor.

These *in situ* hybridization studies have largely confirmed the neuroanatomical distribution of ERα that had been established previously by autoradiographic and immunocytochemical methods (e.g., Jacobs *et al.*, 1996). Some differences were noted among the studies.

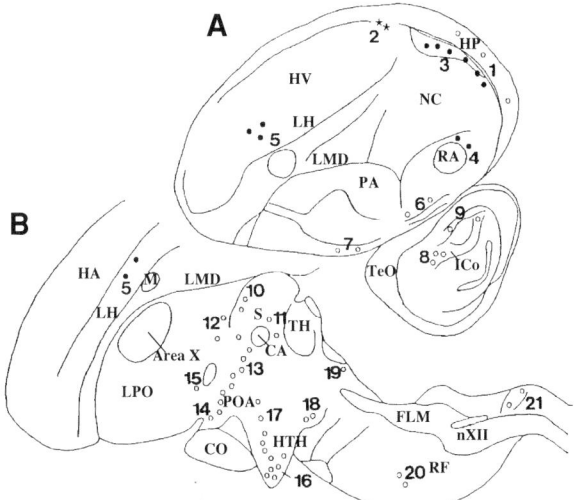

FIGURE 4 Generalized distribution of ERα-in cells in the avian brain. (A) Lateral and (B) medial view of a generic avian brain. Open circles indicate areas expressing ERα common to all species investigated in the orders Anseriformes, Galliformes, Columbiformes, Psittaciformes, Apodiformes, and Passeriformes. Filled circles represent areas expressing ERα that are unique to all (area 3) or to some songbird species (areas 4 and 5). The asterisks indicates an area that contains many ERα expressing cells in songbird species, but only a few in tyrannids and in the budgerigar. 1, hippocampus (HP); 2, hyperstriatum accessorium; 3, neostriatal band along the lateral ventricle including the song-control nucleus high vocal center (HVc); 4, archistriatum around the song-control nucleus robustus archistriatalis (RA); 5, rostral forebrain lateral and rostral to song-control nucleus anterioris magnocellularis (M); 6, cells interspersed with the occipitomesencephalic tract; 7, nucleus taeniae; 8, nucleus intercollicularis (ICo); 9, substantia grisea and fibrosa periventricularis; 10, lateral septum; 11, nucleus commissurae pallii; 12, bed nucleus of the stria terminalis surrounding the nucleus accumbens; 13, nucleus interstitialis; 14, nucleus preopticus medialis; 15, cells lateral to the tractus septomesencephalicus; 16, nucleus infundibuli; 17, nucleus posterior lateralis hypothalami; 18, cells scattered in the dorsolateral hypothalamus; 19, substantia grisea centralis; 20, nucleus raphe and reticular formation (RF); 21, nucleus solitarius. CA, anterior commissure; CO, chiasma opticum; FLM, fasciculus longitudinalis medialis; HA, hyperstriatum accessorium; HTH, hypothalamus; HV, hyperstriatum ventrale; LH; lamina hyperstriatica; LMD, lamina medullaris dorsalis; LPO, lobus parolfactorius; NC, neostriatum caudale; nXII, nucleus nervi hypoglossi; PA, paleostriatum augmentatum; POA, preoptic area; TeO, tectum opticum, TH, thalamus. Modified from Gahr et al. (1993).

For example no ERα mRNA could be detected in the ICo of zebra finches, whereas previous studies identified estrogen-binding sites and ERα-ir cells in this nucleus (K. W. Nordeen et al., 1987; Gahr et al., 1987). Whether this discrepancy relates to a difference in sensitivity between methods or is due to a very rapid turnover of ERα mRNA in ICo specifically is unknown. Similarly, binding assays on microdissected tissue from zebra finches that had been pretreated with the aromatase inhibitor androtatrienedione (ATD) had revealed the presence of estrogen binding in the song-control nuclei area X and MAN of adult male zebra finches (Walters et al., 1988). No ERα mRNA was detected in these nuclei, which also appear to be devoid of ERα-ir cells. The origins of the estrogen binding in these nuclei is therefore unclear.

It is also interesting to note that northern blot analysis indicated the existence of a single transcript for ERα in the zebra finch telencephalon at 4.1 kb, but other transcripts with higher molecular weights were present in the ovary and oviduct (Jacobs et al., 1996). It is important to investigate whether these other transcripts occur in other brain regions such as the diencephalon and how these different transcripts relate to estrogen action.

ERα has also been cloned in another songbird species, the canary (Gahr and Metzdorf, 1997), so probes could be designed to analyze the neuroanatomical distribution of the receptor in this species (Gahr and Metzdorf, 1997; Fusani et al., 2000; Metzdorf et al., 1999). The distribution of ERα mRNA emerging from these studies coincides well with previous immunocytochemical results and with results obtained in another songbird species, the zebra finch, with the exception that ERα mRNA appears to be present in the HVc in canaries but not in zebra finches—in this species, ERα are located around but not in HVc proper.

Dense ERα mRNA labeling overlapping with tyrosine hydroxylase immunoreactivity was also detected in the locus ceruleus and the area ventralis of Tsai of male canaries (Maney et al., 2001). The presence of ERα in these cell groups suggests that sex steroid hormones may affect song production by modulating the catecholaminergic system at the site of synthesis by acting both as androgens (see previous discussion) or as estrogens.

In summary, it appears that the overall distribution of ERα in the avian brain is quite similar to the distribution of AR. ERα are found in diencephalic and limbic structures in all avian species. They are also present in a limited number of telencephalic areas adjacent or overlapping with the song-control nuclei in songbirds. The functional significance of these telencephalic receptors is not fully understood (see later; Schlinger and Brenowitz, Chap. 33 in this volume).

a) Colocalization of Androgen Receptors and Estrogen Receptor α Because the activation of many aspects of reproductive behavior is obtained in birds, as in mammals, by a synergistic action of androgens and estrogens (both types of steroids being eventually derived from the local intracellular metabolism of testosterone; see later), a number of studies have been carried out to research whether both AR and ERα are colocalized in the same neurons. This was shown clearly to be the case in a number of limbic nuclei in mammals, although the degree of colocalization was quite variable from one nucleus to the other (Wood and Newman, 1995a; Gréco et al., 1998). In birds, a single study was, to our knowledge, performed on this question. Gahr (1990) demonstrated by combining immunocytochemistry with H222SPγ and autoradiography using tritiated 5α-dihydrotestosterone that in the canary, many cells in the ICo simultaneously contain both AR and ERα. In other brain nuclei, such as HVc, both types of receptors are present in a large number of cells, but their colocalization in the same cell is actually a very rare event. Based on this study, it appears therefore that the functional synergism between androgens and estrogens can be mediated by the action of both types of steroids on the same neuron as well as by their action on organized neural circuits containing AR and ERα in different cells (intra- vs intercellular interactions). More studies in a greater diversity of animal models would, however, be desirable to determine to what extent the synergism between androgens and estrogens in the activation of reproductive behavior of birds results from the action of both types of steroids on the same or on different but interconnected neurons.

3. Estrogen Receptors, β Subtype

The identification of a second type of ER has raised new issues about the action of estrogens (Kuiper et al., 1996, 1998). This newly identified receptor, ERβ, was found to be present in brain areas not previously thought to be responsive to estrogen (Shughrue et al., 1997). This suggested many questions about the possible function of this newly identified form of ER (Gustafsson, 1999; Patrone et al., 2000). An interesting hypothesis has been proposed by Kuiper et al. (1998) for the differential distribution of the two receptor subtypes in the brain. They suggest that these two receptors provide a way in which estrogen can selectively modulate reproduction (e.g., ovulation and reproductive behaviors) as opposed to nonreproductive events (e.g., learning and memory). They argue that ERα is important for reproduction, whereas ERβ is more important for nonreproductive events. Some data supporting this idea have been collected in mammals. For example, the ERα knockout mice, which have normal levels of ERβ (Shughrue et al., 1997), have major deficiencies in reproductive behavior, whereas the ERβ knockout mice apparently exhibit normal sexual behavior (Krege et al., 1998; Ogawa et al., 1999). For a long time, nothing was know about the potential existence and distribution of ERβ in birds, so their potential significance in the control of behavior was impossible to assess.

In the 1990s, the ERβ was cloned in the Japanese quail (Lakaye et al., 1998; Foidart et al., 1999a) and European starling (Bernard et al., 1999). This permitted the synthesis of specific oligo- and riboprobes that were then used to analyze the neuroanatomical distribution of the mRNA in these two species (Lakaye et al., 1998; Foidart et al., 1999a; Bernard et al., 1999). Three antisense oligonucleotide probes (q1–q3 located in the hinge domain, the amino-terminal domain (NHD), and the liquid-binding domain (LBD) of the ERβ cDNA, respectively) were used for *in situ* hybridization studies in quail (Foidart et al., 1999a). These probes correspond to parts of the quail ERβ sequence that have a minimal homology with the corresponding fragment of the ERα sequence in the chicken or with other known sequences in Genbank. Sections obtained through the rostral to caudal extent of the forebrain were processed by *in situ* hybridization, either with each of these three probes separately or with several combinations of two different probes. In all cases, a similar pattern of ERβ mRNA distribution was observed (see Fig. 5).

An extensive distribution of the ERβ mRNA was detected throughout the rostral to caudal extent of the

the anterior commissure (therefore including the POM and BST). Additional, less numerous populations were present in these embryos in periventricular position at the level of the infundibulum and in the mediobasal hypothalamus at the level of the VMN (Guennoun and Gasc, 1990). An earlier study based on *in vivo* autoradiography also reported the presence of P binding sites in the telencephalon at the level of the hyperstriatum ventrale (Wood-Gush *et al.*, 1977). A similar population of cells that accumulated radioactivity after the injection of tritiated P was also identified in the hyperstriatum ventralis and dorsalis of the duck, *Anas platyrhynchos* (Rhees *et al.*, 1972). This population of cells is, however, not mentioned in the immunocytochemical studies. The source of this discrepancy does not appear to have been identified, but may relate to differences in techniques; autoradiography may have identified binding sites for metabolites of P that are not PR *sensu stricto*. PR-ir were also identified in the brain of male and female ring doves (Askew *et al.*, 1997). The densest clusters of immunoreactive cells were located in the anterior and medial POA, the nucleus paraventricularis magnocellularis, the nucleus hypothalami lateralis, and the tuberal infundibular region.

C. Distribution of Steroid-Metabolizing Enzymes

Studies carried out since the 1970s in a variety of mammalian and avian species have shown that steroids, and in particular Testosterone (T), can be extensively metabolized when they enter their target cells (see reviews by Celotti *et al.*, 1979, 1997; Martini *et al.*, 1990; Poletti *et al.*, 1999; Balthazart, 1983, 1989). This metabolism is highly relevant to the control of reproductive behavior (see also Balthazart, 1989). The metabolites that are formed from the parent steroid either have their own receptors or targets in the brain and regulate the behavior (they mimic and actually cause some or all effects of T at the molecular level) or have no receptor and therefore represent inactivation products for the parent steroid. The ratio of active vs inactive metabolites that are produced can be affected by factors such as the sex, age, season, or hormonal condition of the subjects and this provides a mechanism for the fine adjustment of behavior. In addition, there is an anatomical specialization of these steroid-metabolizing enzymes—their concentration or activity varies from one brain area to the other. The same steroid can therefore act through different neuroendocrine and neurochemical mechanisms in different brain regions.

These general principles hold true, in various degrees, for the three major classes of sex steroids—androgens (e.g., T), estrogens (e.g., E_2), and progestagens (e.g., P). In mammals and in a small number of avian models (mainly poultry), the pathways of T, E_2, and P metabolism in the brain have all been described and their significance for the control of reproductive behavior has been to some extent experimentally studied. In other species of birds, the available knowledge is more restricted and, with a few exceptions, only the metabolism of T and its role in the control of sexual and vocal behavior has been analyzed.

1. Testosterone Metabolism

a) Metabolic Pathways (Aromatase, 5α-reductase, and 5β-reductase) T is the major androgen secreted by the testes in birds, and significant amounts of androstenedione ($\Delta 4$) are found in the circulation of a number of species. In the brain and pituitary gland, as well as in a number of peripheral target structures, T and $\Delta 4$ are extensively metabolized into other steroids that are androgenic, estrogenic, or have no hormonal properties. A number of *in vivo* and *in vitro* studies have described the metabolism of T in the avian brain and a summary of the major pathways identified in the quail, ring dove, and zebra finch brain is presented in Fig. 6 (see Balthazart, 1989, for a more extensive discussion of this problem in a broader context).

In the avian brain, three enzymes catalyze the transformation of T or $\Delta 4$ into behaviorally relevant metabolites: (1) aromatase leads to the production of estrogens (E_2 or estrone, E_1), (2) 5α-reductase produces 5α-DHT, and (3) 5β-reductase leads to the formation of the behaviorally inactive 5β-DHT (or the corresponding compounds if $\Delta 4$ is the substrate). These transformations are thermodynamically irreversible, at least in physiological conditions. In addition, 17β-hydroxysteroid dehydrogenase (17β-HSDH permits the reversible interconversion of T with $\Delta 4$. The 5α- and 5β-DHT can be further metabolized into the corresponding 3α- and 3β-diols under the catalytic action of the 3α- or 3β-HSDH. These transformations are also reversible.

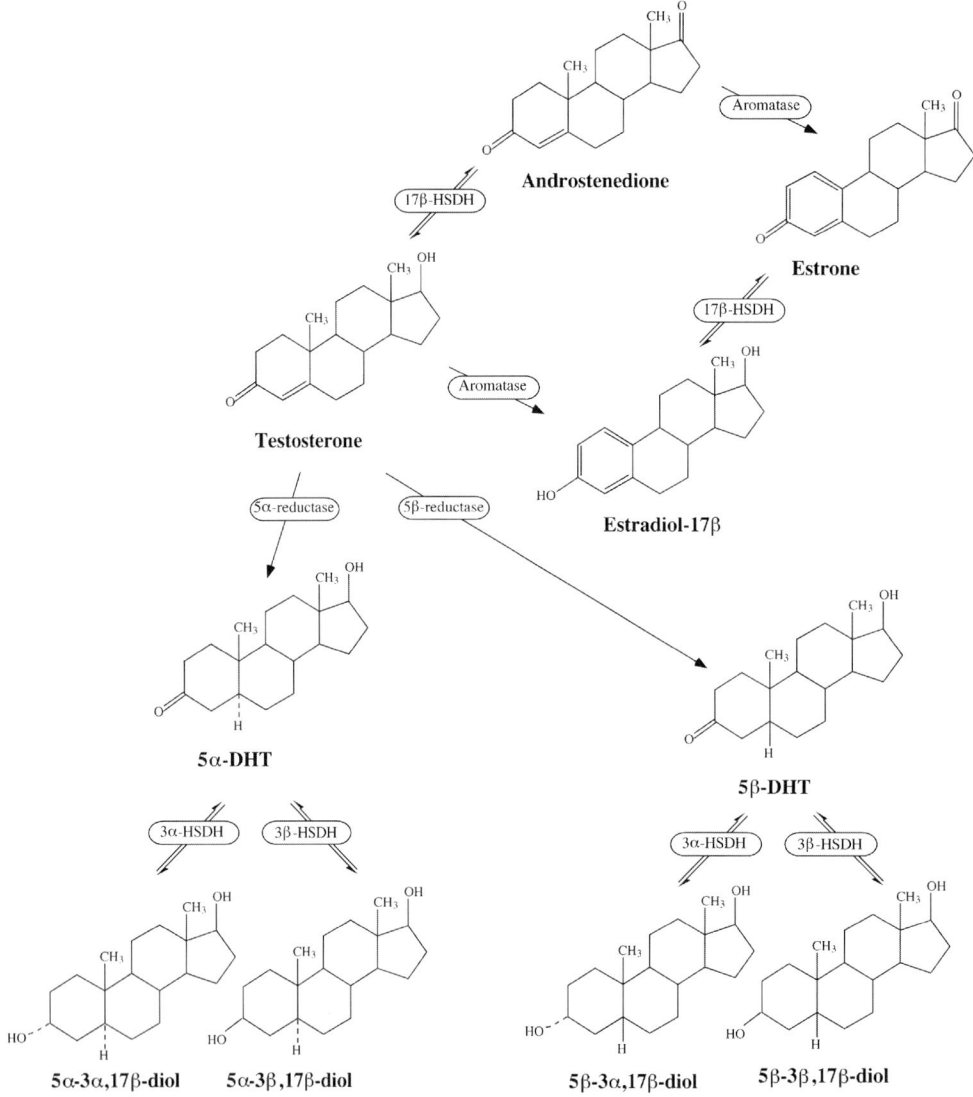

FIGURE 6 Testosterone metabolic pathways identified in the avian brain. Single arrows indicate thermodynamically irreversible transformations; double arrows indicate reversible interconversions. DHT, dihydrotestosterone; 5α(β)-3α(β),17β-diol, 5α(β)-androstane-3α(β),17β-diol; 3α(β)-HSDH, 3α(β)-hydroxysteroid dehydrogenase; 17β-HSDH, 17β-hydroxysteroid dehydrogenase. Androstenedione can be metabolized by 3α(β)-HSDH exactly like testosterone (but the metabolites produced are not indicated to preserve the clarity of the figure). Data from Balthazart et al. (1986a). Hutchison and Steimer (1981, 1986); Vockel et al. (1988, 1990a,b); Schlinger and Arnold (1991, 1992a,b).

The formation of all these steroids has been confirmed in the quail, ring dove, and zebra finch brain during *in vitro* experiments (Balthazart *et al.*, 1983; Schumacher *et al.*, 1984; Schumacher and Balthazart, 1987; Hutchison and Steimer, 1981, 1986; Steimer and Hutchison, 1981b; Vockel *et al.*, 1988, 1990b; Schlinger and Arnold, 1991, 1992b). Some or all of these transformations are also known to occur in a wider diversity of species, although the amount of information is more limited. The existence these metabolic pathways has also been confirmed *in vivo* in a limited number of cases by injecting radioactive T into the live animals and measuring the accumulation of radioactive metabolites in a variety of tissues after the sacrifice of the subjects. The presence of an active aromatase and 5β-reductase has in this way been confirmed *in vivo* in ring doves (Hutchison *et al.,* 1986) and in zebra finches (Schlinger and Arnold, 1992a). Other than these few exceptions, most of the available data concerning T metabolism in the avian brain are derived from *in vitro* studies in which brain homogenates were incubated with radioactive substrate before the radioactive metabolites produced were quantified. These data demonstrate the presence of the enzymes in the central nervous system, but the measures of activity obtained in these studies may ignore some regulatory mechanisms that play a key role in the live animal. Some caution should therefore be exercised when using these assay data to interpret physiological phenomena.

By incubating equal amounts of brain homogenate in the presence of increasing amounts of radioactive substrate (i.e., T), it has been possible to obtain estimates of the maximum velocity (Vmax) and of the affinity (Km; high affinity equals low Km) of the T-metabolizing enzymes in the avian brain. In adult birds, an inverse relationship was found between the estimated affinity and Vmax of the three enzymes that irreversibly metabolize T (see Fig. 7). These data indicate that in conditions when a low (nanomolar) concentration of T is available (which is presumably the case most of the time *in vivo*), the steroid is preferentially transformed into estrogens by the aromatase that has a high affinity (low Km) for this substrate. By contrast, if higher amounts of substrate become present, as could happen in a bird that has been injected with exogenous T, then a larger proportion could be inactivated into 5β-reduced steroids that have no marked hormonal activity by themselves (see Section V). The capacity of the 5β-reductase is extremely high compared to the other two enzymes and this enzyme should be able to catalyze the transformation of a huge amount of substrate when it becomes available.

b) Neuroanatomical Localization of Testosterone-Metabolizing Enzymes The distribution of T-metabolizing enzymes has been studied in the avian brain by enzyme assays (the measure of the production of radioactive metabolites during the *in vitro* incubation of brain homogenates) that were performed on brain samples that had been dissected with more or less anatomical specificity (e.g., entire diencephalon, POA, and telencephalon). In a more limited number of cases, this type of assay has also been carried out on specific brain nuclei that had been microdissected by the Palkovits punch technique (the dissection with hollow needles of nuclei from 2- to 300-μm-thick cryostat section; see Palkovits, 1973; Palkovits and Brownstein, 1983). Information of this sort is only available for Japanese quail (Schumacher and Balthazart, 1987; Balthazart *et al.,* 1990f) and zebra finches (Vockel *et al.,* 1990a,b).

In addition, the distribution of aromatase in the avian brain has been analyzed with a cellular level of anatomical resolution by immunocytochemistry and *in situ* hybridization in a few selected species (Balthazart *et al.,* 1990b,e; Foidart *et al.,* 1995; Aste *et al.,* 1998b; Beyer *et al.,* 1994; Shen *et al.,* 1994, 1995; Saldanha *et al.,* 2000b). Similar data are not available for the 5α- and 5β-reductase, which have not been cloned in birds and cannot be identified by immunocytochemistry. Immunocytochemical data on the distribution of the

Enzyme	Km	Vmax
Zebra Finch		
Aromatase	18 nM	200 fmol/mg protein/h
5α-reductase	117 nM	3,333 fmol/mg protein/h
5β-reductase	134 nM	95,000 fmol/mg protein/h
Quail		
Aromatase	15 nM	2,184 fmol/mg protein/h
5α-reductase	114 nM	1,488 fmol/mg protein/h
5β-reductase	473 nM	19,400 fmol/mg protein/h

FIGURE 7 Apparent affinity (Km) and maximum velocity (Vmax) of the three major enzymes that catalyze irreversible transformations of T in the quail and Zebra finch brain. Data from Schumacher *et al.* (1983); Vockel *et al.* (1988).

5α-reductase are, however, available in mammals (see Poletti *et al.*, 1999, for review).

c) Aromatase Activity in Chicken, Ring Doves, and Quail

The first studies of T metabolism in the avian brain were carried out in chicken, ring doves, and Japanese quail (Nakamura and Tanabe, 1974; Steimer and Hutchison, 1980, 1981b; Hutchison and Steimer, 1981; Schumacher *et al.*, 1983, 1984). In these species it was demonstrated that the metabolic pathways described in Fig. 6 are widely distributed in the brain. In general, it was observed that enzymatic transformations leading to the production of behaviorally inactive metabolites, such as the 5β-reductase, are more active in brain areas that do not appear to be directly involved in the control of reproduction (e.g., parts of the telencephalon and the cerebellum), whereas aromatase and 5α-reductase, which produce T metabolites that play an important role in the control of sexual behavior and of GnRH secretion, are particularly active in the hypothalamic and limbic areas that are known to control reproductive behavior and where GnRH neurons are located (Schumacher *et al.*, 1983; Schumacher and Balthazart, 1984a; Steimer and Hutchison, 1980, 1981b).

In quail, a specialization in the distribution of these enzymes was even observed in the POA-hypothalamic area, which could be related to the functional role supposed for the enzymes (Schumacher *et al.*, 1983; Schumacher and Balthazart, 1984a, 1987; Balthazart and Schumacher, 1984a). Aromatase activity is, for example, higher in the POA (a key site for the control of male sexual behavior) than in the hypothalamus, whereas the 5α-reductase activity is higher in the mediobasal and tuberal hypothalamus than in the POA and rostral hypothalamus, which could be related to the high potency of 5α-reduced metabolites of T in the feedback control of gonadotropin secretion (Davies *et al.*, 1980). The posterior hypothalamus appears to be a key area in this control (Davies and Follett, 1975). Conversely, the activity of the 5β-reductase that produces behaviorally inactive metabolites is low in the entire POA-hypothalamus compared to directly adjacent telencephalic areas (Schumacher and Balthazart, 1984a, 1986).

Further refinement in the localization of these enzymes was subsequently obtained in quail by combining ultrasensitive radioenzyme assay techniques with the microdissection method of Palkovits (1973; Palkovits and Brownstein, 1983). High levels of aromatase activity were detected in the POM and VMN (Schumacher and Balthazart, 1987). The 5α-reductase activity was high in a series of hypothalamic nuclei—in decreasing order, the area lateralis hypothalami (LHy), PVN, nucleus preopticus dorsolateralis (PD), and nucleus anterior hypothalami (AM)—and in a few other structures—the bed nucleus of the pallial commissure (BPC) and nucleus septalis medialis (SM). In contrast, the 5β-reductase activity was comparatively low in these hypothalamic and limbic structures, but high in other brain regions such as the nucleus septalis lateralis (SL) or the ventral part of the archistriatum (AV).

d) Aromatase Activity in Zebra Finches

In zebra finches, the activity of the aromatase, 5α-reductase, and 5β-reductase were measured by radioenzyme assays in brain nuclei that had been dissected by the Palkovits punch technique (Vockel *et al.*, 1990a,b) (Fig. 8). 5α-reductase activity was more or less evenly distributed in all brain nuclei that were considered, with the noticeable exception of the RA, in which enzyme activity was twice that found in all other regions. High levels of 5β-reductase activity were found throughout the brain (note the very different scales in the graphs), but especially in the MAN, HVc, and nucleus striae terminalis (nST). These two reductases were even present in two steroid-insensitive regions that had been included in the study as controls, the ectostriatum (E) and the nucleus rotundus (Rt).

High levels of aromatase were observed in the diencephalic and limbic nuclei that are known to express this enzyme in mammals and other avian species, namely the POA, PVM, the nucleus medialis hypothalami posterioris (PMH), nST, and Tn; (homolog to parts of the mammalian amygdala). The activity of aromatase was also found to be markedly affected by the age of the subjects (Fig. 8).

Interestingly, these studies also reported the presence of significant levels of aromatase activity in telencephalic song-control nuclei such as the area X, MAN, HVc, and RA. They also indicated that the area parahippocampalis (APH), which had originally been selected as a control region, was characterized by an extremely high enzymatic activity larger than in any of the diencephalic or limbic nuclei that had been studied (Vockel

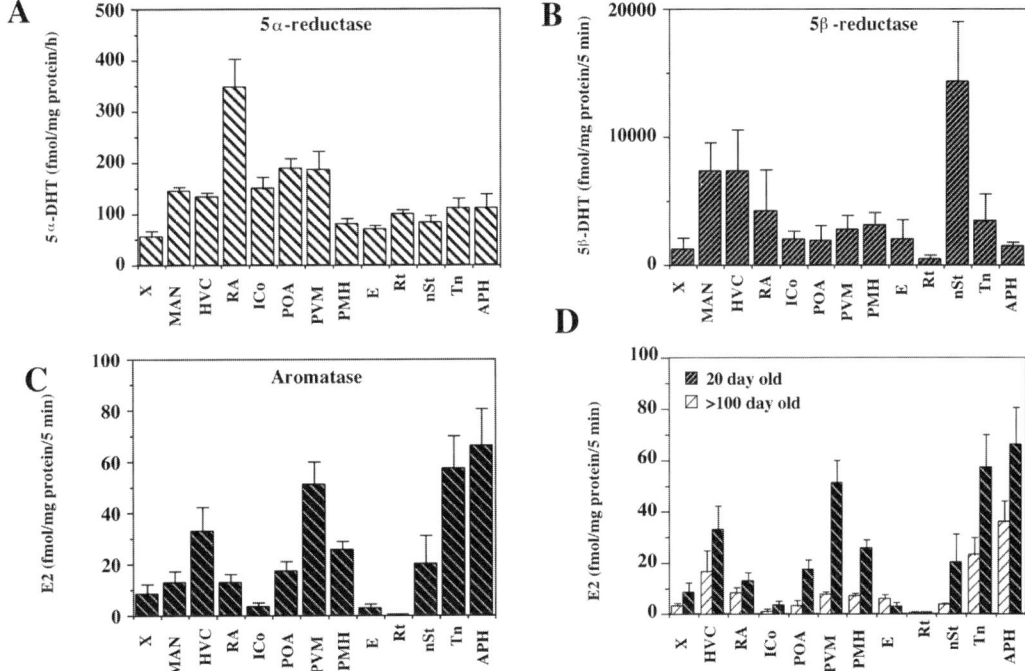

FIGURE 8 Distribution and changes with age of the activity of testosterone-metabolizing enzymes in the zebra finch brain. (A–C) Formation of 5α-DHT (5α reduction), 5β-DHT (5β reduction) and estradiol (aromatization) by different brain nuclei of adult male zebra finches. (D) Comparison of the aromatase activity in different brain nuclei of young (20-day-old) and adult (>100-day-old) male zebra finches. Data represent the mean ± SE of 6–11 replicates in each case. Note that different scales have been used to represent the activity of the three enzymes. APH, area parahippocampalis; E, ectostriatum; HVC, hyperstriatum ventrale, pars caudalis; ICo, nucleus intercollicularis; MAN, nucleus magnocellularis of the anterior neostriatum; nSt, nucleus stria terminalis; PMH, nucleus medialis hypothalami posterioris; POA, nucleus preopticus anterioris; PVM, nucleus periventricularis magnocellularis; RA, nucleus robustus archistriatalis; Rt, nucleus rotundus; Tn, nucleus taeniae; X, area X of lobus parolfactorius. Data from Vockel *et al.* (1988, 1990a).

et al., 1990b). Additional studies confirmed the presence of a very high aromatase activity in the dorsal telencephalon and showed that the enzyme is actually present in the entire roof of the forebrain in the neostriatum, hippocampal, and parahippocampal regions. This high level of telencephalic aromatase activity has been independently confirmed (Schlinger and Arnold, 1991, 1992b), and a series of elegant studies based on the injection of radioactive androgens into the brain or periphery combined with blood collection from the jugulars or carotids has provided experimental evidence indicating that brain aromatase substantially contributes to the circulating levels of estrogens in the zebra finch (Schlinger and Arnold, 1992a, 1993). These data suggested that the song-control nuclei have the capacity to produce the T metabolites E_2 and 5α-DHT, which had been shown, during behavioral experiments, to mimic the effects of T on song production and courtship behavior.

e) Cellular Localization of Aromatase by Immunocytochemistry and In Situ Hybridization The distribution of aromatase protein and mRNA has been described at the cellular level in the zebra finch, canary, quail, and dove brain by ICC (Balthazart *et al.*, 1990b,e, 1996a; Foidart *et al.*, 1995; Beyer *et al.*, 1994; Saldanha *et al.*, 2000a,b); and *in situ* hybridization (ISH; Shen *et al.*, 1994, 1995; Aste *et al.*, 1998b; Metzdorf *et al.*, 1999; Fusani *et al.*, 2000), and this new information has led to a partial revision of these conclusions. In all species, ICC and ISH studies confirmed the presence of aromatase and its mRNA in the diencephalic and limbic regions such as the POA, PVM, PMH, BST, and Tn that are implicated in the control of reproduction and where a high level of enzyme activity had been measured (see Fig. 9). They also identified a high level of aromatase expressed in the hippocampus (e.g., Shen *et al.*, 1995; Saldanha *et al.*, 1998, 2000b).

Unexpectedly however, all telencephalic song-control nuclei of zebra finches and canaries were found to contain only minimal, often undetectable, amounts of the protein or its mRNA (Shen *et al.*, 1994, 1995; Balthazart *et al.*, 1996a; Metzdorf *et al.*, 1999). A small number of weakly aromatase immunoreactive cells was observed in one study in the medial MAN of zebra finches (Balthazart *et al.*, 1996a), but this was not confirmed in subsequent work using a zebra-finch-specific antibody (Saldanha *et al.*, 2000b). ISH similarly failed to detect significant amounts of aromatase mRNA in all song-control nuclei, including MAN (Shen *et al.*, 1995).

The presence of a large amount of aromatase (protein and mRNA) was, however, confirmed in the neostriatum and its distribution characterized. At the level of HVc or in slightly more rostral parts of the telencephalon, aromatase and its mRNA are present in broad areas of the medial neostriatum adjacent to the lateral ventricles. At more caudal levels, the cluster of aromatase-expressing cells extends more medially as a band coursing along the dorsal edge of the lamina archistriatalis dorsalis; they are also present in the ventrolateral aspects of the neostriatum. Based on these detailed anatomical data, it is possible that the aromatase activity that had been detected in HVc and RA by radioenzyme assays performed on nuclei microdissected by the Palkovits punch technique (Fig. 8) originated in a contamination by neostriatal tissue immediately surrounding these nuclei. An alternative explanation is suggested by the finding that aromatase mRNA is present in the nucleus interfacialis (Nif) of canaries (Fusani *et al.*, 2000). Because previous work showed that aromatase activity and immunoreactivity are present in neuronal processes, including axons (Schlinger and Callard, 1989; Naftolin *et al.*, 1996), it is conceivable that a part at least of the aromatase activity that had been originally measured in HVc is located in axons originating in Nif that project to HVc (Fusani *et al.*, 2000).

f) Subcellular Localization of Aromatase   All ICC studies performed so far suggest that the aromatase immunoreactive material is located in cells that have, in general, a neuronal morphology. Double-labeled studies that combine aromatase ICC with a marker of glial or neuronal cells on brain sections have not, however, been performed in birds, so the conclusion that, in the living brain, aromatase is mainly (or exclusively) located in neurons is only based on indirect, partly unreliable evidence. It must be mentioned, however, that in cell cultures derived from embryonic zebra finches brain, evidence has been obtained indicating that aromatase may be located in both neuronal and glial cells (Schlinger *et al.*, 1994). This conclusion was based on experimental manipulations designed to specifically affect the density of neurons or glial cells in these cultures. It was, for example, shown that the addition of the neurotoxin kainic acid to these cultures did not result in a major decline of aromatase activity in parallel with the observed decrease in neuron density (Schlinger *et al.*, 1994). Furthermore, labeling of these cultures by *in situ* hybridization indicated that aromatase-positive cells had in general a glial (astrocyte) morphology. Although these data could still receive alternative explanations, they strongly suggests that, in these cultures, aromatase may be preferentially located in the glial compartment. Why a different situation is apparently observed *in vivo* remains to be understood.

In this context, it should also be mentioned that studies in mammals have indicated that experimental brain lesions induce in their vicinity the expression of aromatase in glial cells (Garcia-Segura *et al.*, 1999b). This finding has been reproduced in zebra finches in which it could be demonstrated that, 1–3 days after a penetrating injury, aromatase immunoreactive glial cells can be observed along the penetration tract (Peterson *et al.*, 2000). The induction of a local production of estrogens into the vicinity of lesioned brain areas could have a significant role in the processes of brain repair. Estrogens are indeed known to play a significant role in various forms of brain plasticity (e.g., Garcia-Segura *et al.*, 1999a). This newly discovered kind of plasticity in aromatase expression could also explain why aromatase seems to be localized in the neuronal or glial compartment in the living brain and in cell cultures, respectively.

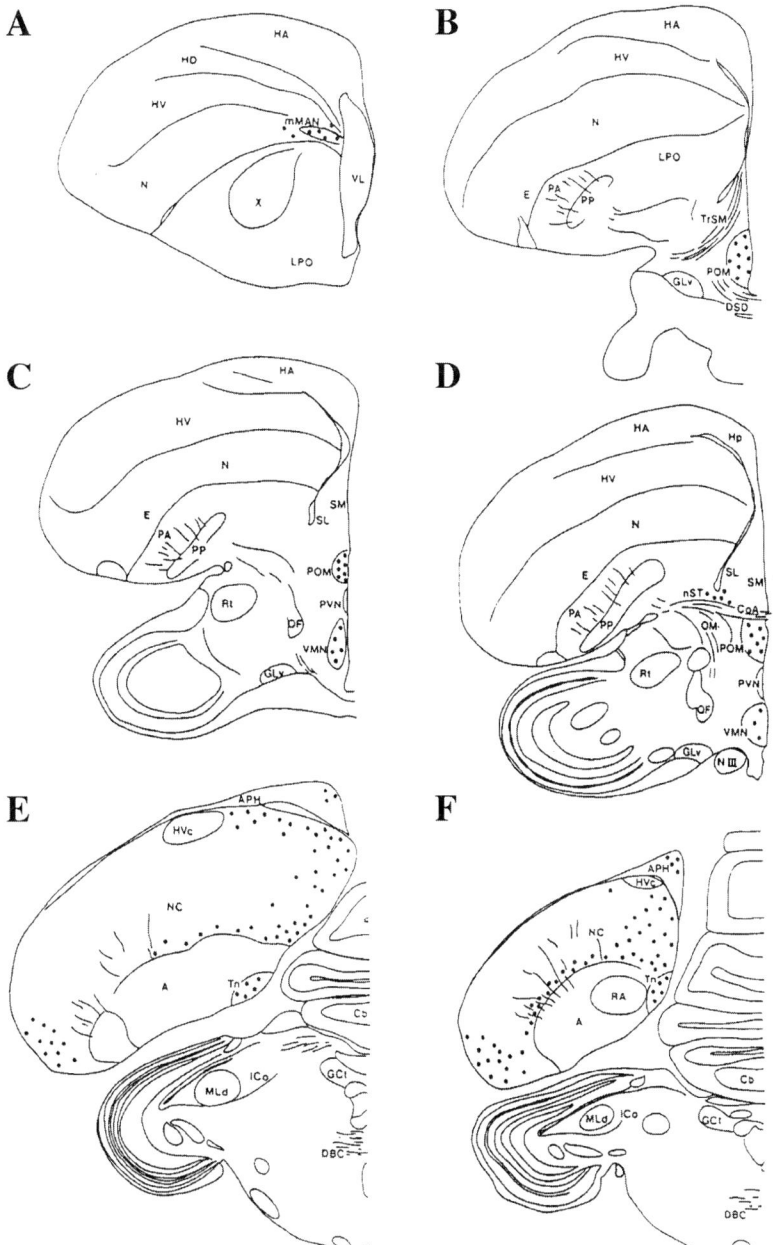

FIGURE 9 Schematic drawings illustrating the distribution of aromatase immunoreactive cells (dots) in the brain of male zebra finches. Panels A–F are presented in rostral to caudal order. A, archistriatum; APH, area parahippocampalis; Cb, cerebellum; CoA, commissura anterioris; DBC, decussatio brachiorum conjunctivorum; DSD, decussatio supraoptica dorsalis; E, ectostriatum; GCt, substantia grisea centralis; GLv, nucleus geniculatus lateralis, pars ventralis; HA, hyperstriatum accessorium; HD, hyperstriatum dorsalis; Hp, hippocampus; HV, hyperstriatum ventralis; HVC, high vocal center (formally hyperstriatum ventralis pars caudale); ICo, nucleus intercollicularis; LPO, lobus parolfactorius; MLd, nucleus mesencephalicus lateralis pars dorsalis; mMAN, medial part of the magnocellular nucleus of the anterior neostriatum; N, neostriatum; NC, neostriatum caudale; nST, nucleus striae terminalis; NIII, nervus oculomotorius; OM, tractus occipitomesencephalicus; PA, paleostriatum augmentatum; POM, nucleus preopticus medialis; PP, paleostriatum primitivum; PVN, nucleus paraventricularis magnocellularis; VL, ventriculus lateralis; QF, tractus quintofrontalis; RA, nucleus robustus archistriatalis; Rt, nucleus rotundus; SL, nucleus septalis lateralis; SM, nucleus septalis medialis; Tn, nucleus taeniae; TrSM, tractus septomesencephalicus; VMN, nucleus ventromedialis hypothalami; X, area X. Adapted from Balthazart et al. (1996a).

Most ICC studies of brain aromatase clearly indicate that the immunoreactive material is essentially localized in the neuronal perikarya, leaving a clear unstained nucleus. However, several studies have revealed that this immunoreactive material is also present in cell processes, including dendrites and the full length of axons (Foidart *et al.*, 1994b). Immunoreactive punctate structures representing presumptive synaptic boutons were also described in that study. It was confirmed by pre-embedding ICC and electron microscopy that numerous axons and synaptic boutons containing aromatase immunoreactive material are indeed present in the POA of the quail, and also of rat, monkey, and even human (Naftolin *et al.*, 1990b, 1996).

In addition, biochemical studies performed in quail, zebra finches, and rats (Schlinger and Callard, 1989; Schlinger and Arnold, 1992b; Steimer, 1988; Roselli, 1995) have indicated the presence of high levels of aromatase activity in synaptosomes (pinched-off synaptic terminals) prepared by differential centrifugation. Two of these studies even indicated that aromatase activity is enriched in purified synaptosomal fractions compared with crude homogenates (Schlinger and Callard, 1989; Steimer, 1988), which indicates that the immunoreactive aromatase identified in presynaptic boutons is functionally active. Taken together, these data suggest that significant amounts of estrogens are produced at the presynaptic level. This local production of estrogens in the close vicinity of synapses may provide steroid signals that could affect brain activity independent of the binding to nuclear receptors acting as transcription factors (i.e., by nongenomic mechanisms). It is known that estrogens are able to modify the electrical activity of the neuronal membranes within seconds after their application, which essentially rules out the possibility of a classic steroid-receptor-mediated effect on protein synthesis (for additional discussion, see Blaustein and Olster, 1989; Schlinger and Callard, 1989; Schumacher, 1990; McEwen, 1994; Ramirez *et al.*, 1996). Some effects of estrogens on brain functioning that appear to be independent of their binding to intracellular receptors have also been described (e.g., Pasqualini *et al.*, 1995; Thompson and Moss, 1994; Mermelstein *et al.*, 1996). Whether the presence of aromatase activity in brain areas, such as part of the zebra finch neostriatum, that are apparently devoid of intracellular estrogen receptors relates to these membrane effects of estrogens is unknown.

g) Anatomical Relationships between Aromatase and Other Steroid-Metabolizing Enzymes with Steroid Receptors   As previously described, the precise mapping of the T-metabolizing enzymes in the avian brain has been performed with a reasonable degree of anatomical specificity (with the Palkovits punch method) in only two species, the Japanese quail and zebra finch. However, these techniques do not provide a cellular level of anatomical resolution. It is therefore difficult to draw precise correlations between the distribution of these enzymes and the distribution of the steroid receptors that are supposed to bind the locally produced metabolite 5α-DHT. The 5β reduced metabolites do not bind or bind with a very low affinity to androgen receptors (Lieberburg and Nottebohm, 1979). Their relationship with these receptors is therefore not physiologically relevant. In addition, the enzyme aromatase has been visualized by immunocytochemistry in a few species and in one case, the relationship of this enzyme to ER was studied at the cellular level by double-labeled immunocytochemistry.

In quail, high levels of 5α-reductase activity were identified in brain nuclei that are known for containing AR (see previous discussion). This is true for the LHy, AM, BPC, and SM. Although these areas are not those that contain the densest populations of AR, these receptors are definitely present and could potentially bind the locally produced 5α-DHT. Whether the 5α-reductase and AR are localized in the same or different neurons has not been investigated, but studies in mammals indicate that a substantial fraction of the brain 5α-reductase is located in glial cells (Melcangi *et al.*, 1990, 1993, 1998, 1999; Poletti *et al.*, 1999).

Most nuclei of the song system are steroid-sensitive and contain, at least, AR, as demonstrated by *in vivo* autoradiography (Ball, 1990; Brenowitz, 1991), binding assays (Harding *et al.*, 1984), immunocytochemistry (Balthazart *et al.*, 1992d), and *in situ* hybridization (Nastiuk and Clayton, 1994, 1995; Gahr and Metzdorf, 1997; Metzdorf *et al.*, 1999). One noticeable exception to this rule is area X, which appears to be devoid of androgen binding sites. Significant 5α-reductase was found in all these nuclei, which suggests that the AR located in the song-control nuclei could be occupied in physiological conditions by T as well as by its metabolite 5α-DHT. This enzymatic activity was particularly low in area X, which fits in well with the absence of androgen binding sites in this nucleus.

It is usually accepted that the 5β-reduced androgens are biologically inactive compounds as far as activation of reproductive behavior is concerned and that the 5β reduction is an inactivation pathway for testosterone (Steimer and Hutchison, 1981a; Hutchison and Steimer, 1981; Balthazart, 1989). Many studies in several species of birds showed that 5β-reductase activity is lower in steroid target areas than in nontarget tissue (reviewed in Balthazart, 1983, 1989). The distribution pattern of the 5β-reductase observed in the zebra finch to some extent contradicts this generalization. If, as expected, the enzyme activity was low in all hypothalamic nuclei as demonstrated previously in other species, it was very high in several nuclei of the song system that are known targets for androgens (MAN, HVc, and to a lesser extent RA). In addition, the lowest production of 5β-DHT was observed in the two nuclei of the visual system, E and Rt, which are not steroid-sensitive (Vockel et al., 1990a,b). The mechanisms underlying this physiological differentiation and its biological meaning are totally unclear. However, it is the case that the 5β-reductase activity that had been detected in HVc and RA by radioenzyme assays performed on nuclei microdissected by the Palkovits punch technique could potentially be influenced by the contamination of the samples by tissue immediately surrounding these nuclei (see Section III.C.1.e).

The relationships between aromatase activity and ER can be evaluated in more detail and this comparison has revealed some striking discrepancies. In both quail and zebra finches, some brain areas such as the POA hypothalamic nuclei (POA, PVM, and PMH) and limbic regions (Tn and nSt) contain ER, as demonstrated by autoradiography (Watson and Adkins-Regan, 1989b; K. W. Nordeen et al., 1987) and immunocytochemistry (Balthazart et al., 1989; Gahr et al., 1987, 1993; Gahr and Konishi, 1988), as well as a high aromatase activity and a high density of aromatase-expressing cells (Balthazart et al., 1990b,e; Saldanha et al., 2000b; Shen et al., 1995). In other brain areas, however, some mismatches can be observed.

The ICo was identified in studies of both quail and zebra finches as a site with dense ER—by autoradiography (Watson and Adkins-Regan, 1989b; K. W. Nordeen et al., 1987), ICC (Balthazart et al., 1989; Gahr et al., 1987, 1993; Gahr and Konishi, 1988), and binding assays on punched nuclei (Walters et al., 1988)—but enzyme assays revealed no or barely detectable levels of enzyme activity and no aromatase-expressing cells can be detected by ICC or ISH (see previous discussion). In contrast, high levels of aromatase activity are observed in a large portion of the dorsal telencephalon (hippocampus, area parahippocampalis, and dorsal neostriatum) of song birds (zebra finch and brown-headed cowbirds), whereas these brain regions are not known as a classical target for steroids. Anatomical studies that have documented the distribution of aromatase and ER in these brain regions also confirm the presence of broad discrepancies between areas expressing the enzyme and the receptor. ER have been demonstrated in a large neostriatal area located under the lateral ventricle at the level of HVc in the zebra finch brain (Gahr et al., 1987), in which high aromatase activity and numerous aromatase-expressing cells are detected. However, aromatase immunoreactive cells and cells expressing aromatase mRNA are found beyond this specific region of the neostriatum, namely in the area dorsal to the lamina archistriatalis dorsalis and in the ventrolateral aspects of the neostriatum, where no ER have been detected so far. These observations therefore raise questions concerning how estrogens locally produced in the dorsal telencephalon may affect, directly or indirectly, the control of reproduction and of singing behavior, given that they are in areas devoid of ER.

In quail, the specific relationship at the cellular level between aromatase and ER was studied by double-labeled immunocytochemistry (Balthazart et al., 1991). Given that the enzyme and the ER usually coexist in the same brain areas (with the exception of the ICo in quail), a parsimonious view of the functional organization of the brain suggested that these two neurochemical markers were present in the same cells (i.e., they were colocalized) so that estrogens produced by aromatase could bind to their specific receptors in order to activate sexual behavior or to exert positive feedback on the synthesis of aromatase (intracrine action).

As expected, double-labeled immunocytochemical studies showed that in the ventromedial and tuberal hypothalamus a large fraction (70–80%) of the aromatase immunoreactive (ARO-ir) cells also contain

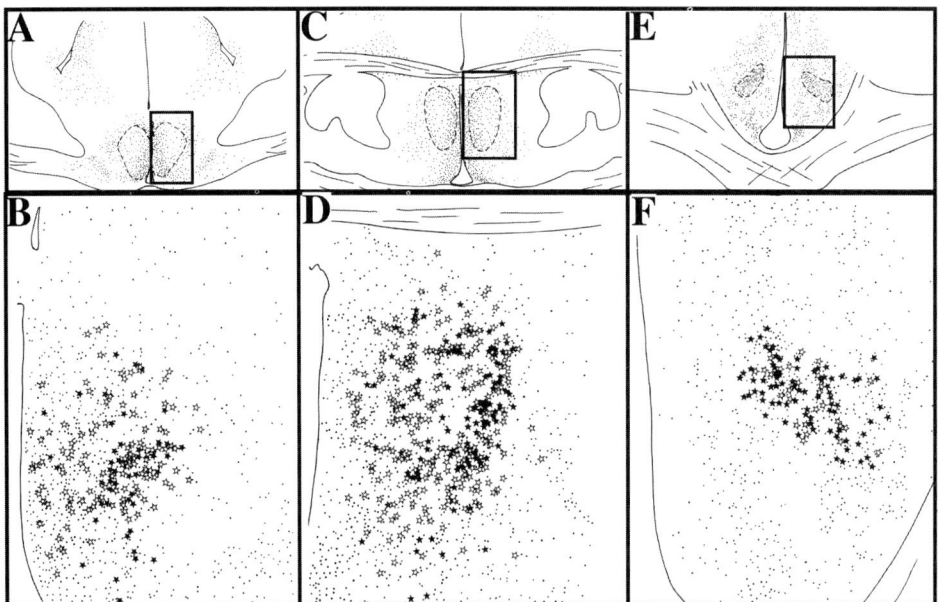

FIGURE 10 *Camera lucida* drawings of quail brain sections that had been double-labeled for aromatase and estrogen receptors at the level of the preoptic area-hypothalamus. (A–B) Rostral part of POM. (C–D) POM at the level of the anterior commissure. (E–F) Mediobasal hypothalamus at the level of the ventromedial nucleus. In sections of the POM (B, D) only a small percentage of cells express aromatase and estrogen receptors at the same time; this colocalization is by contrast very frequent in the caudal hypothalamus at the level of the nucleus inferioris hypothalami (F). In each case, (A–C) indicate the location of the area, which has been magnified. The rectangle defines the enlarged area. Dots, cell labeled for estrogen receptor; open star, cell labeled for aromatase; filled star, cell double-labeled for ER and aromatase. Adapted from Balthazart *et al*. (1991).

immunoreactive ER (Balthazart *et al.*, 1991). Surprisingly, however, very few doubled-labeled cells were found in more rostral groups of ARO-ir cells such as in the POM (only 17% of ARO-ir cells containing demonstrable ER) or the BST(4%) (Fig. 10). Interestingly, a similar organization has been subsequently observed in the brain of developing rats and mice. Using a double-labeled immunocytochemistry technique based on antibodies to aromatase and ER that are different from those used in the quail study, it could be observed in the brain of neonatal rodents that in rostral areas such as the anteromedial preoptic nucleus, BST, and medial amygdaloid nucleus, the majority of ARO-ir cells do not contain ER-ir material, whereas in more caudal structures such as the ventromedial hypothalamic nucleus, the colocalization between aromatase and ER is the rule (Yokosuka *et al.*, 1994; Tsuruo *et al.*, 1995, 1996).

The data therefore indicate that even in brain areas where aromatase and ER coexist, we cannot necessarily assume that they are colocalized in the same cells. This finding raises questions regarding the way in which locally formed estrogens may affect various aspects of reproduction, including the activation of male sexual behavior. These questions are discussed later.

In general, the partial mismatch between the T-metabolizing enzymes and the corresponding steroid receptors raises the question of how T metabolites exert their actions in the brain. It is often assumed that all steroids act in an autocrine fashion and exert their biological effects through binding with intracellular receptors located in the same cell as the enzymes. The presence of aromatase at the presynaptic level (Naftolin *et al.*, 1996) certainly suggests that a paracrine mode of action is also possible. The demonstration that the infusion of radioactive $\Delta 4$ in the zebra finch telencephalon results in increased levels of radioactive estrogen in the jugular blood (Schlinger and Arnold, 1992a, 1993) even suggests an endocrine action for brain aromatase.

This represents without a doubt an exciting discovery in the field and its biological significance should be experimentally evaluated.

2. Estradiol Metabolism

In quail, although most ARO-ir cells in the tuberal hypothalamus contain ER-ir in their nucleus, this colocalization is the exception in the POA and the BST, where the ER can be demonstrated in less than 20% (POA) and 5% (BST) of the ARO-ir cells (Balthazart et al., 1991). This observation therefore questions the mode of action of the estrogens produced by aromatization of T—they probably cannot act in an intracrine fashion because receptors are generally not present in the cells that contain aromatase. An intracrine action mediated by ERβ remains possible, but the experimental data needed to test this idea are not available (see previous discussion).

A paracrine action for locally produced estrogens therefore has to be considered (action on neighboring ER-positive cells after passive diffusion) or alternatively it can be speculated that locally produced estrogens do not exert their effects through the classic genomic mode of action. In addition, light and electron microscopy demonstrates the presence of ARO-ir material in cell processes, including axons and presynaptic terminals (Balthazart et al., 1992c; Balthazart and Foidart, 1993b; Naftolin et al., 1990b, 1996b). It is therefore very likely that estrogens are produced at the presynaptic level in the brain. These estrogens diffuse passively to bind to ER in neighboring cells, but, alternatively, these morphological data could also suggest that E_2 acts directly in the terminals.

It is possible that locally produced estrogens require further metabolization before they exert their biological effects. Many years ago it was shown that, in the mammalian brain, estrogens can be hydroxylated in position 2 or 4, which leads to the formation of catecholestrogens (Fishman, 1976, 1981; MacLusky et al., 1984). The presence of an active 2-hydroxylase activity leading to the production of 2-hydroxy-E_2 has been demonstrated in the quail brain (Balthazart et al., 1994b). This enzymatic activity was measured in very small samples dissected by the Palkovits punch method (Palkovits and Brownstein, 1983) and a relatively precise neuroanatomical localization was therefore possible (Fig. 11). This showed that, in general, the brain nuclei that display a high level of aromatase activity (AA) (Schumacher and Balthazart, 1987; Balthazart et al., 1990f) also contain high levels of 2-hydroxylase activity (Balthazart et al., 1994b) and vice versa. We do not have the anatomical data at the cellular level necessary to tell us whether these two enzymes are colocalized in the same cells but this appears possible based on the available biochemical results. This scenario is actually quite likely based on reports suggesting that these two enzymatic activities are in fact due to the same molecule, which shifts its activity as a function of the substrate concentration or pH (Osawa et al., 1993; Almadhidi et al., 1996). Aromatase and estrogen-2-hydroxylase activities always copurify in a variety of chromatographic systems (including an affinity column based on a monoclonal antibody raised against the placental aromatase). The single band of protein with a molecular weight of 55 kDa (corresponding to aromatase) demonstrates both aromatase and estrogen-2-hydroxylase activities, transfection of Chinese hamster ovarian cells with a human placental aromatase cDNA results in the expression of both activities, and finally reciprocal inhibitions of one or the other activity are observed as a function of the substrate being present (androgens inhibit the hydroxylase activity and estrogens inhibit the aromatase activity) (Osawa et al., 1993). It is therefore difficult to avoid the conclusion that aromatase is also the estrogen-2-hydroxylase that produces catecholestrogens.

The presence of catecholestrogens at the presynaptic level is highly relevant to the control of this behavior. They may directly regulate the activity of catecholaminergic neurotransmitters and in this way affect reproductive behavior by a direct action at the level of nerve terminals, independent of any genomic action (see Section V.B.2.a).

3. Progesterone Metabolism

The central action of progesterone can also be modulated by the intracellular metabolism of the steroid at the level of its target organs, as described for testosterone. In fact, several of the enzymes (e.g., the 5α- and 5β-reductases) that metabolize testosterone are not absolutely substrate-specific and are able to catalyze the same reactions with progesterone as a substrate. In mammals, it is established that in the hypothalamus and other brain areas, progesterone (or 4-pregnene-3,20-dione) can be enzymatically transformed into a

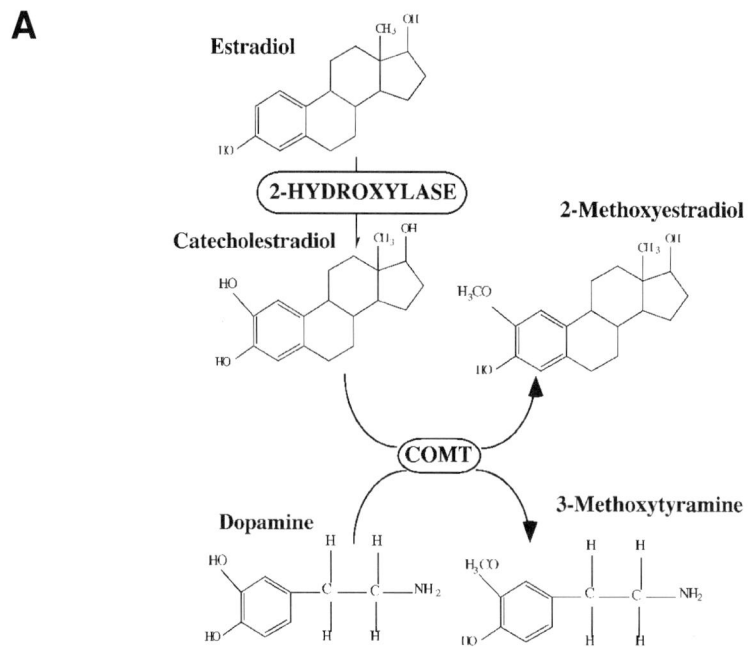
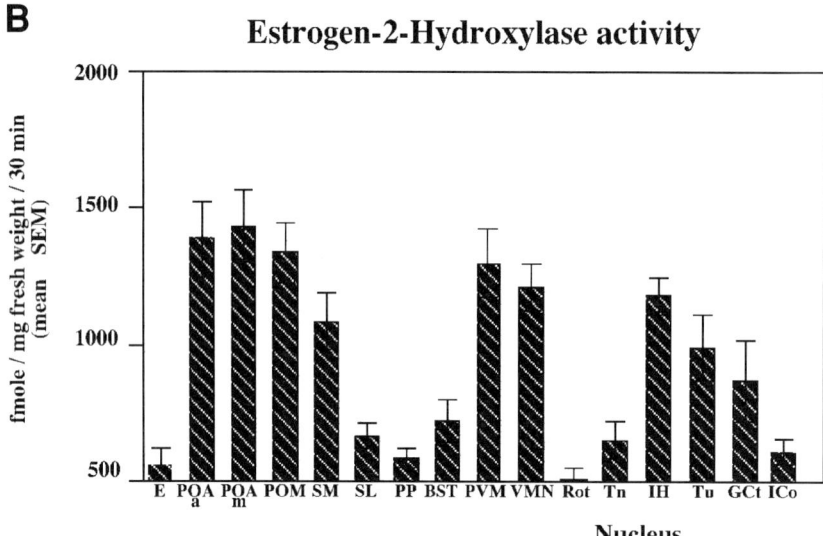

FIGURE 11 Potential interactions of estrogens and dopamine in the control of behavior and distribution of the estrogen-2-hydroxylase activity in the brain of male Japanese quail. (A) Hypothetical model describing possible interactions between catecholestrogens formed by 2- or 4-hydroxylation of estrogens and dopamine. Both substrates compete for the catabolizing enzyme, catechol-O-methyl transferase (COMT) so that an increase in catecholestrogen concentration should lead to an inhibition of the catabolism of dopamine by the COMT, resulting in increased dopaminergic activity. (B) Distribution of the 2-hydroxylase activity in the male quail brain. High levels of activity are specifically present in brain nuclei that also contain high levels of aromatase activity, which indirectly supports the idea that both enzymatic activities are catalyzed by the same protein. BST, bed nucleus of the stria terminalis; E, ectostriatum; GCt, substantia grisea centralis; ICo, nucleus intercollicularis; IH, nucleus inferioris hypothalami; POAa, anterior part of the preoptic area; POAm, medial part of the preoptic area; POM, nucleus preopticus medialis; PP, paleostriatum primitivum; PVM, nucleus paraventricularis magnocellularis; Rot, nucleus rotundus; SL, nucleus septalis lateralis; SM, nucleus septalis medialis; Tn, nucleus taeniae; Tu, tuber; VMN, nucleus ventromedialis hypothalami. Data from Balthazart et al. (1994b).

number of other progestins including 5α-pregnane-3,20 dione or 5α-dihydroprogesterone (5α reduction), 3α-hydroxy-5α-pregnane-20-one (5α,3α-ol), 5α-pregnane-3α,20α-diol (5α-diol), and 20α-hydroxy-4-pregnane-3-one or 20α-dihydroprogesterone (20α-DHP; see Karavolas et al., 1984). These different progestins bind with quite different affinities to the progestin receptor in the brain (Karavolas et al., 1984), so that they can be expected to have very different potencies and properties. Accordingly, functional studies have shown that in mammals these compounds have differential effects on the control of gonadotropin secretion and on the activation of female sexual receptivity (Czaja et al., 1974; Stupnicka et al., 1977; Zanisi et al., 1984).

In birds, only a few studies have been devoted to the brain metabolism of progesterone and its biological significance. Nakamura and Tanabe (1974) confirmed that the chicken brain is able to convert radioactive progesterone into 5α-DHP and 5α,3α-ol. In addition, Sharp and Massa (1980) demonstrated that, as was expected based on studies of testosterone metabolism, the avian brain also produces large amounts of 5β-pregnanes (progestins reduced in 5β position), such as 5β-pregnane-3,20-dione (5β-dihydroprogesterone, 5β-DHP) and 3α-hydroxy-5β-pregnane-20-one (5β,3α-ol). The avian brain is indeed known to metabolize testosterone extensively into compounds of the 5β-androstane series (Balthazart, 1983, 1989) and as previously indicated the enzyme catalyzing this reaction (5β-reductase) only shows a limited specificity and can use both testosterone and progesterone as substrates.

In one study, the progesterone metabolism was analyzed in five areas of the chicken brain obtained by microdissection from the telencephalon (part of the lobus parolfactorius immediately rostral to the POA), the POA, and the hypothalamus. Three metabolites of progesterone were produced in large amounts and were quantified in this study—5β-DHP, its metabolite 5β,3α-ol, and 5α-DHP. The 5β reduction of progesterone was very active, but its 5α reduction was almost undetectable in the lobus parolfactorius. In contrast, an opposite ratio of metabolites (high 5α- but low 5β-reductase activities) was observed throughout the POA and hypothalamus. Significant changes in the activity of these enzymes were also detected as birds stopped egg-laying and started molting, suggesting that this metabolism may have a functional significance (see Balthazart et al., 1988b, for a more detailed description of these data and their functional interpretation). Much work remains to be done to fully understand the behavioral relevance of progesterone metabolism in the avian brain.

IV. NEUROENDOCRINE MECHANISMS MEDIATING THE TRANSDUCTION OF ENVIRONMENTAL INFORMATION

A. Photoperiod

The focus of this section is on reproductive neuroendocrinology given that seasonal variation in reproductive function is the most commonly measured variable in studies of the biology of seasonality in birds. The structure and function of the avian reproductive neuroendocrine system is generally similar to that described, in somewhat more detail, in mammalian and other vertebrate species (Murton and Westwood, 1975; Oksche, 1983; Follett, 1984). Environmental stimuli such as photoperiodic information are processed by various sensory inputs that terminate in the brain. This information must be interpreted and some sort of physiological decision made about the significance of the stimulus. For photoperiodic information, the system is able to measure the length of the photoperiod using a circadian clock of some sort and then interpret its significance based on the previous photoperiodic history the bird has experienced. In other words, as we have seen in previous sections of this review, a short photoperiod of 8L:16D is interpreted very differently if it follows 3–4 weeks of similar photoperiods or 3–4 weeks of much longer photoperiods. Based on this complex interpretation of the significance of a particular photoperiod, a physiological decision is made that results in the stimulation or inhibition of the GnRH neuronal system present in the preoptic region and the hypothalamus. These neurons project to the median eminence, where they release GnRH into the portal blood system and in turn regulate the synthesis and release of the gonadotropins, LH, and FSH, which are synthesized and secreted from the gonadotropes present in the anterior pituitary gland. The gonadotropins then regulate spermatogenesis and steroidogenesis in the gonads (Scanes,

2000). These features of the avian reproductive neuroendocrine system are similar in many respects to the generalized pattern observed in all vertebrate species. We focus here on several important features of this system that are unique to birds.

1. Extraretinal Photoreceptor in Birds

One of the most unusual features of the photoperiodic response in birds, compared to mammals, is that the sensory receptor mediating the response to photoperiod is not in the retina but rather is located in the hypothalamic region of the brain. It was first suggested in the 1930s in ducks (Benoit, 1935) that the photoinduction of gonadal growth in birds did not require the eyes. This was subsequently confirmed in several songbird species such as the white-crowned sparrow and the house sparrow (e.g., McMillan et al., 1975; Yokoyama et al., 1978). Thorough studies by Wilson (1989, 1991) of tree sparrows have led to the conclusive demonstration that neither the eyes nor the pineal gland are needed for the stimulation of gonadal growth by long days, the onset of photorefractoriness in response to long days, or the breaking of refractoriness in response to short days. The exact location of this encephalic photoreceptor remains a mystery. Various studies that compare the different areas of the brain in which the discrete presentation of illumination is effective or ineffective in inducing photostimulation point to the basal hypothalamus and the tuberal hypothalamus as being critical sites mediating the photoperiodic response in birds (see Oliver and Baylé, 1982, for review). An action spectrum for the photoperiodic response in Japanese quail was established by Foster et al. (1985) and indicated that the photopigment mediating the response to photoperiod is very similar to rhodopsin. Immunohistochemical studies revealed opsin-like immunoreactivity in the septum and the tuberal area of the hypothalamus in ring dove, suggesting possible sites for the location of the receptor (Silver et al., 1988). Similar staining that localizes immunoreactive opsin in the septum and tuberal hypothalamus has now been reported in songbird species, including starlings (Saldanha et al., 1994b). The existence of rhodopsin gene expression in the lateral septum of pigeons (Wada et al., 1998) and of various phototransduction molecules (Wada et al., 2000) is consistent with the importance of the septum in this response.

There is strong evidence that the tuberal hypothalamus is at least involved in the transduction of the light signal in quail, whether or not the photoreceptors are located there. Meddle and Follett (1995) demonstrated that rapid and transient activation of the immediate early gene *c-fos* occurred in the quail tuberal hypothalamus soon after photostimulation, and was followed by a rapid rise in plasma LH. Thus, it appears that, in birds, light must pass through the skull and into the hypothalamus for transduction of its signal to occur.

2. Suprachiasmatic Nucleus and the Site of the Biological Clock in Birds

The pineal gland, the eyes, and the hypothalamic suprachiasmatic nucleus (SCN) have all been suggested as sites for the avian biological clock (Cassone and Menaker, 1985). However, in contrast to the situation in mammals, most data suggest a minor role for the pineal gland in the mediation of photoperiodic effects in birds (Follett, 1984; Gwinner, 1986). Also, as noted previously, it has been shown in several avian species that the eyes are not necessary for the exhibition of photoperiodic responses (Follett, 1984; Underwood et al., 1984); neither is the pineal (Wilson, 1991). In mammals it is now clear that the SCN in the hypothalamus is the site of the biological clock involved in photoperiodic time measurement. Many lines of evidence support this assertion, the best being that lesions to this nucleus disrupt responses to photoperiod and that cells in this nucleus rhythmically express genes known to be involved in the regulation of the clock.

Initial studies of the avian circadian system were directed at a medial hypothalamic nucleus lying in the same region as the mammalian SCN (overlying the optic chiasm and adjacent to the third ventricle). The results in quail (Simpson and Follett, 1981), house sparrows (*Passer domesticus*; Takahashi and Menaker, 1982), and Java sparrows (*Padda orzyivora*; Ebihara and Kawamura, 1981) suggested that lesions of this nucleus resulted in the loss of locomotor rhythmicity, but did not disrupt photoperiodic responses (Simpson and Follett, 1981). However, at least in the case of house sparrows, the hypothalamic lesions were large and resulted in a decrease in overall activity level (Takahashi and Menaker,

1982), raising the possibility that the effects were not specific.

One feature of the mammalian SCN is direct input from the retina (Moore, 1973). A clue to the location of the SCN in birds might be to identify the retinorecipient nucleus. The application of sensitive tract-tracing techniques in a number of avian species has identified a retinorecipient region in the lateral hypothalamus in many avian species (Norgren and Silver, 1989) that is sometime referred to as the visual SCN. Only one behavioral study has been directed specifically to this nucleus. Lesions of the lateral hypothalamic retinorecipient nucleus do not affect circadian rhythmicity in pigeons (Ebihara et al., 1987). It is possible that the large hypothalamic lesions of Takahashi and Menaker (1982) in house sparrow included this region. It has been reported that the medial nucleus exhibits the rhythmic expression of the clock gene *Per* and that this expression is regulated by light; no such regulated expression was observed in the visual SCN (Yoshimura et al., 2000). These data strongly indicate that the medial nucleus referred to as the SCN in birds is the site of the biological clock.

3. Steroid Hormone Feedback Effects Are Not Involved in Regulating Response to Photoperiod in Birds

In species such as the European starling, the entire photoperiodic cycle, including changes from photosensitivity to photorefractoriness, can be readily detected in castrated birds using changes in plasma levels of the pituitary gonadotropin hormone LH as the dependent variable indicative of reproductive condition (Dawson and Goldsmith, 1984). There is also evidence in several avian species that the ability of the pituitary gland to respond to stimulation by the hypothalamic-releasing hormone GnRH does not change seasonally or at least does not change in a dramatic fashion (e.g., Balthazart et al., 1980c; Wingfield et al., 1979; Storey and Nicholls, 1983). Because of these findings, several investigators have argued that the major physiological changes that are involved in the various transitions during the reproductive cycle from photosensitivity to photorefractoriness occur in the brain and do not involve changes in steroid feedback sensitivity in the hypothalamic-pituitary-gonadal axis (Nicholls et al., 1988b).

In relation to the photoinduction of gonadal growth, this idea has been most rigorously tested by Wilson (1985a) in the tree sparrow. He developed an experimental paradigm that distinguishes the T feedback-dependent from feedback-independent effects of photostimulation on LH secretion. In castrated tree sparrows, LH levels are much higher in long-day-stimulated birds than in photosensitive birds on short days. First Wilson (1985a) tested whether the administration of an antiandrogen to castrated birds, on long days and short days, increased LH, hypothesizing that castration-resistant androgens may still suppress LH levels. No increase in LH was observed, indicating that the gonadostimulatory effects of long days are at least in part independent of changes in sensitivity to T feedback. In a second series of studies, Wilson (1985a) tested both the minimum concentration of T that is required to suppress LH in castrated birds during the course of photostimulation (the setpoint) and the degree to which a unit of plasma LH changes per unit change in exogenously administered T (the sensitivity of LH to T feedback). From these studies, Wilson (1985a) concluded that long day lengths do reduce the inhibitory effect on LH by increasing the setpoint and decreasing the sensitivity of the T feedback mechanism. Wilson and Donham (1988) have therefore argued that, at the physiological level, the initiation of reproduction in photosensitive birds in response to photostimulation involves both an increase in the photoperiodic drive of gonadotropin secretion by the hypothalamus and, at least in certain species such as the tree sparrow, a photoperiodic reduction in the working of androgen negative feedback on gonadotropin activity.

However, the possible importance of changes in androgen feedback varies among species (Wilson and Donham, 1988), and even in tree sparrows it is undeniably true that the effects of photosensitivity followed by photostimulation involves predominantly a striking change in the drive that the hypothalamus puts on the pituitary gland. In contrast to the onset of photosensitivity, it is generally agreed that the onset of photorefractoriness in birds involves a shut-off of the hypothalamic stimulation of the pituitary and does not involve changes in steroid feedback (Nicholls et al., 1988a,b; Wilson and Donham, 1988). The main evidence supporting this fact is that the long-day induction of photorefractoriness can occur in castrated birds, thus indicating that the state of photorefractoriness is initiated and maintained by T-independent processes (Nicholls et al., 1988b; Wilson and Donham, 1988). Furthermore, as demonstrated in tree sparrows by Wilson (1985b), LH levels in castrated photorefractory tree sparrows were not affected by T replacement nor did the administration of antiandrogens have any effect on plasma LH levels.

4. Roles of Prolactin and Thyroid Hormones in Regulating Photoperiodic Responses in Birds

The onset of photorefractoriness may be the result of an inhibition of GnRH activity signaled by a change in hormone secretion. Such a hormonal signal could act directly on the GnRH neuronal system or act through intermediate agents. As reviewed by Nicholls et al. (1988b), prolactin secretion increases in many species of birds in close temporal association with the onset of photorefractoriness. There is also evidence that there are high densities of prolactin receptors in the brain areas containing GnRH perikarya and terminals in doves and starlings (Buntin and Ruzycki, 1987). It seems that the increased levels of prolactin are the result of the onset of refractoriness rather than the cause (Nicholls et al., 1988b). For example, Goldsmith and Follett (1987) found that the endogenous administration of prolactin or experimentally induced increases in exogenous prolactin could suppress reproductive activity in photosensitive starlings, but that the gonads regrew once the treatment ended. Similarly, intracerebroventricular infusion of prolactin has been found to be potently gonadoinhibitory, but it does not induce photorefractoriness in starlings (Juss and Goldsmith, 1992). Vasoactive intestinal polypeptide (VIP) is the neuropeptide secreted into the portal system that stimulates the release of prolactin in birds (Macnamee et al., 1986; Mauro et al., 1992; Saldanha et al., 1994a; Youngren et al., 1994; El Halawani et al., 1995; Sun and El Halawani, 1995). The immunization of starlings against VIP prevents prolactin release, but does not prevent the onset of photorefractoriness (Dawson and Sharp, 1998). This experiment provides perhaps the best evidence suggesting that seasonal increases in prolactin concentrations in the plasma are simply temporally related to the onset of photorefractoriness, but do not have a causal role.

Hormones secreted by the thyroid gland are more likely candidates to serve as the factors that may regulate GnRH activity in the context of seasonality. It was first demonstrated in 1972 that the thyroid is required for the onset of refractoriness in starlings (Wieselthier and Van Tienhoven, 1972). Similar findings have subsequently been reported for other avian species (Nicholls et al., 1988b). Experimental work in starlings has demonstrated that exogenous thyroxine treatment can block the onset of photosensitivity in photorefractory starlings on short days, including the associated changes in hypothalamic GnRH content (Boulakoud et al., 1991) and that, similarly, in photosensitive birds exogenous thyroxine can induce a decline in GnRH content characteristic of the photorefractory state (Boulakoud and Goldsmith, 1991). These studies involved the administration of pharmacological doses of thyroxine. Is there any evidence that endogenous thyroxine levels regulate physiological responses to photoperiod?

Plasma thyroxin concentrations increase when starlings, quail, or tree sparrows are transferred from short to long days (Dawson, 1984; Sharp and Klandorf, 1981; Reinert and Wilson, 1996; Bentley et al., 1997). Despite the long-day-induced rise in plasma thyroxin concentrations, the best explanation of the available data is that thyroid hormones have a permissive role in the termination of the breeding season of starlings (Bentley et al., 1997), as they do in sheep (Dahl et al., 1995; Thrun et al., 1996, 1997). Thyroxine seems to be acting as a permissive factor for the onset of photorefractoriness in starlings, in that it must be present in the circulation in at least minimal physiological concentrations to terminate breeding. However, when thyroxine is present in physiological concentrations it is not the rate-limiting factor in the onset of photorefractoriness. In this way thyroxine can be envisaged as a link in the chain of events that begins with the perception and transduction of a long-day signal and ends with gonadal regression and change in reproductive state. Data suggest that thyroid hormones may be permissive, in the sense that they allow the production of thyroid-dependent neurotrophins that are involved in the neuronal plasticity that is so characteristic of photorefractoriness in birds (Bentley et al., 1997). It is now necessary to identify the neural sites of thyroid hormone action that generate these effects. These receptor sites may provide insights into the neural circuits that modulate GnRH activity in the context of seasonal breeding.

5. High Nocturnal Concentrations of Melatonin Code for Day Length in Birds, but Do Not Mediate Physiological Responses to Photoperiod

One of the more puzzling aspects of the neuroendocrine responses of birds to photoperiod is the fact that melatonin rhythms seem to play little or no role in mediating these reponses. Birds, like other vertebrate species, clearly possess a pineal melatonin transducer of photic information (Gwinner and Hau, 2000). Melatonin is high during the dark phase of the circadian cycle and therefore provides a code for night length. However, birds do not seem to use seasonal variation in melatonin rhythms to regulate responses to photoperiod, as seasonally breeding mammalian species clearly do. Numerous attempts to demonstrate an effect of pinealectomy on reproduction in birds have failed (Gwinner and Hau, 2000). The avian retina, however, is also a source of melatonin (Underwood et al., 1984). Wilson combined pinealectomy with ocular enucleation in American tree sparrows and found that the complete reproductive cycle was unaffected (Wilson, 1991). It is still possible, however, even in this study, that the circadian melatonin signal was not completely abolished. In Japanese quail, for example, the eyes contribute 33% of circulating melatonin and the pineal contributes 54%, leaving 13% unaccounted for (Underwood et al., 1984). Experiments were also performed on Japanese quail that involved the exogenous injection of melatonin so that relatively long days that would normally stimulate gonadal growth were associated with melatonin patterns indicative of short days. Such an experimental regimen is effective in blocking photostimulation in hamsters, but it failed to block reproductive stimulation in quail, supporting the contention that, unlike mammals, birds do not read the duration of the melatonin signal to measure the dark phase of the circadian cycle (Juss et al., 1993).

B. Visual and Auditory Sensory Inputs on the Reproductive Axis

As reviewed in Section V, it is clear that social stimuli mediated by the visual and auditory systems have dramatic effects on the reproductive neuroendocrine axis in birds. They also obviously control, on a shorter-term basis, the expression of reproductive behaviors. There are many unanswered questions about the neural mechanisms regulating these social effects on endocrine physiology and behavior. However, studies using the immediate-early-gene technique to identify brain areas expressing genes in response to a particular stimulus have been very useful. We review some of these studies in which brain areas expressing immediate early genes in response to social stimuli known to influence endocrine secretions have been studied. We also discuss some lesion and tract-tracing studies that provide insight into the neural pathways that might influence how these stimuli regulate the hypothalamic-hypophyseal-gonadal axis.

1. Induction by Sexual Behavior of the Immediate Early Genes ZENK and fos

The identification of a sexually dimorphic nucleus in the POA of Japanese quail led to major advances in our understanding of the neuroendocrine controls of male sexual behavior (see Section V.B.1). The POM in this species is larger in males than in females (Viglietti-Panzica et al., 1986). Its volume regresses after castration and is restored to values observed in sexually mature males by a 2-week treatment with testosterone (Panzica et al., 1987, 1991). When ovariectomized female quail are treated with testosterone, they develop a POM that is as large as the POM of males (Panzica et al., 1987, 1991), suggesting that the volume difference observed in intact birds only reflects the higher circulating testosterone levels in males (i.e., an activational, but not an organizational, sex difference). The endocrine regulation of the POM volume therefore differs from that of sexually dimorphic brain areas in the preoptic region in other species, such as the rat sexually dimorphic nucleus (Arnold and Gorski, 1984; Tobet and Fox, 1992; Gorski, 1987).

Subsequent experiments revealed that the POM is a necessary and sufficient site of testosterone action for the activation of both the appetitive and consummatory components of male-typical behavior (see Section V). Testosterone action in the POM of castrated males is sufficient to activate sexual responses when suitable stimuli are present. This, however, does not exclude steroids acting in other brain sites to promote behavior expression. Several techniques have been used to investigate these other areas that are involved in the expression of male behavior in response to adequate visual or auditory stimuli.

a) Studies Using Immediate Early Genes In mammals, the detection of immediate early genes (IEGs) (e.g., *c-fos*) has provided an alternative powerful technique to identify brain areas that are activated during the performance of specific behaviors. For example, in gonadally intact male rats sacrificed 1 hour after copulation, significant increases in *fos* immunoreactivity were observed in the medial amygdala, BST, central tegmental field, and medial POA (Robertson *et al.*, 1991; Baum and Everitt, 1992; Baum and Wersinger, 1993; Wersinger *et al.*, 1993; Coolen *et al.*, 1996, 1997). All these brain regions had previously been associated with the display of male sexual behavior in rodents through lesion, electrical stimulation, and steroid implantation studies (Meisel and Sachs, 1994).

i) Fos. An antibody has become available that allows Fos detection in the avian brain (Sharp *et al.*, 1995) and Fos immunocytochemistry was therefore used as an independent tool to identify brain areas implicated in the control of copulatory behavior in male quail (Meddle *et al.*, 1997). Male Japanese quail were allowed to interact freely with adult females and the presence of active sexual behavior, including cloacal contact movements, was confirmed in each case. Control subjects were exposed to a domestic chick (same size as an adult quail) and no sexual behavior was observed. Copulation induced the appearance of Fos immunoreactive cells in the POA, hyperstriatum ventrale, parts of the archistriatum, and ICo. The induction of Fos was observed throughout the rostral to caudal extent of the preoptic region of males from the level of the tractus septomesencephalicus to the level of the anterior commissure, and in the rostral part of the hypothalamus to the level of the supraoptic decussation (Fig. 12). These immunoreactive cells did not lie directly adjacent to the third ventricle, but were located 500–1000 μm from the ventricle wall at the level of the lateral edge of the POM or, in more caudal sections, in a position ventrolateral to the BST. It is unlikely that the Fos induction in males resulted from copulation-induced endocrine changes because copulation did not affect plasma levels of LH or testosterone. It was therefore concluded that the responses were due to copulation-associated somatosensory inputs or to stimuli originating from the female. It is, however, quite interesting to observe that previous studies of mammals had identified a Fos induction after copulation in brain circuits that appears to be specifically activated by genital (penile)-somatosensory or by olfactory-vomeronasal stimuli. Such inputs should play little or no role in birds that have no intromittent organ and in which olfaction is supposed to play little or no role in the control of sexual behavior. A differential Fos expression had therefore been expected, but in fact copulation induced in the quail brain a pattern of Fos expression that is superficially quite similar to what had been observed in rats. The Fos induction in the POA and BST of quail was, however, more restricted and concerned more lateral aspects of these areas than in rats. In particular, Fos induction in the POA did not concern cells that express aromatase, indicating that mating-related stimuli do not affect directly the estrogen-synthesizing neurons (Foidart *et al.*, 1999b). These localized differences in Fos induction also may reflect species differences in the use of olfactory cues or in the nature of the somatosensory feedback that are experienced during sexual interactions.

Interestingly, the induction of Fos expression was also observed in several brain areas such as the ventral hypertsriatum, medial archistriatum, and BST in males that were allowed to express appetitive sexual behavior (watching a female through a narrow window; see section on ZENK, next, and Section V.B.1.b), but were not allowed to copulate (Tlemçani *et al.*, 2000). The data therefore clearly indicate that the IEG expression is not related solely to the control of the copulatory act, but also is related to the processing in a variety of telencephalic association areas of stimuli originating from the female.

ii) ZENK. During additional studies designed to identify brain areas involved in the regulation of male appetitive and consummatory sexual behavior, cells immunoreactive for the protein encoded by another IEG, *ZENK,* were also mapped (Ball *et al.*, 1997). The ZENK protein (also known as egr-1 in mammals) is a zinc finger transcriptional regulator. Castrated male quail chronically treated with testosterone were trained during 12 sessions in a two-chamber test cage to acquire a social proximity response that provides a measure of appetitive sexual behavior. In this procedure, males learn to stay close to, and observe through a window, a female that is later released and allowed to interact freely with the male, which can then express consummatory sexual behavior. Control birds receive a similar training

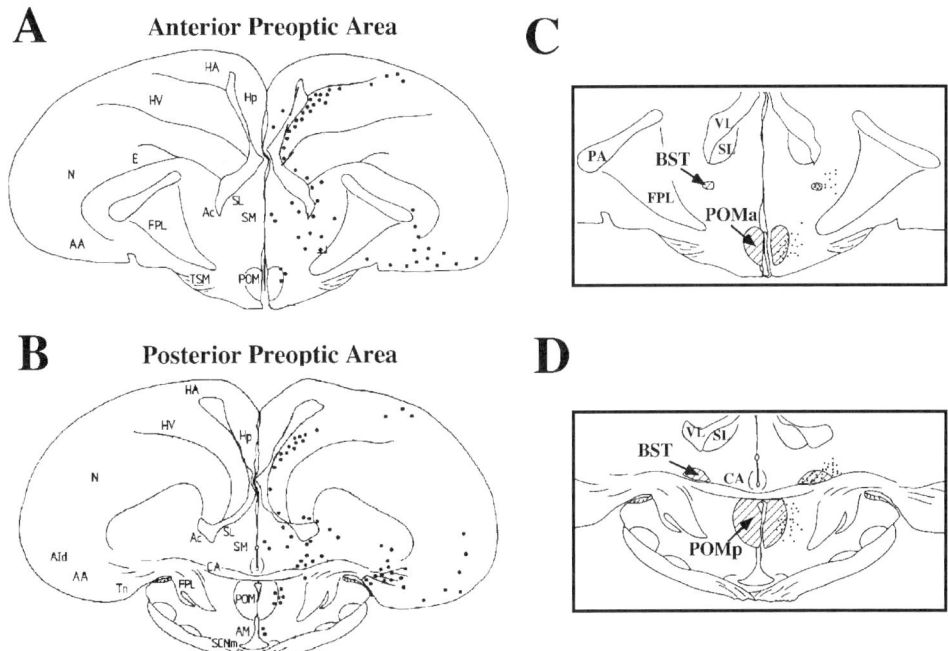

FIGURE 12 (A–B) Schematic drawings of coronal sections in the male quail preoptic area—(A) rostral; (B) caudal—illustrating the anatomical localization of Fos-like immunoreactive immunoreactive cells (dots) that were detected in subjects sacrificed after they had the opportunity to copulate with a sexually mature female quail. (C–D) Schematic representation of distribution of Fos-ir cells in relation with ARO-ir cell groups in the male quail preoptic area. The black dots illustrate the distribution of Fos-ir perikarya and the striped areas represent the two nuclei identified by the presence of dense clusters of ARO-ir cells, namely the POM and BST. AA, archistriatum anterior; Ac, nucleus accumbens; AId, archistriatum intermedium, pars dorsalis; AM, nucleus anterior medialis hypothalami; BST, bed nucleus striae terminalis; CA, commissura anterior; E, ectostriatum; FPL, fasciculus prosencephali lateralis (lateral forebrain bundle); HA, hyperstriatum accessorium; Hp, hippocampus; HV, hyperstriatum ventrale; N, neostriatum; PA, paleostriatum augmentatum; POM, nucleus preopticus medialis; SCNm, nucleus suprachiasmaticus, pars medialis; SL, nucleus septalis lateralis; SM, nucleus septalis medialis; Tn, nucleus taeniae; TSM, tractus septomesencephalicus; VL, ventriculus lateralis. Data from Meddle et al. (1997); Foidart et al. (1999b).

in the chamber, but without being provided free access to a female so that the proximity response was not acquired (Balthazart et al., 1995). After 12 training sessions, males were either allowed to freely copulate with a female in the test cage for 45 min (consummatory sexual behavior group) or allowed to watch a female through the window for 45 min (appetitive sexual behavior group). Control males either remained in their home cage or were placed in the chamber and did not exhibit the proximity response. Birds were then perfused and the ZENK protein was visualized by a standard immunocytochemical procedure employing a polyclonal antibody (Santa Cruz Biotech, Inc) that recognizes a portion of the egr-1 peptide sequence similar in both birds and mammals. Copulatory activity markedly increased the number of ZENK-ir cells in the BST both in the subdivision dorsal to the anterior commissure and at a more caudal level where this structures forms a characteristic V-shape structure. Increases in ZENK-ir cell numbers observed in this area after the expression of appetitive sexual behavior were not statistically significant. By contrast, ZENK-ir cell numbers in the ICo increased in males in all groups placed in the test chamber. These data indicate that induction of the ZENK protein occurs in behavioral contexts related to reproductive behavior; whether this results only from the performance of these behaviors or whether this induction is related to components of these behaviors that involve learning and reward, as has been suggested in other species, is unknown.

b) Measures of 2-Deoxyglucose Uptake The measure by quantitative autoradiography of the $[^{14}C]$-2-deoxyglucose (2-DG) incorporation was also used to investigate the brain circuits functionally involved in the appetitive and consummatory aspects of male sexual behavior of quail (Dermon et al., 1997). As in the experiments already described, castrated male quail chronically treated with testosterone were trained during 12 sessions in a two-chamber test cage to acquire a social proximity response used to measure appetitive sexual behavior. Control birds were trained in the same procedure without physical access to the female and did not learn the social proximity response. Males were then injected IP with 100 μCi/kg of 2-DG and either allowed to freely copulate with a female in the test cage for 45 min (consummatory sexual behavior group) or allowed to watch the female through the window for 45 min (appetitive sexual behavior group). The control group was placed in the test cage for 45 min, as during the training procedure. Brains were processed for autoradiography and 2-DG accumulation was measured by quantitative image analysis. The expression of sexual behaviors modified the 2-DG incorporation in 12 different brain areas. In the consummatory sexual behavior group, 2-DG accumulation was increased compared to controls in the rostral POA, paleostriatum primitivum, nucleus interpeduncularis, ICo, nucleus mesencephalicus lateralis pars dorsalis, nervus oculomotorius, and nucleus lemnisci lateralis, but decreased in the medial part of the hippocampus, tuberculum olfactorium, and nucleus nervi oculomotorii. A different pattern of results was observed in the appetitive sexual behavior group, which showed an increased 2-DG accumulation compared to controls in the hyperstriatum ventrale, neostriatum caudale pars dorsolateralis, nucleus mesencephalicus lateralis pars dorsalis, and nucleus lemnisci lateralis, but a decrease of 2-DG uptake in the tuberculum olfactorium. Local metabolism was similarly affected by the expression of appetitive sexual behavior and consummatory sexual behavior in a few brain areas (nucleus mesencephalicus lateralis pars dorsalis, nucleus lemnisci lateralis, and tuberculum olfactorium), but specific changes appeared to be associated with the expression of appetitive sexual behavior (forebrain associative areas) and consummatory sexual behavior (motor-related and sexually dimorphic areas).

c) Tract-Tracing Studies Illustrating the Connectivity of the Medial Preoptic Nucleus and Bed Nucleus of the Striae Terminalis A full understanding of the mechanism underlying male sexual activity requires the identification of the neural circuitry linked to this behavior and, in particular, of the afferents and efferents of the POM. As a first step in this research, *in vitro* tracing studies with the lipophilic fluorescent tracer DiI demonstrated a number of bidirectional connections between the POM and several hypothalamic and thalamic nuclei, including the nucleus dorsolateralis anterior thalami (Balthazart et al., 1994a).

DiI implantation in aldehyde-fixed tissue demonstrated anterograde projections from the POM to the tuberal hypothalamus, the area ventralis of Tsai, and GCt. Dense networks of fluorescent fibers were also seen in several hypothalamic nuclei, such as the anterior medialis hypothalami, the paraventricularis magnocellularis, and the VMN. A major projection in the dorsal direction was also observed from the POM toward the nucleus septalis lateralis and medialis.

Fluorescent cells were seen in all these areas, demonstrating that the POM receives afferent projections from all these regions. The implantation of DiI into the GCt also revealed massive bidirectional connections with a large number of more caudal mesencephalic and pontine structures. The GCt therefore appears to be an important center connecting anterior levels of the brain to brain-stem nuclei that may be involved in the control of male copulatory behavior. Most of these bidirectional projections could be confirmed by implanting DiI in the identified targets of POM and observing the fluorescent label in POM (cells or fibers) (Balthazart et al., 1994a). After the implantation of DiI in the POM, fluorescent fibers (but no fluorescent cells) were seen in the ICo, suggesting the presence of a unidirectional pathway connecting the POM to ICo. However, no experiment has so far confirmed the existence of this connection by applying a retrograde tracer in ICo.

In vitro tracing with DiI has technical limitations and, in particular, this procedure does not easily identify long-distance projections. Therefore, additional studies were carried out with the tracer cholera toxin B-subunit (CTB) or with red fluorescent latex beads in order to obtain more information on more distant connections of the POM and of the other group of ARO-ir cells centered on the BST (Balthazart and Absil, 1997). This technique confirmed all the connections of the POM that had been identified with DiI. Retrograde-labeled cells were seen, namely in the telencephalon (hippocampus, septum, and archistriatum), hypothalamus (many areas in periventricular position), thalamus, mesencephalon, and pons. CTB tracing confirmed that most of these connections are bidirectional. In addition, a strong input from the rostral part of the Tn to the POM was identified. Furthermore, a large number of retrograde-labeled cells were seen in the major catecholaminergic cell groups, including dopaminergic areas such as the retroruberal field, substantia nigra (SN), and area ventralis of Tsai, and noradrenergic cell groups such as the locus ceruleus and subceruleus (see later).

A significant number of brain areas were identified that appear to project both to the POM and the BST. A number of quantitative differences were, however, observed. Compared to the POM, BST injections of tracer labeled a smaller number of neurons in the septal area and in periventricular position throughout the rostral to caudal extent of the hypothalamus. Many neurons in the VMN were, for example, filled with tracer after injection in the POM, but this nucleus was completely devoid of retrogradely transported tracer after injection into the BST. In contrast, injections of tracer into the BST labeled more cells in the neostriatum, archistriatum, area ventralis of Tsai, SN, locus ceruleus, and subceruleus region than injections into the POM.

Taken together, these data indicate that a large number of brain areas are connected to the POM and activated during the expression of appetitive or consummatory aspects of male sexual behavior. These areas are therefore likely to be involved in the activation of behavior. None of these areas receive, to our knowledge, direct afferent inputs coming from the eyes or ears, but these stimuli could affect behavior by indirect pathways.

The social life of quail, like that of many other avian species, is organized mainly by visual and acoustic cues; olfactory and tactile stimuli are usually considered to play only a minor role (Hinde, 1965; Lehrman, 1965). Based on the tracing studies, two types of sensory information should be able to reach the POM—a steroid-sensitive structure that plays a key role in the integration and activation of male sexual behavior (see Section V.B.1; Fig. 13). The projection from the nucleus dorsolateralis anterior thalami (DLA) to POM appears to have a particular relevance for the processing of visual information. The DLA is a part of the geniculate complex that receives direct retinal input (Breazile and Kuenzel, 1993; Güntürkün, 1991; Güntürkün et al., 1993) and contains a high density of melatonin receptors (Cozzi et al., 1993; Panzica et al., 1994). Therefore, primary visual information could potentially reach the POM through this pathway. Moreover, the cerebrospinal-fluid- (CSF)-contacting neurons of the lateral septal organ and of the tuberal region are frequently considered to be extraretinal photoreceptors (Silver et al., 1988; Silver and Ramos, 1990). These two regions send dense inputs to the POM and these connections could also relay information about the environmental level of light to the dimorphic nucleus. Information about environmental light can therefore reach the POM through different routes—retinal input through DLA or deep photoreceptors through septal region and tuberal hypothalamus.

We do not know whether specific visual information about the mating partner reaches the dimorphic nucleus. The thalamofugal (Güntürkün, 1991; Güntürkün et al., 1993; Horn, 1985) or retinal-thalamic-hyperstriatal (Breazile and Kuenzel, 1993) pathway is connected to POM via nucleus DLA, but it is unlikely that the level of integration of the visual information in the geniculate complex (specifically, DLA) would permit the identification of the female as such. Projections to the POM, originating from telencephalic regions where the final processing of visual information takes place, would be requested for that purpose. A diffuse projection from the hyperstriatum accessorium (part of the visual Wulst) to the POM has been identified by retrograde tracing with CTB or with fluorescent microspheres (Balthazart and Absil, 1997). This connection could convey complex visual information, but more functional studies on the visual Wulst would be needed (Güntürkün, 1991; Güntürkün et al., 1993) and a better definition of its connection to the POM should be established by specific tract-tracing experiments before the significance of this anatomical relation can be established.

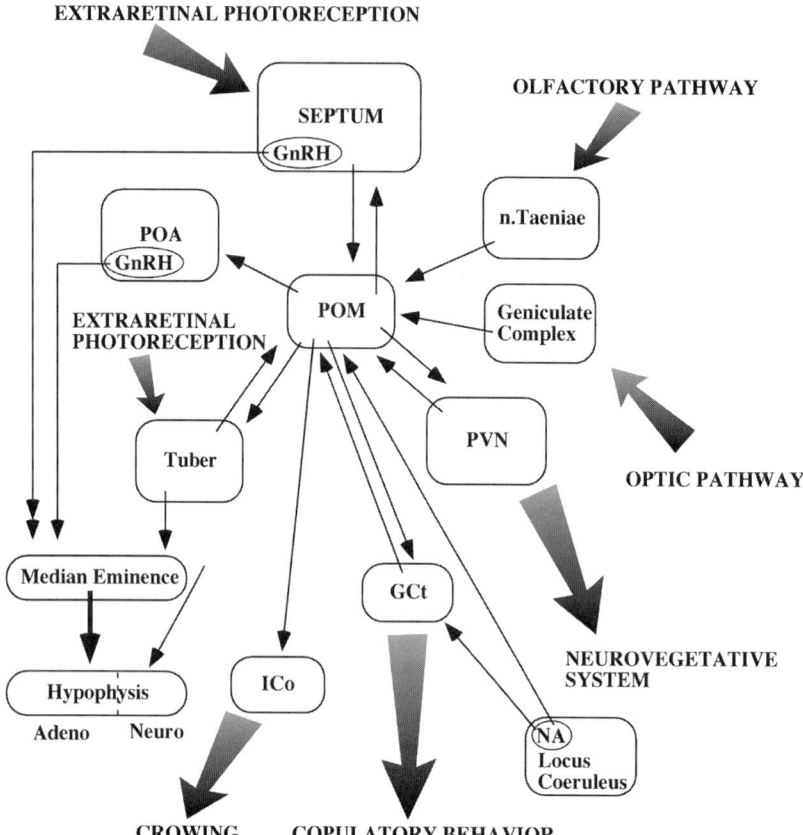

FIGURE 13 Schematic representation of the afferent and efferent connections of the quail medial preoptic nucleus (POM) and their probable functional significance. The figure illustrates the putative presence of visual and olfactory inputs and the outputs to neurovegetative centers, (the PVN) and to nuclei directly connected to the motor control (the GCt and ICo). Visual stimuli could indirectly reach the preoptic area via the thalamic geniculate complex. Light can also be perceived by extraretinal photoreceptors in the septal and tuberal regions. Light perceived in this way affects the activity of the hypothalamic-hypophyseal-gonadal axis, but no specific images (e.g., sexual partner) can be perceived and no direct effect on behavior is therefore possible. The olfactory signal could also potentially reach the POM and affect reproductive behavior via nucleus taeniae. Adapted fom Panzica et al. (1996b).

No direct auditory input to the POM of quail has been so far identified, but recall that visual cues provided by a taxidermic female model are sufficient to stimulate the appetitive and consummatory aspects of sexual behavior of male quail (Domjan and Nash, 1988). It is therefore plausible that auditory stimuli are not implicated in the direct control of male sexual behavior in this species. Cheng et al. (1998) have identified cells in the preoptic region that exhibit auditory responsiveness, especially in association with the presentation of the female's own nest-cooing.

In mammals, olfactory information derived mainly from the accessory olfactory system reaches the POA and appears to play a key role in the activation of male copulatory behavior. The path followed by this chemosensory information has been relatively well documented and includes the corticomedial amygdala and the BST (Segovia and Guillamón, 1993; Meisel and Sachs, 1994). In vivo tracing with CTB has revealed the presence in quail of an important projection from the archistriatum and in particular the Tn to the POM (Absil et al., 1994). The Tn is the avian holomog of parts the mammalian medial amygdala (Zeier and Karten, 1971; Nauta and Karten, 1970; Thompson *et al.*, 1998), which suggests that olfactory inputs could reach the POM of the quail. The importance of olfactory information in the control of behavior in birds is usually considered to be minimal, but a limited number of studies suggest that this widespread idea should perhaps be reconsidered and that the chemical information originating in the female could modulate aspects of the reproductive behavior (Wenzel, 1973; Balthazart and Schoffeniels, 1979). The projection from Tn to POM would then acquire a particular importance.

These studies establish that the POM potentially receives both visual and olfactory information. It must be stressed, however, that the amount of sensory information that reaches the nucleus through these pathways has not been experimentally determined and we do not know what type of cells in POM (e.g., steroid-sensitive or not) are connected to these inputs.

Complex outputs from the POM have also been identified. They namely reach the septum, the PVN and VMN, the tuberal region, the ICo, the GCt, and the area ventralis of Tsai. Most of these structures have been implicated directly or indirectly in the control of copulatory behavior in mammals (Meisel and Sachs, 1994). Many of these regions are also steroid-sensitive in quail (see Section III) and in mammals. They are presumably part of the nervous circuitry that controls copulation. In particular, the connection with the GCt is potentially of utmost importance here. This area is massively connected in a bidirectional way with a large number of more caudal mesencephalic and pontine structures (Balthazart *et al.*, 1994a), and therefore it appears to be an important center connecting anterior levels of the brain to brain-stem nuclei involved in the control of the complex motor output represented in male copulatory behavior. The POM projection to GCt originates primarily from ARO-ir cells, suggesting that these estrogen-producing neurons may play a direct role in the control of behavior (Absil *et al.*, 2001).

2. Song Induction of ZENK

Based on the work of David Clayton and colleagues, starting in the 1980s a number of genes expressed as mRNA in the songbird forebrain were cloned (reviewed in Clayton, 1997). No genes were found that were specific to brain areas involved in regulating song, but several recognized classes of IEG transcription factors were cloned in songbirds (Clayton, 1997). One IEG in particular, ZENK (Mello *et al.*, 1992), named so because it is homologous to genes cloned in other species (ZENK is an acronym for zif-268, egr-1, NGFI-A, krox-24), has been found to be regulated specifically in response to conspecific song in the songbird brain.

The initial observation is that the ZENK mRNA and protein are expressed at high levels relatively rapidly (i.e., in less than 1 hour) in the auditory telencephalon in response to conspecific song (Mello *et al.*, 1992; Mello and Ribeiro, 1998). This expression was especially high in areas of the auditory telencephalon, such as the caudal-medial neostriatum (NCM) and the caudal part of the vertical hyperstriatum (cHV), that had not been previously identified as areas specifically involved in song perception. It is also high in other areas such as the HVc shelf and the RA cup that were previously thought to receive auditory inputs specific to song. The ZENK response is specifically tuned to novel conspecific song. ZENK expression is basal in response to simple tones, but it is twice as high in response to conspecific as opposed to heterospecific song (Mello *et al.*, 1992). Furthermore, repeated presentations of the same conspecific song leads to a cessation of the ZENK response (i.e., habituation), whereas the response to a different conspecific song is still observed (Mello *et al.*, 1995). The ZENK response to song is dependent on early experience; zebra finches raised in social isolation do not exhibit this response (Jin and Clayton, 1997). It is also important to note that the ZENK response is not limited to the laboratory. The playback of song to free-living, wild song sparrows (*Melospiza melodia*) results in the induction of the ZENK mRNA of a magnitude and with a distribution in the brain that is similar to that observed in laboratory-housed zebra finches and canaries (Jarvis *et al.*, 1997).

The ZENK response is clearly coding for complex aspects of song. Ribeiro *et al.* (1998) have demonstrated how the spatial distribution and immunocytochemical labeling intensities of ZENK-expressing neurons in the brain of canaries hearing conspecific song are closely correlated with variation among the syllables in male canary songs. Moreover, in contrast to more classic tonotopic organization schemes that are well documented for auditory forebrain regions in other species, the ZENK expression patterns elicited by various narrow-band syllables (i.e., whistles) are not replicated by presenting pure-tone stimuli that simply match the fundamental frequencies of these conspecific song syllables. Thus, the spatial organization of neuronal populations in NCM observed by Ribeiro et al., correlates primarily with variation in conspecific song. This is significant in that it provides the first indication of a salient organization underlying populations of neurons in the auditory forebrain of birds that corresponds to behaviorally relevant signals.

There are some interesting analogies between the specificity of the ZENK response in the brain and the endocrine response to song in songbirds. For example, a study in female canaries investigated the effects of conspecific (male canary) song on reproductive development in singly-housed female canaries, comparing them to the effects of heterospecific song (male zebra finch song) and no song stimulus (Bentley et al., 2000). As expected, conspecific song enhanced follicular development in canaries exposed to 11L:13D compared to canaries housed in the same photoperiod but exposed to zebra finch song. More unexpectedly, canaries exposed to zebra finch song underwent enhanced follicular development compared to canaries exposed to no song. The same pattern was observed in oviposition following exposure to 18L:6D; conspecific song induced oviposition earlier and at a greater frequency than in the heterospecific and no song groups, with the fewest eggs being laid in the no song group. These results indicate that both conspecific and heterospecific male song can enhance reproductive activity in singly-housed female canaries. If we compare the hormonal effects reported in Bentley et al. (2000) with the effects of heterospecific song on the expression of the IEG *ZENK* (Mello et al., 1992), there is a strong correlation with the ZENK data in terms of the extent of a physiological response to conspecific and heterospecific song. The ZENK response in female canaries to conspecific song is greater than that to heterospecific song, which in turn is greater than the response to no song (Mello et al., 1992). In the Bentley et al. (2000) study there is a very similar gradation of response to conspecific song, heterospecific song, and no song, but using a different physiological measurement. No link between ZENK expression and the subsequent stimulation of the GnRH system has been demonstrated. However, it is possible that ZENK induction in response to song stimulus is an early step that leads to the modulation of the activity of the GnRH system.

3. Pathways from Auditory and Visual Areas to the GnRH System

There is no definitive description of a pathway from visual or auditory sensory areas to the septo-preoptic-infundibular cGnRH-I system that regulates endocrine responses made by the reproductive system to environmental stimuli. However, there are some interesting suggestions, especially for the effects of auditory stimuli on the endocrine system. For example, Cheng and Zuo (1994) have provided evidence for pathways in doves that could mediate the effects of vocal behavior on endocrine secretion in this species (see later). They have suggested that direct projections from the midbrain vocal-control ICo to areas containing GnRH-ir cell bodies in the anterior hypothalamus and other projections from ICo via the auditory thalamus to the VMN could form the neuroanatomical basis of the self-feedback phenomenon that they have described in doves. Wilczynski et al. (1993) have also discovered connections between the auditory thalamus and areas containing GnRH cells in the amphibian brain. Vocal effects on the reproductive system are quite dramatic in songbird species. Midbrain and brain-stem areas controlling vocal behavior are similar in songbird species and nonsongbird species, such as ring doves (Brenowitz, 1991; Ball, 1994). Therefore a similar pathway from the midbrain to the anterior hypothalamus, where GnRH immunoreactive cells are found, could be present in the songbird brain. However, nonsongbird species such as the ring dove do not have a discrete telencephalic network that connects to this midbrain and brain-stem unit (Brenowitz, 1991; Ball, 1990, 1994). The telencephalic portion of the vocal control system is a neural specialization limited to oscines and possibly to members of the parrot order, such as budgerigars (Brenowitz, 1991; Ball, 1994). The involvement of HVc in the perception of song is unique to oscines and the evolution of specialized telencephalic structures such as HVc could well have lead to the occurrence of new and different connections between vocal-control areas and the hypothalamus in songbirds as compared to other avian taxa.

In songbird species such as zebra finches, tract-tracing studies suggest that there are projections from the medial hypothalamus to motor areas in the midbrain controlling vocalizations (Striedter and Vu, 1998). No clear connections from the telencephalic song control system to the hypothalamic GnRH system have been identified in songbirds. However, a connection from the hypothalamus to the telencephalic vocal-control system in zebra finches has been identified by Foster *et al.* (1997). They report that a subregion of the lateral hypothalamus projects to a nucleus in the thalamus that in turn projects to the song-control nucleus mMAN. Nucleus mMAN projects to HVc (Foster *et al.*, 1997). This pathway suggests a way in which hypothalamic inputs can modulate the song system, but unless similar back projections are identified it does not explain how information processed by the song system reaches the GnRH system in the hypothalamus.

C. Seasonal Plasticity in the Gonadotropin-Releasing-Hormone Neuronal System

Another unusual feature of the avian seasonal neuroendocrine response, compared to mammals, is the marked plasticity of the avian GnRH system. First, as reviewed in Section III, recall that the avian brain expresses at least two forms of GnRH. Changes in the septo-preoptic-infundibular cGnRH-I system have been identified as one of the key events involved in the neural control of seasonal breeding (Ball, 1993). Among the first clear pieces of evidence suggesting that the GnRH system should be the focus of the search for neural mechanisms controlling seasonal breeding in birds came from studies of European starlings. Although some of the initial studies of the dynamics of GnRH did not use antisera specific to cGnRH-I or cGnRH-II, most of the later studies did, and it appears that the changes in GnRH content reviewed here are restricted to the septo-preoptic-infundibular cGnRH-I neuronal system. Dawson *et al.* (1985) measured GnRH by radioimmunoassay in dissected hypothalami taken from birds in different seasonal states. They found marked changes in GnRH content associated with different seasonal states. Increases in the hypothalamic content of GnRH provided the first physiological indicator that the experience of short days had induced the dissipation of refractoriness and the development of photosensitivity. Similarly, in juvenile photorefractory starlings exposed to short days, hypothalamic GnRH content increases gradually such that after 6 weeks in short days (which makes them fully photosensitive) the levels of cGnRH I as measured by radioimmunoassay have increased fivefold (Goldsmith *et al.*, 1989).

Work on starlings using immunocytochemistry (Foster *et al.*, 1987) confirmed these findings and provided anatomical details of changes. The hypothalamic distribution of immunoreactive GnRH perikarya and beaded fibers was similar for short-day photosensitive (regressed gonads) and long-day photostimulated (enlarged gonads) starlings. However, photostimulated birds tended to show greater staining of fibers in the median eminence than photosensitive birds, and the photosensitive birds lacked staining in the pineal stalk. This suggested that production of GnRH was similar in these two groups, but transport and presumably release was greater in the photostimulated birds. Immunostaining in long-day photorefractory birds was dramatically lower than in either short-day photosensitive or long-day photostimulated birds. The distribution of perikarya was unaltered, but fewer cells were apparent; those that were visible stained only faintly, and they were smaller in cross-sectional area than in photosensitive or photostimulated birds. Fiber-staining in photorefractory individuals was virtually absent.

The decrease in GnRH content or immunoreactivity associated with the onset of photorefractoriness occurs after the pituitary has shown a marked decline in the release of LH (Goldsmith *et al.*, 1989). It is now clear though that synthesis of the preprocessed GnRH peptide (pro-GnRH) is halted at the time of gonadal regression (Parry *et al.*, 1997) and that the release of the processed peptide (i.e., cGnRH-I) is also terminated or reduced at the same time (Dawson and Goldsmith, 1997). Thus, it appears that the inhibition of GnRH associated with the onset of photorefractoriness in starlings involves at least two steps. First, while GnRH content is still high there is an inhibition of release so that gonadotropin secretion and gonad size decrease. As refractoriness develops a dramatic decline in the amount of GnRH available occurs in the brain as measured by radioimmunoassay or immunocytochemistry. This decline in GnRH content is associated with an increase in neural input to the GnRH perikarya (Parry and Goldsmith, 1993). Ultrastructural studies of GnRH-ir cells in starlings reveals that GnRH cells in long-term refractory birds have a higher number of axosomatic terminals per neuron compared to photosensitive birds or birds that had just gone refractory and were in the process of gonadal regression. Whether this decline in GnRH content results from an increase in inhibitory neural input (perhaps from increases in γ-aminobutyric-acidergic, GABAergic, input) that inhibits transcription of the prepro-GnRH protein or whether this decline is due to changes in posttranslational processing of the prepro-GnRH protein is not known.

As discussed previously, most seasonally breeding birds studied thus far eventually become absolutely refractory to the stimulatory effects of long days (Nicholls et al., 1988b; Wilson and Donham, 1988). In these species, as was just discussed in starlings, refractoriness typically correlates with a dramatic decrease in the amount of GnRH in the hypothalamus, compared to levels in photosensitive and photostimulated birds (reviewed in Ball and Hahn, 1997). In addition to starlings, this centrally mediated down-regulation of reproductive physiology has been detected in garden warblers (*Sylvia borin*; Bluhm et al., 1991), dark-eyed juncos (*Junco hyemalis*; Saldanha et al., 1994a; Deviche et al., 2000), house sparrows (*Passer domesticus*; Hahn and Ball, 1995), American tree sparrows (*Spizella arborea*; Reinert and Wilson, 1996; Wilson and Reinert, 1996), and house finches (*Carpodacus mexicanus*; Cho et al., 1998). Data for one more taxon, Gambel's white-crowned sparrows (*Zonotrichia leucophrys gambelii*), are somewhat ambiguous. The injection of hypothalamic extracts from photosensitive, but not photorefractory, individuals increases plasma gonadotropin levels (Wingfield and Farner, 1993). This finding is consistent with reduced hypothalamic content of GnRH during absolute refractoriness in these birds as well. However, Meddle et al. (1999b) induced elevated plasma gonadotropins in photorefractory Gambel's white-crowned sparrows via systemic injection of the glutamate receptor agonist N-methyl-D-aspartate (NMDA), a secretagogue for GnRH. This finding suggests that sufficient GnRH was present (or inducible) to generate a gonadotropin surge following the onset of photorefractoriness. These findings potentially cast doubt on the earlier interpretation that white-crowned sparrows down-regulate GnRH production during refractoriness, as appears to be the case for all other songbirds studied (see Ball and Hahn, 1997; Hahn et al., 1997). However, the results in Meddle et al. (1999b) are consistent with the idea that a dramatic reduction of GnRH immunoreactivity only occurs during long-term absolute photorefractoriness, following an initial period of inhibited GnRH release without reduced production (as discussed in Ball and Hahn, 1997). Thus, on the whole, the existing data suggest that the hypothalamic-pituitary-gonad axis may be switched off at the hypothalamic level during refractoriness in many species, precluding or greatly reducing reproductive responses to either photic or nonphotic environmental cues.

In contrast to the species that become absolutely photorefractory, Japanese quail show no decline in hypothalamic GnRH when relatively photorefractory (Foster et al., 1988). They also show no change in hypothalamic GnRH content when photostimulated (Creighton and Follett, 1987). In fact, male quail transferred to short days after months of long-day stimulation actually show an increase in hypothalamic GnRH, as if GnRH production continues but secretion ceases and consequently the peptide accumulates in the brain (Foster et al., 1988). These findings suggest that there may be a fundamental difference between the neuroendocrine mechanisms underlying the two forms of photorefractoriness. Because quail are the only birds that are know definitively to exhibit relative photorefractoriness, this idea requires further exploration. However, this difference, if generally true, is of substantial significance to the potential that a species may have for temporal reproductive flexibility. Individuals that maintain active neuroendocrine transduction systems (i.e., GnRH cells containing GnRH) may retain at all times of the year the capacity for rapid stimulation by environmental cues, even if relative photorefractoriness has greatly reduced the net hypothalamic drive due to photoperiod. In contrast, individuals that have switched off GnRH production may be unresponsive to all manner of cues. In other words, species that become absolutely photorefractory display breeding seasons that are more rigidly timed, with little capacity to adjust flexibly their breeding duration, in contrast to species that become only relatively photorefractory. One aspect of the brain that changes markedly as a function of season is the GnRH neuronal system (reviewed in a previous section).

V. MECHANISMS OF STEROID HORMONE ACTION ON REPRODUCTIVE BEHAVIOR

From a mechanistic point of view, behaviors can be viewed as a series of muscular contractions triggered by an organized series of nerve impulses. To activate a behavioral pattern, a hormone therefore has to modify the neural activity and neurotransmission in specific brain areas or neurons. Hormones achieve this goal by modifying the concentration or the activity of neurotransmitters and neuropeptides. Great progress has been achieved since the 1950s in the understanding of how simple molecules such as steroids or peptidergic hormones are able to produce coordinated changes in brain activity that result in the appearance of complex and specific behaviors.

Hormones are essential for the regulation and coordination of a variety of behaviors in appropriate environmental contexts. It must be clearly stated, however, that hormones do not induce behaviors; they only change the probability of their appearance in a particular social situation. In addition, the relationship between hormones and behavior is not unidirectional. In addition to the influence of hormones on behavior, an organism's behavior (or other environmental stimuli) can also alter the endocrine state. For example, in seasonal breeders hormones secreted by the pituitary gland and gonads synchronize the onset of reproductive behavior with the time of year most conducive to reproductive success. In addition, the secretion of these hormones is also influenced by environmental stimuli such as the behavior of conspecifics. This type of relationship has not been investigated in great detail. We describe at the end of this section the few well-established cases in which a clear influence of behavior on the endocrine physiology has been demonstrated.

A. Peripheral vs Central Effects of Steroid Hormones

The brain is the major site of hormone action necessary for the expression of particular behaviors and most of this section is devoted to a review of the way in which these central effects take place. However, it must be kept in mind that hormones have widespread effects in the entire organism and there are at least three ways that hormones act on peripheral tissues that are relevant to behavior control (Hinde, 1970).

First, they can change the nature of the sensory inputs to the brain. Androgens, for example, have marked effects on secondary sexual characters such as the penis in mammals and some species of birds (e.g., ratites and waterfowls; e.g., Balthazart and Hendrick, 1979) and on associated structures such as the cloacal or proctodeal gland in quail and comb in chickens (Adkins and Adler, 1972; Adkins, 1977; Balthazart and Hendrick, 1978). It has been clearly shown that in male rats androgens influence ejaculation by enhancing the sensitivity of the penis (Beach and Levinson, 1950; Larsson et al., 1973). The same type of effect is likely to take place in birds, even though this has never been formally demonstrated. It was observed that in ducks, estradiol benzoate injections increase the frequency of precopulatory behaviors (e.g., the grasping of the female's neck feathers and mounting), but do not increase the frequency of copulation *sensu stricto* (Balthazart and Deviche, 1977). Similar differential effects were observed in rats (Davidson, 1969; Södersten, 1973) and interpreted by referring to the fact that estrogen activates the central component of copulation, but does not promote the development of androgen-dependent sensory structures (papillae) on the penis. This interpretation could also apply to ducks in which estrogens do not affect penile development but in which testosterone or its androgenic metabolite 5α-DHT markedly increase penile size (Balthazart and Deviche, 1977; Balthazart and Hendrick, 1979). Alternative interpretations are possible and the critical experiments directly testing the influences of genital inputs to the brain on the performance of copulatory behaviors have not been carried out; there is no formal demonstration for this type of mechanism in the control of male sexual behavior in birds.

In canaries, nest-building behavior is controlled by a central action of estrogens, but the hormone action is markedly influenced by tactile stimuli received from the nest cup. Characteristics of the nest such as size and texture affect the amount and type of material that are subsequently incorporated. The effectiveness of these stimuli is itself affected by the state of the brood patch. During the nest-building period, the female canary, as do many other birds, loses feathers from her breast where the skin become highly vascularized and more sensitive to tactile stimulation (see Hinde, 1965, for review). These changes in brood-patch sensitivity are themselves under the control of estrogens acting to some extent in synergism with progesterone or prolactin (Steel and Hinde, 1963; Hinde *et al.*, 1963; Hinde, 1965). Therefore estrogens influence nest-building behavior both by a central action and by modifying sensory signals originating in the brood patch.

There is also evidence that in ring doves the effects of prolactin on regurgitation and feeding of young squabs depend, at least in part, on the effects of the hormone on the crop sac—anesthesia of the crop sac leads indeed to a decrease in feeding (Lehrman, 1965; see Kinghammer and Hess, 1964; Lott and Comerford, 1968, for alternative explanations).

Second, hormones such as androgens are known to have an anabolic (trophic) effect on muscles that are ultimately the effector organs of behavior. Effector organs such as the muscles controlling the syrinx (a specialized structure in birds necessary for vocalization; Nottebohm, 1975) are increased by androgens (Luine *et al.*, 1980). Castration also decreases the level of cholinergic activity in the syrinx and this effect is reversed by a treatment with testosterone or 5α-DHT (Luine *et al.*, 1980). Androgens presumably affect song production and quality via these morphological and biochemical changes in the syrinx, as well as by their central action on telencephalic song control nuclei.

Third and finally, hormones are capable of altering the external social signals provided by superficial structures. Many birds exhibit an important sex dimorphism in their plumage and in a number of integumentary derivatives and skin appendages such as the beak, comb, wattles, cloacal gland, and penis (Stettenheim, 1972). These structures are generally under hormonal control and are likely to play an important role as social signals during sexual interactions, but experimental evidence that this is the case is relatively scarce—see, for example, Klint (1980), for the role of male plumage in sexual selection in ducks, Domjan and colleagues (Domjan and Nash, 1988; Nash and Domjan, 1991) for the role of female plumage in the development of appetitive sexual behavior in quail, and Rohwer and colleagues (Rohwer, 1975; Rohwer and Rohwer, 1978) for the correlation between male plumage and social status in Harris's sparrows (*Zonotrichia querula*). By influencing these visual signals, hormones can therefore have profound effects on the expression of sexual behaviors.

It should also be noted that in mammals, hormone-driven changes in olfactory stimuli play an important role in sexual interactions. For example, in rhesus monkeys, intravaginal treatment of a female with estradiol increases the frequency with which she receives mounts from males, probably via changes in the olfactory signal emitted by the female (Michael and Saayman, 1968). No such effect has been formally identified in birds, but it must be noted that contrary to claims made in several textbooks, birds are equipped with a fairly sensitive olfactory system (Wenzel, 1973). Olfactory signals could therefore play a role in the control of a number of behaviors. This could be the case for nest-building in starlings, which appear to select specific types of odorant material to build their nest (e.g., Clark and Mason, 1988), and for sexual behavior in ducks, in which it has been shown that olfactory stimuli play a detectable role in the control of mate selection and mating frequency (Balthazart and Schoffeniels, 1979). The origin of the olfactory signals originating in the female has not been formally identified, but it is worth noting that Jacob *et al.* (1979) demonstrated that the chemical composition of the uropygial-gland (preen gland) secretion is sexually dimorphic and changes in female ducks during the reproductive season. This secretion, which is spread daily over the plumage, could therefore serve as a hormonally controlled olfactory social signal.

In conclusion, it is clear that a hormone-induced modification in social behaviors usually represents more than the consequence of the action of the hormone at the brain level. The peripheral effects of these hormones are likely to be involved in many cases, even if the formal demonstration of this mode of action is often lacking. The central effects nevertheless play a critical role and have been documented best. They are the focus of the following section.

B. Male Sexual Behavior: Appetitive and Consummatory Aspects

Studies of vertebrate male sexual behavior have investigated, independently to a large degree, two types of intracellular chemical communication systems that are involved in the activation of these behaviors. One system includes the gonadal sex steroid hormones, in particular the androgen testosterone. The other system of interest concerns neurotransmitters and neuropeptides of various types, in particular monoaminergic transmitters such as the catecholamines norepinephrine, epinephrine, and dopamine and the indoleamine serotonin. These two types of controls are considered here. One of the major problems that needs to be addressed by scientists working in the field of the physiological control of male sexual behavior involves the elucidation of how these two systems interact. After a consideration of the effects of steroids and neurotransmitters on male sexual behavior, we provide a synthesis of how these systems interact to activate the full behavior in physiological conditions.

1. Site of Steroid Hormone Activation

As discussed previously, male sexual behavior is often divided into arousal and satiety components. Arousal involves the pursuit of females and behavioral and physiological responses to cues provided by distal females. Satiety is attained by the act of copulation itself. This distinction was first formally introduced into the field of behavioral endocrinology in 1956 by Frank Beach who postulated that the physiological control of male sexual behavior involves both a sexual arousal mechanism and an intromission and ejaculatory mechanism. This distinction made by Beach is similar to the distinction between appetitive and consummatory aspects of behavior that was articulated by ethologists such as Tinbergen (1951), Lorenz (1950), and Baerends (1988), who were building on the pioneering work of Craig (1918), among others. The fundamental idea is that some stereotyped behaviors result in a functional outcome that is associated with a reduction in motivation, whereas other more variable behaviors allow an individual to converge on this functional outcome (Timberlake and Silva, 1995). Although dichotomizing behavior in this way is problematic in some cases (Hinde, 1953), the distinction has been useful to both ethologists and experimental psychologists for the elucidation of the mechanisms mediating many motivated behaviors such as ingestive behavior (Timberlake and Silva, 1995). The terms appetitive and consummatory have also been applied to the analysis of rodent male sexual behavior by Everitt (1990).

Research on the neuroendocrine controls of male sexual behavior in birds has focused almost exclusively on the controls of the consummatory aspects. However, some attention was also devoted to the appetitive component of this behavior in one particularly suitable model species, the Japanese quail. These studies are considered in sequence.

a) Consummatory Male Sexual Behavior Given that sexual behavior is activated by testosterone in birds, as in mammals, the localization of AR in the brain was first used as a guide to identify the brain regions where the steroid action could be implicated in behavior control. As explained in Section III, earlier autoradiographic studies, later confirmed by studies using other approaches (immunocytochemistry and *in situ* hybridization), indicated that androgen binding sites in the avian brain are located, as in other vertebrates, mainly in the POA-hypothalamus, in a few other limbic regions (nST and POM) and in the mesencephalic ICo.

In the 1960s, the technique of stereotaxic implantation of steroids in the brain, originally developed by Lisk (1962), indicated that the POA is the most important of these androgen binding sites for the activation of male sexual behavior. Subsequent experimental studies confirmed that in birds, as in other vertebrate classes, the medial part of the POA plays a key role in the activation by steroids of male copulatory behavior.

This role of the POA in birds was first established by experiments analyzing the behavioral effects of stereotaxic implants of T in castrated subjects. It was found that in both ring doves and domestic cockerels such T implants restore full copulatory behavior when placed in the medial POA, but not in other brain sites (Barfield, 1969, 1971; J. B. Hutchison, 1971, 1978). Similar results were later obtained in additional species such as the Japanese quail (Watson and Adkins-Regan, 1989a,c).

The relatively large size of the implants used in these studies did not, however, permit an accurate determination of the site of T action. A significant advance in the understanding of the neural sites controlling male-typical copulatory behavior was made in quail with the identification in this species of a sexually dimorphic nucleus in the POA. The POM in this species is larger in males that shown copulatory behavior in response to T than in females that do not (Viglietti-Panzica *et al.*, 1986; Adkins and Adler, 1972; Balthazart *et al.*, 1983). Furthermore, the volume of POM regresses after castration and is restored to values observed in sexually mature males by a 2-week treatment with T (Panzica et al., 1987, 1991). These data indicated that the volume of this nucleus varies in parallel with copulatory behavior (large volume in sexually active birds; small volume in inactive subjects) even if the correlation is not perfect when sex differences are concerned—the sex difference in copulatory behavior is organizational in nature, whereas the difference in POM volume is not; it simply results from a differential activation by T in adults (Panzica et al., 1987, 1991; Aste et al., 1991; see also Balthazart and Adkins-Regan, Chapter 66).

Subsequent experiments revealed that the POM is a necessary and sufficient site of T action for the activation of copulatory behavior in males. Electrolytic lesions of the POM, but not of the surrounding POA, completely suppress copulatory behavior activated in castrated males by Silastic implants containing T. Conversely, stereotaxic implants filled with T activate all aspects of copulatory behavior in castrated males if their tip is located within the cytoarchitectonic boundaries of the POM, but not if it is located in the adjacent POA (Balthazart and Surlemont, 1990b; Balthazart et al., 1992e). These data clearly indicate that T action in the POM is sufficient to activate copulatory behavior in adult male quail, although they do not rule out the possibility that the action of T at additional sites in the central nervous system may contribute to the behavioral activation under physiological conditions (see also Section IV.B.1 on IEGs). Other studies demonstrated that T must be aromatized in the POM in order to exert its behavioral effects (Watson and Adkins-Regan, 1989c; Balthazart and Surlemont, 1990a; Balthazart et al., 1990a). In particular, it could be shown that stereotaxic implants of aromatase inhibitors in the medial preoptic region significantly inhibit the activation of copulatory behavior produced by a systemic treatment with T of castrated males (see Section V.A.2). This aromatase-dependence of behavior was also used to further refine the analysis of the anatomical sites of steroid action on quail copulatory behavior.

It had been established that ARO-ir neurons are a specific marker for the sexually dimorphic POM in quail and that the number of these immunoreactive cells is markedly increased by a systemic treatment with testosterone. Therefore, aromatase immunocytochemistry was used to map, at a cellular level of resolution, the areas that are destroyed by electrolytic lesions or that are stimulated by the stereotaxic implantation of T in the POA. These measures of the cellular action of T in the POA were then correlated with the behavior of the animals to identify the parts of the POA that are critical in the activation of copulatory behavior (Balthazart et al., 1992e). As expected based on previous studies, electrolytic lesions of the POA disrupted the activation of male sexual behavior by T only if they destroyed a significant part of the POM and, in parallel, reduced the absolute number of ARO-ir neurons in the POM. Conversely, stereotaxic T implants in or close to POM activated sexual behavior and increased the number of ARO-ir cells in the nucleus. Correlative analyses suggested that a part of the POM just rostral to the anterior commissure is critical for the activation of copulatory behavior. The best correlations between the behavioral deficits induced by electrolytic lesions and the size of the lesions was indeed in this area. In addition, high correlations were observed between the behavior activated by T implants and the number of ARO-ir cells that were induced by T in this area rostral to the anterior commissure.

b) Appetitive Male Sexual Behavior As previously explained, most studies on avian sexual behavior were at one time confined to the analysis of the controls of consummatory sexual behavior. A lot of attention has also been devoted to the control by steroids of singing behavior in birds of the passeriformes family. Depending on the species and social context, singing is used either to defend a territory or to attract females. Singing can therefore be considered as a form of appetitive sexual behavior.

Singing is similar to other sexual behaviors in that it is activated by T, presumably acting through both its androgenic and estrogenic metabolites (Harding et al., 1983, 1988a; Walters and Harding, 1988). Songbirds have been shown to possess a complex network of steroid-sensitive nuclei located mainly in the telencephalon that appear to play the key role in the learning and production of song (Stokes et al., 1974; Nottebohm et al., 1976). The coverage of the very active field of research devoted to the analysis of the song system is, however, beyond the scope of this chapter; the relevant literature on this topic is reviewed in Schlinger and Brenowitz (Chap. 33 in this volume).

Recent studies carried out in starlings indicate that the amount of singing produced by males in a reproductive context (presence of a female and of nest material) is also controlled by the medial part of the POA (Riters and Ball, 1999; Riters et al., 2000a). This finding reinforces the result of studies carried out in quail demonstrating that the POA is implicated in the control of appetitive as well as consummatory sexual behavior (see later). How the telencephalic and diencephalic regions interact to control singing remains unclear. Because AR are present in many song-control nuclei and ER are not so widespread and their presence in some nuclei appears to be species specific (e.g., they are present in the HVc of canaries but not zebra finches; Gahr et al., 1987, 1993), it could be speculated that singing is activated by a combination of androgen action in the telencephalic song-control nuclei (HVc and RA) and of estrogen in the POA.

Earlier stereotaxic studies suggested that testosterone may not act only in the POA to activate the full range of reproductive behaviors. In domestic fowl, for example, testosterone propionate implants in the POA and anterior hypothalamus activated sexual behavior, but not aggressive behavior and crowing; courtship behavior (waltzing) was only moderately activated (Barfield, 1964, 1969). A partially successful localization of the sites where androgens activate these behaviors was obtained. Some aggression was displayed in birds bearing implants in the lateral forebrain, in and below the paleostriatum (Barfield, 1965). Waltzing was observed in one bird bearing simultaneously two implants located in the POA and in the lateral forebrain, suggesting that performance of this courtship behavior depends on the simultaneous activation of these two brain sites, apparently mediating aggressive and sexual behaviors. This type of brain control supports the ethological interpretation of courtship, which states that this type of behavior reflects the conflict between aggressive and sexual motivation (Hinde, 1970). No other study has, however, been carried out to test this interpretation, which was based on too few subjects to be considered firmly established.

A significant amount of research was also carried out to identify the neuroendocrine mechanisms controlling appetitive sexual behavior in quail. Appetitive male sexual behavior as applied to quail consists of producing displays that attract a female and the behaviors of searching for and approaching a potential mate the consummatory component includes the actual contact between the sexes culminating in copulation. Making precise distinctions between these two behavioral components can be difficult at times, but in general clear dissociations can usually be discerned.

As part of a long-term research program devoted to explicating the role of learning in the control of sexual behavior, Domjan and his colleagues at the University of Texas (Crawford et al., 1993; Domjan, 1994) developed a variety of behavioral procedures that are appropriate for the investigation of appetitive sexual behavior in quail. These methods include the application of Pavlovian conditioning procedures in which a neutral stimulus such as a gray foam block serves as the conditional stimulus (CS) that is temporally paired with access to a female, which serves as the unconditional stimulus (US). Male quail readily acquire an approach response to a CS when it is paired with a US in this way, and these Pavlovian studies have been useful for the explication of the mechanisms mediating the acquisition and maintenance of a classically conditioned response (see Domjan and Hollis, 1988; Domjan, 1994; Hilliard and Domjan, 1995).

During the course of these studies by Domjan and colleagues, another phenomenon was discovered that they referred to as a learned social proximity response. When males are placed in an arena, they learn to stand in front of a narrow window that provides a view of a female, but only after they have been allowed to copulate at least once with a female who has been released into that arena. The response involves a remarkable change in a male's behavior—after a single copulation, males spend the majority of their time (literally days) standing in front of the window and looking through it at the female (Domjan and Hall, 1986a,b). This response is a form of associative learning, but cannot easily be classified as either a form of classical conditioning or instrumental conditioning (Domjan and Hollis, 1988).

Because this learned response is relatively easy to obtain under laboratory conditions and because it involves aspects of the learning process that normally occurs in male quail when they engage in sexual behavior, we used this procedure as a measure of appetitive male sexual behavior in quail. The procedure appears to be a good indicator of appetitive sexual behavior in that the male seems clearly to be engaging in this behavior in anticipation of copulatory behavior itself. Male quail when isolated in a large arena first pursue a generalized search for females and then, when a female is localized to a particular place, they exhibit a more focused search. Such variable searching behavior is characteristic of an appetitive behavioral response. The learned social proximity response in males appears to be a good example of a focused sexual search and thereby provides a useful measure of appetitive sexual behavior that we can contrast with the stereotyped sequence of the neck grab, mounting, and cloacal contact movements characteristic of the consummatory sexual response. The studies described next use this learned proximity response to assess the neuroendocrine mechanisms mediating appetitive sexual behavior in quail so that we can compare the mechanisms involved in the control of this aspect of sexual behavior with the relatively well-characterized mechanisms mediating consummatory sexual behavior.

We developed for these studies a modification of the learned social proximity response first described by Domjan and Hall (1986a,b) that permits us to quantify relatively quickly appetitive sexual behavior in quail. In this modified procedure, quail are tested for relatively brief periods of time (25 min), so a large number of subjects can be examined each day (Balthazart et al., 1995).

With this method, studies were initiated to investigate whether similar or different brain areas are implicated in the control of the two components of male sexual behavior in quail. Because central T aromatization is a limiting factor in the activation of both appetitive and consummatory male sexual behavior (see Section V.A.2), attention was focused on brain areas that had been shown to contain dense populations of neurons expressing the enzyme aromatase, namely the POM and BST. Castrated male quail chronically treated with T were first trained to acquire the social proximity response used to measure appetitive sexual behavior. After eight training sessions, during which males learned to stay close to and observe through a window a female who was later released and allowed to copulate with the male (Balthazart et al., 1995), males were submitted to bilateral electrolytic lesions aimed at the POM or BST. They were then retested during nine additional sessions for the presence of appetitive and consummatory sexual behavior (Balthazart et al., 1998a). After perfusion, brain aromatase was localized via immunocytochemistry in the brain of these subjects in order to permit an accurate reconstruction of the lesions and of the damage that had been made to these specific cell populations.

As expected based on previous results, lesions affecting the POM ARO-ir cells completely abolished consummatory sexual behavior. However, they also significantly decreased, but did not completely suppress, all measures of appetitive sexual behavior. Lesions aimed at the BST had no effect on appetitive sexual behavior, but moderately decreased consummatory sexual behavior. Histological reconstructions indicated that POM lesions were usually confined to this nucleus and the surrounding lateral POA, whereas lesions aimed at the BST almost always also destroyed a substantial portion of the nucleus accumbens (Ac) as defined in the chicken atlas (i.e., a small cell group adjacent to the ventral tip of the lateral ventricles; Kuenzel and Masson, 1988).

Somewhat surprisingly, the best dissociation between the two components of male sexual behavior resulted from lesions to different subregions of the POM. Damage to a portion of the POM just rostral to the anterior commissure resulted in the complete inhibition of consummatory sexual behavior (as already discussed), whereas damage to parts of the POM just rostral to this region selectively inhibited appetitive sexual behavior (Fig. 14). Interestingly, lesions of the POM also markedly depressed the expression of rhythmic cloacal sphincter movements that are produced by males when visually exposed to a sexually mature female. Therefore, these data strongly suggest that the preoptic region plays an important role in the regulation of motivational as well as performance aspects of male sexual behavior.

In a parallel study, appetitive and consummatory sexual behaviors were measured in castrated males that received T-implants directed at either the POM or BST. Five successive behavior tests assessing the acquisition of the social proximity response indicative of appetitive sexual behavior were performed and immediately followed by a 5-min period during which the males had free access to the females and could express consummatory sexual behavior (Riters et al., 1998). During these five test sessions, only a few birds displayed cloacal contact movements, but these were all males who had T-filled cannulae directly implanted in the POM. In

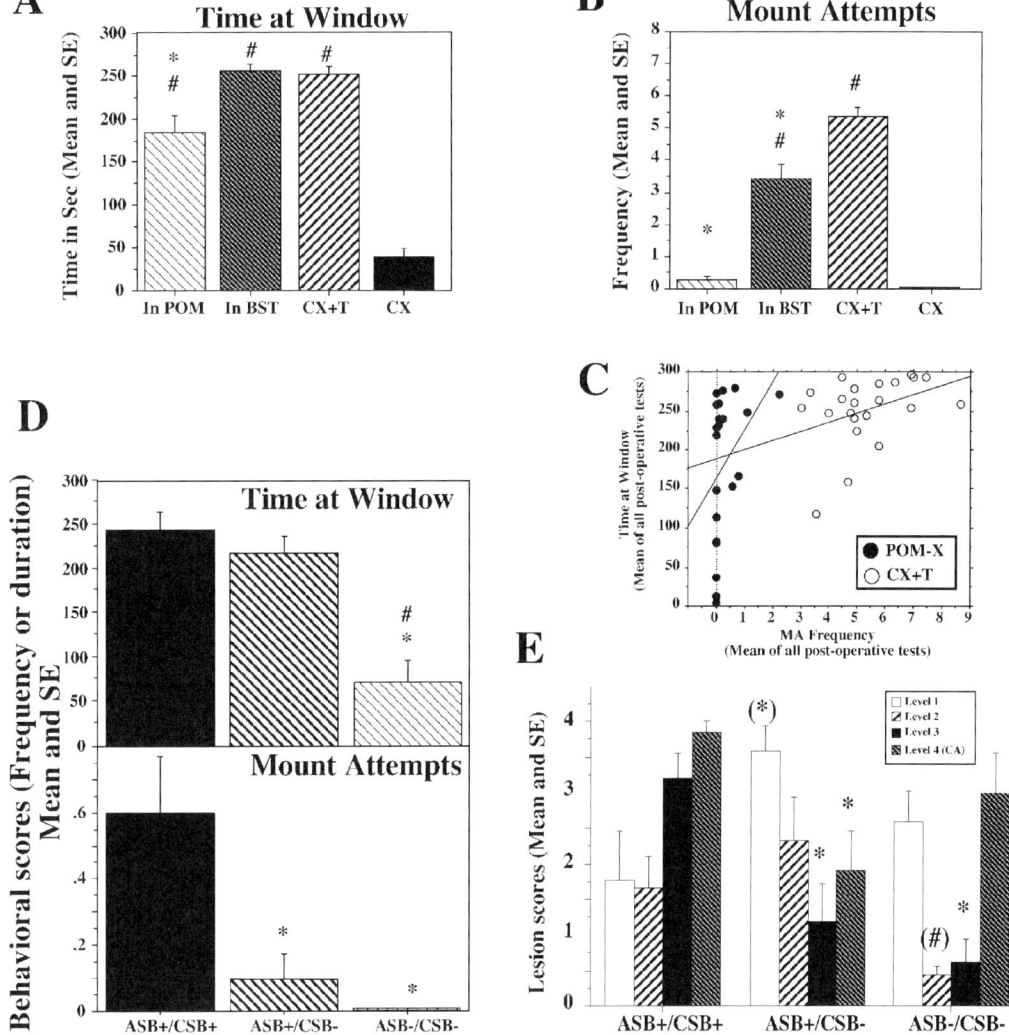

FIGURE 14 Effects of lesions of the medial preoptic nucleus (POM) or bed nucleus striae terminalis (BST) on the testosterone-induced male sexual behavior in quail. (A–B) Means of behavioral scores for the measures of appetitive and consummatory male sexual behavior observed in four groups of castrated male quail that were treated with testosterone (CX + T) and received an electrolytic lesion in the POM or BST or were left untreated as controls (CX). Experimental groups were then compared two by two by Fisher PLSD tests following a significant ANOVA (* indicates $p < 0.05$ by comparison with the CX + T group; # indicates $p < 0.005$ by comparison with the CX group). (C) Relations between a measure of appetitive sexual behavior (time spent at the window watching the female) and a measure of consummatory sexual behavior (mount attempts, MA, frequency) in birds bearing a lesion of the POM and in their control group (CX + T). Correlation coefficients associated with the regression lines indicated in the figure are not significant ($p > 0.05$). These data clearly illustrate the nearly complete inhibition of consummatory sexual behavior, but the quite variable inhibition of appetitive sexual behavior in the lesioned group. (D) Behavioral scores (frequency of mount attempts or time at window) computed for three subgroups of birds bearing a POM lesion defined by the presence of appetitive sexual behavior and of a low level of consummatory sexual behavior (ASB+/CSB+), by the presence of appetitive sexual behavior and the complete absence of consummatory sexual behavior (ASB+/CSB−) or by the strong inhibition of appetitive sexual behavior and the complete absence of consummatory sexual behavior (ASB−/CSB−). The three groups were compared two by two by Fisher PLSD tests following a significant ANOVA (* indicates $p < 0.05$ by comparison with ASB+/CSB+ subgroup and # indicates $p < 0.05$ by comparison with ASB+/CSB− subgroup). (E) Means of the lesion scores observed in at four rostrocaudal levels of the POM in the three subgroups of birds defined by their behavior as shown in (D). Data were analyzed by a separate one-way ANOVA for each rostrocaudal level followed by Fisher PLSD tests comparing groups two by two. The results are shown at the top of the bars: * indicates $p < 0.05$ by comparison with ASB+/CSB+ subgroup and # indicates $p < 0.05$ by comparison with ASB+/CSB− subgroup. Parentheses around a symbol indicates that the corresponding general ANOVA comparing the three subgroups did not detect a significant effect, so that results of the Fisher PLSD tests can only be considered as indicative. CA, anterior commissure. Data from Balthazart et al. (1998a).

addition, males bearing T implants in POM displayed a higher level of mount attempts than any other group and a low number of mount attempts was observed in birds with T implants located just outside of POM. No males in any other group exhibited consummatory sexual behavior. Overall, the males treated with T in the POM also displayed a higher social proximity response (as assessed by the measurement of looking through and spending time in front of the window providing visual access to the female) than birds in any other group. Previous reports had shown that this social proximity response does not develop in birds that fail to or are not allowed to copulate with the female (Balthazart et al., 1995). Accordingly, a closer analysis of the behavior of the birds with implants aimed at the POM (i.e., quail with T in POM, T just outside of POM, and empty implants in or just outside of POM) revealed that the T-treated birds that copulated also displayed a significant elevation in time spent in front of and looking through the window, whereas T-treated birds that failed to copulate showed very low levels of these responses, similar to birds with empty implants.

One potential problem with the use of the social proximity response as a measure of appetitive sexual behavior in quail resides is that the response is learned as a result of being reinforced by the performance of copulatory behavior. This linkage prevents the assessment of appetitive male sexual behavior in subjects that fail to copulate and introduces a possible complication into some experiments, in that it may be difficult at times to discern whether experimental manipulations affect the appetitive sexual behavior per se or the ability of the birds to learn a new response or maintain the previously formed association.

A second behavioral procedure has therefore been developed based on studies conducted by Seiwert, Thompson, Adkins-Regan, and colleagues (Thompson et al., 1995, 1998). Male quail produce a meringue-like foam that is transferred to females during copulation and may enhance the probability that the sperm that is transferred fertilizes the egg (K. M. Cheng et al., 1989). This foam is produced by rhythmic movements of a sexually dimorphic striated cloacal sphincter muscle that is interdigitated with the proctodeal gland (Seiwert, 1994; Seiwert and Adkins-Regan, 1998). These movements are greatly facilitated in males, including sexually naive males, when the stimulus animal is a female, compared to when it is a male (Seiwert and Adkins-Regan, 1992; Seiwert, 1994; Thompson et al., 1995, 1998). These rhythmic cloacal sphincter muscle movements are facilitated nearly 20-fold in castrated males treated with T and provided with visual access to a female, compared to castrated males receiving no T (Balthazart et al., 1998a). These cloacal sphincter muscle movements are reminiscent of noncontact erections described in mammalian species (Sachs, 1995), in that they involve muscle movements that control effector organs associated with consummatory aspects of male sexual behavior in response to sensory cues emitted by a female.

Cloacal sphincter movement were also quantified in birds that had received lesions aimed at the POM as already described. It was found that POM lesion almost completely abolish this aspect of the male appetitive sexual response (Balthazart et al., 1998a) (Fig. 15). In addition, rhythmic cloacal sphincter muscle movements in response to visual access to a female were also observed in birds that had received stereotaxic implants of T in the POM and BST (Riters et al., 1998). Both males with T in the POM and males with T just outside of POM (less than 200–300 μm) displayed some increase in the frequency of cloacal sphincter muscle movements, but a clear response was only observed in a small number of individuals and its magnitude was still much lower than in birds treated systemically with T. This effect was therefore not significant. However, significantly more rhythmic cloacal sphincter muscle movements were observed in T-implanted males that had previously copulated than those that had not, regardless of implant site.

Overall, the results of these experiments involving the electrolytic lesion or the stereotaxic implantation of T in the brain are consistent in indicating that the POM plays an important role in both appetitive and consummatory aspects of male sexual behavior. There may be some specialization in the subregions of the POM that participate in the activation by T of these two components and additional brain sites are likely to be involved. The available results, however, clearly indicate that mechanisms mediating these two components of the behavior are not completely dissociated and that some integration is likely to take place in the POA.

A small population of ARO-ir cells has also been identified in the Tn, an area of the avian forebrain that is the

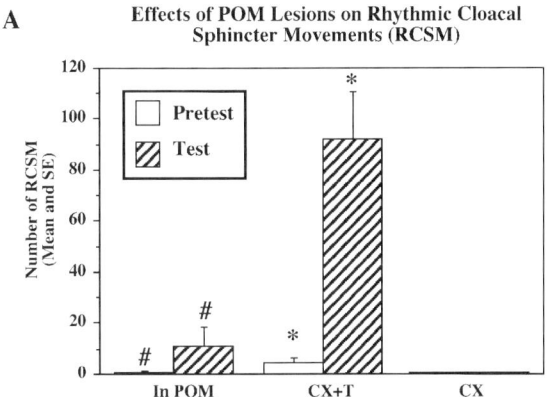

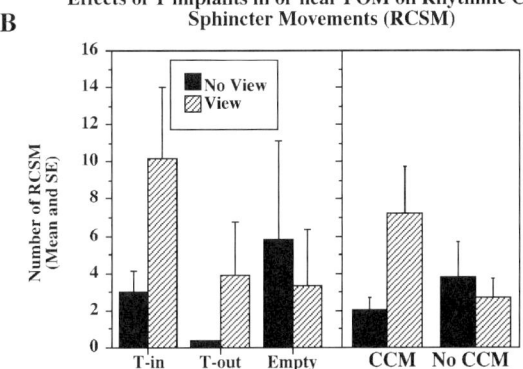

FIGURE 15 (A) Effects of testosterone treatment and of a lesion in the medial preoptic nucleus (POM) on the frequency of rhythmic cloacal sphincter muscles movements (RCSM) in the absence (pretest) or presence (test) of a stimulus female. Fisher PLSD tests were performed to compare the behavior of the three groups of birds in the absence (pretest) and presence (test) of the female (* indicates $p < 0.05$ by comparison with the control (CX) group; # indicates $p < 0.05$ by comparison with the CX + T group). (B) Mean number of RCSM in the absence (No View) or in the visual presence (View) of a female for males bearing a T-filled cannula directly in (T-in) or within 200–300 μm (T-out) of the POM, compared to control males with empty implants in or within 200–300 μm (Empty) of these nuclei. The right part of this panel represents the mean number of RCSM for males that had previously copulated (CCM) compared to those that had never copulated (No CCM) regardless of implant site. Data from Balthazart *et al.* (1998a); Riters *et al.* (1998).

homolog of components of the amygdala in mammals (Zeier and Karten, 1971; Thompson *et al.*, 1998). Bilateral lesions to this nucleus attenuated appetitive measures of male sexual behavior (Thompson *et al.*, 1998). In particular, the bilateral ablation of Tn decreased the speed at which a male approached a female, the time they spent in association with a female, the number of copulations they engaged in during a 5-min interaction with a female, and finally the number of cloacal sphincter muscle movements displayed in the presence of a female. These data thus suggest that, as the amygdala in mammals, the Tn in birds is a component of the neural circuit mediating male sexual behavior and that it is involved in the regulation of both appetitive and consummatory aspects of this behavior (Everitt *et al.*, 1989; Everitt, 1990, 1995; Wood and Newman, 1995b,c).

In the absence of a female, in both laboratory and feral conditions, sexually motivated male quail or cockerels produce a loud broadband two- to three-syllable vocalization referred to as a crow. This vocalization is attractive to female quail (Goodson and Adkins-Regan, 1997), and males who succeed in attracting a mate exhibit a marked reduction in crowing (Wetherbee, 1961). Thus, this display clearly seems to be an example of an appetitive behavior.

Although crowing could potentially provide an easily discernible and sensitive measure, its frequency is highly variable among males and its production can be influenced by a variety of external stimuli that may or may not be specifically relevant to sexual behavior. It is clear, however, that the occurrence of crowing is androgen dependent—this behavior disappears in castrated quail and cockerels and is restored by systemic treatment with T (Adkins, 1977; Adkins and Pniewski, 1978; Davis and Domm, 1943). A number of studies have therefore attempted to identify the brain areas where T acts to activate this vocalization. Although the pathway from the telencephalon to the syrinx that controls vocalizations in songbirds has been the focus of numerous studies (Stokes *et al.*, 1974; Nottebohm *et al.*, 1982; Nottebohm, 1980; see also Schlinger and Brenowitz, Chapter 33 in this volume), it has received much less attention in other avian families (see, however, Gahr, 2000; Jarvis and Mello, 2000; Jarvis *et al.*, 2000). One mesencephalic nucleus, the ICo, which is part of the song-control system in oscines, is present in galliforms. The ICo in chickens and quail also contains AR, as identified by *in vivo* autoradiography and immunocytochemistry (Meyer, 1973; Meyer *et al.*, 1976; Barfield *et al.*, 1978; Watson and Adkins-Regan, 1989b; Balthazart *et al.*, 1992d). Several studies, therefore, researched whether T action in the ICo plays a role in the activation of crowing behavior.

The electrical stimulation of the medial ICo elicited a number of vocalizations, including crows in cockerels and quail (Potash, 1970; Phillips and Youngren, 1971; Armitage and Seller, 1981; Seller, 1981). Conversely, lesions of ICo were shown to decrease or suppress crowing. However, attempts to activate crowing by stereotaxic implants of T in ICo have met with contradictory results. Phillips and Barfield (1977) implanted castrated roosters with testosterone propionate (TP) in the ICo both uni- and bilaterally and also combined ICo implants with TP implants in the POA, but they observed no activation of crowing.

Watson (1989) implanted unilaterally 5α-dihydrotestosterone propionate, (DHTP) in the ICO region of castrated quail, and this elicited crowing vocalizations in some of the treated subjects. However, these implants were fairly large and caused some leakage of the hormone in the peripheral circulation, as attested by a moderate (although not statistically significant) growth of the androgen-dependent cloacal gland. In addition, DHTP implants located outside ICo (e.g., in the GCt) had similar behavioral effects. The anatomical specificity of the crow activation cannot therefore be established based on these results.

Yazaki and collaborators (1995, 1997) confirmed that bilateral electrolytic lesions of ICo eliminate crowing (and distress calls) induced by systemic T in young Japanese quail. In addition, a small amount of T implanted in ICo activated a crow-like vocalization in young quail chicks while at the same time decreasing the occurrences of distress vocalizations. A systemic T treatment was also shown to modulate the crows produced by females following an electrical stimulation of the ICo (Yazaki et al., 1999).

Taken together, these results suggest that in quail, T action in the ICo is critical for the activation of crowing. Interestingly, it was also demonstrated that the stereotaxic implantation of T in the ICo activates crowing with very short latencies (within 1 hour), at least in some subjects. This fast action suggests that the steroid may be affecting behavior by nongenomic actions that do not involve the binding of T to intracellular AR acting as transcription factors. Accordingly, Yazaki et al. (1998) identified and partly purified two proteins (42 and 47 kDa) from quail ICo membranes that appear to bind T in a specific and saturable manner. Whether membrane actions of T in the ICo mediate the fast activation of crowing will have to be tested in future experiments.

In conclusion, the role of androgens in the ICo of galliforms remains somewhat controversial and there is no available explanation for the discrepancy between the results of earlier studies performed on cockerels and the later studies performed on quail. In addition, the nature of the effects of T on crowing may be less direct than is usually admitted. Meyer et al. (1976) have suggested that this uptake could be related to the increase in the persistence in attending to objects that is observed after systemic injections of T (Andrew, 1972a,b; Andrew and Jones, 1992). Andrew (1975) noted that electrical stimulations of the ICo induces calling and alerting in chicks, whereas lesions in the ICo produce a number of behavioral effects, including muteness, impaired visual-targeting behavior, and absence of exploratory pecking at moving targets. Andrew and de Lanerolle (1975) suggested that chicks with ICo lesions treat visual objects as if they were not conspicuous, but no T-implant study has analyzed whether these behavioral deficits are specific to the action of T in the ICo.

In ring doves, the ICo region also accumulates radioactivity after injection of tritiated T (Martinez-Vargas et al., 1974; Kim et al., 1978) and stereotaxic experiments have shown that this area is implicated in the control of vocal behavior. TP implants in the ICo increase the occurrence frequency of nest-coos in castrated male doves, and lesions of this nucleus decrease the nest-cooing frequency (Cohen and Cheng, 1982; Cohen, 1981, 1983). Similarly, estrogen implants in the ICo activate nest-cooing in females (Cohen and Cheng, 1981). These effects play a key role in the control of steroid-mediated behavior in the ring dove reproductive cycle both by synchronizing partners in a pair and, more surprisingly, by self-stimulating ovarian development in the female (Cheng, 1992; see Sections V.B.6 and V.C.6).

2. Role of Steroid Metabolism in the Regulation of Behavior

As previously mentioned, in most vertebrate species and in birds in particular castration suppresses the expression of male sexual behaviors and these behaviors are restored within a few days by treatment with T. Because T is extensively metabolized in the brain of all species that have been investigated, numerous studies have been carried out to evaluate the potential role of this metabolism in the control of male reproductive behavior. As discussed in Section III, T can be irreversibly converted in the avian brain into three types of metabolites—estrogen, 5α reduced androgens, and 5β reduced androstanes. In general, it appears that the first two types of metabolites (acting alone or in synergy) are of paramount importance for the activation of most types of male reproductive behaviors. The behavioral role of 5β reduced metabolites of T is, in contrast, less obvious and contradictory data have been collected at this level.

a) Role of Testosterone Aromatization
i) Activation of male copulatory behavior. In a large number of avian species, it has been demonstrated that the activation of male copulatory behavior by T requires, as in rodents, the aromatization of this androgenic steroid into an estrogen. This conclusion is based on a wide variety of converging experimental evidence collected since the 1970s.

1. The behavioral effects of T in castrated male birds can be mimicked by natural estrogens such as E_2 or by synthetic estrogenic compound such as diethylstilbestrol (Adkins and Pniewski, 1978; Adkins et al., 1980; Cheng and Lehrman, 1975; Hutchison, 1971; Steimer and Hutchison, 1981a; Schumacher and Balthazart, 1983; Harding et al., 1983, 1988b).

2. Aromatizable androgens such as T or androstenedione activate male sexual behavior in castrates, whereas nonaromatizable androgens such as 5α-DHT or methyltrienolone (R1881) have little or no effect at this level (Adkins, 1977; Adkins et al., 1980; Schumacher et al., 1987; Alexandre and Balthazart, 1986; Harding et al., 1983) (Fig. 16).

3. Aromatase inhibitors such as ATD, 4-hydroxyandrostenedione (4OH-A), Fadrozole, or Vorozole markedly inhibit or completely block the activation of male sexual behavior by T (Adkins et al., 1980; Evrard et al., 1989; Walters and Harding, 1988; Schlinger and Callard, 1990; Foidart et al., 1994b; Soma et al., 1999c, 2000). Interestingly, several of these studies demonstrated that the effects of aromatase inhibitors on the behavioral activation by T are completely reversed by the concurrent administration of an estrogen. This clearly

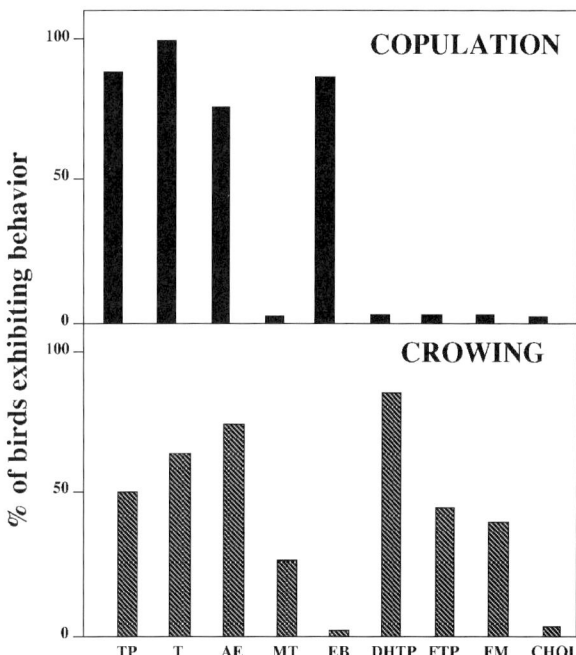

FIGURE 16 Percentage of male quail implanted with steroid-filled Silastic capsules that copulated (exhibited at least one mount; top) or crowed at least once (bottom). AE, androstenedione; CHOL, cholesterol; DHTP, 5α-dihydrotestosterone proprionate; EB, estradiol benzoate; FM, fluoxymesterone; FTP, 6α-fluorotestosterone proprionate; MT, 17α-methyltestosterone; T, testosterone; TP, testosterone proprionate. TP, T, and AE are aromatizable androgen; EB is an estrogen; MT, DHTP, FTP, and FM are nonaromatizable androgens. Data from Adkins et al. (1980).

demonstrates that the effects of aromatase inhibition are specific to estrogen depletion and do not result from nonspecific toxic effects of the drugs.

4. The injection of antiestrogens (tamoxifen or nitromifene citrate, CI-628), which block the access of estrogens to their specific receptors, block testosterone-induced sexual behavior (Adkins and Nock, 1976a; Alexandre and Balthazart, 1986).

Taken together, these data support the hypothesis that the action of T on sexual behavior requires the aromatization of the steroid into an estrogen. This proposition has been called the aromatization hypothesis. A different but related hypothesis is that, at the cellular level, the action of T on male sexual behavior results from the binding of estrogens to ER and from the transcriptional regulation effected by the occupied

ER (the estrogen receptor hypothesis; Yahr, 1979). This view, however, ignores a number of other experimental findings.

1. Exogenous estrogens activate copulatory behavior only when injected at relatively high doses that appear to have toxic effects on the liver (Balthazart *et al.*, 1985; Alexandre and Balthazart, 1986). This high-dose requirement may be explained by the fact that in physiological conditions, the aromatization of T takes place in the brain close to the site of estrogen action on behavior. Therefore, only a limited part of the brain is exposed to potentially high concentrations of estrogens derived from aromatization, whereas the entire organism is exposed to estrogens after a systemic injection. This could potentially explain the toxicity of the systemic treatments as well as the requirement for high doses of systemic estrogens due to intense peripheral catabolism before the hormone reaches its target sites in the brain. It is also possible that these brain-target sites are more easily reached by locally formed estrogens than by estrogens from the peripheral circulation, although no specific experimental data are at present available to support this notion (estrogens are lipophilic compounds that are supposed to cross the blood–brain barrier easily and should have free access to any brain region).

2. Nonaromatizable androgens such as 5α-DHT and the derived 5α-androstanediols or the synthetic androgen methyltrienolone, although they cannot activate a very active copulatory behavior in birds, are not completely devoid of behavioral action. This has been clearly demonstrated in the rat (see Yahr, 1979; Martini, 1982, for discussion), and there is evidence that the same effects are also present in quail (Adkins, 1977; Deviche and Schumacher, 1982; Balthazart *et al.*, 1985; Alexandre and Balthazart, 1986).

3. Antiandrogens such as flutamide are able to reduce (although not completely suppress) T-induced sexual behavior in male quail (Balthazart *et al.*, 1985; Balthazart and Surlemont, 1990a).

Therefore, it seems likely that, although male sexual behavior in most birds depends primarily on the action of estrogens, its full restoration involves, at least in part, some androgen-dependent mechanisms (see also later discussion). The role of androgens as compared to estrogens appears to be relatively small, as indicated by the fact that E_2, alone, but not 5α-DHT alone, activates an intense copulatory behavior in castrated male subjects of many species including, for example, quail and zebra finches.

ii) Appetitive components of male sexual behavior are also activated by estrogenic metabolites of testosterone. Previous work in a variety of birds has demonstrated that the activation of copulatory behavior by T requires the aromatization of the steroid into estrogens (Balthazart, 1989; Balthazart and Foidart, 1993b). Because both the appetitive and the consummatory aspects of male sexual behavior in quail appear to be controlled by T acting at similar, partly overlapping brain sites, it was hypothesized that both components of sexual behavior also depend on the same endocrine mechanisms for their activation in adulthood and in particular that the appetitive aspects are activated by estrogenic metabolites of T. Three types of experiments demonstrated that this is indeed the case using the acquired social proximity response described in Section V.B.1.b as a measure of appetitive behavior.

It was first demonstrated that the learned proximity response can be acquired by castrated birds if they are systemically treated with either the endogenous estrogen E_2 or with a synthetic estrogen, such as diethylstilbestrol (DES). These compounds were found to mimic the behavioral effects of T (Balthazart *et al.*, 1995). A second experiment further demonstrated that once the proximity response is acquired, its expression can be blocked by daily injections of the antiestrogen tamoxifen (Balthazart *et al.*, 1995). Finally, it was demonstrated that the daily injection of an aromatase inhibitor progressively inhibits the social proximity response that has been acquired by castrated birds treated with T (Balthazart *et al.*, 1997c).

In conclusion, these experiments demonstrate that appetitive aspects of male sexual behavior in quail are activated, as is the case for consummatory sexual behavior, by T acting through its estrogenic metabolites. The endocrine specificity is therefore similar, if not identical, for the activation of both aspects of sexual behavior.

As previously discussed, singing in oscines can be considered as an expression of appetitive sexual behavior. It is therefore interesting to observe that the activation of courtship songs in zebra finches and red-winged blackbirds is also mediated by an interaction of androgens and estrogens, with estrogens apparently playing the most important part in this process (Harding *et al.*, 1983, 1988b). The treatment with an aromatase inhibitor (ATD) was also shown in this avian model to inhibit the T-induced singing, which clearly confirmed the estrogen dependence of this behavior (Walters and Harding, 1988).

iii) Localization of the action of estrogenic metabolites in the brain. Given that in quail T acts mainly in the POM to activate sexual behavior in quail, that T acts via its estrogenic metabolites, and that aromatase activity and ER are present in high concentration in the POM, it was hypothesized that T actually is aromatized and estrogens acts in this nucleus to activate sexual behavior. This could be confirmed by a set of experimental studies based on the stereotaxic implantation of estrogens, aromatase inhibitors and antiestrogens in the medial part of the POA.

It was originally found that implants of estrogens (E_2 or the synthetic estrogen DES) in the medial POA activate copulatory behavior in castrated quail as do systemic treatments with the same compounds (Watson and Adkins-Regan, 1989a; Balthazart and Surlemont, 1990a). A second set of studies showed that, conversely, the implantation in the medial POA of an aromatase inhibitor (Vorozole or R76713) or of an antiestrogen (tamoxifen) inhibits the activation of sexual behavior by a systemic treatment with T (Watson and Adkins-Regan, 1989c; Balthazart *et al.*, 1990a; Balthazart and Surlemont, 1990a).

These studies indicated that the T aromatization and estrogen action related to the activation of male sexual behavior take place in the POA. Additional work correlating the specific location of small implants filled with ATD with the behavioral effects further demonstrated that, as could be expected based on anatomical data (all preoptic ARO-ir cells are located in the POM), the aromatization supporting copulatory behavior takes place specifically in the POM. ATD implants located in the POM markedly (and significantly) inhibit male sexual behavior in castrated quail treated systemically with T. In contrast, implants located in the POA but outside the POM are not effective—behavior is expressed at the same level as in control birds with cholesterol implants (Balthazart and Surlemont, 1990a).

iv) Mode of action of locally produced estrogens. The data presented so far clearly demonstrate that estrogens produced locally in the POM by the aromatization of T are a key factor in the activation of male copulatory behavior in quail (Balthazart and Surlemont, 1990a,b; Adkins *et al.*, 1980; Balthazart *et al.*, 1990a,c). These behavioral effects of T are blocked by the concurrent injection of antiestrogens (Adkins and Nock, 1976a; Alexandre and Balthazart, 1986; Balthazart and Surlemont, 1990a), which suggests that the locally formed estrogens must interact with ER to activate behavior, although alternative interpretations are possible. It has indeed been demonstrated that antiestrogens can affect actions of estrogens on brain physiology, independent of the nuclear ER (Hiemke and Ghraf, 1984; Gray and Ziemian, 1992).

We had expected that ER would be colocalized with aromatase, at least in the POM, where the biological role of the locally produced E_2 is well established. The simplest and most parsimonious model explaining the local production and action of estrogens indeed implied that both the metabolism and action take place in a single cell (intracrine action). Because such a colocalization between ER and aromatase was observed in only 17% of the ARO-ir cells in the POM (Balthazart *et al.*, 1991; see Section III), additional hypotheses had to be formulated.

Three main groups of not mutually exclusive mechanisms can, in theory, be invoked to explain the behavioral effects of E_2 derived from local aromatization (Fig. 17). It is first possible that the few cells that contain at the same time ER and aromatase mediate the activation of male sexual behavior, whereas the rest of the POM does not. Given the multiple roles of the medial POA in vertebrates, it is indeed likely that the entire population of the POM neurons is not implicated in the behavioral activation. In this scenario, the control of behavior is effected by genomic activation in an intracrine mode (estrogens are produced and exert their effects in the same cell). Consistent with this interpretation, it has indeed been shown that most of ARO-ir cells that simultaneously contain ER are localized in the dorsolateral part of the POM (Balthazart *et al.*, 1991; Foidart *et al.*, 1996), a subregion of the nucleus that appears to be closely associated with behavioral activation (Panzica *et al.*, 1996b). This mode of action provides, however,

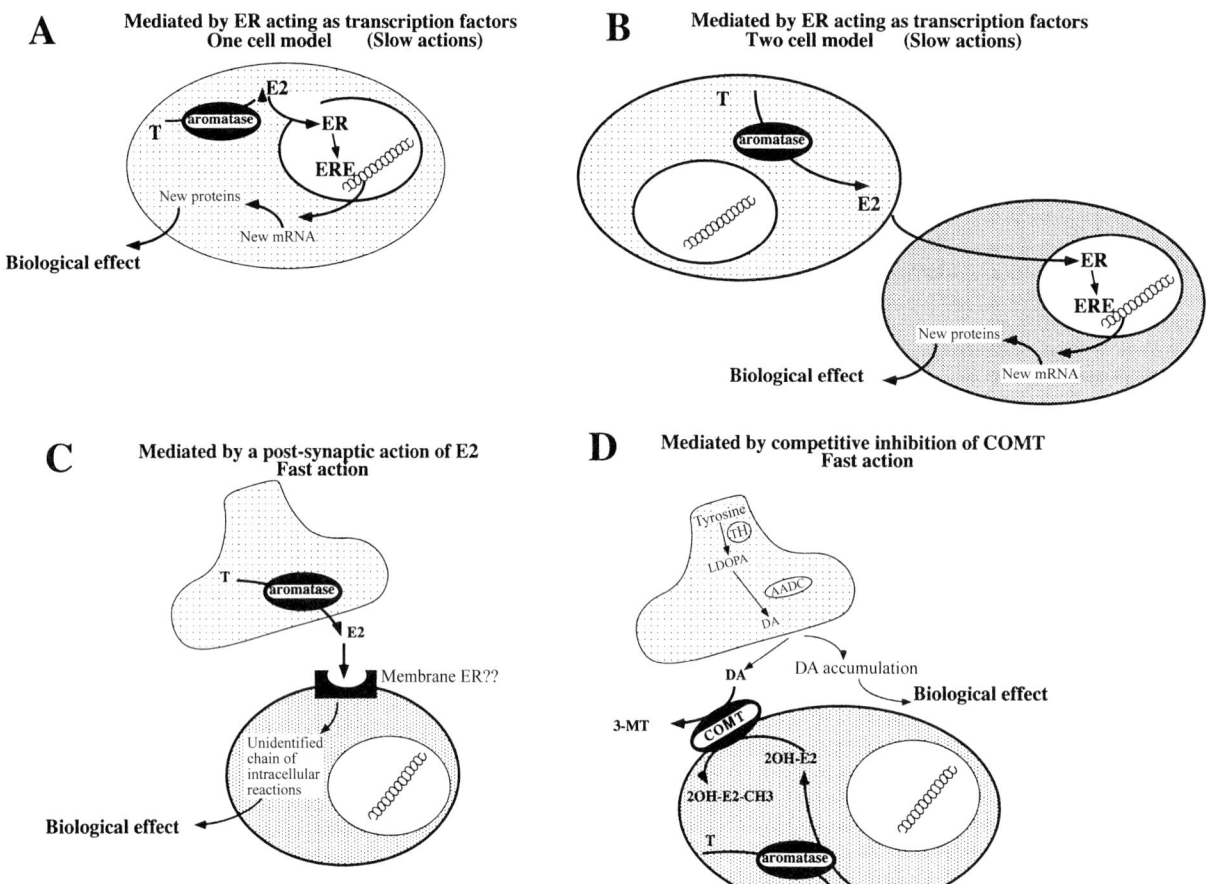

FIGURE 17 Schematic models describing the various ways in which estrogens formed locally in the brain by aromatization of testosterone could modify the expression of sexual behavior. In all panels, the cell or cell structure (axon terminal) containing aromatase and producing estrogens is dotted and the cell or cell structure where locally produced estrogens act is lightly shaded. (A) Estrogens bind to intracellular receptors (ER) that act as transcription factors at the DNA level by interacting with estrogen responsive elements (ERE). This leads to an increased synthesis of new mRNA and proteins that are ultimately responsible for the biological effects of E_2 in the cell where it was produced. This mode of action can take place in brain areas where ERs are colocalized with aromatase (e.g., the VMN; intracrine action), but it is impossible where this colocalization is not observed (POM and BST). (B) Estrogens produced locally in ER-negative neurons could diffuse to adjacent cells (paracrine action) that are ER-positive and produce biological effects by acting as transcription activators. (C) E_2 produced at the presynaptic level could exert its biological effects by acting directly at the level of the postsynaptic membranes. Mechanisms mediating this type of effects remain somewhat unclear and the definitive identification of membrane receptors for E_2 has not been completed. However, estrogens have been shown to exert important actions on cell membranes in the brain, including synaptogenesis and synaptic plasticity. An alternative mechanism of aromatase action at the synaptic level is also suggested by reports that aromatase, in addition to its role in the metabolism of androgens to estrogens, catalyzes a variety of enzymatic reactions such as the 6- or 7-hydroxylation of estrogens, the O-deethylation of 7-ethoxycoumarin or the removal of a methyl group from various substrates including cocaine (Osawa et al., 1993, 1994, 1997). Aromatase acting as an N-demethylase could have important effects on neurotransmitter metabolism and availability at the synaptic level. (D) Estrogens can be metabolized to produce catechol estrogens and there is evidence suggesting that this enzymatic reaction is catalyzed by aromatase itself acting as a bifunctional enzyme (Osawa et al., 1993). Catechol estrogens are the most powerful known competitive inhibitors of catechol O-methyl transferase (COMT) and have been proposed to block the metabolism of catecholamines in this manner, leading to their accumulation in the synaptic cleft and therefore to an enhancement of their action. This could represent another way through which estrogens locally produced in the brain, and in particular in axon terminals, could exert biological actions without binding to nuclear receptors.

no suggestion for a possible role of the large majority of ARO-ir neurons in POM.

A second possibility also assumes that locally produced estrogens act at the genomic level as transcription factor (they bind to nuclear ER), but in a paracrine fashion. ER positive cells are present in a large number in the POM (even if they do not correspond to ARO-ir cells; Balthazart *et al.*, 1989, 1991). It is therefore possible that estrogens produced by local aromatization of T passively diffuse through the intercellular space to neighboring cells and act in these cells after binding to the nuclear ER. The presence of ERβ in the POM is also consistent with this idea (Lakaye *et al.*, 1998; Foidart *et al.*, 1999a).

Finally, a third possibility, or more precisely group of possibilities, no longer implicates the binding of estrogens to nuclear ER but rather contemplates other nonconventional modes of steroid action. A number of independent observations support this type of explanation. In quail and in rats, biochemical studies have demonstrated the presence of high levels of aromatase activity in synaptosomes (pinched off synaptic terminals) prepared by differential centrifugation (Schlinger and Callard, 1989; Steimer, 1988; see also Section III). In addition, it has been shown by preembedding immunocytochemistry and electron microscopy that numerous synaptic boutons containing ARO-ir material are present in the POA of the quail as well as in the rat, monkey, and human (Naftolin *et al.*, 1990b, 1996; Balthazart *et al.*, 1990d). This suggests that significant amounts of estrogens are produced at the presynaptic level. These may be responsible for effects that would not be mediated by the nuclear ER but rather would involve a nongenomic action of the steroid (Schumacher, 1990; McEwen, 1994). This could include the previously described synaptogenic or synaptolytic effects of gonadal steroids (Naftolin and Brawer, 1978; Naftolin *et al.*, 1990a; Panzica *et al.*, 1985). Estrogens also appear to be responsible for the fluctuations of the postsynaptic membrane organization during the ovarian cycle (Naftolin *et al.*, 1990a), and they interfere with the binding of catecholamines to the synaptic membrane (Inaba and Kamata, 1979). Their synthesis at the synapse level is therefore functionally very relevant (see Section V.B.4.c.iii on rapid changes in aromatase activity).

Alternatively, it is possible that locally produced estrogens require further metabolism before they may exert their biological effects. It has been shown that in the brain estrogens can be hydroxylated in position 2 or 4, which leads to the formation of catecholestrogens (MacLusky *et al.*, 1984). The presence of an active 2-hydroxylase activity leading to the production of 2-hydroxy-estradiol has been demonstrated in the quail brain (Balthazart *et al.*, 1994b). Interestingly, the brain nuclei that display a high level of AA (Schumacher and Balthazart, 1987; Balthazart *et al.*, 1990f) also contain high levels of 2-hydroxylase activity (Balthazart *et al.*, 1994b) and vice versa. We do not have anatomical data at the cellular level that would tell us whether these two enzymes are colocalized in the same cells, but this appears possible based on the available biochemical results. This is also quite probable based on a report suggesting that these two enzymatic activities are due to the same protein, which shifts its activity as a function of the substrate concentration or pH (Osawa *et al.*, 1993).

Catecholestrogens are methylated by the enzyme catechol-O-methyl transferase (COMT). They compete at this level with the endogenous catecholamine, dopamine (DA). The methylation of DA into methoxytyramine represents one major catabolic pathway for this amine and it can therefore be expected that the presence of high concentrations of catecholestrogens exerts a competitive inhibition on the methylation of DA by the COMT activity, resulting in a buildup of DA concentration (Timmers *et al.*, 1988; Timmers and Lambert, 1989). More generally, it has been shown in a variety of model systems that catecholestrogens are able to modulate the synthesis, metabolism, and binding of catecholamines (MacLusky *et al.*, 1984; McEwen and Krey, 1984). Because it is well established that catecholamines, and in particular DA, represent a significant part of the neurochemical signals that control male sexual behavior (Crowley *et al.*, 1989; Meyerson *et al.*, 1979, 1985; Dohanich *et al.*, 1985; Meisel and Sachs, 1994; Bitran and Hull, 1987; Blackburn *et al.*, 1992; Crowley and Zemlan, 1981; Barclay and Cheng, 1985, 1992; Barclay *et al.*, 1992; Ottinger *et al.*, 1988; Edens, 1987; see also later), the presence of catecholestrogens at the presynaptic level is highly relevant to the control of this behavior. Their presence in the synaptic zone might directly regulate the activity of these neurotransmitters and these data bring additional support to the idea that estrogens produced at the presynaptic level could affect reproductive behavior by a direct action on the catecholamines metabolism at the level of nerve terminals, independent of any genomic action.

b) Role of Testosterone 5α Reduction As explained previously in detail, estrogenic metabolites of T play a major role in the activation of most aspects of male reproductive behavior. Many experiments have also identified a significant direct role of androgens in this process. In the brain, T can be transformed into a number of 5α reduced metabolites such as 5α-DHT and the two corresponding diols 5α-androstane-3α,17β-diol, and 5α-androstane-3β,17β-diol. T and 5α-DHT both bind with similar high affinities to the AR and in this way are able to activate the transcription of androgen-dependent genes.

In quail, two aspects of the behavioral repertoire of the male are efficiently activated by 5α-DHT. Castrated subjects treated with this steroid exhibit the precopulatory display, strutting and emit crowing vocalizations with frequencies similar to those observed in T-treated birds (Adkins, 1977; Schumacher and Balthazart, 1983). This observation, however, does not demonstrate that 5α reduction is required for the activation of these behaviors. It has been difficult, for technical reasons, to determine whether such effects of androgens in physiological conditions on behavior are due to the direct action of T or to the action of its metabolite 5α-DHT. The blockade of AR does not permit a differentiation of the actions of these two steroids; effective and specific inhibitors of the 5α-reductase activity were not available for a long time. One experiment attempted to answer this question in quail by injecting T-treated castrates with the 5α-reductase inhibitor 17β-N,N-diethylcarbamoyl-4-methyl-4-aza-5α-androstan-3-one (4MA; Alexandre and Balthazart, 1986). 4MA injections did not inhibit in a significant manner the activation of male copulatory behavior by T and, furthermore, when 4MA injections were combined with injections of the aromatase inhibitor ATD, behavior was not inhibited more than in birds injected with ATD alone (Alexandre and Balthazart, 1986). Newer inhibitors of 5α-reductase activity have become available, but their behavioral effects have not been tested in birds to the best of our knowledge. Additional studies with these compounds are needed to assess the specific behavioral significance of 5α-reduction of T in birds.

In general, the treatment of castrated birds with 5α-DHT alone activates little or no male copulatory behavior (Adkins, 1977; Adkins and Pniewski, 1978; Schumacher and Balthazart, 1983; Harding et al., 1983; Cheng and Lehrman, 1975). Some variability was observed, however, between experiments testing the behavioral effects of 5α-DHT. In mammals, large differences are commonly observed between species or even between strains of the same species. Similarly, in quail some studies found that 5α-DHT has no effect at all on copulatory behavior (Adkins, 1977; Adkins and Pniewski, 1978; Schumacher and Balthazart, 1983), whereas in other studies treatment for several weeks of castrated males with high doses of 5α-DHT restored sexual activity in a small but reproducible percentage of the birds (Deviche and Schumacher, 1982; Balthazart et al., 1985). It is difficult to ascertain whether this small percentage of reactive birds relates to individual differences in the steroid-specificity of behavioral activation (changes in the balance between estrogen- and androgen-dependence) or some other processes such as a differential catabolism of 5α-DHT. Several studies have shown that 5α-DHT is rapidly metabolized by the liver and the brain into several other compounds including large amounts of 5α-androstane-3α,17β-diol and 5α-androstane-3β,17β-diol (Deviche et al., 1987). These two diols have only limited androgenic effects as far as the activation of male sexual behavior is concerned so that they could be considered a relative inactivation pathway for 5α-DHT. In rats 5α-androstane-3β,17β-diol binds with a relatively high affinity to the ER (Vreeburg et al., 1975; Thieuland et al., 1981, 1982), and this could explain why this compound, as well as its parent steroid 5α-DHT, are able to activate some copulatory behavior in rats (Baum and Vreeburg, 1976) as well as in quail (Balthazart et al., 1985; see also Thieuland et al., 1983; for further discussion on this topic).

i) Interaction of estrogens and androgens. Although it is widely accepted that activation by T of male sexual behavior in most (if not all) avian species critically depends on its aromatization into an estrogen, most experiments attempting to activate behavior directly by a systemic treatment with estrogens used very high, probably nonphysiological levels of hormone. In view of the fact that E_2 binds with a low but nevertheless substantial affinity to the AR in the brain (Sheridan,

1983; Harding *et al.,* 1984; Lieberburg and Nottebohm, 1979; Bonneau *et al.,* 1987), this activation by estrogens could be of little biological relevance.

It has been shown in a large number of species that the effects of low doses of E_2, behaviorally ineffective by themselves, are markedly increased by a concurrent treatment with 5α-DHT (e.g., Adkins and Pniewski, 1978; Balthazart *et al.,* 1985; Harding *et al.,* 1983; see Martini, 1982; Melcangi *et al.,* 1999, for review on this topic in mammals). In mammals, this finding was originally interpreted by suggesting that 5α-DHT is responsible for the morphological development of peripheral structures involved in copulation (e.g., the penis), whereas estrogens were acting centrally on the behavior per se. This interpretation is, however, unlikely in birds that have, in general, no intromittant organ (with the exception of a few families, such as ducks) and nevertheless show a synergistic activation of copulatory behavior by estrogens and 5α-DHT. Furthermore, it has been shown in a few species that central action of estrogens and androgens are implicated in the activation of behavior. In rats it is indeed possible to facilitate copulatory behavior by brain implants of 5α-DHT in subjects receiving systemic subthreshold doses of estrogens (Baum *et al.,* 1982).

There is, therefore, compelling evidence that both estrogen and androgen in the brain are implicated in the activation of male sexual behavior. Estrogens derived from T aromatization occupy estrogen-binding sites, but it remains unclear whether androgen binding sites are occupied in physiological conditions by 5α-DHT or its parent hormone T due to the lack of good 5α-reductase inhibitors (see previous comment).

The existence of this central synergism between estrogens and androgens raises the question of the localization of the two types of receptors and of their anatomical relationship at the cellular level. However, this problem has not been studied in detail. Although it is clear that estrogens act mainly at the level of the medial POA to activate copulation, the site of androgenic stimulation has not been specifically identified. It is only known that in quail the implantation of the antiandrogen flutamide in the POA interferes with the behavioral activation induced by systemic T (Balthazart and Surlemont, 1990a). Similarly, in songbirds, the respective sites of androgen and estrogen action required for the activation of song (Harding *et al.,* 1983; Walters and Harding, 1988) remain completely unknown. Few of the song-control nuclei contain at the same time both AR and ER (this is only the case in ICo and in the HVc of canaries, but not of zebra finches; Gahr *et al.,* 1987, 1993), so an action on two distinct brain areas must probably be considered. The fact that lesions of the medial POA, a classic site for estrogen action, markedly decrease the amount of singing produced by male European starlings in a reproductive context (the presence of a female and of nest material; Riters and Ball, 1999) raises the hypothesis that singing in oscines may be controlled by the synergistic action of estrogens acting in the POA and androgens acting directly in the telencephalic song-control nuclei (e.g., the HVc and RA). This proposition, supported by circumstantial correlative evidence (Riters and Ball, 1999; Riters *et al.,* 2000a), has not been directly tested experimentally.

If androgens and estrogens activate behaviors at the same brain sites, we should determine whether they do so by acting on the same cells containing both types of receptors or on adjacent cells whose projections then interact functionally. To discriminate between these two alternative mechanisms, a limited number of studies in mammals and birds have analyzed simultaneously in the same brain sections the distribution of AR and ER. In hamsters and rats, it was found by double-labeled immunocytochemistry that a limited number of neurons located in brain areas that control sexual behavior (e.g., the POA, BST, and amygadala) do indeed contain the two types of receptors (Wood and Newman, 1995a; Gréco *et al.,* 1998). Limited information on this topic is available in birds. In the canary, it was shown by ER immunocytochemistry combined with *in vivo* autoradiography for 5α-DHT that many neurons in ICo contain both AR and ER. This colocalization was extremely rare in other brain areas (Gahr, 1990). Additional studies are needed to determine the cellular mechanisms responsible for the synergistic actions of E_2 and 5α-DHT.

Alternative indirect modes of interactions between these two steroids are also possible. It has been suggested, based on experiments carried out in rats, that estrogens inhibit the rapid catabolism of 5α-DHT into the corresponding diols, which are very weak androgens by themselves. This hypothesis was based on the observation that the aromatase inhibitor ATD inhibits male sexual behavior, but that the behavior can be restored by the simultaneous administration of the 5α-reductase inhibitor 4-MA (Södersten and Gustafsson, 1980b; Södersten et al., 1985, 1986). In this interpretation, E$_2$ derived from T aromatization inhibited the catabolism of 5α-DHT, and 4-MA played the same role in the absence of endogenous estrogens following administration of ATD. It must be mentioned, however, that E$_2$ was never identified as a potent 5α-reductase inhibitor except when present at very high, probably nonphysiological doses (Södersten et al., 1986). Furthermore, the behavioral effects of 4-MA in ATD-treated subjects could not be reproduced in quail (Alexandre and Balthazart, 1986), which throws additional doubts on this hypothesis. This hypothesis also implies that the activation of sexual behavior is mediated at the cellular level by the interaction of an androgen with AR (estrogens only serve as a 5α-DHT catabolism inhibitor). This then explains why the nonaromatizable synthetic androgen R1881 was shown in some experiments to activate a significant level of copulatory behavior in castrated subjects (Mammals: Baum, 1979; Södersten and Gustafsson, 1980a; Birds: Alexandre and Balthazart, 1986). Some behavioral activation has also been detected in quail after systemic treatment with 5α-DHT (Deviche and Schumacher, 1982; Balthazart et al., 1985; see previous discussion). The specificity of action of methyltrienolone has, however, been questioned. This compound is never able to restore copulatory behavior to its full precastration level, and, furthermore, it does so only at very high doses, which raises the possibility of a pharmacological interaction with receptors other than the AR (see Balthazart, 1989, for discussion and references). Evidence for this theory has been obtained; behaviorally effective doses of R1881 were found to reduce cytosolic estrogen binding sites by as much as 91% (Nyby and Simon, 1987). Although R1881 has no interaction with ER *in vitro* (Raynaud et al., 1980), it seems capable of interaction with ER *in vivo*.

In conclusion, despite much research carried out since the discovery of brain aromatization of T (Naftolin et al., 1972, 1975), we do not understand in detail how androgens and estrogens interact to activate male reproductive behavior in birds or in mammals. More research on this topic is desirable.

c) Role of Testosterone 5β Reduction The avian brain is also characterized by its capacity to transform T into 5β-reduced metabolites, mainly 5β-dihydrotestosterone (5β-DHT, an isomer of 5α-DHT) and the corresponding diols (essentially 5β-androstane-3α, 17β-diol). An active 5β-reductase activity has been identified in the brain of all avian species that have been studied—starling (Massa et al., 1977), chicken (Nakamura and Tanabe, 1974; Balthazart and Hirschberg, 1982), quail (Balthazart et al., 1979), ring dove (Hutchison and Steimer, 1981), zebra finch (Balthazart et al., 1986b), and Lapland longspur (*Calcarius lapponicus*; Soma et al., 1999a). The activity of this enzyme is in contrast low or nondetectable in mammals with exception of the golden hamster, (*Mesocricetus auratus*; Callard et al., 1978b, 1979).

Quantitatively, 5β reduction is the most active metabolic pathway that metabolizes T in the avian brain and 5β-reduced metabolites routinely represent 80–90% of the compounds produced during standard *in vitro* incubation with radioactive T. Interestingly, 5β-DHT appears to be devoid of any hormonal activity in most biological systems. 5β-DHT does not depress plasma gonadotropin levels nor stimulate the growth of secondary sexual characteristics such as the cloacal gland of quail and the comb of chicken (Adkins, 1977; Davies et al., 1980; Massa et al., 1980; Mori et al., 1974; Balthazart and Hirschberg, 1979). This compound also has no activational effect on male reproductive behavior in quail (Adkins, 1977) or doves (Hutchison and Steimer, 1981; Steimer and Hutchison, 1981a; Cohen and Cheng, 1982; Silver et al., 1979). In addition, 5β-DHT has no effect of the sexual differentiation of copulatory behavior in quail—injection of 2 mg 5β-DHT into quail eggs on day 9 of incubation (i.e., during the sensitive period when the injection of T or E$_2$ completely demasculinizes male-typical copulatory behavior: see Balthazart and Adkins-Regan, Chapter 66) has no effect on the reproductive behavior of birds hatched from these eggs (Schumacher et al., 1989). Taken together, these facts suggest that the 5β reduction of testosterone represents an inactivation shunt for the hormone that regulates the concentration of the active hormone in the target cells (Steimer and Hutchison, 1981a).

This interpretation is consistent with kinetic data indicating that the affinity of 5β-reductase for its substrate testosterone is 5–30 times lower than the affinity of the other metabolizing enzymes that produce active metabolites (aromatase and 5α-reductase). In contrast 5β-reductase has a much higher capacity (5–100 times) than the two other enzymes (Schumacher et al., 1984). When limiting concentrations of T are available, as in most physiological conditions, the formation of active metabolites (E_2 and 5α-DHT) are therefore favored, but, if too much substrate becomes available, the activity of this inactivation shunt becomes functionally important.

In contrast to these data, some limited androgenic effects of 5β-DHT were identified on the growth of the quail cloacal gland or growth of the chicken comb when the compound was injected in large doses (Balthazart and Hirschberg, 1979; Balthazart et al., 1981; Deviche et al., 1982). Some copulatory behavior was also observed in quail that had been injected with 5β-DHT in combination with subthreshold doses of T (Deviche et al., 1982). These effects can presumably be explained by the low affinity of 5β-DHT for the AR (Lieberburg and Nottebohm, 1979).

More surprisingly, it was observed that in young domestic chickens (Gallus domesticus) injections or subcutaneous Silastic implants of 5β-DHT are as efficient as T in activating the sexual responses elicited in the hand test situation described by Andrew (1975). In this test, the researcher's hand is first presented to the chick at the level of the breast and then suddenly lowered to floor level. The behavioral repertoire shown in these conditions consists of all the responses normally seen in adult cocks and includes mounting on the hand, crouching, treading, circling, and pelvic thrust. All these behaviors were induced by 5β-DHT with the same frequencies as in other chicks treated in parallel with T (Balthazart and Hirschberg, 1979; Balthazart et al., 1981). Surprisingly, the effects of 5β-DHT in this test were not blocked by the concurrent administration of the antiandrogen cyproterone acetate at a dosage that completely abolished the effects of T (Balthazart et al., 1981).

The discrepancy between this high behavioral effectiveness of 5β-DHT in the chick's hand test and its nearly complete inactivity in other animal models could be explained by the specific test situation in which the birds do not have to approach the stimulus (the hand is lowered in front of the chick), contrary to what happens in a normal situation (i.e., 5β-DHT could activate the copulatory reflex, but not the approach response and in general the appetitive aspects of sexual behavior). Alternatively, the discrepancy could also relate to the young age of the chick, associated with an immature blood–brain barrier (i.e., allowing 5β-DHT to enter the brain, although it could not do so in adults) or an immature less specific AR (that binds 5β-DHT more efficiently than the adult receptor; see Balthazart et al., 1981, for a more detailed discussion). There are no data that would allow us to discriminate between these interpretations. Based on all the available evidence, the behavioral effects observed in young chicks should be considered an exception, and it should be accepted that 5β-androstanes are devoid of androgenic, in particular behavioral, activity in birds. These compounds are not biologically inactive, however. In young animals, 5β-androstanes play a key role in hematopoiesis (Levere et al., 1967; Irving et al., 1976; Garavini and Cristofori, 1984).

d) Behavioral Effects Mediated by Changes in Brain Testosterone Metabolism The activity of brain T-metabolizing enzymes is affected by diverse factors, such as individual differences, the age or sex of the subjects, and their endocrine conditions. These metabolic changes are often correlated with differences in behavior and presumably play a causal role in the control of these behaviors. In particular, changes in aromatase, 5α-reductase, and 5β-reductase activities in specific brain regions seem to play a key role in the control of processes such as the sexual differentiation of reproductive behavior, sexual maturation, and puberty. These data are reviewed here.

i) Individual differences in behavior and brain metabolism of testosterone. The causation of individual differences in behavior is poorly understood. Although the previous history of an individual and other developmental factors presumably contribute to the explanation of these differences, the endocrine system should also play a significant part in their control. However, in a large number of studies it has been impossible to relate individual levels of reproductive behaviors that are known to be androgen-dependent to plasma levels of T (Balthazart and Schumacher, 1985; Balthazart, 1989). It is generally assumed that this lack of correlation is due to the fact that T circulates in adult males at levels that are more than sufficient to activate behavior and that, ultimately, the behavioral effects of T are modulated in association with their action in the brain (Nelson, 2000). Individual differences in intracellular metabolism (relative activation and inactivation) could then obscure the relationship of the behavior with plasma T levels and play a causal role in the genesis of the behavioral differences.

This idea was first illustrated in a study by Dessi-Fulgheri et al. (1976) showing that individual levels of fighting behavior in mice are positively correlated with the activity of the 17β-hydroxysteroid dehydrogenase in the brain, whereas a negative correlation was observed between the behavior and the aromatizing enzyme in the brain. The fighting behavior was by contrast not related to plasma T or E_2 levels. This prompted us to investigate whether similar correlations could be observed in quail.

An initial experiment demonstrated that, in a group of 20 male quail transferred from short days to long stimulating days, there is no correlation between the measures of reproductive behavior and plasma T but significant correlations are observed between behavior and aspects of the brain T metabolism. Aggressive actions were negatively correlated with the 5β-reductase activity in the hypothalamus (Balthazart et al., 1979). In two other experiments, several aggressive and sexual behaviors were quantified during three different tests (Delville et al., 1984a). The individual variations among all types of behaviors in the different situations were strongly correlated, indicating the existence of stable interindividual differences. In one experiment, the behavioral measures were significantly correlated with plasma T, but they were not in the other experiment performed under slightly different conditions. In both experiments, significant correlations were found between behavior and the hypothalamic 5β-reductase activity (the production of 5β-DHT and 5β-diol), but in the first experiment these correlations were positive, whereas they were negative in the second. These correlations were specific in that they were observed with the metabolism in the anterior but not posterior hypothalamus. These data suggest that individual variations in behavior are related to some aspects of T metabolism in the brain, particularly the 5β-reductase activity in the hypothalamus. The significance of these relationships is difficult to establish due the variations observed among experiments. The negative correlations between hypothalamic 5β-reductase and behavior could have a causal meaning so that birds would be behaviorally more active when their brain inactivates T less efficiently (5β-reduced compounds are behaviorally inactive). The experiment showing the reverse correlation is difficult to interpret in this context, although potential explanations have been proposed that could be experimentally tested (Delville et al., 1984a). Overall, the existence of these correlations, independent of their direction, points to a biologically relevant role of brain T metabolism. Whether behavioral differences are caused by differences in brain T metabolism or the correlations indicate the effects of the behavioral activity on the metabolism is, however, unclear. Studies carried out in ring doves clearly indicate that both types of causal links are likely to be functionally important (see Section V.B.6).

ii) *Sexual differentiation of behavior.* In Japanese quail, a series of studies have investigated the ontogeny of the brain metabolism of T and its relations with the development and sexual differentiation of male reproductive behavior. Masculine sexual behavior is strongly differentiated in quail (see Balthazart and Adkins-Regan, Chapter 66). Testosterone treatment restores copulation in castrated males, but is without effect in females (Adkins, 1975; Balthazart et al., 1983). Adkins and collaborators established that this differential responsiveness to the activating effects of T results from the demasculinization of female embryos by ovarian steroids. Males are usually considered the neutral or anhormonal sex because their phenotype apparently develops in the (relative) absence of hormonal control (Adkins-Regan, 1983). These conclusions are based on the finding that estradiol benzoate (EB) injection into male eggs demasculinizes the future adults (they do not copulate in response to T; Adkins, 1975, 1979), whereas the blockage of estrogen action or production in female embryos by the injection of an antiestrogen or an aromatase inhibitor prevents their demasculinization (Adkins, 1976; Balthazart et al., 1992a).

Surprisingly, TP injections also demasculinize male embryos (Adkins, 1975; Adkins-Regan et al., 1982). Knowing that the embryonic testes and adrenal glands secrete significant amounts of T (Ottinger and Bakst, 1981; Schumacher et al., 1988b) raises the intriguing question as to why males are not demasculinized by their testicular secretions. The demasculinization of male embryos requires larger doses of androgen than of estrogen—2 μg of E_2, estrone, or estriol injected on day

9 of incubation significantly decrease the copulatory behavior of male quail, but the same dose of T is not effective (Whitsett *et al.,* 1977). This differential sensitivity is confirmed by detailed dose-response experiments—the critical doses for demasculinizing male copulatory behavior are 1 and 500 μg for EB and TP, respectively (Adkins, 1979).

It can therefore be inferred that physiological plasma levels of T are too low to demasculinize male embryos. However, the analysis of T metabolism in the brain identified an additional mechanism that contributes to prevent the demasculinization of male embryos by their endogenous androgens. A series of experiments by Adkins-Regan *et al.* (1982) showed that the T-induced demasculinization requires T aromatization. This is supported by the observations that aromatizable androgens (T, TP, and androstenedione), but not nonaromatizable ones (5α-DHTP and androsterone), are active agents in the demasculinization process; that the antiestrogen tamoxifen blocks the T-induced demasculinization; and that ATD, an aromatase inhibitor, inhibits the TP-induced, but not the EB-induced, demasculinization.

Considering that rates of aromatization in the brain are extremely low (a few femtomoles per milligram of tissue per hour) in 4-day-old chick (Callard *et al.,* 1978a,b), in newly hatched or adult quail or ring doves (Steimer and Hutchison, 1980; Schumacher *et al.,* 1984; Hutchison and Schumacher, 1986), and in embryonic quail (Schumacher *et al.,* 1988a), it can be expected that the activity of the enzyme is a limiting step in the demasculinization induced by T. This would explain the requirement for large doses of exogenous hormones and protect male embryos from their endogenous secretions.

In the avian brain, T is also reduced into 5β-androstanes (mainly 5β-DHT and 5β-diol). Based on the available data, it appears that these compounds are devoid of androgenic activity in adult birds (see previous discussion Balthazart, 1983, 1989), and 5β-DHT is also apparently devoid of differentiating effects in the quail (Schumacher *et al.,* 1989). It is thus usually considered that 5β-reductase is an inactivation pathway for T that controls in the target cells the biological activity of the hormone. Interestingly, the 5β-reductase activity is extremely high in the hypothalamus of male quail throughout embryonic life (Balthazart and Ottinger, 1984). This enzymatic activity is at least 10 times higher in the embryos than in the adults and only decreases when birds reach sexual maturity at 4–5 weeks posthatching. This is relatively specific to the hypothalamus—the 5β-reductase activity decreases markedly in the cerebellum around hatching and even earlier in the cloacal gland, a sexually dimorphic androgen target organ (Sachs, 1967) that also differentiates under the influence of embryonic steroids (Adkins, 1975, 1979; Adkins-Regan *et al.,* 1982; Schumacher and Balthazart, 1984b). Considering that 5β reduction irreversibly transforms T into behaviorally inactive compounds that are also not aromatizable, the high enzymatic activity present in the embryonic hypothalamus should protect males from being behaviorally demasculinized by converting aromatizable androgens to nonaromatizable metabolites.

iii) Sexual development during ontogeny. In domestic cockerels, sexual maturation is contingent with a sharp decrease of the 5β-reductase activity in the brain and pituitary gland (Massa and Sharp, 1981). In Japanese quail, experiments were carried out to research whether the changes described in cockerels were anatomically and biochemically specific (i.e., do they occur in neuroendocrine structures only and do they specifically affect the 5β-reductase?). T metabolism was studied in the hypothalamus, hyperstriatum, pituitary gland, and cloacal gland in quail of different ages between hatching and sexual maturity (Balthazart and Schumacher, 1984b). A sharp decrease in 5β-reductase activity was observed in the brain but not in the pituitary or cloacal gland. This change also appeared specific to 5β-reductase and did not affect the 5α reduction of T.

Based on these data, it was then speculated that the relative insensitivity of young birds to the activation of reproductive behaviors by T (see, e.g., Schleidt, 1970) could result from the presence in their brain of an active 5β-reductase causing a very rapid inactivation of the hormone. For a number of technical reasons (see Balthazart *et al.,* 1984a, for detail) this idea cannot be tested directly. However, it is possible to obtain a measure of the relative action of T in adult and young quail by comparing, in both age groups, the behavioral and morphological effects of T with those of 5α-DHT. Both T and 5α-DHT activate crowing and promote cloacal gland growth in adult castrated quail.

Because 5β-reductase activity decreases with age in the brain but not in the cloacal gland, 5β-androstanes have little or no androgenic action in quail (see previous discussion) and 5α-DHT is protected from inactivation by 5β-reductase, whereas T is not, it could be predicted that 5α-DHT should be relatively more potent than T for activating crowing in young quail than in adult quail, whereas no such age-related difference would be found in the activation of cloacal gland growth. Experimental data confirmed this prediction (Balthazart et al., 1984a).

A number of reports had previously established that T and 5α-DHT stimulate crowing and cloacal gland growth in adult quail with approximately the same efficiency when hormones are given in unesterified form (Balthazart et al., 1980b; Deviche and Schumacher, 1982; Wada, 1982; Schumacher and Balthazart, 1983). In contrast, we found that in young quail 5α-DHT is largely more potent than T in the induction of crowing, but that this difference was not observed in the activation of cloacal gland growth. These observations are best explained by referring to the fact that 5β-reductase inactivates T more in the brain of young than adult quail and that 5α-DHT is protected from this inactivation (see Balthazart et al., 1984a, for a more detailed discussion). Therefore, developmental changes in 5β-reductase activity probably play an important role in the control of T action.

The changes in 5β-reductase activity as a function of age appear to be a common feature of birds and have also been demonstrated in ring doves (Hutchison and Hutchison, 1985) and in zebra finches (Balthazart et al., 1986b), in addition to the cockerel and quail already mentioned. In parallel, the 5α-reductase and aromatase activities are generally lower in young birds than in adults. This conclusion is supported by studies on one precocial (quail) and two altricial species (ring dove and zebra finch). In contrast, brain aromatase activity appears to be high during the perinatal period of mammals (Canick et al., 1984). The biological implications of this taxonomic difference are unknown. Kinetic studies carried out with quail hypothalamic tissue suggest that differences between chicks and adult metabolic enzymes are not caused by ontogenetic changes in affinity of the enzymes for their substrate. The apparent Km for each enzymatic activity is similar in adult and newly hatched quail (Hutchison and Schumacher, 1986). The age-related changes in enzyme activity therefore presumably reflect differences in the amount of enzyme expressed in young and adult subjects. This is in contrast with data obtained in zebra finches in which the Km of 5β-reductase and aromatase seem to decrease (increased affinity) between hatching and adulthood (Vockel et al., 1988). In this case, the change in enzymatic activity may be related to changes in the structure of the enzymes or in their molecular environment (the presence of age-specific competitors or activators). Whether this difference between quail and zebra finches represents a general difference between precocial and altricial species and has biological consequences for the control of behavior remains to be determined.

iv) Sex differences and sexual differentiation. T metabolism in the brain also contributes to the explanation of sex differences in behavioral responsiveness to T. In mammals and birds, the process of sexual differentiation results in two types of adults with profound differences in their behavioral responses to steroids, in particular to T. The same treatment with T often elicits more vigorous and more frequent copulatory behavior in castrated males than in ovariectomized females. In some species such as the Japanese quail, females are almost completely insensitive to the activating effects of T on male sexual behavior (Adkins and Adler, 1972; Adkins, 1975). Numerous studies have been devoted to the analysis of the mechanisms that may underly this differential sensitivity to T (e.g., the distribution of steroid receptors, modulation of neurotransmitter levels, or turnover). In particular, experiments were conducted to research whether the sexually differentiated responses to T result from a sexually differentiated neural metabolism (the production of more active metabolites and less inactive metabolites in males than in females). Data supporting this interpretation were obtained in a few model systems. In many mammalian and avian species, the POA-hypothalamic aromatase activity is higher in males than in females—in mammals (Naftolin et al., 1972, 1975; Reddy et al., 1974; Roselli et al., 1985; Tobet et al., 1985) and birds (Schumacher and Balthazart, 1984a, 1986; Schlinger and Callard, 1987; Vockel et al., 1988, 1990b).

By contrast, very few sex differences in 5α-reductase activity have been identified in brain areas that could be directly related to the behavioral sex differences.

This enzymatic activity shows major changes during ontogeny (see previous discussion), but the patterns are usually quite similar in males and females. Using a microdissection of the hypothalamic and adjacent areas, Schumacher and Balthazart (1986) demonstrated the presence in the anterior hypothalamus of a higher 5α-reductase activity in males than in females. This study also showed that the 5β-reductase activity is higher in females than in males for brain regions located in the lobus paraolfactorius and in POA.

Together, these data support the hypothesis that the behavioral insensitivity of females to activating effects of T results from an insufficient transformation of the steroid into active metabolites or from an excessive inactivation by 5β reduction. These studies were, however, performed on gonadally intact animals, so enzymatic differences observed in the brain could result from the exposure to a different hormonal milieu. Most of the sex differences in T metabolism detected so far indeed consist in a higher aromatase activity in males, and it is established that aromatase activity is inducible by T (see later). Therefore, the higher aromatase in males may only reflect their higher levels of plasma T. Accordingly, gonadectomy not only decreases aromatase activity, but also suppresses its dimorphism in all species investigated—for example, in rats (Roselli et al., 1985) and quail (Schumacher and Balthazart, 1986). One study, however, analyzed the sex differences of T metabolism in male and female quail that were either gonadally intact or had been gonadectomized and treated or not treated with exogenous T (Schumacher and Balthazart, 1986). The sex difference in 5β-reductase activity that had been found in intact birds was confirmed in this study, but disappeared in gonadectomized birds and was not restored by the treatment with T. Similarly, the sex difference in 5α-reductase activity that was present in the anterior hypothalamus of gonadally intact subjects is only the result of a differential induction by T. The 5α-DHT production in this brain region was decreased by castration in males and increased by T treatment in both sexes. However, this regulation by T of the 5α-reductase activity in the brain probably plays no part in the control of male sexual behavior because 5α- reductase activity is no longer different in males and females after treatment with the same dose of T, even though their behavior remains dimorphic.

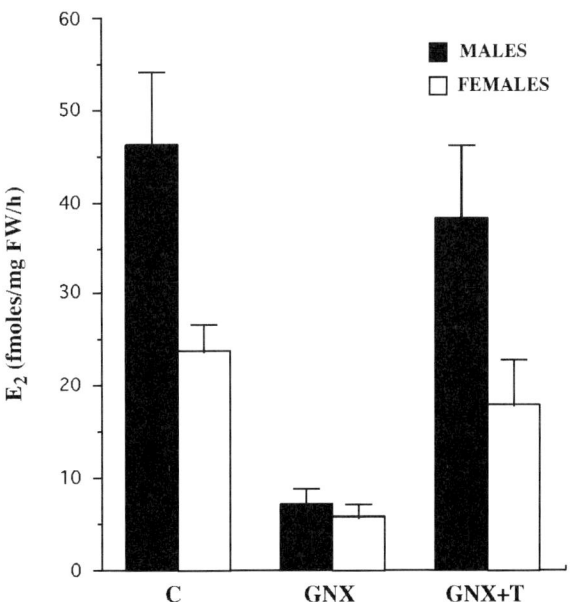

FIGURE 18 Sexual dimorphism and control by steroids of aromatase activity (AA) in the quail POA. The figure illustrates the mean levels of AA measured in sexually mature birds (C), in gonadectomized birds (GNX), and in GNX birds treated with testosterone (GNX + T). In control birds, AA is higher in males than in females; it is reduced to basal levels by gonadectomy and induced differentially in males and females by a same treatment with T. Data from Schumacher and Balthazart (1986).

In contrast, the study of aromatase identified a stable sex difference that is presumably implicated in the control of behavior (see Fig. 18). The higher AA previously observed in the POA of males compared with females disappeared in gonadectomized animals and AA was reduced to similar baseline levels in both sexes. However, the induction of enzymatic activity by T was significantly larger in males than in females. Kinetic experiments confirmed that in T-treated males and females AA is higher in males for all concentration of substrate between 10 and 80 nM, although the affinity (Km) of the enzyme is similar in both sexes. This suggests that males and females differ by the quantity of aromatase that is present in their POAs, but that the characteristics of the enzyme are the same in both sexes (Schumacher and Balthazart, 1986). This differential induction of aromatase by T can be observed for a wide range of T dosages administered to the subjects in vivo (Balthazart et al., 1986a, 1990c). Interestingly, the sexually differentiated inducibility of the aromatase by T does not seem to be established during the early posthatching period when the mechanisms regulating the copulatory behavior are not themselves fully differentiated (Schumacher and Balthazart, 1984b; Schumacher and Hutchison, 1986). Considering that the activation of copulatory behavior by T requires its aromatization into E_2, the enzymatic difference observed in the quail POA should contribute to the causation of the behavioral sex differences in response to T. It must, however, be noted that this enzymatic difference alone cannot explain the difference in behavior because the treatment of ovariectomized females with estrogens, which should bypass the enzymatic limitation, is not effective for inducting male-typical copulatory behavior (Schumacher and Balthazart, 1983).

v) Seasonal changes and changes related to photoperiod. In wild birds living in the temperate zone, which exhibit pronounced annual breeding cycles, there is an associated cycle in the activity of T-metabolizing enzymes, especially aromatase. This correlation provides additional evidence for a functional implication of these enzymes in the control of reproductive behavior. These effects can either be direct in that they modify T action in the POA–anterior hypothalamus or indirect, in which case they affect the secretion of hormonal steroids via a change in their feedback action on the hypothalamus-pituitary axis. These changes are well documented in a number of avian species, but also in some mammals whose reproduction is heavily dependent on photoperiod, such as hamsters.

In the European starling (*Sturnus vulgaris*), as in other songbirds, song is regulated by a network of steroid-sensitive nuclei in the telencephalon, but also influenced by steroid action in the diencephalon (Riters and Ball, 1999). In starlings, serum T concentrations are highest at the onset of breeding in spring when males sing to attract females for reproduction. Outside the breeding season, T is undetectable; however, males continue to sing at high levels. This suggests that singing outside the breeding season might not be T-dependent, although it appears to be so in the spring. Alternatively, singing when T concentrations are low might continue to be regulated by T due to an increased sensitivity of the brain to the action of the steroid. Such a change in sensitivity to T may result from increased steroid receptor concentrations in the brain or from changes in the intracellular T metabolism leading to an increased production of active metabolites. Bottoni and Massa (1981) showed that the 5α- and 5β-reductases of T by the hypothalamus and pituitary gland are quite different in the breeding season (May) compared to the beginning (July) and the end of the photorefractory period (November during fall singing). Specifically, the formation of 5β-androstanes by the hypothalamus was greater in May than in July or November. The opposite changes were detected in the pituitary gland. These enzymatic changes have, unfortunately, no obvious role in the control of reproduction.

One study analyzed the seasonal changes for a full year in the activity of four brain T-metabolizing enzymes—aromatase; 5α-reductase; 5β-reductase; and 17β-HSDH, which converts E_2 into estrone or T into androstenedione (Riters *et al.*, 2000b). Regional differences in the magnitude and timing of seasonal changes in each of these enzymes were demonstrated. Aromatase activity was highest in each brain region during the breeding season. Peak activity levels for 17β-HSDH and 5α-reductase activities were observed at the onset of the breeding season, with smaller peaks detected outside the breeding season in July in the telencephalon. In addition to these peaks in enzyme activity obviously related to the breeding season, a high AA was observed in the telencephalon throughout fall and winter. During the same period, 5β-reductase activity was minimal in the telencephalon. Taken together, these results support the idea that seasonal changes in the activity of T-metabolizing enzymes that produce androgenic and estrogenic metabolites or that inactivate T play a significant role in determining seasonal changes in behavior and reproductive physiology. These data are also compatible with the idea that singing in male starlings outside the breeding season continues to be regulated by steroids because the brain sensitivity to T action varies as a consequence of changes in intracellular metabolism.

Similarly, in Lapland longspur, an arctic breeding species, it was found that the 5β-reductase activity is high throughout the telencephalon (compared to the diencephalon) and changes in a region-specific manner during the breeding cycle. The changes observed in brain 5β-reductase activity could not, however, explain the discrepancy observed between the changes in time of plasma T and territorial aggression in males (increases in plasma T during the spring are not correlated with aggression in this species, contrary to behaviour observed in temperate-zone species; Soma *et al.*, 1999a).

In Japanese quail, short photoperiods, which inhibit all reproductive processes, induce a decrease in hypothalamic aromatase and 5α-reductase activities (the production of behaviorally active metabolites), but an increase in the production of 5β-androstanes (Schlinger *et al.*, 1984; Callard, 1984). These enzymatic changes should amplify the effects on behavior of the variations in plasma T resulting from the exposure to short days. In general, it seems that the hypothalamic aromatase is modulated to a larger extent that the reductases. In red grouse (*Lagopus lagopus scoticus*), AA in the anterior and posterior hypothalamus is directly related to gonadal function during a photoinduced reproductive cycle (Sharp *et al.*, 1986). Enzyme activity increases within 3 weeks of transfer to long days and stays high for approximately 1 month, during which birds are reproductively active. When they become photorefractory and as a consequence gonadal activity declines, the AA returns to baseline level. These enzymatic changes are probably controlled directly by variations in plasma T (because T induces brain AA), but they should amplify the behavioral effects of T by increasing the production of active estrogenic metabolites. Similar controls are also present in photoperiodic mammals (Campbell *et al.*, 1978; Callard *et al.*, 1983; Morin and Zucker, 1978).

vi) Aging. Aging in animals and humans coincides with a decrease in sexual activity associated with a host of endocrine modifications including changes in the patterns of secretion of T and pituitary gonadotropins. These phenomena are also observed in Japanese quail, in which a marked decrease in copulatory behavior is observed after approximately 1 year of age. In older quail, two subpopulations can be distinguished that either show or do not show copulatory behavior in standard test situations (Ottinger *et al.*, 1983). In parallel, T metabolism in the POA–anterior hypothalamus is also affected by age and these changes are differential in sexually active and inactive birds. The 5α-reductase activity increases markedly in old active males, but does not change or slightly decreases in old inactive birds compared to young control subjects. There is also a general decrease in 5β-reductase with age, but this change is not different in active and inactive birds (Balthazart *et al.*, 1984b). Considering that 5α-DHT is an active metabolite of T that activates copulatory behavior and sexual displays in combination with E_2 (5β-DHT is devoid of behavioral effects), the enzymatic changes observed in aging animals can be considered to be neuroendocrine adaptations (the production of more active and less inactive metabolites) that could be causally related to the maintenance of sexual activity in old birds.

A host of studies have therefore shown that the metabolism of T in the brain varies as a function of the age, sex, and endocrine condition of a subject. These changes correlate with changes in behavior and, more specifically, with changes in the effectiveness of T action on behavior. Based on the behavioral effects of the metabolites, it can be expected that this intracellular metabolism of T and its variations amplify or inhibit the effects of T on behavior. A direct experimental test of this idea is, however, available in a limited number of cases only.

3. Control of the Activity of Steroid-Metabolizing Enzymes

Given the key role played by several steroid-metabolizing enzymes, in particular by aromatase, in the control of reproductive behavior, a large number of experiments have been carried out to investigate the factors that control the activity of these enzymes. A very large fraction of these studies were devoted to the controls of preoptic AA and these are reviewed here.

The activity of brain aromatase in birds varies markedly as a function of the sex of the subjects, their age, the photoperiod they are exposed to, and the social condition in which the birds are living. Most of these changes are mediated by changes in the circulating levels of T. Castration reduces the POA-hypothalamic AA to basal levels in all species investigated so far and treatment with exogenous T restores the enzymatic activity to levels normally seen in sexually mature males. AA in other brain regions seems, however, to be less sensitive to variations in plasma T, and in some cases (e.g., in the songbirds telencephalon) the mechanisms that control the activity of this enzyme have not been fully identified.

a) Neuroanatomically Specific Control by Testosterone of Brain Aromatase Activity High levels of AA have been measured in the brain areas that are implicated in the activation of male copulatory behavior in a few avian species such as the ring dove, quail, and zebra finch (see Section III for details). The highest levels of AA are actually located in the medial part of the POA where T action is necessary and sufficient to activate sexual behavior in males exposed to the adequate stimuli from a female.

In quail, biochemical studies combining ultrasensitive radioenzymatic assays with microdissection by the punch technique of Palkovits (Palkovits and Brownstein, 1983) have identified a very high level of AA in the POM—AA is higher in this nucleus than in all other brain areas that were investigated (Schumacher and Balthazart, 1987). AA in POM is also significantly higher in males than in females (Schumacher and Balthazart, 1986) and it is controlled by the circulating levels of T—a decrease is observed after castration, but enzyme activity is restored to levels typical of sexually mature males after 2 weeks of treatment with T (Schumacher and Balthazart, 1986; Balthazart *et al.*, 1990c). These sex differences and T-induced changes in enzyme activity parallel differences observed in the copulatory behavior of corresponding subjects—males but not females show male-typical copulatory responses and it is well established that castration suppresses and T treatment restores copulatory behavior (see previous discussion). Therefore, these correlations provide additional support to the idea that the preoptic AA represents a limiting step in the activation by T of this behavior.

Subsequently, immunocytochemistry and *in situ* hybridization studies demonstrated that in several species (e.g., quail, dove, zebra finch, starling) the POM is clearly outlined by a dense population of cells expressing high levels of aromatase. Because the POM has been identified as a key area for the activation of male sexual behavior, detailed studies were carried out in quail to analyze by semiquantitative anatomical methods the controls of these ARO-ir neurons. A sex difference in the number of preoptic ARO-ir cells (males > females) could in this way be located in the posterior part of the POM at the level of the anterior commissure. In addition, it was shown that very few ARO-ir elements are present in the POM of castrated males, but that their number dramatically increases after a 2-week treatment with T. This increase was particularly important also in the caudal part of the nucleus (Foidart *et al.*, 1994a; Balthazart *et al.*, 1996d). These changes in the number of positive cells presumably reflect the differences in enzymatic activity that had been identified before (males > females; control + T males > control males) and suggest that these resulted from a change in the amount of enzyme present in the POA (see Balthazart and Foidart, 1993a,b, for additional discussion).

This notion is further supported by studies in which the concentration of aromatase mRNA was quantified by reverse transcriptase-polymerase chain reaction (RT-PCR) in subjects placed in various endocrine conditions. The aromatase mRNA concentration in the POA was significantly reduced by castration and displayed a four-fold increase after treatment with T (Harada *et al.*, 1992). This suggests that T affects AA primarily by changing the concentration of the enzyme, presumably through an increased transcription of its mRNA. Alternative mechanisms, including the stabilization of the preexisting mRNA, the modulation of mRNA translation, or the direct regulation of the enzymatic activity, cannot be completely excluded, but they should only play a minor role in aromatase control (see Balthazart and Foidart, 1993b; Panzica *et al.*, 1996b, for more detail). It is clear that the major part of the control by T of AA takes place at the pretranslational level.

The anatomical data also showed that the changes and sex differences in aromatase concentration are more prominent in the caudal than in the rostral part of the POM. This suggests that this part of the nucleus may play a more critical role in the control of aromatase-dependent responses such as male copulatory behavior. As previously described, this notion has received direct experimental support from the detailed analysis of the behavioral effects of restricted electrolytic lesions aimed at the POM. Lesions of the caudal POM are more closely associated with a deficit in copulatory behavior than are more rostral lesions (Balthazart *et al.*, 1998a).

b) Preoptic Aromatase Activity Is Controlled by Testosterone Mainly through Its Estrogenic Metabolites Given the causal relationships that link aromatase to sexual behavior, studies were carried out to analyze the endocrine specificity of aromatase induction. These have consistently demonstrated that both in quail and ring doves the endocrine specificity of aromatase induction is similar to the specificity of sexual behavior. Aromatase can be most efficiently increased by a combined action of estrogens (e.g. E_2 or DES) and androgens (e.g. DHT or methyltrienolone), but the role of estrogens is always more important than the role of androgenic metabolites (Adkins and Pniewski, 1978; Adkins et al., 1980; Schumacher and Balthazart, 1983; Balthazart et al., 1985; Hutchison and Steimer, 1986; Hutchison et al., 1989). High doses of estrogens alone produce a significant induction of aromatase, but this is not the case for DHT, which acts only to synergize with E_2 and increase its effects. These relationships have been documented at the levels of the enzymatic activity (Hutchison and Steimer, 1986; Schumacher et al., 1987), of the number of ARO-ir cells (Harada et al., 1993; Balthazart et al., 1994c), and of the aromatase mRNA concentration (Harada et al., 1993). Taken together, these data clearly show that estrogens produced locally in the brain by the aromatization of T play a key role both in the control of male sexual behavior and in the control of AA and aromatase synthesis.

c) Estrogen Effects on Aromatase Activity and Synthesis Are Indirect It is in general accepted that most effects of steroids are genomic and mediated through binding with specific intracellular (nuclear) receptors. A parsimonious view of the functional organization of the brain suggested therefore that estrogens would increase the synthesis of aromatase mRNA by binding to ER and activating transcription directly in the nucleus of aromatase cells. Consistent with this view, double-labeled immunocytochemical studies showed that in the ventromedial and tuberal hypothalamus a large fraction (70–80%) of the ARO-ir cells also contain ER-ir (Balthazart et al., 1991). However, very few doubled-labeled cells were found in more rostral groups of ARO-ir cells such as the POM (only 17% of ARO-ir cells containing ER) or the BST (4%). A similar neuroanatomical specialization in the colocalization of aromatase and ER has also been detected in rodents, suggesting that this represents a common feature of vertebrates (Yokosuka et al., 1994; Tsuruo et al., 1995, 1996).

These anatomical data strongly suggest that the simplistic view implying that locally produced estrogens act in the cell where they were synthesized to stimulate the transcription of aromatase (intracrine process) has to be reconsidered. Estrogen production and estrogen action presumably do not take place in the same cells. It is possible that the E_2 produced by aromatization diffuses to adjacent neurons that contain ER and acts at this level by a paracrine action—brain areas containing ARO-ir cells also contain ER-ir cells even if these two markers are not colocalized (Balthazart et al., 1991). Alternatively, the estrogens produced in the brain may be returned to the general blood circulation (or to local circuits of blood vessels) as already demonstrated in the zebra finch (*Taeniopygia guttata;* Schlinger and Arnold, 1992a, 1993) and in this way affect ER-positive cells located at a distance from the ARO-ir cells. In both cases, however, these mechanisms imply the existence of a nervous (micro)circuit with at least one synaptic connection in the control of aromatase synthesis by steroids.

This notion is indirectly supported by data derived from measurements of AA in neuronal *in vitro* cultures. Although it is well established in both mammals and birds that androgens and estrogens acting alone or in synergy exert a very marked stimulatory effect on AA and aromatase expression (Roselli et al., 1987; Roselli and Resko, 1989; Roselli, 1991; Balthazart et al., 1990f; Schumacher et al., 1987; Harada et al., 1992, 1993), it has been impossible to demonstrate this effect *in vitro* in neuronal cells cultures derived from embryonic rats and mice (Lephart et al., 1992; Abe-Dohmae et al., 1994) or quail (J. Balthazart and C. Balthazart-Raze, unpublished; M. Baillien and J. Balthazart, unpublished). This could reflect the incomplete maturity of the cellular elements present in these cultures, but, alternatively, this may simply be due to the disruption in culture of the (local) circuitry implicated in the aromatase control. Based on the anatomical data previously presented, we are inclined to believe that the second of these interpretations may be correct.

It is also interesting to note that despite the fact that several studies have been devoted to the aromatase gene (*CYP19*), none of them has identified estrogen responsive elements (ERE) on that gene. Different promoters located on exon 1 are used to regulate aromatase transcription in different human tissues, and the promoters used in the brain have been identified in a few mammalian species (Simpson et al., 1994; Lephart, 1996; Honda et al., 1994, 1996) but little information is, to our knowledge, available on this topic in avian species (Ramachandran et al., 1999). It is still possible that an ERE is located at a significant distance upstream from the *CYP19* gene and that this has so far prevented its identification, but the negative data obtained may also be taken as evidence suggesting that estrogens do not regulate aromatase expression in a direct manner. It has also become clear that ER can affect transcription by mechanisms that do not involve ERE consensus sequences (e.g., via binding to an activator protein 1 (AP1) consensus sequence, e.g., Paech et al., 1997). Taken together these data support the notion that estrogens produced by aromatization of T in the brain do not bind to ER located in the same cells to regulate the enzyme concentration in an intracrine mode of action.

This conclusion was formulated before the discovery in mammals of ERβ. The absence of colocalization between aromatase and ER concerns only the classic receptor, ERα. ERβ has now been cloned in at least two avian species, the Japanese quail and European starling, and the corresponding mRNA has been shown by in situ hybridization to be present in all brain areas that contains high densities of aromatase cells, in particular the POM and BST (Lakaye et al., 1998; Foidart et al., 1999a; Bernard et al., 1999). These studies were based on film autoradiography and do not provide a cellular level of localization. It is not known whether ERβ is colocalized with aromatase in these areas or is mostly located in adjacent neurons, as previously demonstrated for ERα.

Therefore, other modes of regulation have been considered and, in particular, experimental evidence has been accumulated indicating that aromatase concentrations in the POA-hypothalamus are controlled by afferent catecholaminergic inputs on aromatase cells. This evidence is reviewed Section V.B.4.c.

4. Steroid–Neurotransmitter Interactions

Steroids have been shown to modify neurotransmissions and consequently reproductive behavior in a variety of ways (McEwen, 1981; Feder, 1984; McEwen et al., 1987; Etgen et al., 1992). Among the many neurotransmitters regulated by T, DA appears to be an important transmitter for the control of male sexual behavior (Blackburn et al., 1992; Bitran and Hull, 1987; Hull, 1995; Hull et al., 1999). The general conclusion that originally emerged from a series of studies by several different laboratories is that DA facilitates male sexual behavior in rats and other mammals. The administration of dopaminergic agonists decreases the latency to initiate copulatory behavior and reduces the number of intromissions required for ejaculation. DA antagonists have also been reported consistently to disrupt both the initiation and the rate of copulatory behavior. These effects involve both the D1 and the D2 dopamine receptor subtypes. The neuroanatomical location of these effects has not been fully investigated, but it is clear that the POA is, at least, one effective site for the actions of these drugs on male sexual behavior (Blackburn et al., 1992; Meisel and Sachs, 1994). Some of these conclusions have been extended to a few species of birds, although a number of differences appear to exist. With the available evidence, it is difficult to determine whether discrepancies concern the few species that were investigated or the two vertebrate classes in general.

It is unclear how DA (or other neurotransmitters and neuropeptides) and T interact in the regulation of male sex behavior. Three possibilities have been discussed, illustrated schematically for DA in Fig. 19. First, changes in dopaminergic activity might be one of the neurochemical events that form part of the cascade of changes induced in the brain by T. It is known that in mammals, T alters DA turnover in the POA and hypothalamus (Simpkins et al., 1980, 1983; Hull et al., 1995) and affects dopaminergic transmission in the nigrostriatal pathway (Alderson and Baum, 1981). ER have also identified in dopaminergic neurons, namely in the nucleus periventricularis and in the zona incerta (Sar, 1984; Grant and Stumpf, 1975; Batailler et al., 1992). In birds ER also have been detected in dopaminergic areas and in a few limited cases specifically in dopaminergic neurons (Maney et al., 2001; Bailhache et al., 1991; T. Bailhache, and J. Balthazart, unpublished data), and this may represent the anatomical substrate for this regulation. Major changes in the turnover of the catecholamines DA and norepinephrine (NE) have also been described following the treatment of male zebra finches with androgens, estrogens, or both (Barclay and Harding, 1988, 1990). Accordingly, based on pharmacological experiments, specific behavioral roles for NE in the control of male sexual behavior in quail (Balthazart et al., 1988a; Balthazart and Ball, 1989) or of singing in songbirds (Barclay et al., 1992, 1996) have been suggested.

Second, it could also be the case that DA influences copulatory behavior independently of the actions of steroids; in others words, there could be several systems regulating male sexual behavior and only subsets of these are modified by steroids.

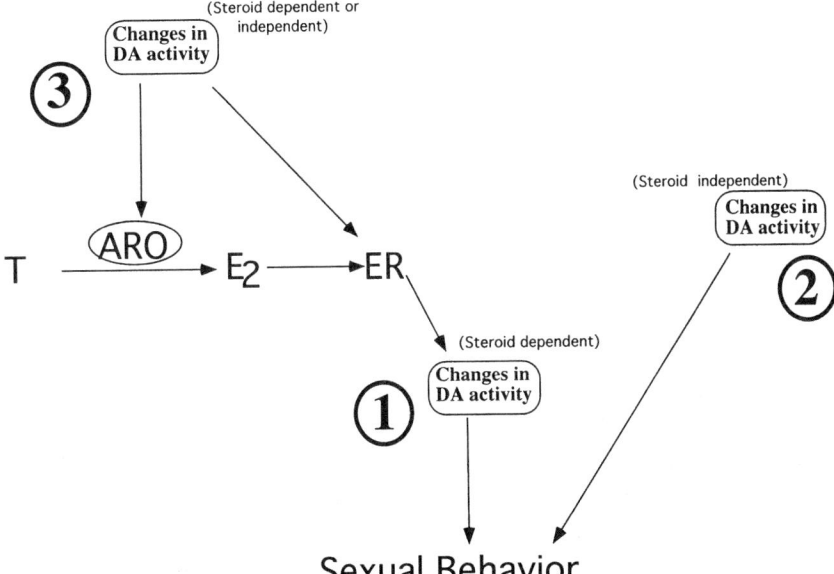

FIGURE 19 Diagram of the possible interactions of the neurotransmitter dopamine (DA) and estrogen-sensitive mechanisms that control the activation of male sexual behavior. Three possibilities are presented. (1) Changes in dopaminergic activity may be one of the neurochemical events that form part of the cascade of changes induced in the brain by steroids. (2) DA could influence copulatory behavior independently of the actions of steroids. (3) DA could modify the environment that steroids act on by changing, for example, the expression or activity of aromatase (ARO) or the concentration of estrogen receptors (ER). Adapted from Balthazart and Ball (1992).

Third, DA could modify the environment that T acts on. There is a substantial literature suggesting that in mammals DA regulates *in vivo* estrogen binding in the brain and pituitary gland (Gietzen *et al.,* 1983; Thompson *et al.,* 1983; see Dohanich *et al.,* 1985; Nock and Feder, 1981, for reviews). However the magnitude of these effects and their physiological relevance are questionable because only small increases ($\leq 10\%$) in the concentration of cytosol ER could be observed after the injection of the DA agonist apomorphine, and these treatments did not alter the level of nuclear ER accumulating after the injection of a saturating dose of E_2 (Blaustein and Turcotte, 1987). It is also possible that DA modulates brain AA because the D1 dopaminergic receptor uses cyclic adenonsine monophosphate (cAMP) as second messenger and cAMP is well recognized as a control factor for aromatase (see later). These hypotheses are not mutually exclusive. The dopaminergic system consists of several anatomically distinct cell groups that are also functionally differentiated. It is well established that many of these cell groups innervate steroid-sensitive brain areas.

Little experimental evidence is available that would permit us to discriminate among these hypotheses, especially in birds. Work on quail suggests, however, that the first and third of these hypotheses (DA as a part of the cascade of neurochemical events controlled by T and DA affecting T action in the brain) are critically involved in the activation of male sexual behavior and in the control of sex dimorphism.

a) Behavioral Effects of Pharmacological Manipulations of Catecholaminergic Systems

i) Effects of dopamine agonists and antagonists on appetitive and consummatory sexual behavior in quail. Neuropharmacological studies in rodents suggest that DA stimulates male sexual motivation and copulatory performance, but different dopaminergic inputs appear to be involved in different aspects of male sexual behavior. It is, for example, established that DA released in the medial POA enhances the rate and efficiency of copulation and facilitates genital reflexes, whereas DA released in the nucleus accumbens enhances general responsiveness to motivational stimuli associated with preparatory or appetitive aspects of male sexual behavior (Hull, 1995; Hull et al., 1999).

Pharmacological studies in quail also support the idea that changes in dopaminergic activity could play a key role in the activation of sexual behavior in this species. A first study confirmed that pharmacological manipulation of the DA system affects male sexual behavior, but found, in contrast to what has been described in rodents, that the general dopaminergic agonist apomorphine inhibits consummatory sexual behavior in this species (Absil et al., 1994). Apomorphine is a nonselective dopamine agonist that appears to act primarily on D1-like receptors at low doses; at higher doses its effects result predominantly from an interaction with D2-like receptors. The discrepancy between the effects of apomorphine in quail and in rodents could therefore be explained by a higher ratio of D2 to D1 receptors in birds compared to mammals (Richfield et al., 1987).

This possibility was tested by comparing the behavioral effects of apomorphine with the effects of two indirect dopaminergic agonists, nomifensine and amfonelic acid, which increase dopaminergic transmission by the inhibition of dopamine reuptake or by promoting dopamine release (Castagna et al., 1997). These compounds should not display a dose-dependent differential effect on D1 and D2 receptors. In addition, the role of dopamine in the control of appetitive sexual behavior was investigated because it was suspected, based on the studies already described, that appetitive and consummatory male sexual behavior may be regulated by at least partly different neural circuits. The behavioral effects of these pharmacological manipulations of dopaminergic transmission were investigated in castrated male Japanese quail that were chronically treated with exogenous T (subcutaneous Silastic implants). Appetitive male sexual behavior was measured by the learned social proximity response that has been described before. The stimulus female was subsequently released into the cage to evaluate copulatory behavior per se. Apomorphine inhibited in a dose-dependent manner both appetitive and consummatory components of sexual behavior. The behavioral profiles of the two indirect agonists that were tested in similar conditions were, however, substantially different. Nomifensine decreased appetitive sexual behavior, but increased the frequency of mount attempts, a consummatory sexual behavior. In contrast, amfonelic acid increased aspects of both the appetitive (looking through the window) and consummatory behaviors (mount-attempt and cloacal-movement frequencies). Therefore in quail, as in rodents, increases in dopaminergic tone appear to facilitate both appetitive and consummatory aspects of male sexual behavior. The inhibitory effects of apomorphine presumably reflect its predominant action at the level of D2-like receptors in quail, whereas in rats this compound acts primarily on D1-like receptors at low doses and only interacts with D2-like receptor at higher doses.

This interpretation was then tested by studying, with the same experimental protocols, the behavioral effects of specific D1 and D2 dopaminergic receptor agonists and antagonists in castrated male Japanese quail that were chronically treated with exogenous T (subcutaneous Silastic implants). The effects of five compounds were tested—one D1 (SKF38393) and two D2 (PPHT or N-0434 and quinpirole or LY171555) agonists, and one D1 (SCH23390) and one D2 (Spiperone) antagonist (Fig. 20).

All compounds were tested at a low and a high dose (100 μg/kg and 1 mg/kg, respectively, for all drugs, except spiperone for which the doses were 2 and 10 mg/kg). A consistent effect of all drugs on consummatory sexual behavior was observed; this aspect of sexual behavior was stimulated by the D1 agonist, but inhibited by the D2 agonists (Balthazart et al., 1997d). Antagonists consistently displayed the opposite effects (inhibition of behavior by D1 antagonist and stimulation by D2 antagonists). Far fewer effects of the treatments were detected on the two measures of appetitive behavior. The time spent in front of the window providing visual access to a female was decreased by the two D2 agonists, but not affected by the other treatments. These data therefore demonstrate that, as in rodents, male copulatory behavior in quail is stimulated by the action of dopamine at the level of its D1 receptors but inhibited by activation of D2. The partial dissociation observed between the effects of the same treatments on the appetitive and consummatory aspects of sexual

	D1+ SKF 38393	D1- SCH 23390	D2+ PPHT (N-0434)	D2+ QUINPIROLE LY171555	D2- SPIP
Appetitive sexual behavior (Time, look)	-	-	↙	↙	-
Consummatory sexual behavior (MA)	↗	↙	↙	↙	↗

FIGURE 20 Qualitative summary of the effects of various dopaminergic drugs on measures of appetitive sexual behavior (time spent in front of the window providing a visual access to a female and the number of looks through window) and of consummatory sexual behaviors (mount attempts, MA) in castrated male quail treated with exogenous testosterone. D1- and D2-like compounds were tested. + sign indicates agonists; − sign indicates antagonists; SPIP, spiperone. Arrows directed toward the top or bottom of the graph, respectively, indicate significant increases or decreases in the behavior measured after injection of the corresponding compound. Data from Balthazart et al. (1997d).

behavior suggests that these two behavioral systems may be controlled by the action of dopamine on different neuronal networks.

It is of interest to note here that the behavioral pharmacology of dopamine appears to be similar in quail and in rats (the facilitation of sexual responses following increases in dopaminergic tone) despite the very different temporal organization of sexual behavior in these two species. In quail, the entire copulatory sequence from neck grab (NG) to cloacal contact movements (CCM) is usually observed within minutes or even seconds after a male and a female have been placed in the same arena. In contrast, a copulatory sequence in rats usually lasts for a longer time (10–20 min) and includes a series of mounts and intromissions that only culminate in ejaculation after repeated intromissions have occurred. This sequence of mounts and intromissions is associated with a progressive rise in dopamine levels, as assessed by both *in vivo* voltametry (Mas *et al.*, 1995a,b) or *in vivo* dialysis (Pfaus *et al.*, 1990; Wenkstern *et al.*, 1993; Sachs *et al.*, 1992), in the POA and nucleus accumbens of male rats. Because DA agonists facilitate the performance of copulatory behavior including ejaculation, the progressive increase in DA release during successive mounts and intromissions has been interpreted as a neurochemical change that is required to trigger ejaculation (Blackburn *et al.*, 1992; Hull, 1995; Hull *et al.*, 1997). We do not known whether DA release in the brain is increased during the performance of a copulatory sequence in quail, but it appears from the temporal considerations that a rise in DA activity may not be required for the completion of a successful cloacal contact and ejaculation in quail (ejaculation is often observed after as little as 5 seconds of interaction between a male and a female).

The role of DA action in the brain has often been assumed to mediate the rewarding aspect of a behavior, and the facilitatory role of DA on ejaculation in rats was considered to be one aspect of this reward system. The argument is that the rise in DA in the POA and nucleus accumbens makes intromissions progressively more rewarding and that this in turn leads to ejaculation. A reinterpretation of DA action has been proposed claiming that the major role played by this transmitter in association with rewarding events is to increase arousal and focus attention on the relevant rewarding stimuli (Wickelgren, 1997; Spanagel and Weiss, 1999). In the case of sexual behavior, DA would, according to this interpretation, focus attention toward stimuli originating from the female. This process could well be occurring in both quail and rats and provide one explanation for the similarity in the behavioral pharmacology of dopamine in these two species. The slower copulatory sequence in rats, compared to quail, may be related to the difference in genital anatomy (the presence of an intromittent organ in rats but not quail) leading to a major difference in the temporal organization of the behavior, but DA action would otherwise still be quite similar and possibly related in part to the focusing of attentional processes.

ii) Effects of noradrenergic transmission on reproductive behavior. Less evidence is available that supports the notion that the noradrenergic system is also implicated in the control of male reproductive behavior in birds. This is probably due, in large part, to the fact that systemic treatments with noradrenergic agonists or antagonists (contrary to what is observed with dopaminergic compounds) produce a diversity of nonspecific effects (e.g., on blood pressure, intestinal transport, body temperature, and awakeness) that prevent the assessment of specific effects on male sexual behavior. Any experiment must therefore be based on the stereotaxic injection of these drugs into the relevant brain sites. This technically more challenging approach has hardly been used in birds. A few experiments have, however, made use of the specific noradrenergic neurotoxin N-(2-chloroethyl)-N-ethyl-2-bromobenzylamine hydrochloride (DSP4), which causes long-lasting, fairly specific depletions of the central noradrenergic innervation while sparing its peripheral counterpart (more accurately both central and peripheral noradrenergic inputs are affected; however, regeneration occurs in the periphery, but not centrally, so in the long term the noradrenergic depletion is exclusively central).

One series of studies in quail indicated that a single DSP4 injection causing a significant depletion of NE concentration in all brain areas including the POA-hypothalamus, and in the POM specifically, markedly increases the activating effects of T on male copulatory behavior (Balthazart *et al.*, 1988a; Balthazart and Ball, 1989). These studies suggest that NE may exert a chronic inhibitory effect on the expression of this behavior. It has in parallel been shown that the POA, and more specifically the POM, of quail is characterized by a higher NE concentration in females than in males (Ottinger *et al.*, 1986; Ottinger and Balthazart, 1987). This higher concentration of NE in females may therefore contribute to the sex difference in copulatory behavior (inhibited more by NE in females than in males; see Balthazart and Adkins-Regan, Chapter 66).

The notion that NE exerts an inhibitory effect on the expression of male sexual behaviors is also supported by studies in ring doves. Barclay and Cheng (1992) demonstrated that male doves treated with either 6-hydroxydopamine or the dopamine β-hydroxylase inhibitor U-14,624, two compounds that both depleted NE levels in the POA-hypothalamus, showed increased levels of bow-cooing and nest-cooing displays. Conversely, males treated with compounds that elevated the brain noradrenergic transmission, such as tyramine or desipramine, showed decreased levels of these two displays. These data therefore suggest that in doves, as in quail, NE exerts a central inhibition on the expresion of male reproductive behaviors.

These catecholaminergic inputs therefore represent one possible way that steroids may influence song learning (Marler *et al.*, 1988) and production (Harding *et al.*, 1983; Bottjer and Johnson, 1997; Schlinger, 1997). However, this hypothesis has not been investigated in great detail. Studies conducted mainly in mammals demonstrate that catecholamines modulate a variety of complex behaviors and cognitive processes. Arousal and attentional processes, which appear to be implicated in the learning, perception, and production of song, are affected by NE and, in particular, by projections arising from the locus ceruleus (Sara, 1985; Aston-Jones *et al.*, 1999; Waterhouse *et al.*, 1988; Cole and Robbins, 1989; Woodward *et al.*, 1991). NE also seems to modulate higher cognitive processes such as memory (Sara, 1985) and selective attention (Shelley *et al.*, 1997; Robbins, 1997).

In songbirds, two studies have analyzed the effects of the noradrenergic neurotoxin DSP4 on song production (Barclay *et al.*, 1992, 1996). These experiments suggest that the DSP4-induced decrease of NE levels in the brain and, in particular, in song-control nuclei leads to a significant suppression of courtship singing, but does not affect song structure. This decreased singing behavior results from an increased latency between the introduction of the female into the male's cage and the first song. According to the authors of these studies, this increased latency may be the result of deficits in attention processes.

It was shown that NE plays a key role in the modulation of the auditory responsiveness of RA neurons by afferent inputs from HVc (Dave *et al.*, 1998). RA neurons display weaker auditory responses in awake than in anesthetized zebra finches, and, interestingly, sleep is also associated with more vigorous and complex auditory responses in RA. These sleep-associated changes in response strength may result from an action of NE in the HVc as suggested by the observation that local NE injections into the HVc produced similar changes in responsiveness. This catecholaminergic neuromodulation may therefore control motor access to the auditory feedback that is required for song learning and maintenance.

In addition, it has been shown that the expression of the IEG *ZENK* in the anterior forebrain vocal pathway (area X; dorsolateral nucleus of the anterior thalamus, DLM; and lMAN) varies as a function of the social context in which song is produced. It has been postulated that the ascending catecholaminergic projections to these nuclei are implicated in this context-dependent activation of brain activity (Jarvis *et al.*, 1998; Hessler and Doupe, 1999a,b). Taken together, these studies therefore indicate that NE should have an important role in the control of the song.

Central dopaminergic neurons also appear to be involved in arousal-like processes. However, the processes controlled by DA are radically different from those controlled by the locus ceruleus neurons. The main function of the ascending dopaminergic systems is to energize or activate behavior in response to cues that signal the availability of incentives or reinforcers (Robbins, 1997). Midbrain dopaminergic pathways also modulate motor control and motivation (DeLong and Georgopoulos, 1981; Wise and Rompre, 1989; Koob, 1992; Salamone, 1992; Aosaki *et al.*, 1994), and DA could also be implicated in the control of higher cognitive processes such as working memory (Sawaguchi and Goldman-Rakic, 1991; Castner *et al.*, 2000). To our knowledge, no specific research has been conducted to study the role of the dopaminergic system in song learning and song production. A striking increase of the catecholaminergic innervation of the song-control nuclei is observed in zebra finches during early song learning (Soha *et al.*, 1996), and the telencephalic nuclei Nif and HVc, implicated mainly in song production, become strongly immunoreactive for tyrosine hydroxylase (TH) as the song becomes fully mature. These anatomical data suggest that DA could modulate different parameters of song production such as the stereotypy, frequency, speed, and intensity. These relationships should be analyzed by specific experiments.

b) Effects of Steroids on Catecholaminergic Activity Consistent with the idea that changes in catecholamine activity could represent a significant part of the cascade of neurochemical events triggered by T that results in the expression of aspects of male sexual behavior (e.g., copulation and singing), a number of studies have shown, as also demonstrated in mammals, that steroids affect the activity of catecholamines in the avian brain. All these studies evaluated the brain catecholaminergic activity by the turnover of DA and NE that was measured by the decrease of the brain concentration of these two amines following the blockage of their resynthesis after an injection of the TH inhibitor α-methyl-*p*-tyrosine (αMPT). The amine depletion in these conditions is assumed to reflect its use and therefore its release. Although absolute levels measured in this way are probably severely affected by important errors (the method assumes, for example, that the use of amines remains constant after the inhibition of their synthesis, which is known to be an oversimplification; see Weiner, 1974, for further discussion), the relative values obtained in different physiological situations allows useful comparisons.

The most complete studies on this topic have been carried out in zebra finches in which it could be shown that T as well as its androgenic or estrogenic metabolites exert profound and anatomically specific effects on the turnover of catecholamines. It was shown that several hypothalamic and song-control nuclei contain significant levels of NE and DA and that in most of these nuclei the steady state levels or turnover rates of NE or DA (measured by the αMPT-depletion method) are markedly affected by a treatment with androstenedione that is known to activate high levels of singing behavior (Barclay and Harding, 1988). The endocrine specificity of this response was tested in a second set of study comparing the effects on NE and DA levels and turnover of a treatment with E_2 or 5α-DHT, alone or in combination (Barclay and Harding, 1990). Catecholaminergic activity (baseline and turnover) was found to be affected by the steroids in 64% of the cases in three hypothalamic and six vocal-control nuclei that were studied (area X, MAN, HVc, RA, DM, and Nif). In parallel with behavioral data, catecholamines were affected more by treatments that provided both androgenic and estrogenic stimulation (E_2 + DHT) than by either treatment alone. However, all hormone-induced changes in noradrenergic function were estrogen-mediated, whereas more variability was present in the response of dopaminergic systems and the effects of androgen alone were quite frequent at this level. Catecholaminergic activity in the song-control nuclei was also affected by the age of the subjects, with dramatic changes taking place during ontogeny in parallel with the critical periods for song learning and sexual differentiation of reproductive behavior and of the song-control system (Harding et al., 1998). Taken together, these data clearly indicate that the brain catecholaminergic activity is markedly affected by steroids in zebra finches in parallel with the development and expression of singing behavior. The changes in catecholaminergic activity appear to represent one of the important ways through which steroids affect the organization and activation of behavior.

NE, DA, and their turnover have also been measured in the brains of male and female quail in several studies, using either spectrofluorometric assays (Ottinger et al., 1986; Ottinger and Balthazart, 1987) or HPLC coupled with electrochemical detection (Balthazart et al., 1992b). These studies identified only limited effects of gonadectomy whether associated or not associated with steroid treatments on the catecholaminergic activity, but a number of sex differences (presumably reflecting long-term effects of steroids) were, in contrast, observed. Physiological studies further indicate that some of these sex differences may be organizational in nature.

Spectrofluorometric assays first identified the presence of high concentrations of NE and DA in the POA (Ottinger et al., 1986). This study also showed that the NE concentration in the POA is slightly but significantly higher in females than in males.

This sex dimorphism in NE concentration was confirmed in a following study using HPLC (Balthazart et al., 1992b). The higher sensitivity of this method also allowed to dissect smaller brain samples by the Palkovits punch method (Palkovits, 1973; Palkovits and Brownstein, 1983) and to show that the sexually differentiated NE concentration is specifically present in the POM. The existence of this sex difference is also supported by immunocytochemical studies showing that the area covered by dopamine-β-hydroxylase immunoreactive (DBH-ir) fibers in the medial POA is wider in females than in males (Bailhache and Balthazart, 1993). This difference in the POM was not affected by gonadectomy whether associated or not associated with a subsequent treatment with T (Balthazart et al., 1992b). These manipulations, however, affected the NE turnover in other brain areas, such as the tuberal hypothalamus. Furthermore, an interaction between the sex of the birds and their reaction to castration and T treatment was observed in the POM where gonadectomy tends to increase NE turnover in males but decrease it in females (Balthazart et al., 1992b).

No reliable sex difference in the baseline level of DA could be detected in the POA, but turnover studies showed that the disappearance of DA after one injection of the TH inhibitor αMPT was much faster in males than in females in the POA (Ottinger and Balthazart, 1987) and specifically in the POM (Balthazart et al., 1992b). This measure was sexually differentiated in sexually mature subjects, but also in birds that had been gonadectomized and implanted with Silastic implants filled with T or left empty as controls.

Usually, no depletion of DA was found in females after an αMPT injection, whereas a rapid decrease was seen in males. However, some decrease was seen in T-treated ovariectomized females (still lower than in males undergoing the same treatment), indicating an effect of the steroid treatment on the dopaminergic activity. The fact that the sex difference in DA turnover was observed in males and females placed in similar endocrine conditions (e.g., in gonadectomized subjects) strongly supports the idea that this difference is organizational in nature, but this notion has not been experimentally tested so far. This potentially organized sex difference could have an important physiological and behavioral significance. It is well established that DA stimulates male copulatory behavior in rats (Meisel and Sachs, 1994; Blackburn et al., 1992; Bitran and Hull, 1987) as well as in quail (see previous discussion). A sexually differentiated control by DA could therefore be part of the mechanisms that mediate the sex difference in quail behavior.

In summary, it appears that the catecholaminergic activity is affected by steroids in the avian brain, as has been previously established in mammals. This conclusion, however, is based on only a small number of studies in birds and additional work should be performed to fully characterize this type of steroid effect.

c) Effects of Catecholamines on Steroid-Sensitive Systems As previously mentioned, there are many ways through which catecholamines (or other transmitters) and steroids may interact to activate reproductive behavior. One of these possible mechanisms assumes that catecholamines affect steroid (T) action in the brain. Although it is of possible widespread significance, the manner by which neurotransmitters and neuropeptides can modify the action of the hormone has not been studied in much detail, especially in birds.

i) Steroid receptors. The neurochemical environment can exert an influence on steroid action in two obvious ways. One way is through the up- and down-regulation of steroid receptor concentration or binding affinity. Steroids apparently modify reproductive events by acting through a nuclear receptor (McEwen and Pfaff, 1985). Several neurotransmitters have been shown to regulate the binding of steroids to their receptors in the mammalian brain. Pharmacological manipulation of both the dopaminergic and noradrenergic system leads to significant changes in E_2 binding in the brain, and it has for example been reported that the administration of DA agonists such as apomorphine increases the binding of E_2 (Gietzen et al., 1983; Thompson et al., 1983; Blaustein and Olster, 1989). Surprisingly, the direct activation of a steroid receptor by DA also appears to be possible (Power et al., 1991). This type of interaction has, however, not been formally identified in any avian model to this date.

ii) Aromatase concentrations. The data available clearly indicate that T increases aromatase activity in the POA of all species of higher vertebrates examined. This induction of enzyme activity reflects an increase in the concentration of the enzyme and of its mRNA, clearly suggesting an increased transcription (Harada et al., 1992). In mammals, this effect appears to be largely mediated by an interaction of T or its 5α reduced metabolites with AR (Roselli et al., 1987; Roselli and Resko, 1984), whereas in birds aromatase induction appears to be largely mediated by an action of estrogens derived from T aromatization (a feedback effect of the product of enzyme on the enzyme itself; Schumacher et al., 1987; Hutchison and Steimer, 1986). A parsimonious explanation of this control assumes that estrogens, formed by aromatization in one neuron, interact in the cell nucleus of the same cell with nuclear ER to induce the synthesis of new enzyme molecules. The anatomical data already described strongly suggest, however, that this is not the case, at least in the POA. A control exerted via a transsynaptic mechanism has therefore been contemplated.

The second messenger, cAMP, is known to modulate gene expression through the phosphorylation of transcriptional activator proteins (Schwartz and Kandel, 1991). In particular, it has been previously demonstrated in mammals that cAMP regulates AA in a number of tissues (Verhoeven et al., 1979; Verhoeven, 1980; Cardinali et al., 1982; Mendelson et al., 1984), including the brain (Callard, 1981). In the few cases in which the time course of this effect was analyzed, it appeared that the cAMP-induced increase in AA develops gradually over several days, so it is likely to be due to a progressive increase in enzyme concentration (Mendelson et al., 1984; Callard, 1981). We can thus speculate that a transmitter or neuropeptide that uses cAMP as second messenger could be part of the brain circuit that controls aromatase synthesis and activity. It is known that the effects of DA and NE at the level of some receptor subtypes are mediated by this second messenger (Etgen and Petitti, 1986; Etgen et al., 1992; Gingrich and Caron, 1993). Furthermore, previous neurochemical studies have identified, by HPLC coupled with electrochemical detection, large concentrations of the two neurotransmitters (especially NE) in the POM (Balthazart et al., 1988a; Balthazart and Ball, 1989) and high densities of α_2 adrenergic receptors localized in the POM (Ball et al., 1989; Balthazart and Ball, 1989). Attention was therefore focused on these catecholamines.

Anatomical studies combining immunocytochemistry for aromatase and for the catecholamine-synthesizing enzymes TH and DBH identified dense networks of TH-ir and DBH-ir fibers in the brain regions that contain ARO-ir cells not colocalized with ER, namely in the POM and BST (Bailhache and Balthazart, 1993). In these areas, ARO-ir cells were found in close association with TH-ir and DBH-ir fibers and punctate structures that in some cases were completely surrounding the ARO-ir cells, forming basket-like structures (Bailhache et al., 1991; see Fig. 21).

The origin of this catecholaminergic innervation was studied by combining injections of retrograde tracers in the POM or BST with immunocytochemistry for TH (Balthazart and Absil, 1997). The TH-ir innervation of the POM and BST originates from a variety of dopaminergic cell groups. A quantitative analysis of these data revealed that the dopaminergic inputs to POM originate primarily in the area ventralis of Tsai (A10 group) and in a dopaminergic cell group located at the ventromedial corner of the anterior hypothalamus (this

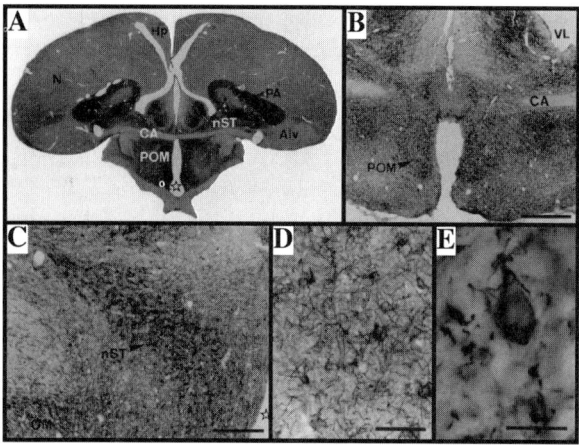

FIGURE 21 Photomicrographs illustrating the interactions between aromatase immunoreactive (ARO-ir) cells and tyrosine hydroxylase immunoreactive (TH-ir) fibers in the rostral forebrain of male quail. (A) Low magnification of a section at the level of the anterior commissure (CA), illustrating the clusters of ARO-ir cells in the medial preoptic nucleus (POM) and rostral portion of the nucleus striae terminalis (BST). Both clusters are completely surrounded by TH-ir fibers. (B–C) Medium enlargements demonstrating that TH-ir fibers can be observed in close proximity of ARO-ir cells both in the POM (B) and BST (C). (D) High magnification of the weakly immunoreactive aromatase cells in the neostriatum, illustrating their anatomical relationship with TH-ir fibers. (E) High magnification of one ARO-ir cell from the BST closely associated with TH-ir fibers and punctate structures. Magnification bars, (B) 500 μm, (C) 200 μm, (D) 50 μm, and (E) 20 μm. Modified from plates in Balthazart et al. (1998b). **See insert for a color version of this figure.**

cell group appears to be homologous to the anteroventral periventricular nucleus, AVPv, described by Simerly et al., 1985), whereas inputs to the BST are derived primarily from dopaminergic cells located in the substantia nigra (A9 cell group) and to a lesser extent in the retrorubral field (A8) and in the area ventralis of Tsai. Lighter inputs originating in the noradrenergic cell groups were also observed.

The functional significance of these inputs for the control of AA was tested in a series of experiments. In a first study, systemic injections of the noradrenergic neurotoxin DSP4 that significantly depleted brain NE concentrations (Balthazart et al., 1988a; Balthazart and Ball, 1989) also increased, in parallel, the preoptic aromatase activity. This suggested that NE chronically inhibits this enzymatic activity (Balthazart and Ball, 1989). A significant enhancement of the effects of T on male copulatory behavior was also observed in these DSP4-treated males, indicating that the NE-induced change in aromatase has indeed functional consequences.

The DBH fibers originating from the locus ceruleus, which are in close contact with ARO-ir cells in the POM and BST (Bailhache et al., 1991), presumably represent the morphological signature of this regulation. It is also interesting to observe that in the POM, the NE concentration and the density of DBH-ir fibers are significantly higher in female than in male quail (Balthazart et al., 1992b; Bailhache and Balthazart, 1993). On the contrary, AA is lower in females than in males. If NE inhibits AA in the quail brain, then the higher concentration of NE in females may explain the sex difference in enzymatic activity (it would be inhibited more by NE in females than males).

It is already known that noradrenergic agonists modulate AA in the pineal gland (Cardinali et al., 1982) and in the testes (Verhoeven, 1980), and similar controls may take place in the mammalian hypothalamus (Canick et al., 1987; Raum and Swerdloff, 1981; Raum et al., 1984). Given that the noradrenergic activity in the brain appears to be under the control of estrogens (McEwen and Krey, 1984), an estrogen-sensitive noradrenergic transmission might represent the neuroanatomical substrate underlying the regulation of AA by estrogen.

In another study, castrated testosterone-treated male quail were chronically injected with the TH inhibitor αMPT and this treatment produced, after 3 days, a significant inhibition of AA (Balthazart et al., 1996c). It is known, however, that a chronic treatment with αMPT decreases both NE (which presumably inhibits AA in the quail brain, based on the DSP4 experiments described) and DA (Balthazart et al., 1992b). It can therefore be expected that a selective dopaminergic inhibition leads to an even larger decrease in enzymatic activity, and these data are therefore consistent with the notion that DA up-regulates brain aromatase, in particular in the POM (see Balthazart and Ball, 1992, for additional discussion).

It is also interesting to note that turnover studies identified a sex difference in the DA turnover in the quail brain. The disappearance of DA after one injection of αMPT was much faster in males than in females in the POA (Ottinger and Balthazart, 1987), and in the POM in particular (Balthazart *et al.*, 1992b). This measure was sexually differentiated in gonadally intact adult subjects, but also in birds that had been gonadectomized and treated or not treated with Silastic implants of T (Balthazart *et al.*, 1992b). The fact that the sex difference in DA turnover was still observed in birds placed in the same endocrine conditions (gonadectomized and T-treated) supports the idea that this difference is organizational in nature. This sex difference could also be implicated in the control of AA. As previously discussed, the intracellular second messenger of D1-like dopaminergic receptors, cAMP (Gingrich and Caron, 1993), is known to modulate AA in several tissues including the brain (Verhoeven *et al.*, 1979; Verhoeven, 1980; Cardinali *et al.*, 1982; Callard, 1981; Mendelson *et al.*, 1984), and the admittedly limited pharmacological data described here support the idea that this control also takes place in the quail POA (the stimulation of the adenylate cyclase by DA acting on the D1 receptor subtype would increase AA). The higher DA turnover in males compared to females should then lead to a higher stimulation of aromatase, which fits with the data. These links are, however, based in part on data collected in other species, mostly in mammals, and additional experiments involving the pharmacological manipulation of the dopaminergic and noradrenergic systems followed by a measure of AA should be performed in birds to further test these ideas.

Finally in a third experiment, castrated T-treated males received a unilateral injection of 6-hydroxydopamine (6-OHDA, 10 μg) into the POA (Balthazart *et al.*, 1997c). The birds were sacrificed 1 day later and the AA was measured separately in the POA in the side receiving the injection and in the contralateral side. TH activity was also measured in these samples by a radioenzyme assay based on the release of tritiated water from 3,5-[^{3}H]-L-tyrosine in order to quantify the extent of the catecholaminergic lesion. A significant decrease in AA was observed in the POA on the injection side where TH activity was also markedly diminished. Although the mean 6-OHDA-induced decrease in AA was of modest amplitude, it was statistically significant and it was also significantly correlated ($r = 0.629$; $p < 0.05$) with the depletion in TH activity. A major diminution in AA was always observed in subjects that had a clear decrease in TH activity. These results therefore provide evidence for a direct control of aromatase concentration and activity by catecholamine neurotransmitters, consistent with the anatomical data indicating the presence of an apparent TH innervation on ARO-ir cells (see Balthazart *et al.*, 1998b; Balthazart and Ball, 1998a, for a more detailed discussion of this regulation of aromatase by catecholamines).

Taken together, anatomical data demonstrate that ARO-ir cells receive dense catecholaminergic inputs and preliminary pharmacological evidence suggests that these inputs could be implicated in the control of the synthesis (and consequently activity) of the enzyme. Further studies should test these causal relationships. It is interesting to note that such a control of aromatase would be reminiscent of that described in much more detail for the regulation of GnRH-producing neurons. Although steroids exert a strong influence on the synthesis and release of GnRH, neurons producing this peptide usually contain no ER (Shivers *et al.*, 1983; Herbison and Theodosis, 1992; Herbison *et al.*, 1993; see, however, Butler *et al.*, 1999; Skynner *et al.*, 1999, for evidence apparently contradicting this idea), and they are controlled by an estrogen-sensitive neuronal network that involves several neurotransmitters and neuropeptides (Barraclough and Wise, 1982; Weiner *et al.*, 1988; De Vries, 1990).

iii) Rapid changes in aromatase activity. The experiments described indicate the presence of regulations by catecholamines of AA in the quail brain. Because these effects were observed after 1 to several days of modification of the catecholaminergic activity, it was assumed that the enzymatic changes result from a modification of the enzyme concentration. It is indeed known that NE and DA are able to modify intracellular cAMP concentration, which can in turn modulate the phosphokinase A activity (PKA) resulting in a change of the cAMP response-element binding protein (CREB) phosphorylation level and subsequent modifications of transcription (Abe-Dohmae *et al.*, 1996, 1997).

In addition, the possible existence of a direct modulation of aromatase activity by DA and NE was also investigated. AA was measured during *in vitro* incubations of quail hypothalamic homogenates by the production of tritiated water from [1β-^{3}H]-androstenedione (Baillien and Balthazart, 1997). Norepinephrine and prazosin (an α1-adrenergic antagonist) had no or very limited effect on AA. However, in contrast, DA (10^{-6} to 10^{-3} M) and some D1 and D2 receptor agonists

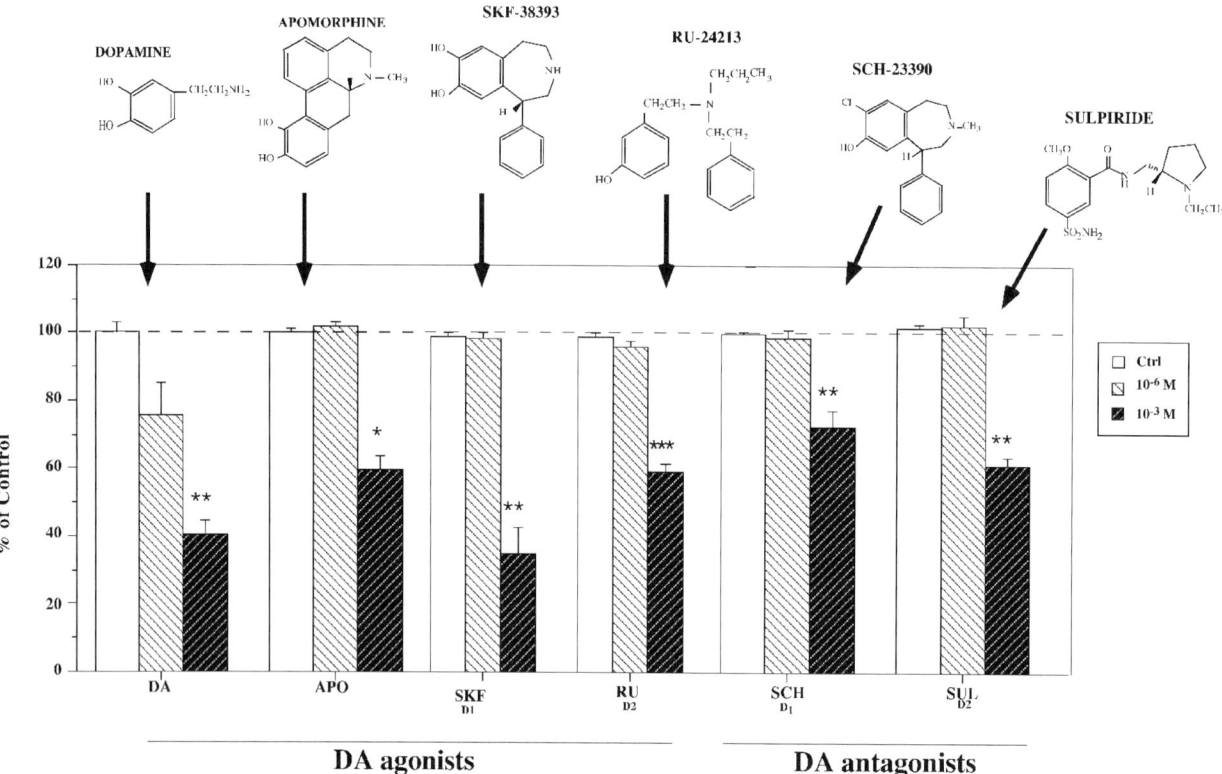

FIGURE 22 Effects of dopamine (DA), general DA agonist apomorphine (APO) and of specific DA agonists—SKF (SKF-38393, D1); RU (RU-24213, D2)—and antagonists—SCH (SCH-23390, D1); SUL (sulpiride, D2)—on aromatase activity measured in homogenates of the quail preoptic area–hypothalamus. Triplicate assays were performed during two to four independent experiments and results (mean ± standard errors) are expressed as percentage of their respective control. Comparison of each dose with the corresponding control condition was performed when appropriate by Student's t-tests for matched samples adapted for post hoc analyses using as the basis for comparison the relevant mean square of the ANOVA carried out previously (* indicates $p < 0.05$; ** indicates $p < 0.01$). Data from Baillien and Balthazart (1997).

(apomorphine, D1 and D2; SKF-38393, D1; and RU-24213, D2) depressed aromatase activity by 40–70% at the 10^{-3} M concentration. One D1 (SCH-23390) and one D2 (sulpiride) receptor antagonist also produced a major inhibition of AA, whereas other antagonists (spiperone, D2; and pimozide, D2) either had no significant effect or only produced moderate decreases in AA. The inhibitory effect of the agonists was not antagonized by the less active antagonists SCH-23390 (D1) or spiperone (D2). These results suggest that the inhibitory effects of DA or dopaminergic compounds are not mediated through binding to DA receptors. It appears likely that these drugs inhibit AA by a direct effect on the enzyme, as suggested by the competitive nature of DA and SKF-38393 inhibition of AA (Ki 59 and 84 μM, respectively; Fig. 22).

Although this direct inhibition of the enzyme activity may appear surprising, note that previous studies have shown that aromatase is actually a multifunctional enzyme that catalyzes a variety of reactions such as 2- and 6-hydroxylations and N-demethylation of various substrates (Osawa et al., 1994, 1997; Toma et al., 1996). Dopamine could therefore act as an alternative substrate for aromatase and in this way compete with T and prevent its transformation into estrogens. This mechanism may represent an important physiological pathway through which neurotransmitters could rapidly affect steroid-dependent processes such as the neural synthesis of estrogens. This would provide a means by which environmental stimuli could affect reproductive behavior and physiology. The physiological significance of this finding in vivo is under study and has been discussed elsewhere (Balthazart and Ball, 1998a).

These effects raised the question of how DA could actually interact with aromatase. It is generally accepted that aromatase is located in the neuronal perikarya at the level of the rough endoplasmic reticulum, whereas DA is released extracellularly and is not supposed to enter its target cells. It is conceivable that in homogenates the cellular compartmentalization is lost so that DA could actually acts as a substrate for aromatase as suggested by Osawa and colleagues (1994); it would compete with androgens and in this way inhibit their aromatization. The competitive nature of the inhibition (Baillien and Balthazart, 1997) speaks in favor of this mechanism. However, this mode of action appears less likely in an intact cell system in which aromatase is supposed to be primarily intracellular whereas DA is an extracellular signal that acts at the level of the membrane of its target cells. It is possible that DA is synthesized in aromatase cells, but no colocalization between TH and aromatase has been detected in the quail brain except perhaps in a small cell group of the rostroventral hypothalamus (Bailhache et al., 1991; Balthazart et al., 1998b). This interpretation is therefore not supported by experimental evidence.

To test whether the rapid inhibition of aromatase activity is still observed in systems that preserve the cellular compartments, additional experiments were carried out on hypothalamic explants maintained in suitable *in vitro* conditions (Baillien and Balthazart, 2000). An *in vitro* culture system was designed allowing the survival of hypothalamic explants and the continuous measure of their aromatase activity every 5 min for 1 hour (Balthazart et al., 2001a). In this system, AA, assessed by the production of tritiated water from [1β-^{3}H]-androstenedione, was shown to increase during the first 15 min and then to remain stable during the following 45 min. DA (1 mM), SKF-38393 (D1 agonist, 0.5 mM), PPHT (D2 agonist, 0.5 mM), SCH-23390 (D1 antagonist, 0.5 mM), and sulpiride (D2 antagonist, 0.5 mM) were added after 20 min and withdrawn after 30 min. High concentrations of all effectors were used to ensure that physiological levels of these compounds could reach the aromatase cells located in the explants within 5 min. All compounds were shown to induce a rapid significant inhibition of AA (40–50%) that was fully reversible (Baillien and Balthazart, 2000; Balthazart et al., 2001b). DA only produced a smaller inhibition ($\pm 20\%$), probably due to its degradation before reaching the POM, which contains most of the AA. Nomifensin (0.5 mM), an inhibitor of DA reuptake, also produced a reliable and reversible inhibition of AA, demonstrating that the physiological accumulation of DA in the synaptic cleft rapidly modulates the activity of the enzyme.

These data seem to exclude actions mediated through D1 or D2 receptors because DA agonists as well as antagonists have similar effects. They also indicate that DA can rapidly affect the neural aromatase activity, presumably via a nongenomic control of the enzyme, given the rapid appearance of the effects (less than 5 min). Finally, these experiments show that the interaction of DA and aromatase still takes place when intra- and extracellular compartments are kept intact. One report has shown that after the transfection of cells in culture, aromatase can be expressed, in part, at the cell surface (Amarneh and Simpson, 1996) and could therefore be accessible to DA action. Whether this is true in neurons remains to be ascertained. Alternatively, we can also postulate that the rapid effects of DA on AA are mediated transsynaptically after DA acts on an interneuron that is not itself aromatase positive. We should then explain why this system remains functional in hypothalamic homogenates that should not preserve this cellular arrangement.

Irrespective of the cellular mechanisms that mediate this effect of DA on AA, these data indicate that the catecholaminergic system is able to modulate steroid action in the avian brain. Because the catecholaminergic activity is itself directly affected by the environment and, in particular, by social interactions, this mode of control of steroid action could represent one of the important ways through which behavior performance is fine-tuned to the external circumstances.

d) Other Transmitter and Peptidergic Systems and Their Behavioral Significance A limited number of studies have also investigated the possible involvement of other transmitters and neuropeptides in the control of reproductive behavior of birds. A very substantial portion of these studies were devoted to vasotocin and will be reviewed first. The more limited information concerning other peptidergic system will then be discussed.

i) Vasotocin. The neurohypophyseal nonapeptide arginine-vasotocin (AVT) is a nonmammalian homolog of the antidiuretic hormone arginine-vasopressin (AVP; Acher *et al.,* 1970, 1985; Moore, 1992). AVP was originally named based on its action in the control of osmoregulation and blood pressure, but this hormone is also implicated in thermoregulation, in learning and memory, and in the control of various aspects of social and sexual behavior. Like its mammalian homolog, AVT is also involved in the control of aspects of reproduction such as oviposition (Koike *et al.,* 1988; Rice *et al.,* 1985; Shimada *et al.,* 1986), male sexual behavior (Kihlström and Danninge, 1972; Bernroider and Leutgeb, 1994; Goodson *et al.,* 1996; Leutgeb, 1995), and vocalizations (Voorhuis *et al.,* 1991).

The anatomical distribution of AVT cells and fibers has been investigated by immunocytochemistry in the brain of several avian species (Kiss *et al.,* 1987; Voorhuis *et al.,* 1988; Voorhuis and de Kloet, 1992; for reviews see Korf *et al.,* 1988; Viglietti-Panzica and Panzica, 1991). In Japanese quail (*Coturnix japonica*) specifically, AVT immunoreactive (AVT-ir) cells and fibers are present in various parts of the hypothalamus (Bons, 1980; Viglietti-Panzica, 1986; Viglietti-Panzica *et al.,* 1994) and in extrahypothalamic areas, such as the BST, septum, and various nuclei of the mesencephalic, pontine, and bulbar regions (Panzica *et al.,* 1988; Viglietti-Panzica *et al.,* 1992). Studies have identified sex differences in the AVT innervation of quail brain areas that are directly (medial POA and POM, Viglietti-Panzica *et al.,* 1994) or indirectly (septal region or BST, Viglietti-Panzica *et al.,* 1992; Aste *et al.,* 1995) involved in the regulation of sexual behavior (Panzica *et al.,* 1996b). These studies also demonstrated that this innervation is controlled by T—it decreases or disappears after castration, but is restored to the level seen in sexually mature birds by a treatment with exogenous T (Viglietti-Panzica *et al.,* 1992, 1994; Panzica *et al.,* 1996a).

In quail (Panzica *et al.,* 1998) and chickens (Jurkevich *et al.,* 2000), it has also been demonstrated that the sex difference in AVT innervation of the POM and BST are largely organizational in nature. The treatment of ovariectomized females with T does not result in a significant increase of the AVT-ir innervation of these nuclei. However, experimental manipulations of the embryonic endocrine milieu causes permanent changes in the vasotocinergic innervation of the POM and BST. Fertilized quail eggs of both sexes were injected on day 9 of incubation either with EB (25 μg, a treatment that suppresses the capacity to show copulatory behavior in adulthood) or with the aromatase inhibitor R76713 (10 μg, a treatment that makes adult females behaviorally responsive to T) or with the solvents as a control (C). At 3 weeks posthatching, all subjects were gonadectomized and later implanted with Silastic capsules filled with T. Two weeks later all birds were perfused and brain sections were processed for AVT immunocytochemistry. Despite the similarity of the adult endocrine conditions of the subjects (all birds were gonadectomized and treated with T Silastic implants, providing the same plasma level of steroid), major qualitative differences were observed in the density of AVT-ir structures in the POM of the different groups. Dense immunoreactive structures (fibers and a few cells) were observed in the POM of C males but not females, EB males had completely lost this immunoreactivity (and lost the capacity to display copulatory behavior), and, conversely, R76713 females displayed a male-typical AVT-ir system in the nucleus (and they also displayed high levels of copulatory behavior). Similar changes in immunoreactivity were seen in the BST and in the lateral septum (AVT-ir fibers only in this case), but not in the magnocellular vasotocinergic system. These neurochemical changes closely parallel the effects of the embryonic treatments on male copulatory behavior (see Balthazart and Adkins-Regan, Chapter 66). The vasotocinergic system of the POM can therefore be considered an accurate marker of the sexual differentiation of brain circuits mediating this behavior.

Close anatomical relationships have also been observed in the quail brain between AVT-ir fibers and neurons that contain aromatase, the enzyme that catalyzes the transformation of T into E_2 and therefore plays a critical role in the activation of male sexual behavior (Balthazart and Foidart, 1993b; Balthazart *et al.,* 1996c; Panzica *et al.,* 1996b). In most brain regions that contain dense populations of ARO-ir cells, such as the POM, the BST, and the mediobasal and tuberal hypothalamus (Balthazart *et al.,* 1990e; Foidart *et al.,* 1995), a dense cluster of AVT-ir fibers is observed and these AVT-ir fibers come in close contact with ARO-ir elements, suggesting the presence of a physiologically relevant innervation (Balthazart *et al.,* 1997b).

Taken together, these behavioral and neuroanatomical data suggest possible functional relationships among AVT, aromatase, and male sexual behavior in quail. Because the AVT-ir innervation of areas such as the POM or the septum is T-sensitive, it was speculated that changes in AVT activity may be a part of the biochemical cascade of neurochemical events initiated by T through which this steroid activates male sexual behavior and crowing in quail. This notion was tested by injecting sexually mature male quail that had been previously castrated and treated with standardized amounts of exogenous T with either AVT or an AVT receptor antagonist, specific for the V1 receptor subtype. AVT was originally injected systemically and produced marked behavioral effects. The effects of these treatments on appetitive and consummatory aspects of male sexual behavior were separately assessed in these studies because previous work in mammals and quail suggested that these two components of male sexual behavior may be controlled by neural mechanisms that are at least partly different (Everitt and Stacey, 1987; Everitt *et al.*, 1989; Everitt, 1990; Balthazart and Ball, 1997; Balthazart *et al.*, 1996b; Castagna *et al.*, 1997).

The appetitive and consummatory components of sexual behavior, as well as the occurrence frequency of crows, were inhibited in a dose-dependent manner by injections of AVT (Castagna *et al.*, 1998). Opposite effects were observed after injection of the V1 receptor antagonist, dPTyr(Me)AVP. Additional experiments comparing the intramuscular (IM) and the intracerebroventricular (ICV) injections of these compounds were then carried out and these studies demonstrated that lower doses of AVT are more active after central than after systemic injection and that the effects of systemic injections of AVT are blocked by a central injection of dPTyr(Me)AVP. The behavioral inhibition was associated with a modified diuresis after systemic injection, but not central injection. These results provide direct evidence that AVT affects male sexual behavior in quail by a direct action on the brain, independent of its peripheral action on diuresis (Castagna *et al.*, 1998).

It is important to notice that the pharmacological manipulations described here suggest that AVT may inhibit the expression of appetitive and consummatory aspects of male sexual behavior in quail, whereas the anatomical data indicate that a high degree of AVT expression (dense AVT-ir fibers and a high level of AVT mRNA) is, rather, associated with physiological situations in which these behaviors are expressed (higher AVT expression in males than in females, in T-treated birds than in castrates, and in sexually mature males than in older subjects). It had originally been anticipated that the increase in AVT production is part of a cascade of biochemical events triggered by T in the brain that result in the activation of male sexual behavior. The behavioral studies summarized here make this interpretation impossible, but alternative explanations can be offered.

Based on studies carried out in mammals (De Vries, 1995), it is unlikely that increases in the density of AVT-ir fibers after T treatment reflect a blockade of the peptide release resulting in its accumulation in fibers and terminals (see Castagna *et al.*, 1998, for further discussion). This interpretation is also supported by the fact that T increases in parallel the AVT mRNA concentration as observed by *in situ* hybridization (Aste *et al.*, 1997). Alternatively, we could postulate that a single injection of exogenous AVT decreases rather than increases the AVT activity in specific brain areas because the injected compound is quickly metabolized, at the same time strongly and persistently inhibiting the secretion of the endogenous peptide. This interpretation, however, does not take into account the fact that inhibitions of sexual behavior were observed almost immediately after the injection of AVT and disappeared in approximately 30 min. We therefore suggest that the T-induced increase in AVT-ir should not be considered to be one of the central consequence of the T action that leads to the activation of male sexual behavior but rather reflects the development of a mechanism that is implicated in the maintenance of behavioral homeostasis.

When male sexual behavior is activated (high levels of circulating T), a negative control mechanism may need to be established in order to organize the distribution of behavioral occurrences on a short-term basis (i.e., birds should not be sexually active all the time). This mechanism is obviously not needed in castrates that are behaviorally inactive. A steroid-sensitive neuropeptidergic innervation would provide an adequate support for such a control, which could be directly sensitive to environmental stimuli. On a long-term basis, changes in steroid levels would establish the anatomical substrate of the behavioral control (control of the synthesis of AVT and possibly of the growth of

AVT-containing fibers); on short-term basis, environmental and social stimuli could regulate the release of AVT from its terminals and in this way switch off behavior for limited periods of time. This interpretation could be tested by additional studies, including the identification of the brain areas (e.g., POM, septum, and BST) in which AVT exerts its behavioral effects and the analysis of environmental stimuli that are potentially able to modulate AVT release at these specific anatomical sites.

In addition, we also note that a number of pharmacological experiments in other bird species have provided rather conflicting results. Whether AVT enhances or inhibits the expression of steroid-dependent behavior seems to be quite variable and a function of the species under study, time of the year and so on. One early study showed that the injection of AVT into intact sexually mature pigeons or cocks produces a short-term increase in the frequency of copulatory acts (Kihlström and Danninge, 1972), but Bernroider and Leutgeb (1994) presented data in an abstract suggesting that AVT decreases motivational aspects of sexual learning in quail. Two studies also reported that central AVT injections stimulate courtship behavior and aggression. In zebra finches, the infusion in the septum of an AVT antagonist significantly decreased the expression of three aggressive behaviors (pecks, beak fences, and chases), whereas AVT injections facilitated beak fencing (Goodson and Adkins-Regan, 1999). Directed song, a courtship behavior, was not affected by these treatments despite the fact that a previous study reported an inhibition of courtship following the peripheral administration of AVT (Harding and Rowe, 1997). This effect was reversed by a treatment with T, suggesting that AVT effects were mediated by the inhibition of T secretion. In contrast, ICV injections of AVT in female white-crowned sparrows were reported to facilitate the expression of song and a variety of other vocalizations (Maney et al., 1997a).

Many of these experiments point to a stimulatory role of AVT on reproductive behavior in birds, whereas an inhibition of male sexual behavior was observed in quail. It is difficult to make direct comparisons among the studies because they were carried out in different species and under very different experimental conditions (different seasons, endocrine conditions, etc). One study, for example, has suggested that seasonal variations might explain these changes in AVT action because injections of an AVT analog activated singing in canaries in the early fall, but inhibited this behavior during the winter (Voorhuis et al., 1991). No general theory has been offered to explain why AVT stimulates aspects of reproductive behavior in some species, but inhibits the same or similar behaviors in other species. Additional studies on a variety of animal models are needed to understand these discrepancies.

ii) Other neuropeptides. In many avian species, the presence of a large number of other neuropeptides has been demonstrated in steroid-sensitive areas of the brain that are known to participate in the control of aggressive and sexual behavior. It has also been shown in a number of selected cases that the expression of these peptides is either sexually differentiated or modified by treatment with sex steroids that are able to activate in parallel reproductive behaviors (e.g., neurotensin, opioids, and VIP). It can therefore be hypothesized that many of these peptides participate to the control of male sexual behaviors. However, this hypothesis has not been studied in great detail and only a few rather anecdotal studies are available to support this notion. It has, for example, been shown that distress vocalizations are decreased by opioid peptides in domestic chicks (Panksepp et al., 1978) and that injection of VIP into the septum of male zebra finches significantly reduces the incidence of aggressive pecks (Goodson and Adkins-Regan, 1999). In addition, according to one report in an abstract, the administration into the third ventricle of LHRH activates male copulatory behavior in castrated male quail (Ottinger et al., 1988). However, the available data do not permit us to build an organized picture of the role of neuropeptides in the control of male reproductive behavior in birds.

5. Rapid Actions of Steroids and the Rapid Regulation of Aromatase Activity

Studies of aromatase based on the measure of the enzymatic activity, on the semiquantitative evaluation of the aromatase protein (number of ARO-ir cells in the POM), and on the quantification of the aromatase mRNA by RT-PCR indicate that T similarly increases these three independent measures of the enzyme, suggesting that the increase in aromatase mRNA levels is the main or only mechanism implicated in the regulation by T of the enzyme activity (Balthazart and Foidart, 1993b). However, the magnitude of the T effect increases as we progress from DNA transcription to the enzymatic activity (372% for mRNA, 497% for the protein, and 645% for the enzyme activity). This might only represent experimental artifacts related to the different methods that were used to collect these data, but, alternatively, these discrepancies could indicate that additional mechanisms under the control of T modulate the translation of the mRNA into a protein and the enzymatic activity of the protein.

a) Modifications of Estrogen Production Do Not Necessarily Involve Changes in Aromatase Synthesis and Concentration   Estrogens have generally been viewed as slow-acting messengers that act via changes in gene transcription. These effects are consistent with mechanisms that regulate the local production of estrogens by aromatase in a slow manner (via changes in enzyme concentration). However, studies suggest that in rats the estrogenic metabolites of T may activate aspects of male sexual behavior rapidly at the membrane level, whereas androgenic metabolites act more slowly via genomic mechanisms (Cross and Roselli, 1999; see, however, Benten *et al.*, 1999, for the rapid membrane effects of T). This observation that estrogens in the male brain may act rapidly on cell membranes is consistent with evidence based on the female brain (and peripheral tissues) indicating that effects of estrogens may be quite rapid and mediated by effects on the cell membrane in some cases (e.g., Pasqualini *et al.*, 1995; Ramirez *et al.*, 1996; Moss *et al.*, 1997; Joëls, 1997; Herbison, 1998; Gu *et al.*, 1999; Brubaker and Gay, 1999; McEwen and Alves, 1999; Schumacher *et al.*, 1999). In quail nongenomic effects of estrogens on behavior have not been positively identified. However, copulatory behavior appears and disappears rapidly in response to changing stimulus conditions. Given that the activation of this behavior is clearly dependent on estrogenic metabolites of T, it is possible to entertain the idea that the rapid regulation of this behavior could be mediated by rapid changes in the action of estrogen.

These rapid effects of estrogens on behavior and other aspects of brain physiology raise important questions about the regulation of estrogen synthesis via the regulation of the enzyme aromatase in the brain (Balthazart and Ball, 2000). Little is known about how AA is physiologically regulated in particular brain areas. However, if estrogen is acting rapidly on a cell membrane we would expect estrogen availability to also be regulated rapidly. Little attention has been paid so far to the idea that AA could be rapidly affected by the neurochemical cellular environment in a manner that would not involve changes in enzyme concentration (see, however, Bellino and Holben, 1989, for such a study on placental aromatase).

The regulation of activity modifies enzymatic effects more rapidly than the regulation of enzyme concentration. The activity of many enzymes, such as TH, the rate-limiting enzyme in catecholamine synthesis, is rapidly modified by conformational changes in the enzyme molecule, including phosphorylations, that are produced in the presence of suitable concentrations of ATP and the divalent cation Mg^{2+} (Albert *et al.*, 1984; Daubner *et al.*, 1992). These phosphorylations are catalyzed by specific kinases that transfer the terminal phosphate group from ATP to the hydroxyl moiety of amino acid residues (tyrosine, threonine, and serine) of the enzymatic protein. Mg^{2+} is required for this reaction, which makes kinase activity critically dependent on the Mg^{2+} intracellular concentration. Given that previous studies have implicated divalent cations in the control of AA—Ca^{2+} (Onagbesan and Podie, 1989; Hochberg *et al.*, 1986) and Mg^{2+} (Steimer and Hutchison, 1991)—and because several consensus sites of phosphorylation are present in the mammalian and avian aromatase sequences (e.g., Harada, 1988; Corbin *et al.*, 1988; Means *et al.*, 1989; McPhaul *et al.*, 1988; Shen *et al.*, 1994; Harada *et al.*, 1992), we investigated whether Ca^{2+} concentrations or ATP and Mg^{2+} concentrations such as those used to obtain maximal changes in TH activity (Ames *et al.*, 1978) affected AA in male quail brain homogenates (Balthazart *et al.*, 2001b).

b) Calcium-Dependent Rapid Changes in Aromatase Activity in Brain Homogenates   Aliquots of hypothalamic homogenates were preincubated for 0 or 15 min in the presence of 1 mM ATP, 5 mM $MgCl_2$ (Mg), or 0.1 mM sodium orthovanadate (VAN; a general phosphatase inhibitor), separately or in combinations, before AA was measured in the samples (Fig. 23). AA was not affected by a 15-min preincubation in the control condition nor after the addition of ATP alone. VAN moderately inhibited AA measured after 15 min of preincubation. AA measured in the presence of Mg

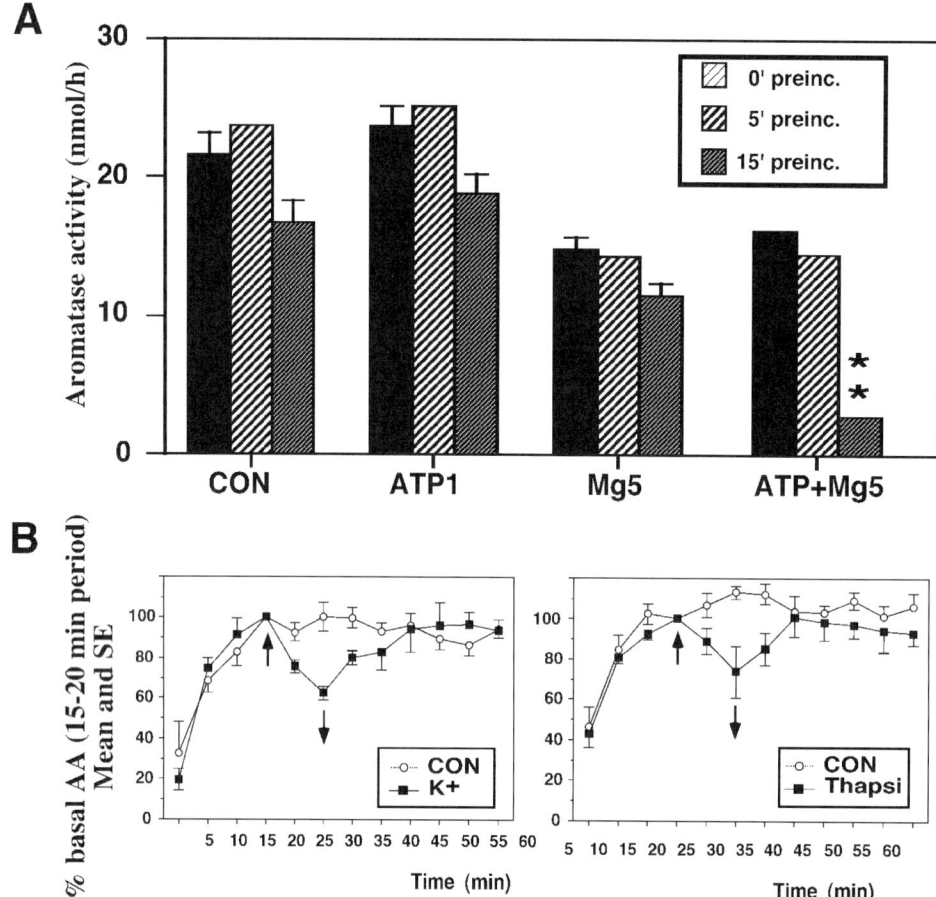

FIGURE 23 Rapid changes in aromatase activity observed in the quail preoptic area–hypothalamus in conditions that modify protein phosphorylations. (A) Aromatase activity measured in preoptic area–hypothalamus homogenates after a preincubation for 0, 5, or 15 min at 37°C in the presence of 1 mM ATP, 5 mM $MgCl_2$, 1 mM ATP + 5 mM $MgCl_2$ or in control (CON) conditions. Asterisks at the top of the 15-min bars indicate the results of post hoc t-tests comparing in each treatment the enzymatic activity with 0 or 15 min preincubation. (B) Aromatase activity in paired preoptic area–hypothalamus explants incubated in vitro and exposed for 10 min (up arrow) (left) to a depolarization by K^+ (concentration was raised to 75 mM with simultaneous decrease of the Na^+ concentration) or (right) to thapsigargin (8 μM in 1% DMSO, controls also containing 1% DMSO in this specific experiment). Normal saline was restored at 30 min (down arrow). All data are means ± SE or tritiated water production in individual samples ($n = 5$ in each case) expressed in percentage of basal release, defined as the mean activity during the period preceding the experimental manipulation (15–20 min). Adapted from Balthazart et al. (2001a).

was lower than in control conditions, but no effect of the duration of preincubation could be detected. In the presence of both ATP and Mg, AA did not differ from samples containing Mg alone at the 0 min preincubation time, but was significantly depressed after 15 min (16.9% of control values). This inhibition was further enhanced by the addition of the phosphatase inhibitor (ATP + Mg + VAN, 6.2% of control values), although the magnitude of this effect was limited due to the very low level of enzyme activity remaining in the presence of ATP and Mg alone.

Additional experiments demonstrated that the presence of free Ca^{2+} is necessary for aromatase inhibition to occur. A significant decrease in AA was observed in preincubation conditions, corresponding to increases in Ca^{2+} availability. The combination of ATP with Mg again induced a very marked decrease of AA, further amplified by the addition of Ca^{2+}. This enzymatic inhibition was completely abolished in the presence of 2 mM EGTA (which chelates free Ca^{2+} present in the homogenates), clearly indicating the Ca^{2+} dependence of the aromatase inactivation by ATP and Mg.

Parametric experiments testing the influence of Mg^{2+} and Ca^{2+} concentrations on AA in the presence or absence of ATP identified a dose-dependent inhibition of AA and demonstrated that the Mg^{2+} and Ca^{2+} concentrations at which these changes in AA are detected correspond to the normal intracellular concentrations that are observed in physiological conditions. These observations are consistent with the fact that *in vivo* Mg^{2+} is a limiting factor for the activity of kinases that are directly responsible for the phosphorylation of proteins.

c) Effects of Calcium and Neurotransmitters on Aromatase Activity in Hypothalamic Explants In order to investigate whether this Ca^{2+}-dependent inhibition of aromatase plays a functional role in intact neurons, paired left and right explants of POA-hypothalamus were incubated *in vitro* in oxygenated glucose-saline in the presence of 25 nM [1β-^{3}H]-androstenedione and cumulative AA in these explants was measured every 30 min by quantifying the amount of tritiated water that had been released (Balthazart *et al.*, 2001b). One hemiexplant (the left or the right one, selected randomly) always served as the control and the matched other half was submitted to experimental treatments designed to regulate the free intracellular Ca^{2+} concentration. Every 30 min, the incubation medium was aspirated with a syringe and replaced by fresh medium containing [1β-^{3}H]-androstenedione. Withdrawn samples were immediately cooled in an ice bath and further processed to isolate the tritiated water produced by aromatization from the remaining radioactive steroids as previously described (Baillien and Balthazart, 1997). This allowed a continuous measure of AA in the blocks (Balthazart *et al.*, 2001b).

AA measured in these *in vitro* conditions remained relatively stable over a 5-hour period, although a slow but regular decline was observed. The complete removal of Ca^{2+} in the incubation medium for a duration of 60 min did not affect enzyme activity, indicating that the functional properties of membranes in cells containing aromatase remained intact in these conditions. In contrast, a rise in extracellular K^+ concentration immediately and markedly inhibited AA. We hypothesized that the K^+-induced enzymatic inhibition resulted from a Ca^{2+} influx produced by the massive depolarization. Consistent with this interpretation, this inhibition was significantly reduced when the K^+-induced depolarization was produced in hypothalamic blocks that were incubated in a Ca^{2+}-free medium.

A massive depolarization is also likely to release neurotransmitters and, accordingly, the addition of ionotropic excitatory amino acid receptors agonists (NMDA, AMPA, and Kainate) markedly depressed AA. These data indicated that AA in hypothalamic brain explants can be modulated by treatments that influence intracellular Ca^{2+} concentration. However, these studies only quantified changes in AA every 30 min and the actual time course of these enzymatic changes was therefore not assessed. In addition, no recovery of AA had been observed in explants that had been depolarized by K^+ for 60 min, which suggested that Ca^{2+} inactivates aromatase in an irreversible manner. Additional experiments were conducted to assess the time course of changes in AA induced by the K^+ depolarization. When AA was measured every 5 min, a transient (10-min) rise in K^+ concentration resulted in a significant inhibition of AA within 5 min, but this effect of a transient depolarization was fully reversible (Fig. 23B).

Nearly identical results were obtained when brain explants were exposed for 10 min to thapsigargin, a lactone known for its capacity to modify intracellular pools of Ca^{2+}. The increase in intracellular Ca^{2+} concentration presumably induced by this compound resulted in a significant decrease in AA. Although the effects of thapsigargin on the sarcoplasmic Ca^{2+}-ATPase are considered to be irreversible (Taylor and Broad, 1998), a full recovery of AA was observed after removal of the drug, presumably following the Ca^{2+} reuptake by thapsigargin-insensitive intracellular stores (Neusser *et al.*, 1999) or its extrusion from the cells by a Ca-ATPase or the reduction of Ca^{2+} influx (Taylor and Broad, 1998).

d) Functional Implications In summary, the data described illustrate two radically different ways through

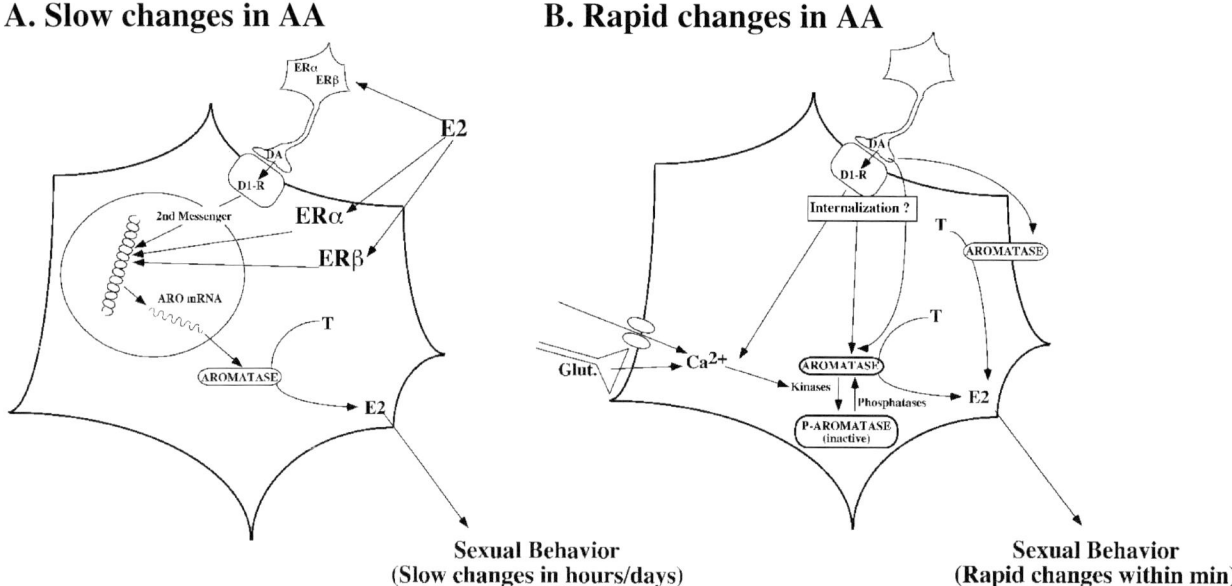

FIGURE 24 Diagram of the possible mechanisms that control in a (A) slow or (B) rapid manner the activity of the steroid-metabolizing enzyme aromatase (ARO) as they relate to the activation of male reproductive behavior by testosterone (T). Controls by estrogens and by the catecholamine dopamine (DA) are considered. The two panels illustrate the slow controls that are presumably mediated by changes in aromatase transcription and more rapid effects that do not apparently relate to changes in enzyme concentration. (A) Aromatase concentration, and presumably transcription, can be up-regulated by the action of estradiol directly on an aromatase-expressing cell via binding to one of the two forms of estrogen receptor, ERα or ERβ. Aromatase transcription could also be controlled indirectly by estradiol acting on catecholaminergic estrogen-sensitive neurons. Dopaminergic projections on the aromatase cells could then control the activity of second messenger systems (e.g., AMP) regulating aromatase transcripton as illustrated here for the action of DA via its binding to receptors of the D1 subtype D1-R. (B) DA and other transmitters such as glutamate could mediate rapid changes in aromatase activity independent of changes in enzyme concentration. DA could interact directly with intracellular aromatase or with aromatase located at the cell membrane level. How DA could be internalized in aromatase cells is unclear. DA could also modify aromatase activity less directly by interfering with the glutamate (Glut.) or Ca^{2+}-dependent phosphorylations of the enzyme. Changes in aromatase activity can be mediated by calcium-dependent phosphorylations of the enzyme (reversible transformation of aromatase in phosphorylated aromatase) that render it inactive. These phosphorylation processes are presumably catalyzed by various kinases. Conversely, phosphatases that catalyze dephosphorylation of the enzymatic protein should enhance enzymatic activity. Adapted from Balthazart et al. (2001b).

which the synthesis of estrogens in the brain can be regulated (Fig. 24A) and two ways in which estrogens could affect reproductive behavior. A host of studies have shown that the activity of the preoptic aromatase can be increased by T acting in quail via its locally produced estrogenic metabolites. These changes in enzymatic activity are relatively slow and only reach their maximum after several hours or days. This rate of control is fully consistent with the well-characterized genomic action of estrogen in the brain. Estrogens, as do other sex steroid hormones, act as transcription factors and regulate the transcription of specific proteins. These effects can be direct, via the binding to ER that subsequently modulate the activity of genes that contain an ERE (or another type of consensus site) or indirectly through the regulation of other genes such as the immediate early genes *fos* or *jun* that then regulate the genes controlled by AP1 sequences.

However, during the 1990s, more rapid electrophysiological or neurochemical effects of estrogens were described and it was reported that estrogenic metabolites of aromatizable androgens act rapidly in the male rat brain to facilitate male-typical behavior (Cross and Roselli, 1999). The data described demonstrate that in the presence of ATP and Mg^{2+}, conditions that are known to promote the phosphorylation of a variety of enzymes, a dramatic inhibition of AA is detected within minutes. Also note that the ionic changes that affect brain AA are of a physiological magnitude. This strongly supports the physiological relevance of the observed effects.

A massive depolarization presumably induced by a K^+ shock markedly suppresses AA measured in hypothalamic tissue blocks maintained *in vitro*. This inhibition was significantly reduced when no Ca^{2+} was present, suggesting that the K^+ depolarization affects AA via changes in Ca^{2+} influx and that the effects of Ca^{2+} identified in brain homogenates do actually take place in intact neurons. Glutamate receptors of the NMDA and non-NMDA subtypes have been identified in the quail POA-hypothalamus and the kainate receptor appears to be the most prominent of the non-NMDA subtype (De la Torre *et al.*, 1998). Agonists directed against both the NMDA and non-NMDA excitatory amino acid receptor subtypes rapidly inhibited AA in the hypothalamic blocks. Excitatory amino acid receptors are intrinsic ion channels that are permeable to Na^+ and K^+ as well as Ca^{2+} (MacDermott *et al.*, 1986; Ascher and Nowak, 1988; Hollmann *et al.*, 1991). They could mediate Ca^{2+} influxes in aromatase cells. Based on pharmacological experiments, it seems possible that K^+ effects were mediated by a presynaptic release of transmitters such as glutamate (Wu and Saggau, 1997). These effects of the K^+ depolarization or of the glutamatergic agonists were observed with latencies as short as 5 minutes and were fully reversible. Together, these *in vitro* data based on continuous measures of AA in POA-hypothalamus explants indicate that a K^+ depolarization or the stimulation of excitatory amino acid receptors have a profound effect on brain AA that could be mediated by changes in intracellular Ca^{2+} concentration.

As we have described in detail, similar rapid inhibitions of AA are also observed in hypothalamic homogenates and in hypothalamic explants exposed to dopaminergic agonists and antagonists. The pharmacological data available seem to exclude an effect of these dopaminergic compounds that would be mediated by the dopaminergic receptors that are located at the level of neuronal membranes. Whether these effects are also mediated by rapid variations in intracellular calcium or by other mechanisms is under investigation.

Although the experimental manipulations described resulted in inhibitions of AA, it is quite possible that fast changes in brain function due to rapid effects of estrogens are the result of an up-regulation of AA. There are at least two not mutually exclusive ways in which such an up-regulation could occur. On the one hand, if the phosphorylation of aromatase leads to a decrease in its activity, the dephosphorylation of the same sites in the molecule should up-regulate the enzymatic activity. On the other hand, the incubation conditions that have been employed were selected because they are associated with maximal enzymatic activities. It is conceivable that in these conditions, aromatase is largely dephosphorylated and has a maximal enzymatic activity that cannot be further increased. This interpretation is consistent with the fact that incubations were carried out in phosphate-free media because our preliminary experiments suggested that phosphate buffers inhibit AA. Under physiological conditions it is likely that the relative activities of phosphatases and kinases can up- and down-regulate, respectively, AA.

Rapid changes in the availability of locally produced estrogens can therefore take place in the brain based on variation in neurotransmitter activity. Biochemical and immunocytochemical studies have shown that aromatase is present in presynaptic boutons in quail (see Section III). Estrogens could therefore be produced in locally high concentration and act in a paracrine fashion on postsynaptic membranes (see also Fig. 17). Accumulating evidence demonstrates that, in addition to their relatively slow genomic effects (i.e., their action as transcription factors after binding to intracellular receptors), estrogens can rapidly (milliseconds to minutes) modulate electrical properties of neurons and the activity of various chemical messengers (Pasqualini *et al.*, 1995; Mermelstein *et al.*, 1996; Ramirez *et al.*, 1996; Moss *et al.*, 1997; Joëls, 1997; Herbison, 1998; Gu *et al.*, 1999; Brubaker and Gay, 1999; McEwen and Alves, 1999). In particular, it has been established that estrogen injections affect precopulatory behaviors (anogenital sniffing and mount attempts) in rats within 15 min (Cross and Roselli, 1999), suggesting the participation of nongenomic mechanisms to the behavioral activation. But the mechanisms regulating estrogen availability, which must also be changing rapidly, have not been investigated. Rapid changes in AA regulated electrophysiologically resulting in changing levels of estrogens at the presynaptic level provide a novel mechanism for such a rapid control of estrogen availability in the brain.

6. Effects of Behavior on Endocrine Physiology

The relationship between hormones and behavior is often viewed as unidirectional, with hormones affecting in a more or less specific manner the expression of behaviors. The reverse causal link, although less studied, is known to exist in birds as well as in mammals. The effects of behavioral activity on the endocrine state actually represent an important control mechanism for reproductive cycles and help the ensuring the synchronization of reproductive stages between males and females. The best-documented example of how behavioral interactions can affect the endocrine physiology has probably been obtained in ring doves (Lehrman, 1965; Cheng, 1979). In male doves, a rise in plasma androgens levels is observed within 4 hours after pairing with an intact female and androgen levels remain high for approximately 5 days (Feder *et al.*, 1977). The factors controlling this endocrine reaction have been examined in a series of experiments manipulating the stimuli from the females that are accessible to the male (O'Connell *et al.*, 1981a). Males exposed to ovariectomized females had lower androgen levels than males exposed to intact females, indicating that the female gonadal condition (and presumably behavior) influences the male endocrine response. Deaf males also had lower androgen increases than normal males when exposed to an intact female, indicating the auditory cues play a role in the control of the androgen response. The presence of a glass partition between the male and the female did not, however, influence the response and a similar rise in plasma androgens was seen in males exposed to a female with or without a glass separation. Contact cues from the mating situation therefore appear to be of no importance. Additional studies also analyzed the factors that maintain the higher levels of circulating androgens of males once they have been established by the interaction with a sexually competent female (O'Connell *et al.*, 1981b). These levels were not affected (decreased nor increased) if a new female was provided everyday—plasma androgens returned to baseline level after 7–9 days at a time when incubation normally begins. If the male's nest was regularly destroyed or no nest material was provided, males retained, in contrast, a higher level of plasma androgens compared to males that were able to build a complete nest. Exposure to a courting female also maintained higher androgen levels than exposition to an incubating female. There is, therefore, a complex interaction between stimuli emanating from the female and her behavior and from the nest that control the changes in plasma androgens during the first phase of the reproductive cycle of the ring dove. The rise in plasma androgens induced by the interaction with the female is also indirectly responsible for the behavioral transition observed during the cycle. The intracerebral metabolism of these androgens into estrogens by the enzyme aromatase plays a key limiting role at this level.

When a male ring dove is paired with a female, the male directs predominantly aggressive courtship (bow-cooing and chasing) toward its partner. After a few days, these displays are progressively replaced by nest-oriented behaviors such as nest-cooing and wing-flipping (Lovari and Hutchison, 1975; Cheng, 1979). All these behaviors are activated by testicular secretions—they are absent in castrated males and can be restored by T treatment. However, the aggressive components of courtship can be activated by nonaromatizable androgens, whereas the nest-oriented courtship requires either estrogens or aromatizable androgens (Hutchison, 1970; Cheng and Lehrman, 1975; Adkins-Regan, 1981).

The shift from androgen-dependent to estrogen-dependent behaviors is not paralleled by modifications of the plasma concentration of E_2 during the breeding cycle (Korenbrot *et al.*, 1974). E_2 was actually not detected in the plasma of the males at any stage in the reproductive cycle, but in view of the low levels of circulating estrogens in male birds and the relative lack of sensitivity of the assay used in that study, this is probably an experimental artifact. The behavioral transition between aggressive and nest-oriented courtship is actually controlled by estrogens formed in the target areas in the brain. Steimer and Hutchison (1981b) demonstrated that the conversion of T to E_2 in the POA of the ring dove is markedly increased by T. This provides a molecular mechanism that could control the behavioral transition from aggressive to nest-oriented courtship. As already described, the interaction with the female results in a massive surge of plasma T (Feder *et al.*, 1977; O'Connell *et al.*, 1981a). This T peak roughly coincides with the behavioral transition. Dudley *et al.* (1984) showed that 24 hours after the introduction of a female dove into the cage of a male, there is a twofold increase in AA confined to the ventromedial POA. This increase in enzyme activity is sustained until day 5 of courtship and presumably provides the estrogens needed to activate the estrogen-dependent nest-oriented behavior. The preoptic aromatase activity then declines during the incubation phase of the cycle (Lea and Armstrong, 1986). The preoptic aromatase system thus appears to play an important role in modulating the action of androgens during the cycle of the ring dove. Together with the injection and implant experiments that demonstrate the steroid specificity of the various components of courtship behaviors (Hutchison, 1970, 1971; Cheng and Lehrman, 1975; Adkins-Regan, 1981), this transition represents one of the best examples illustrating the critical role played by the neural metabolism of T in the control of behavior.

Like ring doves, male white-crowned sparrows have higher plasma levels of LH and of T if caged with an E_2-treated female that displays numerous courtship postures than males caged alone or with a cholesterol-implanted nonreceptive female (Wingfield and Farner, 1980; Moore, 1983); similar observations have now been reported in quite a few species (Wingfield and Moore, 1987).

In contrast, in Japanese quail the reproductive physiology of the male is stimulated by long photoperiods and no additional increase in plasma T can be induced by exposure and sexual interactions with sexually mature females (Delville et al., 1984b). However, it could be shown that sexual maturation occurs more rapidly in young males exposed to marginally stimulating photoperiods if they are raised in the presence of females (Delville et al., 1984b). The endocrine response to the presence of females therefore varies with the species considered and may depend on the importance of photoperiodic cues in determining the endocrine physiology as well as on the social-system characteristic of the species (e.g., the presence or absence of territorial aggression and monogamy vs polygamy; Wingfield and Moore, 1987).

Finally, note that the nature of the specific stimuli that affect the endocrine physiology of male subjects has rarely been determined. In the ring dove example, the experimental analysis has dissected the female sensory cues that are important in causing the increase the plasma T levels in the male. However, it is unclear whether the increase in plasma T results from the perception of the stimuli originating in the female or from the performance of behaviors in response to these stimuli. Detailed experimental analyses carried out in female doves strongly suggest that both aspects could play an important role (see later) and more work on this topic is warranted.

7. Is a General Model of the Hormonal Control of Male Sexual Behavior Emerging?

The experiments on the physiology of male sexual behavior presented demonstrate that: (1) T, acting especially through its estrogenic metabolites, is necessary for the activation of male sexual behavior; (2) the administration of DA agonists and antagonists can profoundly affect male sexual behavior, as has been observed in other vertebrates; and (3) several interconnected brain areas that serve as targets for the effects of T or receive catecholaminergic inputs are involved in the regulation of these behaviors. But how do these two systems interact physiologically? One obvious possible mechanism is that T can stimulate male sexual behavior via the modification of dopaminergic transmission (Fig. 25). This could involve the modification of synthesis and release of DA or change in the sensitivity of brain areas to DA via the modification of the receptor number or affinity. In quail two other possible ways in which catecholamines can modify aromatase have been identified. One is a long-acting mechanism that involves the activation of DA receptors followed by the alteration of the genomic expression of aromatase. The other is a more rapid mechanism that does not appear to be receptor-mediated and presumably involves the direct interaction of DA with aromatase. This last mechanism represents a functional form of cross talk between the steroid-sensitive systems (i.e., the aromatase cells) on the one hand and the DA system, on the other hand. This interaction presumably does not involve a receptor protein but rather consists of a substrate competition for an enzyme. It should therefore be called functional cross talk rather than cross talk *sensu stricto*.

The ways in which DA and T appear to be interacting are schematically presented in Fig. 25. The center of the diagram illustrates the pathway (from left to right) by which T is metabolized by the action of ARO in circumscribed areas of the brain into an estrogen such as E_2.

The possible modulation of ARO by DA is noted by the arrow going from the top of the figure to the ARO step. Two possible mechanisms are proposed—a slow

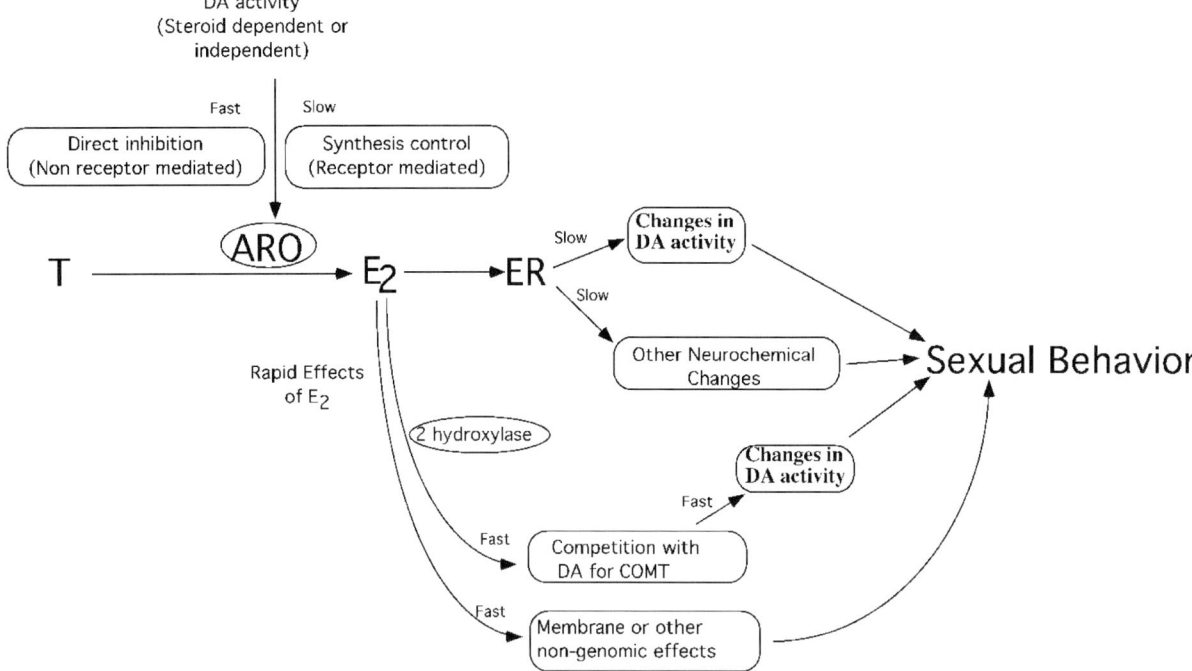

FIGURE 25 Diagram of the possible interactions of the neurotransmitter dopamine (DA), the steroid-metabolizing enzyme aromatase (ARO), and the estrogens as they relate to the activation of male reproductive behavior by testosterone (T). Two types of steroid actions that could result in behavioral changes are considered—slow effects that are presumably mediated by interaction with nuclear receptors and changes in gene transcription and more rapid effects that do not involve genomic effects and should result from more direct interactions of steroids with the neuronal physiology, presumably at the neuronal membrane level. Modified from Balthazart et al. (1998b).

mechanism that involves DA cells projecting to ARO-ir cells and the activation of DA receptors initiating a biochemical cascade that results in a change in the synthesis of ARO, for which there is *in vivo* evidence; and a fast (seconds to minutes) mechanism that involves the intracellular interaction between DA and AA that appears to be independent of DA receptor activation, for which there is *in vitro* evidence.

The estrogens bind to an intracellular ERα or ERβ. The ligand-activated ER can then act genomically to induce changes in protein synthesis that ultimately result in changes in DA activity or in other neurochemical systems that are required for the activation of male sexual behavior. These changes are denoted slow because they involve genomic activation and take hours to days to complete. Locally produced E_2 could also influence behavior through rapid actions that do not involve an interaction with the ER. Evidence for this nongenomic mode of action is not available in birds, but data in mammals indicate that estrogens produce rapid effects at the membrane level (Mermelstein et al., 1996; Ramirez et al., 1996; Joëls, 1997) and modify precopulatory behavior within 15–35 min after injection (Cross and Roselli, 1999). Two possible ways that this could happen are illustrated by the arrows coursing down from E_2 in the diagram. These rapid effects include the interaction with cell membranes (no such mechanisms have been definitively identified for E_2 in birds yet) and the possible metabolism of E_2 to a catecholestrogen via the enzyme 2-hydroxylase and the resulting substrate competition with DA for the enzyme COMT. The change in DA that results from this latter interaction could lead to a change in behavior. There is evidence in some vertebrate species for the substrate competition between DA and catecholestrogens for COMT, but the possible behavioral consequences of this are unknown. It has been shown that 2-hydroxylation of estrogens takes place in the avian brain (Balthazart et al.,

1994b). The potential role of hydroxylated estrogens on DA neurotransmission should therefore be analyzed experimentally.

In conclusion, although it has been known for many years that both the gonadal sex steroid hormone T and the catecholamine neurotransmitter DA influence male sexual behavior, the nature of any possible interaction between these chemical messenger systems has been largely unexplored. The role of other transmitters and neuropeptides is even less well understood. When such an interaction is discussed, the assumption made by most researchers appears to be that T promotes sexual behavior by influencing the action of DA. This is a perfectly plausible hypothesis given that pharmacological manipulations of DA can have relatively rapid effects on sexual behavior and T acting through its androgenic and estrogenic metabolites is well known to modify neurotransmission of many types of neurotransmitters including catecholamines. Although this is a plausible model, it remains largely untested. However, data have been collected from rodent species that support this idea (Simpkins et al., 1980, 1983; Alderson and Baum, 1981). It has been shown that when exposed to a female, castrated rats exhibit an attenuation in DA release compared to intact controls (Hull et al., 1995, 1999). Thus, the modulation of DA release by T may be one part of the causal chain of events that activate this behavior, but is it the only way these two systems interact?

Studies of the activation of male sexual behavior in quail have revealed additional ways in which these two systems could interact to influence this behavior. Dopaminergic afferent inputs to regions rich in aromatase-positive neurons appear to enhance AA. Thus, DA can also promote male sexual behavior by promoting the conversion of T to E_2, a critical step for the activation of male reproductive behavior in many species. A surprising and novel interaction between DA and T has also been described in quail. This again involves the enzyme aromatase, but in this case DA and aromatase are thought to interact in a relatively fast (seconds to minutes) manner, independently of DA receptors and perhaps even ER. These rapid effects include the possibility that locally produced estrogen in high concentrations could result in cell membrane effects significant for behavior (no such mechanisms have been definitively identified for E_2) and the possible metabolism of E_2 to a catecholestrogen via the enzyme 2-hydroxylase and the resulting substrate competition with DA for the enzyme COMT. In both these cases, the interrelation of DA and aromatase is on the time course we would expect of pharmacological manipulations of neurotransmitter systems rather than genomically mediated effects of sex steroid hormones. These novel interactions, both slow acting and fast acting, need to be tested in other species, but they could provide important new insights into our understanding of male sexual behavior, both from the perspective of basic research and from the perspective of the interpretation of clinical interventions.

C. Female Sexual Behavior

Very surprisingly, much less research has been devoted to the experimental analysis of the endocrine control of female sexual behavior in birds (with the exception of poultry). This contrasts markedly with the situation in mammals in which the female receptive response, the lordosis, has been the subject of intense investigations (quantitatively more than the masculine sexual behavior) since the 1960s. The reason for the preference for the study of females in mammals and males in birds is unclear, but may be related to the fact that the lordosis response in rodents is an easily quantifiable behavior that can be reliably elicited in standardized conditions (e.g., with a flank palpation by the experimenter; see Pfaff, 1980, 1999).

1. Activation of Receptivity and Proceptivity

The limited amount of data available clearly indicates that the expression of female sexual behavior in birds critically depends on the steroid secretions from the ovary, mainly of estrogens with a potential synergistic role of progestagens. In 1913, Goodale observed that ovariectomized hens show "no sex instincts." Davis and Domm (1943) confirmed that, contrary to sexually mature females, bilaterally ovariectomized hens do not squat in response to the male's approach. Similar observations are reported in quail—females that have been functionally ovariectomized by exposure to short-day photoperiods (Adkins, 1973) cease laying within 2 weeks and lose all signs of sexual receptivity (Adkins and Adler, 1972; Noble, 1972; Adkins, 1973). Surgical ovariectomy leads to the same behavior deficits (Delville and Balthazart, 1987).

The removal of the left ovary in female ring doves, the only one that is normally active in most bird species (Lofts and Murton, 1973; Murton and Westwood, 1975), rapidly leads to the disappearance of female courtship behaviors such as wing-flipping and nest-cooing that are normally shown by females in response to male courtship (Cheng and Lehrman, 1975; Cheng, 1979). These behaviors slowly reappear after a period of 6–8 weeks, but it has been shown that the behavioral recovery is associated with a compensatory hypertrophy of the right ovary. The surgical ablation of this regenerated gonad leads to the complete and definitive suppression of these behaviors (Cheng, 1973a,b).

The treatment of ovariectomized females with estrogens alone was shown in several avian species to restore sexual behaviors to the level typical of sexually mature subjects. Early experiments performed in the 1940s indicated that administration of estrogens to bilaterally ovariectomized poulards induces squatting behavior (Allee and Collias, 1940; Davis and Domm, 1943). Subsequent research in Japanese quail confirmed this conclusion—injections of E_2 at a daily dose of 0.05–0.1 mg/day effectively restored receptive behavior in females that had been functionally ovariectomized by exposure to short days (Adkins and Adler, 1972). These effects of estrogens were blocked by the concurrent administration of the antiestrogen CI-628 (Adkins and Nock, 1976b). Squatting was similarly induced in 87% of female quail maintained in constant darkness (a condition that suppresses ovarian activity) by the injection of 0.2 mg/day of EB (Noble, 1972), whereas this behavior was restored to intact levels in surgically ovariectomized quail by 2 weeks of injections with 0.1 mg/day of EB (Delville and Balthazart, 1987). This study also confirmed that the squatting behavior observed in gonadally intact sexually mature females is estrogen-dependent—this behavior can be markedly inhibited by injections of the antiestrogen tamoxifen (Delville and Balthazart, 1987). In ring doves, estrogen alone (0.05 mg/day) also restored the sexual behavior of females, including wing flipping and nest coos (Cheng, 1973b).

A large number of studies on a diversity of songbird species have confirmed and expanded the notion that injections of exogenous estrogens activate most if not all components of female sexual behavior and in particular squatting, the best indicator of female receptivity. This activation of squatting by estrogens has been demonstrated in song sparrows (*Melospiza melodia;* Searcy and Marler, 1981; O'Loghlen and Beecher, 1997), white crowned sparrows (Moore, 1982, 1983) and red-winged blackbirds (Searcy and Capp, 1997; see also Wingfield and Silverin, Chapter 31). In canaries in particular, estrogens markedly affect the sexual responses of the female to vocal stimuli produced by the male. Females that are nearing ovulation or that have been treated with exogenous estrogen produce copulation solicitation displays (CSDs)—squatting accompanied by rapid vibrations of the wings—when exposed to males songs or to tapes of these songs (Nagle *et al.,* 1993; Leboucher *et al.,* 1994, 1998b). These CSDs are no longer observed in females housed in short days, which cause ovarian regression and therefore lower plasma estrogen levels. The supression of estrogen production by the injection of the aromatase inhibitor Fadrozole leads to a similar reduction of behavioral expression (Leboucher *et al.,* 1998b).

In some mammals, the behavioral effects of estrogens on female receptivity are enhanced by a treatment with progesterone, whereas in other species this synergism is not observed and estrogens alone are fully effective in activating receptive behavior. Based on the species that have been studied, it seems that E_2 alone may induce sexual receptivity in species with induced ovulation (e.g., rabbits, ferrets, cats, prairie voles, and collared and brown lemmings), whereas an additional participation of progesterone is required for the full display of receptivity in many species of spontaneous ovulators (e.g., rats, hamsters, guinea pigs, and goats; Bakker and Baum, 2000). A limited number of experiments have addressed the same question in birds and researched whether progesterone has any behavioral effects by itself or synergizes with E_2 to activate squatting. All experiments carried out indicate little or no behavioral activation following injections of progesterone alone—for example, quail (Adkins and Adler, 1972) and doves (Cheng and Silver, 1975). Furthermore, in several experiments, no or little additional effects of the concurrent administration of progesterone could be detected in estrogen-treated females (in quail; Noble, 1972). The inhibitory effects of progesterone on estradiol-induced female receptivity have also been reported in turkey hens (El Halawani *et al.,* 1986). Similarly, in canaries injections of progesterone inhibit the CSDs expressed by females in response to the playback of male song (Leboucher et al., 2000).

Large doses of estrogens were often used in the earlier experments performed in birds, and the negative conclusions concerning the lack of synergistic effects of progesterone on the E_2-induced female behavior could be related to the excessive (supraphysiological) stimulation by estrogens. Some of the earlier experiments on quail were also performed in females that had been functionally ovariectomized by exposure to short days (Adkins, 1973). It was therefore impossible to make sure that low levels of circulating progesterone were not already present in the experimental females before treatment with exogenous progesterone. It could be speculated that the lack of effect of the injected progesterone was an artifact of the experimental situation. However, other studies in quail that used a more physiological threshold of estrogens in ovariectomized females reached the same conclusion—no or little significant additive effect of progesterone can be identified in the activation of female receptivity by estrogens (Delville and Balthazart, 1987). It must be stressed that progesterone of adrenal origin may still be present in ovariectomized birds, so it is still not absolutely certain that progesterone plays no role in the control of female receptivity. Given that a clear synergism between E_2 and progesterone can be observed in the activation of nest-building in subjects that are not adrenalectomized (see next), it appears likely that progesterone is not implicated in a physiological manner in the activation of female receptive behavior in birds. This conclusion seems to apply to species that are essentially induced ovulators (e.g., canaries and ring doves) as well as to species which regularly ovulate even in the absence of a male (e.g., Japanese quail). The correlation that has been suggested based on mammalian studies between the type of ovulation control and the effectiveness or lack of effect of progesterone in the control of sexual receptivity therefore does not seem to hold in birds based on the small number of species that have been studied in enough detail. Additional work on a broader variety of species is needed.

2. Nest-Building

There is a broad diversity in the type of nests that are built by birds (Drent, 1975) and in the amount of time that females, males or both invest in this activity. Some species just lay their eggs on the ground and do not take care of them (e.g., Japanese quail; incubation was bred out of this domestic species) or drop them in the nest of other species (e.g., old world cuckoos and cowbirds). Other species build very elaborate structures and spent a considerable amount of time in this activity. The building of the nest can be done by the female alone—as in ducks (McKinney, 1969) and canaries (Hinde, 1958)—or in cooperation with her mate—as in ring doves (Lehrman, 1963). Exceptionally, in some species, the nest is built by the male alone—as in red-billed queleas (Morel and Bourlière, 1956).

The endocrine bases of this behavior have been studied in great detail in a few species. Most of the work has focused on females, but in a small number of cases the males have also been considered and some sex differences in the endocrine control of nest building have been identified. In addition, studies performed mainly in canaries and ring doves have demonstrated that even if adequate endocrine stimuli are present, the performance of nest-building is markedly affected by the social and physical environment (see later). Nest-building also markedly influences the physiology of the hypothalamic-pituitary-gonadal axis, and this behavior therefore plays an important role in the timing of ovulation in the female, as illustrated mainly by work in ring doves (see Cheng, 1979; Balthazart, 1983, for details).

Studies in domestic hens demonstrate that nest-building is controlled by hormones secreted by the postovulatory follicle (Wood-Gush and Gilbert, 1964, 1970) and, accordingly, the behavior can be activated by treatments with exogenous E_2 and progesterone (Wood-Gush and Gilbert, 1973). A number of old studies in a variety of species also indicate that androgens can increase nest-building behavior in the female as well as in the male when both sexes participate—as in black-crowned night herons (Noble and Wurm, 1940) and budgerigars (Brockway, 1969b). However E_2 is often, if not always, more effective than T and it can be suspected that the effects of T are mediated by its central aromatization into an estrogen (see Sections V.B.4.c and V.B.5). This idea has not been explicitly tested. The roles of estrogens and progestagens in the activation of nest-building behavior have been studied in great detail in ring doves and canaries.

a) Ring Doves In doves, the male usually selects the nest material and brings it to the nest site where the female incorporates it in the nest. The readiness to build is not observed when a male and a female are first paired together; it develops progressively after a few days of courtship. There is during this period a marked growth of the ovarian follicles in the female, which suggests an endocrine basis for the nest-building behavior. This idea has been independently confirmed by the observation that nest-building behavior can be induced by the injection of exogenous hormones. Injections of TP or EB activate the gathering of nest material in castrated male doves (Martinez-Vargas, 1974) and a combined estrogen plus progesterone treatment is very effective for eliciting nest-building activity in ovariectomized female doves (Cheng, 1973b). Treatment with either hormone in isolation produces only minor effects (Cheng, 1973b; Cheng and Silver, 1975).

Interestingly, hormone treatment of females with estrogens and progestins also faciliates the behavior in the untreated male mate (Martinez-Vargas and Erickson, 1973; Cheng and Silver, 1975), indicating that social factors play a significant role in addition to the endocrine factors. This does not mean, however, that hormones play no role in the control of nest-building in the male; this social facilitation is indeed not observed in castrated males. It seems therefore that sexually intact males are physiologically ready to participate in nest building on exposure to the adequate social stimuli. Additional controls of the nest-building activity are also exerted by the nest itself (White, 1975a,b,c; Cheng and Balthazart, 1982).

b) Canaries Major interactions between the nest condition and hormonal factors have also been identified in canaries (see Hinde, 1965; Hinde and Steel, 1966). In this species, the female usually builds the nest almost alone (Hinde, 1965); the male makes no real contribution and is only seen unfrequently picking up material, but he never incorporates it into the nest cup (Hinde, 1958). During the nest building period, however, the male actively courts the female, feeds her, and copulates with her. These behaviors have been shown to enhance the female's building behavior.

Nest-building activity in canaries culminates 2–3 days before egg-laying, suggesting a specific relationship with the endocrine state of the subjects (Hinde, 1965). Accordingly, injections of EB into females during the winter, at a time when no nest-building is normally observed, induce active building in some subjects. The doses of EB that had to be injected to obtain this behaviroal activation were, however, very high and toxic. Furthermore, no additional activation was observed when females were concurrently injected with progesterone. In an elegant suite of experiments, Hinde and coworkers established how endocrine stimuli of a more physiological nature interact with the environment (in particular the lighting regime and the nest cup condition). This resulted in a detailed model that takes into account all factors controlling reproduction in the canary (see Hinde, 1965, for review). In this model, small physiological doses of estrogens acting in synergy with progesterone are the key hormonal stimuli that activate nest-building. The endocrine control of this behavior is therefore similar in doves and canaries. In addition, canaries develop a brood patch in response to estrogen and the increased skin sensitivity plays a key role in determining the nest-building activity. There is also a marked intereaction between hormones and the day length in the activation of nest-building—estrogens are by far more effective in subjects exposed to long day lengths than in subjects exposed to short day lengths (see Hinde, 1965; Balthazart, 1983, for more detail).

3. Correlations of Behavioral and Endocrine Changes

A number of studies have also demonstrated that the steroids that are supposed to activate various aspects of female behavior based on ovariectomy and hormone replacement studies (mostly E_2 and progesterone) vary in the plasma in parallel with changes in behavior. These covariations have mostly been identified during the course of the annual cycle of reproduction, but a few studies also indicate correlations on a shorter-term basis (e.g., during the daily cycle). Field studies clearly illustrate in a diversity of species that the frequencies of female reproductive behavior peak during the spring at a time when maximal levels of plasma estrogens are detected (see Wingfield and Silverin, Chapter 31).

In ring doves, work by Lehrman and coworkers showed well before the advent of sensitive assays for plasma hormones that the development of sexual receptivity and nest-building behavior in females is related to the maturation of the ovarian follicles (reviewed in Cheng, 1979). Radioimmunoassays of plasma E_2 and of the gonadotropic hormones LH and FSH have further refined this correlation (Korenbrot et al., 1974; Cheng and Follett, 1976). They also demonstrated that experimental manipulations affecting the maturation of the ovarian follicle and the secretion of sex steroids and gonadotropic hormones affect in parallel the expression of female behaviors, which suggests a causal nature for these correlations (Cheng and Balthazart, 1982; see also Section V.C.6).

In female quail, the frequency of squatting (a sign of sexual receptivity) and the percentage of male approaches that are followed by squatting increase at the end of the day, approximately 11–13 hr after lights on (in a photoperiod of 16L:8D). In some cases, this increased receptivity is associated with a significant decrease of the frequency of male avoidance. The increased receptivity at the end of the day does not appear to be directly caused by the oviposition and does not result directly from changes in the behavior of the male stimuli. This interpretation is supported by the observation that the increase in receptivity takes place at the same time after lights on (but different clock times) in two groups of females that were raised in two different photoperiods (shifted by 6 hr) and tested with a same group of males raised in one of the two photoperiods. The increase in receptivity coincides with an increase in plasma E_2 and progesterone. Considering that this behavior is suppressed by ovariectomy, it has been argued that the daily changes in receptivity could be controlled by the hormonal changes associated with the ovulatory cycle (Delville et al., 1986). Plasma levels of E_2 and progesterone similarly change during the daily ovulatory cycle of domestic hens (Shodono et al., 1975; Johnson and van Tienhoven, 1980), and it can be expected that these endocrine changes also affect the receptivity of the hen during the day.

4. Sites of Action of Sex Steroid Hormones

Little research has been concerned in birds on the identification of the brain sites and circuitry involved in the control of female reproductive behaviors. In ring doves, Gibson and Cheng (1979) produced electrolytic lesions in various parts of the POA-hypothalamus of ovariectomized EB-treated females. They noted that a significant decline in courtship behavior is induced only by lesions affecting the posterior medial hypothalamus. Also, intracranial implants of EB are most effective in activating courtship if placed in the posterior medial hypothalamus (at the level of the VMN). Little or no courtship (sexual crouch or nest soliciting) is observed when these implants are placed in the POA or anterior hypothalamus (Gibson and Cheng, 1979). These data indicate that, as in mammals (Barfield et al., 1983; Pleim et al., 1989), the VMN is a key site for estrogen action on female sexual behavior. This notion is consistent with the fact that this nucleus contains a high numbers of neurons expressing ERα (Martinez-Vargas et al., 1975; Watson and Adkins-Regan, 1989b; Balthazart et al., 1989; Gahr et al., 1993) and ERβ (Foidart et al., 1999a). Studies also demonstrate that the expression of female sexual behavior is associated with the induction of the IEG *c-fos* in the VMN of quail (Meddle et al., 1999a). How this nucleus is incorporated into a full circuitry integrating sensory inputs and motor outputs is poorly understood. Additional studies are needed to evaluate the role of the VMN in other species.

A few studies have also attempted to identify the brain areas where steroids need to act in order to activate nest-building in ring doves. As previously mentioned, sexually active males are ready to gather nest material when introduced to a female treated with estrogen, but castrated males do not respond to the female unless they are themselves treated with E_2 or T. Stereotaxic implants of T in the POA, anterior hypothalamus, and area of the ventral neostriatum intermediale were effective in reinstating the collection and gathering of nest material in castrated males. Implants in other brain areas were not active (Erickson and Hutchison, 1977). There is, therefore, a large overlap between the brain areas that are involved in males in the activation by T of courtship and copulation, on the one hand, and of nest-building, on the other hand. It also plausible that the same brain areas are implicated in the activation of nest-building by steroids in females, but this idea has not been, to the best of our knowledge, experimentally tested.

5. Steroid–Neurotransmitter Interactions

In mammals, in addition to its effects at the pituitary level, GnRH acts in various brain sites that appear to include the VMN, POA and GCt. These effects result in a modulation of the induction of female sexual receptivity in E_2-primed rats (Moss and Dudley, 1989, 1990; Dudley and Moss, 1991). Detailed studies using various forms of GnRH and GnRH fragments indicate that structural changes in the molecule at the N-terminal portion, drastically affect the pituitary activity, but do not modify the behavioral activity of the molecule. By contrast, some C-terminal fragments are not active at the pituitary level, but they facilitate female sexual behavior. No behavioral effect could be detected in rat after treatment with chicken GnRH (cLHRH-I; Moss and Dudley, 1989). Little information is available about the potential role of luteinizing hormone releasing hormone (LHRH) in the control of reproductive behavior of birds. It must however be mentioned that mammalian GnRH (mLHRH) enhances the expression of female sexual behavior in ring doves that have been primed with estrogens (Cheng, 1977). Furthermore, studies in estrogen-primed female white-crowned sparrows demonstrate that injections into the third ventricle of cGnRH-II increase the display of copulation solicitations with a latency of 30 min (Maney et al., 1997b). No effect of cGnRH-I was observed in these conditions. Therefore, it appears likely that various forms of GnRH exert behavioral effects by acting as transmitters in the brain in birds, as in mammals, and further studies on this topic are certainly warranted.

6. Effects of Behavior Performance on Endocrine State

The female endocrine physiology can also, as in males, be influenced by behavioral interactions with a partner (see also Section IV.B). In female quail, for example, ovarian development can be stimulated by exposure to male vocalizations (Guyomarc'h et al., 1981; Guyomarc'h and Guyomarc'h, 1982). It has also been shown in several avian species that the interactions with a male or the presence of a nest and of nest material can substantially advance ovarian follicular maturation and egg-laying (see also Section IV.B).

Experimental studies on the reproductive cycle of ring doves have clearly demonstrated that the behavior of each member in a pair has profound influences on the behavior and reproductive physiology of the other member (Cheng, 1979). When male and female ring doves are placed in a same cage, they perform a highly predictable sequence of courtship displays that culminate in egg-laying. On the basis of a suite of elegant studies, Lehrman and collaborators suggested that a combination of visual and acoustic cues emanating from the male courtship stimulate the female hypothalamus and promote the secretion of GnRH, which in turn enhances the secretion by the pituitary of gonadotropic hormones. The actions of these hormones at the ovarian level then cause the female's follicles to develop and she eventually ovulates (Lehrman, 1965; Friedman, 1977). Subsequent studies carried out when sensitive radioimmunoassays became available fully demonstrate the validity of this hypothesis.

However, a series of very carefully planned experiments have accumulated evidence that leads to a partial reinterpretation of this effect. Although, it is still correct that male courtship stimulates female courtship and, in particular, her display of nest-coos, it is the female's own nest-cooing that activates GnRH secretion in the female hypothalamus (Cheng, 1986). In this revised model, it is therefore the female's own behavior (obviously influenced by the male) that controls the female ovarian development and, under appropriate experimental circumstances, follicle development should take place in the absence of the male provided the female still produces nest-coos. This hypothesis of self-stimulation in female doves is supported by a large amount of converging evidence that has been reviewed in detail (Cheng, 1992). We briefly discuss here only the most important of the experimental data supporting the self-stimulation hypothesis.

In one type of experiment, it was demonstrated that females exposed to the male courtship show little or no follicular development if they are prevented from performing nest-coos themselves. The final outcome of these experiments appeared to be independent of the way in which females were prevented from cooing and that included devocalization by severing of the hypoglosal nerves, deflating the interclavicular sac, or lesioning the midbrain ICo (Cohen and Cheng, 1979, 1981; Cheng et al., 1988) (Fig. 26). These three methods all produced a clear deficits in the female's nest-cooing behavior, and they all blocked follicular development. It is important to note, however, and these devocalized females were still courted actively by the males, indicating that the failure of follicular development was caused by a change in the behavior of the female, not the male.

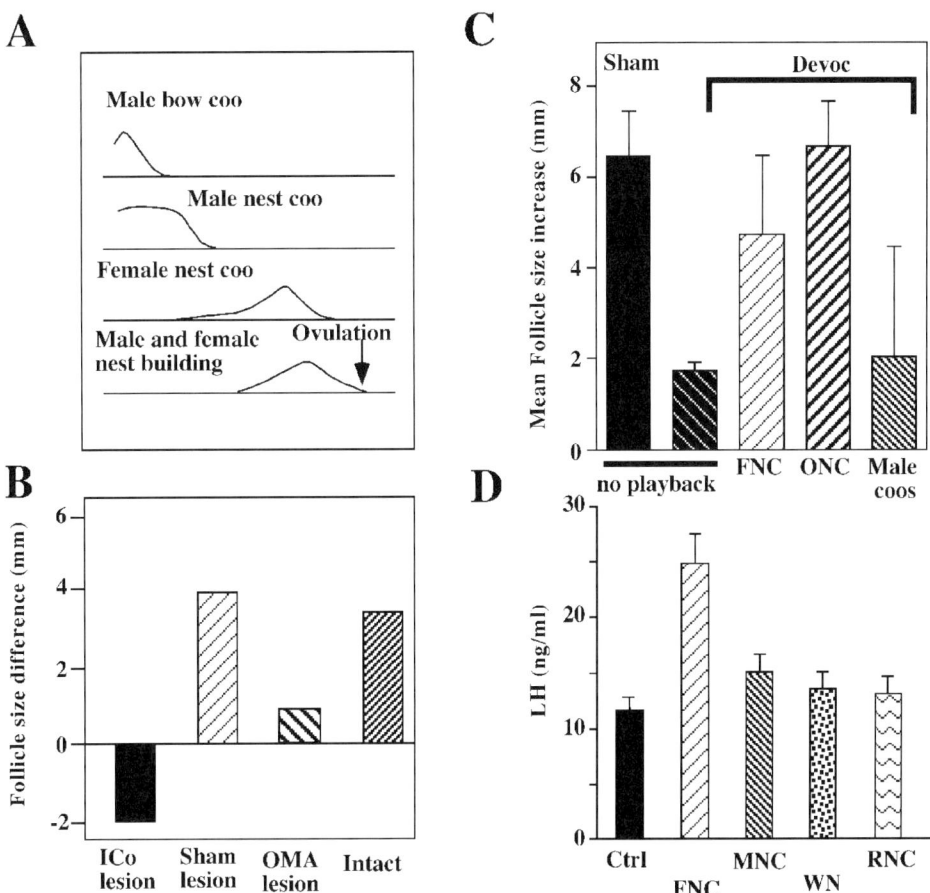

FIGURE 26 Self-stimulation of ovarian development in female ring doves. (A) Behavioral changes in the reproductive cycle of ring doves. When paired with a female, the male originally performs large numbers of bow-coos that are then followed by nest-coos. The female nest-coos are produced a few days later and then both sexes start building the nest. Ovulation of the two eggs takes place soon after the completion of nest building. (B) Effects of devocalization by lesion of the intercollicular nucleus (ICo) on the ovarian development of females exposed to stimulus males. The median change in the diameter of the largest ovarian follicle is presented from the time of lesion to the time of autopsy 28 days later. Follicles of ICo-lesioned birds were smaller than those of birds receiving a sham lesion, a lesion in other midbrain areas (OMA) or no lesion (intact). (C) Mean increment in follicle size (diameter in millimeters) of devocalized (hypoglossal nerves section) and sham-operated females hearing different types of coos (FNC, female nest coos, ONC, female own nest coos or male coos). (D) Mean pituitary LH levels in female doves exposed to different acoustic stimuli. Ctrl, no sound stimulation; FNC, female nest-coos; MNC, male nest-coos; RNC, reversed nest-coos (coos played in reverse order); WN, white noise. The FNC group shows a significantly higher level than all other groups. Data from Cheng (1992); Cheng et al. (1998).

In another experiment, attempts were made to promote follicular development by specific vocalizations. Females that had been devocalized by section of the hypoglossal nerves were exposed to the broadcast in sound-proof chambers of tapes containing male coos, female nest-coos, or nest-coos produced by the experimental female before devocalization (own coos). The increase in ovarian follicle size was found to be greater in females hearing their own coos than in females hearing other female's coos. Males vocalizations were even less effective, which clearly contradicts the older idea that male vocalizations directly stimulate the female's endocrine responses (Cheng et al., 1988). Additional experiments designed to test this self-stimulation hypothesis all converge to support this notion (Cheng, 1992). They certainly do not exclude that the stimulation of the female ovarian development could be due in part to a direct action of stimuli emanating from the male courtship, but they clearly indicate that the female's own coos have a key role. Part of their effect may be due to the performance of the behavior and part to the proprioceptive feedback associated with the behavior (see Cheng, 1992, for further discussion).

The neural substrate mediating these effects has also been identified to some extent. In particular, neuroanatomical tract-tracing studies identified pathways that potentially convey the auditory stimuli related to nest-cooing from the auditory areas to the hypothalamic region where the activity of GnrH neurons can be modulated. There are massive hypothalamic afferent projections originating in the shell region of the auditory thalamic nucleus (Durand et al., 1992) and minor projections originating in the midbrain vocal-control nucleus (Cheng and Zuo, 1994).

The biological significance of these inputs was demonstrated by electrophysiological and neuroendocrine studies showing that neural activity can be demonstrated electrophysiologically in the POA and anterior hypothalamic area, that receive projections from the auditory thalamic relay when birds hear species specific vocalizations and that this activity correlates with increases in LH concentration induced by hearing species-typical coos (Cheng et al., 1998). It was even found that LH increments are significantly greater when females hear female nest-coos than when they hear male nest-coos (Fig. 26D), which fully supports the results of the behavioral studies described here. There is, therefore, a direct functional linkage between the neural processing of vocal input and the gonadal growth induced by nest-coos as a result of increased secretion of LH.

The phenomenon of self-stimulation, documented in great detail in doves, may also exist in many other species. Evidence suggesting that this may be the case has been compiled by Cheng (1992). This literature clearly elaborates the functional interpretation of vocalizations that should no longer be considered only to be communication signals between individuals but could, in addition, have evolved as a mean to adjust the endocrine physiology of a subject to its social environment.

7. Behavioral Endocrinology of Female Sexual Behavior: Toward a Synthesis

In birds, the relatively limited number of experiments that have investigated the endocrine controls of reproductive behaviors in the female indicate that, as in mammals, the ovarian steroids E_2 and progesterone play a prominent role. At the cellular level, it appears that the same mechanisms should mediate the action of steroids in females and in males. In males, however, the most important steroid, T, undergoes an active metabolism at the level of its target brain areas and changes in this metabolism seem to play an important role in the control of the behavioral activation. In contrast in females, the most active steroid, E_2 acts directly in the brain and this action does not appear to be controlled by intracellular enzymes. The transformation of estrogen into catechol-estrogens could, however, be implicated, as in mammals (Rodriguez-Sierra and Blake, 1983), in the activation of some aspects of the behavioral repertoire, but this possibility has not been investigated in birds to our knowledge. Progesterone, like T, can undergo an active intracellular metabolism and be transformed into 5α- and 5β-reduced compounds that have behavioral effects that are different from those of the parent steroid. This possibility has not been investigated in detail in birds (see Balthazart et al., 1988b).

In the avian female, E_2 and progesterone presumably modulate the action of various neurotransmitters and neuropeptides, as demonstrated in female mammals and illustrated previously for the male in a number of avian species, but the experimental studies supporting these principles are relatively scarce. It is clear, however, that GnRH synergises with estrogens to activate female receptivity in birds as in mammals.

Studies in ring doves have best documented the bidirectional interactions between behavior and endocrine physiology and the notion of self-stimulation has been elaborated based on the detailed analysis of the experimental situations that promote follicular development. These studies should inspire additional work on the interrelationships between hormones, the brain, and behavior.

D. Parental Behavior

1. Correlations between Hormonal Changes during the Reproductive Cycle and Behavior

Based on studies of a variety of domesticated and feral species, a generalized avian endocrine profile can be described that mediates the transitions from courtship behavior to nest-building to incubation to the care of the young (Silver, 1978; Wingfield and Farner, 1980; Balthazart, 1983; Goldsmith, 1983; Wingfield et al., 1987; Silverin, 1988; Gratto-Trevor et al., 1990; Buntin, 1996). In both males and females, gonadal steroids such as the estrogens, androgens, and progestins and the pituitary gonadotropins, LH and FSH, tend to be high during the courtship and the nest-building period, regardless of the role played by either sex in nest-building. If either or both sexes engage in parental care, the transition to incubation that occurs during egg-laying involves a decline in the gonadal steroids and the gonadotropins and a rise in prolactin (see Wingfield and Farner, 1980; Balthazart, 1983; Goldsmith, 1983; Buntin, 1996, for reviews). One exception to this rule for the decline in sex steroids applies to progesterone in male birds, which in several species does not appear to change during the transition to incubation (e.g., Ball and Wingfield, 1987; Silver et al., 1974) and in some cases even increases (Fivizzani et al., 1986). In species with polygynous mating systems such as the red-winged blackbird (*Agelaius phoeniceus*), in which the male does not make the transition to incubation, the decline in androgens is not observed (e.g., Beletsky et al., 1989). In most avian species, a rise in plasma levels of prolactin is correlated with the onset and maintenance of incubation behavior (see Goldsmith, 1983; Lea, 1987; Buntin, 1996, for reviews). If only one sex incubates, levels of prolactin in that sex are generally far higher than in the other during incubation (Goldsmith, 1983; Gratto-Trevor et al., 1990). However, this correlation between gonadal steroid decline and rising prolactin and the onset of incubation is not perfect. For example, in apparently monogamous songbirds (passerines), males do not incubate or incubate very little (all members of the Suborder Passeres lack brood patches). But, it has been shown in three songbird species, the European starling (*Sturnus vulgaris*), the white-crowned sparrow (*Zonotrichia leucophrys*), and the song sparrow (*Melospiza melodia*), that T nonetheless declines just prior to incubation and prolactin rises during incubation. However, in every case, the male prolactin levels are lower than those measured in females (Dawson and Goldsmith, 1982; Hiatt et al., 1987; Wingfield and Goldsmith, 1990). In these species, as in most passerines, these males subsequently feed their altricial nestlings after they hatch. In general, although there appears to be a good correlation between the combination of declining plasma levels of the sex steroids and the gonadotropins and rising prolactin levels with the onset of incubation, this correlation is clearer in females than in male birds.

2. Prolactin and Parental Care in Pigeons and Doves

One well-studied exception to this pattern among biparental monogamous species occurs in the Columbiformes. As illustrated by the ring dove, both parents engage in parental care and both parents exhibit a decline in the plasma levels of the gonadal steroids prior to the onset of incubation (Silver, 1978; Cheng, 1979; Buntin, 1996). However, prolactin levels do not rise until incubation is under way (day 5 of a 14-day incubation period; reviewed by Lea, 1987; Buntin, 1996). This variant in the pattern of prolactin secretion is thought to be associated with the fact that ring doves, as do all columbiformes, possess a crop sac in which they produce a milky substance fed to the young. This crop is well known to be prolactin-dependent and it grows near the end of incubation to insure that it is fully developed in time to feed the squab; it appears to be costly to develop the crop sac early in incubation.

3. Experimental Studies of the Role Played by Steroid Hormones and Prolactin in Mediating the Transition from Courtship to Parental Care

Studies that have investigated in detail the causal role that these hormones play in the control of parental care using the standard methods of hormone removal and replacement have generally been limited to domesticated species that breed in captivity, such as ring doves, canaries, domestic chickens (*Gallus domesticus*), and turkeys (*Meleagris gallopavo*). This review does not cover in detail all the experimental work resulting from these studies, and the reader is referred to the available reviews (Silver, 1978; Cheng, 1979; Balthazart, 1983; Lea, 1987; El Halawani et al., 1990; Buntin, 1996).

In female ring doves E_2 and progesterone are essential for nest-building to occur and for the transition to incubation behavior (Cheng and Silver, 1975). It was demonstrated early on that implanting progesterone directly into diencephalic brain sites promotes the onset of incubation (Komisaruk, 1967). In female turkeys it is clear that E_2 and progesterone acting in synergy with prolactin are essential for the onset of incubation (El Halawani et al., 1986), whereas in doves, which possess an unusual pattern of prolactin secretion, this hormone seems to be important for the maintenance but not the onset of incubation (Buntin, 1986; Lea, 1987). Males have been studied less intensively, but the results for ring doves suggest that males are affected more by situational and stimulus factors than by endocrine physiology than are females (Silver, 1978; Balthazart, 1983).

Studies of nondomesticated species in the field have generally been limited to manipulating plasma levels of hormones by administering hormone implants. Most of this work has been done on males and it suggests that maintaining high T levels by implanting intact males with capsules containing the hormone is incompatible with parental care (Silverin, 1980; Hegner and Wingfield, 1987; Oring et al., 1989).

Experimental studies of prolactin in nondomesticated species are rare because of the difficulty in manipulating this hormone, which is secreted by the pituitary. Pedersen (1989) administered prolactin to intact free-living female willow ptarmigan (*Lagopus lagopus*) and found that there was no increase in incubation constancy, but that there was a slight increase in their sitting-tightness and in their distraction display rate when flushed off the nest. As reviewed in the previous section, studies in feral birds that correlate hormone levels and parental care, in general, reveal hormone profiles consistent with the notion that prolactin acts synergistically with the sex steroids to stimulate the onset of incubation.

Declining prolactin levels have been related to the termination of the incubation of infertile eggs or to the termination of the brooding of the young in ring doves (Silver, 1984). Silver (1984), however, found no evidence that prolactin was involved in the maintenance or termination of the parental feeding of the young in this species. Studies of free-living species such as the semipalmated sandpiper (*Calidris pusilla;* Gratto-Trevor et al., 1990) and the pied flycatcher (*Ficedula hypoleuca;* Silverin and Goldsmith, 1990) were both unable to find a relationship between plasma prolactin levels and the decline in brooding. Although further study is necessary, it is possible that the termination of parental care, unlike its onset, is mediated primarily by nonhormonal factors, as has been argued to be the case in certain mammalian species (e.g., Reisbick et al., 1975).

4. Hormonal Basis of Parental Care in Brood Parasites and Polyandrous Species

Field endocrinologic investigations have been conducted on two groups that might be considered behavioral exceptions to the generic avian pattern. These are the brood parasitic brown-headed cowbirds (*Molothrus ater*) and the sex-role-reversed polyandrous species such as the spotted sandpiper (*Actitis macularia*), Wilson's phalarope (*Phalaropus tricolor*), and the red-necked phalarope (*Phalaropus lobatus*). These studies are mentioned briefly here (see also Wingfield and Silverin, Chap. 31 in this volume). Studies of both these groups of birds have failed to reveal the major endocrine deviations that we might expect. Cowbirds possess a sex-steroid-hormone profile and a pattern of gonadotropin secretion over the course of the breeding cycle not unlike nesting species (Dufty and Wingfield, 1986). These brood parasites are essentially locked into the sexual phase of the nesting cycle and their endocrine profiles reflect this. However, they do show a seasonal pattern in prolactin secretion that is reminiscent of nesting species (Dufty et al., 1986). Similarly field endocrinologic investigations of the sex-role-reversed species did not reveal a major reversal in the pattern of the gonadotropins or the gonadal steroids (Fivizzani et al., 1986; Fivizzani and Oring, 1986; Oring et al., 1986b). The pattern of prolactin secretion in these species was also not anomalous. Although plasma levels of prolactin are higher in males than in females during the incubation and brooding periods, this is to be expected because males, depending on the species, engage in either all or most of the incubation and brooding (Oring et al., 1986a,b; Gratto-Trevor et al., 1990). Thus, major changes in the reproductive behavior of a species do not appear to be accompanied by a radical reorganization of endocrine secretions. The physiological factors influencing these behavioral differences should be sought in the neural sites that the hormones act on to activate behavior.

5. Studies of the Neural Basis of Parental Care in Birds

The neural regulation of parental care in avian species has not been extensively investigated. Studies of the localization of prolactin receptors in a variety of species have been helpful in localizing possible sites where prolactin might act to facilitate the onset of incubation behavior (Buntin, 1996). Not surprisingly, given its importance in maternal behavior in mammalian species (Numan, 1994), the preoptic region has emerged as a critical site for prolactin's action in relation to avian parental care based on these binding studies (Buntin, 1996). Lesions to the preoptic region in ring doves specifically disrupt prolactin-induced parental feeding but spares prolactin-induced hyperphagia (Slawski and Buntin, 1995). In accord with this finding is the fact that expression of the IEG, c-*fos* is enhanced in the preoptic region of doves in association with 2 weeks of incubation behavior (Sharp *et al.*, 1996). In Wilson's phalarope, a sex-role-reversed species, prolactin binding does not differ qualitatively between the males who incubate and the females who do not, but there is an up-regulation of prolactin receptors in the POA in incubating males, further implicating this brain region in the regulation of incubation behavior. However, many questions concerning the neuroendocrine basis of sex and species diversity of parental care patterns in birds remain.

VI. CONCLUSION

In this chapter we have documented in some detail the neuroendocrine regulation of reproduction and reproductive cycles in avian species. Studies in birds have provided an excellent illustration of many important concepts in the field of behavioral and environmental endocrinology. These studies have been especially valuable in elucidating the regulation of breeding cycles by photoperiod and other environmental variables. Work in avian species has also shown how social interactions can have profound effects on neuroendocrine physiology. Because we know a large amount about the natural history of avian species, mechanistic studies concerning the neuroendocrine integration of environmental stimuli can be readily related to the ecological context in which such interactions between neuroendocrine physiology and various stimuli in the environment normally occur. Many species-typical avian reproductive behaviors have been described in detail and the neural circuit regulating these behaviors has been reasonably well studied in several cases. This combination of a good description of the behavior with the knowledge of the neural sites involved in regulating the behavior has provided neuroendocrinologists with excellent opportunities to study how hormones, especially steroid hormones, regulate neural circuits that activate reproductive behaviors. Studies of steroid hormone action in defined neural circuits has allowed for a link between investigations at the cellular level of analysis and behavioral activation by steroid hormones. One notable result of avian studies has been the ability to anatomically localize steroid-metabolizing enzymes and study the physiology of the enzyme systems in relation to the presence of sex-steroid-hormone receptors in defined neural circuits. Avian studies have been particularly helpful for the investigation of the enzyme aromatase due to the fact that it is present in high concentrations in avian neural tissue and therefore can be more easily localized with immunocytochemical methods than is the case in mammalian species. Overall, such studies have also been helpful in clarifying cellular properties of the steroid-responsive neural substrate in the context of hormone action in relation to the activation of various behaviors.

Important questions remain at both the cellular and molecular levels of analysis and at the systems neuroscience level of analysis. At the cellular level, more needs to be learned about the consequences of steroid hormone action. What genes are regulated by steroids and how does this result in changes in behavior? The firm foundation we have based on avian studies should be very useful in guiding such investigations. At the systems level, questions remain about the neuroanatomical pathways that project from various sensory receptors to the neuroendocrine system. The way in which experience during ontogeny and context in adulthood influence the ability of these pathways to regulate the neuroendocrine system is also an important question for future research. It is our hope that this chapter will inspire a new generation of researchers to take advantage of avian species in the pursuit of such investigations.

References

Abe-Dohmae, S., Tanaka, R., and Harada, N. (1994). Cell type- and region-specific expression of aromatase mRNA in cultured brain cells. *Mol. Brain Res.* **24**, 153–158.

Abe-Dohmae, S., Takagi, Y., and Harada, N. (1996). Neurotransmitter-mediated regulation of brain aromatase: Protein kinase C- and G-dependent induction. *J. Neurochem.* **67**, 2087–2095.

Abe-Dohmae, S., Takagi, Y., and Harada, N. (1997). Autonomous expression of aromatase during development of mouse brain is modulated by neurotransmitters. *J. Steroid Biochem. Mol. Biol.* **61**, 299–306.

Absil, P., Das, S., and Balthazart, J. (1994). Effects of apomorphine on sexual behavior in male quail. *Pharmacol., Biochem. Behav.* **47**, 77–88.

Absil, P., Riters, L. V., and Balthazart, J. (2001). Preoptic aromatase cells project to the mesencephalic central gray in the male Japanese quail (*Coturnix japonica*). *Horm. Behav.* (**submitted** for publication).

Acher, R., Chauvet, J., and Chauvet, M. T. (1970). Phylogeny of the neurohypophysial hormones. The avian active peptides. *Eur. J. Biochem.* **17**, 509–513.

Acher, R., Chauvet, J., Chauvet, M. T., and Hurpet, D. (1985). Evolution of neurohypophysial hormones and their precursors. In "Current Trends in Comparative Endocrinology" (B. Lofts and W. N. Holmes, eds.), pp. 1147–1152. Hong Kong University Press, Hong Kong.

Adkins, E. K. (1973). Functional castration of the female japanese quail. *Physiol. Behav.* **10**, 619–621.

Adkins, E. K. (1975). Hormonal basis of sexual differentiation in the Japanese quail. *J. Comp. Physiol. Psychol.* **89**, 61–71.

Adkins, E. K. (1976). Embryonic exposure to an antiestrogen masculinizes behavior of female quail. *Physiol. Behav.* **17**, 357–359.

Adkins, E. K. (1977). Effects of diverse androgens on the sexual behavior and morphology of castrated male quail. *Horm. Behav.* **8**, 201–207.

Adkins, E. K. (1979). Effect of embryonic treatment with estradiol or testosterone on sexual differentiation of the quail brain. *Neuroendocrinology* **29**, 178–185.

Adkins, E. K., and Adler, N. T. (1972). Hormonal control of behavior in the Japanese quail. *J. Comp. Physiol. Psychol.* **81**, 27–36.

Adkins, E. K., and Nock, B. L. (1976a). The effects of the antiestrogen CI-628 on sexual behavior activated by androgen and estrogen in quail. *Horm. Behav.* **7**, 417–429.

Adkins, E. K., and Nock, B. L. (1976b). Behavioral responses to sex steroids of gonadectomized and sexually regressed quail. *J. Endocrinol.* **68**, 49–55.

Adkins, E. K., and Pniewski, E. E. (1978). Control of reproductive behavior by sex steroids in male quail. *J. Comp. Physiol. Psychol.* **92**, 1169–1178.

Adkins, E. K., Boop, J. J., Koutnik, D. L., Morris, J. B., and Pniewski, E. E. (1980). Further evidence that androgen aromatization is essential for the activation of copulation in male quail. *Physiol. Behav.* **24**, 441–446.

Adkins-Regan, E. (1981). Effect of sex steroids on the reproductive behavior of castrated male ring doves (*Streptopelia* sp.). *Physiol. Behav.* **26**, 561–565.

Adkins-Regan, E. (1983). Sex steroids and the differentiation and activation of avian reproductive behavior. In "Hormones and Behavior in Higher Vertebrates" (J. Balthazart and R. Gilles, eds.), pp. 219–228. Springer-Verlag, Berlin.

Adkins-Regan, E. K., Pickett, P., and Koutnik, D. (1982). Sexual differentiation in quail: Conversion of androgen to estrogen mediates testosterone-induced demasculinization of copulation but not other male characteristics. *Horm. Behav.* **16**, 259–278.

Albert, K. A., Helmer-Matyjek, E., Nairn, A. A., Müller, T. H., Haycock, J. W., Greene, L. A., Goldstein, M., and Greengard, P. (1984). Calcium/phospholipid-dependent protein kinase (protein kinase C) phosphorylates and activates tyrosine hydroxylase. *Proc. Natl. Acad. Sci. U.S.A.* **81**, 7713–7717.

Alderson, L. M., and Baum, M. J. (1981). Differential effects of gonadal steroids on dopamine mesolimbic and nigrostriatal pathways of the male rat brain. *Brain Res.* **218**, 189–206.

Alexandre, C., and Balthazart, J. (1986). Effects of metabolism inhibitors, antiestrogens and antiandrogens on the androgen and estrogen induced sexual behavior in Japanese quail. *Physiol. Behav.* **38**, 581–591.

Allee, W. C., and Collias, N. (1940). The influence of estradiol on the social organization of flocks of hens. *Endocrinology (Baltimore)* **27**, 87–94.

Almadhidi, J., Moslemi, S., Drosdowsky, M. A., and Séralini, G. E. (1996). Equine cytochrome P450 aromatase exhibits an estrogen 2-hydroxylase activity *in vitro*. *J. Steroid Biochem. Mol. Biol.* **59**, 55–61.

Amarneh, B. A., and Simpson, E. R. (1996). Detection of aromatase cytochrome P450, 17α-hydroxylase cytochrome P450 and NADPH:P450 reductase on the surface of cells in which they are expressed. *Mol. Cell. Endocrinol.* **119**, 69–74.

Ames, M. M., Lerner, P., and Lovenberg, W. (1978). Tyrosine hydroxylase: Activation by protein phosphorylation and end product inhibition. *J. Biol. Chem.* **253**, 27–31.

Amoss, M. R., Burges, R., Blackwell, R., Vale, W., Fellows, R., and Guillemin, R. (1971). Purification, amino acid composition and N-terminus of the hypothalamic luteinizing hormone releasing hormone factor (LRF) of ovine origin. *Biochem. Biophys. Res. Commun.* **44**, 205–210.

Andersson, M. (1994). "Sexual Selection." Princeton University Press, Princeton, NJ.

Andrew, R. (1975). Effects of testosterone on the behaviour of the domestic chick. I. Effects present in males but not in females. *Anim. Behav.* **23**, 139–155.

Andrew, R. J. (1972a). Changes in search behaviour in male and female chicks, following different doses of testosterone. *Anim. Behav.* **20**, 741–750.

Andrew, R. J. (1972b). Recognition processes and behaviour, with special reference to effects of testosterone on persistence. *Adv. Study Behav.* **4**, 175–208.

Andrew, R. J. (1975). Midbrain mechanisms of calling and their relation to emotional states. *In* "Neural and Endocrine Aspects of Behavior in Birds" (P. Wright, P. G. Caryl, and D. M. Vowles, eds.), pp. 275–304. Elsevier, Amsterdam.

Andrew, R. J., and de Lanerolle, N. (1975). The effects of muting lesions on emotional behavior and behavior normally associated with calling. *Brain, Behav. Evol.* **10**, 377–399.

Andrew, R. J., and Jones, R. B. (1992). Increased distractability in capons: An adult parallel to androgen-induced effects in the domestic chick. *Behav. Processes* **26**, 201–210.

Aosaki, T., Graybiel, A. M., and Kimura, M. (1994). Effect of the nigrostriatal dopamine system on acquired neural responses in the striatum of behaving monkey. *Science* **265**, 412–414.

Appeltants, D., Absil, P., Balthazart, J., and Ball, G. F. (2000a). Identification of the origin of catecholaminergic inputs to HVc in canaries by retrograde tract tracing combined with tyrosine hydroxylase immunocytochemistry. *J. Chem. Neuroanat.* **18**, 117–133.

Armitage, S. E., and Seller, T. J. (1981). Midbrain regions involved in call production of Japanese quail. *Experientia* **37**, 847–848.

Armstrong, E. G. (1947). "Courtship and Display Amongst Birds." Linsay Drummond, London.

Arnold, A. P. (1979). Hormone accumulation in the brain of the zebra finch after injection of various steroids and steroid competitors. *Soc. Neurosci. Abstr.* **5**, 437.

Arnold, A. P., and Gorski, R. A. (1984). Gonadal steroid induction of structural sex differences in the central nervous system. *Annu. Rev. Neurosci.* **7**, 413–442.

Arnold, A. P., and Saltiel, A. (1979). Sexual difference in pattern of hormone accumulation in the brain of a song bird. *Science* **205**, 702–705.

Arnold, A. P., Nottebohm, F., and Pfaff, D. W. (1976). Hormone concentrating cells in vocal control areas of the brain of the zebra finch (*Poephila guttata*). *J. Comp. Neurol.* **165**, 487–512.

Ascher, P., and Nowak, L. (1988). The role of divalent cations in the N-methyl-D-aspartate responses of mouse central neurones in culture. *J. Physiol. (London)* **399**, 247–266.

Askew, J. A., Georgiou, G. C., Sharp, P. J., and Lea, R. W. (1997). Localization of progesterone receptor in brain and pituitary of the ring dove: Influence of breeding cycle and estrogen. *Horm. Behav.* **32**, 105–113.

Aste, N., Panzica, G. C., Viglietti-Panzica, C., and Balthazart, J. (1991). Effects of in ovo estradiol benzoate treatments on sexual behavior and size of neurons in the sexually dimorphic medial preoptic nucleus of Japanese quail. *Brain Res. Bull.* **27**, 713–720.

Aste, N., Panzica, G. C., Viglietti-Panzica, C., Absil, P., Balthazart, J., Mühlbauer, E., and Grossman, R. (1995). The vasotocin system of the nucleus of the stria terminalis in the Japanese quail. *Soc. Neurosci. Abstr.* **21**, 357.

Aste, N., Viglietti-Panzica, C., Balthazart, J., and Panzica, G. C. (1997). Testosterone modulation of peptidergic pathways in the septo-preoptic region of male Japanese quail. *Poul. Avian Biol. Rev.* **8**, 77–93.

Aste, N., Balthazart, J., Absil, P., Grossmann, R., Mülhbauer, E., Viglietti-Panzica, C., and Panzica, G. C. (1998a). Anatomical and neurochemical definition of the nucleus of the stria terminalis in Japanese quail (*Coturnix japonica*). *J. Comp. Neurol.* **396**, 141–157.

Aste, N., Panzica, G. C., Viglietti-Panzica, C., Harada, N., and Balthazart, J. (1998b). Distribution and effects of testosterone on aromatase mRNA in the quail forebrain: A non-radioactive in situ hybridization study. *J. Chem. Neuroanat.* **14**, 103–115.

Aston-Jones, G., Rajkowski, J., and Cohen, J. (1999). Role of locus coeruleus in attention and behavioral flexibility. *Biol. Psychiatry* **46**, 1309–1320.

Baerends, G. P. (1988). Ethology. *In* "Steven's Handbook of Experimental Psychology" (R. C. Atkinson, R. J. Herrnstein, G. Lindzey, and R. D. Luce, eds.), 2nd ed., Vol. 1, pp. 765–830. Wiley, New York.

Bailhache, T., and Balthazart, J. (1993). The catecholaminergic system of the quail brain: Immunocytochemical studies of dopamine b-hydroxylase and tyrosine hydroxylase. *J. Comp. Neurol.* **329**, 230–256.

Bailhache, T., Foidart, A., Surlemont, C., Harada, N., and Balthazart, J. (1991). Catecholaminergic innervation of aromatase and estrogen receptor-immunoreactive cells in the quail brain. *Soc. Neurosci. Abstr.* **17**, 269.

Baillien, M., and Balthazart, J. (1997). A direct dopaminergic control of aromatase activity in the quail preoptic area. *J. Steroid Biochem. Mol. Biol.* **63**, 99–113.

Baillien, M., and Balthazart, J. (2000). A rapid dopaminergic control of aromatase activity in quail POA-hypothalamic explants. *Abstr. 7th Int. Symp. Avian Endocrinol.*, Abstr. No. 11.06.

Baker, J. R. (1938). The evolution of breeding seasons. *In* "Evolution: Essays on Aspects of Evolutionary Biology" (G. B. DeBeer, ed.), pp. 161–177. Clarendon Press, Oxford.

Bakker, J., and Baum, M. J. (2000). Neuroendocrine regulation of GnRH release in induced ovulators. *Front. Neuroendocrinol.* **21**, 220–262.

Ball, G. F. (1990). Chemical neuroanatomical studies of the steroid-sensitive songbird vocal control system: A comparative approach. *In* "Hormones, Brain and Behavior in Vertebrates" (J. Balthazart, ed.), Vol. 1, pp. 148–167. Comp. Physiol Vol. 8, Karger, Basel.

Ball, G. F. (1993). The neural integration of environmental information by seasonally breeding birds. *Am. Zool.* **33**, 185–199.

Ball, G. F. (1994). Neurochemical specializations associated with vocal learning and production in songbirds and budgerigars. *Brain, Behav. Evol.* **44**, 234–246.

Ball, G. F., and Bentley, G. E. (2000). Neuroendocrine mechanisms mediating the photoperiodic and social regulation of seasonal reproduction in birds. *In* "Reproduction in Context" (K. Wallen and J. Schneider, eds.), pp. 129–158. MIT Press, Cambridge MA.

Ball, G. F., and Hahn, T. P. (1997). GnRH neuronal ststems in birds and their relation to the control of seasonal reproduction. *In* "GnRH Neurons. Gen to Behavior" (I. S. Parhar and Y. Sakuma, eds.), pp. 325–342. Brain Shuppan, Tokyo.

Ball, G. F., and Wingfield, J. C. (1987). Changes in plasma levels of luteinizing hormone and sex steroid hormones in relation to multiple-broodedness and nest-site density in male starlings. *Physiol. Zool.* **60**, 191–199.

Ball, G. F., Nock, B., McEwen, B. S., and Balthazart, J. (1989). Distribution of α_2-adrenergic receptors in the brain of the Japanese quail as determined by quantitative autoradiography: Implications for the control of sexually dimorphic reproductive processes. *Brain Res.* **491**, 68–79.

Ball, G. F., Juss, T. S., and Parry, D. M. (1992). Immunohistochemical localization of cGnRH I and cGnRH II in the brains of photosensitive and photorefractory European starlings and Japanese quail. *Soc. Neurosci. Abstr.* **18**, 117.

Ball, G. F., Besmer, H. R., Hahn, T. P., Proudman, J. A., Ottinger, M. A., and McCarthy, M. M. (1995). Localization of cGnRH-I and PRE-PRO-GnRH-I mRNA in laying and refractory turkey hens. *Soc. Neurosci. Abstr.* **21**, 100.

Ball, G. F., Tlemçani, O., and Balthazart, J. (1997). Induction of the Zenk protein after sexual interactions in male Japanese quail. *NeuroReport* **8**, 2965–2970.

Ball, G. F., Bernard, D. J., Foidart, A., Lakaye, B., and Balthazart, J. (1999). Steroid sensitive sites in the avian brain: Does the distribution of the estrogen receptor a and b types provide insight into their function? *Brain, Behav. Evol.* **54**, 28–40.

Balthazart, J. (1983). Hormonal correlates of behavior. *Avian Biol.* **7**, 221–365.

Balthazart, J. (1989). Steroid metabolism and the activation of social behavior. *Adv. Comp. Environ. Physiol.* **3**, 105–159.

Balthazart, J., and Absil, P. (1997). Identification of catecholaminergic inputs to and outputs from aromatase-containing brain areas of the Japanese quail by tract tracing combined with tyrosine hydroxylase immunocytochemistry. *J. Comp. Neurol.* **382**, 401–428.

Balthazart, J., and Ball, G. F. (1989). Effects of the noradrenergic neurotoxin DSP-4 on luteinizing hormone levels, catecholamine concentrations, a_2-adrenergic receptor binding, and aromatase activity in the brain of the Japanese quail. *Brain Res.* **492**, 163–175.

Balthazart, J., and Ball, G. F. (1992). Is dopamine interacting with aromatase to control sexual behavior in male quail? *Poult. Sci. Rev.* **4**, 217–233.

Balthazart, J., and Ball, G. F. (1997). Neuroendocrine regulation of appetitive and consummatory aspects of male sexual behavior in Japanese quail. *In* "Perspectives in Avian Endocrinology" (R. Etches and S. Harvey, eds.), pp. 241–255. Society for Endocrinology, Bristol, UK.

Balthazart, J., and Ball, G. F. (1998a). New insights into the regulation and function of brain estrogen synthase (aromatase). *Trends Neurosci.* **21**, 243–249.

Balthazart, J., and Ball, G. F. (1998b). The Japanese quail as a model system for the investigation of steroid-catecholamine interactions mediating appetitive and consumatory aspects of male sexual behavior. *Annu. Rev. Sex Res.* **9**, 96–176.

Balthazart, J., and Ball, G. F. (2000). Fast regulation of steroid biosynthesis: A further piece in the neurosteroid puzzle. *Trends Neurosci.* **23**, 57–58.

Balthazart, J., and Deviche, P. (1977). Effect of exogenous hormones on the reproductive behavior of adult male domestic ducks. I. Behavioral effects of intramuscular injections. *Behav. Processes* **2**, 129–146.

Balthazart, J., and Foidart, A. (1993a). Neural bases of behavioral sex differences in quail. *In* "The Development of Sex Differences and Similarities in Behavior" (M. Haug, R. E. Whalen, C. Aron, and K. L. Olsen, eds.), pp. 51–75. Kluwer Academic Publishers, Dordrecht, The Netherlands.

Balthazart, J., and Foidart, A. (1993b). Brain aromatase and the control of male sexual behavior. *J. Steroid Biochem. Mol. Biol.* **44**, 521–540.

Balthazart, J., and Hendrick, J. C. (1978). Steroidal control of plasma luteinizing hormone, comb growth and sexual behavior in male chicks. *J. Endocrinol.* **77**, 149–150.

Balthazart, J., and Hendrick, J. C. (1979). Effects of exogenous gonadotropic and steroid hormones on the social behavior and gonadal maturation of male domestic ducks. *Arch. Int. Physiol. Biochem.* **87**, 741–761.

Balthazart, J., and Hirschberg, D. (1979). Testosterone metabolism and sexual behavior in the chick. *Horm. Behav.* **12**, 253–263.

Balthazart, J., and Hirschberg, D. (1982). Effects of several androgens on testosterone metabolism in the brain and crest of male chicks. *IRCS Med. Sci.* **10**, 377–378.

Balthazart, J., and Ottinger, M. A. (1984). 5β-reductase activity in the brain and cloacal gland of male and female embryos of the Japanese quail (*Coturnix coturnix japonica*). *J. Endocrinol.* **102**, 77–81.

Balthazart, J., and Schoffeniels, E. (1979). Pheromones are involved in the control of sexual behavior in birds. *Naturwissenschaften* **66**, 55–56.

Balthazart, J., and Schumacher, M. (1984a). Organization and activation of behavior in quail: Role of testosterone metabolism. *J. Exp. Zool.* **232**, 595–604.

Balthazart, J., and Schumacher, M. (1984b). Changes in testosterone metabolism by the brain and cloacal gland during sexual maturation in the Japanese quail. *J. Endocrinol.* **100**, 13–18.

Balthazart, J., and Schumacher, M. (1985). Role of testosterone metabolism in the activation of sexual behavior in birds. *In* "Neurobiology. Current Comparative Approaches" (R. Gilles and J. Balthazart, eds.), pp. 121–140. Springer-Verlag, Berlin.

Balthazart, J., and Surlemont, C. (1990a). Androgen and estrogen action in the preoptic area and activation of copulatory behavior in quail. *Physiol. Behav.* **48**, 599–609.

Balthazart, J., and Surlemont, C. (1990b). Copulatory behavior is controlled by the sexually dimorphic nucleus of the quail POA. *Brain Res. Bull.* **25**, 7–14.

Balthazart, J., Massa, R., and Negri-Cesi, P. (1979). Photoperiodic control of testosterone metabolism, plasma gonadotrophins, cloacal gland growth, and reproductive behavior in the Japanese quail. *Gen. Comp. Endocrinol.* **39**, 222–235.

Balthazart, J., Blaustein, J. D., Cheng, M. F., and Feder, H. H. (1980a). Hormones modulate the concentration of cytoplasmic progestin receptors in the brain of male doves (*Streptopelia risoria*). *J. Endocrinol.* **86**, 251–261.

Balthazart, J., Bottoni, L., and Massa, R. (1980b). Effects of sex steroids on testosterone metabolism, plasma gonadotropins, cloacal gland growth and reproductive behavior in Japanese quail. *Boll. Zool.* **47**, 185–192.

Balthazart, J., Willems, J., and Hendrick, J. C. (1980c). Changes in pituitary responsiveness to luteinizing hormone-releasing hormone during an annual cycle in the domestic duck, *Anas platyrhynchos* L. *J. Exp. Zool.* **211**, 113–123.

Balthazart, J., Malacarne, G., and Deviche, P. (1981). Stimulatory effects of 5β-dihydrotestosterone on the sexual behavior in the domestic chick. *Horm. Behav.* **15**, 246–258.

Balthazart, J., Schumacher, M., and Ottinger, M. A. (1983). Sexual differences in the Japanese quail: Behavior, morphology and intracellular metabolism of testosterone. *Gen. Comp. Endocrinol.* **51**, 191–207.

Balthazart, J., Schumacher, M., and Malacarne, G. (1984a). Relative potencies of testosterone and 5α-dihydrotestosterone on crowing and cloacal gland growth in the Japanese quail (*Coturnix coturnix japonica*). *J. Endocrinol.* **100**, 19–23.

Balthazart, J., Turek, R., and Ottinger, M. A. (1984b). Altered brain metabolism of testosterone is correlated with reproductive decline in aging quail. *Horm. Behav.* **18**, 330–345.

Balthazart, J., Schumacher, M., and Malacarne, G. (1985). Interaction of androgens and estrogens in the control of sexual behavior in male Japanese quail. *Physiol. Behav.* **35**, 157–166.

Balthazart, J., Devos, F., Dohet, A., Foidart, A., Hugla, J. L., Radermaker, F., and Schumacher, M. (1986a). The induction of aromatase and sexual behavior by testosterone in male and female Japanese quail: A dose-response study. *IRCS Med. Sci.* **14**, 1188–1189.

Balthazart, J., Schumacher, M., and Pröve, E. (1986b). Brain testosterone metabolism during ontogeny in the Zebra finch. *Brain. Res.* **378**, 240–256.

Balthazart, J., Libioulle, J. M., and Sante, P. (1988a). Stimulatory effects of the noradrenergic neurotoxin DSP4 on sexual behavior in male quail. *Behav. Processes* **17**, 27–44.

Balthazart, J., Verheyen, G., Schumacher, M., and Decuypere, E. (1988b). Changes in progesterone metabolism in the chicken hypothalamus during induced egg laying stop and molting. *Gen. Comp. Endocrinol.* **72**, 282–295.

Balthazart, J., Gahr, M., and Surlemont, C. (1989). Distribution of estrogen receptors in the brain of the Japanese quail: An immunocytochemical study. *Brain Res.* **501**, 205–214.

Balthazart, J., Evrard, L., and Surlemont, C. (1990a). Effects of the non-steroidal aromatase inhibitor, R76713 on testosterone-induced sexual behavior in the Japanese quail (*Coturnix coturnix japonica*). *Horm. Behav.* **24**, 510–531.

Balthazart, J., Foidart, A., and Harada, N. (1990b). Immunocytochemical localization of aromatase in the brain. *Brain Res.* **514**, 327–333.

Balthazart, J., Foidart, A., and Hendrick, J. C. (1990c). The induction by testosterone of aromatase activity in the preoptic area and activation of copulatory behavior. *Physiol. Behav.* **47**, 83–94.

Balthazart, J., Foidart, A., Surlemont, C., Harada, N., Leranth, C., and Naftolin, F. (1990d). Immunocytochemical localization of aromatase and estrogen receptors in the brain. *Soc. Neurosci. Abstr.* **16**, 1313.

Balthazart, J., Foidart, A., Surlemont, C., Vockel, A., and Harada, N. (1990e). Distribution of aromatase in the brain of the Japanese quail, ring dove, and zebra finch: An immunocytochemical study. *J. Comp. Neurol.* **301**, 276–288.

Balthazart, J., Schumacher, M., and Evrard, L. (1990f). Sex differences and steroid control of testosterone-metabolizing enzyme activity in the quail brain. *J. Neuroendocrinol.* **2**, 675–683.

Balthazart, J., Foidart, A., Surlemont, C., and Harada, N. (1991). Neuroanatomical specificity in the colocalization of aromatase and estrogen receptors. *J. Neurobiol.* **22**, 143–157.

Balthazart, J., De Clerck, A., and Foidart, A. (1992a). Behavioral demasculinization of female quail is induced by estrogens: Studies with the new aromatase inhibitor, R76713. *Horm. Behav.* **26**, 179–203.

Balthazart, J., Foidart, A., Sante, P., and Hendrick, J. C. (1992b). Effects of α-methyl-para-tyrosine on monoamine levels in the Japanese quail: Sex differences and testosterone effects. *Brain Res. Bull.* **28**, 275–288.

Balthazart, J., Foidart, A., Surlemont, C., Harada, N., and Naftolin, F. (1992c). Neuroanatomical specificity in the autoregulation of aromatase-immunoreactive neurons by androgens and estrogens: An immunocytochemical study. *Brain Res.* **574**, 280–290.

Balthazart, J., Foidart, A., Wilson, E. M., and Ball, G. F. (1992d). Immunocytochemical localization of androgen receptors in the male songbird and quail brain. *J. Comp. Neurol.* **317**, 407–420.

Balthazart, J., Surlemont, C., and Harada, N. (1992e). Aromatase as a cellular marker of testosterone action in the preoptic area. *Physiol. Behav.* **51**, 395–409.

Balthazart, J., Dupiereux, V., Aste, N., Viglietti-Panzica, C., Barrese, M., and Panzica, G. C. (1994a). Afferent and efferent connections of the sexually dimorphic medial preoptic nucleus of the male quail revealed by in vitro transport of DiI. *Cell Tissue Res.* **276**, 455–475.

Balthazart, J., Stoop, R., Foidart, A., Granneman, J. C. M., and Lambert, J. G. D. (1994b). Distribution and regulation of estrogen-2-hydroxylase in the quail brain. *Brain Res. Bull.* **35**, 339–345.

Balthazart, J., Stoop, R., Foidart, A., and Harada, N. (1994c). Synergistic control by androgens and estrogens of aromatase in the quail brain. *NeuroReport* **5**, 1729–1732.

Balthazart, J., Reid, J., Absil, P., Foidart, A., and Ball, G. F. (1995). Appetitive as well as consummatory aspects of male sexual behavior in quail are activated by androgens and estrogens. *Behav. Neurosci.* **109**, 485–501.

Balthazart, J., Absil, P., Foidart, A., Houbart, M., Harada, N., and Ball, G. F. (1996a). Distribution of aromatase-immunoreactive cells in the forebrain of zebra finches (*Taeniopygia guttata*): Implications for the neural action of steroids and nuclear definition in the avian hypothalamus. *J. Neurobiol.* **31**, 129–148.

Balthazart, J., Castagna, C., and Ball, G. F. (1996b). Differential effects of D1 and D2 dopamine receptor agonists and antagonists on appetitive and consummatory aspects of male sexual behavior in Japanese quail. *Soc. Neurosci. Abstr.* **22**, 158.

Balthazart, J., Foidart, A., Absil, P., and Harada, N. (1996c). Effects of testosterone and its metabolites on aromatase-immunoreactive cells in the quail brain: Relationship with the activation of male reproductive behavior. *J. Steroid Biochem. Mol. Biol.* **56**, 185–200.

Balthazart, J., Tlemçani, O., and Harada, N. (1996d). Localization of testosterone-sensitive and sexually dimorphic aromatase-immunoreactive cells in the quail preoptic area. *J. Chem. Neuroanat.* **11**, 147–171.

Balthazart, J., Absil, P., Baillien, M., and Ball, G. F. (1997a). Morphological and pharmacological evidence for a dopaminergic regulation of aromatase in the quail preoptic area. *Abstr. 1st Meet. Soc. Behav. Neuroendocrinol.*, p. 26, Baltimore, MD.

Balthazart, J., Absil, P., Viglietti-Panzica, C., and Panzica, G. C. (1997b). Vasotocinergic innervation of areas containing aromatase-immunoreactive cells in the quail forebrain. *J. Neurobiol.* **33**, 45–60.

Balthazart, J., Castagna, C., and Ball, G. F. (1997c). Aromatase inhibition blocks the activation and sexual differentiation of appetitive male sexual behavior in Japanese quail. *Behav. Neurosci.* **111**, 381–397.

Balthazart, J., Castagna, C., and Ball, G. F. (1997d). Differential effects of D1 and D2 dopamine-receptor agonists and antagonists on appetitive and consummatory aspects of male sexual behavior in Japanese quail. *Physiol. Behav.* **62**, 571–580.

Balthazart, J., Absil, P., Gérard, M., Appeltants, D., and Ball, G. F. (1998a). Appetitive and consummatory male sexual behavior in Japanese quail are differentially regulated by subregions of the preoptic medial nucleus. *J. Neurosci.* **18**, 6512–6527.

Balthazart, J., Foidart, A., Baillien, M., Harada, N., and Ball, G. F. (1998b). Anatomical relationships between aromatase and tyrosine hydroxylase in the quail brain: Double-label immunocytochemical studies. *J. Comp. Neurol.* **391**, 214–226.

Balthazart, J., Foidart, A., Houbart, M., Prins, G. S., and Ball, G. F. (1998c). Distribution of androgen receptor-immunoreactive cells in the quail forebrain and their relationship with aromatase immunoreactivity. *J. Neurobiol.* **35**, 323–340.

Balthazart, J., Baillien, M., and Ball, G. F. (2001a). Rapid and reversible inhibition of brain aromatase activity. *J. Neuroendocrinol.* **13**, 61–71.

Balthazart, J., Baillien, M., and Ball, G. F. (2002). Interactions between aromatase (estrogen synthase) and dopamine in the control of male sexual behavior in quail. *Comp. Biochem. Physiol.* (in press).

Baptista, L. F., and Petrinovich, L. (1986). Egg production in hand-raised White-crowned sparrows *Condor* **88**, 379–380.

Barclay, S. R., and Cheng, M.-F. (1985). The role of alpha adrenergic system in the male ring dove's courtship behavior. *Soc. Neurosci. Abstr.* **11**, 736.

Gibson, M. J., and Cheng, M.-F. (1979). Neural mediation of estrogen-dependent courtship behavior in female ring doves. *J. Comp. Physiol. Psychol.* **93**, 855–867.

Gietzen, D. W., Hope, W. G., and Woolley, D. E. (1983). Dopaminergic agonists increase [^{3}H]estradiol binding in hypothalamus of female rats, but not males. *Life Sci.* **33**, 2221–2228.

Gingrich, J. A., and Caron, M. G. (1993). Recent advances in the molecular biology of dopamine receptors. *Annu. Rev. Neurosci.* **16**, 299–321.

Godden, P. M., Luck, M. R., and Scanes, C. G. (1977). The effect of luteinizing hormone-releasing hormone and steroids on the release of LH and FSH from incubated turkey pituitary cells. *Acta Endocrinol. (Copenhagen)* **85**, 713–717.

Goldsmith, A. R. (1983). Prolactin in avian reproductive cycles. *In* "Hormones and Behaviour in Higher Vertebrates" (J. Balthazart, E. Pröve, and R. Gilles, eds.), pp. 375–387. Springer-Verlag, Berlin.

Goldsmith, A. R., and Follett, B. K. (1987). The termination of seasonal breeding in starlings: Is prolactin involved? *Endocr. Soc. Abst.* **890**, 243.

Goldsmith, A. R., Ivings, W. E., Pearce-Kelly, A. S., Parry, D. M., Plowman, G., Nicholls, T. J., and Follett, B. K. (1989). Photoperiodic control of the development of the LHRH neurosecretory system of European starlings (*Sturnus vulgaris*) during puberty and the onset of photorefractoriness. *J. Endocrinol.* **122**, 255–268.

Goodale, H. D. (1913). Castration in relation to secondary sexual characters in brown leghorns. *Am. Nat.* **47**, 159–169.

Goodson, J. L., and Adkins-Regan, E. (1997). Playback of crows of male Japanese quail elicits female phonotaxis. *Condor* **99**, 990–993.

Goodson, J. L., and Adkins-Regan, E. (1999). Effect of intraseptal vasotocin and vasoactive intestinal polypeptide infusions on courtship song and aggression in the male zebra finch (*Taeniopygia guttata*). *J. Neuroendocrinol.* **11**, 19–25.

Goodson, J. L., Greenwood, V. R., and Adkins-Regan, E. (1996). The central control of courtship and aggression in male zebra finches (*Taeniopygia guttata*): Effect of vasotocin infusions. *Soc. Neurosci. Abstr.* **22**, 2068.

Gorski, R. A. (1987). Sexual differentiation of the brain: Mechanisms and implications for neuroscience. *In* "From Message to Mind" (S. S. Easter, Jr., K. F. Barald, and B. M. Carlson, eds.), pp. 256–271. Sinauer Assoc., Sunderland, MA.

Gowaty, P. A. (1994). Architects of sperm competition. *Trends Ecol. Evol.* **9**, 160–161.

Gowaty, P. A. (1996). Battles of the sexes and the origins of monogamy. *In* "Partnerships in Birds" (J. L. Black, ed.), Oxford Ser. Ecol. Evol., pp. 21–52. Oxford University Press, Oxford.

Grant, L. D., and Stumpf, W. E. (1975). Hormone uptake sites in CNS biogenic amines systems. *In* "Anatomical Neuroendocrinology" (W. E. Stumpf and L. D. Grant, eds.), pp. 445–463. Karger, Basel.

Gratto-Trevor, C. L., Oring, L. W., Fivizzani, A. J., El Halawani, M. E., and Cooke, F. (1990). The role or prolactin in parental care in a monogamous and a polyandrous shorebird. *Auk* **107**, 718–729.

Gray, J. M., and Ziemian, L. (1992). Antiestrogen binding sites in brain and pituitary of ovariectomized rats. *Brain Res.* **578**, 55–60.

Gréco, B., Edwards, D. A., Michael, R. P., and Clancy, A. N. (1998). Androgen receptors and estrogen receptors are colocalized in male rat hypothalamic and limbic neurons that express Fos immunoreactivity induced by mating. *Neuroendocrinology* **67**, 18–28.

Gu, Q., Korach, K. S., and Moss, R. L. (1999). Rapid action of 17β-estradiol on kainate-induced currents in hippocampal neurons lacking intracellular estrogen receptors. *Endocrinology (Baltimore)* **140**, 660–666.

Guennoun, R., and Gasc, J.-M. (1990). Estrogen-independent and estrogen-induced progesterone receptors, and their regulation by progestins in the hypothalamus and pituitary of the chick embryo: An immunohistochemical study. *Dev. Brain Res.* **55**, 151–159.

Güntürkün, O. (1991). The functional organization of the avian visual system. *In* "Neural and Behavioural Plasticity" (R. J. Andrew, ed.), pp. 92–105. Oxford University Press, Oxford.

Güntürkün, O., Miceli, O., and Watanabe, M. (1993). Anatomy of the avian thalamofugal pathway. *In* "Vision, Brain and Behavior in Birds" (H. P. Zeigler and H. J. Bischof, eds.), pp. 115–135. MIT Press, Cambridge, MA.

Gustafsson, J. Å. (1999). Estrogen receptor β—a new dimension in estrogen mechanism of action. *J. Endocrinol.* **163**, 379–383.

Guyomarc'h, C., and Guyomarc'h, J. C. (1982). La stimulation du développement sexuel des femelles de caille japonaise, *Coturnix coturnix japonica*, par des chants de mâles: Mise en évidence de période privilégiées dans le nycthémère. *C. R. Seances Acad. Sci., Sér. 3* **295**, 37–40.

Guyomarc'h, C., Guyomarc'h, J. C., and Garnier, D. H. (1981). Influence de la perception de vocalisations de mâles sur la reproduction chez les femelles de *Coturnix coturnix japonica*. *Biol. Behav.* **6**, 167–182.

Gwinner, E. (1975). Die circannuale Periodik der Fortphlanzungsaktivität bein Star (*Sturnus vulgaris*) unter dem Einfluss gleich- un andersgeschlechtiger Artgenossen. *Z. Tierpsychol.* **38**, 34–43.

Gwinner, E. (1986). "Circannual Rhythms." Springer-Verlag, Berlin.

Gwinner, E. (1996). Circannual clocks in avian reproduction and migration. *Ibis* **138**, 47–63.

Gwinner, E., and Hau, M. (2000). The pineal gland, circadian rhythms and photoperiodism. *In* "Sturkies Avian Physiology" (G. C. Whittow, ed.), 5th ed., pp. 557–568. Academic Press, San Diego, CA.

Gwinner, E., and Scheuerlein, A. (1999). Photoperiodic responsiveness of equatorial and temperate-zone stonechats. *Condor* **101**, 347–359.

Hahn, T. P., and Ball, G. F. (1995). Changes in brain GnRH associated with photorefractoriness in house sparrows (*Passer domesticus*). *Gen. Comp. Endocrinol.* **99**, 349–363.

Hahn, T. P., Boswell, T., Wingfield, J. C., and Ball, G. F. (1997). Temporal flexibility in avian reproduction: Patterns and mechanisms. *In* "Current Ornithology" (V. Nolan, Jr., E. D. Ketterson, and C. F. Thompson, eds.), Vol. 14, pp. 39–80. Plenum Press, New York.

Hamner, W. M. (1963). Diurnal rhythms an dphotoperiodism in testicular recrudescence of the House Finch. *Science* **142**, 1294–1295.

Hamner, W. M. (1971). On seeking an alternative to the endobenous reproductive rhythm hypothesis in birds. *In* "Biochronometry" (M. Menaker, ed.) pp. 448–461. National Academy of Sciences, Washington, DC.

Hamner, W. M., and Enright, J. T. (1967). Relationships between photoperiodism and circadian rhythms of activity in the house finch. *J. Exp. Biol.* **46**, 211–227.

Harada, N. (1988). Cloning of a complete cDNA encoding human aromatase: Immunochemical identification and sequence analysis. *Biochem. Biophys. Res. Commun.* **156**, 725–732.

Harada, N., Yamada, K., Foidart, A., and Balthazart, J. (1992). Regulation of aromatase cytochrome P-450 (estrogen synthetase) transcripts in the quail brain by testosterone. *Mol. Brain Res.* **15**, 19–26.

Harada, N., Abe-Dohmae, S., Loeffen, R., Foidart, A., and Balthazart, J. (1993). Synergism between androgens and estrogens in the induction of aromatase and its messenger RNA in the brain. *Brain Res.* **622**, 243–256.

Harding, C. F., and Rowe, S. A. (1997). Vasotocin treatment inhibits courtship behavior in male zebra finches: Concomitant androgen treatment inhibits this effect. *Soc. Neurosci. Abstr.* **23**, 2135.

Harding, C. F., Sheridan, K., and Walters, M. J. (1983). Hormonal specificity and activation of sexual behavior in male zebra finches. *Horm. Behav.* **17**, 111–133.

Harding, C. F., Walters, M. J., and Parsons, B. (1984). Androgen receptor levels in hypothalamic and vocal control nuclei in the male zebra finch. *Brain Res.* **306**, 333–339.

Harding, C. F., Walters, M. J., Collado, D., and Sheridan, K. (1988). Hormonal specificity and activation of social behavior in male red-winged blackbirds. *Horm. Behav.* **22**, 402–418.

Harding, C. F., Barclay, S. R., and Waterman, S. A. (1998). Changes in catecholamine levels and turnover rates in hypothalamic, vocal control, and auditory nuclei in male zebra finches during development. *J. Neurobiol.* **34**, 329–346.

Hattori, A., Ishii, S., and Wada, M. (1986). Effects of two kinds of chicken luteinizing hormone-releasing hormone (LH-RH), mammalian LH-RH and its analogues on the release of LH and FSH in Japanese quail and chicken. *Gen. Comp. Endocrinol.* **64**, 446–455.

Hau, M., Wikelski, M., and Wingfield, J. C. (1998). A neotropical forest bird can measure the slight changes in tropical photoperiod. *Proc. R. Soc. London, Ser. B* **265**, 89–95.

Hau, M., Wikelski, M., and Wingfield, J. C. (2000). Visual and nutritional food cues fine-tune timing of reproduction in a neotropical rainforest bird. *J. Exp. Zool.* **286**, 494–504.

Hegner, R. E., and Wingfield, J. C. (1987). Effects of experimental manipulation of testosterone levels on parental investment and breeding success in male house sparrows. *Auk* **104**, 462–469.

Herbison, A. E. (1998). Multimodal influence of estrogen upon gonadotropin-releasing hormone neurons. *Endocr. Rev.* **19**, 302–330.

Herbison, A. E., and Theodosis, D. T. (1992). Localization of oestrogen receptors in preoptic neurons containing neurotensin but not tyrosine hydroxylase, cholecystokinin or luteinizing hormone-releasing hormone in the male and female rat. *Neuroscience* **50**, 283–298.

Herbison, A. E., Robinson, J. E., and Skinner, D. C. (1993). Distribution of estrogen receptor-immunoreactive cells in the preoptic area of the ewe: Co-localization with glutamic acid decarboxylase but not luteinizing hormone-releasing hormone. *Neuroendocrinology* **57**, 751–759.

Hessler, N. A., and Doupe, A. J. (1999a). Social context modulates singing-related neural activity in the songbird forebrain. *Nat. Neurosci.* **2**, 209–211.

Hessler, N. A., and Doupe, A. J. (1999b). Singing-related neural activity in a dorsal forebrain-basal ganglia circuit of adult zebra finches. *J. Neurosci.* **19**, 10461–10481.

Hiatt, E. S., Goldsmith, A. R., and Farner, D. S. (1987). Plasma levels of prolactin and gonadotropins during the reproductive cycle of white-crowned Sparrows (*Zonotrichia leucophrys*). *Auk* **104**, 208–217.

Hiemke, C., and Ghraf, R. (1984). Interaction of non-steroidal antiestrogens with dopamine receptor binding. *J. Steroid Biochem.* **21**, 663–667.

Hilliard, S., and Domjan, M. (1995). Effects on sexual conditionning of devaluating the US through satiation. *Q. J. Exp. Psychol.* **48B**, 84–92.

Hinde, R. A. (1953). Appetitive behavior, consummatory act, and the hierarchical organization of behaviour—with special reference to the great tit *(Parus major). Behaviour* **5**, 189–224.

Hinde, R. A. (1958). The nest building behavior of domesticated canaries. *Proc. Zool. Soc. London* **131**, 1–48.

Hinde, R. A. (1965). Interaction of internal and external factors in integration of canary reproduction. *In* "Sex and Behavior" (F. A. Beach, ed.), pp. 381–415. J Wiley, New York.

Hinde, R. A. (1970). "Animal Behavior," 2nd ed. McGraw-Hill, New York.

Hinde, R. A., and Steel, E. A. (1966). Integration of reproductive behavior in female canaries. *Symp. Soc. Exp. Biol.* **20**, 401–426.

Hinde, R. A., and Steel, E. A. (1978). The influence of daylength and male vocalizations on the estrogen-dependent behavior of female canaries and bugerigars, with discussion of data from other species. *Adv. Study Behav.* **8**, 39–73.

Hinde, R. A., Bell, R. Q., and Steel, E. (1963). Changes in sensitivity of the canary brood patch during the natural breeding cycle. *Anim. Behav.* **11**, 553–560.

Hochberg, Z., Bick, T., Pelman, R., Brandes, J. M., and Barzilai, D. (1986). The dual effect of calcium on aromatization by cultured human trophoblast. *J. Steroid Biochem.* **24**, 1217–1219.

Hoffman, G. E., Melnyk, V., Hayes, T., Bennett-Clarke, C., and Fowler, E. (1978). Immunocytology of LHRH neurons. *In* "Brain-endocrine Interactions. III. Neural Hormones and Reproduction" (D. E. Scott, G. P. Kozlowski, and A. Weindl, eds.), pp. 67–82. Karger, Basel.

Holberton, R. L., and Able, K. P. (1992). Persistence of circannual cycles in a migratory bird held in constant dim light. *J. Comp. Physiol. A* **171**, 477–481.

Hollmann, M., Hartley, M., and Heineman, S. (1991). Ca2+ permeability of KA-AMPA-gated glutamate receptor channels depends on subunit composition. *Nature (London)* **252**, 851–853.

Honda, S. I., Harada, N., and Takagi, Y. (1994). Novel exon 1 of the aromatase gene specific for aromatase transcripts in human brain. *Biochem. Biophys. Res. Commun.* **198**, 1153–1160.

Honda, S. I., Harada, N., and Takagi, Y. (1996). The alternative exons 1 of the mouse aromatase cytochrome *P*-450 gene. *Biochim. Biophys. Acta Gene. Struct. Expression* **1305**, 145–150.

Horn, G. (1985). "Memory, Imprinting, and the Brain." Clarendon Press, Oxford.

Hull, E. M. (1995). Dopaminergic influences on male rat sexual behavior. *In* "Neurobiological Effects of Sex Steroid Hormones" (P. E. Micevych and R. P. Hammer, Jr., eds.), pp. 234–253. Cambridge University Press, Cambridge, UK.

Hull, E. M., Du, J. F., Lorrain, D. S., and Matuszewich, L. (1995). Extracellular dopamine in the medial preoptic area: Implications for sexual motivation and hormonal control of copulation. *J. Neurosci.* **15**, 7465–7471.

Hull, E. M., Du, J. F., Lorrain, D. S., and Matuszewich, L. (1997). Testosterone, preoptic dopamine, and copulation in male rats. *Brain Res. Bull.* **44**, 327–333.

Hull, E. M., Lorrain, D. S., Du, J. F., Matuszewich, L., Lumley, L. A., Putnam, S. K., and Moses, J. (1999). Hormone-neurotransmitter interactions in the control of sexual behavior. *Behav. Brain Res.* **105**, 105–116.

Husmann, D. A., and McPhaul, M. J. (1991). Localization of the androgen receptor in the developing rat gubernaculum. *Endocrinology (Baltimore)* **128**, 383–387.

Husmann, D. A., Wilson, C. M., McPhaul, M. J., Tilley, W. D., and Wilson, J. D. (1990). Antipeptide antibodies to two distinct regions of the androgen receptor localize the receptor protein to the nuclei of target cells in the rat and human prostate. *Endocrinology (Baltimore)* **126**, 2359–2368.

Hutchison, J. B. (1970). Differential effects of testosterone and oestradiol on male courtship behavior in the Barbary dove *(Streptopelia risoria). Anim. Behav.* **18**, 41–51.

Hutchison, J. B. (1971). Effects of hypothalamic implants of gonadal steroids on courtship behavior in Barbary doves *(Streptopelia risoria). J. Endocrinol.* **50**, 97–113.

Hutchison, J. B. (1978). Hypothalamic regulation of male sexual responsiveness to androgen. *In* "Biological Determinants of Sexual Behavior" (J. B. Hutchison, ed.), pp. 277–319. J Wiley, Chichester.

Hutchison, J. B., and Hutchison, R. E. (1985). Phasic effects of hormones in the avian brain during behavioural development. *In* "Neurobiology. Current Comparative Approaches" (R. Gilles and J. Balthazart, eds.), pp. 105–120. Springer, Berlin.

Hutchison, J. B., and Schumacher, M. (1986). Development of testosterone-metabolizing pathways in the avian brain: Enzyme localization and characteristics. *Dev. Brain Res.* **25**, 33–42.

Hutchison, J. B., and Steimer, T. (1981). Brain 5β-reductase. A correlate of behavioral sensitivity to androgen. *Science* **213**, 244–246.

Hutchison, J. B., and Steimer, T. (1986). Formation of behaviorally effective 17β-estradiol in the dove brain: Steroid control of preoptic aromatase. *Endocrinology (Baltimore)* **118**, 2180–2187.

Hutchison, J. B., Steimer, T., and Hutchison, R. E. (1986). Formation of behaviorally active estrogen in the dove brain:

Induction of preoptic aromatase by intracranial testosterone. *Neuroendocrinology* **43**, 416–427.

Hutchison, J. B., Joris, S., Hutchison, R. E., and Steimer, T. (1989). Steroid control of sexual behavior and brain aromatase in the dove: Effects of nonaromatizable androgens, methyltrienolone (R1881), and 5α-dihydrotestosterone. *Horm. Behav.* **23**, 542–555.

Hutchison, R. E. (1978). Hormonal differentiation of sexual behavior in Japanese quail. *Horm. Behav.* **11**, 363–387.

Inaba, M., and Kamata, K. (1979). Effect of estradiol-17β and other steroids on noradrenaline and dopamine binding to synaptic membrane fragments of rat brain. *J. Steroid Biochem.* **11**, 1491–1497.

Irving, R. A., Mainwaring, W. I. P., and Spooner, P. M. (1976). The regulation of haemoglobin synthesis in cultured chick blastoderms by steroids related to 5β-androstane. *Biochem. J.* **154**, 81–93.

Jacob, J., Balthazart, J., and Schoffeniels, E. (1979). Sex differences in the chemical composition of uropygial gland waxes in domestic ducks. *Biochem. Syst. Ecol.* **7**, 149–153.

Jacobs, E. C., Arnold, A. P., and Campagnoni, A. T. (1996). Zebra finch estrogen receptor cDNA: Cloning and mRNA expression. *J. Steroid Biochem. Mol. Biol.* **59**, 135–145.

Jarvis, E. D., and Mello, C. V. (2000). Molecular mapping of brain areas involved in parrot vocal communication. *J. Comp. Neurol.* **419**, 1–31.

Jarvis, E. D., Schwabl, H., Ribeiro, S., and Mello, C. V. (1997). Brain gene regulation by territorial singing behavior in freely ranging songbirds. *NeuroReport* **8**, 2073–2077.

Jarvis, E. D., Scharff, C., Grossman, M. R., Ramos, J. A., and Nottebohm, F. (1998). For whom the bird sings: Context-dependent gene expression. *Neuron* **21**, 775–788.

Jarvis, E. D., Ribeiro, S., Da Silva, M. L., Ventura, D., Vielliard, J., and Mello, C. V. (2000). Behaviourally driven gene expression reveals song nuclei in hummingbird brain. *Nature (London)* **406**, 628–632.

Jin, H., and Clayton, D. F. (1997). Localized changes in immediate-early gene regulation during sensory and motor learning in zebra finches. *Neuron* **19**, 1049–1059.

Joëls, M. (1997). Steroid hormones and excitability in the mammalian brain. *Front. Neuroendocrinol.* **18**, 2–48.

Johnson, A. L. (2000). Reproduction in the female. In "Sturkie's Avian Physiology" (G. C. Whittow, ed.), pp. 569–596. Academic Press, San Diego, CA.

Johnson, A. L., and van Tienhoven, A. (1980). Plasma concentrations of six steroids and LH during the ovulatory cycle of the hen. *Biol. Reprod.* **23**, 386–393.

Johnson, F., Sablan, M. M., and Bottjer, S. W. (1995). Topographic organization of a forebrain pathway involved with vocal learning in zebra finches. *J. Comp. Neurol.* **358**, 260–278.

Jozsa, R., and Mess, B. (1982). Immunohistochemical localization of the luteinizing hormone releasing hormone (LHRH)-containing structures in the central nervous system of the domestic fowl. *Cell Tissue Res.* **227**, 451–458.

Jurkevich, A., Grossman, R., Rimeikene, R., and Köhler, A. (2000). Parallelism in sexual differentiation between the extrahypothalamic vasotocin system and male-typical behavior of chickens. *Trab. Inst. Cajal Invest. Biol.* **77**, 210–212.

Juss, T. S., and Goldsmith, A. R. (1992). Intracerebroventricular prolactin is potently gonado-inhibitory but does not induce photorefractoriness. *Abstr. Ser., 5th Int. Symp. Avian Endocrinol.*, Edinburgh, Scotland, Abstr. P88, p. 95.

Juss, T. S., Meddle, S. L., Servant, R. S., and King, V. M. (1993). Melatonin and photoperiodic time measurement in Japanese quail (*Coturnix coturnix japonica*). *Proc. R. Soc. London, Ser. B* **254**, 21–28.

Karavolas, H. J., Bertics, P. J., Hodges, D., and Rudie, N. (1984). Progesterone processing in neuroendocrine structures. In "Metabolism of Hormonal Steroids in the Neuroendocrine Structures" (L. Martini, ed.), Vol. 13, pp. 149–170. Raven Press, New York.

Katz, I. A., Millar, R. P., and King, J. A. (1990). Differential regional distribution and release of two forms of gonadotropin-releasing hormone in the chicken brain. *Peptides (N.Y.)* **11**, 443–450.

Kawashima, M., Kamiyoshi, M., and Tanaka, K. (1978). A cytoplasmic progesterone receptor in the hen pituitary and hypothalamic tissues. *Endocrinology (Baltimore)* **102**, 1207–1213.

Kawashima, M., Kamiyoshi, M., and Tanaka, K. (1979). Cytoplasmic progesterone receptor concentrations in the hen hypothalamus and pituitary: Difference between laying and nonlaying hens and chnages during the ovulatory cycle. *Biol. Reprod.* **20**, 581–585.

Kihlström, J. E., and Danninge, I. (1972). Neurohypophysial hormones and sexual behavior in males of the domestic fowl (*Gallus domesticus* L.) and the pigeon (*Columbia livia* Gmel). *Gen. Comp. Endocrinol.* **18**, 115–120.

Kim, Y. S., Stumpf, W. E., Sar, M., and Martinez-Vargas, M. C. (1978). Estrogen and androgen target cells in the brain of fishes, reptiles, and birds: Phylogeny and ontogeny. *Am. Zool.* **18**, 425–433.

Kinghammer, E., and Hess, E. H. (1964). Parental feeding in ring doves (*Streptopelia roseogrisea*): Innate or learned. *Z. Tierpsychol.* **21**, 338–347.

Kiss, J. Z., Voorhuis, T. A. M., van Eekelen, J. A. M., de Kloet, E. R., and de Wied, D. (1987). Organization of vasotocin-immunoreactive cells and fibers in the canary brain. *J. Comp. Neurol.* **263**, 347–364.

Klint, T. (1980). Influence of male nuptial plumage on mate selection in female mallard. *Anim. Behav.* **28**, 1230–1238.

Koenig, W. D., and Mumme, R. L. (1987). "Population Ecology of the Cooperatively Breeding Acorn Woodpecker." Princeton University Press, Princeton, NJ.

Koike, T. I., Shimada, K., and Cornett, L. E. (1988). Plasma levels of immunoreactive mesotocin and vasotocin during oviposition in chickens: Relationship to oxytocic action of the peptides in vitro and peptide interaction with myometrial membrane binding sites. *Gen. Comp. Endocrinol.* **70**, 119–126.

Komisaruk, B. R. (1967). Effects of local brain implants of progesterone on reproductive behavior in ring doves. *J. Comp. Physiol. Psychol.* **64**, 219–224.

Konishi, M. (1985). Birdsong: From behavior to neuron. *Annu. Rev. Neurosci.* **8**, 125–170.

Konishi, M., Emlen, S. T., Ricklefs, R. E., and Wingfield, J. C. (1989). Contributions of bird studies to biology. *Science* **246**, 465–472.

Koob, G. F. (1992). Drugs of abuse: Anatomy, pharmacology and function of reward pathways. *Trends Pharmacol. Sci.* **13**, 177–184.

Korenbrot, C. C., Schomberg, D. W., and Erickson, C. J. (1974). Radioimmunoassay of plasma estradiol during the breeding cycle of ring doves (*Streptopelia risoria*). *Endocrinology (Baltimore)* **94**, 1126–1132.

Korf, H. W., Panzica, G. C., Viglietti-Panzica, C., and Oksche, A. (1988). Pattern of peptidergic neurons in the avian brain: Clusters-local circuitries-projections. *Basic Appl. Histochem.* **32**, 55–75.

Krege, J. H., Hodgin, J. B., Couse, J. F., Enmark, E., Warner, M., Mahler, J. F., Sar, M., Korach, K. S., Gustafsson, J. A., and Smithies, O. (1998). Generation and reproductive phenotypes of mice lacking estrogen receptor b. *Proc. Natl. Acad. Sci. U.S.A.* **95**, 15 677–15 682.

Kreutzer, M. L., and Vallet, E. (1991). Differences in the responses of captive female canaries to variation in conspecific and heterospecific songs. *Behaviour* **117**, 106–116.

Kroodsma, D. E. (1976). Reproductive development in a female song bird: Differential stimulation by quality of male song. *Science* **192**, 574–575.

Kroodsma, D. E., and Byers, B. E. (1991). The function(s) of bird song. *Am. Zool.* **31**, 318–328.

Kuenzel, W. J., and Blähser, S. (1991). The distribution of gonadotropin-releasing hormone (GnRH) neurons and fibers throughout the chick brain (*Gallus domesticus*). *Cell Tissue Res.* **264**, 481–495.

Kuenzel, W. J., and Masson, M. (1988). "A Stereotaxic Atlas of the Brain of the Chick (*Gallus domesticus*)." Johns Hopkins University Press, Baltimore, MD.

Kuiper, G. G. J. M., Enmark, E., Pelto-Huikko, M., Nilsson, S., and Gustafsson, J.-Å. (1996). Cloning of a novel estrogen receptor expressed in rat prostate and ovary. *Proc. Natl. Acad. Sci. U.S.A.* **93**, 5925–5930.

Kuiper, G. G. J. M., Shughrue, P. J., Merchenthaler, I., and Gustafsson, J.-Å. (1998). The estrogen receptor b subtype: A novel mediator of estrogen action in neuroendocrine systems. *Front. Neuroendocrinol.* **19**, 253–286.

Lack, D. (1968). "Ecological Adaptations for Breeding in Birds." Methuen, London.

Lakaye, B., Foidart, A., Grisar, T., and Balthazart, J. (1998). Partial cloning and distribution of estrogen receptor beta in the avian brain. *NeuroReport* **9**, 2743–2748.

Larsson, K., Södersten, P., and Beyer, C. (1973). Sexual behavior of male rats treated with estrogen in combination with dihydrotestosterone. *Horm. Behav.* **4**, 289–299.

Lea, R. W. (1987). Prolactin and avian incubation: A comparison between Galliformes and Columbiformes. *Sitta* **1**, 117–141.

Lea, R. W., and Armstrong, D. G. (1986). Chnages in aromatase activity in the brain of the male ring dove (*Streptopelia risoria*) during the breeding cycle. *Comp. Biochem. Physiol.* **4**, 693–698.

Leboucher, G., Kreutzer, M., and Dittami, J. (1994). Copulation-solicitation displays in female canaries (*Serinus canaria*): Are oestradiol implants necessary? *Ethology* **97**, 190–197.

Leboucher, G., Depraz, V., Kreutzer, M., and Nagle, L. (1998a). Male song stimulation of female reproduction in canaries: Features relevant to sexual displays are not relevant to nest-building or egg-laying *Ethology* **104**, 613–624.

Leboucher, G., Béguin, N., Mauget, R., and Kreutzer, M. (1998b). Effects of fadrozole on sexual displays and reproductive activity in the female canary. *Physiol. Behav.* **65**, 233–240.

Leboucher, G., Béguin, N., Lacroix, A., and Kreutzer, M. (2000). Progesterone inhibits female courtship behavior in domestic canaries (*Serinus canaria*). *Horm. Behav.* **38**, 123–129.

Lehrman, D. S. (1959). Hormonal responses to external stimuli in birds. *Ibis* **101**, 478–495.

Lehrman, D. S. (1963). The reproductive behavior of ring doves. *Sci. Am.* **11**, 433–438.

Lehrman, D. S. (1965). Interaction between internal and external environments in the regulation of the reproductive cycle of the ring dove. In "Sex and Behavior" (F. A. Beach, ed.), pp. 355–380. J Wiley, New York.

Lehrman, D. S., and Friedman, M. (1969). Auditory stimulation of oavarian activity in the ring dove (*Streptopelia risoria*). *Anim. Behav.* **17**, 494–497.

Lehrman, D. S., Wortis, R. P., and Brody, P. (1961). The presence of the mate and of nesting material as stimuli for the development of incubation behavior and for gonadotropin secretion in the ring dove (*Streptopelia risoria*). *Endocrinology (Baltimore)* **68**, 507–516.

Leinhart, R. (1927). Contribution à l'étude de l'incubation. *C. R. Seances Soc. Biol. Ses. Fil.* **97**, 1296–1297.

Lephart, E. D. (1996). A review of brain aromatase cytochrome P450. *Brain. Res. Rev.* **22**, 1–26.

Lephart, E. D., Simpson, E. R., and Ojeda, S. R. (1992). Effects of cyclic AMP and androgens on *in vitro* brain aromatase enzyme activity during prenatal development in the rat. *J. Neuroendocrinol.* **4**, 29–35.

Leutgeb, S. (1995). Social preference in the Japanese quail (*Coturnix coturnix japonica*): Hormonal modulation. Thesis, University of Salzburg.

Levere, R. D., Kappas, A., and Granick, S. (1967). Stimulation of hemoglobin synthesis in chick blastoderm by certain 5β-androstane and 5α-pregnane steroids. *Proc. Natl. Acad. Sci. U.S.A.* **58**, 985–990.

Levin, R. N., and Wingfield, J. C. (1992). The hormonal control of territorial aggression in tropical birds. *Ornis Scand.* **23**, 284–291.

Lewis, J. W., Ryan, S. M., Arnold, A. P., and Butcher, L. L. (1981). Evidence for catecholamine projection to area X in the zebra finch. *J. Comp. Neurol.* **196**, 347–354.

Lieberburg, I., and Nottebohm, F. (1979). High-affinity androgen binding proteins in synrigeal tissues of songbirds. *Gen. Comp. Endocrinol.* **37**, 286–293.

Ligon, J. D. (1998). "The Evolution of Avian Breeding Systems." Oxford University Press, Oxford.

Lincoln, G. A., Racey, P. A., Sharp, P. J., and Klandorf, H. (1980). Endocrine changes associated with spring and autumn sexuality of the Rook, *Corvus frugilegus*. *J. Zool.* **190**, 137–153.

Lisk, R. D. (1962). Diencephalic placement of estradiol and sexual receptivity in the female rat. *Am. J. Physiol.* **203**, 493–496.

Lofts, B., and Murton, R. K. (1973). Reproduction in birds. *Avian Biol.* **3**, 1–107.

Lofts, B., Murton, R. K., and Westwood, N. J. (1966). Gonad cycles and the evolution of breeding seasons in British Columbidae *J. Zool.* **150**, 249–272.

Lorenz, K. (1950). The comparative method in studying innate behavior patterns. *Symp. Soc. Exp. Biol.* **4**, 221–268.

Lott, D. F., and Brody, P. N. (1966). Support of ovulation in the ring dove by auditory and visual stimuli. *J. Comp. Physiol. Psychol.* **62**, 311–313.

Lott, D. G., and Comerford, S. (1968). Hormonal initiation of parental behavior in inexperienced ring doves. *Z. Tierpsychol.* **25**, 71–75.

Lovari, S., and Hutchison, J. B. (1975). Behavioural transitions in the reproductive cycle of Barbary doves (*Streptopelia risoria*). *Behaviour* **53**, 126–150.

Lubahn, D. B., Joseph, D. R., Sar, M., Tan, J.-A., Higgs, H. N., Larson, R. E., French, F. S., and Wilson, E. M. (1988). The human androgen receptor: Complementary deoxyribonuclei acid cloning, sequence analysis and gene expressin in prostate. *Mol. Endocrinol.* **2**, 1265–1275.

Lücke, J., and Haase, E. (1980). Autoradiographische Untersuchungen am Gehirn von Bergfinken (*Fringilla montifringilla* L.) nach injektion von 3H-Testosteron. *J. Hirnforsch.* **21**, 369–380.

Luine, V., Nottebohm, F., Harding, C. F., and McEwen, B. S. (1980). Androgen affects cholinergic enzymes in syringeal motor neurons and muscles. *Brain Res.* **192**, 89–107.

MacDermott, A. B., Mayer, M. L., Westbrook, G. L., Smith, S. J., and Baker, J. L. (1986). NMDA-receptor activation increases cytoplasmic calcium concentration in cultured spinal cord neurones. *Nature (London)* **321**, 519–522.

MacLusky, N. J., Philip, A., Hurlburt, C., and Naftolin, F. (1984). Estrogen metabolism in neuroendocrine structures. *In* "Metabolism of Hormonal Steroids in the Neuroendocrine Structures" (F. Celotti, F. Naftolin, and L. Martini, eds.), pp. 103–116. Raven Press, New York.

Macnamee, M. C., Sharp, P. J., Lea, R. W., Sterling, R. J., and Harvey, S. (1986). Evidence that vasoactive intestinal polypeptide is a physiological prolactin-releasing factor in the bantam hen. *Gen. Comp. Endocrinol.* **62**, 470–478.

Maney, D. L., Goode, C. T., and Wingfield, J. C. (1997a). Intraventricular infusion of arginine vasotocin induces singing in a female songbird. *J. Neuroendocrinol.* **9**, 487–491.

Maney, D. L., Richardson, R. D., and Wingfield, J. C. (1997b). Central administration of chicken gonadotropin-releasing hormone-II enhances courtship behavior in a female sparrow. *Horm. Behav.* **32**, 11–18.

Maney, D. L., Schoech, S. J., and Wingfield, J. C. (1999). Environmental endocrinology and the timing of reproduction: Interaction of photoperiod and temperature. *Proc. 22nd Int. Ornithol. Congr.*, Durban.

Maney, D. L., Bernard, D. J., and Ball, G. F. (2001). Gonadal steroid receptor mRNA in catecholaminergic nuclei of the canary brainstem. *Neurosci. Lett.* **31**, 189–192.

Marivoet, S., Hertogen, M., Verhoeven, G., and Heyns, W. (1990). Antibodies against synthetic peptides recognize the human and rat androgen receptor. *J. Steroid Biochem.* **37**, 39–45.

Marler, P., Peters, S., Ball, G. F., Dufty, A. M., and Wingfield, J. C. (1988). The role of sex steroids in the acquisition and production of birdsong. *Nature (London)* **336**, 770–772.

Martinez-Vargas, M. C. (1974). Nest building in the ring dove (*Streptopelia risoria*): Hormonal and social factors. *Behaviour* **50**, 123–151.

Martinez-Vargas, M. C., and Erickson, C. J. (1973). Social and hormonal determinants of nest building in the ring dove (*Streptopelia risoria*). *Behaviour* **45**, 12–37.

Martinez-Vargas, M. C., Sar, M., and Stumpf, W. E. (1974). Brain targets for androgens in the dove (*Streptopelia risoria*). *Am. Zool.* **14**, 1285.

Martinez-Vargas, M. C., Stumpf, W. E., and Sar, M. (1975). Estrogen localization in the dove brain. Phylogenetic considerations and implications for nomenclature. *In* "Anatomical Neuroendocrinology," (W. E. Stumpf and P. P. Grant, eds.), pp. 166–175. Karger, Basel.

Martinez-Vargas, M. C., Stumpf, W. E., and Sar, M. (1976). Anatomical distribution of estrogen target cells in the avian CNS: A comparison with the mammalian CNS. *J. Comp. Neurol.* **167**, 83–104.

Martini, L. (1982). The 5α-reduction of testosterone in the neuroendocrine structures. Biochemical and physiological implications. *Endocr. Rev.* **3**, 1–25.

Martini, L., Celotti, F., Lechuga, M. J., Melcangi, R. C., Motta, M., Negri-Cesi, P., Poletti, A., and Zoppi, S. (1990). Androgen metabolism in different target tissues. *Ann. N.Y. Acad. Sci.* **595**, 184–198.

Mas, M., Fumero, B., and González-Mora, J. L. (1995a). Voltammetric and microdialysis monitoring of brain monoamine neurotransmitter release during sociosexual interactions. *Behav. Brain Res.* **71**, 69–79.

Mas, M., Fumero, B., Perez-Rodriguez, I., and González-Mora, J. L. (1995b). The neurochemistry of sexual satiety. An experimental model of inhibited desire. *In* "The Pharmacology of Sexual Function and Dysfunction" (J. Bancroft, ed.), pp. 115–131. Elsevier Science, Amsterdam.

Massa, R., and Sharp, P. J. (1981). Conversion of testosterone to 5β-reduced metabolites in the neuroendocrine tissues of the maturing cockerel. *J. Endocrinol.* **88**, 263–269.

Massa, R., Cresti, L., and Martini, L. (1977). Metabolism of testosterone in the anterior pituitary and in the central nervous system of the European starling. *J. Endocrinol.* **75**, 347–354.

Massa, R., Davies, D. T., and Bottoni, L. (1980). Cloacal gland of the Japanese quail: Androgen dependence and metabolism of testosterone. *J. Endocrinol.* **84**, 223–230.

Mauro, L. J., Youngren, O. M., Proudman, J. A., Phillips, R. E., and El Halawani, M. E. (1992). Effects of reproductive status, ovariectomy, and photoperiod on vasoactive intestinal peptide in the female turkey hypothalamus. *Gen. Comp. Endocrinol.* **87**, 481–493.

Mayr, E. (1963). "Animal Species and Evolution." Harvard University Press, Cambridge, MA.

McCracken, K. G. (2000). The 20-cm spiny penis of the Argentine lake Duck (*Oxyura vittata*). *Auk* **117**, 820–825.

McEwen, B. S. (1981). Neural gonadal steroid actions. *Science* **211**, 1303–1311.

McEwen, B. S. (1994). Steroid hormone actions on the brain: When is the genome involved? *Horm. Behav.* **28**, 396–405.

McEwen, B. S., and Alves, S. E. (1999). Estrogen actions in the central nervous system. *Endocr. Rev.* **20**, 279–307.

McEwen, B. S., and Krey, L. C. (1984). Properties of estrogen-sensitive neurons: Aromatization, progestin receptor induction and neuroendocrine effects. *In* "Metabolism of Hormonal Steroids in the Neuroendocrine Structures" (F. Celotti, F. Naftolin, and L. Martini, eds.), pp. 117–128. Raven Press, New York.

McEwen, B. S., and Pfaff, D. W. (1985). Hormone effects on hypothalamic neurons: Analyzing gene expression and neuromodulator action. *Trends Neurosci.* 105–110.

McEwen, B. S., Jones, K. J., and Pfaff, D. W. (1987). Hormonal control of sexual behavior in the female rat: Molecular, cellular and neurochemical studies. *Biol. Reprod.* **36**, 37–45.

McKinney, F. (1969). The behavior of ducks. *In* "The Behavior of Domestic Animals" (E. S. E. Hafez, ed.), pp. 593–626. Baillière, Tindall & Cassell, London.

McMillan, J. P., Underwood, H. A., Elliot, J. A., Stetson, M. H., and Menaker, M. (1975). Extra-retinal light perception. 4. Further evidence that eyes do not participate in photoperiodic photoreception. *J. Comp. Physiol. A* **97**, 205–214.

McNeil, T. H., Kozlowski, G. P., Abel, J. H., Jr., and Zimmerman, E. A. (1976). Neurosecretory pathways in the mallard duck (*Anas platyrhynchos*) brain: Localization by aldehyde fuchsin and immunoperoxidase techniques for neurophysin (NP) and gonadotropin releasing hormone (Gn-RH). *Endocrinology (Baltimore)* **99**, 1323–1332.

McPhaul, M. J., Noble, J. F., Simpson, E. R., Mendelson, C. R., and Wilson, J. D. (1988). The expression of a functional cDNA encoding the chicken cytochrome P-450$_{arom}$ (aromatase) that catalyzes the formation of estrogen from androgen. *J. Biol. Chem.* **263**, 16358–16363.

Means, G. D., Mahendroo, M. S., Corbin, C. J., Mathis, J. M., Powell, F. E., Mendelson, C. R., and Simpson, E. R. (1989). Structural analysis of the gene encoding human aromatase cytochrome P-450, the enzyme responsible for estrogen biosynthesis. *J. Biol. Chem.* **264**, 19385–19391.

Meddle, S. L., and Follett, B. K. (1995). Photoperiodic activation of *fos*-like immunoreactive protein in neurones within the tuberal hypothalamus of Japanese quail. *J. Comp. Physiol. A* **176**, 79–89.

Meddle, S. L., King, V. M., Follett, B. K., Wingfield, J. C., Ramenofsky, M., Foidart, A., and Balthazart, J. (1997). Copulation activates Fos-like immunoreactivity in the male quail forebrain. *Behav. Brain Res.* **85**, 143–159.

Meddle, S. L., Foidart, A., Wingfield, J. C., Ramenofsky, M., and Balthazart, J. (1999a). Effects of sexual interactions with a male on Fos-like immunoreactivity in the female quail brain. *J. Neuroendocrinol.* **11**, 771–784.

Meddle, S. L., Maney, D. L., and Wingfield, J. C. (1999b). Effects of N-methyl-D-aspartate on luteinizing hormone release and Fos-like immunoreactivity in the male white-crowned sparrow (*Zonotrichia leucophrys gambelii*). *Endocrinology (Baltimore)* **140**, 5922–5928.

Meijer, T., Dukstra, C. D., and Daan, S. (1988). Female condition and reproduction. Effects of food manipulation in free-living and captive kestrels. *Ardea* **76**, 141–154.

Meijer, T., Nienaber, U., Langer, U., and Trillmich, F. (1999). Temperature and timing of egg-laying of European starlings. *Condor* **101**, 124–132.

Meisel, R. L., and Sachs, B. D. (1994). The physiology of male sexual behavior. *In* "The Physiology of Reproduction" (E. Knobil and J. D. Neill, eds.), Vol. 2, pp. 3–105. Raven Press, New York.

Melcangi, R. C., Celotti, F., Ballabio, M., Castano, P., Massarelli, R., Poletti, A., and Martini, L. (1990). 5α-reductase activity in isolated and cultured neuronal and glial cells of the rat. *Brain Res.* **516**, 229–236.

Melcangi, R. C., Celotti, F., Castano, P., and Martini, L. (1993). Differential localization of the 5α-reductase and the 3α-hydroxysteroid dehydrogenase in neuronal and glial cultures. *Endocrinology (Baltimore)* **132**, 1252–1259.

Melcangi, R. C., Poletti, A., Cavarretta, I., Celotti, F., Colciago, A., Magnaghi, V., Motta, M., Negri-Cesi, P., and Martini, L. (1998). The 5α-reductase in the central nervous system: Expression and modes of control. *J. Steroid Biochem. Mol. Biol.* **65**, 295–299.

Melcangi, R. C., Magnaghi, V., and Martini, L. (1999). Steroid metabolism and effects in central and peripheral glial cells. *J. Neurobiol.* **40**, 471–483.

Mello, C., Vicario, D. S., and Clayton, D. F. (1992). Song presentation induces gene expression in the songbird forebrain. *Proc. Natl. Acad. Sci. U.S.A.* **89**, 6818–6822.

Mello, C., Nottebohm, F., and Clayton, D. (1995). Repeated exposure to one song leads to a rapid and persistent decline in an immediate early gene's response to that song in zebra pinch telencephalon. *J. Neurosci.* **15**, 6919–6925.

Mello, C. V., and Ribeiro, S. (1998). ZENK protein regulation by song in the brain of songbirds. *J. Comp. Neurol.* **393**, 426–438.

Mello, C. V., Pinaud, R., and Ribeiro, S. (1998). Noradrenergic system of the zebra finch brain: Immunocytochemical study of dopamine-b-hydroxylase. *J. Comp. Neurol.* **400**, 207–228.

Mendelson, C. R., Smith, M. E., Cleland, W. H., and Simpson, E. R. (1984). Regulation of aromatase activity of cultured adipose stromal cells by catecholamines and adrenocorticotropin. *Mol. Cell. Endocrinol.* **37**, 61–72.

Mermelstein, P. G., Becker, J. B., and Surmeier, D. J. (1996). Estradiol reduces calcium currents in rat neostriatal neurons via a membrane receptor. *J. Neurosci.* **16**, 595–604.

Metzdorf, R., Gahr, M., and Fusani, L. (1999). Distribution of aromatase, estrogen receptor, and androgen receptor mRNA in the forebrain of songbirds and nonsongbirds. *J. Comp. Neurol.* **407**, 115-129.

Meyer, C. C. (1973). Testosterone concentration in the male chick brain: An autoradiographic survey. *Science* **180**, 1381–1382.

Meyer, C. C., Parker, D. M., and Salzen, E. A. (1976). Androgen-sensitive midbrain sites and visual attention in chicks. *Nature (London)* **259**, 689–690.

Meyerson, B. J., Palis, A., and Sietniks, A. (1979). Hormone-monoamine interactions and sexual behavior. *In* "Endocrine Control of Sexual Behavior" (C. Beyer, ed.), pp. 389–405. Raven Press, New York.

Meyerson, B. J., Malmnäs, C. O., and Everitt, B. J. (1985). Neuropharmacology, neurotransmitters, and sexual behavior in mammals. *In* "Handbook of Behavioral Neurobiology" (N. Adler, D. Pfaff, and R. W. Goy, eds.), Vol. 7, pp. 495–536. Plenum Press, New York.

Michael, R. P., and Saayman, G. S. (1968). Differential effects on behavior of the subcutaneous and intravaginal administration of oestrogen in the rhesus monkey. *J. Endocrinol.* **41**, 231–246.

Mikami, S. (1986). Immunocytochemistry of the avian hypothalamus and adenohypophysis. *Int. Rev. Cytol.* **103**, 189–248.

Mikami, S., Yamada, S., Hasegawa, Y., and Miyamoto, K. (1988). Localization of avian LHRH-immunoreactive neurons in the hypothalamus of the domestic fowl, *Gallus domesticus* and the Japanese quail, *Coturnix coturnix*. *Cell Tissue Res.* **251**, 51–58.

Millam, J. R., Craig-Veit, C. B., Adams, T. E., and Adams, B. M. (1989). Avian gonadotropin-releasing hormones I and II in brain and other tissues in turkey hens. *Comp. Biochem. Physiol. A* **94A**, 771–776.

Millam, J. R., Faris, P. L., Youngren, O. M., El Halawani, M. E., and Hartman, B. K. (1993). Immunohistochemical localization of chicken gonadotropin-releasing hormones I and II (cGnRH I and II) in turkey hen brain. *J. Comp. Neurol.* **333**, 68–82.

Millar, R. P., and King, J. A. (1984). Structure-activity relations of LHRH in birds. *J. Exp. Zool.* **232**, 425–430.

Millar, R. P., del Milton, R. C., Follett, B. K., and King, J. A. (1986). Receptor binding and gonadotropin-releasing activity of a novel chicken gonadotropin-releasing hormone ([His5, Trp7, Tyr8]GnRH) and a D-Arg6 analog. *Endocrinology (Baltimore)* **119**, 224–231.

Miyamoto, K., Hasegawa, Y., Nomura, M., Igarashi, M., Kangawa, K., and Matsuo, H. (1984). Identification of the second gonadotropin-releasing hormone in chicken hypothalamus: Evidence that gonadotropin secretion is probably controlled by two distinct gonadotropin-releasing hormones in avian species. *Proc. Natl. Acad. Sci. U.S.A.* **81**, 3874–3878.

Moller, A. P., and Birkhead, T. R. (1993). Certainty of paternity covaries with paternal care in birds. *Behav. Ecol. Sociobiol.* **33**, 261–268.

Moore, F. L. (1992). Evolutionary precedents for behavioral actions of oxytocin and vasopressin. *Ann. N.Y. Acad. Sci.* **652**, 156–165.

Moore, M. (1982). Hormonal response of free-living male white-crowned sparrows to experimental manipulation of female sexual behavior. *Horm. Behav.* **16**, 323–329.

Moore, M. (1983). Effect of female sexual displays on the endocrine physiology and behavior of male white-crowned sparrows. *J. Zool.* **199**, 137–148.

Moore, R. Y. (1973). Retinohypothalamic projection in mammals: A comparative study. *Brain Res.* **49**, 403–409.

Morel, G., and Bourlière, F. (1956). Recherches écologiques sur les *Quelea quelea* (L.) de la basse vallée du Sénégal. II. La reproduction. *Alauda* **24**, 97–122.

Mori, K., and Striedter, G. (1992). Neurons in field L of budgerigars prefer species specific calls to white noise. *Soc. Neurosci. Abstr.* **18**, 527.

Mori, M., Suzuki, K., and Tamaoki, B.-I. (1974). Testosterone metabolism in rooster comb. *Biochim. Biophys. Acta* **337**, 118–128.

Morin, L. P., and Zucker, I. (1978). Photoperiodic regulation of copulatory behavior in the male hamster. *J. Endocrinol.* **77**, 249–258.

Morrell, J. I., Kelley, D. B., and Pfaff, D. W. (1975). Sex steroid binding in the brain of vertebrates. In "Brain-endocrine Interactions II" (K. M. Knigge, D. E. Scott, H. Kobayashi, S. Miura, and S. Ishii, eds.), pp. 230–256. Karger, Basel.

Morton, M. L., Pereyra, M. E., and Baptista, L. F. (1985). Photoperiodically induced ovarian growth in the white-crowned sparrow (*Zonotrichia leucophrys gambelii*) and its augmentation by song. *Comp. Biochem. Physiol.* **80A**, 93–97.

Moss, R. L., and Dudley, C. A. (1989). Neuropeptides and the social aspects of female reproductive behavior in the rat. In "Molecular and Cellular Basis of Social Behavior in Vertebrates" (J. Balthazart, ed.), pp. 209–237. Springer-Verlag, Berlin.

Moss, R. L., and Dudley, C. A. (1990). Differential effects of an luteinizing-hormone-releasing hormone (LHRH) antagonist analogue on lordosis behavior induced by LHRH and the LHRH fragment Ac-LHRH[5-10]. *Neuroendocrinology* **52**, 138–142.

Moss, R. L., Gu, Q., and Wong, M. (1997). Estrogen: Nontranscriptional signaling pathway. *Recent Prog. Horm. Res.* **52**, 33–69.

Mosselman, S., Polman, J., and Dijkema, R. (1996). ER beta: Identification and characterization of a novel human estrogen receptor. *FEBS Lett.* **392**, 49–53.

Murton, R. K., and Westwood, N. J. (1975). Integration of gonadotrophin and steroid secretion, spermatogenesis and behavior in the reproductive cycle of male pigeon. In "Neural and Endocrine Aspects of Behavior in Birds" (P. Wright, P. G. Caryl, and D. M. Vowles, eds.), pp. 51–89. Elsevier, Amsterdam.

Murton, R. K., and Westwood, N. J. (1977). "Avian Breeding Cycles." Clarendon Press, Oxford.

Muske, L. E., and Moore, F. L. (1988). The nervus terminalis in amphibians: Anatomy, chemistry and relationship with the hypothalamic gonadotropin-releasing hormone system. *Brain, Behav. Evol.* **32**, 141–150.

Naftolin, F., and Brawer, J. R. (1978). The effect of estrogens on hypothalamic structure and function. *Am. J. Obstet. Gynecol.* **132**, 758–765.

Naftolin, F., Ryan, K. J., and Petro, Z. (1972). Aromatization of androstenedione by the anterior hypothalamus of adult male and female rats. *Endocrinology (Baltimore)* **90**, 295–298.

Naftolin, F., Ryan, K. J., Davies, I. J., Reddy, V. V., Flores, F., Petro, Z., Kuhn, M., White, R. J., Takaoka, Y., and Wolin, L. (1975). The formation of estrogens by central neuroendocrine tissues. *Recent Prog. Horm. Res.* **31**, 295–319.

Naftolin, F., Garcia-Segura, L. M., Keefe, D., Leranth, C., MacLusky, N. J., and Brawer, J. R. (1990a). Estrogen effects on the synaptology and neural membranes of the rat hypothalamic arcuate nucleus. *Biol. Reprod.* **42**, 21–28.

Naftolin, F., Leranth, C., and Balthazart, J. (1990b). Ultrastructural localization of aromatase immunoreactivity in hypothalamic neurons. *Endocr. Soc. Abstr.* **669**, 192.

Naftolin, F., Horvath, T. L., Jakab, R. L., Leranth, C., Harada, N., and Balthazart, J. (1996). Aromatase immunoreactivity in axon terminals of the vertebrate brain—An immunocytochemical study on quail, rat, monkey and human tissues. *Neuroendocrinology* **63**, 149–155.

Nagle, L., Kreutzer, M. L., and Vallet, E. M. (1993). Obtaining copulation solicitation displays in female canaries without estradiol implants. *Experientia* **49**, 1022–1023.

Nakamura, T., and Tanabe, Y. (1974). In vitro metabolism of steroid hormones by chicken brain. *Acta Endocrinol. (Copenhagen)* **75**, 410–416.

Nash, S., and Domjan, M. (1991). Learning to discriminate the sex of conspecifics in male Japanese quail (*Coturnix coturnix japonica*): Tests of "biological constraints." *J. Exp. Psychol.* **17**, 342–353.

Nastiuk, K. L., and Clayton, D. F. (1994). Seasonal and tissue-specific regulation of canary androgen receptor messenger ribonucleic acid. *Endocrinology (Baltimore)* **134**, 640–649.

Nastiuk, K. L., and Clayton, D. F. (1995). The canary androgen receptor mRNA is localized in the song control nuclei of the brain and is rapidly regulated by testosterone. *J. Neurobiol.* **26**, 213–224.

Nauta, W. J. H., and Karten, H. J. (1970). A general profile of the vertebrate brain with sidelights on the ancestry of the cerebral cortex. *In* "The Neurocience. Second Study Program" (F. O. Schmidt, ed.), pp. 7–26. Rockefeller University Press, New York.

Nelson, R. J. (2000). "An Introduction to Behavioral Endocrinology." Sinauer Assoc., Sunderland, MA.

Neusser, M., Golinski, P., Zhu, Z., Zidek, W., and Tepel, M. (1999). Thapsigargin-insensitive calcium pools in vascular smooth muscle cells. *Clin. Exp. Hypertens.* **21**, 395–405.

Nicholls, T. J., Follett, B. K., Goldsmith, A. R., and Pearson, H. (1988a). Possible homologies between photorefractoriness in sheep and birds: The effect of thyroidectomy on the length of the ewe's breeding season. *Reprod. Nutr. Dev.* **28**, 375–385.

Nicholls, T. J., Gollsmith, A. R., and Dawson, A. (1988b). Photorefractoriness in birds and comparison with mammals. *Physiol. Rev.* **68**, 133–176.

Noble, G. K., and Wurm, M. (1940). The effect of testosterone propionate on the black-crowned night heron. *Endocrinology (Baltimore)* **26**, 837–850.

Noble, R. (1972). The effects of estrogen and progesterone on copulation in female quail (*Coturnix coturnix japonica*) housed in contnuous dark. *Horm. Behav.* **3**, 199–204.

Noble, R. (1973). Hormonal control of receptivity in female quail (*Coturnix coturnix japonica*). *Horm. Behav.* **4**, 61–72.

Nock, B., and Feder, H. H. (1981). Neurotransmitter modulation of steroid action in target cells that mediate reproduction and reproductive behavior. *Neurosci. Biobehav. Rev.* **5**, 437–447.

Nordeen, E. J., Nordeen, K. W., and Arnold, A. P. (1987). Sexual differentiation of androgen accumulation within the zebra finch brain through selective cell loss and addition. *J. Comp. Neurol.* **259**, 393–399.

Nordeen, K. W., Nordeen, E. J., and Arnold, A. P. (1986). Estrogen establishes sex differences in androgen accumulation in zebra finch brain. *J. Neurosci.* **6**, 734–738.

Nordeen, K. W., Nordeen, E. J., and Arnold, A. P. (1987). Estrogen accumulation in zebra finch song control nuclei: Implications for sexual differentiation and adult activation of song behavior. *J. Neurobiol.* **18**, 569–582.

Norgren, R. B., Jr., and Lehman, M. N. (1991). Neurons that migrate from the olfactory epithelium in the chick express luteinizing hormone-releasing hormone. *Endocrinology (Baltimore)* **128**, 1676–1678.

Norgren, R. B., Jr., and Silver, R. (1989). Retinohypothalamic projections and the suprachiasmatic nucleus in birds. *Brain, Behav. Evol.* **34**, 73–83.

Norgren, R. B., Lippert, J., and Lehman, M. N. (1991). Luteinizing hormone-releasing hormone in the pigeon terminal nerve and olfactory bulb. *Neurosci. Lett.* **135**, 201–204.

Nottebohm, F. (1975). Vocal behavior in birds. *Avian Biol.* **5**, 287–332.

Nottebohm, F. (1980). Brain pathways for vocal learning in birds: A review of the first 10 years. *Prog. Psychobiol. Physiol. Psychol.* **9**, 85–214.

Nottebohm, F. (1989). From bird song to neurogenesis. *Sci. Am.* **260**, 74–79.

Nottebohm, F., and Arnold, A. P. (1976). Sexual dimorphism in the vocal control areas in the song bird brain. *Science* **194**, 211–213.

Nottebohm, F., and Nottebohm, M. (1971). Vocalizations and breeding behavior of surgically deafened ring doves, *Streptopelia risoria*. *Anim. Behav.* **19**, 313–327.

Nottebohm, F., Stokes, T. M., and Leonard, C. M. (1976). Central control of song in the canary, *Serinus canarius*. *J. Comp. Neurol.* **165**, 457–486.

Nottebohm, F., Kelley, D. B., and Paton, J. A. (1982). Connections of vocal control nuclei in the canary telencephalon. *J. Comp. Neurol.* **207**, 344–357.

Nottebohm, F., Alvarez-Buylla, A., Cynx, J., Kirn, J., Ling, C. Y., Nottebohm, M., Suter, R., Tolles, A., and Williams, H. (1990). Song learning in birds: The relation between perception and production. *Philos. Trans. R. Soc. London, Ser. B* **329**, 115–124.

Numan, M. (1994). Maternal behavior. *In* "The Physiology of Reproduction" (E. Knobil and J. D. Neil, eds.), 2nd ed., Vol. 2, pp. 221–302. Raven Press, New York.

Nyby, J. G., and Simon, N. G. (1987). Nonaromatizable androgens may stimulate a male mouse reproductive behavior by binding to estrogen receptors. *Physiol. Behav.* **39**, 147–151.

O'Connell, M. E., Reboulleau, C., Feder, H. H., and Silver, R. (1981a). Social interactions and androgen levels in birds. I. Female characteristics associated with increased plasma androgen levels in the male ring dove (*Streptopelia risoria*). *Gen. Comp. Endocrinol.* **44**, 454–463.

O'Connell, M. E., Silver, R., Feder, H. H., and Reboulleau, C. (1981b). Social interactions and androgen levels in birds. II. Social factors associated with a decline in plasma androgen levels in male ring doves (*Streptopelia risoria*). *Gen. Comp. Endocrinol.* **44**, 464–469.

Ogawa, S., Chan, J., Chester, A. E., Gustafsson, J. Å., Korach, K. S., and Pfaff, D. W. (1999). Survival of reproductive behaviors in estrogen receptor b gene-deficient (bERKO) male and female mice. *Proc. Natl. Acad. Sci. U.S.A.* **96,** 12 887–12 892.

Oksche, A. (1983). Reflections on the structural basis of avian neuroendocrine systems. *In* "Avian Endocrinology: Environmental and Ecological Perspectives" (S. Mikami, K. Homma, and M. Wada, eds.), pp. 3–10. Springer-Verlag, Berlin.

Oliver, J., and Baylé, J. D. (1982). Brain photoreceptors for the photo-induced testicular response in birds. *Experientia* **38,** 1021–1029.

O'Loghlen, A. L., and Beecher, M. D. (1997). Sexual preferences for mate song types in female song sparrows. *Anim. Behav.* **53,** 835–841.

Onagbesan, O. M., and Podie, M. J. (1989). Calcium-dependent stimulation of estrogen secretion by FSH from theca cells of the domestic hen (*Gallus domesticus*). *Gen. Comp. Endocrinol.* **75,** 177–186

Oring, L. W. (1982). Avian mating systems. *Avian Biol.* **6,** 1–92.

Oring, L. W., Fivizzani, A. J., and El Halawani, M. E. (1986a). Changes in plasma prolactin associated with laying and hatch in the Spotted Sandpiper. *Auk* **103,** 820–822.

Oring, L. W., Fivizzani, A. J., El Halawani, M. E., and Goldsmith, A. R. (1986b). Seasonal changes in prolactin and luteinizing hormone in the polyandrous Spotted Sandpiper, *Actitis macularia*. *Gen. Comp. Endocrinol.* **62,** 394–403.

Oring, L. W., Fivizzani, A. J., and El Halawani, M. E. (1989). Testosterone-induced inhibition of incubation in the spotted sandpiper (*Actitis mecularia*). *Horm. Behav.* **23,** 412–423.

Osawa, Y., Higashiyama, T., Shimizu, Y., and Yarborough, C. (1993). Multiple functions of aromatase and the active site structure; Aromatase is the placental estrogen 2-hydroxylase. *J. Steroid Biochem. Mol. Biol.* **44,** 469-480.

Osawa, Y., Higashiyama, T., and Yarborough, C. (1994). Diverse functions of aromatase cytochrome P-450: Catecholestrogen synthesis, cocaine N-demethylation, and other selective drug metabolisms. *In* "Cytochrome P450. 8th International Conference" (M. C. Lechner, ed.), pp. 893–896. John Libbey Eurotext, Paris.

Osawa, Y., Higashiyama, T., Toma, Y., and Yarborough, C. (1997). Diverse function of aromatase and the N-terminal sequence deleted form. *J. Steroid Biochem. Mol. Biol.* **61,** 117–126.

Ottinger, M. A., and Bakst, M. R. (1981). Peripheral androgen concentrations and testicular morphology in embryonic and young male Japanese quail. *Gen. Comp. Endocrinol.* **43,** 170–177.

Ottinger, M. A., and Balthazart, J. (1987). Brain monoamines in Japanese quail: Effects of castration and steroid replacement therapy. *Behav. Processes* **14,** 197–216.

Ottinger, M. A., Duchala, C. S., and Masson, M. (1983). Age-related reproductive decline in the male Japanese quail. *Horm. Behav.* **17,** 197–207.

Ottinger, M. A., Schumacher, M., Clarke, R. N., Duchala, C. S., and Balthazart, J. (1986). Comparison of monoamine concentrations in the brains of adult male and female Japanese quail. *Poult. Sci.* **65,** 1413–1420.

Ottinger, M. A., Cortes-Burgos, L., and Rawlings, C. S. (1988). Noradrenergic agonists and LHRH stimulate male reproductive behavior in Japanese quail. *Soc. Neurosci. Abstr.* **14,** 529.

Paech, K., Webb, P., Kuiper, G. G. J. M., Nilsson, S., Gustafsson, J. Å., Kushner, P. J., and Scanlan, T. S. (1997). Differential ligand activation of estrogen receptors ERa and ERb ar AP1 sites. *Science* **277,** 1508–1510.

Palkovits, M. (1973). Isolated removal of hypothalamic or other brain nuclei of the rat. *Brain Res.* **59,** 449–450.

Palkovits, M., and Brownstein, M. J. (1983). Microdissection of brain areas by the punch technique. *In* "Brain Microdissection Techniques" (A. C. Cuello, ed.), pp. 1–36. Wiley, New York.

Panksepp, J., Vilberg, T., Bean, N. J., Coy, D. H., and Kastin, A. J. (1978). Reduction of distress vocalization in chicks by opiate-like peptides. *Brain Res. Bull.* **3,** 663–667.

Panzica, G. C., Malacarne, G., De Bernochi, A., and Viglietti-Panzica, G. C. (1985). Effects of steroid hormones on the neuropil of the hypothalamic paraventricular nucleus of male chickens. *Cell Tissue Res.* **240,** 169–174.

Panzica, G. C., Viglietti-Panzica, C., Calcagni, M., Anselmetti, G. C., Schumacher, M., and Balthazart, J. (1987). Sexual differentiation and hormonal control of the sexually dimorphic preoptic medial nucleus in quail. *Brain Res.* **416,** 59–68.

Panzica, G. C., Calcagni, M., Ramieri, G., and Viglietti-Panzica, C. (1988). Extrahypothalamic distribution of vasotocin-immunoreactive fibers and perikarya in the avian central nervous system. *Basic Appl. Histochem.* **32,** 89–94.

Panzica, G. C., Viglietti-Panzica, C., Sanchez, F., Sante, P., and Balthazart, J. (1991). Effects of testosterone on a selected neuronal population within the preoptic sexually dimorphic nucleus of the Japanese quail. *J. Comp. Neurol.* **303,** 443–456.

Panzica, G. C., Fraschini, F., Aste, N., Lucini, V., Viglietti-Panzica, C., Cozzi, B., and Stankov, B. (1994). The density of melatonin receptors is dependent upon the prevailing photoperiod in the Japanese quail (*Coturnix japonica*). *Neurosci. Lett.* **173,** 111–114.

Panzica, G. C., Garcia-Ojeda, E., Viglietti-Panzica, C., Thompson, N. E., and Ottinger, M. A. (1996a). Testosterone effects on vasotocinergic innervation of sexually dimorphic medial preoptic nucleus and lateral septum during aging in male quail. *Brain Res.* **712,** 190–198.

Panzica, G. C., Viglietti-Panzica, C., and Balthazart, J. (1996b). The sexually dimorphic medial preoptic nucleus of quail: A key brain area mediating steroid action on male sexual behavior. *Front. Neuroendocrinol.* **17**, 51–125.

Panzica, G. C., Castagna, C., Viglietti-Panzica, C., Russo, C., Tlemçani, O., and Balthazart, J. (1998). Organizational effects of estrogens on brain vasotocin and sexual behavior in quail. *J. Neurobiol.* **37**, 684–699.

Parry, D. M., and Goldsmith, A. R. (1993). Ultrastructural evidence for changes in synaptic input to the hypothalamic luteinizing hormone-releasing hormone neurons in photosensitive and photorefractory starlings. *J. Neuroendocrinol.* **5**, 387–395.

Parry, D. M., Goldsmith, A. R., Millar, R. P., and Glennie, L. M. (1997). Immunocytochemical localization of GnRH precursor in the hypothalamus of European starlings during sexual maturation and photorefractoriness. *J. Neuroendocrinol.* **9**, 235–243.

Pasqualini, C., Olivier, V., Guibert, B., Frain, O., and Leviel, V. (1995). Acute stimulatory effect of estradiol on striatal dopamine synthesis. *J. Neurochem.* **65**, 1651–1657.

Patrone, C., Pollio, G., Vegeto, E., Enmark, E., De Curtis, I., Gustafsson, J. Å., and Maggi, A. (2000). Estradiol induces differential neuronal phenotypes by activating estrogen receptor α or β. *Endocrinology (Baltimore)* **141**, 1839–1845.

Pedersen, H. C. (1989). Effects of exogenous prolactin on parental behaviour in free-living female willow ptarmigan *Lagopus, l. lagopus. Anim. Behav.* **38**, 926–934.

Perrins, C. M. (1970). The timing of birds breeding seasons. *Ibis* **112**, 242–255.

Perrins, C. M., and Birkhead, T. (1983). "Avian Ecology." Blackie, Glasgow and London.

Peterson, R. S., Saldanha, C. J., Mills, R., and Schlinger, B. A. (2000). Aromatase is rapidly transcribed and translated in glia following neural injury in the zebra finch. *Soc. Neurosci. Abstr.* **26**, 512.

Pfaff, D. W. (1976). The neuroanatomy of sex hormone receptors in the vertebrate brain. In "Neuroendocrine Regulation of Fertility" (T. C. Anand-Kumar, ed.), pp. 30–45. Karger, Basel.

Pfaff, D. W. (1980). "Estrogens and Brain Function: Neural Analysis of a Hormone-Controlled Mammalian Reproductive Behavior." Springer-Verlag, New York.

Pfaff, D. W. (1999). "Drive. Neurobiological and Molecular Mechanisms of Sexual Motivation." MIT Press, Cambridge, MA.

Pfaus, J. G., Damsma, G., Nomikos, G. G., Wenkstern, D. G., Blaha, C. D., Phillips, A. G., and Fibiger, H. C. (1990). Sexual behavior enhances central dopamine transmission in the male rat. *Brain Res.* **530**, 345–348.

Pfaus, J. G., Smith, W. J., and Coopersmith, C. B. (1999). Appetitive and consummatory sexual behaviors of female rats in bilevel chambers—I. A correlational and factor analysis and the effects of ovarian hormones. *Horm. Behav.* **35**, 224–240.

Phillips, R. E., and Barfield, R. J. (1977). Effects of testosterone implants in midbrain vocal areas of capons. *Brain Res.* **122**, 378–381.

Phillips, R. E., and Youngren, O. M. (1971). Brain stimulation and species-typical behaviour: Activities evoked by electrical stimulation of the brains of chickens (*Gallus gallus*). *Anim. Behav.* **19**, 757–779.

Pleim, E. T., Brown, T. J., MacLusky, N. J., Etgen, A. M., and Barfield, R. J. (1989). Dilute estradiol implants and progestin receptor induction in the ventromedial nucleus of the hypothalamus: Correlation with receptive behavior in female rats. *Endocrinology (Baltimore)* **124**, 1807–1812.

Poletti, A., Celotti, F., Maggi, R., Melcangi, R. C., Martini, L., and Negri-Cesi, P. (1999). Aspects of hormonal steroid metabolism in the nervous system. In "Neurosteroids: A New Regulatory Function in the Nervous System" (E. E. Baulieu, P. Robel, and M. Schumacher, eds.), pp. 97–123. Humana Press, Totowa, NJ.

Polikarpova, E. (1940). Influence of external factors upoin the development of the sexual gland of the sparrow. *Dokl. Nauk SSSR* **27**, 91–95.

Potash, L. M. (1970). Vocalizations elicited by electrical brain stimulation in *Coturnix coturnix japonica. Behaviour* **31**, 149–167.

Power, R. F., Mani, S. K., Codina, J., Conneely, O. M., and O'Malley, B. W. (1991). Dopaminergic and ligand-independent activation of steroid hormone receptors. *Science* **254**, 1636–1639.

Ramachandran, B., Schlinger, B. A., Arnold, A. P., and Campagnoni, A. T. (1999). Zebra finch aromatase gene expression is regulated in the brain through an alternate promoter. *Gene* **240**, 209–216.

Ramirez, V. D., Zheng, J. B., and Siddique, K. M. (1996). Membrane receptors for estrogen, progesterone, and testosterone in the rat brain: Fantasy or reality. *Cell. Mol. Neurobiol.* **16**, 175–198.

Raum, W. J., and Swerdloff, R. S. (1981). The role of hypothalamic adrenergic receptors in preventing testosterone-induced androgenization in the female rat brain. *Endocrinology (Baltimore)* **109**, 273–278.

Raum, W. J., Marcano, M., and Swerdloff, R. S. (1984). Nuclear accumulation of estradiol derived from the aromatization of testosterone is inhibited by hypothalamic beta-receptor stimulation in the neonatal female rat. *Biol. Reprod.* **30**, 388–396.

Raynaud, J. P., Bouton, M. M., Moguilevsky, M., Ojasoo, T., Philibert, D., Beck, G., Labrie, F., and Mornon, J. P. (1980).

Steroid hormone receptors and pharmacology. *J. Steroid Biochem.* **12**, 143–157.

Reddy, V. V. R., Naftolin, F., and Ryan, K. J. (1974). Conversion of androstenedione to estrone by neural tissues from fetal and neonatal rats. *Endocrinology (Baltimore)* **94**, 117–121.

Reinert, B. D., and Wilson, F. E. (1996). The thyroid and the hypothalamus-pituitary-ovarian axis in American tree sparrows (*Spizella arborea*). *Gen. Comp. Endocrinol.* **103**, 60–70.

Reinke, H., and Wild, J. M. (1998). Identification and connections of inspiratory premotor neurons in songbirds and budgerigar. *J. Comp. Neurol.* **391**, 147–163.

Reisbick, S., Rosenblatt, J. S., and Mayer, A. D. (1975). Decline of maternal behavior in the virgin and lactating rat. *J. Comp. Physiol. Psychol.* **89**, 722–732.

Rhees, R. W., Abel, J. H., and Haack, D. W. (1972). Uptake of tritiated steroids in the brain of the duck (*Anas platyrhynchos*). An autoradiographic study. *Gen. Comp. Endocrinol.* **18**, 292–300.

Ribeiro, S., Cecchi, G. A., Magnasco, M. O., and Mello, C. V. (1998). Toward a song code: Evidence for a syllabic representation in the canary brain. *Neuron* **21**, 359–371.

Rice, G. E., Arnason, S. S., Arad, Z., and Skadhauge, E. (1985). Plasma concentrations of arginine vasotocin, prolactin, aldosterone, and corticosterone in relation to oviposition and dietary NaCl in the domestic fowl. *Comp. Biochem. Physiol.* **81A**, 769–777.

Richfield, E. K., Young, A. B., and Penney, J. B. (1987). Comparative distribution of dopamine D-1 and D-2 receptors in the basal ganglia of turtles, pigeons, rats, cats, and monkeys. *J. Comp. Neurol.* **262**, 446–463.

Ricklefs, R. E. (1983). Avian postnatal development. *Avian Biol.* **7**, 1–83.

Riddle, O., Bates, R. W., and Lahr, E. L. (1935). Prolactin induces broodiness in fowl. *Am. J. Physiol.* **111**, 352–360.

Riters, L. V., and Ball, G. F. (1999). Lesions to the medial preoptic area affect singing in the male European starling (*Sturnus vulgaris*). *Horm. Behav.* **36**, 276–286.

Riters, L. V., Absil, P., and Balthazart, J. (1998). Effects of brain testosterone implants on appetitive and consummatory components of male sexual behavior in Japanese quail. *Brain Res. Bull.* **47**, 69–79.

Riters, L. V., Eens, M., Pinxten, R., Duffy, D. L., Balthazart, J., and Ball, G. F. (2000a). Seasonal changes in courtship song and the medial preoptic area in male European starlings (*Sturnus vulgaris*). *Horm. Behav.* **38**, 250–261.

Riters, L. V., Baillien, M., Eens, M., Pinxten, R., Foidart, A., Ball, G. F., and Balthazart, J. (2001). Seasonal variation in androgen-metabolizing enzymes in the diencephalon and telencephalon of the male european starling (*Sturnus vulgaris*). *J. Neuroendocrinol.* **13**, 985–997.

Robbins, T. W. (1997). Arousal systems and attentional processes. *Biol. Psychol.* **45**, 57–71.

Robertson, G. S., Pfaus, J. G., Atkinson, L. J., Matsumura, H., Phillips, A. G., and Fibiger, H. C. (1991). Sexual behavior increases c-*fos* expression in the forebrain of the male rat. *Brain Res.* **564**, 352–357.

Rodriguez-Sierra, J. F., and Blake, C. A. (1983). Catechol oestyrogens: Their contraceptive effects and possible involvement in some reproductive processes of the rat. *In* "Hormones and Behavior in Higher Vertebrates" (J. Balthazart, E. Pröve, and R. Gilles, eds.), pp. 40–55. Springer-Verlag, Berlin.

Rohwer, S. (1975). The social significance of avian winter plumage variability. *Evolution (Lawrence, Kans.)* **29**, 593–610.

Rohwer, S., and Rohwer, F. C. (1978). Status signaling in Harris' sparrows: Experimental deceptions achieved. *Anim. Behav.* **26**, 1012–1022.

Roselli, C. E. (1991). Synergistic induction of aromatase activity in the rat brain by estradiol and 5α-dihydrotestosterone. *Neuroendocrinology* **53**, 79–84.

Roselli, C. E. (1995). Subcellular localization and kinetic properties of aromatase activity in rat brain. *J. Steroid Biochem. Mol. Biol.* **52**, 469–477.

Roselli, C. E., and Resko, J. A. (1984). Androgens regulate brain aromatase activity in adult male rats through a receptor mechanism. *Endocrinology (Baltimore)* **114**, 2183–2189.

Roselli, C. E., and Resko, J. A. (1989). Testosterone regulates aromatase activity in discrete brain areas of male rhesus macaques. *Biol. Reprod.* **40**, 929–934.

Roselli, C. E., Horton, L. E., and Resko, J. A. (1985). Distribution and regulation of aromatase activity in the rat hypothalamus and limbic system. *Endocrinology (Baltimore)* **117**, 2471–2477.

Roselli, C. E., Horton, L. E., and Resko, J. A. (1987). Time-course and steroid specificity of aromatase induction in rat hypothalamus-preoptic area. *Biol. Reprod.* **37**, 628–633.

Rowan, W. (1929). Experiments in bird migration I. Manipulation of the reproductive cycle: Seaonal histological changes in the gonads. *Proc. Boston Soc. Nat. Hist.* **39**, 151–208.

Rozenboim, I., Silsby, J. L., Tabibzadeh, C., Pitts, G. R., Youngren, O. M., and El Halawani, M. E. (1993). Hypothalamic and posterior pituitary content of vasoactive intestinal peptide and gonadotropin-releasing hormones I and II in the turkey hen. *Biol. Reprod.* **49**, 622–626.

Runfedlt, S., and Wingfield, J. C. (1985). Experimentally prolonged sexual activity in female sparrows delays termination of reproductive activity in their untreated mates. *Anim. Behav.* **33**, 403–410.

Sachs, B. D. (1967). Photoperiodic control of the cloacal gland of the Japanese quail. *Science* **157**, 201–203.

Sachs, B. D. (1995). Context-sensitive variation in the regulation of erection. *In* "The Pharmacology of Sexual Function and Dysfunction" (J. Bancroft, ed.), pp. 97–108. Elsevier, Amsterdam.

Sachs, B. D., Akasofu, K., and McEldowney, S. S. (1992). Interaction of apomorphine and copulatory behavior in the penile-erection/stretching-yawning syndrome. *Soc. Neurosci. Abstr.* **18**, 1071.

Salamone, J. D. (1992). Complex motor and sensori-motor functions of striatal and accumbens dopamine: Involvement in instrumental behavior processes. *Psychopharmacology* **107**, 160–174.

Saldanha, C. J., Deviche, P. J., and Silver, R. (1994a). Increased VIP and decreased GnRH expression in photorefractory dark-eyed juncos (*Junco hyemalis*). *Gen. Comp. Endocrinol.* **93**, 128–136.

Saldanha, C. J., Leak, R. K., and Silver, R. (1994b). Detection and transduction of daylength in birds. *Psychoneuroendocrinology* **19**, 641–656.

Saldanha, C. J., Popper, P., Micevych, P. E., and Schlinger, B. A. (1998). The passerine hippocampus is a site of high aromatase: Inter- and intraspecies comparisons. *Horm. Behav.* **34**, 85–97.

Saldanha, C. J., Schultz, J. D., London, S. E., and Schlinger, B. A. (2000a). Telencephalic aromatase but not a song circuit in a sub-oscine passerine, the golden-collared manakin (*Manacus vitellinus*). *Brain, Behav. Evol.* **56**, 29–37.

Saldanha, C. J., Tuerk, M. J., Kim, Y. H., Fernandes, A. O., Arnold, A. P., and Schlinger, B. A. (2000b). Distribution and regulation of telencephalic aromatase expression in the zebra finch revealed with a specific antibody. *J. Comp. Neurol.* **423**, 619–630.

Sar, M. (1984). Estradiol is concentrated in tyrosine hydroxylase-containing neurons of the hypothalamus. *Science* **223**, 938–940.

Sar, M., Lubahn, D. B., French, F. S., and Wilson, E. M. (1990). Immunohistochemical localization of the androgen receptor in rat and human tissues. *Endocrinology (Baltimore)* **127**, 3180–3186.

Sara, S. J. (1985). Noradrenergic modulation of selective attention: Its role in memory retrieval. *Ann. N.Y. Acad. Sci.* **444**, 178–193.

Sawaguchi, T., and Goldman-Rakic, P. S. (1991). Dopamine receptors in prefrontal cortex: Involvement in working memory. *Science* **251**, 947–950.

Scanes, C. G. (2000). Pituitary gland. *In* "Sturkies Avian Physiology" (G. C. Whittow, ed.), pp. 437–460. Academic Press, San Diego, CA.

Schally, A. V., Arimura, A., and Baker, Y. (1971). Isolation and properties of the FSH and LH-releasing hormone. *Biochem. Biophys. Res. Commun.* **43**, 393–399.

Schleidt, W. M. (1970). Precocial sexual behavior in turkeys (*Meleagris gallopavo* L.). *Anim. Behav.* **18**, 760–761.

Schlinger, B. A. (1997). Sex steroids and their actions on the birdsong system. *J. Neurobiol.* **33**, 619–631.

Schlinger, B. A., and Arnold, A. P. (1991). Brain is the major site of estrogen synthesis in a male songbird. *Proc. Natl. Acad. Sci. U.S.A.* **88**, 4191–4194.

Schlinger, B. A., and Arnold, A. P. (1992a). Circulating estrogens in a male songbird originate in the brain. *Proc. Natl. Acad. Sci. U.S.A.* **89**, 7650–7653.

Schlinger, B. A., and Arnold, A. P. (1992b). Plasma sex steroids and tissue aromatization in hatchling zebra finches: Implications for the sexual differentiation of singing behavior. *Endocrinology (Baltimore)* **130**, 289–299.

Schlinger, B. A., and Arnold, A. P. (1993). Estrogen synthesis *in vivo* in the adult zebra finch: Additional evidence that circulating estrogens can originate in brain. *Endocrinology (Baltimore)* **133**, 2610–2616.

Schlinger, B. A., and Callard, G. V. (1987). A comparison of aromatase, 5α- and 5β-reductase activities in the brain and pituitary of male and female quail (*Coturnix c. japonica*). *J. Exp. Zool.* **242**, 171–180.

Schlinger, B. A., and Callard, G. V. (1989). Localization of aromatase in synaptosomal and microsomal subfractions of quail (*Coturnix coturnix japonica*) brain. *Neuroendocrinology* **49**, 434–441.

Schlinger, B. A., and Callard, G. V. (1990). Aromatization mediates aggressive behavior in quail. *Gen. Comp. Endocrinol.* **79**, 39–53.

Schlinger, B. A., Scanes, C., Randhawa, M., and Callard, G. V. (1984). Distribution of aromatase activity in quail brain (*C.c. japonica*): Effects of photoperiod and castration. *J. Steroid Biochem.* **20**, 1571.

Schlinger, B. A., Amur-Umarjee, S., Shen, P., Campagnoni, A. T., and Arnold, A. P. (1994). Neuronal and non-neuronal aromatase in primary cultures of developing zebra finch telencephalon. *J. Neurosci.* **14**, 7541–7552.

Schumacher, M. (1990). Rapid membrane effects of steroid hormones: An emerging concept in neuroendocrinology. *Trends Neurosci.* **13**, 359–362.

Schumacher, M., and Balthazart, J. (1983). The effects of testosterone and its metabolites on sexual behavior and morphology in male and female Japanese quail. *Physiol. Behav.* **30**, 335–339.

Schumacher, M., and Balthazart, J. (1984a). Sexual dimorphism of the hypothalamic metabolism of testosterone in the Japanese quail (*Coturnix coturnix japonica*). *Prog. Brain Res.* **61**, 53–61.

Schumacher, M., and Balthazart, J. (1984b). The postnatal demasculinization of sexual behavior in the Japanese quail. *Horm. Behav.* **18**, 298–312.

Schumacher, M., and Balthazart, J. (1986). Testosterone-induced brain aromatase is sexually dimorphic. *Brain Res.* **370**, 285–293.

Schumacher, M., and Balthazart, J. (1987). Neuroanatomical distribution of testosterone metabolizing enzymes in the Japanese quail. *Brain Res.* **422**, 137–148.

Schumacher, M., and Hutchison, J. B. (1986). Testosterone induces hypothalamic aromatase during early development in quail. *Brain Res.* **377**, 63–72.

Schumacher, M., Contenti, E., and Balthazart, J. (1983). Testosterone metabolism in discrete areas of the hypothalamus and adjacent brain regions of male and female Japanese quail. *Brain Res.* **278**, 337–340.

Schumacher, M., Contenti, E., and Balthazart, J. (1984). Partial characterization of testosterone-metabolizing enzymes in the quail brain. *Brain Res.* **305**, 51–59.

Schumacher, M., Alexandre, C., and Balthazart, J. (1987). Interactions des androgènes et des oestrogènes dans le contrôle de la reproduction. *C. R. Seances Acad. Sci. Sér. 3* **305**, 569–574.

Schumacher, M., Hutchison, R. E., and Hutchison, J. B. (1988a). Ontogeny of testosterone-inducible brain aromatase activity. *Brain Res.* **441**, 98–110.

Schumacher, M., Sulon, J., and Balthazart, J. (1988b). Changes in serum concentrations of steroids during embryonic and post-hatching development of male and female Japanese quail (*Coturnix coturnix japonica*). *J. Endocrinol.* **118**, 127–134.

Schumacher, M., Hendrick, J. C., and Balthazart, J. (1989). Sexual differentiation in quail: Critical period and hormonal specificity. *Horm. Behav.* **23**, 130–149.

Schumacher, M., Coirini, H., Robert, F., Guennoun, R., and El-Etr, M. (1999). Genomic and membrane actions of progesterone: Implications for reproductive physiology and behavior. *Behav. Brain Res.* **105**, 37–52.

Schwab, R. G., and Lott, D. F. (1969). Testis growth and regression in Starlings (*Strunus vulgaris*) as a function of the presence of females. *J. Exp. Zool.* **171**, 39–42.

Schwartz, J. H., and Kandel, E. R. (1991). Synaptic transmission mediated by second messengers. *In* "Principles of Neural Science" (E. R. Kandel, J. H. Schwartz, and T. M. Jessel, eds.), pp. 173–193. Am. Elsevier, New York.

Scott, D. M., and Ankney, C. D. (1980). Fecundity of the brown-headed cowbird in southern Ontario. *Auk* **97**, 677–683.

Searcy, W. A., and Capp, M. S. (1997). Estradiol dosage and the sollicitation display assay in red-winged blackbirds. *Condor* **99**, 826–828.

Searcy, W. A., and Marler, P. (1981). A test for responsiveness to song structure and programming in female sparrows. *Science* **213**, 926–928.

Segovia, S., and Guillamón, A. (1993). Sexual dimorphism in the vomeronasal pathway and sex differences in reproductive behaviors. *Brain Res. Rev.* **18**, 51–74.

Seiwert, C. M. (1994). "The Neuromuscular System Controlling Foam Production in Japanese Quail: An Investigation of Structure and Function." Cornell University, Ithaca, NY.

Seiwert, C. M., and Adkins-Regan, E. (1992). Social facilitation of sphincter cloacae muscle movement in male Japanese quail. *Soc. Neurosci. Abstr.* **18**, 894.

Seiwert, C. M., and Adkins-Regan, E. (1998). The foam production system of the male Japanese quail: Characterization of structure and function. *Brain, Behav. Evol.* **52**, 61–80.

Seller, T. J. (1981). Midbrain vocalization centers in birds. *Trends Neurosci.* **4**, 301–303.

Sharp, P. J., and Klandorf, H. (1981). The interaction between day length and the gonads in the regulation of levels of plasma thyroxine and triiodothyronine in the Japanese quail. *Gen. Comp. Endocrinol.* **45**, 504–512.

Sharp, P. J., and Massa, R. (1980). Conversion of progesterone to 5α- and 5β-reduced metabolites in the brain of the hen and its potential role in the induction of the preovulatory release of luteinizing hormone. *J. Endocrinol.* **86**, 459–464.

Sharp, P. J., Haase, E., and Fraser, H. M. (1975). Immunofluorescent localization of sites binding anit-synthetic LHRH serum in the median eminence of the greenfinch (*Chloris chloris* L.). *Cell Tissue Res.* **162**, 83–91.

Sharp, P. J., Armstrong, D. G., and Moss, R. (1986). Changes in aromatase activity in the neuroendocrine tissues of red grouse (*Lagopus lagopus scoticus*) in relation to the development of long-day refractoriness. *J. Endocrinol.* **108**, 129–135.

Sharp, P. J., Dunn, I. C., Main, G. M., Sterling, R. J., and Talbot, R. T. (1990a). Gonadotropin releasing hormones: Distribution and function. *In* "Endocrinology of Birds" (M. Wada, S. Ishii, and C. G. Scanes, eds.), pp. 31–43. Springer-Verlag, Berlin.

Sharp, P. J., Talbot, R. T., Main, G. M., Dunn, I. C., Fraser, H. M., and Huskisson, N. S. (1990b). Physiological roles of chicken LHRH-I and -II in the control of gonadotrophin release in the domestic chicken. *J. Endocrinol.* **124**, 291–299.

Sharp, P. J., Li, Q., Talbot, R. T., Barker, P., Huskisson, N., and Lea, R. W. (1995). Identification of hypothalamic nuclei involved in osmoregulation using fos immunocytochemistry in the domestic hen (*Gallus domesticus*), Ring dove (*Streptopelia risoria*), Japanese quail (*Coturnix japonica*) and Zebra finch (*Taenopygia guttata*). *Cell Tissue Res.* **282**, 351–361.

Sharp, P. J., Li, Q., Georgiou, G., and Lea, R. W. (1996). Expression of fos-like immunoreactivity in the hypothalamus of the ring dove (*Streptopelia risoria*) at the onset of incubation. *J. Neuroendocrinol.* **8**, 291–298.

Shelley, A. M., Catts, S. V., Ward, P. B., Andrews, S., Mitchell, P., Michie, P., and McConaghy, N. (1997). The effect of decreased catecholamine transmission on ERP indices of selective attention. *Neuropsychopharmacology* **16**, 202–210.

Shen, P., Campagnoni, C. W., Kampf, K., Schlinger, B. A., Arnold, A. P., and Campagnoni, A. T. (1994). Isolation and characterization of a zebra finch aromatase cDNA: In situ hybridization reveals high aromatase expression in brain. *Mol. Brain Res.* **24**, 227–237.

Shen, P., Schlinger, B. A., Campagnoni, A. T., and Arnold, A. P. (1995). An atlas of aromatase mRNA expression in the zebra finch brain. *J. Comp. Neurol.* **360**, 172–184.

Sheridan, P. J. (1983). Androgen receptors in the brain: What are we measuring? *Endocr. Rev.* **4**, 171–178.

Sherry, D. F. (1989). Food storing in the paridae. *Wilson. Bull.* **101**, 289–304.

Sherwood, N. M., Wingfield, J. C., Ball, G. F., and Dufty, A. M. (1988). Identity of GnRH in passerine birds: Comparison of GnRH in song sparrow (*Melospiza melodia*) and starling (*Sturnus vulgaris*) with 5 vertebrate GnRHs. *Gen. Comp. Endocrinol.* **69**, 341–351.

Shimada, K., Neldon, H., and Koike, T. I. (1986). Arginine vasotocin (AVT) release in relation to uterine contractility in the hen. *Gen. Comp. Endocrinol.* **64**, 362–367.

Shivers, B. D., Harlan, R. E., Morrell, J. I., and Pfaff, D. W. (1983). Absence of oestradiol concentration in cell nuclei of LHRH-immunoreactive neurones. *Nature (London)* **304**, 345–347.

Shodono, M., Nakamura, T., Tanabe, Y., and Wakabayashi, K. (1975). Simultaneous determinations of oestradiol-17 beta, progesterone and luteinizing hormone in the plasma during the ovulatory cycle of the hen. *Acta Endocrinol. (Copenhagen)* **78**, 565–573.

Shughrue, P., Scrimo, P., Lane, M., Askew, R., and Merchenthaler, I. (1997). The distribution of estrogen receptor-b mRNA in forebrain regions of the estrogen receptor—a knockout mouse. *Endocrinology (Baltimore)* **138**, 5649–5652.

Silver, R. (1978). The parental behavior of ring doves. *Am. Sci.* **66**, 209–215.

Silver, R. (1984). Prolactin and parenting in the pigeon family. *J. Exp. Zool.* **232**, 617–625.

Silver, R., and Ramos, C. (1990). Vasoactive intestinal polypeptide in avian reproduction. *In* "Hormones, Brain and Behavior in Vertebrates" (J. Balthazart, ed.), Vol. 1, pp. 191–204. Karger, Basel.

Silver, R., Reboulleau, C., Lehrman, D. S., and Feder, H. H. (1974). Radioimmunoassay of plasma progesterone during the reproductive cycle of male and female ring doves (*Streptopelia risoria*). *Endocrinology (Baltimore)* **94**, 1547–1554.

Silver, R., O'Connell, M., and Saad, R. (1979). The effects of androgens on the behavior of birds. *In* "Endocrine Control of Sex Behavior" (C. Beyer, ed.), pp. 223–279. Raven Press, New York.

Silver, R., Andrews, H., and Ball, G. F. (1985). Parental care in an ecological perspective: A quantitative analysis of avian subfamilies. *Am. Zool.* **25**, 823–840.

Silver, R., Witkovsky, P., Horvath, P., Alones, V., Barnstable, C. J., and Lehman, M. N. (1988). Coexpression of opsin- and VIP-like immunoreactivity in CSF-contacting neurons of the avian brain. *Cell Tissue Res.* **253**, 189–198.

Silver, R., Ramos, C., Machuca, H., and Silverin, B. (1992). Immunocytochemical distribution of GnRH in the brain of adult and posthatching great tit Parus major and ring dove *Streptopelia roseogrisea*. *Ornis Scand.* **23**, 222–232.

Silverin, B. (1980). Effects of long-acting testosterone treatment of free-living pied flycatchers, *Ficedula hypoleuca*, during the breeding period. *Anim. Behav.* **28**, 906–912.

Silverin, B. (1988). Endocrine aspects of avian mating systems. *Proc. 19th Int. Ornithol. Cong.*, Vol. 2, pp. 1676–1684.

Silverin, B., and Goldsmith, A. R. (1990). Plasma prolactin concentrations in breeding pied flycatchers (*Ficedula hypoleuca*) with an experimentally prolonged brooding period. *Horm. Behav.* **24**, 104–113.

Silverin, B., and Viebke, P. A. (1994). Low temperatures affect the photoperiodically induced LH and testicular cycles differently in closely related species of tits (*Parus* sp.). *Horm. Behav.* **28**, 199–206.

Silverman, A. J., Livine, I., and Witkin, J. W. (1994). The gonadotropin-releasing hormone (GnRH) neuronal systems: Immunocytochemistry and in situ hybridization. *In* "The Physiology of Reproduction" (E. Knobil and J. D. Neil, eds.), 2nd ed., pp. 1683–1709. Raven Press, New York.

Simerly, R. B., Swanson, L. W., and Gorski, R. A. (1985). The distribution of monoaminergic cells and fibers in a periventricular preoptic nucleus involved in the control of gonadotropin release: Immunohistochemical evidence for a dopaminergic sexual dimorphism. *Brain Res.* **330**, 55–64.

Simpkins, J. W., Kalra, P. S., and Kalra, S. P. (1980). Inhibitory effects of androgens on preoptic area dopaminergic neurons in castrated rats. *Neuroendocrinology* **31**, 177–181.

Simpkins, J. W., Kalra, S. P., and Kalra, P. S. (1983). Variable effects of testosterone on dopamine activity in several microdissected regions in the preoptic area and medial basal hypothalamus. *Endocrinology (Baltimore)* **112**, 665–669.

Simpson, E. R., Mahendroo, M. S., Means, G. D., Kilgore, M. W., Hinshelwood, M. M., Graham-Lorence, S., Amarneh, B., Ito, Y., Fisher, C. R., Michael, M. D., Mendelson, C. R., and Bulun, S. E. (1994). Aromatase cytochrome P450, the enzyme responsible for estrogen biosynthesis. *Endocr. Rev.* **15**, 342–355.

Simpson, S. M., and Follett, B. K. (1981). Pineal and hypothalamic pacemakers: Their role in regulating circadian rhythmicity in Japanese quail. *J. Comp. Physiol. A* **144**, 381–389.

Skynner, M. J., Sim, J. A., and Herbison, A. E. (1999). Detection of estrogen receptor a and b messenger ribonucleic acids in adult gonadotropin-releasing hormone neurons. *Endocrinology (Baltimore)* **140**, 5195–5201.

Slawski, B. A., and Buntin, J. D. (1995). Preoptic area lesions disrupt prolactin-induced parental feeding behavior in ring doves. *Horm. Behav.* **29**, 248–266.

Smith, G. T., Brenowitz, E. A., and Prins, G. S. (1996). Use of PG-21 immunocytochemistry to detect androgen receptors in the songbird brain. *J. Histochem. Cytochem.* **44**, 1075–1080.

Södersten, P. (1973). Estrogen-activated sexual behavior in male rats. *Horm. Behav.* **4**, 247–256.

Södersten, P., and Gustafsson, J.-Å. (1980a). Activation of sexual behavior in castrated rats with the synthetic androgen 17β-hydroxy-17α-methyl-estra-4,9,11-triene-3-one (R1881). *J. Endocrinol.* **87**, 279–283.

Södersten, P., and Gustafsson, J. A. (1980b). A way in which estradiol might play a role in the sexual behavior of male rats. *Horm. Behav.* **14**, 271–274.

Södersten, P., Eneroth, P., Mode, A., and Gustafsson, J.-Å. (1985). Mechanisms of androgen-activated sexual behaviour in rats. *In* "Neurobiology" (R. Gilles and J. Balthazart, eds.), pp. 48–59. Springer-Verlag, Berlin.

Södersten, P., Eneroth, P., Hansson, T., Mode, A., Johansson, D., Naslund, B., Liang, T., and Gustafsson, J. A. (1986). Activation of sexual behaviour in castrated rats: The role of oestradiol. *J. Endocrinol.* **111**, 455–462.

Soha, J. A., Shimizu, T., and Doupe, A. J. (1996). Development of the catecholaminergic innervation of the song system of the male zebra finch. *J. Neurobiol.* **29**, 473–489.

Sohrabji, F., Nordeen, K. W., and Nordeen, E. J. (1989). Projections of androgen-accumulating neurons in a nucleus controlling avian song. *Brain Res.* **488**, 253–259.

Soma, K. K., Bindra, R. K., Gee, J., Wingfield, J. C., and Schlinger, B. A. (1999a). Androgen-metabolizing enzymes show region-specific changes across the breeding season in the brain of a wild songbird. *J. Neurobiol.* **41**, 176–188.

Soma, K. K., Hartman, V. N., Wingfield, J. C., and Brenowitz, E. A. (1999b). Seasonal changes in androgen receptor immunoreactivity in the song nucleus HVc of a wild bird. *J. Comp. Neurol.* **409**, 224–236.

Soma, K. K., Sullivan, K., and Wingfield, J. (1999c). Combined aromatase inhibitor and antiandrogen treatment decreases territorial aggression in a wild songbird during the nonbreeding season. *Gen. Comp. Endocrinol.* **115**, 442–453.

Soma, K. K., Sullivan, K. A., Tramontin, A. D., Saldanha, C. J., Schlinger, B. A., and Wingfield, J. C. (2000). Acute and chronic effects of an aromatase inhibitor on territorial aggression in breeding and nonbreeding male song sparrows. *J. Comp. Physiol. A* **186**, 759–769.

Spanagel, R., and Weiss, F. (1999). The dopamine hypothesis of reward: Past and current status. *Trends Neurosci.* **22**, 521–527.

Steel, E. A., and Hinde, R. A. (1963). Hormonal control of brood patch and oviduct development in domesticated canaries. *J. Endocrinol.* **26**, 11–24.

Steimer, T. (1988). Aromatase activity in rat brain synaptosomes. Is an enzyme associated with the neuronal cell membrane involved in mediating non-genomic effects of androgens. *Eur. J. Neurosci., Suppl.*, p. 9.

Steimer, T., and Hutchison, J. B. (1980). Aromatization of testosterone within a discrete hypothalamic area associated with the behavioral action of androgen in the male dove. *Brain Res.* **192**, 586–591.

Steimer, T., and Hutchison, J. B. (1981a). Metabolic control of the behavioral action of androgens in the dove brain: Testosterone inactivation by 5β-reduction. *Brain Res.* **209**, 189–204.

Steimer, T., and Hutchison, J. B. (1981b). Androgen increases formation of behaviorally effective oestrogen in dove brain. *Nature (London)* **292**, 345–347.

Steimer, T., and Hutchison, J. B. (1991). Micromethods for the in vitro study of steroid metabolism in the brain using radiolabelled tracers. *In* "Neuroendocrine Research Methods" (B. Greenstein, ed.), Vol. 2, pp. 875–919. Harwood Academic Publishers, Chur, Switzerland.

Sterling, R. J., and Sharp, P. J. (1982). The localization of LH-RH neurones in the diencephalon of the domestic hen. *Cell Tissue Res.* **222**, 283–298.

Sterling, R. J., Gasc, J. M., Sharp, P. J., Tuohimaa, P., and Baulieu, E. E. (1987). The distribution of nuclear progesterone receptor in the hypothalamus and forebrain of the domestic hen. *Cell Tissue Res.* **248**, 201–205.

Stettenheim, P. (1972). The integument of birds. *Avian Biol.* **2**, 1–63.

Stokes, T. M., Leonard, C. M., and Nottebohm, F. (1974). The telencephalon, diencephalon, and mesencephalon of the canary, *Serinus canaria*, in stereotaxic coordinates. *J. Comp. Neurol.* **156**, 337–374.

Storey, C. R., and Nicholls, T. J. (1983). Responses of photosensitive and photorefractory intact and castrated male canaries *Serinus canarius* to treatment with synthetic mammalian luteinizing releasing-hormone. *Ibis* **125**, 228–234.

Striedter, G. F., and Vu, E. T. (1998). Bilateral feedback projections to the forebrain in the premotor network for singing in zebra finches. *J. Neurobiol.* **34,** 27–40.

Stuchbury, B. J., Rhymer, J., and Morton, E. S. (1994). Extrapair paternity in hooded warblers. *Behav. Ecol.* **5,** 384–392.

Stumpf, W. E., and Sar, M. (1978). Anatomical distribution of estrogen, androgen, progestin, corticoid and thyroid hormone target sites in the brain of mammals: Phylogeny and ontogeny. *Am. Zool.* **18,** 435–445.

Stupnicka, E., Massa, R., Zanisi, M., and Martini, L. (1977). Role of anterior pituitary and hypothalamic metabolism of progesterone in the control of gonadotropin secretion. *Prog. Reprod. Biol.* **2,** 88–95.

Sun, S. S., and El Halawani, M. E. (1995). Protein kinase-C mediates chicken vasoactive intestinal peptide-stimulated prolactin secretion and gene expression in turkey primary pituitary cells. *Gen. Comp. Endocrinol.* **99,** 289–297.

Takahashi, J. S., and Menaker, M. (1982). Role of the suprachiasmatic nuclei in the circadian system of the house sparrow. *J. Neurosci.* **2,** 815–822.

Takeda, H., Chodak, G., Mutchnik, S., Nakamoto, T., and Chang, C. (1990). Immunohistochemical localization of androgen receptors with mono- and polyclonal antibodies to androgen receptor. *J. Endocrinol.* **126,** 17–25.

Tan, J.-A., Joseph, D. R., Quarmby, V. E., Lubahn, D. B., Sar, M., French, F. S., and Wilson, E. M. (1988). The rat androgen receptor: Primary structure, autoregulation of its messenger ribonucleic acid, and immunocytochemical localization of the receptor protein. *Mol. Endocrinol.* **2,** 1276–1285.

Taylor, C. W., and Broad, L. M. (1998). Pharmacological analysis of intracellular Ca^{2+} signalling: Problems and pitfalls. *Trends Pharmacol. Sci.* **19,** 370–375.

Tchernichovski, O., Schwabl, H., and Nottebohm, F. (1998). Context determines the sex appeal of male zebra finch song. *Anim. Behav.* **55,** 1003–1010.

Thieuland, M. L., Samperez, S., and Jouan, P. (1981). Evidence of 5α-androstane-3β,17β-diol binding to the estrogenreceptor in the cytosol of male rat pituitary. *Endocrinology (Baltimore)* **108,** 1552–1560.

Thieuland, M. L., Benie, T., and Jouan, P. (1982). Ontogeny of 5α-androstane-3β,17β-diol and 17β-estradiol binding to cytoplasm and nuclei of the male rat pituitary. *Endocrinology (Baltimore)* **110,** 1300–1307.

Thieuland, M. L., Benie, T., Michaud, S., Klein, H., and Vessieres, A. (1983). Binding and effects of 5α-androstane-3β,17β-diol in the male rat pituitary. *J. Steroid. Biochem.* **19,** 241–246.

Thompson, M. A., Wooley, D. E., Gietzen, D. W., and Conway, S. (1983). Catecholamine synthesis inhibitors acutely modulate [^{3}]estradiol binding by specific brain areas and pituitary in ovariectomized rats. *Endocrinology (Baltimore)* **113,** 855–865.

Thompson, R. R., Goodson, J. L., Ruscio, M. G., and Adkins-Regan, E. (1995). Damage to the telencephalic nucleus taeniae disrupts sexual approach behavior in male Japanese quail. *Soc. Neurosci. Abstr.* **21,** 1463.

Thompson, R. R., Goodson, J. L., Ruscio, M. G., and Adkins-Regan, E. (1998). Role of the archistriatal nucleus taeniae in the sexual behavior of male Japanese quail (*Coturnix japonica*): A comparison of function with the medial nucleus of the amygdala in mammals. *Brain, Behav. Evol.* **51,** 215–229.

Thompson, T. L., and Moss, R. L. (1994). Estrogen regulation of dopamine release in the nucleus accumbens: Genomic- and nongenomic-mediated effects. *J. Neurochem.* **62,** 1750–1756.

Thrun, L. A., Dahl, G. E., Evans, N. P., and Karsch, F. J. (1996). Time-course of thyroid-hormone involvement in the development of anestrus in the ewe. *Biol. Reprod.* **55,** 833–837.

Thrun, L. A., Dahl, G. E., Evans, N. P., and Karsch, F. J. (1997). A critical period for thyroid hormone action on seasonal changes in reproductive neuroendocrine function in the ewe. *Endocrinology (Baltimore)* **138,** 3402–3409.

Timberlake, W., and Silva, K. M. (1995). Appetitive behavior in ethology, psychology, and behavior systems. In "Perspectives in Ethology Behavioral Design" (N. S. Thompson, ed.), Vol. 2, pp. 211–253. Plenum Press, New York.

Timmers, R. J. M., and Lambert, J. G. D. (1989). Catechol-o-methyltransferase in the brain of the male african catfish, Clarias gariepinus; distribution and significance for the metabolism of catecholstrogens and dopamine. *Fish Physiol. Biochem.* **7,** 201–210.

Timmers, R. J. M., Granneman, J. C. M., Lambert, J. G. D., and van Oordt, P. G. W. J. (1988). Estrogen-2-hydroxylase in the brain of the male African catfish, *Clarias gariepinus. Gen. Comp. Endocrinol.* **72,** 190–203.

Tinbergen, N. (1951). "The Study of Instinct." Clarendon Press, Oxford.

Tlemçani, O., Ball, G. F., D'Hondt, E., Vandesande, F., Sharp, P. J., and Balthazart, J. (2000). Fos induction in the Japanese quail brain after expression of appetitive and consummatory aspects of male sexual behavior. *Brain Res. Bull.* **52,** 249–262.

Tobet, S. A., and Fox, T. O. (1992). Sex differences in neuronal morphology influenced hormonally throughout life. In "Handbook of behavioral neurobiology" (A. A. Gerall, H. Moltz, and I. L. Ward, eds.), Vol. 11, pp. 41–83. Plenum Press, New York.

Tobet, S. A., Baum, M. J., Tang, H. B., Shim, J. H., and Canick, J. A. (1985). Aromatase activity in the perinatal forebrain: Effects of age, sex and intrauterine position. *Dev. Brain Res.* **23,** 171–178.

Toma, Y., Higashiyama, T., Yarborough, C., and Osawa, Y. (1996). Diverse functions of aromatase: O-deethylation of 7-ethoxycoumarin. *Endocrinology (Baltimore)* **137,** 3791–3796.

Tremblay, G. B., Tremblay, A., Copeland, N. G., Gilbert, D. J., Jenkins, N. A., Labrie, F., and Giguère, V. (1997). Cloning, chromosomal localization, and functional analysis of the murine estrogen receptor beta. *Mol. Endocrinol.* **11**, 353–365.

Trivers, R. L. (1972). Parental investment and sexual selection. In "Sexual Selection and the Descent of Man" (B. G. Campbell, ed.), pp. 136–179. Aldine, Chicago.

Tsuruo, Y., Ishimura, K., and Osawa, Y. (1995). Presence of estrogen receptors in aromatase-immunoreactive neurons in the mouse brain. *Neurosci. Lett.* **195**, 49–52.

Tsuruo, Y., Ishimura, K., Hayashi, S., and Osawa, Y. (1996). Immunohistochemical localization of estrogen receptors within aromatase-immunoreactive neurons in the fetal and neonatal rat brain. *Anat. Embryol.* **193**, 115–121.

Underwood, H. S., Binkley, S., Siopes, T., and Mosher, K. (1984). Melatonin rhythms in the eyes, pineal bodies, and blood of Japanese quail (*Coturnix coturnix japonica*). *Gen. Comp. Endocrinol.* **56**, 70–81.

Van Gils, J., Absil, P., Grauwels, L., Moons, L., Vandesande, F., and Balthazart, J. (1993). Distribution of luteinizing hormone-releasing hormones I and II (LHRH-I and -II) in the quail and chicken brain as demonstrated with antibodies directed against synthetic peptides. *J. Comp. Neurol.* **334**, 304–323.

Van Laar, J. H., Voorhorst-Ogink, M. M., Zegers, N. D., Boersma, W. J. A., Claassen, E., Van der Korput, J. A. G. M., De Winter, J. A. R., Van der Kwast, T. H., Mulder, E., Trapman, J., and Brinkmann, A. O. (1989). Characterization of polyclonal antibodies against the N-terminal domain of the human androgen receptor. *Mol. Cell. Endocrinol.* **67**, 29–38.

Verhoeven, G. (1980). Effect of neurotransmitters and follicle-stimulating hormone on the aromatization of androgens and the production of 3′,5′-monophosphate by cultured testicular cells. *J. Steroid Biochem.* **12**, 315–322.

Verhoeven, G. P., Dierckx, P., and de Moor, P. (1979). Stimulation effect of neurotransmitters on the aromatization of testosterone by Sertoli cell-enriched cultures. *Mol. Cell. Endocrinol.* **13**, 241–253.

Viglietti-Panzica, C. (1986). Immunohistochemical study of the distribution of vasotocin reacting neurons in avian diencephalon. *J. Hirnforsch.* **27**, 559–566.

Viglietti-Panzica, C., and Panzica, G. C. (1991). Peptidergic neurons in the avian brain. *Ann. Sci. Nat. Zool. Biol. Anim.* **12**, 137–155.

Viglietti-Panzica, C., Panzica, G. C., Fiori, M. G., Calcagni, M., Anselmetti, G. C., and Balthazart, J. (1986). A sexually dimorphic nucleus in the quail preoptic area. *Neurosci. Lett.* **64**, 129–134.

Viglietti-Panzica, C., Anselmetti, G. C., Balthazart, J., Aste, N., and Panzica, G. C. (1992). Vasotocinergic innervation of the septal region in the Japanese quail: Sexual differences and the influence of testosterone. *Cell Tissue Res.* **267**, 261–265.

Viglietti-Panzica, C., Aste, N., Balthazart, J., and Panzica, G. C. (1994). Vasotocinergic innervation of sexually dimorphic medial preoptic nucleus of the male Japanese quail: Influence of testosterone. *Brain Res.* **657**, 171–184.

Vockel, A., Pröve, E., and Balthazart, J. (1988). Changes in the activity of testosterone-metabolizing enzymes in the brain of male and female zebra finches during the post-hatching period. *Brain Res.* **463**, 330–340.

Vockel, A., Pröve, E., and Balthazart, J. (1990a). Effects of castration and testosterone treatment on the activity of testosterone-metabolizing enzymes in the brain of male and female zebra finches. *J. Neurobiol.* **21**, 808–825.

Vockel, A., Pröve, E., and Balthazart, J. (1990b). Sex- and age-related differences in the activity of testosterone-metabolizing enzymes in microdissected nuclei of the zebra finch brain. *Brain Res.* **511**, 291–302.

Voorhuis, T. A. M., and de Kloet, E. R. (1992). Immunoreactive vasotocin in the zebra finch brain (*Taeniopygia guttata*). *Dev. Brain Res.* **69**, 1–10.

Voorhuis, T. A. M., Kiss, J. Z., de Kloet, E. R., and de Wied, D. (1988). Testosterone-sensitive vasotocin-immunoreactive cells and fibers in the canary brain. *Brain Res.* **442**, 139–146.

Voorhuis, T. A. M., de Kloet, E. R., and de Wied, D. (1991). Effect of a vasotocin analog on singing behavior in the canary. *Horm. Behav.* **25**, 549–559.

Vreeburg, J. T. M., Schretlen, P. J. M., and Baum, M. J. (1975). Specific, high affinity binding of 17β-estradiol in cytosols from several brain regions and pituitary of intact and castrated adult male rats. *Endocrinology (Baltimore)* **97**, 969–977.

Wada, M. (1982). Effects of sex steroids on calling, locomotor activity, and sexual behavior in castrated male Japanese quail. *Horm. Behav.* **16**, 147–157.

Wada, M. (1993). Low temperature and short days together induce thyroid activation and suppression of LH release in Japanese quail. *Gen. Comp. Endocrinol.* **90**, 355–363.

Wada, Y., Okano, T., Adachi, A., Ebihara, S., and Fukada, Y. (1998). Identification of rhodopsin in the pigeon deep brain. *FEBS Lett.* **42**, 53–56.

Wada, Y., Okano, T., and Fukada, Y. (2000). Phototransduction molecules in the pigeon deep brain. *J. Comp. Neurol.* **428**, 138–144.

Walters, M. J., and Harding, C. F. (1988). The effects of an aromatization inhibitor on the reproductive behavior of male zebra finches. *Horm. Behav.* **22**, 207–218.

Walters, M. J., McEwen, B. S., and Harding, C. F. (1988). Estrogen receptor levels in hypothalamic and vocal control nuclei in the male zebra finch. *Brain Res.* **459**, 37–43.

Warren, R. P., and Hinde, R. A. (1961). Does the male stimulate oestrogen secretion in female canaries? *Science* **133**, 1354–1355.

Waterhouse, B. D., Sessler, F. M., Cheng, J.-T., Woodward, D. J., Azizi, S. A., and Moises, H. C. (1988). New evidence for a gating action of norepinephrine in central neuronal circuits of mammalian brain. *Brain Res. Bull.* **21**, 425–432.

Watson, J. T. (1989). Neuroanatomical localization of endocrine control of reproductive behavior in the Japanese quail (*Coturnix japonica*). Ph.D. Thesis, Cornell University, Ithaca, NY.

Watson, J. T., and Adkins-Regan, E. (1989a). Activation of sexual behavior by implantation of testosterone propionate and estradiol benzoate into the preoptic area of the male Japanese quail (*Coturnix japonica*). *Horm. Behav.* **23**, 251–268.

Watson, J. T., and Adkins-Regan, E. (1989b). Neuroanatomical localization of sex steroid-concentrating cells in the Japanese quail (*Coturnix japonica*): Autoradiography with [^{3}H]-testosterone, [^{3}H]-estradiol, and [^{3}H]-dihydrotestosterone. *Neuroendocrinology* **49**, 51–64.

Watson, J. T., and Adkins-Regan, E. (1989c). Testosterone implanted in the preoptic area of male Japanese quail must be aromatized to activate copulation. *Horm. Behav.* **23**, 432–447.

Weindl, A., and Sofroniew, M. V. (1982). Peptide neurohormones and cirumventricular organs in the pigeon. *Front. Horm. Res.* **9**, 88–104.

Weiner, N. (1974). A critical assessment of methods for the determination of monoamine synthesis turnover rates in vivo. *Adv. Biochem. Pharmacol.* **12**, 143–159.

Weiner, R. I., Findell, P. R., and Kordon, C. (1988). Role of classic and peptide neuromediators in the neuroendocrine regulation of LH and prolactin. *In* "The Physiology of Reproduction" (E. Knobil, J. Neill, *et al.*, eds.), pp. 1235–1281. Raven Press, New York.

Wenkstern, D., Pfaus, J. G., and Fibiger, H. C. (1993). Dopamine transmission increases in the nucleus accumbens of male rats during their first exposure to sexually receptive female rats. *Brain Res.* **618**, 41–46.

Wenzel, B. M. (1973). Chemoreception. *Avian Biol.* **3**, 389–415.

Wersinger, S. R., Baum, M. J., and Erskine, M. S. (1993). Mating-induced FOS-like immunoreactivity in the rat forebrain: A sex comparison and a dimorphic effect of pelvic nerve transection. *J. Neuroendocrinol.* **5**, 557–568.

Westneat, D. F. (1990). Genetic parentage in indiog buntings: A study using DNA fingerprinting. *Behav. Ecol. Sociobiol.* **27**, 67–76.

Westneat, D. F., Sherman, P. W., and Morton, M. L. (1990). The ecology and evolution of extra-pair copulations in birds. *Curr. Ornithol.* **7**, 331–369.

Wetherbee, D. K. (1961). Investigations of the life history of the common Coturnix. *Am. Midl. Nat.* **65**, 168–186.

White, S. J. (1975a). Effects of stimuli emanating from the nest on the reproductive cycle in the ring dove. I. Pre-laying behavior. *Anim. Behav.* **23**, 854–868.

White, S. J. (1975b). Effects of stimuli emanating from the nest on the reproductive cycle in the ring dove. II. Building during the pre-laying period. *Anim. Behav.* **23**, 869–882.

White, S. J. (1975c). Effects of stimuli emanating from the nest on the reproductive cycle in the ring dove. III. Building inthe post-laying period and effects on the success of the cycle. *Anim. Behav.* **23**, 883–888.

Whitsett, J. M., Irvin, E. W., Edens, F. W., and Thaxton, J. P. (1977). Demasculinization of male Japanese quail by prenatal estrogen treatment. *Horm. Behav.* **8**, 254–263.

Wickelgren, I. (1997). Getting the brain's attention. *Science* **278**, 35–37.

Wieselthier, A. S., and Van Tienhoven, A. (1972). The effect of thyroidectomy on testicular size and on the photorefractory period in the starling (*Sturnus vulgaris* L.). *J. Exp. Zool.* **179**, 331–338.

Wilczynski, W., Allsion, J. D., and Marler, C. A. (1993). Sensory pathways linking social and environmental cues to endocrine control regions of amphibian forebrains. *Brain, Behav. Evol.* **42**, 252–264.

Wild, J. M. (1997). Neural pathways for the control of birdsong production. *J. Neurobiol.* **33**, 653–670.

Wilson, F. E. (1985a). Androgen feedback-dependent and -independent control of photoinduced LH secretion in male tree sparrows (*Spizella arborea*). *J. Endocrinol.* **105**, 141–152.

Wilson, F. E. (1985b). An androgen-independent mechanism maintains photorefractoriness in male tree sparrrows (*Spizella arborea*). *J. Endocrinol.* **107**, 137–143.

Wilson, F. E. (1989). Extraocular control of photorefractoriness in American tree sparrows (*Spizella arobrea*). *Biol. Reprod.* **41**, 111–116.

Wilson, F. E. (1991). Neither retinal nor pineal photoreceptors mediate photoperiodic control of seasonal reproduction in American tree sparrows (*Spizella arborea*). *J. Exp. Zool.* **259**, 117–127.

Wilson, F. E., and Donham, R. S. (1988). Daylength and control of seasonal reproduction in male birds. *In* "Processing of Environmental Information in Vertebrates" (M. H. Stetson, ed.), pp. 101–120. Springer-Verlag, Berlin.

Wilson, F. E., and Reinert, B. D. (1996). The timing of thyroid-dependent programming in seasonally breeding male American tree sparrows (*Spizella arborea*). *Gen. Comp. Endocrinol.* **103**, 82–92.

Wingfield, J. C. (1980). Fine temporal adjustments of reproductive function. *In* "Avian Endocrinology" (A. Epple and M. H. Stetson, eds.), pp. 367–389. Academic Press, New York.

Wingfield, J. C. (1983). Environmental and endocrine control of reproduction: An ecological approach. In "Avian Endocrinology: Environmental and Ecological Perspectives" (S. I. Mikami, K. Homma, and M. Wada, eds.), pp. 265–288. Springer-Verlag, Berlin.

Wingfield, J. C., and Farner, D. S. (1976). Avian endocrinology—field investigations and methods. *Condor* **78**, 570–573.

Wingfield, J. C., and Farner, D. S. (1980). Control of seasonal reproduction in temperate-zone birds. *Prog. Reprod. Biol.* **5**, 62–101.

Wingfield, J. C., and Farner, D. S. (1993). Endocrinology of reproduction in wild species. *Avian Biol.* **9**, 163–327.

Wingfield, J. C., and Goldsmith, A. R. (1990). Plasma levels of prolactin and gonadal steroids in relation to multiple-brooding and renesting in free-living populations of the song sparrow, *Melospiza melodia. Horm. Behav.* **24**, 89–103.

Wingfield, J. C., and Kenagy, G. J. (1991). Natural regulation of reproductive cycles. In "Vertebrate Endocrinology: Fundamental and Biomedical Implications" (P. Pang and M. Schreibman, eds.), Vol. 4, Part B, pp. 181–241. Academic Press, San Diego, CA.

Wingfield, J. C., and Moore, M. C. (1987). Hormonal, social, and environmental factors in the reproductive biology of free-living male birds. In "Psychobiology of Reproductive Behavior: An Evolutionary Perspective" (D. Crews, ed.), pp. 148–175. Prentice-Hall, Englewood Cliffs, NJ.

Wingfield, J. C., Crim, J. W., Mattocks, P. W., and Farner, D. S. (1979). Responses of photosensitive and photorefractory male white-crowned sparrows (*Zonotrichia leucophrys gambelii*) to synthetic mammalian luteinizing hormone releasing hormone (Syn-LHRH). *Biol. Reprod.* **21**, 801–806.

Wingfield, J. C., Ball, G. F., Dufty, A. M., Hegner, R. E., and Ramenofsky, M. (1987). Testosterone and aggression in birds: Tests of the "challenge" hypothesis. *Am. Sci.* **75**, 602–608.

Wingfield, J. C., Hahn, T. P., Levin, R., and Honey, P. (1992). Environmental predictabiligy and control of gonadal cycles in birds. *J. Exp. Zool.* **261**, 214–231.

Wingfield, J. C., Hahn, T. P., Wada, M., and Schoech, S. J. (1997). Effects of day length and temperature on gonadal development, body mass, and fat depots in white-crowned sparrows, *Zonotrichia leucophrys pugetensis. Gen. Comp. Endocrinol.* **107**, 44–62.

Wise, R. A., and Rompre, P. P. (1989). Brain dopamine and reward. *Annu. Rev. Psychol.* **40**, 191–225.

Wood, R. I., and Newman, S. W. (1995a). Androgen and estrogen receptors coexist within individual neurons in the brain of the Syrian hamster. *Neuroendocrinology* **62**, 487–497.

Wood, R. I., and Newman, S. W. (1995b). Integration of chemosensory and hormonal cues is essential for mating in the male Syrian hamster. *J. Neurosci.* **15**, 7261–7269.

Wood, R. I., and Newman, S. W. (1995c). The medial amygdaloid nucleus and medial preoptic area mediate steroidal control of sexual behavior in the male Syrian hamster. *Horm. Behav.* **29**, 338–353.

Wood-Gush, D. G. M., and Gilbert, A. B. (1964). The control of the nesting behavior of the domestic hen. II. The role of the ovary. *Anim. Behav.* **12**, 451–453.

Wood-Gush, D. G. M., and Gilbert, A. B. (1970). The nesting behavior of hens with ovarian transplants. *Anim. Behav.* **18**, 52–54.

Wood-Gush, D. G. M., and Gilbert, A. B. (1973). Some hormones involved in the nesting behavior of hens. *Anim. Behav.* **21**, 98–103.

Wood-Gush, D. G. M., Langley, G. A. S., Leitch, A. F., Gentle, M. J., and Gilbert, A. B. (1977). An autoradiographic study of sex steroids in the chicken telencephalon. *Gen. Comp. Endocrinol.* **31**, 161–168.

Woodward, D. J., Moises, H. C., Waterhouse, B. D., Yeh, H. H., and Cheun, J. E. (1991). Modulatory actions of norepinephrine on neural circuits. *Adv. Exp. Med. Biol.* **287**, 193–208.

Wu, L. G., and Saggau, P. (1997). Presynaptic inhibition of elicited neurotransmitter release. *Trends Neurosci.* **20**, 204–212.

Yahr, P. (1979). Data and hypotheses in tales of dihydrotestosterone. *Horm. Behav.* **13**, 92–96.

Yazaki, Y., Matsushima, T., and Aoki, K. (1995). The role of the mesencephalic call region in the Japanese quail chick. In "Nervous Systems and Behavior. Proceedings of the 4th International Congress of Neuroethology" (M. Burrows, T. Matheson, P. L. Newland, and H. Schuppe, eds.), pp. 319. Thieme, Stuttgart and New York.

Yazaki, Y., Matsushima, T., and Aoki, K. (1997). Testosterone modulates calling behavior in Japanese quail chicks. *Zool. Sci.* **14**, 219–225.

Yazaki, Y., Yamamoto, K., Matsushima, T., and Aoki, K. (1998). Non-genomic action of testosterone mediates avian vocal behavior. *Proc. Jpn. Acad.* **74**, 132–135.

Yazaki, Y., Matsushima, T., and Aoki, K. (1999). Testosterone modulates stimulation-induced calling behavior in Japanese quails. *J. Comp. Physiol. A* **184**, 13–19.

Yokosuka, M., Okamura, H., and Hayashi, S. (1994). Immunohistochemical detection of estrogen receptor and aromatase in the developing rat brain. *Neurosci. Res., Suppl.* **19**, S127.

Yokoyama, K., Farner, D. S. (1976). Photoperiodic responses in bilaterally enucleated female white-cronwed sparrows, *Zonotrichia lechophrys gambelii. Gen. Comp. Endocrinol.* **30**, 528–533.

Yokoyama, K., Oksche, A., Darden, T., and Farner, D. S. (1978). The sites of encephalic photoreception in photoperiodic induction of the growth of the testis in the white-crowned sparrow. *Cell Tissue Res.* **189**, 441–467.

Yoshimura, T., Suzuki, Y., Makino, E., Yasuo, S., Yokota, Y., and Ebihara, S. (2000). Molecular analysis of avian circadian clock. *Abstr. 7th Annu. Meet., Soc. Res. Biol. Rhythms.*

Youngren, O. M., Silsby, J. L., Rozenboim, I., Phillips, R. E., and El Halawani, M. E. (1994). Active immunization with vasoactive intestinal peptide prevents the secretion of prolactin induced by electrical stimulation of the turkey hypothalamus. *Gen. Comp. Endocrinol.* **95**, 330–336.

Zanisi, M., Messi, E., and Martini, L. (1984). Physiological role of 5α-reduced metabolites of progesterone. *In* "Metabolism of Hormonal Steroids in the Neuroendocrine Structures" (L. Martini, ed.), Vol. 13, pp. 171–183. Raven Press, New York.

Zeier, H., and Karten, H. J. (1971). The archistriatum of the pigeon: Organization of afferent and efferent connections. *Brain Res.* **31**, 313–326.

Zenone, P. G., Sims, M. E., and Erickson, C. J. (1979). Male ring dove behavior and the defense of genetic paternity. *Am. Nat.* **114**, 615–626.

Zigmond, R. E., Nottebohm, F., and Pfaff, D. W. (1973). Androgen-concentrating cells in the midbrain of a songbird. *Science* **179**, 1005–1007.

Zigmond, R. E., Detrick, R. A., and Pfaff, D. W. (1980). An autoradiographic study of the localization of androgen concentrating cells in the chaffinch. *Brain Res.* **182**, 369–381.

Neural and Hormonal Control of Birdsong

Barney A. Schlinger
Department of Physiological Science and Laboratory of Neuroendocrinology
Brain Research Institute
University of California
Los Angeles, California 90095

Eliot A. Brenowitz
Departments of Psychology and Zoology
Virginia Merrill Bloedel Hearing Research Center
University of Washington
Seattle, Washington 98195

Birdsong is a complex learned behavior performed by the oscine passerine birds. Birds sing in reproductive and aggressive contexts, but there is great diversity in song behavior across species, seasons, and sexes. Song learning and production are controlled by a collection of neural circuits, the song-control system, that is unique to this group of birds. The growth, maturation, and adult function of this circuit depends on hormonal signals, especially the reproductive steroid hormones. This chapter reviews studies of the neural control of song and functions of endocrine systems that influence the song-control system. They reveal how sex steroids can influence the development of motor and learning pathways and then stimulate plasticity of these circuits to modify song throughout adult life. Much of the observed behavioral diversity can be accounted for by age, sex, and seasonal differences in the neural distribution of steroid receptors or in the gonadal secretion of sex steroids. Songbirds may also synthesize steroids in nongonadal sites and use nontraditional steroids or cellular mechanisms to control song. The evolution in songbirds of multiple mechanisms to synthesize and respond to sex steroids contributes to a growing body of work expanding traditional concepts about the relationship between hormones, brain, and behavior.

I. INTRODUCTION

Birdsong is a complex form of acoustic communication performed by a vast number of individuals belonging to a large number of bird species. It is perhaps one of the most conspicuous hormone-dependent vertebrate behaviors of the natural world. A great deal is known about the neural circuitry underlying the learning and expression of song and how steroid hormones influence this circuitry, both during development and in adulthood, to define the quality, quantity, and timing of the songs that are ultimately expressed by adult birds. This system has become one of the best available to evaluate how the hormonal signaling molecules act on the central nervous system to control a complex vertebrate behavior.

The hormonal basis of birdsong was suspected quite early, when field ornithologists noted a relationship between the seasonal incidence of song and reproduction (Andrews, 1969; Armstrong, 1973; Catchpole and Slater, 1995). Since the late 1970s, research on this model has proliferated and investigations in the field have been supplemented with sophisticated analyses of hormone effects on song behavior, on the architecture of neural circuits, on neuronal gene expression, on neuronal replacement, and on neuronal electrophysiology.

Some of this research indicates that gonadal steroids alone may not fully organize or activate the song system. Consequently, a second significant research focus has been analyses of the synthesis, secretion, and metabolism of the hormones that are suspected of controlling song. In this chapter, we focus specifically on the role that the sex steroid hormones play in controlling anatomical and functional properties of the neural song system. We also describe the anatomical and functional properties of the endocrine systems that produce the neuroactive sex steroids. Numerous reviews already exist that provide separate coverage of avian endocrine systems, song behavior, and the neurobiology of song (Wingfield and Farner, 1993; Catchpole and Slater, 1995; Arnold, 1997; Bottjer and Johnson, 1997; Brenowitz, 1997; Schlinger, 1997, 1998; Ball, 2000). In the present review, we synthesize these three areas of investigation, with an emphasis on recent developments in the field.

A. Avian Systematics

There are approximately 9000 species of living birds. Approximately 5300 species belong to the order Passeriformes, which consists of the oscine suborder (the songbirds) and the suboscine suborder, which includes such birds as flycatchers, antbirds, cotingas, and pittids. The order is considered to be a single evolutionary lineage derived from a common ancestor (i.e., monophyletic), and the oscines and suboscines are each viewed as monophyletic lineages within the Passeriformes (Raikow, 1982; Sibley *et al.*, 1988). There are approximately 4000 species of songbirds, essentially all of which use vocalizations for communication. Within this large group of species, there is extensive taxonomic diversity in various aspects of vocal behavior including the timing of vocal learning, patterns of song production across the sexes, the number of songs that are learned (i.e., repertoire size), and the seasonality of song behavior. This diversity presents rich opportunities for comparative studies of the relationship between the structure and function of brain regions and song behavior.

B. Anatomy of the Song System and Mechanism of Song Production

Song behavior in songbirds is regulated by a discrete network of interconnected nuclei. Two pathways are

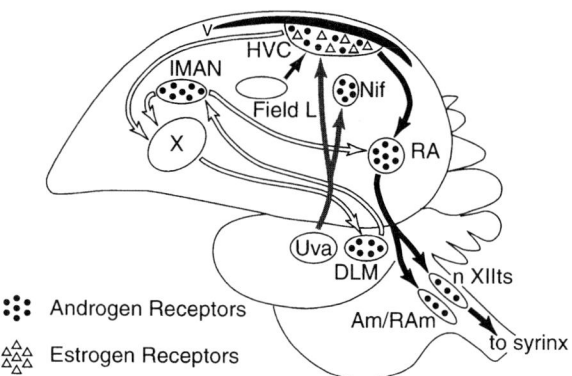

FIGURE 1 Sagittal schematic of the songbird brain showing projections of major nuclei in the song system and the distribution of steroid receptors. The descending motor pathway (black and dark grey arrows) controls the production of song. The dark grey arrows indicate inputs to HVc from the thalamic nucleus Uva and the neostriatal nucleus Nif. The black arrows indicate the descending projections from HVc in the neostriatum to RA in the archistriatum and thence to the vocal nucleus nXIIts, the respiratory nucleus RAm, and the laryngeal nucleus Am in the medulla. The white arrows indicate the anterior forebrain pathway that is essential for song learning. It indirectly links HVc to RA via area X in the parolfactory lobe, DLM in the thalamus, and lMAN in the neostriatum. lMAN also projects to area X. Field L is an auditory region in the neostriatum that projects to HVc (light grey arrow). Am, nucleus ambiguus; DLM, medial portion of the dorsolateral nucleus of the thalamus; HVc, high vocal center; lMAN, lateral portion of the magnocellular nucleus of the anterior neostriatum; Nif, nucleus interface; RA, robust nucleus of the archistriatum; RAm, nucleus retroambigualis; Uva, nucleus uvaeformis; V, ventricle; X, area X; nXIIts, tracheosyringeal part of the hypoglossal nucleus.

involved in song learning and production (Fig. 1). The motor pathway controls the production of song. This circuit consists of projections from the thalamic nucleus uvae formis (Uva) and the neostriatal nucleus interface (Nif) to the neostriatal nucleus HVc (also known as the high or higher vocal center). HVc projects to the robust nucleus of the archistriatum (RA) in the telencephalon, and RA projects both to the dorsomedial part of the intercollicular nucleus (ICo) in the midbrain (not shown in Fig. 1) and to the tracheosyringeal part of the hypoglossal motor nucleus in the brainstem (nXIIts). Motor neurons in nXIIts send their axons to the muscles of the sound-producing organ, the syrinx. When these motorneurons are stimulated, the syringeal muscles contract and move the medial and lateral labia into the expiratory airstream; this sets the labia into vibration to produce sound. The contraction of the syringeal muscles also changes the shape and length of the vocal tract, which can influence the frequency composition of sounds produced by the labia (Suthers *et al.*, 1999). The projection from RA onto the motor neurons in nXIIts is myotopically organized (Vicario, 1991). Neuronal activity in the premotor nuclei HVc and RA is synchronized with the production of sound by the syrinx (Yu and Margoliash, 1996). If nuclei in the motor pathway are inactivated, a bird may adopt appropriate posture and beak movements, but does not produce song (Nottebohm *et al.*, 1976).

RA also projects to nucleus retroambigualis (RAm) and nucleus ambiguus (Am) in the medulla. RAm contains many respiratory-related neurons that fire in phase with expiration. Am contains motoneurons that innervate the larynx. This pattern of descending projections from RA may be important for the coordination of syringeal, respiratory, and laryngeal muscle activity during song production. Birds only produce sound during expiration.

The second, anterior forebrain pathway is believed to be essential for song learning and recognition. This pathway consists of projections from the HVc to area X and then to the medial portion of the dorsolatenal nucleus of the thalamus (DLM), from the DLM to the lateral portion of the magnocellular nucleus of the anterior neostriatum (lMAN), and finally to the RA. In addition, lMAN neurons that project to the RA send collaterals to area X, thus providing the potential for feedback in this pathway. The projections in this pathway are topographically organized (Bottjer and Johnson, 1997). The inactivation of lMAN, DLM, or area X in adults apparently does not disrupt previously crystallized song, whereas the same lesions in juveniles prevent the development of normal song (Bottjer *et al.*, 1984; Sohrabji *et al.*, 1990; Scharff and Nottebohm, 1991; Hasema and Bottjer, 1992). Juvenile males with lesions of area X persist in producing songs that are plastic in structure, as though they are unable to crystallize. In contrast, if the lMAN is lesioned in juvenile males, they produce songs with aberrant but stable structure. Observations in adult island canaries (*Serinus canarius*), which can develop new songs as adults, appear consistent with results from juvenile zebra finches; lesions of the lMAN made in adult male canaries in mid-September, when song is seasonally plastic in structure, lead to a progressive decline in syllable diversity (Nottebohm *et al.*, 1990).

C. Song System of Male and Female Birds

Sexual patterns of song behavior vary extensively across songbird species. At one extreme are species such as the zebra finch and Carolina wren (*Thryothorus ludovicianus*), in which only males normally sing (Nottebohm and Arnold, 1976; Nealen and Perkel, 2000). At the other extreme are species such as the bay wren (*Thryothorus nigricapillus*) and buff-breasted wren (*Thryothorus leucotis*), in which males and females contribute equally to antiphonal song duets (Farabaugh, 1982; Levin, 1996a). Between these extremes are species in which female song is present but is typically less complex in structure and occurs less commonly than does male song. Examples of such species include the canary and the rufous-and-white wren (*Thryothorus rufalbus*) (Farabaugh, 1982; Pesch and Guttinger, 1985).

The variation among species in sexual patterns of song behavior is accompanied by a concomitant variation in the neural song-control system. In species in which only males sing, there are extreme sexual dimorphisms in the structure of the song nuclei. In female zebra finches, for example, there is not a well-defined area X, the remaining forebrain nuclei are much smaller, and HVc neurons do not form synaptic connections with RA neurons (Nottebohm and Arnold, 1976; Konishi and Akutagawa, 1985). Comparable patterns of sexual dimorphism are observed in the brains of other species in which only males sing (MacDougall-Shackleton and Ball, 1999; Nealen and Perkel, 2000). In those species in which females are able to sing, however, the brains of males and females have the same network of song nuclei (Nottebohm and Arnold, 1976; Brenowtz *et al.*, 1985; Brenowitz and Arnold, 1986; Brenowitz, 1997).

The degree to which the sexes of any species differ in the size of the song nuclei corresponds closely with the extent to which they differ in the complexity of song behavior. This relationship can be seen clearly when we compare closely related species that differ in the degree of sex differences in the occurrence and complexity of song behavior. An example of such a comparative analysis is illustrated in Fig. 2. It shows the male-to-female ratios of the volume of HVc in four species of wrens in the same taxonomic family (Certhiidae). In the marsh

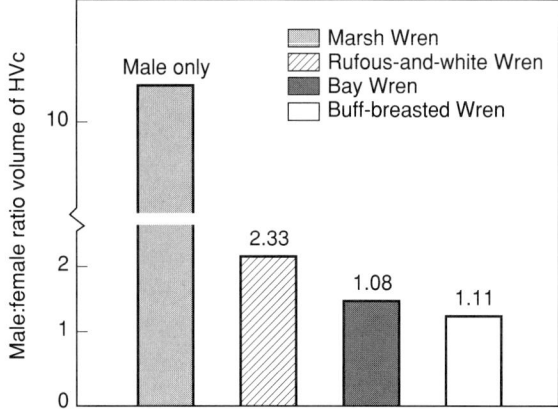

FIGURE 2 Male:female ratios for the volume of the song-control nucleus HVc in the marsh wren, rufous-and-white wren, bay wren, and buff-breasted wren. The labels above the bars refers to sex differences in song behavior for each species. In the marsh wren, only males sing. The label numbers above the bars for the other three species indicates the male:female ratio in the number of song types produced. This figure demonstrates that the extent of sexual dimorphism in the size of HVc is correlated with the extent to which the sexes of a species differ in the complexity of song behavior.

wren, only males sing (Brenowitz et al., 1994). Female rufous-and-white wrens of Central America routinely sing in duets with males, but males sing about twice as many different types of songs as do females (Farabaugh, 1982). In two other species of Central American wrens that sing duets, the bay wren and buff-breasted wren, there are no sex differences in the number of song types produced (Farabaugh, 1982; Levin, 1996b). As we proceed from the marsh wrens to the bay and buff-breasted wrens in this group, we find, therefore, a decreasing incidence of sex differences in song behavior.

Several interesting observations emerge from comparisons of the neural song-control systems of these four wren species. In the marsh wren, the nonsinging females have a much smaller HVc (and RA) and do not have a well-defined area X. In the rufous-and-white wren we see an intermediate degree of sexual dimorphism in the size of HVc and the other song nuclei that parallels the intermediate degree of sex difference in song behavior. In the bay and buff-breasted wrens, we find no sex differences in either the song nuclei of the brain or song behavior. The same pattern is observed for the number of neurons in these regions (Brenowitz et al., 1985, 1994; Brenowitz and Arnold, 1986; Brenowitz, 1997). This and other comparative analyses (MacDougall-Shackleton and Ball, 1999), therefore, support the hypothesis that the degree of sexual dimorphism present in the neural song-control system is related to the extent to which the sexes differ in the complexity of their song behavior.

D. Functional Significance of Birdsong

Song serves two main functions in birds (reviewed by Catchpole and Slater, 1995). It can play an important role in aggressive behavior, usually between members of the same sex. This function of song is most often seen in defense of a territory. The second main function of song occurs in the context of courtship. In most songbird species, males use song to attract females to their territories. Females may select among potential mates on the basis of individual song characteristics. The male's song may directly stimulate reproductive behavior in females. In addition to these two main functions, song may act in other behavioral contexts. For example, song may be important in mediating dominance behavior among members of a social group.

E. Song and the Seasons

Breeding occurs seasonally in most species of birds that live in temperate and subtropical latitudes. It generally occurs at times of the year when the resources necessary for successfully rearing offspring are most abundant. In such species, song is also seasonal in occurrence. Males sing at high rates early in the breeding season when they first establish territories. Once males have mated with one or more females, the rate of song production drops considerably. Outside the breeding season, males may sing only occasionally or not at all.

In tropical latitudes (23.5° N to 23.5° S), seasonal cycles in environmental factors are not as pronounced as at other latitudes. The availability of critical resources for rearing young birds, therefore, does not vary as much with season in the tropics. A consequence of this relative lack of seasonality is that breeding in many tropical species may occur at almost any time of the year. Birds of such species may defend territories and attempt to attract new mates throughout the year, and song production is often much less seasonal in occurrence than in temperate and subtropical species.

F. Song Learning

Vocal behavior occurs widely throughout the 23 taxonomic orders of birds. Song in the oscine Passeriformes is distinctive, however, because it is a learned behavior. Vocal learning is known to also occur only in two other groups of birds, the parrots and a species of hummingbird. If a young songbird is raised in isolation from other birds, he never produces a normal song (Thorpe, 1958; Marler, 1970). Some species of birds learn to sing only if they are exposed to song (either from a live tutor or from a tape recorder) during their first year of life. We refer to these species as age-limited learners. Male swamp sparrows, for example, must hear song between 10 and 60 days after hatching (Marler and Peters, 1982). With repeated exposure to the tutor song, males form a sensory memory or template of the song. At approximately 8 months of age, males first start to translate this sensory template into a motor program during the sensorimotor phase of song learning. Initially, a male sparrow emits sounds that bear only a remote resemblance to the tutor song. This first phase of subsong is marked by the production of crude sounds that are highly variable in structure. The young male improves his vocal performance during the next few months. With practice, he comes to produce more polished sounds that bear a closer resemblance to the tutor song. This period of plastic song begins at about 10 months of age and is marked by variability in the order in which song syllables are combined. Over the next 1–2 months, the male continues to improve his performance so that by 12 months of age he produces a crystallized song that has a well-defined invariant structure. This progressive improvement in performance of singing depends on the bird being able to hear himself sing. If a bird is deafened before the onset of subsong, he never develops the ability to produce normal song (Konishi, 1985).

In contrast to age-limited learners, other bird species are able to develop new songs even as adults beyond their first year. These species are referred to as open-ended learners. An example is the canary. A young male canary begins to produce subsong approximately 40 days after hatching (Nottebohm, 1987). Plastic song begins at approximately 60 days. A male starts to produce stereotyped adult song by approximately 8 months of age. Throughout the first breeding season, song remains stable in structure. After the breeding season ends, however, the song becomes extremely variable. In the late summer and early fall, the adult male's vocalizations are similar to those of juvenile subsong. During this period, some song syllables are lost from the bird's repertoire, others are modified, and new syllables may be added. The result is that by his second breeding season, the number of song syllables in a male's repertoire may increase by up to 40%.

G. General Anatomy and Function of the Hypothalamic-Pituitary-Gonadal Axis in Adult and Developing Songbirds

There is little unique about the hypothalamic-pituitary-gonadal (HPG) axis of songbirds compared to other vertebrates. Hypothalamic gonadotropin-releasing hormone (GnRH) stimulates anterior pituitary release of gonadotropins (luteinizing hormone, LH, and follicle-stimulating hormone, FSH) that stimulate gonadal growth, the secretion of several reproductive hormones including the sex steroids (testosterone, T, and estradiol, E_2), and the maturation and release of gametes (Marshall, 1961; Kobayashi, 1973; Lofts, 1973; Sherwood et al., 1988; Wingfield and Farner, 1993). Sex steroid synthesis occurs predominantly in the interstitial or Leydig cells of the testes and in the granulosa and theca cells of the ovarian follicle; hence, these cells are the targets of the pituitary gonadotropins. These steroids feed back onto the brain and pituitary to complete the axis circuit.

Many songbirds breed seasonally in response to changes in environmental cues such as photoperiod and food availability. In these species, the brain plays a considerable role in integrating environmental and internal cues, then activating the pituitary and gonads under appropriate conditions and allowing the reproductive system to regress when environmental conditions are not suited for breeding (Farner, 1986; Wingfield and Kenagy, 1991). In general, when the testes are stimulated by gonadotropins, the Leydig cells are large, numerous, and exhibit morphological properties consistent with steroidogenesis (Chan and Lofts, 1974; Lam and Farner, 1976; Rohss and Silverin, 1983;

Silverin and Sharp, 1996). However, circulating T levels do not always correlate well with blood levels of gonadotropins, or with testis size or Leydig cell morphology (e.g., Morton et al., 1990), suggesting that testicular steroid production is controlled by multiple mechanisms. Gonadotropins also stimulate a population of ovarian follicles that includes hypertrophy of the theca and granulosa cell layers and morphological changes associated with steroidogenesis (Lofts, 1973). Between the nonbreeding and breeding seasons, songbird ovaries may increase in size 175-fold and the testes 360-fold (Marshall, 1961; Lofts, 1973).

In many species, song production changes in parallel with the reproductive system, probably as a result of the concomitant flux in reproductive hormones. Thus, by accurately gauging environmental and social conditions, the brain allows for the expression of song at the most appropriate times of the year. There is evidence that the brain might respond to changing conditions and directly regulate song expression by routes independent of the HPG axis, but the underlying mechanisms are not well understood (Bernard et al., 1997; Smith et al., 1997b). Melatonin from the pineal gland, for example, may regulate song independently of gonadal hormones (Gahr and Kosar, 1996; Bentley et al., 1999).

We know very little about the HPG axis of developing birds, but given that gonadal steroids might play an important role in the growth of song-control neural circuitry (see later), the state of the HPG axis at this time has important implications for song. In a few species, plasma sex steroids have been measured after hatching (Hutchison et al., 1984; Weichel et al., 1986; Williams et al., 1987; Adkins-Regan et al., 1990; Schlinger et al., 1992; Silverin and Sharp, 1996), but the role of the brain and pituitary in regulating the developing gonads and the synthesis and secretion of sex steroid hormones is poorly understood. In the great tit (*Parus major*), although sex steroids are present in blood of nestlings at hatching, it is likely that the HPG axis only becomes fully functional after about 9 days posthatching (Silverin and Sharp, 1996). Castration of nestling 9-day-old males does not stimulate an increase in circulating LH, as would be expected if steroidal negative feedback on brain and pituitary GnRH and gonadotropin secretion was functional. Moreover, prior to day 9, GnRH neurons may not be positioned properly in the hypothalamus for activation of pituitary gonadotropes (Silver et al., 1992) and, at least in males, Leydig cells may still be in an immature state (Silverin and Sharp, 1996). Nevertheless, LH was found to circulate in parallel with gonadal steroids of both male and female nestlings, suggesting that the pituitary might exert some control over gonadal steroidogenesis at early ages, despite the immature morphology of the steroidogenic cells (Silverin and Sharp, 1996). It is unclear, therefore, whether the steroids in blood are from the gonads and, if they are, whether they are secreted upon stimulation by the brain and pituitary or produced by the gonads autonomously.

Gonadal steroids do not only activate song and other reproductive behaviors, but they also feed back onto the songbird brain, and possibly the pituitary, to regulate the secretion of GnRH and the gonadotropins (Lofts, 1973). In males it is likely that testicular androgens are first converted into estrogens in the hypothalamus and that it is the estrogens that serve to feedback negatively on GnRH release. Treatment with antiandrogens does not cause gonadotropin levels to rise (Searcy and Wingfield, 1980). By contrast, the treatment of intact male songbirds with drugs that inhibit aromatization causes androgen levels in blood to rise dramatically, suggesting the interruption of the negative feedback control of testicular androgen production (Schlinger et al., 1999; Soma et al., 2000a).

II. RELATIONSHIP OF SONG TO GONADAL HORMONES

A. Adult Song Expression

1. Studies Relating Reproductive Cycles to the Production of Birdsong

Singing activity is matched to annual reproductive cycles of songbirds (Armstrong, 1973; Catchpole and Slater, 1995). This is seen most clearly in birds breeding at high latitudes; reproduction is constrained to the late spring and early summer and song production is also generally maximal at this time. As previously stated, song functions in two major capacities, in aggressive territorial defense and in mate attraction and stimulation. Thus, song production often begins quite early in the breeding season soon after arrival on the breeding grounds by migrants, or even in mid- to late winter by residents. Song then continues until territories are established, mates are secured, and nesting is well underway, when singing decreases. If breeding fails or the opportunity arises for additional mating attempts song production may increase again (Armstrong, 1973; Slagsvold, 1977; Lampe and Espmark, 1987; Rost, 1992; Wada et al., 1999).

Although this general pattern of song activity holds true for many species, when song expression is examined on a finer scale, a more complex picture emerges. Song production can vary in a circadian pattern, often with maximal production at dawn and a second peak in the evening. Across the breeding cycle, some species sing different songs or vary elements of individual songs, suggesting that these songs have unique functions (Shiovitz, 1975; Richards, 1981; Kroodsma et al., 1989; Catchpole and Slater, 1995; Smith et al., 1997a). Some species sing similar amounts year round; others sing throughout the year but vary the amount of song with stages of reproduction (Nice, 1943; Lack, 1946; Armstrong, 1973; Silverin et al., 1986; Wingfield and Hahn, 1994). Arctic or high-altitude-breeding birds with very constrained breeding seasons may sing in significant amounts for only a few days or weeks (Hunt et al., 1995). Many species sing during periods of reproduction (spring and summer) and have a second phase of singing in the autumn, apparently as they establish winter territories and initiate the attraction of mates (Logan, 1992). In some species, only males sing, whereas in others females also sing, and the seasonal patterns of their song production can be as complex as those of males (Lack, 1946; Lowther, 1962; Beletsky, 1983; Ritchison, 1983, 1986; DeVoogd et al., 1995).

This pronounced diversity of song production underscores the principle that although sex steroid hormones may be critical for some aspect of the generation of song, there are likely to be multiple neural and hormonal signals that collectively influence song production. Moreover, the involvement of each of these mechanisms is likely to differ across species. Defining the specific role of sex steroids in the organization and activation of song has been a difficult task, contrasting somewhat from the more direct function of sex steroids in organizing and activating copulatory behaviors in rodents (Arnold and Schlinger, 1993).

2. Studies Relating Direct Measures of Circulating Hormones with Production of Birdsong

The complexity of song behavior notwithstanding, there is still considerable evidence that sex steroids do activate song expression. Some evidence comes from correlations between song output and levels of sex steroid hormones in blood, in particular plasma T levels. In some species, song is expressed only by adult males with elevated levels of circulating androgens and not by juveniles or females with low levels of circulating androgen. When androgens are elevated in young birds, they may sing (Silverin et al., 1986). In males, T levels generally rise at the onset of the breeding season, remain elevated as the birds breed, and then decline as reproduction terminates. An activational role for T is presumed to be important because song production often follows a strikingly similar pattern (Rost, 1990, 1992; Schwabl and Kriner, 1991; Smith et al., 1997a; Wada et al., 1999). Other sex steroids fluctuate seasonally in blood of male songbirds, such as dihydrotestosterone (DHT), E_2, and progesterone. DHT often circulates coordinately with T (Wingfield and Farner, 1993), so it may also contribute to song expression. Which steroids in blood naturally activate song is not known. Moreover, the ways in which the brain integrates sex steroid levels with additional stimuli to modulate song output is poorly understood.

3. Experimental Evidence Directly Linking Reproductive Hormones and Birdsong—Gonadectomy or Photoperiod-induced Gonadal Regression and Steroid Replacement

Experimental studies support the hypothesis derived from field observations that sex steroids, particularly T, regulate song behavior. The castration of males decreases or eliminates singing (Nottebohm, 1969, 1980b; Pröve, 1974; Arnold, 1975b; Heid et al., 1985), and T treatment of castrated or intact males can increase song production (Nottebohm, 1969, 1980b; Pröve, 1974; Arnold, 1975b; Searcy and Wingfield, 1980; Heid et al., 1985; Kroodsma, 1986; Hunt, 1997). In some species, adult females can be stimulated to sing by treatments with T (Shoemaker, 1939; Baldwin et al., 1940; Herrick and Harris, 1957; Baker and Cunningham, 1983). Song types can be influenced differently by sex steroids. Zebra finches, for example, sing two song types—directed song is thought to serve as a stimulus to females during courtship, whereas undirected song is produced in the absence of females. Directed song is thought to be more sensitive to stimulation by circulating androgens (Walters *et al.*, 1991) and, for full expression, may also require estrogens (see later).

4. Evidence of Gonad-Independent Song Expression

Although song is produced at the highest rate during periods of intense reproductive activity when gonadal sex steroids are elevated, songs are also produced during nonreproductive periods. As discussed previously, song is used, in part, in aggressive contexts, especially in territorial defense (Lack, 1946; Catchpole and Slater, 1995). Territory defense is most conspicuous during the breeding season, but many species use songs to defend territories year round, to defend separate feeding territories in the nonbreeding season, or to attract mates during the nonbreeding season (Lack, 1946; Hoelzel, 1986; Dittami, 1987; Kelsey, 1989; Dittami and Gwinner, 1990; Logan and Wingfield, 1990; Levin and Wingfield, 1992; Schwabl, 1992; Morton, 1996). There is some indication that plasma sex steroids can be elevated briefly at times to stimulate song production, especially in early autumn as defense of nonbreeding territories or the creation of dominance hierarchies are initiated (Lincoln *et al.*, 1980; Dawson, 1983; Schlinger, 1987; Silverin *et al.*, 1989; Rost, 1992). There is also evidence, however, for song production at times when the traditional circulating sex steroids, such as E_2, T, and DHT, are basal (Dittami and Gwinner, 1990; Logan and Wingfield, 1990; Gwinner *et al.*, 1994; Wingfield and Hahn, 1994; Smith *et al.*, 1997a).

In one subspecies of the North American song sparrow (*Melospiza melodia*), males and females actively defend feeding territories year round with a wide range of aggressive behaviors, including songs (Wingfield and Hahn, 1994). Simulated territorial intrusions were used to study aggression in these birds and involved placing a live caged male song sparrow into a territory together with tape-recorded song playbacks. In both the breeding and nonbreeding seasons, territorial birds responded within seconds, approached the caged bird, sang, and made hovering or darting flights toward the intruder. The only differences seen across the seasons were that during the nonbreeding season territories may have included one or more birds of the same or opposite sex (Wingfield and Monk, 1992) and that song rate and quality were reduced compared to the breeding season (Wingfield and Monk, 1994; Smith *et al.*, 1997a).

When observed during the breeding season, this kind of territorial aggression in many animals is associated with enlarged testes and elevated levels of circulating T (Wingfield and Marler, 1988). In nonbreeding song sparrows, however, the testes are regressed, and T, DHT, and E_2 are all present at basal levels in blood (<0.1 ng/ml; Wingfield and Hahn, 1994a; Smith *et al.*, 1997a; Soma and Wingfield, 1999). Furthermore, if these nonbreeding sparrows are castrated, they remain aggressive and continue to sing (Wingfield 1994).

We can conclude from these kinds of data that sex steroids do not control song or territorial aggression outside of the breeding season. In some cases, however, drugs that block sex steroid synthesis or sex steroid action significantly inhibit territorial aggression and song of nonbreeding birds. In one case, treatment for 30 days with a combination of androstratrienedione (ATD), an inhibitor of aromatase, and flutamide, an androgen-receptor blocker, inhibited all measures of winter territorial aggression (Soma *et al.*, 1999b). This experiment was particularly interesting because there is good evidence that T-induced aggression in breeding birds is mediated, at least in part, by local aromatization to E_2 (Archawaranon and Wiley, 1988; Schlinger and Callard, 1991; Walters and Harding, 1988). Treatments with flutamide alone did not reduce aggression in winter European robins (*Erithecus rubecula*; Schwabl and Kriner, 1991), perhaps because estrogens activate aggression in winter.

This conclusion is supported by studies in which nonbreeding song sparrows were treated with fadrozole, a potent aromatase inhibitor in songbirds (Wade *et al.*, 1994; Soma *et al.*, 2000a,b). The treatment of song sparrows for 10 days with fadrozole alone significantly reduced territorial aggression, an effect that was completely reversed by simultaneous treatment with a subcutaneous implant of E_2 (Soma *et al.*, 2000b) (Fig. 3). This result strongly supports the conclusion that sex steroids, specifically E_2, activate singing in winter song sparrows, despite basal levels of sex steroids in blood. In

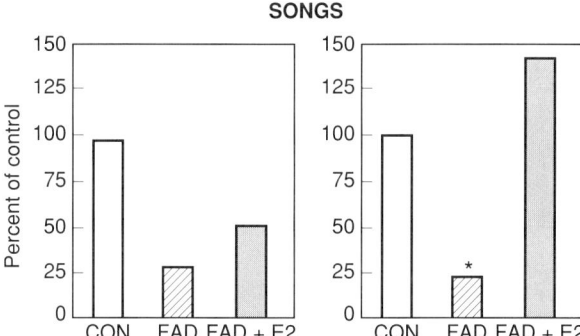

FIGURE 3 Effects of chronic (~10 days) fadrozole (FAD; an aromatase inhibitor) or fadrozole + E_2 treatment on song of adult male song sparrows stimulated by simulated territorial intrusions during the autumn nonbreeding season. Data are expressed as a percentage of the control mean. Compared to controls (CON), fadrozole significantly reduced aggression (not shown) and the rate of song ($*$, $p < 0.05$). From Soma et al. (2000a), with permission.

a second study, fadrozole reduced song within 24 hr after the start of treatment (Soma et al., 2000a). This kind of relatively rapid behavioral loss associated with estrogen removal is consistent with a the view that E_2 might act in part by a relatively rapid cellular mechanism to stimulate nonterritorial aggression and song. The paradoxical observation that E_2 activates winter aggression when circulating E_2 and its immediate androgenic substrates are basal suggests that the functional E_2 is not derived from the periphery but instead is synthesized directly in the brain. This issue is discussed more fully later.

B. Development of the Song System

1. Studies Relating Sex Steroids to Sexually Dimorphic Development of the Song System

In some songbirds, there is unequal performance of song between males and females, and measures of song-system morphology and biochemistry can correlate with vocal output. An extreme example is the zebra finch, a species in which adult males sing regularly, but adult females never sing. The song system of the male is substantially more developed than that of the female (Nottebohm and Arnold, 1976). (Gurney, 1981, 1982; Gurney and Konishi, 1980) reported that estrogens, and to a lesser degree androgens, stimulated masculine growth of the song system when they were injected into very young (posthatching) females. These effects of sex steroids are considerable, affecting not only the overall volumes of HVc, RA, area X, and lMAN, but also the numbers, sizes, biochemical properties, and connectivity of neurons in these nuclei (Arnold, 1992).

Estrogens may influence masculine growth of the song system by stimulating the synthesis, transport, and secretion of growth factors. In juvenile male zebra finches, brain-derived neurotrophic factor (BDNF) is synthesized in neurons of HVc and perhaps also lMAN (Johnson et al., 1997; Akutagawa and Konishi, 1998; Dittrich et al., 1999). Some of these neurons project to nucleus RA, where the release of BDNF may influence the formation of connections between these nuclei (Akutagawa and Konishi, 1998; Dittrich et al., 1999), perhaps in part by regulating neuron survival in nucleus RA (Johnson et al., 1997). BDNF expression in juvenile zebra finches appears to depend on estrogens. The treatment of males with E_2 prior to day 35 (when BDNF is normally first elevated in HVc) causes a transient increase in BDNF expression (Dittrich et al., 1999). This observation suggests that E_2 is naturally responsible for the up-regulation of BDNF seen in HVc of males at this time. E_2 appears to act even earlier to establish the estrogen-dependent increase in BDNF. BDNF in HVc is not up-regulated by E_2 in juvenile females, unless they are also treated with E_2 shortly after hatching (Dittrich et al., 1999), at ages when estrogens have their most potent and permanent masculinizing effects on song-system growth (Adkins-Regan and Ascenzi, 1987). These results establish an important relationship between E_2 and BDNF, one that may remain important in the adult brain in species that retain significant neural plasticity throughout life (Rasika et al., 1999).

The effectiveness of sex steroid treatments in masculinizing the song system of female zebra finches does not prove, however, that sex steroids normally stimulate masculine song system growth in males. Tests of this hypothesis have yielded ambiguous results (Schlinger, 1998) that are intriguing because the data both lend support for and argue against a significant role for sex steroids in song-system development. One possibility is that sex steroids act in synergy with nonsteroidal signals to produce a fully masculine song system (Schlinger, 1998; Gahr and Metzdorf, 1999).

Ideas derived from studies of any one species may be inadequate to fully describe the mechanisms used to create song systems if more than one mechanism is involved in the process of brain sexual differentiation. Studies of other species, therefore, would be useful, particularly of species in which song is expressed to different degrees by males and females. In some species, such as the canary, females can be stimulated to sing as adults, unlike female zebra finches. Normally, the song system of adult males canaries is much more fully developed than that of adult females. If treated with T, however, adult females can sing (Shoemaker, 1939; Baldwin et al., 1940; Herrick and Harris, 1957), and their song system shows marked growth as well (DeVoogd and Nottebohm, 1981). Hormonal effects on early song-system development have been examined in only one other bird, the European starling *(Sturnus vulgaris)*. This species offers a nice contrast to the zebra finch because both male and female starlings sing as adults, but females less so, and the volumes of the female song nuclei are about half the size of males (Bernard et al., 1993; Casto and Ball, 1996). These birds differ markedly from zebra finches in that the treatment of developing females with E_2 has minimal effects, only slightly masculinizing some song nuclei (Casto and Ball, 1996). The mechanisms controlling growth of the neural circuitry in this species remain unknown. Perhaps sex steroids act on the embryonic starling brain to stimulate growth of the song system. Alternatively, the song system may grow to masculine and feminine proportions independently of sex steroids. Clearly, much research remains to be done to answer these questions. This controversy is covered in greater detail elsewhere (Arnold, Chapter 63). In this section, we focus on what we know about the endocrine physiology of developing birds with respect to song-system development.

2. Measures of Endogenous Gonadal Steroids and Steroid Production and Song-System Development

To evaluate the endocrine basis of song-system development, concentrations of sex steroids have been measured in the blood of a few species at ages when the song system is presumably sensitive to their organizational actions. Songbirds are, for the most part, quite small and only small amounts of blood can, therefore, be collected from a given individual bird during posthatching ages of brain maturation. Sampling multiple birds and pooling blood is consequently often necessary. The practical difficulties of obtaining an adequate number of hatchlings mandates using a captive breeding songbird. For these reasons, the zebra finch has emerged as the leading model because it breeds prolifically in captivity and reaches sexual maturity at an early age (approximately 90 days posthatching).

Three studies measured plasma sex steroids in the blood of zebra finches in the first 3 weeks after hatching (Hutchison et al., 1984; Adkins-Regan et al., 1990; Schlinger and Arnold, 1992b), when the song system is apparently most sensitive to the organizational actions of these hormones (Adkins-Regan et al., 1994). Although all these studies found no significant differences in circulating androgens between males and females, they showed little agreement otherwise. Most noteworthy was evidence obtained by Hutchison and his colleagues (1984) that males had a surge of E_2 in their blood in the first week after hatching that was not seen in females. This result seemed to make sense at the time, because experiments with females showing that E_2 masculinized the song system (see previous discussion) suggested that males should have a sexually dimorphic estrogenic signal at this time. A second study, however, found no significant E_2 surge in young males (Adkins-Regan et al., 1990). A third study found a somewhat similar increase in estrone (E_1) in young males, but levels of E_1 were never significantly different from females nor was E_2 ever elevated (Schlinger and Arnold, 1992b). In summary, based on measures of circulating hormones, we are unable to conclude that there is a sexually dimorphic blood-borne estrogenic signal that might be responsible for masculinizing the neural song system of developing male zebra finches.

Indeed, subsequent studies investigating the steroidogenic potential of developing zebra finch tissues suggest that males lack the ability to synthesize significant amounts of estrogens peripherally (Cam and Schlinger, 1998; Freking et al., 2000). Males might still synthesize more estrogen than females, but might do so in the brain itself (see later).

3. Evidence Pointing to Gonad-Independent Sexual Differentiation of the Brain

In both birds and mammals, gonadal hormones are thought to be the key for sexually dimorphic phenotypic development, including the development of the brain (Goy and McEwen, 1980; Adkins, 1981; Arnold and Gorski, 1984; Balthazart and Ball, 1995; Schlinger, 1998). If male zebra finches do not secrete more estrogens or more aromatizable androgens than do females during sexual differentiation of the song system (Adkins-Regan et al., 1990; Schlinger and Arnold, 1992b; Cam and Schlinger, 1998; Freking et al., 2000), however, then the masculine state might develop independently of the gonads, perhaps by brain-autonomous mechanisms in males. A variety of studies now support this conclusion (see Arnold, Chap. 63 in this volume for thorough review). Some studies are quite convincing. For example, females treated very early in development with an aromatase inhibitor fail to grow ovaries but instead grow testes (up to 99% testicular tissue). Because they make sperm, and probably also male-typical steroids, they appear to be functional testes, residing in the body of genetic females (Wade and Arnold, 1996; Wade et al., 1996, 1997, 1999; Gong et al., 1999). Invariably, the neural song system of these birds is feminine, in keeping with their genetic sex but not their gonadal sex.

These results suggest that the gonads may not be required for sex-specific growth of the song system. But how do we interpret these results in light of the evidence that estrogens and androgens can masculinize properties of the song system of females? Several conclusions can be reached, including the possibility that sexual differentiation is only partly independent of gonadal steroids (discussed elsewhere). Another possibility is that sex steroids remain important for song-system growth, but they are not derived from the gonads. Evidence for adrenal and neural steroidogenesis (discussed later) lends some support for this hypothesis.

C. Song Learning

Sex steroids may also be important for song learning (Nottebohm, 1969), perhaps signaling the onset and termination of critical periods for learning. Interestingly, estrogens and androgens may have unique and opposing functions that might coordinate the maintenance of plasticity (estrogen) for new song learning and the termination of plasticity (androgen) to fix memory circuits to ensure appropriate song output (Bottjer and Johnson, 1997). A role for estrogen in plasticity associated with song learning was suspected initially when E_2 was found to circulate at high levels in the blood of juvenile song sparrows and swamp sparrows (Marler et al., 1987, 1988) at ages when birds are acquiring new song memories. E_2 levels then declined when the birds began to vocalize as young adults. Estrogen was further implicated in the song-learning process when blood levels of E_2 were observed to correlate with the degree of song learned by individual swamp sparrows (Marler et al., 1987). It is somewhat surprising to find sex steroids elevated at these ages, when the birds are not yet reproductive and are thought to be beyond the ages when steroids organize neural circuits. Conceivably the song system is uniquely sensitive to sex steroids, including during periods of song learning that extend for relatively prolonged periods of juvenile life. This suggests that the endocrine system has also evolved extended steroidogenesis to meet the demands of the appropriate steroid-dependent neural circuits.

Androgens, but not estrogens, seem responsible for fixing the learned components of song so they are available for the construction of stereotyped song output. If birds are castrated or treated with drugs that block androgen action, abnormal songs are produced that lack stereotypy (Arnold, 1975a; Kroodsma, 1986; Bottjer and Hewer, 1992). By contrast, if birds are treated with T before song learning is complete, an abnormal song is also generated, but in this case because the song crystallizes prematurely (Korsia and Bottjer, 1991; Whaling et al., 1995). The sources(s) of each type of sex steroid, androgen or estrogen, reaching song-learning neural circuits at the appropriate developmental stage is unknown. Enzymes that inactivate T or that potentiate the actions of T are expressed in the brains of juvenile songbirds in or around these learning circuits (Saldanha et al., 1999). But whether the gonads or other tissues synthesize and secrete androgens at these ages is unknown.

III. STEROID SENSITIVITY OF THE SONG SYSTEM

A. Evidence for Steroid Sensitivity of the Song-Control System

As previously discussed, gonadal steroid hormones have important effects on the development of the song circuits and the activation of song behavior. These hormones are also critical for seasonal changes in the morphology of the adult song circuits, as discussed later. The presence of gonadal steroid receptors in most of the song nuclei is consistent with the idea that these hormones act directly on the song nuclei to exert these effects.

B. Presence of Androgen Receptors and Estrgen Receptors in Song Nuclei of Adults

As do other vertebrates, songbirds have androgen receptors (AR) and estrogen receptors (ER) in diencephalic and mesencephalic structures, as well as in limbic regions of the telencephalon such as the hippocampus. Songbirds also evolved abundant expression of hormone receptors in nonlimbic regions of the telencephalon. AR are expressed at high levels in HVc, RA, lMAN, medial MAN (mMAN), and Nif in the telencephalon, and also in the midbrain vocal region ICo, nXIIts in the brain stem, and the muscles of the vocal production organ, the syrinx (Fig. 1). The presence of AR in these regions was first demonstrated with *in vivo* and *in vitro* steroid-binding methods (Arnold *et al.*, 1976; Arnold and Saltiel, 1979; Lieberburg and Nottebohm, 1979) and, subsequently, with immunocytochemistry (ICC) (Balthazart *et al.*, 1992; Smith *et al.*, 1996). The expression of the mRNA for the AR was shown in these nuclei using *in situ* hybridization methods (Nastiuk and Clayton, 1994; Gahr *et al.*, 1996; Gahr and Metzdorf, 1997; Bernard *et al.*, 1999; Metzdorf *et al.*, 1999). The message for AR is also expressed in the caudomedial neostriatum (NCM), a region thought to be involved in song memories, and in brain-stem respiratory nuclei that are connected to vocal nuclei (Gahr and Wild, 1997; Metzdorf *et al.*, 1999).

AR mRNA was reported to be expressed in low levels in area X of the song system in one study (Bernard *et al.*, 1999), but was not observed there in another study (Metzdorf *et al.*, 1999). The AR protein has not been detected in this nucleus with either steroid-binding methods or ICC (Arnold *et al.*, 1976; Balthazart *et al.*, 1992; Smith *et al.*, 1996). It is possible that steroid-binding methods are not sensitive enough to detect low levels of AR (Arnold, 1980), but ICC methods are less subject to this limitation.

ER are not as widely distributed in the song system as are AR. ER are present in HVc and ICo of all species of songbirds examined, as shown by both *in vivo* steroid-binding methods and ICC (Gahr *et al.*, 1987, 1993; Nordeen *et al.*, 1987; Brenowitz and Arnold, 1989). The abundance of ER in the HVc varies among species, however. In zebra finches, ER are sparsely distributed in HVc proper, with only approximately 4% of cells labeled following injection of ^{3}H-E$_2$ (Nordeen *et al.*, 1987). In the bay wren, approximately 30% of HVc cells are estrogen (E) targets (Brenowitz and Arnold, 1989). ER-containing (ER+) cells are not distributed uniformly throughout HVc; they are most common in the mediocaudal region and rarer in the laterorostral portion. ER are more abundant in paraHVc, a song-control area just medial to caudal HVc (Nordeen *et al.*, 1987; Johnson and Bottjer, 1995). NCM also contains ER+ neurons (Hidalgo *et al.*, 1995; Gahr and Metzdorf, 1997).

Walters *et al.* (1988) reported that area X has low levels of ER. They treated castrated male zebra finches with ATD, an inhibitor of E synthesis, and performed *in vitro* binding assays of ER levels in tissue punches taken from area X. Neither the ER protein nor mRNA have been detected in area X by other studies using *in vivo* steroid-binding methods, ICC, or *in situ* hybridization techniques (Gahr *et al.*, 1987; Nordeen *et al.*, 1987; Brenowitz and Arnold, 1989; Bernard *et al.*, 1999; Metzdorf *et al.*, 1999).

C. Steroid Sensitivity of Discrete Cell Populations in Song Nuclei

In the HVc, AR are expressed in both RA- and area X-projecting neurons (Sohrabji *et al.*, 1989). This distribution of AR is consistent with the evidence already discussed that androgens influence both song development, regulated by the projection to the anterior forebrain pathway via area X, and the motor production of song, regulated by the descending motor pathway via the RA (Bottjer and Johnson, 1997). The RA-projecting neurons in HVc are exclusively androgen-accumulating. The area X-projecting neurons in HVc contain either AR or ER (Johnson and Bottjer, 1993, 1995), but individual X-projecting neurons express only one of these receptor types (Gahr, 1990).

In the bay wren, approximately two-thirds of the cells in the HVc are T targets, and one-third are E targets (Brenowitz and Arnold, 1985, 1989). Given Gahr's (1990) observation that individual HVc neurons express only one receptor type, the androgen- and estrogen-accumulating cells in the bay wren may represent different populations of neurons.

The paraHVc in canaries and zebra finches contains a high density of E target cells, but no androgen target cells (Nordeen et al., 1987; Johnson and Bottjer, 1995). This region has many area X-projecting neurons, and these neurons have ER but no AR in the finches (Nordeen et al., 1987).

In the lMAN of zebra finches both RA-projecting and nonprojecting neurons have AR (Korsia and Bottjer, 1989). A higher proportion of the projecting neurons than nonprojecting neurons are androgen targets.

D. Development of Steroid Receptors in Song Nuclei

The proportion of HVc cells that contain AR in young male zebra finches increases rapidly during the period of song learning (Bottjer, 1987). Gahr and Metzdorf (1999) reported that AR mRNA is first expressed in HVc of finches at day 9 posthatching (P9) and that the area of AR-expressing cells is already larger in males than females at this time. They also reported that this sex difference develops in steroid-free slice cultures of the caudal forebrain taken at P5, when HVc appears to have not yet received input from any of its afferent nuclei. Perlman and Arnold (2001), however, reported that AR mRNA is expressed widely throughout the brain, including the neostriatum in which HVc resides, on P1. They may have been able to detect expresson earlier than Gahr and Metzdorf (1999) because they used a more sensitive ^{33}P-riboprobe (vs ^{35}S) and used a larger cRNA (1.252 vs 0.759 kb). Given that sex differences in plasma androgens have not been observed in zebra finches prior to P5, Gahr and Metzdorf concluded that the initial sex difference in the expression of AR mRNA in HVc occurs independently of gonadal steroids. An alternative hypothesis, however, is that the regulation of AR mRNA expression is influenced by plasma E. High circulating levels of E occur during the first week after hatching (Hutchison et al., 1984; Schlinger and Arnold, 1992b), although it is not clear whether these levels differ between the sexes. Support for this alternative explanation comes from the observation that treating hatchling female zebra finches with E_2 increases AR accumulation in HVc (Nordeen et al., 1986).

AR mRNA begins to be expressed in mMAN after P8 (Gahr and Metzdorf, 1999). At this age, mMAN has not yet established synaptic connections with HVc.

Gahr and Metzdorf (1997) reported that ER mRNA is first expressed in the HVc at P15 in the zebra finches and at P30 in canaries. Cells in the caudal neostriatum expressed ER mRNA starting at P5–6. Jacobs et al. (1999), however, observed expression of ER mRNA in the HVc of zebra finches starting at P10. They suggested that they may have been able to detect the expression earlier than Gahr and Metzdorf (1997) because they used a ^{33}P-riboprobe (vs ^{35}S), used a larger cRNA (2.8 vs 0.93 kb), and a longer exposure time (4 weeks vs 1–2 weeks).

In zebra finches, Jacobs et al. (1999) observed the early expression of ER mRNA in the archistriatum, where the song nucleus RA resides. The ER mRNA was absent in the archistriatum at P18, but by P25 was expressed in cells in and dorsal to RA. The timing of this expression coincides with the establishment of synaptic connections between HVc and RA in males; by P15 the HVc axons form transient connections with neurons dorsal to the RA, and from P25-35 there is a massive ingrowth of these axons into the RA in males but not females (Konishi and Akutagawa, 1985; Mooney and Rao, 1994). ER mRNA is not expressed in the RA of adult canaries (Gahr and Metzdorf, 1997; Metzdorf et al., 1999).

E. Colocalization of Steroid Receptors and Neurotransmitters

Gonadal steroids interact with various neurotransmitter systems in the song-control circuits. Tyrosine hydroxylase (TH), the rate-limiting enzyme in catecholamine (CA) synthesis, and the transmitters norepinephrine (NE) and dopamine (DA) are all present in HVc, RA, Nif, area X, and lMAN in zebra finches (Barclay and Harding, 1988, 1990; Sakaguchi and Saito, 1989; Bottjer, 1993; Soha et al., 1996). NE and DA, their receptors, and the synthetic enzymes are present in higher levels in male than female finches (Bottjer, 1993). The castration of male finches decreased NE and DA levels and turnover in RA and area X, and treatment with either the aromatizable androgen androstenedione or a combination of DHT and E_2 reinstated CA function (Barclay and Harding, 1988, 1990). In the RA, E_2 alone increased NE levels. In area X, E_2 produced lower levels of NE than did DHT, but higher levels of DA than did DHT.

Receptors for N-methyl-D-aspartate (NMDA) are present in several song nuclei (Kubota and Saito, 1991; Mooney and Konishi, 1991, 1992; Aamodt et al., 1992). The binding of the NMDA receptor (NR) antagonist MK-801 in lMAN is greater in P30 male zebra finches beginning to learn song than in adults producing stereotyped song (Aamodt et al., 1992, 1995). Juvenile male finches in which MK-801 was injected to block NR on the days on which they were exposed to a song tutor showed little evidence of song learning as adults, whereas males injected on the days following tutoring learned song normally (Aamodt et al., 1996). The mRNA for the NR subunit 2B (NR2B) in lMAN is expressed at twice the level in P30 male finches as in adult males, and the binding of the NR2B-associated ligand ^{3}H-ifenprodil shows a similar developmental decrease (Basham et al., 1999). The treatment of P20 male finches with androgen, which accelerates song development, decreased NR2B mRNA expression in lMAN at P35, relative to age-matched controls (Singh et al., 2000). Concomitent with the developmental change in NR subtype is an increase with age in the decay rate of NMDA excitatory postsynaptic currents (EPSC) in the lMAN (White et al., 1999). The treatment of fledgling (P21–32) and juvenile (P38–49), but not adult (>P90), male finches with T accelerated the increase in decay rate of the NMDA-EPSC and increased dendritic length and spine density in the lMAN (White et al., 1999). Taken together, these different results suggest that circulating androgens may limit sensitive periods for song learning by altering synaptic transmission in the song nuclei.

F. Seasonal Changes and Regulation of Steroid Sensitivity

There are pronounced seasonal changes in the morphology of song nuclei in adults of every seasonally breeding species examined (Nottebohm, 1981; Ball, 2000; Tramontin and Brenowitz, 2000). The entire volumes of several song nuclei including the HVc, area X, RA, and nXIIts are larger during the spring breeding season than during the autumn and winter. In the most extreme case, the volume of the HVc in spotted towhees (*Pipilo maculatus*) nearly triples during the breeding season (Smith, 1996). lMAN, however, does not change in volume between seasons (Smith et al., 1997a,b; Brenowitz et al., 1998; Tramontin et al., 1998; Soma et al., 1998).

The seasonal change in the HVc volume is primarily due to a large increase in neuron number (e.g., Nottebohm, 1987; Brenowitz et al., 1991; Smith et al., 1997a,c; Tramontin et al., 1998, 2000). In one study of wild song sparrows (*Melospiza melodia*), for example, the neuron number in the HVc increased from approximately 150,000 in late autumn to 250,000 in early spring (Smith et al., 1997a). The breeding season increase in the neuron number results from ongoing neurogenesis in the songbird brain (e.g., Goldman and Nottebohm, 1983; Kirn and Nottebohm, 1993; Alvarez-Buylla and Kirn, 1997; Tramontin and Brenowitz, 1999). The HVc in adults continues to incorporate new RA-projecting neurons and interneurons that replace older dying cells (Paton et al., 1985; Kirn and Nottebohm, 1993). This neuronal turnover is seasonally regulated and is greatest during the nonbreeding season (Kirn et al., 1994; Tramontin and Brenowitz, 1999). Elevated plasma gonadal steroid levels seem to decrease the turnover and increase the survival of HVc neurons, thus increasing their number during the breeding season (Rasika et al., 1994; Hidalgo et al., 1995; Tramontin and Brenowitz, 1999).

The cellular basis of volumetric growth of RA differs from that seen in HVc. Neuron number does not change seasonally in RA, but neuron size, spacing, dendritic arborizations, and the sizes of pre- and postsynaptic profiles are greater in the breeding season (DeVoogd et al., 1985; Brenowitz et al., 1991; Hill and DeVoogd, 1991; Smith et al., 1997a,c; Tramontin et al., 1998; Tramontin and Brenowitz, 2000). These seasonal patterns of dendritic change suggest that synaptic efficacy in RA is enhanced during the breeding season (DeVoogd and Nottebohm, 1981).

Several lines of evidence suggest that T (or its active metabolites) is the primary physiological cue that mediates the seasonal changes in the song nuclei. As previously discussed, gonadal steroid receptors are present in the HVc, RA, lMAN, mMAN, DLM, and nXIIts. Seasonal patterns of circulating T correlate positively with the seasonal growth pattern of the song nuclei (Nottebohm, 1981; Smith, 1996; Smith et al., 1997a; Brenowitz et al., 1998; Soma et al., 1998; Tramontin and Brenowitz, 1999). Castration severely attenuates the seasonal growth of the song regions (Bernard et al., 1997; Gulledge and Deviche, 1997; Smith et al., 1997b). Exogenous T induces growth of the song nuclei in castrated males and in nonbreeding males in the fall and winter (Nottebohm, 1980b; Johnson and Bottjer, 1993; Rasika et al., 1994; Bernard and Ball, 1997; Smith et al., 1997b; Wennstrom et al., 2001). It is interesting that even though lMAN expresses high levels of ARs, it does not undergo seasonal changes in morphology in response to seasonal changes in plasma T.

T appears to induce growth of the adult song circuits by acting directly on the HVc, which then stimulates the growth of the efferent nuclei via transsynaptic effects. The HVc grows rapidly in response to exposure to breeding levels of T, whereas the RA and area X grow more slowly (Smith et al., 1997a; Ball, 2000; Tramontin et al., 2000). Unilateral lesion of the HVc selectively blocks the growth of the ipsilateral, but not contralateral, RA and area X in response to exposure to breeding T levels and photoperiod (Brenowitz and Lent, 2000). Implanting T adjacent to the HVc unilaterally stimulates the growth of the ipsilateral, but not contralateral, HVc, RA, and area X (Brenowitz and Lent, 2000). Implanting T adjacent to RA, however, does not stimulate growth of any song nuclei. These results suggest that direct T stimulation of HVc is both necessary and sufficient for growth of the song control circuits. It is notable that RA does not grow in response to high plasma T in the absence of afferent input from the HVc, even though RA neurons have abundant ARs. Also noteworthy is the observation that nXIIts grows in response to systemic T implants even when the ipsilateral the HVc is lesioned and does not grow when T is implanted adjacent to the ipsilateral HVc. These results may indicate that nXIIts, which has high levels of AR, does not require an intact HVc to grown in response to high plasma T. T may act directly on the motor neurons of nXIIts or on the AR-containing syringeal muscles innervated by these neurons, which might then have a retrograde trophic effect on the motor neurons.

The trophic effect of T on the HVc may be mediated, at least partially, through BDNF. The treatment of adult female canaries with T increases protein synthesis and BDNF-like immunoreactivity in the HVc (Konishi and Akutagawa, 1981; Rasika et al., 1999). The infusion of BDNF into the parenchyma adjacent to the HVc mimics the effects of T, increasing neuronal survival in the HVc and increasing its volume. Also, infusing neutralizing antibodies to BDNF blocks the effects of T on neuronal survival in and volumetric growth of the HVc (Rasika et al., 1999). It will be interesting to determine whether BDNF or other growth factors similarly influence the effects of gonadal steroids on seasonal growth of the song circuits.

Seasonal growth of the HVc may be stimulated by the direct actions of T or by its active androgenic or estrogenic metabolites. In adult female canaries exogenous 5α-DHT and E_2 delivered together stimulated greater dendritic growth in RA than did either metabolite alone (DeVoogd and Nottebohm, 1981). E_2 promoted the survival and decreased neuronal turnover in the HVc of adult male canaries (Hidalgo et al., 1995). Wild male song sparrows implanted with osmotic pumps that released the aromatase inhibitor fadrozole during the breeding season had significantly smaller HVcs than did controls implanted with saline-filled pumps (A. D. Tramontin K. K. Soma, J. C. Wingfield, and E. A. Brenowitz, unpublished observation); sparrows treated with fadrozole plus E_2 in the fall had significantly larger HVcs than did control birds treated with fadrozole and saline. Together these results suggest that estrogenic metabolites may contribute to seasonal growth of the song nuclei.

The sensitivity of the HVc to gonadal steroids varies seasonally. At the end of the breeding season, birds become refractory to the stimulatory effects of long days and the testes regress, plasma gonadal steroid levels decrease, and feather molt occurs (Nicholls et al., 1988). During this photorefractory period, the production of AR and ER in the HVc is decreased (Soma et al., 1998; Gahr and Metzdorf, 1999). Immunostaining for the AR in the HVc of male white-crowned sparrows (*Zonotrichia leucophrys*) is more intense and labels more cells during the breeding season than in the fall (Fig. 4; Soma et al., 1998). The activity of 5β-reductase, which catalyzes the conversion of T to the inactive metabolite 5β-DHT, increases at the onset of photorefractoriness

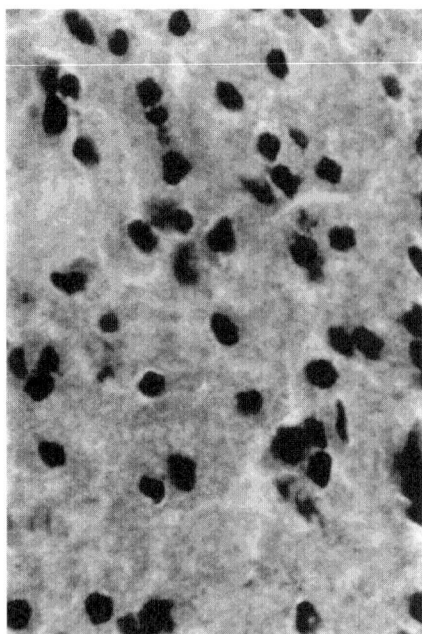 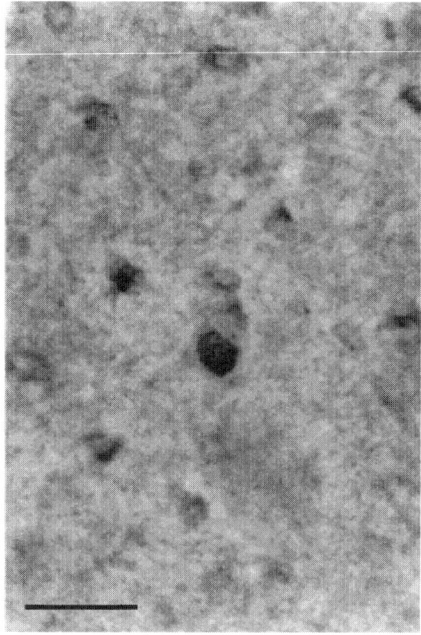

SPRING **AUTUMN**

FIGURE 4 Seasonal changes in androgen-receptor-cell density and staining intensity in the HVc of Gambel's white-crowned sparrows. Note that birds in autumn have fainter staining in cell nuclei. Scale bar, 20 μm. Reprinted from Soma *et al.* (1998), by permission of Wiley-Liss, Inc., a subsidiary of John Wiley & Sons, Inc.

in the hyperstriatum of starlings (Bottoni and Massa, 1981). In photorefractory starlings, treatment with exogenous T does not increase HVc volume (Bernard and Ball, 1997). T does induce the growth of the HVc in photorefractory white-crowned sparrows (Wennstrom *et al.*, 2001), however, suggesting that there are species differences in seasonal patterns of sensitivity to the trophic effects of T.

The seasonal growth of the song nuclei can be modulated by factors other than photoperiodic stimulation of T secretion. In the laboratory, social cues from sexually receptive female white-crowned sparrows enhanced the photo-induced growth of two song nuclei in their male cagemates (Tramontin *et al.*, 1998). The HVc and RA were 20% and 15% larger, respectively, in males housed with females in long spring-like days than in males housed similarly without females.

One of the most striking forms of seasonal plasticity in the song-control system of adults is the ongoing incorporation of new neurons into the HVc. As much as 1.5% of the HVc neurons in an adult female canary are generated per day (Goldman and Nottebohm, 1983).

Paton and Nottebohm (1984) demonstrated that HVc cells labeled by ^{3}H-thymidine show synaptic and action potentials and respond to auditory stimuli. This was the first definitive proof that the newly generated cells are neurons and that they are incorporated into functional circuits. These new neurons in the HVc include many interneurons. At least half of the new HVc neurons project to the RA, however. The survival of these new neurons varies with season. Most neurons born in the spring die within 4 months. Most neurons born in the fall, however, survive at least 8 months (Kirn *et al.*, 1991; Nottebohm *et al.*, 1994).

These seasonal patterns of neuronal survival are correlated with seasonal changes in the levels of gonadal steroids. The highest rates of HVc neuronal death are preceded by decreases in T levels. Each peak of neuronal death is followed by a peak of new neuron addition when T levels begin to rise again (Kirn *et al.*, 1994). Decreases in plasma T may therefore lead to cell death, which creates vacancies for the subsequent incorporation of new neurons. The subsequent increases of T may provide trophic support that maintains these new neurons (Alvarez-Buylla and Kirn, 1997). Support for a trophic role of T comes from the observation that treating adult female canaries with T after a ^{3}H-thymidine injection triples the number of labeled neurons incorporated into the HVc (Rasika *et al.*, 1994). Hormone treatment does not alter the rate of cell birth in the ventricular zone (Brown *et al.*, 1993; Rasika *et al.*, 1994; Hidalgo *et al.*, 1995). It therefore seems that hormones influence postmitotic events (Burek *et al.*, 1995). Hormones could affect, for example, the migration, differentiation, establishment of synaptic connections, and survival of new neurons.

The functional significance of seasonal neuron recruitment to the adult HVc is not clear. It may be related to the ability to learn new songs in adulthood (Nottebohm, 1987). The seasonal changes in the HVc neuronal turnover are correlated with seasonal changes in song behavior. Canaries produce new song elements at the highest rate during the nonbreeding season when song syllables are produced with less temporal and spectral stereotypy (Nottebohm *et al.*, 1986). These peak periods of song learning coincide with peaks in the incorporation of new neurons to the HVc (Kirn *et al.*, 1994). This correlation between song plasticity and neuronal recruitment suggests that seasonal patterns of neuronal replacement in the HVc may provide the neural substrate for seasonal song learning in adult birds; the incorporation of new naïve neurons into functional circuits may be a source of plasticity for this adult learning (Nottebohm, 1989; Alvarez-Buylla *et al.*, 1992; Kirn *et al.*, 1994; Alvarez-Buylla and Kirn, 1997). Seasonal changes in the recruitment of new neurons to the HVc are also observed, however, in the song sparrow, a species that does not learn new songs in adulthood (Tramontin and Brenowitz, 1999). As in the canary, the sparrow neuronal recruitment in the HVc is greater during the nonbreeding season and sparrow song structure becomes less stereotyped then (Smith *et al.*, 1997a). This increased variability of songs in the nonbreeding season, however, does not lead to the development of new song patterns in song sparrows. This observation indicates that seasonal changes in neuronal recruitment might be necessary, but not sufficient, for adult song learning.

An alternative functional hypothesis is that the incorporation of new neurons in the adult HVc is related to song perception (Nottebohm *et al.*, 1990). As previously discussed, the HVc neurons receive auditory input and show selective responses to conspecific song. Lesions of the HVc disrupt the behavioral perception of song (Brenowitz, 1991a). Neuronal addition may provide plasticity for acquiring new perceptual memories of songs each year, which is important in the contexts of males learning to recognize the songs of their territorial neighbors and females learning to recognize the songs of their mate.

A third functional hypothesis is that neuronal turnover in HVc may be a compromise adaptation between two conflicting selective pressures (Nottebohm, 1989). On the one hand, birds are relatively long-lived and this favors a brain large enough to enable the formation and storage of new memories throughout life. On the other hand, flight imposes severe energetic constraints that favor minimizing body (and brain) weight, as shown by the evolution of hollow bones that contain air sacs. Incurring the metabolic costs of neuronal replacement seasonally may represent a strategy for balancing these factors.

G. Comparative Studies of Steroid Receptors in the Song System

Using *in vivo* steroid-binding techniques, the distribution of T target cells in the HVc has been compared between the sexes in zebra finches, canaries, rufous-and-white wrens, and bay wrens (Arnold and Saltiel, 1979; Brenowitz and Arnold, 1985, 1992; Brenowitz *et al.*, 1996; Brenowitz, 1997). In the zebra finch, males have both a greater relative proportion and absolute number of T target cells in the HVc than do females, who cannot sing (Table 1). In canaries, rufous-and-white wrens, and bay wrens, females can sing and we see no sex difference in the proportion of T target cells in the HVc. The extent to which the sexes in these three species differ in the number of T target cells in HVc, however, is correlated with the degree of sexual dimorphism in the complexity of song behavior. The greatest sex difference is found in canaries, an intermediate degree of sex difference is seen in rufous-and-white wrens, and no sex difference is present in bay wrens.

This comparative analysis may indicate that song can only be learned or produced if an adequate proportion of cells in the song nuclei is hormone sensitive. Increases in song complexity above a minimal level may

TABLE 1
Comparison of Male:Female Ratios for Song Behavior and Frequency and Total Number of Testosterone Target Cells in HVc

	Zebra finch[a]	Canary[b]	Rufous- and white-wren[c]	Bay wren[d]
Song repertoire	M only	M >>> F	M > F	M = F
T targets (%)	2.84[e]	1.17	0.98	0.99
T targets (number)	8.34[e]	4.30[e]	2.52[e]	1.20

[a] Data from Arnold and Saltiel (1979); Nordeen *et al.* (1987); Grisham and Arnold (1995).
[b] Data from Pesch and Guttinger (1985); Nottebohm (1980a); Brenowitz and Arnold (1992).
[c] Data from Brenowitz *et al.* (1996); Farabaugh (1982).
[d] Data from Brenowitz and Arnold (1985) and Levin (1996a,b).
[e] Male and female values are significantly different ($p < 0.05$; two-tailed t test).

be related to an increase in the absolute number of steroid-sensitive cells in the song nuclei rather than to an increase in the proportion of such cells (Brenowitz *et al.*, 1996). The comparison between canaries and rufous-and-white wrens may be especially informative in this regard. Female canaries have the same proportion of hormone target cells in the song nuclei as males, but female song is much simpler in complexity and given less often than is male song. The number of hormone-sensitive cells in female canary song nuclei may be close to the minimum necessary to produce any song. On the other hand, female rufous-and-white wrens sing routinely and individual song renditions have syllabic structures comparable to those of males (Farabaugh, 1982). These females only produce about half as many different types of songs as do males, however. Correlated with the greater relative complexity of song behavior in female rufous-and-white wrens than in female canaries, the magnitude of the sex difference in the number of hormone target cells in the song nuclei is only approximately one-half as large for the wrens as it is for canaries.

The hypothesis that increases in song complexity are related to increases in the number of, but not the proportion of, hormone-sensitive cells in the song nuclei can be tested experimentally. If adult female canaries are implanted with T, their song nuclei increase in size and they sing more complex songs than do normal females (Nottebohm, 1980b). This T treatment results in an increase in the absolute number of T target cells in the HVc, but does not alter the proportion of these cells in the HVc, RA, or lMAN (Brenowitz and Arnold, 1990; Bottjer and Maier, 1991). This result supports the hypothesis and illustrates how comparative studies can generate hypotheses that we can test experimentally.

The limited comparative studies performed suggest that bird lineages other than the songbirds do not have gonadal steroid receptors in nonlimbic telencephalic regions. This is true even for the parrots, which are capable of vocal learning (Ball *et al.*, 1990; Brenowitz, 1991a; Gahr *et al.*, 1993; Metzdorf *et al.*, 1999). Gonadal steroid receptors in telencephalic vocal regions therefore do not appear to be a necessary precondition for vocal learning. The presence of steroid receptors in the song nuclei of songbirds may be related to the sexual differentiation of these regions or to the seasonal nature of song and reproduction in most species. As previously discussed, song production is closely related to breeding activity in most songbirds. The regression of the song nuclei in adult birds outside the breeding season, when plasma steroid levels become basal, might provide a mechanism for reducing the energy demands imposed by these areas of the brain outside the breeding season. The oxidative capacity of song nuclei, as measured by cytochrome oxidase activity, is increased by treatment of nonbreeding birds with T (Wennstrom *et al.*, 2000). Additional comparative studies are necessary to clarify the evolutionary origin of the hormone-sensitive song-control system seen in songbirds.

IV. EVOLUTION OF THE SONG SYSTEM

Vocal learning occurs in parrots and hummingbirds as well as in songbirds (Nottebohm, 1972; Baylis, 1982; Kroodsma, 1982; Kroodsma and Baylis, 1982;

R. J. Dooling *et al.*, 1987; Baptista and Schuchmann, 1990; R. D. Dooling *et al.*, 1992). It is of interest to ask whether these other orders have vocal-control systems comparable to those of songbirds and, if so, were these neural circuits inherited from a common ancestor (i.e., homologous), or did they evolve independently (i.e., homoplasous)?

The brain of one parrot species, the budgerigar (*Melopsittacus undulatus*), has been studied in detail (Paton *et al.*, 1981; Hall *et al.*, 1994; Stricter, 1994; Cookson *et al.*, 1996; Breath *et al.*, 1997; Duran *et al.*, 1997). These birds have a vocal-control system that has some general similarities to that of songbirds.

1. In both groups, the descending vocal motor pathway consists of connections between nuclei in the same two anatomical divisions of the forebrain (the neostriatum and the archistriatum), which in turn project to nXIIts in the brain stem. Lesions of these nuclei disrupt vocal behavior in budgerigars (Eaton *et al.*, 1994; Eaton and Breath, 1996) and songbirds (Brenowitz *et al.*, 1997).

2. There are auditory inputs to these areas of the brain in budgerigars and songbirds.

3. The parrots have three brain nuclei that share similarities with area X, DLM, and lMAN found in the anterior forebrain pathway of songbirds. The budgerigar nuclei are found in the same regions of the brain, and they are similarly interconnected. Furthermore, the budgerigar nucleus that shares similarities with lMAN projects to the region that has similarities to RA, as in the oscine brain.

4. The distributions of choline acetyltransferase and acetylcholinesterase are similar in budgerigar and oscine vocal-control nuclei.

The budgerigar and songbird vocal-control circuits differ in numerous ways, however.

1. The absolute positions of the nuclei in the budgerigar forebrain are very different from those in the oscine brain; the oscine HVc is located in the dorsomedial caudal telencephalon, whereas the budgerigar "HVc" is adjacent to the lateral edge of the caudal telencephalon.

2. The projection from the RA to nXIIts is bilateral in budgerigars, but is largely ipsilateral in oscines.

3. The primary functional source of auditory input to the budgerigar vocal-control system is the nucleus basalis in the telencephalon, whereas it is subdivisions L1 and L3 of the telencephalic auditory region field L in oscines (Margoliash *et al.*, 1994).

4. Unlike songbirds, the region that has similarities to area X is not connected to the region similar to the HVc in the budgerigar.

5. The budgerigar vocal-control nuclei lack receptors for steroid hormones, which occur throughout the oscine song system (Ball, 1990; Gahr *et al.*, 1993).

6. Muscarinic cholinergic receptors occur in the oscine HVc, but are absent from the similar region in the budgerigar (Ball *et al.*, 1990).

Jarvis *et al.* (2000) used patterns of mRNA expression of the transcriptional regulator gene *ZENK* to identify regions of the forebrain that seem to be related to vocal behavior in two hummingbird species. They identified discrete nuclei with song-related *ZENK* mRNA activity in similar regions of the forebrain as seen in songbirds and budgerigars, including the anterior and caudolateral neostriatum (the location of the songbird lMAN, HVc, and Nif), the archistriatum (the location of the songbird RA), paleostriatum (the location of songbird area X), and associated regions of the hyperstriatum. These authors have not yet conducted tract-tracing studies and the connectional relationships among these regions of the hummingbird brain and the vocal-production organ are therefore unknown. Pharmacological studies also remain to be conducted on these species, so the occurrence of different neurotransmitters in these regions is unknown. The analysis of two other hummingbird species failed to detect ER in the caudolateral telencephalon, where the HVc is found in songbirds (Gahr *et al.*, 1993).

The comparison of vocal systems in the brains of songbirds, budgerigars, and hummingbirds is interesting both for the similarities and differences between these groups. It is striking that all three groups show vocal-related nuclei in the same general regions of the forebrain. The specific location of nuclei in these regions, however, differs among the three groups. Using a much-debated phylogeny of birds by Sibley *et al.* (1988), Jarvis *et al.* (2000) suggest that there has been a trend toward a shift in the location of the posterior forebrain vocal structures from more anterolateral to posteromedial positions, going from the oldest group (parrots) to the more recent group (songbirds).

The overall similarities observed among these three groups argue against the idea that their vocal-control systems evolved independently *de novo* in each group. On the other hand, the numerous specific differences observed among the vocal systems of these three groups are inconsistent with the idea that these systems were inherited directly from a shared common ancestor. If this were the case, then we might expect to observe comparable vocal-control systems in other intermediary avian lineages. Well-defined forebrain vocal nuclei have not thus far been described in other avian groups, however. The groups that have been studied include the Galliformes (jungle fowl, guinea fowl, and pheasants), Columbiformes (pigeons and doves), and suboscine Passeriformes (Karten and Hodos, 1967; Bonke et al., 1979; Kroodsma and Konishi, 1991). It should be noted, however, that only a few species have been examined in any of these groups.

A parsimonious explanation of the similarities and differences observed among the songbird, parrot, and hummingbird vocal systems may be that they evolved by independent elaboration of circuits already present in a rudimentary form in ancestral birds (Ulinski and Margoliash, 1990; Brenowitz, 1991b, 1997; Margoliash et al., 1994). Margoliash and colleagues have suggested that both the oscine and budgerigar vocal systems can be viewed as elaborations of the general pattern of reptile-bird forebrain organization. For the auditory system, this general organization consists of projections of the thalamic auditory nucleus ovoidalis onto a structure between the intermediate and caudal neostriatum. This auditory-recipient neostriatal structure then projects onto the caudal neostriatum, which in turn projects to the archistriatum. The archistriatum projects to the vocal motor neurons in the brain stem. Consistent with this model, Kroner and Gunturkun (1999) reported that in pigeons, the caudolateral neostriatum (where the HVc is located in songbirds) projects rostrally to the basal ganglia (the location of the songbird area X) and hyperstriatum, and rostrally to the archistriatum (the location of the songbird RA). According to this scenario, songbirds, parrots, and hummingbirds each evolved specialized forebrain vocal-control circuits from this common ancestral substrate, which accounts for their overall similarities. The specific differences in the vocal circuits, however, reflect historical accidents in the way in which the basic elements of the ancestral substrate were elaborated by each group. This model could be tested by a broadscale phylogenetic analysis examining further examples of both vocal learners and nonlearners in a systematic way.

The available evidence suggests that the hormone-sensitive song system present in songbirds is unique to this group, and the question arises as to when in the phyletic lineage leading to modern oscines did this neural system first arise? This system might have first appeared with the origin of the passeriform order. In this case, we might expect to find vocal-control nuclei in at least a rudimentary form in members of the suboscine suborder. Although a comprehensive search has yet to be conducted, preliminary studies of species in four suboscine families have not detected any forebrain song nuclei. Nissl-staining techniques did not reveal cytoarchitectonically distinct clusters of cells comparable to the HVc, RA, LMAN, or area X in the brains of four tyrannid flycatchers (Nottebohm, 1980a; Kroodsma and Konishi, 1991; T. J. DeVoogd, unpublished data), the furnarid or ovenbirds (*Asthenes hudsoni* and *Synallaxis frontalis*; Nottebohm, 1980a), the piprid or manakin (*Manacus vitellinus*; Saldanha et al., 2000a,b), or the thamnophilid slaty antshrike (*Thamnophilus punctuatus*; E. A. Brenowitz, unpublished data). There is also no evidence of steroid hormone receptors in regions of the brain where the HVc, RA, and lMAN are found in oscines (Gahr et al., 1993; E. A. Brenowitz, unpublished data). Clearly, more comprehensive analyses of the brains of suboscine birds, including tract-tracing studies, are required, but the available data suggest that these birds lack a forebrain vocal-control system similar to that of the oscines.

We can tentatively conclude, pending more studies of suboscine brains, that the hormone-sensitive song system arose only with the origin of the oscine lineage. This network of forebrain song nuclei has been observed in at least 60 songbird species in 10 families and the two major songbird divisions Corvida and Passerida (classification of Sibley et al., 1988; for review, see Brenowitz and Kroodsma, 1996). Steroid hormone receptors have been searched for and detected in the forebrain song nuclei of 19 oscine species (see Brenowitz and Kroodsma, 1996).

This comparative analysis suggests that the steroid-sensitive forebrain song system is found among all branches of the oscine lineage. Traits that are widely distributed in the branches of a monophyletic lineage such as the oscine birds are likely to have evolved early in the phylogeny of that lineage. By this reasoning, the song system appears to have evolved very early in the evolution of the songbird lineage. It is intriguing to speculate that the initial development of this hormone-sensitive neural system was a definitive event in the evolutionary origin of the songbirds (Brenowitz and Kroodsma, 1996). A more systematic phylogenetic analysis of how song is controlled among passerine birds could indicate more clearly when and how the songbird song system evolved.

The inspection of the song system in various songbird groups shows that this neural system is very uniform in morphology and chemical properties across taxa. There is extreme diversity, however, within and among taxa in different aspects of song behavior, as already discussed. Three attributes of the song system may enable the production of extreme behavioral diversity by this highly conserved network of brain nuclei (Brenowitz and Kroodsma, 1996).

1. The network appears to function exclusively in controlling song-related behavior. The devotion of the song system to song behavior allows more flexibility in the evolutionary modification of such factors as neuron number and developmental timing of the brain circuits than might be true if this network also functioned in contexts other than song.
2. Steroid hormones have pronounced influences on the development and activation of these circuits. The patterns of hormone secretion and metabolism show extensive diversity across avian taxa in such aspects as developmental timing, seasonality, and sex. This diversity implies that hormone secretion and metabolism are evolutionarily flexible traits. Relatively small changes in hormone release and metabolism, in turn, can have large effects on song-control networks and song behavior.
3. Song is a learned behavior and is thus subject to rapid modification via cultural evolution.

These three attributes together may provide the plasticity that has enabled the diverse expression of song behavior across groups.

V. SUPPLY OF ACTIVE STEROIDS TO STEROID-SENSITIVE NEURAL STRUCTURES

A. Steroid Synthesis by the Gonads

A simplified view of the hormonal control of behavior starts with sex-steroid synthesis and release by the gonads of reproductively active adult animals, followed by the activation of reproductive and aggressive behaviors by these steroids acting on intranuclear steroid receptors in specific target neurons. Studies investigating the organization and activation of song suggests that more complex processes may be used to supply active steroids to song-control circuits, including steroid synthesis at nongonadal sites and the use of sex steroids other than the most commonly studied, T and E_2. Wherever they are formed, all steroids are originally derived from cholesterol, which can be synthesized in steroidogenic cells, or removed from the circulation. Much of what is known about the enzymes and transporters involved in steroidogenesis comes from work on mammalian systems. Given the importance of understanding reproductive processes in poultry (chickens, domesticated turkeys, and quail), however, work on mammals has been extended to these nonsongbird species (for review, see Saito and Shimada, 1997). Much less is known about these enzymes in songbirds (Lofts and Murton, 1973; Freking et al., 2000).

It is important to recognize that several of the enzymes in these reactions are members of the very large family of cytochrome P450 enzymes that mediate a vast number of reactions in a variety of animal tissues (Miller, 1988). These enzymes require coenzyme electron donors for their proper function, and virtually nothing is known about these enzymes in nonmammalian species. This is unfortunate because some of the enzyme-mediated transformations that may have critical importance in songbirds may be modulated by the coenzyme concentrations and not by the cytochrome P450 enzymes themselves. Future studies of these

TABLE 2
Steroidogenic and Steroid Metabolic Enzyme Nomenclature

Previous or full name	Current or abbreviated name	Principal conversions[a]
Side-chain cleavage Cytochrome P450scc	CYP11A1	Cholesterol to Preg
3β-Hydroxysteroid dehydrogenase/isomerase	3β-HSD	Preg to Prog DHEA to AE
17α-Hydroxylase 17α-Hydroxylase/C17-20lyase Cytochrome P45017α	CYP17	Preg to DHEA (via 17α-OH-Preg) Prog to AE (via 17α-OH-Prog)
Aromatase Estrogen synthetase Cytochrome P450arom	CYP19	AE to E_1 T to E_2
17β-Hydroxysteroid dehydrogenase (oxydoreductase)	17β-HSD	AE to T E_1 to E_2
5α-Reductase	5α-Reductase	T to 5α-DHT P to 5α-Prog P-Prog
5β-Reductase	5β-Reductase	T to 5β-DHT P to 5β-Prog P-Prog

[a] AE, androstenedione; DHEA, dehydroepiandrosterone; DHT, dihydrotestosterone; E_1, estrone; E_2, estradiol; Preg, Pregnenolone; Prog, progesterone; T, testosterone.

coenzymes, especially with regard to adrenal and neural sex steroidogenesis, may gain appreciable importance. To simplify the terminology of this complex of enzymes and their genes, the names of some of these enzymes have been modified. In this review, we use the accepted terminology (Table 2). This may be confusing to some readers, especially because the names of some enzymes are particularly familiar (such as aromatase). We limit the scope of our review to those enzymes that we believe are most important in songbird biology.

The enzyme-catalyzed reactions that convert cholesterol into steroids initially, and the principal steroidal substrates and products that are produced by the vertebrate gonads, are listed in Table 2. Cholesterol is first converted into pregnenolone by the cytochrome P450 side-chain cleavage enzyme (CYP11A1). Two enzymes act on pregnenolone, either catalyzing its conversion into the active progestin progesterone by the enzyme 3β-hydroxysteroid dehydrogenase/isomerase (3β-HSD) or converting it into the androgen dehydroepiandrosterone (DHEA) by the cytochrome P450 17α-hydroxylase/C17-20lyase enzyme (CYP17) via the 17α-OH-pregnenolone intermediate. DHEA can be acted on by 3β-HSD, forming androstenedione (AE) or AE can be derived from progesterone by the actions of CYP17 via the intermediate 17α-OH-progesterone. AE can be converted into the more active androgen T by the enzyme 17β-hydroxysteroid dehydrogenase (17β-HSD). Finally, T can be converted into the active estrogen E_2 by the actions of the enzyme cytochrome P450 aromatase (CYP19).

Through the expression of some or all of these enzymes in individual cells, the dominant sex steroids—progesterone, T and E_2—are formed. The Leydig cells of the testes and the granulosa and thecal cells of the ovaries are the principle sites of gonadal sex steroid synthesis, accomplishing this role by the expression of one or more of these enzymes. The activity of these cells and their expression of steroidogenic enzymes are not static. During periods of reproductive activity and under the control of pituitary gonadotropins, each of these cell types undergoes some degree of maturation, including the increased expression of one or more of these enzymes. In the case of the ovary, as each individual follicle matures there may be specific changes in the expression of enzymes in keeping with the need to produce differential amounts of progestins, androgens, and estrogens.

The dominant sex steroids produced by the testes of songbirds are the androgens, T, and 5α-DHT (Wingfield

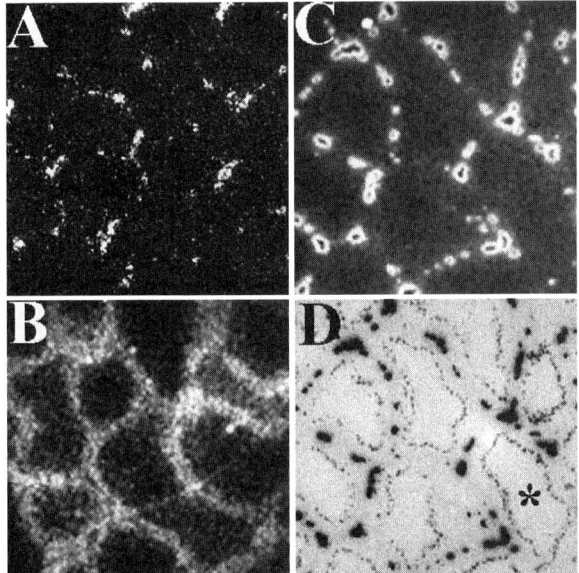

FIGURE 5 Expression of steroidogenic enzymes in the testis of an adult zebra finch. (A–C) Darkfield images showing hybridization of ^{33}P-labeled chicken cDNA probes to CYP11A1, 3β-HSD, and CYP17. (D) Brightfield image of CYP17 hybridization. The lumen of a seminiferous tubule is depicted with an asterisk; interstitial spaces with Leydig cells are present between the tubules where hybridization signal is darkest. Note CYP11A1 and CYP17 are expressed in Leydig cells, whereas 3β-HSD is also expressed in cells of the seminiferous tubule, probably Sertoli cells. From Freking et al. (2000), with permission.

and Farner, 1993). The Leydig cell, located in the interstitial spaces between the seminiferous tubules, is the dominant sex-steroid-producing cell in the testes of birds (Fig. 5). In the zebra finch, all of the enzymes required to produce androgens (CYP11A1, 3β-HSD, and CYP17) are expressed in Leydig cells (Freking et al., 2000). Cells in the seminiferous tubule, most likely Sertoli cells, also appear to express 3β-HSD, (Freking et al., 2000), so it is possible that Sertoli cells also synthesize some sex steroids. Apparently, Leydig cells express little if any CYP19, but CYP19 immunoreactivity has been detected in zebra finch spermatozoa (Saldanha et al., 2000b). Thus, the adult zebra finch testes secrete androgens, but little to no estrogen, and Leydig cells are probably steroidogenically most important.

The hormonal control of song in female songbirds is poorly understood, but might require androgens produced by the ovaries. In a mature chicken follicle, the granulosa cells appear to express CYP11A1 and 3β-HSD and, thus, secrete progestins; whereas the theca predominantly express CYP17 and CYP19 and, thus, make androgens and estrogens from substrate produced by the granulosa (Porter et al., 1989). The expression of these enzymes fluctuates in follicles as they mature in a respective clutch, so that small and intermediate follicles also synthesize sex steroids. It is likely that most androgen is produced in smaller follicles because they express more CYP17 than their larger counterparts (Saito and Shimada, 1997).

In the mature follicles of the zebra finch, CYP11A1 and 3β-HSD appear to be expressed in both the granulosa and theca (Freking et al., 2000); theca otherwise resemble that of chickens in expressing both CYP17 and CYP19 (Freking et al., 2000). These results suggest that both the granulosa and theca synthesize pregnenolone and progestins, but that the theca synthesize androgens and estrogens. As in other species, follicular maturation is associated with the changing expression of steroidogenic enzymes. CYP17 is expressed in both many small and large follicles, so it possible that, as in the hen, androgens may be produced by these smaller follicles, which may then stimulate song in some females.

B. Alternate Sites of Sex Steroid Synthesis

There are several documented cases in which the castration or ovariectomy of male and female songbirds does not eliminate sex steroids from the bloodstream. For example, Marler et al. (1988) found considerable E_2 in the blood of castrated juvenile male song and swamp sparrows, and the levels of E_2 resembled those found in the blood of intact juvenile song sparrows. Adkins-Regan et al. (1990) found E_2 in the blood of castrated or ovariectomized adult zebra finches, in some cases exceeding levels found in intact birds. These studies suggest that there are alternate sites of sex steroid production, the most likely being the adrenal glands. As previously described, there are also a variety of situations in which behaviors that we know or assume to be steroid-dependent are expressed by birds (especially songbirds) when the plasma levels of sex steroids are basal. These results suggest that steroids might be synthesized in the brain itself. This idea, considered unlikely in the 1990s, is recognized as a possible mechanism for the supply of steroids to neural circuits. Work in mammals, amphibia, and some birds, including songbirds, suggests that the brain may be an important site of steroid production (Baulieu, 1997; Mensah-Nyagan et al., 1999; Tsutsui and Ukena, 1999; Zwain and Yen, 1999; Compagnone and Mellon, 2000; Schlinger et al., 2001; Holloway and Clayton, 2001). These ideas are discussed more fully next.

1. Adrenals

Glucocorticoids (corticosterone in birds) and mineralocorticoids (aldosterone) are the principal steroids secreted by the adrenals of most vertebrates. Corticosteroids, in particular, can significantly influence a variety of neural systems, but we know nothing about the sites of action of these steroids in the songbird brain. Corticosteroids probably do influence song production. For example, during periods of stress, birds may transiently terminate reproduction and associated reproductive behaviors, including song. These effects on song are likely to be indirect, via effects on sex steroid production by the gonads. Nevertheless, given that corticosteroids can rapidly terminate reproduction in amphibians (Orchinik et al., 1994) and also rapidly affect activity levels in songbirds (Breuhner et al., 1998), they may also directly impact song circuits. In addition to these kinds of effects, we also know that corticosteroids have important effects on some brain regions associated with learning and memory in mammals (McEwen, 1999). Given the importance of learning in proper song production, it would not be surprising if corticosteroids impacted song-learning circuits during development. Clearly, studies investigating the distribution of glucocorticoid and mineralocorticoid receptors in the songbird brain are needed, as are studies directly investigating their effects on song learning and performance.

The adrenals of some vertebrates are also capable of synthesizing and secreting sex steroids, sometimes in significant amounts. In mammals, cells in the fasciculata and reticularis zones of the adrenal cortex express CYP17. This enzyme is necessary for the synthesis of cortisol, the dominant mammalian glucocorticoid, but adrenal CYP17 sometimes also catalyzes the formation of androgens in large amounts (Pepe and Albrecht, 1990). This enzyme catalyzes two sequential but separable reactions, 17α-hydroxylation and C17-20lyase. Cortisol is derived from 17α-progesterone, but cleavage of the C17–C20 bond of this metabolite produces androstenedione. Thus, the adrenals secrete cortisol if the CYP17 reaction is terminated midway, but secretes androgens if the reaction proceeds fully to completion. Control of this sequence probably involves the regulation of several conditions, including the phosphorylation state of CYP17 and the abundance of suitable electron donors (Miller et al., 1997). Consequently, although the expression of CYP17 in the adrenals is a necessary first step, factors that might ultimately dictate glucocorticoid vs androgen production are diverse.

Adrenocortical physiology also differs considerably across taxa. In birds, corticosterone is the dominant glucocorticoid. It is not hydroxylated at the C17 position; thus, CYP17 is not required for glucocorticoid production in birds. Given the paucity of cortisol in birds, if CYP17 is found in the avian adrenals, its function may be to make androgens. CYP11A1 and 3β-HSD have been detected in the songbird adrenals (Schlinger and Arnold, 1992b; Cam and Schlinger, 1998; Freking et al., 2000) suggesting they have the capacity to make progesterone. CYP17 activity (Schlinger et al., 1999) and mRNA expression (Freking et al., 2000) have also been found, although at low levels. Thus, songbirds adrenals probably secrete some progesterone and possibly also some androgen into the circulation. CYP19 has not been detected (Schlinger and Arnold, 1991; Freking et al., 2000), so it is unlikely that the adrenals are a significant source of circulating estrogen. Given that DHEA can be produced in large amounts by the adrenals of some mammals and has been identified in the blood of songbirds (Soma et al., 2000c), it is possible that adrenal synthesis of DHEA may be important in songbirds. DHEA can be metabolized into active androgens and estrogens by cells cultured from the songbird telencephalon via the activities of 3β-HSD and CYP19 (Vanson et al., 1996). This raises the intriguing possibility that adrenal DHEA could activate androgen- or estrogen-dependent neural targets, including the activation of song.

Although these studies of zebra finches are enlightening, it is likely that other songbird species demonstrate different patterns of adrenal steroidogenic enzyme expression resulting in the synthesis and secretion of sex steroids or steroidal precursors with actions on the brain. For example, DHEA produced in the adrenals could serve as a novel substrate for the formation of active androgens or estrogens in the brain, which could then stimulate song behavior during nonreproductive periods when T is not produced by the gonads (see previous discussion).

2. Brain

As already discussed, when sex-steroid-dependent behaviors are expressed but the hormones cannot be found in blood, it is possible they are made in the brain itself. Just as in the gonads or adrenals, steroid synthesis involves the expression and activity of a series of steroidogenic enzymes, usually in close proximity to one another. There is good evidence that steroidogenic enzymes are expressed in the avian brain (Tsutsui and Schlinger, 2001), including in the brains of songbirds (Vanson et al., 1996; F. Freking and B. A. Schlinger, unpublished). All the essential enzymes for progestin, androgen, and estrogen synthesis have been identified in the songbird brain. Using reverse tranceriptase-polymerase chain reaction (RT-PCR), CYP11A1, CYP17, and CYP19 have been amplified from the telencephalons and cerebella of zebra finches, both during development (1, 3, 5, 9, and 20 days posthatching) and in adulthood (F. Freking and B. A. Schlinger, unpublished).

Perhaps the strongest evidence for *de novo* steroid-synthesis in the avian brain comes from recent studies by Holloway and Clayton (2001). They found E_2 in media removed as much as 3 weeks after slice-cultures were prepared from the developing zebra finch telencephalon. The concentration of E_2 varied over time and was always greater than the small amount of progesterone added to the steroid-deficient media. Their results suggest direct synthesis of E_2 by the songbird telencephalon. They also investigated the development of a major connection between two telencephalic song control nuclei, HVC and RA, a connection that develops in males but not in females. This connection developed *in vitro* in males, but not females, was induced to develop in females by exogenous E_2 and was blocked in males by administration of the aromatase inhibitor fadrozole (Holloway and Clayton, 2001). These results lead to the conclusion that male slices synthesized more E_2 *de novo* than did the female slices, and that this E_2 caused the formation of the male HVC-RA connection. Whether this process occurs *in vivo* is unknown, but these are exciting observations that impact our thinking of brain sexual differentiation and the function of neurosteroids (Schlinger et al., 2001).

Although we have focused on the synthesis of the traditional sex steroids, those that bind to intranuclear receptors and regulate gene expression, it is also possible that steroids synthesized in brain have different actions. Some conjugates of pregnenolone and DHEA or metabolites of progesterone have been shown to influence neural function by directly influencing neurotransmitter receptors (Lambert et al., 1995). Such steroids are thought to be produced in the mammalian brain, representing a functional end point to neurosteroidogenesis (Baulieu, 1998). Although there is no known function for these compounds in regulating singing behaviors, 5α- and 5β-reduced isoforms of allopregnanolone act on γ-aminobutyric acid A (GABA$_A$) receptors and strongly potentiate GABA-induced Cl$^-$ currents on neurons cultured from the developing zebra finch telencephalon (Carlisle et al., 1998) and induce anesthesia in zebra finches when injected *in vivo* (L. Pumphrey and B. A. Schlinger, unpublished). Thus, if they are produced naturally in the songbird brain, they may influence some behaviors, including song.

C. Steroid Metabolism in Brain: Evidence for a Role in Song-System Development, Song Learning, and Song Expression

Although steroid synthesis by the brain itself may be a pathway for hormonal control of some song-related neural circuits at some discrete times, presumably gonadal sex steroids remain the dominant hormonal influences on these circuits. Nevertheless, steroids synthesized peripherally are most likely modified before they reach these circuits in active forms. In particular, brain metabolism of circulating androgens probably plays a critical role in regulating androgen action on song learning and song expression. Three principal androgen-metabolizing enzymes have been identified in the avian brain–CYP19 (aromatase), which as we have already discussed, converts T into E_2; 5α-reductase, which converts T into the active androgen 5α-DHT; and 5β-reductase, which converts T into the largely inactive 5β-DHT. The roles of these enzymes in regulating behavior of nonsongbird species have been described in detail elsewhere (Hutchison and Steimer, 1984; Schlinger and Callard, 1991; Balthazart et al.,

1996b). In these species, steroids act at the level of the hypothalamus and preoptic areas (HPOA) to activate aggressive and reproductive behaviors, and the metabolism of T into active metabolites locally in the HPOA is essential for behavioral activation. Songs are used in both reproductive and aggressive contexts, so we expect that steroids acting on the HPOA might influence song expression. This conclusion has been supported by studies showing the lesions to the medial preoptic nucleus (POM) disrupted song expression in starlings (Riters and Ball, 1999). Thus, in addition to areas in and around song-control circuits, steroid metabolism in the POM may be of considerable importance in controlling song. We discuss the each enzyme in the songbird brain with respect to its possible control of various neural circuits that may ultimately influence song output.

1. Aromatase

Given the numerous documented roles of estrogen in regulating the development and function of the neural song-control circuitry, CYP19 has been the focus of numerous studies in a variety of species. The most extensively studied has been the zebra finch, in which aromatase has been measured using biochemical assays of enzyme activity in brain homogenates (Vockel *et al.*, 1990a,b; Schlinger and Arnold, 1991, 1992b), *in vivo* (Schlinger and Arnold, 1992a, 1993) and in cell culture (Schlinger *et al.*, 1994, 1995; Wade *et al.*, 1995), immunocytochemically with antiaromatase antibodies (Balthazart *et al.*, 1990, 1996a; Saldanha *et al.*, 2000b), and using a variety of molecular techniques (Shen *et al.*, 1994, 1995; Jacobs *et al.*, 1999; Ramachandran *et al.*, 1999). Estrogens play a key role in the expression of courtship songs in this species (Walters *et al.*, 1991); these estrogens are probably produced locally in the brain.

The expression of an aromatase gene is a highly conserved feature of the vertebrate central nervous system (CNS). In species other than the teleost fish, in which aromatase is expressed at extremely high levels in the adult brain (Callard *et al.*, 1990), this enzyme is often expressed in a few discrete sites, typically in the HPOA, involved in the control of reproductive behavior and feedback regulation of reproductive function. This pattern is observed in a variety of nonpasseriform bird species including Columbiformes (doves), Galliformes (chickens, quail, and grouse), Charadriiformes (sandpipers), and Psittaciformes (budgerigars) (Hutchison and Steimer, 1984; Schlinger *et al.*, 1989; Balthazart, 1990; Saldanha *et al.*, 1998; Metzdorf *et al.*, 1999). A strikingly different pattern has been found in the oscine songbirds in which aromatase is expressed at quite high levels in many regions of the brain, in addition to the more conserved sites found in other birds (Schlinger, 1997).

Aromatase activity can be measured in virtually all regions of the brain of juvenile and adult males and females (Vockel *et al.*, 1990a,b), and overall this adds up to a significant quantity of enzyme (Schlinger and Arnold, 1991). More detailed studies of aromatase immunoreactivity and of aromatase gene expression (Shen *et al.*, 1994, 1995; Balthazart *et al.*, 1996a; Saldanha *et al.*, 2000b) defined the neuroanatomic distribution of aromatase-expressing cells in brain. Outside of a few aromatase-positive cells in the mMAN, it is striking that few if any cell bodies expressing aromatase are present in the principal song nuclei, including structures that express ER, such as the HVc. Thus, estrogens reaching these estrogen-sensitive song circuits may not be produced in the nuclei themselves, at least by cells that are part of the song-control circuitry. It is possible, however, that estrogens that impact these estrogen-sensitive circuits are made locally. Aromatase-positive cells reside in shelf regions adjacent to the HVc and RA, and some of these send projections into these nuclei that may form terminal field-like clusters around some neurons (Fig. 6; Saldanha *et al.*, 2000b). Thus, neurons outside the song system may locally regulate steroid actions in song nuclei by sending enzyme-rich projections to steroid-dependent sites.

Aromatase is also expressed widely in the brains of juveniles, in a pattern generally resembling that seen in adults, with a few notable exceptions (Jacobs *et al.*, 1996). As in adult zebra finches, there is little to no aromatase expression in song-control nuclei other than mMAN between posthatching days 5–25. About 3 weeks after hatching, however, aromatase is strongly up-regulated in the archistriatum, especially the area surrounding the RA. Jacobs *et al.* also found aromatase expression in or near regions through which growing axons from song nuclei travel to reach other song-control nuclei. They speculated that estrogens formed

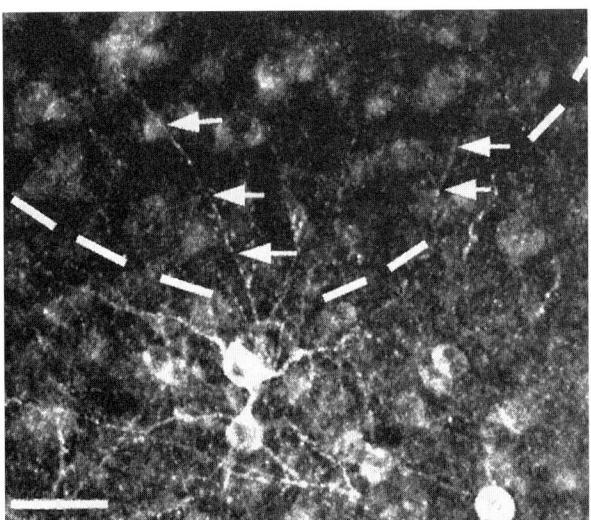

FIGURE 6 Darkfield photomicrograph of aromatase-positive neurons in the shelf region of nucleus HVc. The dashed line depicts the border of HVc. Note the beaded fibers from the aromatase-positive neuron in the shelf region extending into the neuropil of HVc. The pale gray stain of cell bodies results from counterstaining with thionin. From Saldanha *et al.* (2000b), with permission. Copyright © 2000, Wiley-Liss, Inc., a subsidiary of John Wiley & Sons, Inc.

locally might help guide the proper growth of these circuits.

These patterns observed in zebra finches appear to be highly conserved across other species of oscine songbirds. Similarly high levels, particularly in the caudomedial neostriatum, have been found in adult brown-headed cowbirds (*Molothrus ater*; Saldanha and Schlinger, 1997), canaries (*Serinus canarius*; Metzdorf *et al.*, 1999; Fusani, 2000; Saldanha *et al.*, 1998), white-crowned sparrows (*Zonotrichia leucophrys*; Schlinger *et al.*, 1992), house sparrows (*Passer domesticus*; Saldanha *et al.*, 1998), pied flycatchers (*Ficedula hypoleuca*; Foidart *et al.*, 1998), and Lapland longspurs (*Calcarius lapponicus*; Soma *et al.*, 1999a); and in developing mountain chickadees (*Parus gambeli*), house sparrows, white-breasted nuthatches (*Sitta pygmaea*), and house wren (*Troglodytes aedon*; Saldanha *et al.*, 1999). These results contrast with the pattern detected in nonpasseriform species, in which CYP19 is typically low to undetectable outside the diencephalon and one archistriatal nucleus, the nucleus taeniae (e.g., Saldanha *et al.*, 1998). These species differences suggest that high CYP19 expression is associated with the growth of the neural circuitry controlling song in the oscine Passeriformes. However, fairly high levels of CYP19 have also been found in the telencephalon of a suboscine that lacks a visible song-control system (Saldanha *et al.*, 2000a). This observation suggests that high telencephalic aromatase is a characteristic of the passeriform brain, but is not necessarily associated with song. High aromatase in an early passeriform species may have been a preadaptation for the evolution of new estrogen-dependent neural systems, including the song system of the oscine songbirds.

Strikingly, most aromatase expressed in the songbird forebrain is not colocalized with ER, in contrast to what is typically seen in limbic brain regions of songbirds and other species. An exception is a thin band of cells expressing both ER subunit α (ERα) and aromatase in a region of the neostriatum and ventral hyperstriatum bordering the lateral ventricle (Jacobs *et al.*, 1999; Metzdorf *et al.*, 1999). If locally formed estrogens are acting via ERα, it is not clear why aromatase is distributed so widely in the telencephalon. It is possible that estrogens might be acting via ERβ, which has been found in the caudal neostriatum of European starlings (Bernard *et al.*, 1999); this region is rich in aromatase in most songbirds (Schlinger, 1997). The caudal neostriatum also has cells expressing AR, as do several other brain areas that express aromatase (such as the hippocampus) (Metzdorf *et al.*, 1999). It is possible that aromatase functions in these areas to eliminate androgens (by converting them to estrogens) to reduce their binding to AR. Aromatase in the telencephalon has a very high affinity for T, high enough to exclude T from entering other metabolic reactions (Schlinger *et al.*, 1995; and see later).

Some clues as to the role of aromatase in discrete brain regions come from studies showing neuroanatomically restricted regulation of this enzyme. In captive zebra finches and in wild-caught pied flycatchers, there is little evidence for changes in telencephalic aromatase with changes in plasma sex steroid levels or with changes across the breeding cycle (Vockel *et al.*, 1990b; Foidart *et al.*, 1998). In canaries, however, aromatase in the medial caudal neostriatum is high in April and significantly lower in the autumn, with no other obvious differences (Fusani *et al.*, 2000). In male Lapland longspurs, aromatase undergoes substantial changes in several telencephalic regions across display, mate guarding, and incubation phases of the breeding cycle when plasma T levels are high, medium, and low, respectively (Soma et al., 1999a). In both the caudal telencephalon and the rostral hypothalamus, aromatase activity is highest during the display and mate guarding phases, whereas the hippocampus shows the reverse pattern. Aromatase in the rostral telencephalon is highest during the mate guarding phase, but the dorsal and ventromedial telencephalon shows no significant changes. These data suggest that aromatase can experience relatively fine-scale regulation throughout the songbird brain. Apparently, maximal estrogen production occurs in the caudal telencephalon and rostral hypothalamus during the display phase when birds are singing the most. Locally produced estrogens may be acting in these regions to stimulate song behavior.

The mechanisms underlying these regionally different patterns of regulation are unknown. In primary cell cultures of the whole telencephalon from developing zebra finches, aromatase is down-regulated by E_2 and up-regulated by cyclic adenosine monophosphate (cAMP) (Frecking et al., 1998). Specific down-regulation by estrogen *in vivo*, however, has been detected only in the zebra finch hippocampus (C. J. Saldanha et al., 2000). Regulation of intracellular cAMP levels by neurotransmitters or trophic factors may play an important role in the changing levels of aromatase detected in other brain areas.

The aromatase expressed in primary cell culture preparations of the developing zebra finch telencephalon, diencephalon, and cerebellum is unusually high (Schlinger et al., 1994, 1995; Wade et al., 1995). Interestingly, under these *in vitro* conditions aromatase is present in glia as well as in neurons, where the expression is expected (Schlinger et al., 1994). Although it is possible that glia express some CYP19 *in vivo*, astrocytes around sites of neural injury in rodents and songbirds up-regulate CYP19 (Garcia-Segura et al., 1999; Peterson et al., 2000), so enzyme activity in cell culture conditions may be more reflective of the injury state than the natural condition.

2. 5α-Reductase

In many tissues, the action of circulating T as an effective androgen (by binding to and activating androgen receptors) is fully established only after it undergoes conversion into 5α-DHT by the enzyme 5α-reductase (e.g., Wilson et al., 1995). This enzyme is widely distributed in the brains of many vertebrates, including throughout the telencephalon of all songbird species studied (Bottoni and Massa, 1981; Vockel et al., 1990a,b; Saldanha et al., 1999; Soma et al., 1999a). However, studies of this enzyme in the songbird brain have relied solely on measures of activity, so they lack the kind of neuroanatomical and cellular resolution provided by procedures such as ICC or *in situ* hybridization that might provide clues as to its role in controlling song.

If the binding of locally produced 5α-reduced metabolites of T were important in the androgen-dependent activation of song, we could make the following predictions: (1) 5α-reductase is higher in song nuclei than in other telencephalic brain regions, (2) it is higher in male birds that sing than in females who do not, and (3) it is higher during periods of song learning or song expression. 5α-reductase activity was detected in microdissected song nuclei of adult and developing zebra finches (Vockel et al., 1990a,b), and activity was higher in the MAN, HVc, and RA of adult males than of females. 5α-reductase activity may be particularly important in the RA because elsewhere in the song system, enzyme activity was no greater than in other brain regions. In young birds, activity in song-control nuclei was not sexually dimorphic, suggesting that 5α-reductase is not important for song learning. Although these studies reveal some overlap with AR, most areas with 5α-reductase lack intranuclear sex steroid receptors, suggesting that this enzyme may have alternate functions in the brain. As previously discussed, 5α-reductase can also act on progesterone, and some 5α-reduced metabolites of progesterone can bind to and modulate $GABA_A$ channels in the songbird brain (Carlisle et al., 1998). Thus, 5α-reductase may be expressed in songbird brain to metabolize progestins.

Although 5α-reductase may be expressed differently in adult males than in females (Vockel et al., 1990a,b), it is not clear why this pattern of expression is observed. This enzyme appears to experience limited regulation in the songbird telencephalon. In zebra finches, castration and T treatment had no effect on telencephalic 5α-reductase (Vockel et al., 1990b). Similarly, significant changes across the breeding cycle were detected only in the caudal telencephalon and hippocampus, but not other brain areas, of wild male Lapland longspurs (Soma et al., 1999a). In primary cell cultures derived from the telencephalon of developing zebra finches, 5α-reductase activity was unaffected by treatment with cAMP or several sex steroids—E_2, T, 5α-DHT, and 5β-DHT (Freking et al., 1998). Thus, the factors that might produce higher 5α-reductase in song nuclei of male zebra finches are unknown. In summary, although it is likely that 5α-reductase plays some role in regulating androgen-dependent song expression in songbirds, there is no direct experimental evidence establishing such a role.

3. 5β-Reductase

5β-reductase is generally considered the major androgen catabolic reaction in the avian brain (Hutchison and Steimer, 1981), but there is also little direct evidence that brain 5β-reductase, regulates the hormonal control of song. Like 5α-reductase, it is found throughout the telencephalon of every songbird examined (Bottoni and Massa, 1981; Soma et al., 1999a; Vockel et al., 1990a,b; Saldanha et al., 1999); it is usually the most abundant androgen-metabolizing enzyme, sometimes exceeding aromatase and 5α-reductase by several orders of magnitude (Vockel et al., 1990a,b; Saldanha et al., 1999). In the adult longspur telencephalon, 5β-reductase activity was relatively low, compared to the other enzymes (Soma et al., 1999a). The significance of such species differences are unknown. Despite the abundance of this enzyme in the brains of most birds, its affinity for T is relatively low (Schlinger et al., 1995). When T is added to telencephalic cell cultures that express all three enzymes, estrogens and 5β-reduced metabolites are formed in relatively large amounts, but only small amounts of 5α-reduced metabolites are formed (Schlinger et al., 1995). This suggests that brain 5β-reductase may interfere with the 5α-reduction of T but not with its aromatization.

In the adult zebra finch telencephalon, 5β-reductase is generally expressed in higher levels in females than in males (Vockel et al., 1990a). No other species has been examined carefully for sex differences in the telencephalon. Adult female zebra finches do not sing as adults if treated with T, so 5β-reductase might play an important role in inactivating T in adult females. It would be interesting to see if 5β-reductase is less active in the telencephalons of females of other species, such as canaries, that can be stimulated to sing as adults with T. 5β-reductase is also generally present at higher levels in the developing brain, decreasing into adulthood (Vockel et al., 1990a). Especially high levels of 5β-reductase were found in the anterior neostriatum (containing the lMAN, mMAN, and area X) of several juvenile songbirds—approximately 10-fold higher than 5α-reductase and 750-fold higher than aromatase (Saldanha et al., 1999). It is possible that 5β-reductase inactivates T in the anterior forebrain at this time, preserving the neural plasticity underlying song acquisition that typically occurs at these ages.

There is little other evidence to suggest that 5β-reductase is subject to substantial regulation in the songbird telencephalon. In starlings, more 5β-reduced metabolites were formed in the adult male hyperstriatum in summer and fall than in spring (Bottoni and Massa, 1981), suggesting that T down-regulates 5β-reductase in this brain region. However, castration and T treatment had no effect on 5β-reductase in the telencephalons of adult male zebra finches (Vockel et al., 1990b). Similarly, in telencephalic cell cultures, various sex steroids and cAMP had no effect on 5β-reductase activity (Freking et al., 1998). In wild-caught longspurs, only the caudal telencephalon showed changes in 5β-reductase across the breeding cycle, being elevated during the mate guarding phase when plasma T levels were intermediate (Soma et al., 1999a). The significance of this observation, however, is not clear. Much like 5α-reductase, additional studies are required to adequately assess the role that brain 5β-reductase might play in regulating the hormonal control of song. 5β-reductase can also act on progesterone, and some 5β-reduced metabolites of progesterone can bind to and modulate $GABA_A$ channels in the songbird brain (Carlisle et al., 1998). Thus, 5β-reductase may also be expressed in songbird brain to metabolize progestins.

VI. CONCLUSION AND DIRECTIONS FOR FUTURE RESEARCH

The avian song-control system is an excellent model for studying interactions among neural circuits, steroid hormones, and learned behavior. The extensive species diversity observed in different aspects of song learning and behavior provides rich material for comparative studies as a means of testing hypotheses about hormonal influences on the development of the song circuits and song behavior, as well as on plasticity of the adult song system. Variation among species in the sexual patterns of song behavior is accompanied by concomitant variation in the anatomy of the song system. The mechanisms underlying the sexual differentiation of the song system remain an open question. The relative contributions of hormonal and genetic factors to sexually dimorphic development of the song circuits will no doubt be one of the central issues addressed in future studies. Related to this issue is the question of whether the mechanisms that regulate the development of the song circuits in sexually dimorphic species such as the zebra finch also apply to species such as the duetting wrens in which females develop a male-like song system.

There remain multiple questions about the nature of the basic endocrine mechanisms responsible for controlling song. Are traditional androgens and estrogens, such as T, DHT, and E_2, the only active signaling molecules controlling song, or do songbirds also use nontraditional steroids such as DHEA or neuroactive progestins, such as allopregnanolone? When birds are stressed, can adrenal glucocorticoids regulate singing behavior by direct actions on the song system? Investigators may need to measure a more complete set of steroids in the blood of songbirds when evaluating the hormonal basis of song or song learning. The possibility that additional steroids act on the song system also raises questions about their site of synthesis. Are the sex steroids that act on the song system produced only by the gonads or can steroids synthesized by the adrenals or the brain control the development of the song system or stimulate singing in nonbreeding birds? In order to fully account for steroid actions on the brains of different bird species at different times, measures of sex steroids in blood may need to be complemented with studies examining steroid synthesis in other tissues.

We may also need to examine steroid synthesis or metabolism in the brain on a finer scale. Can steroid synthesis or metabolism at the synapse control the endocrine environment around specific neurons of the neural song system? These enzymes might be present in synaptic terminals of neurons projecting into auditory-processing areas or into the song-control system. If so, then these neurons may transmit both electrochemical and steroidal information into the song system, a novel way to couple endocrine and neuronal signaling. Studies examining the ultrastructure of steroid synthesis and metabolism in the song system level will be important.

Finally, it is also important that we consider whether these various steroids control song by binding to traditional intranuclear AR and ER and changing neuronal gene expression or whether there is any involvement of membrane receptors and intracellular second messenger systems as well. It is highly likely that steroids regulate the function of some cells in the song-control system by directly altering intracellular concentrations of cAMP or by changing levels of protein phosphorylation. Elucidating the convergent effects of steroids on the biochemistry and molecular biology of the song system should be an important focus of future studies. Experiments should also be designed to explore whether ERβ is an important receptor-mediated pathway in the songbird brain.

Songbirds are unique among vertebrates in having high concentrations of steroid receptors in nonlimbic regions of the forebrain. The functional role of these telencephalic hormone receptors is not fully understood. In both juvenile and adult brains, lesions of the HVc block the steroid-induced growth of the RA, even though this target nucleus contains high levels of AR. This observation suggests that there is an interaction between steroid hormones and transynaptic trophic effects in the song circuits. The nature of this interaction should be addressed in future studies. Emerging evidence suggests that steroids interact with growth factors during development of the song system, and it would be interesting to know whether such interactions also influence plasticity in adult brains.

Investigators are in the early stages of exploring how steroids interact with neurotransmitter systems to influence song learning and the development of the song circuits. Continued studies of this topic are essential to understand the functional effects of steroids on the song system. The adult song-control system is characterized by extensive plasticity. Many questions remain to be addressed in future studies. What are the functional consequences of seasonal changes in the morphology of the song nuclei and of ongoing neuronal incorporation into the HVc? What factors regulate the extensive seasonal changes of neuron number in the HVc? What are the electrophysiological correlates of seasonal changes in morphology and hormone sensitivity? Is there an interaction between steroid hormones and growth factors in regulating the morphological changes in adult brains?

Little is known about the evolution of telencephalic vocal-control systems in different avian lineages, and this represents an important area for future research. Were the vocal-control systems observed in songbirds, parrots, and hummingbirds independently evolved, inherited from common ancestors, or independently elaborated from ancestral precursors? When in the phylogenetic history of the songbirds did the hormone-sensitive forebrain circuits first arise? Why do the songbirds seem to be the only vertebrates to have evolved abundant expression of hormone receptors in nonlimbic telencephalic regions in adults? Research programs that use the techniques of phylogenetic systematics to address such evolutionary questions will greatly increase our understanding of this extraordinary model.

References

Aamodt, S. M., Kozlowski, M. R., Nordeen, E. J., and Nordeen, K. W. (1992). Distribution and developmental change in [3H]MK-801 binding within zebra finch song nuclei. *J. Neurobiol.* **23**(8), 997–1005.

Aamodt, S. M., Nordeen, E. J., and Nordeen, K. W. (1995). Early isolation from conspecific song does not affect the normal developmental decline of N-methyl-D-aspartate receptor binding in an avian song nucleus. *J. Neurobiol.* **27**(1), 76–84.

Aamodt, S. M., Nordeen, E. J., and Nordeen, K. W. (1996). Blockade of NMDA receptors during song model exposure impairs song development in juvenile zebra finches. *Neurobiol. Learn. Mem.* **65**(1), 91–98.

Adkins, E. K. (1981). Early organization effects hormones. *In* "Neuroendocrinology of Reproduction: Physiology and Behavior" (N. T. Adler, ed.), pp. 159–228. Plenum Press, New York.

Adkins-Regan, E., and Ascenzi, M. (1987). Social and sexual behavior of male and female zebra finches treated with oestradiol during the nestling period. *Anim. Behav.* **35**, 1100–1112.

Adkins-Regan, E., Abdelnabi, M., Mobarak, M., and Ottinger, M. A. (1990). Sex steroid levels in developing and adult male and female zebra finches (*Poephila guttata*). *Gen. Comp. Endocrinol.* **78**(1), 93–109.

Adkins-Regan, E., Mansukhani, V., Seiwert, C., and Thompson, R. (1994). Sexual differentiation of brain and behavior in the zebra finch: Critical periods for effects of early estrogen treatment. *J. Neurobiol.* **25**(7), 865–877.

Akutagawa, E., and Konishi, M. (1998). Transient expression and transport of brain-derived neurotrophic factor in the male zebra finch's song system during vocal development. *Proc. Natl. Acad. Sci. U.S.A.* **95**(19), 11429–11434.

Alvarez-Buylla, A., and Kirn, J. R. (1997). Birth, migration, incorporation, and death of vocal control neurons in adult songbirds. *J. Neurobiol.* **33**(5), 585–601.

Alvarez-Buylla, A., Ling, C. Y., and Nottebohm, F. (1992). High vocal center growth and its relation to neurogenesis, neuronal replacement and song acquisition in juvenile canaries. *J. Neurobiol.* **23**(4), 396–406.

Andrews, R. J. (1969). The effects of testosterone on avian vocalizations. *In* "Bird Vocalizations" (R. A. Hinde, ed.), p. 97. Cambridge University Press, London and New York.

Archawaranon, M., and Wiley, R. H. (1988). Control of aggression and dominance in white-throated sparrows by testosterone and its metabolites. *Horm. Behav.* **22**(4), 497–517.

Armstrong, E. A. (1973). "A Study of Bird Song." Dover, New York.

Arnold, A. P. (1975a). The effects of castration on song development in zebra finches (*Poephila guttata*). *J. Exp. Zool.* **191**(2), 261–278.

Arnold, A. P. (1975b). The effects of castration and androgen replacement on song, courtship, and aggression in zebra finches (*Poephila guttata*). *J. Exp. Zool.* **191**(3), 309–326.

Arnold, A. P. (1980). Quantitative analysis of sex differences in hormone accumulation in the zebra finch brain: Methodological and theoretical issues. *J. Comp. Neurol.* **189**(3), 421–436.

Arnold, A. P. (1992). Developmental plasticity in neural circuits controlling birdsong: Sexual differentiation and the neural basis of learning. *J. Neurobiol.* **23**(10), 1506–1528.

Arnold, A. P. (1997). Sexual differentiation of the zebra finch song system: Positive evidence, negative evidence, null hypotheses, and a paradigm shift. *J. Neurobiol.* **33**(5), 572–584.

Arnold, A. P., and Gorski, R. A. (1984). Gonadal steroid induction of structural sex differences in the central nervous system. *Annu. Rev. Neurosci.* **7**, 413–442.

Arnold, A. P., and Saltiel, A. (1979). Sexual differences in pattern of hormone accumulation in the brain of the songbird. *Science* **205**, 702–705.

Arnold, A. P., and Schlinger, B. A. (1993). Sexual differentiation of brain and behavior: The zebra finch is not just a flying rat. *Brain Behav. Evol.* **42**(4–5), 231–241.

Arnold, A. P., Nottebohm, F., and Pfaff, D. W. (1976). Hormone concentrating cells in vocal control and other areas of the brain of the zebra finch (*Poephila guttata*). *J. Comp. Neurol.* **165**(4), 487–511.

Baker, M. C., and Cunningham, M. A. (1983). Vocal learning in White-crowned sparrows: Sensitive phase and song dialects. *Behav. Ecol. Sociobiol.* **13**, 259–269.

Baldwin, F. M., Goldin, H. S., and Metfessel, M. (1940). Effects of testosterone propionate on female Roller Canaries under complete song isolation. *Proc. Soc. Exp. Biol. Med.* **44**(2), 373–375.

Ball, G. F. (1990). Chemical neuroanatomical studies of the steroid sensitive songbird vocal control system—a comparative approach. In "Hormones, Brain, and Behavior in Vertebrates: Comparative Physiology" (J. Balthazart, ed.), Vol. 8, pp. 148–167. Springer-Verlag, Berlin.

Ball, G. F. (2000). Neuroendocrine basis of seasonal changes in vocal behavior among songbirds. In "Neural Mechanisms of Communication" (M. Hauser and M. Konishi, eds.), pp. 213–253. MIT Press, Cambridge, MA.

Ball, G. F., Nock, B., Wingfield, J. C., McEwen, B. S., and Balthazart, J. (1990). Muscarinic cholinergic receptors in the songbird and quail brain: A quantitative autoradiographic study. *J. Comp. Neurol.* **298**(4), 431–442.

Balthazart, J. (1990). Brain aromatization of testosterone regulates male reproductive behavior in birds. *Prog. Clin. Biol. Res.* **342**(1), 92–98.

Balthazart, J., and Ball, G. F. (1995). Sexual differentiation of brain and behavior in birds. *Trends Endocrinol. Metab.* **6**, 21–29.

Balthazart, J., Foidart, A., Surlemont, C., Vockel, A., and Harada, N. (1990). Distribution of aromatase in the brain of the Japanese quail, ring dove, and zebra finch: An immunocytochemical study. *J. Comp. Neurol.* **301**(2), 276–288.

Balthazart, J., Foidart, A., Wilson, E. M., and Ball, G. F. (1992). Immunocytochemical localization of androgen receptors in the male songbird and quail brain. *J. Comp. Neurol.* **317**(4), 407–420.

Balthazart, J., Absil, P., Foidart, A., Houbart, M., Harada, N., and Ball, G. F. (1996a). Distribution of aromatase-immunoreactive cells in the forebrain of zebra finches (*Taeniopygia guttata*): Implications for the neural action of steroids and nuclear definition in the avian hypothalamus. *J. Neurobiol.* **31**(2), 129–148.

Balthazart, J., Tlemçani, O., and Ball, G. F. (1996b). Do sex differences in the brain explain sex differences in the hormonal induction of reproductive behavior? What 25 years of research on the Japanese quail tells us. *Horm. Behav.* **30**(4), 627–661.

Baptista, L. F., and Schuchmann, K.-L. (1990). Song learning in the Annas hummingbird (*Calypte anna*). *Ethology* **84**(1), 15–26.

Barclay, S. R., and Harding, C. F. (1988). Androstenedione modulation of monoamine levels and turnover in hypothalamic and vocal control nuclei in the male zebra finch: Steroid effects on brain monoamines. *Brain Res.* **459**(2), 333–343.

Barclay, S. R., and Harding, C. F. (1990). Differential modulation of monoamine levels and turnover rates by estrogen and/or androgen in hypothalamic and vocal control nuclei of male zebra finches. *Brain Res.* **523**(2), 251–262.

Basham, M. E., Sohrabji, F., Singh, T. D., Nordeen, E. J., and Nordeen, K. W. (1999). Developmental regulation of NMDA receptor 2B subunit mRNA and ifenprodil binding in the zebra finch anterior forebrain. *J. Neurobiol.* **39**(2), 155–167.

Baulieu, E. E. (1997). Neurosteroids: Of the nervous system, by the nervous system, for the nervous system. *Recent Prog. Horm. Res.* **52**(4, Suppl.), 1–32.

Baulieu, E. E. (1998). Neurosteroids: A novel function of the brain. *Psychoneuroendocrinology* **23**(8), 963–987.

Baylis, J. (1982). Avian vocal mimicry: Its function and evolution. In "Acoustic Communication in Birds" (D. E. Kroodsma and E. Miller, eds.), Vol. 2D, pp. 51–83. Academic Press, London.

Beletsky, L. D. (1983). Aggressive and pair-bonded maintenance songs of female red-winged blackbirds (*Agelaius phoeniceus*). *Z. Tierpsychol.* **62**, 47–54.

Bentley, G. E., Van't Hof, T. J., and Ball, G. F. (1999). Seasonal neuroplasticity in the songbird telencephalon: A role for melatonin. *Proc. Natl. Acad. Sci. U.S.A.* **96**(8), 4674–4679.

Bernard, D. J., and Ball, G. F. (1997). Photoperiodic condition modulates the effects of testosterone on song control nuclei volumes in male European starlings. *Gen. Comp. Endocrinol.* **105**(2), 276–283.

Bernard, D. J., Casto, J. M., and Ball, G. F. (1993). Sexual dimorphism in the volume of song control nuclei in European starlings: Assessment by a Nissl stain and autoradiography for muscarinic cholinergic receptors. *J. Comp. Neurol.* **334**(4), 559–570.

Bernard, D. J., Wilson, F. E., and Ball, G. F. (1997). Testis-dependent and-independent effect photoperiod on volumes of song control nuclei in American tree sparrows. *Brain Res.* **760**(1–2), 163–169.

Bernard, D. J., Bentley, G. E., Balthazart, J., Turek, F. W., and Ball, G. F. (1999). Androgen receptor, estrogen receptor alpha, and estrogen receptor beta show distinct patterns of expression in forebrain song control nuclei of European starlings. *Endocrinology (Baltimore)* **140**(10), 4633–4643.

Bonke, B., Bonke, D., and Scheich, H. (1979). Connectivity of the auditory forebrain nuclei in the guinea fowl. *Cell in Tissue Res.* **200**, 101–121.

Bottjer, S. W. (1987). Ontogenetic changes in the pattern of androgen accumulation in song-control nuclei of male zebra finches. *J. Neurobiol.* **18**(2), 125–139.

Bottjer, S. W. (1993). The distribution of tyrosine hydroxylase immunoreactivity in the brains of male and female zebra finches. *J. Neurobiol.* **24**(1), 51–69.

Bottjer, S. W., and Hewer, S. J. (1992). Castration and antisteroid treatment impair vocal learning in male zebra finches. *J. Neurobiol.* **23**(4), 337–353.

Bottjer, S. W., and Johnson, F. (1997). Circuits, hormones, and learning: Vocal behavior in songbirds. *J. Neurobiol.* **33**(5), 602–618.

Bottjer, S. W., and Maier, E. (1991). Testosterone and the incidence of hormone target cells in song-control nuclei of adult canaries. *J. Neurobiol.* **22**(5), 512–521.

Bottjer, S. W., Miesner, E. A., and Arnold, A. P. (1984). Forebrain lesions disrupt development but not maintenance of song in passerine birds. *Science* **224**, 901–903.

Bottoni, L., and Massa, R. (1981). Seasonal changes in testosterone metabolism in the pituitary gland and central nervous system of the European starling (*Sturnus vulgaris*). *Gen. Comp. Endocrinol.* **43**(4), 532–536.

Brauth, S. E., Heaton, J. T., Shea, S. D., Durand, S. E., and Hall, W. S. (1997). Functional anatomy of forebrain vocal control pathways in the budgerigar. *Ann. N.Y. Acad. Sci.* **807**, 368–385.

Breath, S. E., Eaton, J. T., Shea, S. D., Duran, S. E., and Hall, W.S. (1997). Functional anatomy of forebrain vocal control pathways in the budgerigar. *Ann. N.Y. Acad. Sci.* **807**, 368–385.

Brenowitz, E. A. (1991a). Altered perception of species-specific song by female birds after lesions of a forebrain nucleus. *Science* **251**, 303–305.

Brenowitz, E. A. (1991b). Evolution of the vocal control system in the avian brain. *Semin. Neurosci.* **3**, 399–407.

Brenowitz, E. A. (1997). Comparative approaches to the avian song system. *J. Neurobiol.* **33**(5), 517–531.

Brenowitz, E. A., and Arnold, A. P. (1985). Lack of sexual dimorphism in steroid accumulation in vocal control brain regions of duetting song birds. *Brain Res.* **344**(1), 172–175.

Brenowitz, E. A., and Arnold, A. P. (1986). Interspecific comparisons of the size of neural song control regions and song complexity in duetting birds: Evolutionary implications. *J. Neurosci.* **6**(10), 2875–2879.

Brenowitz, E. A., and Arnold, A. P. (1989). Accumulation of estrogen in a vocal control brain region of a duetting song bird. *Brain Res.* **480**(1–2), 119–125.

Brenowitz, E. A., and Arnold, A. P. (1990). The effects of systemic androgen treatment on androgen accumulation in song control regions of the adult female canary brain. *J. Neurobiol.* **21**(6), 837–843.

Brenowitz, E. A., and Arnold, A. P. (1992). Hormone accumulation in song regions of the canary brain. *J. Neurobiol.* **23**(7), 871–880.

Brenowitz, E. A., and Kroodsma, D. E. (1996). The neuroethology of birdsong. *In* "Ecology and Evolution of Acoustic Communication in Birds" (D. E. Kroodsma and E. H. Miller, eds.), pp. 269–281. Cornell University Press, Ithaca, NY.

Brenowitz, E. A., and Lent, K. (2000). Intracerebral implants of testosterone induce seasonal-like growth of adult avian song control circuits. *Soc. Neurosci. Abstr.* **26**, (1268).

Brenowitz, E. A., Arnold, A. P., and Levin, R. N. (1985). Neural correlates of female song in tropical duetting birds. *Brain Res.* **343**(1), 104–112.

Brenowitz, E. A., Nalls, B., Wingfield, J. C., and Kroodsma, D. E. (1991). Seasonal changes in avian song nuclei without seasonal changes in song repertoire. *J. Neurosci.* **11**(5), 1367–1374.

Brenowitz, E. A., Nalls, B., Kroodsma, D. E., and Horning, C. (1994). Female marsh wrens do not provide evidence of anatomical specializations of song nuclei for perception of male song. *J. Neurobiol.* **25**(2), 197–208.

Brenowitz, E. A., Arnold, A. P., and Loesche, P. (1996). Steroid accumulation in song nuclei of a sexually dimorphic duetting bird, the rufous and white wren. *J. Neurobiol.* **31**(2), 235–244.

Brenowitz, E. A., Margoliash, D., and Nordeen, K. W. (1997). An introduction to birdsong and the avian song system. *J. Neurobiol.* **33**(5), 495–500.

Brenowitz, E. A., Baptista, L. F., Lent, K., and Wingfield, J. C. (1998). Seasonal plasticity of the song control system in wild Nuttall's white-crowned sparrows. *J. Neurobiol.* **34**(1), 69–82.

Breuhner, C. W., Greenberg, A. L., and Wingfield, J. C. (1998). Noninvasive corticosterone treatment rapidly increases activity in Gambel's white-crowned sparrows (*Zonotrichia leucophrys gambelli*). *Gen. Comp. Endocrinol.* **111**, 386–394.

Brown, S. D., Johnson, F., and Bottjer, S. W. (1993). Neurogenesis in adult canary telencephalon is independent of gonadal hormone levels. *J. Neurosci.* **13**(5), 2024–2032.

Burek, M. J., Nordeen, K. W., and Nordeen, E. J. (1995). Estrogen promotes neuron addition to an avian song-control nucleus by regulating post-mitotic events. *Dev. Brain Res.* **85**(2), 220–224.

Callard, G. V., Schlinger, B. A., Pasmanik, M., and Corina, K. (1990). Aromatization and estrogen action in brain. *Prog. Clin. Biol. Res.* **342**, 105–111.

Cam, V., and Schlinger, B. A. (1998). Activities of aromatase and 3β-hydroxysteroid dehydrogenase $\Delta(4)$-$\Delta(5)$ isomerase in whole organ cultures of tissues from developing zebra finches. *Horm. Behav.* **33**(1), 31–39.

Carlisle, H. J., Hales, T. G., and Schlinger, B. A. (1998). Characterization of neuronal zebra finch GABA(A) receptors: Steroid effects. *J. Comp. Physiol. A* **182**(4), 531–538.

Casto, J. M., and Ball, G. F. (1996). Early administration of 17β-estradiol partially masculinizes song control regions and alpha2-adrenergic receptor distribution in European starlings (*Sturnus vulgaris*). *Horm. Behav.* **30**(4), 387–406.

Catchpole, C. K., and Slater, P. J. B. (1995). "Bird Song: Biological Themes and Variations." Cambridge University Press, Cambridge, UK.

Chan, K. M. B., and Lofts, B. (1974). The testicular cycle and androgen biosynthesis in the tree sparrow, Passer montanus saturatus. *J. Zool.* **172**, 47–66.

Compagnone, N. A., and Mellon, S. H. (2000). Neurosteroids: Biosynthesis and function of these novel neuromodulators. *Front. Neuroendocrinol* **21**(1), 1–56.

Cookson, K. K., Hall, W. S., Eaton, J. T., and Breath, S. E. (1996). Distribution of choline acetyl transferase and acetylcholinesterase in vocal control nuclei of the budgerigar. *J. Comp. Neurol.* **369**, 220–235.

Dawson, A. (1983). Plasma gonadal steroid levels in wild starlings (*Sturnus vulgaris*) during the annual cycle and in relation to the stages of breeding. *Gen. Comp. Endocrinol.* **49**(2), 286–294.

DeVoogd, T. J., and Nottebohm, F. (1981). Gonadal hormones induce dendritic growth in the adult avian brain. *Science* **214**, 202–204.

DeVoogd, T. J., Nixdorf, B., and Nottebohm, F. (1985). Synaptogenesis and changes in synaptic morphology related to acquisition of a new behavior. *Brain Res.* **329**(1–2), 304–308.

DeVoogd, T. J., Houtman, A. M., and Falls, J. B. (1995). White-throated sparrow morphs that differ in song production rate also differ in the anatomy of some song-related brain areas. *J. Neurobiol.* **28**(2), 202–213.

Dittami, J. P. (1987). A comparison of breeding and moult cycles and life histories in two tropical species: The blue-eared glossy starling *Lamprotornis chalybaeus* and Rupppell's long-tailed glossy starling *L. purpuropterus*. *Ibis* **129**, 69–85.

Dittami, J. P., and Gwinner, E. (1990). Endocrine correlates of seasonal reproduction and territorial behaviour in some tropical passerines. *In* "Endocrinology of Birds: Molecular to Behavioural" (M. Wada, ed.), pp. 225–233. Springer-Verlag, Berlin.

Dittrich, F., Feng, Y., Metzdorf, R., and Gahr, M. (1999). Estrogen-inducible, sex-specific expression of brain-derived neurotrophic factor mRNA in a forebrain song control nucleus of the juvenile zebra finch. *Proc. Natl. Acad. Sci. U.S.A.* **96**(14), 8241–8246.

Dooling, R. J., Gephart, B., Price, P., McHale, C., and Breath, S. (1987). Effects of deafening on the contact call of the budgerigar. *Anim. Behav.* **35**, 1264–1266.

Dooling, R. J., Brown, S. D., Klump, G. M., and Okanoya, K. (1992). Auditory perception of conspecific and heterospecific vocalizations in birds: Evidence for special processes. *J. Comp. Psychol.* **106**(1), 20–28.

Durand, S. E., Eaton, J. T., Amateau, S.K., and Breath, S. E. (1997). Vocal control pathways through the anterior forebrain of a parrot. *Ann. N.Y. Acad. Sci.* **337**, 179–206.

Eaton, J. T., and Breath, S. E. (1996). Effects of vocal archistriatal lesions and early deafening on vocal development in the budgerigar. *Soc. Neurosci. Abstr.* **22**, 694.

Eaton, J. T., Breath, S. E., and Liang, W. (1994). Lesions of the telencephalic vocal control nuclei in the budgerigar disrupt both calls and warble song. *Neurosci. Abstr.* **20**, 164.

Farabaugh, S. M. (1982). The ecological and social significance of duetting. *In* "Acoustic Communication in Birds" (D. E. Kroodsma and E. Miller, eds.), Vol. 2, pp. 85–124. Academic Press, London.

Farner, D. S. (1986). Generation and regulation of annual cycles in migratory passerine birds. *Am. Zool.* **26**, 493–501.

Foidart, A., Silverin, B., Baillien, M., Harada, N., and Balthazart, J. (1998). Neuroanatomical distribution and variations across the reproductive cycle of aromatase activity and aromatase-immunoreactive cells in the pied flycatcher (*Ficedula hypoleuca*). *Horm. Behav.* **33**(3), 180–196.

Freking, F., Ramachandran, B., and Schlinger, B. A. (1998). Regulation of aromatase, 5α- and 5β-reductase in primary cell cultures of developing zebra finch telencephalon. *J. Neurobiol.* **36**(1), 30–40.

Freking, F., Nazairians, T., and Schlinger, B. A. (2000). The expression of the sex steroid-synthesizing enzymes CYP11A1, 3β-HSD, CYP17, and CYP19 in gonads and adrenals of adult and developing zebra finches. *Gen. Comp. Endocrinol.* **119**(I), 140–151.

Fusani, L., Van't Hof, T., Hutchison, J. B., and Gahr, M. (2000). Seasonal expression of androgen receptors, estrogen receptors, and aromatase in the canary brain in relation to circulating androgens and estrogens. *J. Neurobiol.* **43**, 254–268.

Gahr, M. (1990). Localization of androgen receptors and estrogen receptors in the same cells of the songbird brain. *Proc. Natl. Acad. Sci. U.S.A.* **87**(23), 9445–9448.

Gahr, M., and Kosar, E. (1996). Identification, distribution, and developmental changes of a melatonin binding site in the song control system of the zebra finch. *J. Comp. Neurol.* **367**(2), 308–318.

Gahr, M., and Metzdorf, R. (1997). Distribution and dynamics in the expression of androgen and estrogen receptors in vocal control systems of songbirds. *Brain Res. Bull.* **44**(4), 509–517.

Gahr, M., and Metzdorf, R. (1999). The sexually dimorphic expression of androgen receptors in the song nucleus hyperstriatalis ventrale pars caudale of the zebra finch develops independently of gonadal steroids. *J. Neurosci.* **19**(7), 2628–2636.

Gahr, M., and Wild, J. M. (1997). Localization of androgen receptor mRNA-containing cells in avian respiratory-vocal nuclei: An in situ hybridization study. *J. Neurobiol.* **33**(7), 865–876.

Gahr, M., Flügge, G., and Guttinger, H. R. (1987). Immunocytochemical localization of estrogen-binding neurons in the songbird brain. *Brain Res.* **402**(1), 173–177.

Gahr, M., Guttinger, H. R., and Kroodsma, D. E. (1993). Estrogen receptors in the avian brain: Survey reveals general distribution and forebrain areas unique to songbirds. *J. Comp. Neurol.* **327**(1), 112–122.

Gahr, M., Metzdorf, R., and Aschenbrenner, S. (1996). The ontogeny of the canary HVc revealed by the expression of androgen and oestrogen receptors. *NeuroReport* **8**(1), 311–315.

Garcia-Segura, L. M., Wozniak, A., Azcoitia, I., Rodriguez, J. R., Hutchison, R. E., and Hutchison, J. B. (1999). Aromatase expression by astrocytes after brain injury: Implications for local estrogen formation in brain repair. *Neuroscience* **89**(2), 567–578.

Goldman, S. A., and Nottebohm, F. (1983). Neuronal production, migration, and differentiation in a vocal control nucleus of the adult female canary brain. *Proc. Natl. Acad. Sci. U.S.A.* **80**(8), 2390–2394.

Gong, A., Freking, F. W., Schlinger, B. A., Arnold, A. P., and Wingfield, J. (1999). Pre-hatching inhibition of aromatase activity masculinizes syringeal and gonadal tissue but not the song system in zebra finch females. *Gen. Comp. Endocrinol.* **115**, 346–353.

Goy, R., and McEwen, B. S. (1980). "Sexual Differentiation of the Brain." MIT Press, Cambridge, MA.

Grisham, W., and Arnold, A. P. (1995). A direct comparison of the masculinizing effects of testosterone, androstenedione, estrogen, and progesterone on the development of the zebra finch song system. *J. Neurobiol.* **26**(2), 163–170.

Gulledge, C. C., and Deviche, P. (1997). Androgen control of vocal control region volumes in a wild migratory songbird (*Junco hyemalis*) is region and possibly age dependent. *J. Neurobiol.* **32**(4), 391–402.

Gurney, M. E. (1981). Hormonal control of cell form and number in the zebra finch song system. *J. Neurosci.* **1**(6), 658–673.

Gurney M. E. (1982). Behavioral correlates of sexual differentiation in the zebra finch song system. *Brain Res.* **231**(1), 153–172.

Gurney, M., and Konishi, M. (1980). Hormone-induced sexual differentiation of brain and behavior in zebra finches. *Science* **208**, 1380–1383.

Gwinner, E., Rodl, T., and Schwabl, H. (1994). Pair territoriality of wintering stonechats: Behavior, function, and hormones. *Behav. Ecol. Sociobiol.* **34**, 321–327.

Hall, W. S., Breath, S. E., and Eaton, J. T. (1994). Comparison of the effects of lesions in nucleus basalis and field "L" in vocal learning and performance in the budgerigar. *Brain, Behav. Evol.* **44**, 133–148.

Halsema, K., and Bottjer, S. (1992). Chemical lesions of a thalamic nucleus disrupt song development in male zebra finches. *Soc. Neurosci. Abstr.* **18**, 1052.

Heid, P., Guttinger, H. R., and Pröve, E. (1985). The influence of castration and testosterone replacement on the song architecture of canaries (*Serinus canaria*). *Z. Tierpsychol.* **69**, 224–236.

Herrick, E. H., and Harris, J. O. (1957). Singing female canaries. *Science* **125**, 1299–1300.

Hidalgo, A., Barami, K., Iversen, K., and Goldman, S. A. (1995). Estrogens and non-estrogenic ovarian influences combine to promote the recruitment and decrease the turnover of new neurons in the adult female canary brain. *J. Neurobiol.* **27**(4), 470–487.

Hill, K. M., and DeVoogd, T. J. (1991). Altered day length affects dendritic structure in a song-related brain region in red-winged blackbirds. *Behav. Neural Biol.* **56**(3), 240–250.

Hoelzel, A. R. (1986). Song characteristics and response to playback of male and female Robins *Erithacus rubecula*. *Ibis* **128**, 115–127.

Holloway, C. C., and Clayton, D. E. (2001). Estrogen synthesis in the male brain triggers development of the avian song control pathway in vitro. *Nat. Neurosci.* **4**, 170–175.

Hunt, K. (1997). Testosterone, estrogen, and breeding behavior in an Arctic bird, the Lapland longspur. Ph.D. Dissertation, University of Washington, Seattle.

Hunt, K., Wingfield, J. C., Astheimer, L. B., Buttemer, W. A., and Hahn, T. P. (1995). Temporal patterns of territorial behavior and circulating testosterone in the Lapland longspur and other arctic passerines. *Am. Zool.* **35**, 274–284.

Hutchison, J. B., and Steimer, T. (1981). Brain 5β-reductase: A correlate of behavioral sensitivity to androgen. *Science* **213**(4504), 244–246.

Hutchison, J. B., and Steimer, T. (1984). Androgen metabolism in the brain: Behavioral correlates. *Prog. Brain Res.* **61**(3), 23–51.

Hutchison, J. B., Wingfield, J. C., and Hutchison, R. E. (1984). Sex differences in plasma concentrations of steroids during the sensitive period for brain differentiation in the zebra finch. *J. Endocrinol.* **103**(3), 363–369.

Jacobs, E. C., Arnold, A. P., and Campagnoni, A. T. (1999). Developmental regulation of the distribution of aromatase- and estrogen-receptor-mRNA-expressing cells in the zebra finch brain. *Dev. Neurosci.* **21**(6), 453–472.

Jarvis, E. D., Ribeiro, S., da Silva, M. L., Ventura, D., Vielliard, J., and Mello, C.V. (2000). Behaviourally driven gene expression reveals song nuclei in hummingbird brain. *Nature (London)* **406**, 628–632.

Johnson, F., and Bottjer, S. W. (1993). Hormone-induced changes in identified cell populations of the higher vocal center in male canaries. *J. Neurobiol.* **24**(3), 400–418.

Johnson, F., and Bottjer, S. W. (1995). Differential estrogen accumulation among populations of projection neurons in the higher vocal center of male canaries. *J. Neurobiol.* **26**(1), 87–108.

Johnson, F., Hohmann, S. E., DiStefano, P. S., and Bottjer, S. W. (1997). Neurotrophins suppress apoptosis induced by deafferentation of an avian motor-cortical region. *J. Neurosci.* **17**(6), 2101–2111.

Karten, H., and Hodos, W. (1967). "A Stereotaxic Atlas of the Brain of the Pigeon." Johns Hopkins Press, Baltimore, MD.

Kelsey, M. G. (1989). A comparison of the song and territorial behavior of a long distance migrant, the marsh warbler *Acrocephalus palustris*, in summer and winter. *Ibis* **131**, 403–414.

Kirn, J. R., and Nottebohm, F. (1993). Direct evidence for loss and replacement of projection neurons in adult canary brain. *J. Neurosci.* **13**(4), 1654–1663.

Kirn, J. R., Alvarez-Buylla, A., and Nottebohm, F. (1991). Production and survival of projection neurons in a forebrain vocal center of adult male canaries. *J. Neurosci.* **11**(6), 1756–1762.

Kirn, J. R., O'Loughlin, B., Kasparian, S., and Nottebohm, F. (1994). Cell death and neuronal recruitment in the high vocal center of adult male canaries are temporally related to changes in song. *Proc. Natl. Acad. Sci. U.S.A.* **91**(17), 7844–7848.

Kobayashi, H., and Wada, M. (1973). Neuroendocrinology in birds. "Avian Biol." **3**, 287–347.

Konishi, M. (1985). Birdsong: From behavior to neuron. *Annu. Rev. Neurosci.* **8**, 125–170.

Konishi, M., and Akutagawa, E. (1981). Androgen increases protein synthesis within the avian brain vocal control system. *Brain Res.* **222**(2), 442–446.

Konishi, M., and Akutagawa, E. (1985). Neuronal growth, atrophy and death in a sexually dimorphic song nucleus in the zebra finch brain. *Nature (London)* **315**, 145–147.

Korsia, S., and Bottjer, S. W. (1989). Developmental changes in the cellular composition of a brain nucleus involved with song learning in zebra finches. *Neuron* **3**(4), 451–460.

Korsia, S., and Bottjer, S. W. (1991). Chronic testosterone treatment impairs vocal learning in male zebra finches during a restricted period of development. *J. Neurosci.* **11**, 2362–2371.

Kroner, S. and Gunturkun, O. (1999). Afferent and efferent connections of the caudolateral neostriatum in the pigeon: A retro- and anterograde pathway tracing study. *J. Comp. Neurol.* **407**, 228–260.

Kroodsma, D. E. (1982). Song repertoires: Problems in their definition and use. *In* "Acoustic Communication in Birds" (D. E. Kroodsma and E. Miller, eds.), Vol. 2, pp. 125–146. Academic Press, London.

Kroodsma, D. E. (1986). Song development by castrated marsh wrens. *Anim. Behav.* **34**(5), 1572–1575.

Kroodsma, D. E., and Baylis, J. R. (1982). Appendix: A world survey of evidence for vocal learning in birds. *In* "Acoustic Communication in Birds" (D. E. Kroodsma and E. Miller, eds.), Vol. 2, pp. 311–337. Academic Press, London.

Kroodsma, D. E., and Konishi, M. (1991). A suboscine bird (eastern phoebe, *Sayornis phoebe*) develops normal song without auditory feedback. *Anim. Behav.* **42**(3), 477–487.

Kroodsma, D. E., Bereson, R. C., Byers, B. E., and Minear, E. (1989). Use of song types by the chestnut-sided warbler: Evidence for both intra-and inter-sexual functions. *Can. J. Zool.* **67**, 447–456.

Kubota, M., and Saito, N. (1991). NMDA receptors participate differentially in two different synaptic inputs in neurons of the zebra finch robust nucleus of the archistriatum in vitro. *Neurosci. Lett.* **125**(2), 107–109.

Lack, D. (1946). "The Life of the Robin." Witherby, London.

Lam, F., and Farner, D. S. (1976). The ultrastructure of the cells of Leydig in the white- crowned sparrow (*Zonotrichia leucophrys gambelii*) in relation to plasma levels of luteinizing hormones and testosterone. *Cell Tissue Res.* **169**, 93–109.

Lambert, J. J., Belelli, D., Hill-Venning, C., and Peters, J. A. (1995). Neurosteroids and GABA$_A$ receptor function. *Trends Pharmacol. Sci.* **16**, 295–303.

Lampe, H. M., and Espmark, Y. O. (1987). Singing activity and song pattern of the Redwing *Turdus iliacus* during the breeding season. *Ornis Scand.* **18**, 179–185.

Levin, R. N. (1996a). Song behavior and reproductive strategies in a duetting wren, *Thryothorus nigricapillus*: I. Removal experiments. *Anim. Behav.* **52**, 1093–1106.

Levin, R. N. (1996b). Song behavior and reproductive strategies in a duetting wren, *Thryothorus nigricapillus*: II. Playback experiments. *Anim. Behav.* **52**, 1107–1117.

Levin, R. N., and Wingfield, J. C. (1992). The hormonal control of territorial aggression in tropical birds. *Ornis Scand.* **23**, 284–291.

Lieberburg, I., and Nottebohm, F. (1979). High-affinity androgen binding proteins in syringeal tissues of songbirds. *Gen. Comp. Endocrinol.* **37**(3), 286–293.

Lincoln, G. A., Racey, P. A., Sharp, P. J., and Klandorf, H. (1980). Endocrine changes associated with spring and autumn sexuality of the rook, *Corvus frugilegus*. *J. Zool.* **190**, 137–153.

Lofts, B., and Murton, R. K. (1973). Reproduction in birds. *Avian Biol.* **3**, 1–107.

Logan, C. A. (1992). Testosterone and reproductive adaptations in the autumnal territoriality of Northern Mockingbirds *Mimus polyglottos*. *Ornis Scand.* **23**, 277–283.

Logan, C. A., and Wingfield, J. C. (1990). Autumnal territorial aggression is independent of plasma testosterone in mockingbirds. *Horm. Behav.* **24**(4), 568–581.

Lowther, J. K. (1962). Color and behavioral polymorphism in the white throated sparrow, *Zonotrichia albicollis* (Gmelin). Ph. D. Thesis, University of Ontario.

MacDougall-Shackleton, S. A., and Ball, G. F. (1999). Comparative studies of sex differences in the song-control system of songbirds. *Trends Neurosci.* **22**(10), 432–436.

Margoliash, D., Fortune, E. S., Sutter, M. L., Yu, A. C., Wren-Hardin, B. D., and Dave, A. (1994). Distributed representation in the song system of oscines: Evolutionary implications and functional consequences. *Brain, Behav. Evol.* **44**(4–5), 247–264.

Marler, P. (1970). A comparative approach to vocal learning: Song development in white-crowned sparrows. *J. Comp. Physiol., Psychol., Suppl.* **71**, 1–25.

Marler, P., and Peters, S. (1982). Developmental overproduction and selective attrition: New processes in the epigenesis of birdsong. *Dev. Psychobiol.* **15**(4), 369–378.

Marler, P., Peters, S., and Wingfield, J. (1987). Correlations between song acquisition, song production, and plasma levels of testosterone and estradiol in sparrows. *J. Neurobiol.* **18**(6), 531–548.

Marler, P., Peters, S., Ball, G. F., Dufty, A. M. *et al.* (1988). The role of sex steroids in the acquisition and production of birdsong. *Nature (London)* **336**, 770–772.

Marshall, A. J. (1961). Breeding seasons and migration. *In* "Biology and Comparative Physiology of Birds" (A. J. Marshall, ed.), Vol. 2, pp. 307–339. Academic Press, New York.

McEwen, B. S. (1999). Stress and the aging hippocampus. *Front. Neuroendocrinol.* **20**(1), 49–70.

Mensah-Nyagan, A. G., Do-Rego, J. L., Beaujean, D., Luu-The, V., Pelletier, G., and Vaudry, H. (1999). Neurosteroids: Expression of steroidogenic enzymes and regulation of steroid biosynthesis in the central nervous system. *Pharmacol. Rev.* **51**(1), 63–81.

Metzdorf, R., Gahr, M., and Fusani, L. (1999). Distribution of aromatase, estrogen receptor, and androgen receptor mRNA in the forebrain of songbirds and nonsongbirds. *J. Comp. Neurol.* **407**(1), 115–129.

Miller, W. L. (1988). Molecular biology of steroid hormone synthesis. *Endocr. Rev.* **9**(3), 295–318.

Miller, W. L., Auchus, R. J., and Geller, D. H. (1997). The regulation of 17, 20 lyase activity. *Steroids* **62**, 133–142.

Mooney, R., and Konishi, M. (1991). Two distinct inputs to an avian song nucleus activate different glutamate receptor subtypes on individual neurons. *Proc. Natl. Acad. Sci. U.S.A.* **88**, 4075–4079.

Mooney, R. (1992). Synaptic basis for developmental plasticity in a birdsong nucleus. *J. Neurosci.* **12**(7), 2464–2477.

Mooney, R., and Rao, M. (1994). Waiting periods versus early innervation: The development of axonal connections in the zebra finch song system. *J. Neurosci.* **14**, 6532–6543.

Morton, E. S. (1996). A comparison of vocal behavior among tropical and temperate passerine birds. *In* "Ecology and Evolution of Acoustic Communication in Birds" (D. E. Kroodsma, and E. Miller, eds.), pp. 258–268. Cornell University Press, Ithaca, NY.

Morton, M. L., Pereya, L. E., Burns, D. M., and Allan, N. (1990). Seasonal and age related changes in plasma testosterone in mountain white-crowned sparrows. *Condor* **92**, 166–173.

Nastiuk, K. L., and Clayton, D. F. (1994). Seasonal and tissue-specific regulation of canary androgen receptor messenger ribonucleic acid. *Endocrinology (Baltimore)* **134**(2), 640–649.

Nealen, P. M., and Perkel, D. J. (2000). Sexual dimorphism in the song system of the Carolina wren *Thryothorus ludovicianus*. *J. Comp. Neurol.* **418**(3), 346–360.

Nice, M. M. (1943). Studies in the life history of song sparrow II. The behavior of the song sparrow and other passerines. *Trans. Linn. Soc. N.Y.* **6**, 1–388.

Nicholls, T. J., Goldsmith, A. R., and Dawson, A. (1988). Photorefractoriness in birds and comparison with mammals. *Physiol. Rev.* **68**(1), 133–176.

Nordeen, K. W., Nordeen, E. J., and Arnold, A. P. (1986). Estrogen establishes sex differences in androgen accumulation in zebra finch brain. *J. Neurosci.* **6**(3), 734–738.

Nordeen, K. W., Nordeen, E. J., and Arnold, A. P. (1987). Estrogen accumulation in zebra finch song control nuclei: Implications for sexual differentiation and adult activation of song behavior. *J. Neurobiol.* **18**(6), 569–582.

Nottebohm, F. (1969). The critical period for song learning. *Ibis* **111**, 386–387.

Nottebohm, F. (1972). The origins of vocal learning. *Am. Nat.* **106**, 116–140.

Nottebohm, F. (1980b). Testosterone triggers growth of brain vocal control nuclei in adult female canaries. *Brain Res.* **189**(2), 429–436.

Nottebohm, F. (1981). A brain for all seasons: Cyclical anatomical changes in song control nuclei of the canary brain. *Science* **214**, 1368–1370.

Nottebohm, F. (1987). Plasticity in adult avian central nervous system: Possible relation between hormones, learning, and brain repair. *In* "Handbook of Physiology" (F. Plum ed.), Sect. 1, pp. 85–108. Williams and Wilkins, Baltimore, MD.

Nottebohm, F. (1989). From bird song to neurogenesis. *Sci. Am.* **260**(2), 74–79.

Nottebohm, F., and Arnold, A. P. (1976). Sexual dimorphism in vocal control areas of the songbird brain. *Science* **194**(4261), 211–213.

Nottebohm, F., Stokes, T. M., and Leonard, C. M. (1976). Central control of song in the canary, *Serinus canarius*. *J. Comp. Neurol.* **165**(4), 457–486.

Nottebohm, F., Kaspasian, S., and Pandazis, C. (1981). Brain Space for a learned task. *Brain Res.* **213**, 99–109.

Nottebohm, F., Nottebohm, M. E., and Crane, L. (1986). Developmental and seasonal changes in canary song and their relation to changes in the anatomy of song-control nuclei. *Behav. Neural Biol.* **46**(3), 445–471.

Nottebohm, F., Alvarez-Buylla, A., Cynx, J., Kirn, J., Ling, C. Y., Nottebohm, M., Sutter, R., Toles, A., and Williams, H. (1990). Song learning in birds: The relation between perception and production. *Philos. Trans. R. Soc. London, Ser. B* **329**, 115–124.

Nottebohm, F., O'Loughlin, B., Gould, K., Yohay, K., and Alvarez-Buylla, A. (1994). The life span of new neurons in a song control nucleus of the adult canary brain depends on time of year when these cells are born. *Proc. Natl. Acad. Sci. U.S.A.* **91**(17), 7849–7853.

Orchinik, M., Murray, T. F., and Moore, F. L. (1994). Steroid modulation of $GABA_A$ receptors in an amphibian brain. *Brain Res.* **646**(2), 258–266.

Paton, J. A., and Nottebohm, F. N. (1984). Neurons generated in the adult brain are recruited into functional circuits. *Science* **225**, 1046–1048.

Paton, J. A., Manogue, K. R., and Nottebohm, F. (1981). Bilateral organization of the vocal control pathway in the budgerigar, *Melopsittacus undulatus*. *J. Neurosci.* **1**(11), 1279–1288.

Paton, J. A., O'Loughlin, B. E., and Nottebohm, F. (1985). Cells born in adult canary forebrain are local interneurons. *J. Neurosci.* **5**(11), 3088–3093.

Pepe, G. J., and Albrecht, E. D. (1990). Regulation of the primate fetal adrenal cortex. *Endocr. Rev.* **11**(1), 151–176.

Pesch, A., and Guttinger, H. R. (1985). Der Gesang des weiblichen Kanarienvogels. *J. Ornithol.* **126**, 108–110.

Perlman, W. R., and Arnold, A. P. (2001). Androgen receptor mRNA expression in hatchling zebra finch brain. *Soc. Neurosci. Abs.* **27**, 368.

Peterson, R. S., Saldanha, C. J., and Schlinger, B. A. (2001). Rapid upregulation of aromatase mRNA and protein following neural injury in the zebra finch (*Taeniopygia guttata*). *J. Neuroendocrinol.* **13**, 317–323.

Porter, T. E., Hargis, B. M., Silsby, J. L., and Halawani, M. E. (1989). Differential steroid production between theca interna and theca externa cells: A three-cell model for follicular steroidogenesis in avian species. *Endocrinology (Baltimore)* **125**, 109–116.

Pröve, E. (1974). Der Einfluss von Kastration und Testeronsubstitution auf das Sexualverhalten mannlicher Zebrafinken (*Taeniopygia guttata castonotis* Gould). *J. Ornithol.* **115**, 338–347.

Raikow, R. J. (1982). Monophyly of the passeriformes: Test of a phylogenetic hypothesis. *Auk* **99**, 431–445.

Ramachandran, B., Schlinger, B. A., Arnold, A. P., and Campagnoni, A. T. (1999). Zebra finch aromatase gene expression is regulated in the brain through an alternate promoter. *Gene* **240**(1), 209–216.

Rasika, S., Nottebohm, F., and Alvarez-Buylla, A. (1994). Testosterone increases the recruitment and/or survival of new high vocal center neurons in adult female canaries. *Proc. Natl. Acad. Sci. U.S.A.* **91**(17), 7854–7858.

Rasika, S., Alvarez-Buylla, A., and Nottebohm, F. (1999). BDNF mediates the effects of testosterone on the survival of new neurons in an adult brain. *Neuron* **22**(1), 53–62.

Richards, D. G. (1981). Altering and message components in songs of Rufous-sided Towhees. *Behaviour* **76**, 223–249.

Ritchison, G. (1983). The function of singing in female black-headed grosbeaks (*Pheucticus melanocephalus*) family group maintenance. *Auk* **100**, 105–116.

Ritchison, G. (1986). The singing behavior of female northern cardinals. *Condor* **88**, 156–159.

Riters, L. V., and Ball, G. F. (1999). Lesions to the medial preoptic area affect singing in the male European starling (*Sturnus vulgaris*). *Horm. Behav.* **36**(3), 276–286.

Rohss, M., and Silverin, B. (1983). Seasonal variations in the ultrastructure of the Leydig cells and plasma levels of luteinizing hormone and steroid hormones in juvenile and adult male great tits, *Parus major*. *Ornis Scand.* **14**, 202–212.

Rost, R. (1990). Hormones and behavior: A joint examination of studies on seasonal variation in song production and plasma levels of testosterone in the Great Tit *Parus major*. *J. Ornithol.* **131**, 403–411.

Rost, R. (1992). Hormones and behavior: A comparison of studies on seasonal changes in song production and testosterone plasma levels in the Willow Tit *Parus montanus*. *Ornithol. Fenn.* **69**, 1–6.

Saito, N., and Shimada, K. (1997). Control of ovarian steroidogenesis: Gene expression of steroidogenic enzymes. In "Perspectives in Avian Endocrinology" (S. Harvey and R. J. Etches, eds.), Vol. 1, pp. 193–200. Journal of Endocrinology Ltd., Bristol.

Sakaguchi, H., and Saito, N. (1989). The acetylcholine and catecholamine contents in song control nuclei of zebra finch during song ontogeny. *Dev. Brain Res.* **47**(2), 313–317.

Saldanha, C. J., Schultz, J. D., London, S., and Schlinger, B. A. (2000a). Telencephalic aromatase, but not a song system, in a sub-oscine passerine, the golden collared manakin. *Brain, Behav. Evol.* **56**, 29–37.

Saldanha, C. J., and Schlinger, B. A. (1997). Estrogen synthesis and secretion in the brown-headed cowbird (*Molothrus ater*). *Gen. Comp. Endocrinol.* **105**, 390–401.

Saldanha, C. J., Clayton, N. S., and Schlinger, B. A. (1999). Androgen metabolism in the juvenile oscine forebrain: A cross-species analysis at neural sites implicated in memory function. *J. Neurobiol.* **40**(3), 397–406.

Saldanha, C. J., Tuerek, M. J., Kim, Y.-H., Fernandes, A. O., Arnold, A. P., and Schlinger, B. A. (2000b). Distribution and regulation of telencephalic aromatase expression in the zebra finch revealed with a specific antibody. *J. Comp. Neurol.* **423**, 619–630.

Scharff, C., and Nottebohm, F. (1991). A comparative study of the behavioral deficits following lesions of various parts of the zebra finch song system: Implications for vocal learning. *J. Neurosci.* **11**(9), 2896–2913.

Schlinger, B. A. (1987). Plasma androgens and aggressiveness in captive winter white-throated sparrows (*Zonotrichia albicollis*). *Horm. Behav.* **21**(2), 203–210.

Schlinger, B. A. (1997). Sex-steroids and their actions on the bird song system. Invited review. *J. Neurobiol.* **35**, 619–631.

Schlinger, B. A. (1998). Sexual differentiation of avian brain and behavior: Current views on gonadal hormone-dependent and independent mechanisms. Invited review. *Annu. Rev. Physiol.* **60**, 407–429.

Schlinger, B. A., and Arnold, A. P. (1991). Brain is the major site of estrogen synthesis in a male songbird. *Proc. Natl. Acad. Sci. U.S.A.* **88**(10), 4191–4194.

Schlinger, B. A., and Arnold, A. P. (1992a). Circulating estrogens in a male songbird originate in the brain. *Proc. Natl. Acad. Sci. U.S.A.* **89**(16), 7650–7653.

Schlinger, B. A., and Arnold, A. P. (1992b). Plasma sex steroids and tissue aromatization in hatchling zebra finches—Implications for the sexual differentiation of singing behavior. *Endocrinology (Baltimore)* **130**(1), 289–299.

Schlinger, B. A., and Arnold, A. P. (1993). Estrogen synthesis in vivo in the adult zebra finch: Additional evidence that circulating estrogens can originate in brain. *Endocrinology (Baltimore)* **133**(6), 2610–2616.

Schlinger, B. A., and Callard, G. V. (1991). Brain-steroid interactions and the control of aggressive behavior in birds. *In* "Neuroendocrine Perspectives" (R. M. MacLeod and E. Muller, eds.), Vol. 9, pp. 1–43. Springer-Verlag, New York.

Schlinger, B. A., Fivizzani, A., and Callard, G. V. (1989). Aromatase, 5α- and 5β-reductase in brain, pituitary and skin of the sex-role reversed Wilson's phalarope. *J. Endocrinol.* **122**, 573–581.

Schlinger, B. A., Slotow, R. H., and Arnold, A. P. (1992). Plasma estrogens and brain aromatase in winter white-crowned sparrows. *Ornis Scand.* **23**, 292–297.

Schlinger, B. A., Amur Umarjee, S., Shen, P., Campagnoni, A. T., and Arnold, A. P. (1994). Neuronal and non-neuronal aromatase in primary cultures of developing zebra finch telencephalon. *J. Neurosci.* **14**(12), 7541–7552.

Schlinger, B. A., Amur Umarjee, S., Campagnoni, A. T., and Arnold, A. P. (1995). 5β-reductase and other androgen-metabolizing enzymes in primary cultures of developing zebra finch telencephalon. *J. Neuroendocrinol.* **7**(3), 187–192.

Schlinger, B. A., Lane, N. I., Grisham, W., and Thompson, L. (1999). Androgen synthesis in a songbird: A study of Cyp17 (17α-hydroxylase/C17,20-lyase) activity in the zebra finch. *Gen. Comp. Endocrinol.* **113**(1), 46–58.

Schlinger, B., Soma, K., and London, S. E. (2001). Neurosteroids and brain sexual differentiation. *Trends Neurosci.* **24**, 429–431.

Schwabl, H. (1992). Winter and breeding territorial behaviour and levels of reproductive hormones of migratory European robins. *Ornis Scand.* **23**, 271–276.

Schwabl, H., and Kriner, E. (1991). Territorial aggression and song of male European robins (*Erithacus rubecula*) in autumn and spring: Effects of antiandrogen treatment. *Horm. Behav.* **25**(2), 180–194.

Searcy, W. A., and Wingfield, J. C. (1980). The effects of androgen and antiandrogen on dominance and aggressiveness in male red-winged blackbirds. *Horm Behav.* **14**(2), 126–135.

Shen, P., Campagnoni, C. W., Kampf, K., Schlinger, B. A., Arnold, A. P., and Campagnoni, A. T. (1994). Isolation and characterization of a zebra finch aromatase cDNA: *In situ* hybridization reveals high aromatase expression in brain. *Mol. Brain Res.* **24**, 227–237.

Shen, P., Schlinger, B. A., Campagnoni, A. T., and Arnold, A. P. (1995). An atlas of aromatase mRNA expression in the zebra finch brain. *J. Comp. Neurol.* **360**, 172–184.

Sherwood, N. M., Wingfield, J. C., Ball, G. F., and Dufty, A. M. (1988). Identity of gonadotropin-releasing hormone in passerine birds: Comparison of GnRH in song sparrow (*Melospiza melodia*) and starling (*Sturnus vulgaris*) with five vertebrate GnRHs. *Gen. Comp. Endocrinol.* **69**(3), 341–351.

Shiovitz, K. (1975). The process of species-specific song recognition in the Indigo Bunting (*Passerina cyanea*) and its relationship to the organization of avian acoustic behavior. *Behaviour* **55**, 128–179.

Shoemaker, H. H. (1939). Effect of testosterone propionate on the behavior of the female canary. *Proc. Soc. Exp. Biol. Med.* **41**, 299–302.

Sibley, C., Ahlquist, J., and Monroe, B. J. (1988). A classification of the living birds of the world based on DNA-DNA hybridization studies. *Auk* **105**, 409–423.

Silver, R., Ramos, C., Machuca, H., and Silverin, B. (1992). Immunocytochemical distribution of GnRH in the brain of adult and posthatching Great Tit *Parus major* and Ring Dove *Streptopelia roseograsea*. *Ornis Scand.* **23**, 222–232.

Silverin, B., and Sharp, P. (1996). The development of the hypothalamic-pituitary-gonadal axis in juvenile Great Tits. *Gen. Comp. Endocrinol.* **103**(2), 150–166.

Silverin, B., Viebke, P., and Westin, J. (1986). Seasonal changes in plasma levels of LH and gonadal steroids in free-living Willow Tits *Parus montanus. Ornis Scand.* **17,** 230–236.

Silverin, B., Viebke, P. A., and Westin, J. (1989). Hormonal correlates of migration and territorial behavior in juvenile Willow Tits during autumn. *Gen. Comp. Endocrinol.* **75**(1), 148–156.

Singh, T. D., Basham, M. E., Nordeen, E. J., and Nordeen, K. W. (2000). Early sensory and hormonal experience modulate age-related changes in NR2B mRNA within a forebrain region controlling avian vocal learning. *J. Neurobiol.* **44,** 82–94.

Slagsvold, T. (1977). Bird song activity in relation to breeding cycle, spring weather, and environmental phrenology. *Ornis Scand.* **8,** 197–222.

Smith, G. T. (1996). Seasonal plasticity in the song nuclei of wild rufous-sided towhees. *Brain Res.* **734,** 79–85.

Smith, G. T., Brenowitz, E. A., and Prins, G. S. (1996). Use of PG-21 immunocytochemistry to detect androgen receptors in the songbird brain. *J. Histochem. Cytochem.* **44**(9), 1075–1080.

Smith, G. T., Brenowitz, E. A., Beecher, M. D., and Wingfield, J. C. (1997a). Seasonal changes in testosterone, neural attributes of song control nuclei, and song structure in wild songbirds. *J. Neurosci.* **17**(15), 6001–6010.

Smith, G. T., Brenowitz, E. A., and Wingfield, J. C. (1997b). Roles of photoperiod and testosterone in seasonal plasticity of the avian song control system. *J. Neurobiol.* **32**(4), 426–442.

Smith, G. T., Brenowitz, E. A., and Wingfield, J. C. (1997c). Seasonal changes in the size of the avian song control nucleus HVc defined by multiple histological markers. *J. Comp. Neurol.* **381**(3), 253–261.

Soha, J. A., Shimizu, T., and Doupe, A. J. (1996). Development of the catecholaminergic innervation of the song system of the male zebra finch. *J. Neurobiol.* **29**(4), 473–489.

Sohrabji, F., Nordeen, K. W., and Nordeen, E. J. (1989). Projections of androgen-accumulating neurons in a nucleus controlling avian song. *Brain Res.* **488**(1–2), 253–259.

Sohrabji, F., Nordeen, E. J., and Nordeen, K. W. (1990). Selective impairment of song learning following lesions of a forebrain nucleus in the juvenile zebra finch. *Behav. Neural Biol.* **53**(1), 51–63.

Soma, K. K., and Wingfield, J. C. (1999). Endocrinology of aggression in the nonbreeding season. *Proc. 22nd Int. Ornithol. Congr.,* Durban.

Soma, K. K., Hartman, V. N., Wingfield, J. C., and Brenowitz, E. A. (1998). Seasonal changes in androgen receptor immunoreactivity in the song nucleus HVc of a wild bird. *J. Comp. Neurol.* **409,** 224–236.

Soma, K. K., Bindra, R. K., Gee, J., Wingfield, J. C., and Schlinger, B. A. (1999a). Androgen-metabolizing enzymes show region-specific changes across the breeding season in the brain of a wild songbird. *J. Neurobiol.* **41**(2), 176–188.

Soma, K. K., Sullivan, K., and Wingfield, J. C. (1999b). Combined aromatase inhibitor and antiandrogen treatment decreases territorial aggression in a wild songbird during the nonbreeding season. *Gen. Comp. Endocrinol.* **115,** 442–453.

Soma, K. K., Sullivan, K. A., Tramontin, A. D., Saldanha, C. J., Schlinger, B. A., and Wingfield, J. C. (2000a). Acute and chronic effects of an aromatase inhibitor on territorial aggression in breeding and nonbreeding male song sparrows. *J. Comp. Physiol. A* **186,** 759–769.

Soma, K. K., Tramontin, A. D., and Wingfield, J. C. (2000b). Oestrogen regulates male aggression in the non-breeding season. *Proc. R. Soc. London, Ser. B* **267,** 1089–1096.

Soma, K. K., Wissman, A. M., Brenowitz, E. A., and Wingfield, J. C. (2000c). Effects of dehydroepiandrosterone (DHEA) on behavior and neuroanatomy of a songbird. *Soc. Neurosci. Abstr.* **26,** 1762.

Stricter, G. (1994). The vocal control pathways in budgerigars differ from those in songbirds. *J. Comp. Neurol.* **343,** 35–56.

Suthers, R. A., Goller, F., and Pytte, C. (1999). The neuromuscular control of birdsong. *Philos. Trans. R. Soc. London, Ser. B* **354,** 927–939.

Thorpe, W. H. (1958). The learning of song patterns by birds, with especial references to the song of the chaffinch. *Ibis* **100,** 535–570.

Tramontin, A. D., and Brenowitz, E. A. (1999). A field study of seasonal neuronal incorporation into the song control system of a songbird that lacks adult song learning. *J. Neurobiol.* **40**(3), 316–326.

Tramontin, A. D., and Brenowitz, E. A. (2000). Seasonal plasticity in the adult brain. *Trends Neurosci.* **23**(6), 251–258.

Tramontin, A. D., Smith, G. T., Breuner, C. W., and Brenowitz, E. A. (1998). Seasonal plasticity and sexual dimorphism in the avian song control system: Stereological measurement of neuron density and number. *J. Comp. Neurol.* **396**(2), 186–192.

Tramontin, A. D., Hartman, V. N., and Brenowitz, E. A. (2000). Breeding conditions induce rapid and sequential growth in adult avian song control circuits: A model of seasonal plasticity in the brain. *J. Neurosci.* **20**(2), 854–861.

Tsutsui, K., and Schlinger, B. A. (2001). Steroidogenesis in the avian brain. *In* "Avian Endocrinology," (A. Dawson and C. M. Chaturvedi, eds.), pp. 59–77. Narosa Publishing, New Delhi.

Tsutsui, K., and Ukena, K. (1999). Neurosteroids in the cerebellar Purkinje neuron and their actions. *Int. J. Mol. Med.* **4,** 49–56.

Ulinski, P. S., and Margoliash, D. (1990). Neurobiology of the reptile-bird transition. *In* "Cerebral Cortex" (E. G. Jones and A. Peters, eds.), pp. 217–265. Plenum Press, New York.

Vanson, A., Arnold, A. P., and Schlinger, B. A. (1996). 3β-hydroxysteroid dehydrogenase/5-4 isomerase and aromatase activity in primary cultures of developing zebra finch telencephalon: Dehydroepiandrosterone as substrate for synthesis of androstenedione and estrogens. *Gen. Comp. Endocrinol.* **102**, 342–350.

Vicario, D. S. (1991). Organization of the zebra finch song control system: II. Functional organization of outputs from nucleus Robustus archistriatalis. *J. Comp. Neurol.* **309**(4), 486–494.

Vockel, A., Pröve, E., and Balthazart, J. (1990a). Sex- and age-related differences in the activity of testosterone-metabolizing enzymes in microdissected nuclei of the zebra finch brain. *Brain Res.* **511**(2), 291–302.

Vockel, A., Pröve, E., and Balthazart, J. (1990b). Effects of castration and testosterone treatment on the activity of testosterone-metabolizing enzymes in the brain of male and female zebra finches. *J. Neurobiol.* **21**(5), 808–825.

Wada, M., Shimizu, T., Kobayashi, S., Yatani, A., Sandaiji, Y., Ishikawa, T., and Takemure, E. (1999). Behavioral and hormonal basis of polygynous breeding in male bush warblers (*Cettia diphone*). *Gen. Comp. Endocrinol.* **116**(3), 422–432.

Wade, J., and Arnold, A. P. (1996). Functional testicular tissue does not masculinize development of the zebra finch song system. *Proc. Natl. Acad. Sci. U.S.A.* **93**(11), 5264–5268.

Wade, J., Schlinger, B. A., Hodges, L., and Arnold, A. P. (1994). Fadrozole: A potent and specific inhibitor of aromatase in the zebra finch brain. *Gen. Comp. Endocrinol.* **94**(1), 53–61.

Wade, J., Schlinger, B. A., and Arnold, A. P. (1995). Aromatase and 5α-reductase activity in cultures of developing zebra finch brain: An investigation of sex and regional differences. *J. Neurobiol.* **27**, 240–251.

Wade, J., Springer, M. L., Wingfield, J. C., and Arnold, A. P. (1996). Neither testicular androgens nor embryonic aromatase activity alters morphology of the neural song system in zebra finches. *Biol. Reprod.* **55**(5), 1126–1132.

Wade, J., Gong, A., and Arnold, A. P. (1997). Effects of embryonic estrogen on differentiation of the gonads and secondary sexual characteristics of male zebra finches. *J. Exp. Zool.* **278**(6), 405–411.

Wade, J., Swender, D. A., and McElhinny, T. L. (1999). Sexual differentiation of the zebra finch song system parallels genetic, not gonadal, sex. *Horm. Behav.* **36**, 141–152.

Walters, M. J., and Harding, C. F. (1988). The effects of an aromatization inhibitor on the reproductive behavior of male zebra finches. *Horm. Behav.* **22**(2), 207–218.

Walters, M. J., McEwen, B. S., and Harding, C. F. (1988). Estrogen receptor levels in hypothalamic and vocal control nuclei in the male zebra finch. *Brain Res.* **459**(1), 37–43.

Walters, M. J., Collade, D., and Harding, C. F. (1991). Oestrogenic modulation of singing in male zebra finches: Differential effects in directed and undirected songs. *Anim. Behav.* **42**, 445–452.

Weichel, K., Schwager, G., Heid, P., Guttinger, H. R., and Pesch, A. (1986). Sex differences in plasma steroid concentrations and singing behavior during ontogeny in canaries (*Serinus canaria*). *Ethology* **73**, 281–294.

Wennstrom, K., Reeves, B., and Brenowitz, E. A. (2001). Testosterone treatment increases the metabolic capacity of adult avian song nuclei. *J. Neurobiol.* **48**, 256–264.

Whaling, C. S., Nelson, D. A., and Marler, P. (1995). Testosterone-induced shortening of the storage phase of song development in birds interferes with vocal learning. *Dev. Psychobiol.* **28**(7), 367–376.

White, S. A., Livingston, F. S., and Mooney, R. (1999). Androgens modulate NMDA receptor-mediated EPSCs in the zebra finch song system. *J. Neurophysiol.* **82**(5), 2221–2234.

Williams, T. D., Dawson, A., Nicholls, T. J., and Goldsmith, A. R. (1987). Reproductive endocrinology of free-living nestling and juvenile starlings, *Sturnus vulgaris*, an altricial species. *J. Zool.* **212**, 619–628.

Wilson, J. D., George, F. W., and Renfree, M. B. (1995). The endocrine role in mammalian sexual differentiation. *Recent Prog. Horm. Res.* **50**(7), 349–364.

Wingfield, J. C. (1994). Regulation of territorial behavior in the sedentary song sparrow, *Melospiza melodia morphna*. *Horm. Behav.* **28**(1), 1–15.

Wingfield, J. C., and Farner, D. S. (1993). Endocrinology of reproduction in wild species. *Avian Biol.* **9**, 163–327.

Wingfield, J. C., and Hahn, T. P. (1994). Testosterone and territorial behavior in sedentary and migratory sparrows. *Anim. Behav.* **47**, 77–89.

Wingfield, J. C., and Kenagy, G. J. (1991). Natural regulation of reproductive cycles. In "Vertebrate Endocrinology: Fundamentals and Biomedical Implications" (M. Schreibman and R. E. Jones, eds.), pp. 181–124. Academic Press, San Diego, CA.

Wingfield, J. C., and Marler, P. (1988). Endocrine basis of communication in reproduction and aggression. In "The Physiology of Reproduction" (E. Knobil and J. Neill, eds.), pp. 1647–1677. Raven Press, New York.

Wingfield, J. C., and Monk, D. (1992). Control and context of year-round territorial aggression in the non migratory Song Sparrow *Zonotrichia melodia morphna*. *Ornis Scand.* **23**, 298–303.

Wingfield, J. C., and Monk, D. (1994). Behavioral and hormonal responses of male song sparrows to estradiol-treated females during the non-breeding season. *Horm. Behav.* **28**(2), 146–154.

Yu, A. C., and Margoliash, D. (1996). Temporal hierarchical control of singing in birds. *Science* **273**, 1871–1875.

Zwain, I. H., and Yen, S. S. C. (1999). Neurosteroidogenesis in astrocytes, oligodendrocytes, and neurons of cerebral cortex of rat brain. *Endocrinology (Baltimore)* **140**(8), 3843–3852.

34

Insect Developmental Hormones and Their Mechanism of Action

James W. Truman and Lynn M. Riddiford
Department of Zoology
University of Washington
Seattle, Washington 98195

I. INTRODUCTION

Insect development is regulated by two families of hormones, the steroid ecdysones and the sesquiterpenoid juvenile hormones (JHs). The ecdysones control the molting of the exoskeleton (cuticle) that is secreted by the underlying epidermis and has both rigid and extensible regions. To accommodate the growth and changes in morphology that accompany metamorphosis, a new exoskeleton is periodically formed followed by the shedding of the old one. These molts are evident during the late stages of embryogenesis and continue through the growth and metamorphic phases of postembryonic life. The adult insect does not molt.

The JHs determine the type of molt that occurs in response to ecdysone. When JH is present, the molt is to another similar stage. When JH is absent, ecdysone causes switches in programs so that a change of form can occur. The JHs may also control polyphenisms such as alternative color morphs in locusts and caste development in social insects such as termites, ants, and bees. In the adult, JH regulates reproductive maturation in females and some males.

In this chapter we review briefly the general endocrine regulation of the postembryonic development in insects and the characteristics of insect hormones and then discuss what is known about their cellular and molecular modes of action. The second part of the review focuses primarily on their roles in the development of the nervous system. Here the primary emphasis is on two model insects, the moth *Manduca sexta* and the fruit fly *Drosophila melanogaster*. More detailed information on insect endocrinology can be found in Nijhout (1994).

II. CHEMISTRY AND SECRETION OF INSECT DEVELOPMENTAL HORMONES

A. Ecdysteroids—Synthesis and Metabolism

The insect molting hormones are steroid hormones that are produced by a pair of glands in the anterior thoracic region. In many insects these glands are called the prothoracic glands, but in the higher flies, such as *Drosophila melanogaster*, they are incorporated into a fused endocrine complex called the ring gland (Fig. 1). The prothoracic glands do not store the hormone, but normally synthesize and secrete the steroid when stimulated by the prothoracicotropic hormone (PTTH). In Lepidoptera this neurosecretory peptide is produced by two pairs of neurons in the far lateral region of the protocerebrum (Fig. 1) (Agui *et al.*, 1979; Mizoguchi, 1990; Gilbert *et al.*, 1996). In many insect

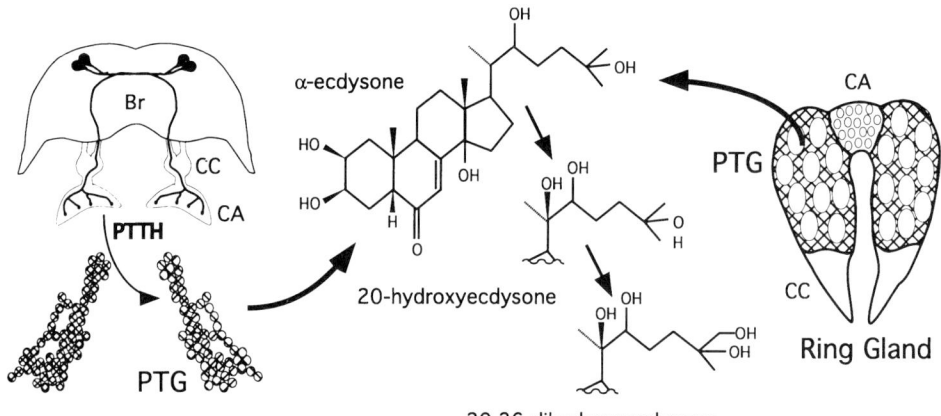

FIGURE 1 Main endocrine organs of larvae of the moth Manduca (left) and the fruit fly Drosophila (right). The main endocrine organs are the corpora cardiaca (CC), the corpora allata (CA), and the prothoracic glands (PTG). In fly larvae, these organs are combined into a compound structure, the ring gland. The PTG is the source of 3-dehydroecdysone and α-ecdysone. α-Ecdysone is converted by peripheral tissues into 20-hydroxyecdysone (the major active hormone) and then inactivated by further hydroxylation to 20,26-dihydroxyecdysone. The initiation of ecdysone secretion from the PTG is through the tropic action of the prothoracicotropic hormone (PTTH), which is released from two pairs of neurosecretory cells in the brain (Br; not shown for the fly system).

larvae, PTTH is released at a time that is determined by the larva reaching a certain size (Nijhout, 1981) and is often confined to a particular temporal gate during the day (Truman, 1972). In the blood-sucking bug *Rhodnius prolixus*, a single, large blood meal signaled via stretch receptors in the abdomen is sufficient to cause PTTH release and the subsequent molt (Wigglesworth, 1940; Steel and Harmsen, 1971; Steel, 1975). Wigglesworth capitalized on the convenience of the *Rhodnius* system to lay the foundation for insect endocrinology.

When stimulated by PTTH, the prothoracic glands synthesize and secrete ecdysones into the hemolymph (Gilbert et al., 1996). The original chemical identification of the molting hormone involved the extraction of a metric ton of pupae of the commercial silkworm *Bombyx mori*. The hormone was found to be a steroid hormone that was termed ecdysone (Butenandt and Karlson, 1954; Hoffmeister and Grützmacher, 1966). A second steroid, 20-hydroxyecdysone (20E, also called β-ecdysone or ecdysterone), was also found in *Bombyx* pupae and later found in crustaceans and a variety of other insects (Hampshire and Horn, 1966; Hoffmeister and Grützmacher, 1966; Horn and Bergamasco, 1985; Rees, 1995). Following the lead of our review (Riddiford et al., 2001), we refer to the class of biologically active molting hormones as ecdysones. The original ecdysone is termed α-ecdysone (Fig. 1).

Insects cannot synthesize the cholesterol ring system, so they are dependent on dietary cholesterol or related plant sterols such as sitosterol for making their ecdysones. Cholesterol is converted to 7-dehydrocholesterol and then, through a set of biochemical steps that are not fully characterized but which involve several P450 hydroxylases (Feyereisen, 1999), forms 3-dehydroecdysone (3dE) or α-ecdysone (Grieneisen, 1994; Rees, 1995). In *Manduca sexta*, 3dE is converted to α-ecdysone after secretion into the hemolymph (Sakurai et al., 1989). In *Drosophila* 3dE and 3-dehydro 20-hydroxyecdysone (3d20E) can activate some specific genes, but whether they are active *in vivo* is not known (Richards, 1978; reviewed by Riddiford, 1993; Gilbert et al., 1996). α-Ecdysone is then converted into 20E by the action of 20-monooxygenase in peripheral tissues such as the midgut and the fat body (Feyereisen, 1999). 20E is generally considered to be the active molting hormone, but α-ecdysone has a range of biological actions that are especially important during the early stages of molting and metamorphosis (Blais and Lafont, 1980; Oberlander, 1985; Champlin and Truman, 1998a,b). The circulating 20E then undergoes further hydroxylation to 20,26-dihydroxyecdysone (20,26E) (Warren and Gilbert, 1986), which does not appear to be biologically active in *Manduca* (Hiruma *et al.*, 1997). The steroid metabolites are further metabolized to polar conjugates, such as steroid phosphates that are then excreted or stored (Rees, 1995).

Two *Drosophila* genes that encode enzymes in the sterol synthesis pathway have been cloned, and mutations in these genes are providing insight into both the ecdysone biosynthesis pathway and the action of the hormone in various developmental pathways. The *disembodied (dib)* gene encodes a cytochrome P450 named CYP302A1, which is in a new subfamily of the P450 cytochromes (Chavez *et al.*, 2000). It is most similar to the 1,25-dihydroxy-vitamin D3 24-hydroxylase and is thought to be located in the mitochondria. In larvae it is found in the prothoracic gland portion of the ring gland, and in the adult, in which these cells have degenerated (Dai and Gilbert, 1991), it is found in the follicle cells of the ovary. In null mutants lacking the Dib protein, both α-ecdysone and 20E remain low during embryonic development, indicating that this enzyme is important in the ecdysteroid biosynthetic pathway. Embryonic development in the *dib* loss-of-function mutant becomes abnormal at stage 14, with anomalies seen in cuticle deposition, midgut development, and head involution, indicating that these events are under the regulation of the embryonic ecdysteroids. The *Drosophila adrenodoxin reductase (dare)* gene encodes an adrenodoxin reductase that is similar to the vertebrate mitochondrial P450 enzyme important for production of reduced nicotinamide adenine dinucleotide phosphate (NADPH) (Freeman *et al.*, 1999). Null *dare* mutants, however, show no embryonic defects, but die during larval molts.

B. Juvenile Hormone—Synthesis and Metabolism

In 1934, Wigglesworth first presented evidence, based on parabiosis experiments with *Rhodnius*, that there was a blood-borne factor from the head that prevented metamorphosis. He also demonstrated that a fused endocrine gland in the head, the corpus allatum, was the source of this inhibitory hormone (Wigglesworth, 1940). This hormone, which later came to be known as the JH, was eventually isolated from the moth *Hyalophora cecropia* and its chemical structure determined as methyl-10,11-epoxy-7-ethyl-3,11-dimethyl-2-*trans*-6-*trans*-tridecadienoate (Röller *et al.*, 1967). This compound, known as JH I (Fig. 2), was soon followed by the identification of related compounds from *H. cecropia* and other insects.

For most insects the active JH is JH III, methyl-10,11-epoxy-3,7,11-trimethyl-2-*trans*-6-*trans*-tridecadienoate (Fig. 2), the epoxidated form of methyl farnesoate (for a review, see Riddiford, 1994). Two of the most

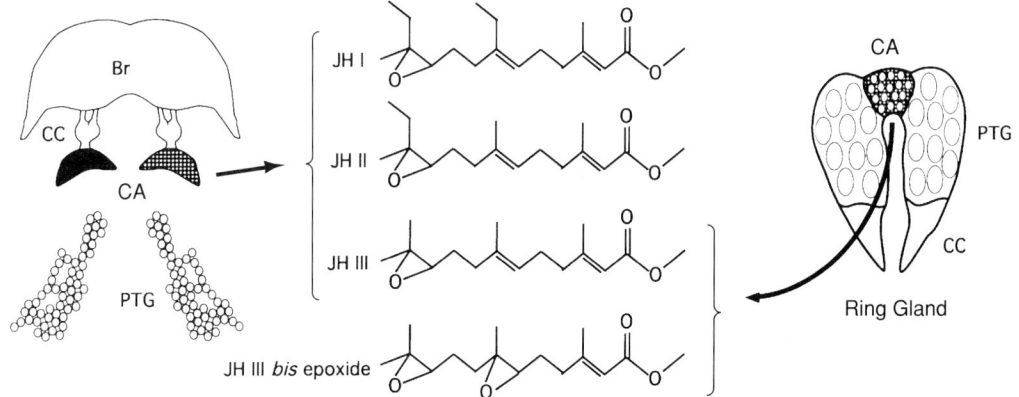

FIGURE 2 The juvenile hormone (JH) system of insect larvae. The diagrams of the *Manduca* (left) and *Drosophila* (right) endocrine systems are as in Fig. 1, with a highlighting of the corpora allata, which secrete the JHs. The Lepidoptera secrete combinations of JH I, II, and III at various times throughout their life. *Drosophila* secrete JH III and JH III *bis* epoxide. Most insects use JH III.

commonly studied groups of insects, however, possess modified forms of the hormone. The corpora allata of larvae of Lepidoptera (moths and butterflies) secrete JH I and JH II, although JH III is the predominant JH found in the adult. In *Drosophila* and other higher Diptera, JH III is also joined by approximately equivalent amounts of JH III-*bis*-epoxide (Richard *et al.*, 1989).

Most insects have paired corpora allata, although in higher flies these glands are also part of the ring gland complex. The regulation of JH synthesis is by both allatotropic and allatostatic neuropeptides from the brain, as well as possibly by direct nervous control (Stay *et al.*, 1994; Tobe and Bendena, 1999; Stay, 2000). JH III is synthesized from mevalonate via the typical farnesol pathway leading to methyl farnesoate that then is converted to JH III by a special microsomal P450 epoxidase located in the corpora allata (Hammock, 1975; Feyereisen *et al.*, 1981; reviewed by Feyereisen, 1999). Presumably in these glands in the higher Diptera, this enzyme has been modified so as to cause a second epoxidation (Feyereisen, 1999). In Lepidoptera, JH I and II are synthesized from a combination of mevalonate and homomevalonate (Schooley and Baker, 1985; Cusson *et al.*, 1996).

JH is catabolized to JH acid by nonspecific hemolymph esterases or by a specific JH esterase (JHE). The latter enzyme appears in the final larval instar and may also appear transiently at the end of the larval and pupal molts (reviewed by Roe and Venkatesh, 1990). JH is also converted to JH diol through action of an epoxide hydrase (Hammock, 1975). Either of these metabolites then may be further degraded to the JH acid diol. These metabolites cannot substitute for JH in either the prevention of metamorphosis or the stimulation of reproductive maturation. A possible exception is the reported role of JH acid in establishing competence for metamorphosis of the fat body and the Verson's glands (Ismail *et al.*, 1998, 2000).

III. HORMONE TITERS

Figure 3 shows the general pattern of JH and ecdysone titers in the hemolymph ("blood") in *Manduca*. Ecdysones are low during the intermolt periods during which growth occurs. When PTTH is released to initiate the molt, the ecdysone titer rises with first α-ecdysone appearing, and then primarily 20E, at the peak levels of approximately 2–10 μg/ml, followed by 20,26E as the total amount of ecdysteroid falls (Warren and Gilbert, 1986; Hiruma *et al.*, 1999; Langelan *et al.*, 2000). In the adult molt the rise of

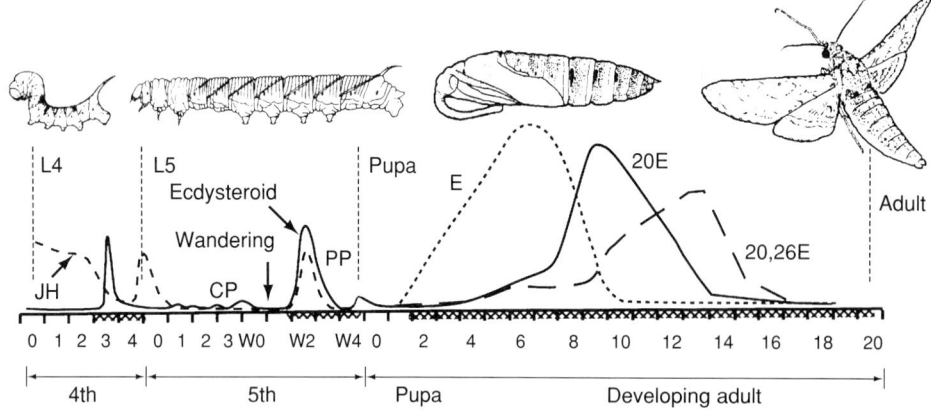

FIGURE 3 The blood titers of juvenile hormone (JH) and various ecdysteroids during L4, L5, pupation, and adult development of *Manduca sexta*. For the L4 and L5, the titer shown is primarily that of 20E (Langelan *et al.*, 2000; Hiruma *et al.*, 1999). Titers of the three major steroids are shown for adult development—E, 20E, and 20,26E. (Warren and Gilbert, 1986). The *x*-axis is separated into days and the crosshatched area shows the time when molts are occurring. 20,26E, 20,26-dihydroxyecdysone; 20E, 20-hydroxyecdysone; CP, commitment peak; E, α-ecdysone; JH, juvenile hormone; L4, fourth larval stage; L5, fifth larval stage; PP, prepupal peak; Wn, days after the start of wandering behavior. Vertical dashed lines show the times of ecdysis (the shedding of the old cuticle at the end of a molt).

α-ecdysone initiates adult development with apolysis, epidermal cell proliferation, and the beginning of scale formation (Nardi and Magee-Adams, 1986). The following peak of 20E then initiates the deposition of the adult cuticle. 20,26E then appears during the second half of adult development (Warren and Gilbert, 1986). The prothoracic glands typically degenerate late in adult development (Dai and Gilbert, 1997, 1999). In the hemolymph, the ecdysones are not known to have carrier proteins and appear only to be catabolized by tissue enzymes (Rees, 1995).

In contrast to the periodic ecdysone surges, JH is secreted throughout most of larval life. In the hemolymph, JH is transported by a JH binding protein (JHBP) that may be of high molecular weight (~500 kDa) in the insects that use JH III, such as locusts and beetles (deKort and Koopmanschap, 1987) and *Drosophila* (Shemshedini and Wilson, 1988), or of low molecular weight in the Lepidoptera that use JH I and JH II (Kramer et al., 1984; Goodman, 1990; Touhara et al., 1993). The JH binding protein both solubilizes the JH and protects it from catabolism by general hemolymph esterases. At the end of each molt and in the final larval instar, a JHE appears (Sanburg et al., 1975; Jones and Click, 1987; Campbell et al., 1998) that can metabolize the JH that is bound to the JHBP and thus clears the hormone from the hemolymph.

The corpora allata cease production of JH in preparation for metamorphosis. In hemimetabolous insects there is no JH during the final nymphal instar. By contrast, in the Holometabola (at least the Lepidoptera and Diptera), JH is present in the hemolymph during the early part of the final larval instar, but then declines in preparation for metamorphosis (Riddiford, 1993, 1994) (Fig. 3). In *Manduca* the corpora allata cease production of JH due to loss of the methyl transferase, but continue to produce JH acid (Bhaskaran et al., 1986), and some tissues such as the wing imaginal discs have a methyl transferase that allows its conversion to JH (Sparagana et al., 1985). Hence, both JH and JH acid are found in the hemolymph (Baker et al., 1987). The JHE in the hemolymph and in the tissues increases as a function of weight during the final larval instar and wipes out the JH in the hemolymph by the time the larva has grown to its final size (Mitsui et al., 1979; Sparks et al., 1983). PTTH is then released (Rountree and Bollenbacher, 1986) to cause ecdysone secretion in the absence of JH, for the first time in the postembryonic life of the insect. This small steroid peak initiates metamorphosis by causing the change from feeding to wandering behavior (Dominick and Truman, 1985) and by the commitment of the various tissues to their metamorphic fates (Riddiford, 1976, 1978; Ohtaki et al., 1986). JH then reappears in the hemolymph during the larval to pupal transition to prevent the precocious adult development of imaginal structures (Kiguchi and Riddiford, 1978; Riddiford, 1994). Just before pupal ecdysis the JHE reappears and eliminates the circulating JH (Sparks et al., 1983). In *Drosophila* JH is present in larvae during the first, second, and early third instars. Circulating JH declines during the late third instar and then transiently peaks just before pupariation (Sliter et al., 1987; Bownes and Rembold, 1987). The JH esterase appears at wandering and then remains through the prepupal period (Campbell et al., 1992, 1998; Khlebodarova et al., 1996).

There is no circulating JH in the pupae of holometabolous insects during the prolonged exposure to ecdysteroids that promotes adult differentiation. In some insects, however, JH reappears at the end of adult development to play a role in adult reproduction (Riddiford, 1994). In the adult the corpora allata resumes the synthesis of JH, although some male moths only produce JH acid (Bhaskaran et al., 1988). Typically JH is critical for reproductive maturation in feeding adult females and also affects the synthesis of male accessory gland products in some insects (Wyatt and Davey, 1996). Although the prothoracic glands degenerate late in metamorphosis, the ecdysones often reappear in the adult, but this time being produced by the follicle cells of the ovary. In mosquitoes and *Drosophila*, the ecdysones cause yolk protein synthesis (Hagedorn and Fallon, 1973; Fallon et al., 1975; Bownes, 1994; Raikhel and Snigirevskaya, 1998; Raikhel et al., 1999) and may also may be critical for driving the final stages of oocyte development, as shown for *Drosophila* (Buszczak et al., 1999; Freeman et al., 1999). Interestingly, although the *dib* gene that encodes an enzyme involved in ecdysone biosynthesis is expressed in follicle cells, flies bearing deletions of *dib* in germ-line clones produce embryos that are similar to those of the zygotic mutants, suggesting that it has no function in oogenesis (Chavez et al., 2000). However, the fecundity was not assessed in these studies. Ecdysone and/or its metabolites are also deposited into the egg for use by the early embryo before the prothoracic glands are developed (Lagueux et al., 1979; Bownes et al., 1988).

IV. HORMONE RECEPTORS

A. Ecdysone Receptor Complex

Molecular approaches to ecdysone receptors (EcR) began with work in *Drosophila* that identified the EcR, a member of the nuclear hormone receptor family (Koelle et al., 1991; see Riddiford et al., 2001, for a review). As shown in Fig. 4, EcR is a typical member of this family, organized into a transactivational A/B region at its N-terminus, followed by a DNA-binding domain (DBD) that possesses two cysteine-cysteine (C_2C_2) zinc fingers, a hinge region, and the ligand-binding domain (LBD). The *ecr* gene of *Drosophila* encodes three distinct receptor isoforms, EcR-A, -B1, and -B2 (Talbot et al., 1993). These share common DBDs and LBDs, but they differ in the transactivational region at the N-terminus (Fig. 4). The A and B isoforms are generated from different promoters, whereas the two B isoforms come from

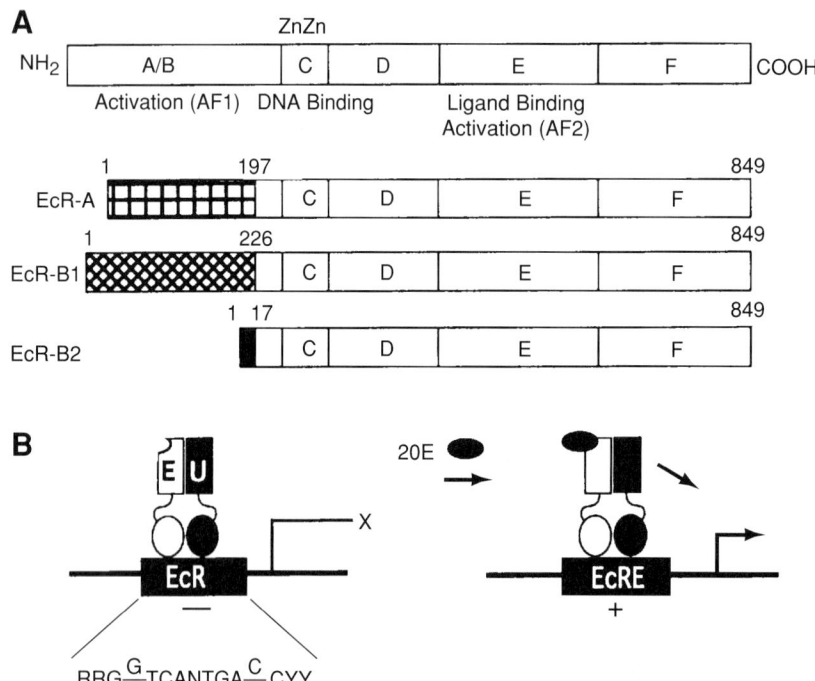

FIGURE 4 The function of nuclear receptors that mediate the action of 20E in insects. (A) Diagram of the protein sequence of a generalized member of the nuclear hormone receptor family. The receptor protein has discrete functional domains—the C domain contains two zinc fingers that are involved in binding to DNA, the E domain is the hormone-binding domain, and both the A/B and E domains contain sites involved in activating the promoters of target genes, the AF1 and AF2 domains, respectively. The *Drosophila* EcR gene encodes three distinct isoforms that differ in their A/B regions, but have identical DNA- and hormone-binding domains. (B) The functional receptor complex is a heterodimer of EcR and ultraspiracle, an orphan nuclear receptor. The EcR-USP dimer binds to specific EcRE. In the absence of ligand, the complex can suppress transcription, but it activates transcription when bound to 20E. The consensus sequence for the EcRE is shown below it. 20E,20-hydroxyecdysone; E and EcR, ecdysone receptor; EcRE, EcR gene response elements; N, any base; R, purine; U and USP, ultraspiracle receptor; Y, pyrimidine (Cherbas and Cherbas, 1996).

alternative splicing. At pupariation, the B1 isoform is predominant in the larval cells that are destined to die or be reprogrammed for metamorphosis, whereas the A isoform is predominant in the imaginal discs. These studies did not determine the localization of the B2 isoform, but subsequent studies with *ecr* null mutants have shown that introduction of the B2 isoform by a heat shock can rescue lethality during embryonic and larval development (Bender *et al.*, 1997; Li and Bender, 2000). Interestingly, both EcR-B1 and EcR-A can also rescue mutants from the early lethality, but only at approximately one-quarter of the efficiency of EcR-B2. Subsequent isolation of EcR from other insects, notably the moths *Manduca sexta* (Fujiwara *et al.*, 1995; Jindra *et al.*, 1996), *Bombyx mori* (Kamimura *et al.*, 1996, 1997), and *Choristoneura fumiferana* (Perera *et al.*, 1999) and the beetle *Tenebrio molitor* (Mouillet *et al.*, 1997) typically show at least two isoforms, one that is A-like and one that is B1-like. A truncated EcR-B2 form has not been found in any insect other than *Drosophila*.

The functional hormone receptor complex is a heterodimer composed of EcR and another member of the nuclear receptor family, ultraspiracle (USP) (Fig. 4; Yao *et al.*, 1992, 1993). This heterodimer is necessary both for binding to the DNA ecdysone response element (EcRE) and for binding ligand, although studies suggest that EcR is the ligand-binding partner (Suhr *et al.*, 1998; Hu, 1998; reviewed in Riddiford *et al.*, 2001). USP is an ortholog of the vertebrate retinoid X receptor (RXR) (Henrich *et al.*, 1990; Oro *et al.*, 1990; Shea *et al.*, 1990), which heterodimerizes with other members of the nuclear receptor family such as the thyroid hormone receptor (TR), the retinoic acid receptor (RAR), the vitamin D receptor, and the peroxisome proliferation activator receptor (PPAR) (Mangelsdorf and Evans, 1995). In ticks, crustaceans, and many insects, the LBD of the insect receptor is very similar (over 70% identity) to that of the vertebrate ortholog (Chung *et al.*, 1998; Guo *et al.*, 1998; Hayward *et al.*, 1999). The LBD has diverged considerably, however, in the Diptera and the Lepidoptera, in which there is only approximately 45–48% identity. The reason for this sudden divergence in the LBD is not known. There is only a single isoform of USP in *Drosophila* (Oro *et al.*, 1992; Henrich *et al.*, 1994), but two isoforms in *Manduca* (Jindra *et al.*, 1997), the midge *Chironomus tentans* (Vögtli *et al.*, 1999), and the mosquito *Aedes aegypti* (Kapitskaya *et al.*, 1996); and two different RXRs in the tick *Amblyomma americanum* (Guo *et al.*, 1998). Both *Manduca* USP isoforms, when transcribed and translated *in vitro*, complex with EcR-B1 and bind to an EcRE, but in the context of a *Manduca* cell line only the EcR-B1–USP-1 dimer binds, not EcR-B1–USP-2 (Lan *et al.*, 1999), indicating that the isoforms in the heterodimeric pair may be critical for particular gene activation. Thus, the USP isoform present at a particular time in development probably determines which genes are activated or inactivated when the hormone appears.

The EcR-USP heterodimer has properties that are shared with its vertebrate counterparts. In the absence of ligand, the EcR-USP complex can bind to the EcRE, where it can suppress basal transcription (Cherbas *et al.*, 1991; Lan *et al.*, 1999). Transcription is then stimulated in response to binding of 20E (Fig. 4). Although there has been considerable discussion about whether EcR can function as a homodimer or as a partner with other members of the nuclear receptor family (Cherbas and Cherbas, 1996; Riddiford *et al.*, 2001), the EcR-USP heterodimer is the only known form for an active ecdysone receptor. It is important to note that USP can heterodimerize with other members of the nuclear receptor family—for example, with *seven-up* (Zelhof *et al.*, 1995) and with hormone receptor 38 (HR38), a homolog of the vertebrate nerve growth factor-induced protein B (NGFI-B/NURR1) (Sutherland *et al.*, 1995; Zhu *et al.*, 2000). In mosquitoes this pairing of USP with AedesHR38 appears to be the mechanism of repression of ecdysone-stimulated gene activation in the previtellogenic female mosquito fat body (Zhu *et al.*, 2000).

B. JH Receptor

The nature of the JH receptor is controversial. Early studies showed that in *Manduca* larval epidermis JH entered the cell and approximately one-third of this was bound in the nuclear fraction (Osir and Riddiford, 1988). Attempts to purify the binding component using photoaffinity-labeled JHs resulted in the isolation of a 29-kDa protein and its gene, called JP29, that had relatively low but specific affinity for JH (Palli *et al.*, 1990, 1994; Charles *et al.*, 1996). This protein is in a family of proteins that includes a lepidopteran hemolymph JHBP (Lerro and Prestwich, 1990) and the *Drosophila* Takeout protein that is thought to be involved with the circadian control of feeding behavior (Sarov-Blat et al., 2000; So et al., 2000). JP29 is found in *Manduca* epidermis during larval life and then disappears as the epidermis is being pupally committed by ecdysone acting in the absence of JH at the end of the feeding stage (Shinoda et al., 1997). It reappears in trace amounts during the onset of adult development.

Because of the structural similarity of JH to some of the retinoids and the finding that some retinoids had weak JH activity in *Manduca* larvae, it was thought that the JH receptor might be one of the retinoid receptors (Palli et al., 1991). Screening a *Manduca* library with the human RAR resulted in the isolation of *Manduca* hormone receptor 3 (MHR3) (Palli et al., 1992), which did not bind JH (S. R. Palli and L. M. Riddiford, unpublished) and later turned out to have higher similarity to the retinoid orphan receptor (ROR) (Giguère et al., 1994). The finding that USP was the RXR homolog (Oro et al., 1990) led to speculation about whether JH is a ligand for the USPs (Talbot et al., 1993; Harmon et al., 1995). The evidence for this possibility is tantalizing, but not conclusive. Jones and Sharp (1997) and Jones and Jones (2000) have found that recombinant *Drosophila* USP binds JH III and JH III bisepoxide, although with a lower affinity (approximately 4×10^{-7} M) than we might expect for a typical hormone–receptor interaction. However, nuclear receptors such as the farnesol X receptor (FXR; in the same subfamily as EcR) that binds bile acids show binding affinities that are even less than this (approximately 10^{-6} M) (Wang et al., 1999; Makashima et al., 1999; Chiang et al., 2000). Bacterially expressed, recombinant USP carries a bacterial phospholipid in its ligand-binding pocket, but neither JH III nor the JH analog methoprene can displace this phospholipid (Billas et al., 2001). JH I acid is predicted to fit into the pocket (Billas et al., 2001), but the biological functions of the JH acid, if they occur, have not been examined conclusively. Consequently, the relationship of USP to JH action needs to be resolved.

A gene associated with JH action is *Methoprene-tolerant* (*Met*; formally known as *Resistance to juvenile hormone (Rst(1)JH)*) gene in *Drosophila* (Wilson and Fabian, 1986). Mutations in this gene render tissues less sensitive to the juvenilizing effects of JH III or JH mimics such as methoprene. Null *Met* mutants are viable and show no defects in larval development or metamorphosis, but the adult females show delayed and greatly reduced vitellogenesis and subsequent oviposition (Wilson and Ashok, 1998). The loss-of-function *Met* mutants have an intracellular JHBP with reduced JH binding activity (Shemshedini and Wilson, 1990). This protein was originally thought to be cytosolic, but studies with an antibody to the recombinant Met protein detects only a nuclear protein in nearly all tissues during development and in the ovarian follicular cells and the male accessory glands (Pursley et al., 2000). This gene encodes a protein that has high similarity with the basic helix-loop-helix PAS family of transcription factors and has most similarity to the aryl hydrocarbon receptor nuclear translocator (ARNT) (Ashok et al., 1998). ARNT is a cytoplasmic protein that complexes with the dioxin receptor (aryl hydrocarbon receptor, AhR) when it binds dioxin or other xenobiotics. The complex tranlocates to the nucleus where the AhR activates genes involved in the metabolism of that xenobiotic (Schmidt and Bradfield, 1996). Exactly how this type of action may be related to JH action is unknown, although Muehleisen et al. (1989) found that dioxin binding in a *Heliothis zea* extract could be competitively inhibited by methoprene or JH I.

In its reproductive actions in *Rhodnius prolixus* and *Locusta migratoria*, JH acts rapidly on the follicle cells of the ovary to cause an increase in the activity of the sodium pump and a consequent shrinking of the cells, thereby allowing the large yolk proteins to pass between the follicle cells to the oocyte (see Wyatt and Davey, 1996, for a review). This action may be mediated by the protein kinase C pathway. A 36-kDa membrane protein from locust follicle cells that was photoaffinity-labeled by JH has been isolated and cloned, but its identity as a membrane receptor for JH has been stymied because the recombinant protein appears to have no JH binding activity (K. G. Davey, personal communication).

V. MOLECULAR MODE OF ACTION OF THE HORMONES

A. Mode of Action of the Ecdysones

Studies of the action of the ecdysones provided the first indication in any system that steroids might act directly on the genome to alter patterns of gene transcription. These studies, carried out in the early 1960s by Clever and Karlson (1960; Clever, 1964), used the salivary glands of the midge (*Chironomus tentans*) and showed that ecdysone rapidly induced puffing (a cytological manifestation of enhanced transcription) of two distinct sites on the giant polytene chromosomes in the salivary glands after the addition of ecdysone to the glands *in vitro*. This set of early puffs then regressed and was followed by a second set of puffs. When the protein synthesis inhibitor cycloheximide was added, the first set of puffs still appeared after hormone treatment, but the second set of puffs was blocked. These puffs were later shown to be sites of mRNA synthesis and thus were the visible indication that ecdysone was acting directly on the DNA to activate particular genes.

In the early 1970s, Ashburner (1973, 1974) repeated these experiments with *Drosophila melanogaster* salivary glands. Here, too, there was a distinct sequence of regions that puffed after exposure of the glands to 20E. A small number of regions puffed within 15–30 minutes of hormone addition, followed by their regression in 3–4 hours and another series of puffs at 3–6 hours of exposure. Again, inhibiting protein synthesis did not block the induction of the early set of puffs but blocked the appearance of the late set. Ashburner *et al.* (1974) proposed a model in which ecdysone and its receptor directly activated a number of early genes, whose protein products then activated a series of late genes and also repressed the early genes. This Ashburner cascade was then verified in the 1990s when *ecr* and the early genes *E74*, *E75*, and *Broad-Complex* (*BR-C*; formally known as *br*) were cloned (Burtis *et al.*, 1990; DiBello *et al.*, 1991; Segraves and Hogness, 1990; reviewed by Thummel, 1996; Richards, 1997; Henrich *et al.*, 1999). These and other ecdysone-induced RNAs appear in the predicted cascade at the end of the final larval instar (Andres *et al.*, 1993; Huet *et al.*, 1993, 1995).

Most of the early genes are transcription factors—*E74*, a member of the ETS oncogene family (Thummel *et al.*, 1990; Burtis *et al.*, 1990), *E75*, a member of the nuclear receptor family (Segraves and Hogness, 1990), and Broad-Complex (*BR-C*), a member of the Broad-Tramtrack-Bric-a-Brac (BTB) family of cysteine 2–histidine 2 (C_2H_2) zinc finger DNA-binding proteins (DiBello *et al.*, 1991). Each of the early genes encodes a number of different protein isoforms generated by alternative splicing or alternative promoters, as in the case of EcR. In the presence of the protein synthesis inhibitor cycloheximide, the transcripts for *E75A* (Segraves and Hogness, 1990) and *BR-C* (Chao and Guild, 1986) increase rapidly in response to 20E *in vitro*. They do not then decrease to low levels as they would normally, indicating that a 20E-induced factor(s) is responsible for their down-regulation. Some 20E-induced early genes are not transcription factors—*E71CD* (formerly known as *eip28/29*; Cherbas *et al.*, 1986, 1991; Andres and Cherbas, 1992); *E63*, which encodes both a member of the EF-hand family of Ca^{+2}-binding proteins (Andres and Thummel, 1995) and a protein with similarity to a mitochondrial import protein (Vaskova *et al.*, 2000); and *E23*, which encodes a protein with similarity to adenosine triphosphate- (ATP)-binding cassette (ABC) transporters (Hock *et al.*, 2000).

The isoforms of the early ecdysone-induced genes have differing sensitivities to 20E. In *Drosophila E74B*, *BR-C* (all four isoforms), *E75C*, and EcR itself all can be activated at nanomolar concentrations of 20E, whereas *E74A*, *E75A*, and *E75B* are activated only at a 10-fold higher concentration with correspondingly higher ED50s (doses effective in 50% of test subjects) (Karim and Thummel, 1991, 1992; Karim *et al.*, 1993). Thus, they classified these early transcripts into two classes—Class I (E74B and EcR) appears first in response to ecdysone and is repressed at the high concentrations at the peak of the ecdysone titer; Class II (E74A, E75A, and E75B) appears only at the higher concentrations of ecdysone and is unaffected by high 20E concentrations *in vitro*. The BR-C transcripts appeared to have characteristics of both classes, attributable to differential promoter sensitivities and to the mix of tissues being examined in this study. Similarly, in *Manduca* abdominal epidermis the EcR and the BR-C transcripts are induced by low levels of 20E (Hiruma *et al.*, 1997, 1999; Zhou *et al.*, 1998a,b). In *Manduca* α-ecdysone synergizes with 20E to induce EcR-B1, although it has no activity by itself (Hiruma *et al.*, 1997). Interestingly, α-ecdysone has no effect on the up-regulation of EcR-A by 20E.

In the ecdysone-induced cascade of transcription factors, there are also genes that are directly induced by 20E but require 20E-induced protein synthesis for their full activation, such as *DHR3* and *MHR3* (Koelle *et al.*, 1992; Palli *et al.*, 1992; Horner *et al.*, 1995) and *E78B* (Huet *et al.*, 1993; Stone and Thummel,

1993)—known as early-late or delayed early genes (Huet *et al.*, 1995; Thummel, 1996; Richards, 1997). Their induction requires exposure to higher levels of 20E (usually $\geq 2 \times 10^{-6}$ M). Their appearance is usually associated with maturational events such as cuticle deposition (Langelan *et al.*, 2000) and eye-pigment deposition (Champlin and Truman, 1998b).

The few late genes, such as *L63*, *L71*, and *L82*, that have been cloned are not transcription factors and may be tissue-specific. The *L71* puff includes seven genes that encode antimicrobial peptides that are found only in the salivary gland (Restifo and Guild, 1986; Wright *et al.*, 1996). This *L71* group is directly regulated by BR-C (Crossgrove *et al.*, 1996). The *L63* gene encodes multiple protein isoforms in the cyclin-dependent kinase (CDK) family (Stowers *et al.*, 2000). The *L82* gene encodes a novel protein that is necessary for development (Stowers *et al.*, 1999). Thus, the early transcription factors are turned on in all tissues, but their effects may be different due to their action together with tissue-specific factors to activate or inactivate tissue-specific genes. For example, the activation of the salivary glue protein gene 4 (*sgs4*) gene at 3C and the three *sgs* genes (*sgs3*, *sgs7*, and *sgs8*) at 68C requires exposure to 20E in an environment that allows protein synthesis (Hansson and Lambertsson, 1989). Both BR-C (for *sgs3*) (von Kalm *et al.*, 1994) and Forkhead, Daughterless, and dAP4 (for *sgs4*) (Lehmann and Korge, 1996; Lehmann *et al.*, 1997; King-Jones *et al.*, 1999) transcription factors have been found necessary for activation.

As the ecdysteroid titer declines, a new series of transcription factors appear, including MHR4 (also called germ-cell nuclear factor related factor, GRF) (Charles *et al.*, 1999; Mouillet *et al.*, 1999; Weller *et al.*, 2001) and βFTZ-F1 (Lavorgna *et al.*, 1991; Sun *et al.*, 1994; Thummel, 1997; Riddiford *et al.*, 1999; Mouillet *et al.*, 1999; Weller *et al.*, 2001) (Fig. 5). MHR4 is directly induced by high 20E, but only appears after a delay due to the presence of 20E-induced inhibitory protein(s) (Hiruma and Riddiford, 2001). Its role is unknown. βFTZ-F1 is encoded by a gene in the 75CD midprepupal puff and requires exposure to 20E followed by its removal (Richards, 1976; Sun *et al.*, 1994; Woodard *et al.*, 1994; Hiruma and Riddiford, 2001). In *Drosophila* βFTZ-F1 is activated by DHR3 and inhibited by the presence of E75B (Kageyama *et al.*, 1997; White *et al.*, 1997; Lam *et al.*, 1997). βFTZ-F1 functions as a competence factor for stage-specific responses, so that some of the transcription factors such as E75A, E74, and E93 are subsequently able to respond to the small prepupal pulse of ecdysteroid (Broadus *et al.*, 1999). The precocious expression of βFTZ-F1 caused the early appearance of E93 mRNA, leading to the degeneration of the salivary glands (Woodard *et al.*, 1994; Baehrecke and Thummel, 1995). In addition, βFTZ-F1 is essential for the activation of one of the pupal cuticle genes, *EDG84A* (Murata *et al.*, 1996) and for normal cuticle deposition at every molt (Yamada *et al.*, 2000) (Fig. 6).

B. Mode of Action of JH

The classic developmental action of JH is its status quo action (Williams, 1961; Riddiford, 1996). Acting in this mode, JH regulates the form of the animal that is undergoing a molt in response to ecdysone. Simply put, if JH is present during the critical early steps of the molt, then the insect assumes the form that it had before; if JH is absent, then it shows a progressive molt—from larva to pupa or from pupa to adult. The commitment to molt to a particular developmental stage occurs at the onset of the ecdysone exposure. This relationship is most evident in the transition from the larval to the pupal stage in *Manduca sexta*. In this case, there are two pulses of ecdysone that cause the larval to pupal transition (Fig. 3). The first is a small peak that evokes a number of behavioral changes such as the cessation of feeding and the onset of searching for an appropriate site for pupation (Dominick and Truman, 1985). It also has profound effects on the developmental capacity of the cells of the larva. It causes the epidermal cells to become committed to develop to the pupal stage (Riddiford, 1976, 1978). Prior to this steroid surge, cells can be directed into a larval molt if provided with JH at the time of a molting ecdysone surge. After the commitment peak, however, the epidermal cells can only make a pupal cuticle, even if subsequently provided with JH. The subsequent formation of the pupal stage comes a few days later when a large surge of ecdysone (the prepupal peak; Fig. 3) causes the formation of the pupal cuticle. The pupal molt is unique in having the commitment step separated in time from the subsequent molting event itself. In both the larval and adult molts, the decision to become a particular stage is followed by the production of the new cuticle. Because the change

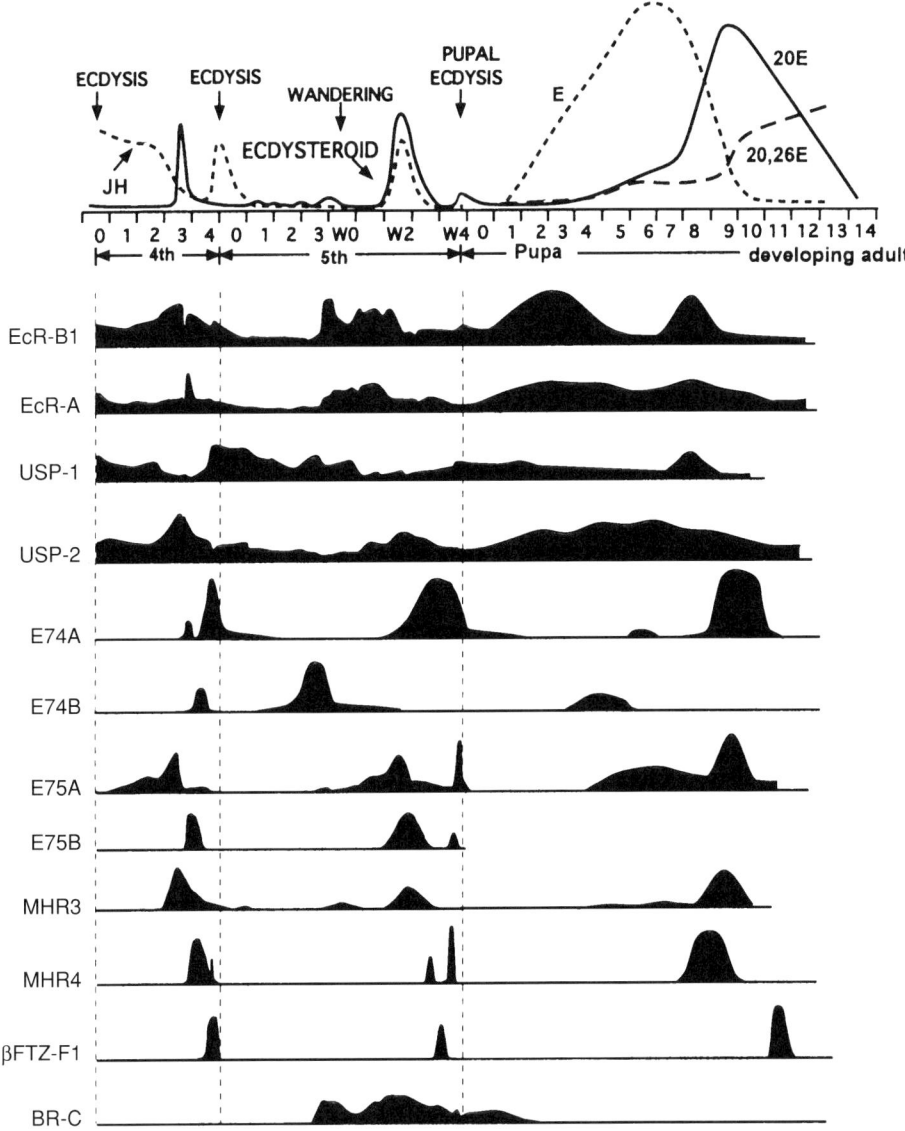

FIGURE 5 An example from the moth *Manduca sexta* of the temporal changes in mRNAs for the components of the ecdysone receptor complex, EcR-USP, and for the major transcription factors that are involved in the ecdysone cascade (E74, E75, MHR3, MHR4, β-FTZ-F1, and BR-C). The mRNAs are from abdominal epidermis taken at various times from the fourth larval stage, the fifth larval stage, the pupa, and the first two-thirds of adult development.

in cellular commitment depends on the presence or absence of JH early in the ecdysone surge, it has been of interest to examine the effects of JH on the early genes that are directly induced by 20E. When *Drosophila* S2 cells are pretreated with methoprene or JH III (Berger *et al.*, 1992), the 20E-induced expression of an hsp27 EcRE-reporter gene construct containing only 15 bp outside the EcRE is suppressed in a dose-responsive manner, but the mechanism of this action is not known. In the epidermis of *Manduca*, the presence of JH during the beginning of the 20E exposure enhances the expression of E75A (Zhou *et al.*, 1998a), but suppresses the appearance of BR-C (Zhou *et al.*, 1998b; Zhou and Riddiford, 2001). These results from *Manduca* suggest

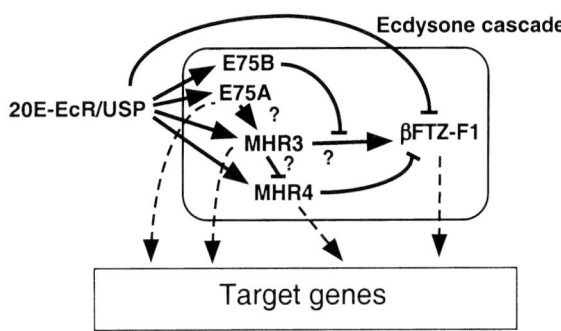

FIGURE 6 A scheme from *Manduca* showing some of the likely relationships of the nuclear receptor members of the ecdysone cascade to one another and to the liganded EcR-USP complex. Interactions between members of the group are probably responsible for the progressive display such as seen in Fig. 5. These transcription factors also act on downstream target genes to help coordinate the processes that occur during the molt.

that high E75A is important for the maintenance of the larval state. For *BR-C*, abundant genetic evidence from *Drosophila* shows that this gene is not needed for larval molting, but that larvae arrest as permanent last-stage larvae if they lack all BR-C function (reviewed by Bayer et al., 1996). Also, some of the effects of JH on *Drosophila* metamorphosis are similar to those of BR-C loss-of-function mutations (Restifo and Wilson, 1998). In *Manduca*, JH treatments that prevent pupal commitment also prevent BR-C expression, supporting the idea that BR-C is a key factor for pupal commitment. It is important to note that once the *BR-C* gene has been activated by 20E at commitment, the return of JH during the pupal molt cannot suppress its continued expression (Zhou and Riddiford, 2001). The molecular basis of these actions of JH is under active investigation.

JH also has developmental actions that are not directly tied to the actions of α-ecdysone or 20E. In *Drosophila*, methoprene or JH III appear to be able to directly up-regulate two genes of unknown function in cultured S2 cells (Dubrovsky et al., 2000). In some insects JH has an important function during larval life of suppressing the formation and growth of imaginal discs. For example, in *Manduca* the cells that make up both the eye primordium (Monsma and Booker, 1996a,b; D. Champlin, L. M. Riddiford, and J. W. Truman, unpublished) and the adult leg primordium (K. Tanaka and J. W. Truman, unpublished) produce larval cuticle during each larval molt. During the final larval instar, however, these cells undergo a premature detachment from the larval cuticle and begin the rapid proliferation that forms the eye and the leg imaginal discs. During the prepupal pulse of ecdysone, these discs then evert to form the pupal molds within which the adult structures form during adult development.

For the penultimate stage eye primordium, the removal of JH by removal of the corpora allata or by culturing the primordium in the absence of hormones causes it to undergo precocious detachment and the proliferation needed to make the imaginal disc (D. Champlin, L. M. Riddiford, and J. W. Truman, unpublished). The readdition of JH to the culture medium can then suppress the ongoing proliferation. Once the eye imaginal disc begins forming, the cells lose their ability to make larval cuticle and they are committed to metamorphic development. After wandering, proliferation is no longer affected by JH but becomes dependent on ecdysone, as discussed later.

VI. CELLULAR ACTIONS OF HORMONES ON THE NERVOUS SYSTEM: *DROSOPHILA* AND *MANDUCA* MODELS

A. Overview of Nervous System Changes during Metamorphosis

On a gross level, the transformation of the central nervous system (CNS) from its larval to its adult form involves the growth of some regions and the regression of others. At a cellular level, these gross changes occur partly through the birth and maturation of adult-specific (imaginal) neurons and the programmed death of larval cells. Many larval neurons, however, escape degeneration. They are carried through metamorphosis and are remodeled to perform new functions in the adult (Fig. 7). These diverse cellular fates are all played out under the control of the ecdysones and JH.

The cellular remodeling of larval neurons during metamorphosis is best understood for the neuromuscular system. There has been considerable work done on both *Manduca* (for reviews, see Levine and Weeks, 1990; Truman, 1992, 1996a,b; Levine et al., 1995) and *Drosophila* (Fernandes and VijayRaghavan, 1993; Fernandes and Keshishian, 1998; Roy and VijayRaghavan, 1999; Truman et al., 1993). In the larva of *Manduca*, the musculature of the body wall is divided

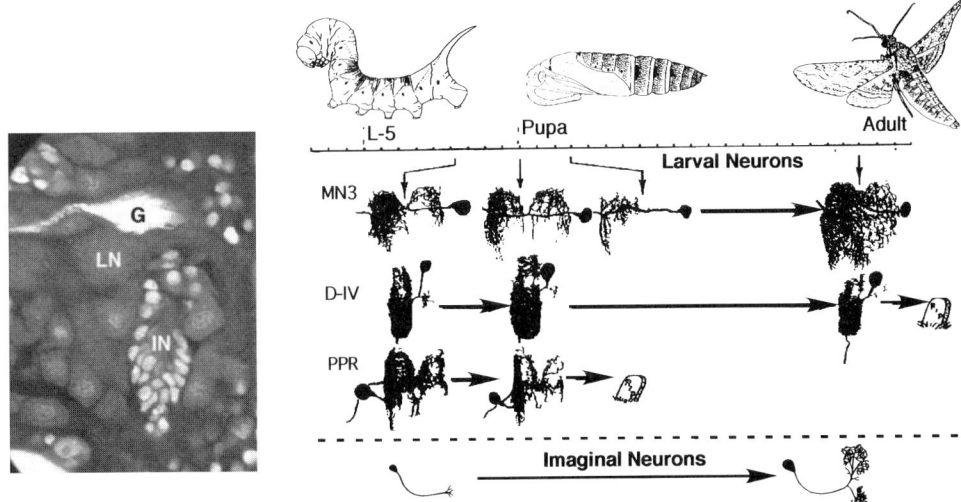

FIGURE 7 A summary of the fates shown by neurons during the course of metamorphosis in the moth *Manduca sexta*. (Left) Confocal optical section through a thoracic ganglion of a fifth instar larva showing the cell bodies of larval neurons (LN), glia (G), and clusters of arrested immature imaginal neurons (IN). (Right) Transition from the fifth stage larva (L-5) to the adult, showing the changes that occur for particular neurons. The motoneuron MN3 shows a regression of dendrites during the larval to pupal transition, followed by the growth of an adult-specific arbor during adult development. The D-IV motoneuron remains unchanged through metamorphosis, but dies after the emergence of the adult. The PPR motoneuron, which supplies the larval-specific proleg, shows dendritic regression during the larval to pupal transition, followed by death. The generalized drawing of an imaginal-specific neuron shows an arrested immature cell in the larva that then undergoes its adult maturation during adult development.

into external and internal muscle groups. During the larval to pupal transition, the external muscles and some internal muscles degenerate, leaving the pupa with only a subset of internal muscles in the abdomen. The motoneurons supplying these persisting internal muscles stay relatively unchanged through metamorphosis and provide a core of functional circuitry to control pupal behavior while the rest of the neuromuscular system is reorganized. Depending on the region of the body, the adult musculature arises during adult development either *de novo* (the legs; Consoulas et al., 1996, 1997) or on templates that form from the remains of the larval external muscles (the abdomen; Truman and Reiss, 1995). Similar to *Manduca*, some adult muscles in *Drosophila* also arise from templates provided by the remains of the larval muscles, although the majority of adult muscles arise without preexisting templates (for reviews, see Bate, 1993; Roy and VijayRaghavan, 1999). For muscles that arise from larval templates, the motoneurons remain in contact with their targets as the muscles regress and then regrow. Associated with the changes in their targets, the neurons show first a dramatic pruning back of their dendritic and axonal arbors. New growth cones then form, spread over the regrowing muscles, and establish adult synaptic contacts. Although most attention in *Manduca* has been directed to the remodeling of form and connectivity patterns of larval neurons, the changes shown by these cells can also involve other cellular properties. For example, the membrane currents of some neurons are altered as the cells shift from being slow to fast motoneurons (Grunewald and Levine, 1998; Duch and Levine, 2000). Also, peptide transmitters or cotransmitters may change during the transition from larva to adult (Tublitz and Loi, 1993; Loi and Tublitz, 1993; Davis et al., 1993).

Although the major strategy on the motor side is one of recycling larval components, the pattern seen on the sensory side is the production of new adult-specific neurons. A large number of sensory neurons arise in the periphery during metamorphosis in conjunction with the development of the adult structures such as the legs, wings, and compound eyes. Most of the interneurons that deal with this expanded sensory input also appear to be adult-specific and arise during larval life from neuronal stem cells (neuroblasts) that are scattered in stereotyped locations in the medial brain and thoracic ganglia (White and Kankel, 1978; Booker and Truman, 1987a; Truman and Bate, 1988; Booker et al., 1996). Although some of these imaginal neurons are born quite early in larval life, they arrest their development and remain as nonfunctional immature neurons until exposed to the hormonal signals that induce metamorphosis (Fig. 7, left).

A prominent feature of the adult brain is the paired optic lobes that process the information from the adult compound eye. The interneurons for each optic lobe arise from extensive inner and outer proliferation zones. Prior to the last larval instar, these proliferation zones expand their population of neuroblasts as these cells undergo repeated symmetrical divisions (Meinertzhagen and Hanson, 1993; Monsma and Booker, 1996a). In the last-stage larva, the neuroblasts then change to an asymmetric pattern of division that results in the production of neurons. For the outer region of the optic lobe, the lamina, contact with the ingrowing photoreceptor axons of the developing eye is required to maintain neurogenesis (Selleck and Steller, 1991; Monsma and Booker, 1996a). Because successive rows of photoreceptor units are added to the eye in a posterior to anterior fashion, this results in a wave of neurogenesis that gradually sweeps across the outer part of the optic lobes.

B. Patterns of Steroid Receptor Expression in the Nervous System

As previously described, the initial description of EcR isoforms in *Drosophila* by Talbot et al. (1993) reported that different tissues showed a dramatic difference in the pattern of EcR isoform expression at the outset of metamorphosis. Larval tissues show a prominent expression of EcR-B1 but relatively little EcR-A, whereas imaginal tissues, such as the imaginal discs, show predominantly EcR-A with little or no EcR-B1. There were some obvious exceptions to this generalization, however, such as a prominent expression of EcR-A in the prothoracic gland portion of the larval ring gland.

The CNS of *Drosophila* has provided the most detailed picture of the fluctuations in EcR-A and EcR-B1 during metamorphosis (Truman et al., 1994). These are summarized in Fig. 8. The two isoforms exhibit

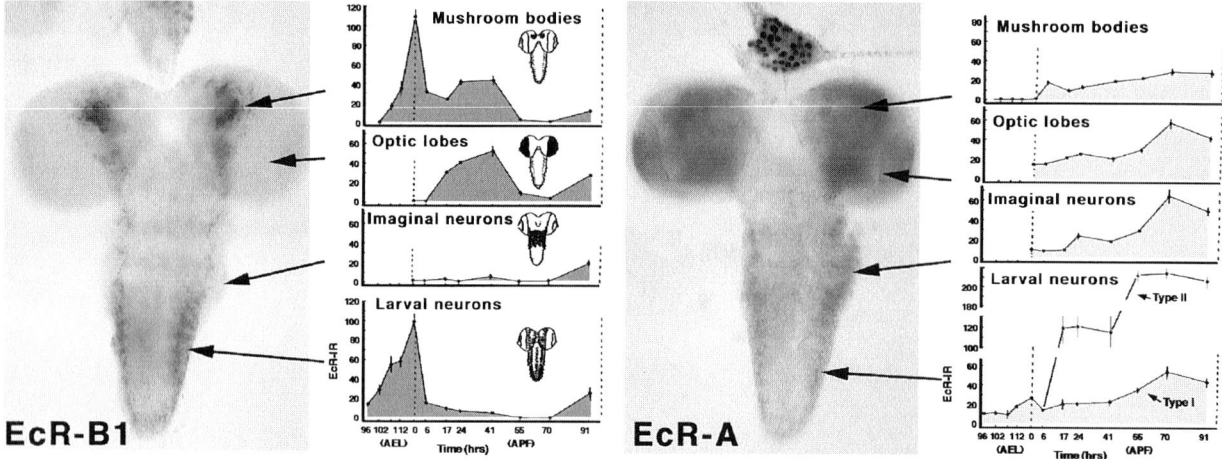

FIGURE 8 Temporal and spatial variation in the expression of the EcR isoforms in the CNS during the course of metamorphosis in *Drosophila*. (Left) EcR-B1 expression. (Right) EcR-A expression. In each case, the photomicrograph shows the distribution of the particular isoform in the CNS at the start of metamorphosis (puparium formation). Included are the two brain lobes that are connected to the fused ganglia from the thoracic and abdominal regions of the body; the endocrine ring gland is located in front of the brain and is at the top of the picture. The graphs show the isoform-specific immunoreactivity as determined by confocal microscopy Major peaks of ecdysteroid occur at pupariation and approximately 24–40 hours after puparium formation (APF). Hours 96–112 AEL (after egg-laying) are during the last larval stage. Data modified from Truman et al. (1994).

a complex pattern of expression that mirrors the diverse origins and cellular fates seen in central neurons through metamorphosis. Neurons show little EcR expression during most of larval growth, consistent with a lack of known developmental effects of ecdysone on these cells in early larval stages. One set of cells that does express EcR-B1 during larval life are the neuroblasts in the medial brain and thoracic part of the CNS and those in the proliferation zones of the optic lobes. Detectable EcR first appears in neurons late in the last (third) larval instar in preparation for metamorphosis. At this point, ecdysone can now evoke the complex developmental responses involved with neuronal growth, remodeling, or death. As shown in Fig. 8, with the notable exception of the type II larval neurons described later, the levels of EcR-A are generally quite similar across the various classes of neurons. The expression of EcR-B1, by contrast, varies markedly from one type of neuron to another and also temporally through metamorphosis. At the outset of metamorphosis, a high level of EcR-B1 expression is seen in many larval neurons and the γ-neurons of the mushroom bodies (Truman et al., 1994; Lee et al., 2000). Both these types of neurons show a pronounced pruning back of larval neurites at this time. After pruning is complete, the larval neurons then down-regulate EcR-B1 and express predominantly or exclusively EcR-A at the time they are showing their adult growth. These remodeling neurons are in interesting contrast to the arrested imaginal neurons, which have no larval processes to prune back and initiate their adult growth at the start of metamorphosis. These cells express only EcR-A at this time. Overall, the EcR-B1 isoform appears to be correlated with a pruning response to ecdysone, whereas EcR-A is associated with neuronal outgrowth in response to steroid. The mutant studies described later confirm the necessity of EcR-B isoforms for the pruning responses.

A brain region in which early EcR-B1 expression is not obviously associated with the pruning of larval neurites is the optic lobes. Although this region consists almost entirely of adult-specific interneurons, these cells begin to show high levels of EcR-B1 by 10 hours after puparium formation and continue to show elevated levels for the next 40 hours of development. Interestingly, this period of development begins with the arrival of the last photoreceptor axons into the optic lobe (Meinertzhagen and Hanson, 1993) and encompasses the time in which there are obvious anteroposterior gradients of development across the optic lobe as the visual interneurons organize themselves into cartridges and columns (Meinertzhagen and Hanson, 1993). These gradients in the optic lobe result from the wave of photoreceptor axon ingrowth from the developing eye imaginal disc. The high levels of EcR-B1 seen in the optic lobe interneurons through this period may be associated with these cells remaining in a plastic phase as they are being organized into their appropriate synaptic units.

One set of larval neurons that deserve special mention are the type II larval neurons (Fig. 8). These cells are unique in that they show enhanced levels of EcR-A starting at approximately 17 hours after pupariation and continuing for the remainder of adult development (Robinow et al., 1993). These larval neurons appear to be associated with ecdysis behavior (the process of shedding the old skin at the end of a molt) and they all degenerate after the emergence of the adult at the end of metamorphosis.

C. Hormonal Regulation of the Development of Imaginal Neurons

It is unlikely that either ecdysone or JH is used to regulate the proliferation of the scattered neuroblasts in the medial brain or ventral ganglia. In both *Drosophila* and *Manduca*, the neuroblasts begin generating neurons early in larval life in a manner that appears unrelated to either the ecdysone or JH titers (Booker and Truman, 1987a; Truman and Bate, 1988). The activation of these stem cells is caused by a nutritional cue associated with larval growth (Britton and Edgar, 1998) but the nature of these cues is unknown.

Although not associated with their birth, hormones are clearly needed for the maturation of the imaginal neurons into mature adult cells (Booker and Truman, 1987b). Prior to the start of the wandering phase, imaginal neurons that have been born earlier in larval life accumulate in clusters of developmentally arrested, immature cells (Fig. 7, left). With the larval to pupal transition, some of the neurons in a cluster degenerate, whereas the remainder show soma enlargement and the start of their maturation into adult neurons. The isolation of larval abdomens prior to the releases of the ecdysone needed for the larval to pupal transition

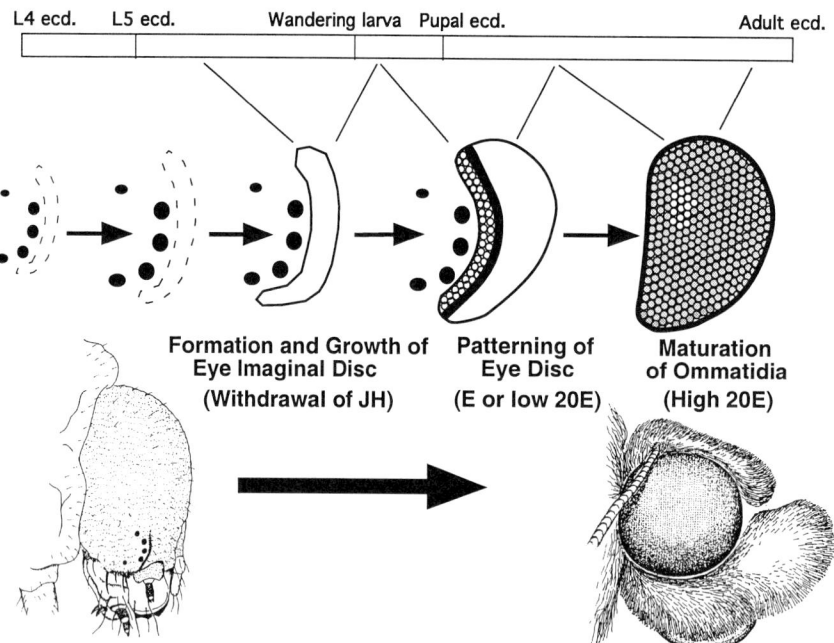

FIGURE 9 The development of the compound eye of *Manduca sexta*. (A) Timeline for the development of the compound eye. At the start of the last larval stage, the decline in the titer of JH allows a crescent-shaped field of cells immediately anterior to the larval eyes to initiate proliferation to form the eye imaginal disc. After the larva stops feeding and begins to search for a site for pupation (the wandering stage), low levels of ecdysteroid support the movement of a morphogenetic wave across the eye disc, resulting in the formation of immature photoreceptor units. The maturation of the structure is then caused by the high levels of ecdysteroids that appear during the differentiation of the adult. (B) Lateral views of the head of the larva and the adult. The eyes of the larva include five to six simple eyes that are located just dorsal to the antenna and mouthparts; the compound eye of the adult is the dominant feature of the head. 20E, 20-hydroxyecdysone; E, α-ecdysone; ecd., time of ecdysis to a particular stage; JH, juvenile hormone.

resulted in the permanent arrest of these cells in the abdominal CNS. However, infusion of 20E into these abdomens to mimic the prepupal ecdysone peak resulted in the same range of developmental responses as seen in control larvae during early metamorphosis. The final maturation of these cells, including the acquisition of their adult transmitter phenotypes, requires the ecdysone surge that causes adult development.

The visual system deserves special mention because of its unusual mode of development. The endocrine regulation of the growth and development of the eye and optic lobe has been intensively studied in *Manduca* (Monsma and Booker, 1996b; Champlin and Truman, 1998b). Larval *Manduca* have a small number of simple eyes, the stemmata, located on the lateral margin of the head (Fig. 9). Just anterior to the stemmata is a crescent of epidermis that is the primordium for the adult eye. During early larval stages, the cells of the eye primordium behave like other larval epidermal cells in that they produce head capsule cuticle at each larval molt, but they differ by remaining diploid. After the entry into the last larval stage, however, JH begins to decline (Fig. 3). This hormone, which has been present through most of larval life, appears to act tonically to prevent the cells of the primordium from transforming into an imaginal disc (D. Champlin, L. M. Riddiford, and J. W. Truman, in preparation). With the decline in JH early in the last instar, the epidermis of the primordium is freed from this suppression and it detaches from the cuticle and begins rapid proliferation. By day 3 or 4 of the last instar, the commitment peak of ecdysone then alters the fate of the general epidermis (Riddiford, 1976, 1978) and also alters the endocrine regulation of the growing imaginal disc. Although the disc continues to grow after seeing this small commitment peak, it no longer can be suppressed by JH treatment.

The commitment peak is followed 2 days later by a large prepupal peak of ecdysone that causes the molt to the pupal stage. For the eye imaginal disc of *Manduca*, this peak causes the formation and progression of the morphogenetic furrow, which forms at the posterior edge of the disc and begins to move anteriorly. Similarly, in the brain at this time, the ecdysone exposure causes the neuroblasts to start their asymmetric cell divisions to produce the visual interneurons (Monsma and Booker, 1996a). *In vitro* studies on both the developing eye (Fig. 10) and the optic lobe showed that the proliferation and patterning processes require the continuing presence of moderate levels of ecdysone (>60 ng 20E/ml). If steroid levels are reduced below this threshold, these processes stop. They resume, however, if steroid levels are brought back into the moderate range. As considered later, the shift of steroid titers to very high levels also terminates proliferation and patterning, but in an irreversible fashion as the tissue is shifted into a program of cellular maturation (Champlin and Truman, 1998a,b). In *Drosophila*, the eye imaginal disc shows a precocious onset of furrow movement in the mid-third larval stage, but furrow progression appears to become dependent on ecdysone signaling by the time metamorphosis begins (Brennan et al., 1998). Interestingly, although dependent on ecdysone, furrow progression and eye differentiation can nevertheless occur in tissue that lacks *ecr* function (Brennan et al., 2001).

Although 20E is generally considered the active ecdysone, α-ecdysone at physiological concentrations can also support the proliferation and patterning of the compound eye and optic lobe in *Manduca*. The most detailed information on the hormonal requirements for proliferation is available for the optic lobe (Champlin and Truman, 1998a). In the absence of α-ecdysone or 20E, the cycling neuroblasts block at the G2 phase of the cell cycle. A suprathreshold pulse of 20E as short as 1.5–2 hours is sufficient to remove the block and send cells though a complete cell cycle, but they then

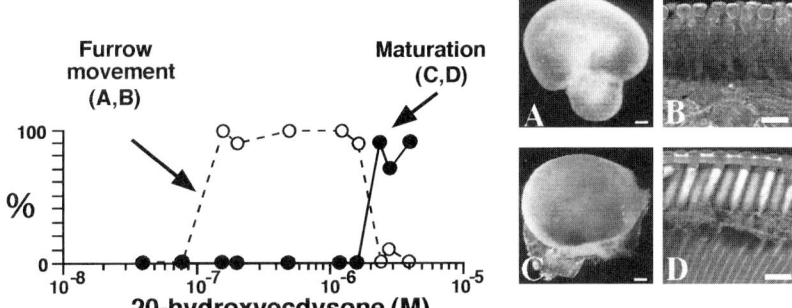

FIGURE 10 Summary of the response of the pupal eye imaginal disc of *Manduca* to treatment with 20E *in vitro*. (Left) Dose–response relationship showing the 20E levels needed to evoke mitosis and movement of the morphogenetic furrow (open circles) and the cellular maturation of the ommatidial units (solid circles). (Right) Photomicrographs of the whole eye disc (A,C) and confocal optical sections of the region posterior to the furrow (B,D). In response to low levels of 20E (A,B), furrow movement occurs across the disc and cells behind the furrow differentiate into the cell types of the ommatidium, including the sensory neurons. (C–D) High concentrations of 20E induce terminal maturation as manifest by the synthesis of the screening pigments (C) and the formation of the cuticular lens, the crystalline cones, and the elongated photoreceptor rhabdomeres (D). Scale bars: 500 μm (A,C); 25 μm (B,D). Data from Champlin and Truman (1998b). **See insert for a color version of this figure.**

arrest at the next G2 phase if steroid continues to be withheld. Therefore, during each cell cycle there is a checkpoint during which the cells assess the state of the steroid concentration. The sustained proliferation in both the eye and optic lobes therefore requires the tonic presence of α-ecdysone or a moderate level of 20E. A candidate for this control point is the transcription of the *Manduca* homolog of *string/CDC2 phosphatase*. This gene is a prominent regulator of the transition from G2 to S phase (Edgar and O'Farrell, 1990). In steroid-dependent cells, its transcription is directly and rapidly induced by exposure to 20E (D. T. Champlin and J. W. Truman, unpublished).

The developing eye and the optic lobes initiate cellular maturation when 20E levels are raised to concentrations above 1000 ng/ml. Only 20E is effective in initiating these high threshold effects. In the brain, these levels of 20E arrest neurogenesis and cause the death of the remaining neuroblasts (Champlin and Truman, 1998a). In the eye, they cause the irreversible arrest of the furrow; patterned cells behind the furrow mature into functional components of the ommatidium— showing the production of the crystalline cone, synthesis of screening pigments, production of photosensitive microvillae in the photoreceptors, and so on (Fig. 10). The unpatterned cells in the imaginal disc in front of the furrow make a naked adult-like cuticle (Champlin and Truman, 1998b). Unlike the tonic responses to moderate levels of steroid, high levels of steroid act as a phasic signal to evoke a developmental program that can continue even if steroid is then withdrawn.

It is important to note that once proliferation and patterning has begun in the eye and the optic lobes, these tissues can be shifted into the program of cellular maturation at any time if the 20E titer is shifted above 1000 ng/ml. Therefore, the size of the adult structure that forms in response to high 20E exposure depends on the length of time that the eye disc is exposed to moderate steroid levels. This is especially obvious in the compound eye in which precocious exposure to high 20E levels results in the formation of a miniature eye (Champlin and Truman, 1998b). A second important point is that, although JH is no longer able to stop the proliferation of the eye imaginal disc after commitment, it can still influence how the imaginal disc responds to 20E. During the larval to pupal transition, the 20E concentration rises to levels that should arrest furrow movement and cause maturation of the ommatidia. This response to high 20E is suppressed, however, by the reappearance of JH during the prepupal peak of ecdysone. If the return of JH is prevented by the surgical removal of the corpora allata, the prepupal peak of 20E induces the premature maturation of the compound eye and we find a pupa with a crescent of adult compound eye (Kiguchi and Riddiford, 1978; Champlin and Truman, 1998b).

Different groups of direct-response genes are associated with the response to low vs high concentrations of 20E. High levels of 20E (over 1000 ng/ml) induce the expression of the orphan receptors, such as MHR3 and E75B (D. T. Champlin and J. W. Truman, 1998b, also unpublished) in the optic lobe of *Manduca*. In *Drosophila* and *Manduca*, these genes are an early part of the ecdysone cascade that can then continue in the absence of steroid. The activation of this regulatory network by high levels of 20E probably accounts for the ballistic nature of the developmental response that then continues even when steroid is withdrawn. In *Drosophila*, lower levels of steroid induce the E74B transcription factor, but not as part of a self-regulating cascade (Karim and Thummel, 1992). As with the developmental response seen in *Manduca*, the maintained expression of E74B requires the sustained presence of 20E.

The mechanism by which 20E, working through EcR-USP, regulates developmental patterning may differ from how it induces maturational responses. Work on *Drosophila* wing imaginal discs that had clonal patches of cells that lacked USP function showed that without USP there was no expression of genes that are early in the ecdysone cascade, such as E75B and DHR3. However, certain late-gene products, such as βFTZ-F1 and BR-C-Z1, were expressed prematurely and precocious metamorphic development was evident for the cells in the clone. Similar studies on the eye imaginal disc of *Drosophila* likewise showed that the lack of USP resulted in an advancement of the morphogenetic furrow over surrounding wild-type tissue (Zelhof *et al.*, 1997). Interestingly, when the wing imaginal discs were maintained *in vitro* in the absence of ecdysone, the wild-type tissue arrested its development but the *usp* null patches went ahead with early metamorphic development despite the lack of 20E (Fig. 11) (Schubiger and Truman, 2000).

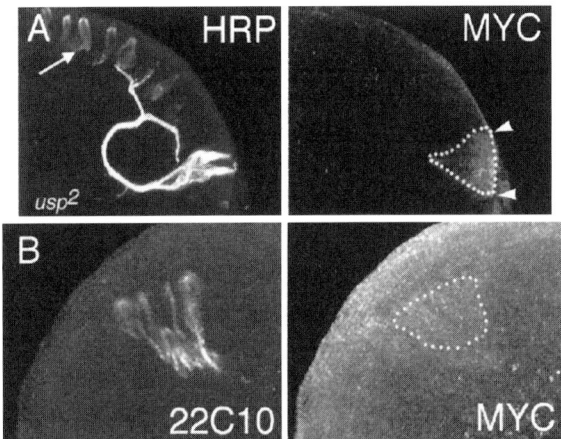

FIGURE 11 The effect of the lack of USP on the birth and development of sensory neurons in the early metamorphic wing of *Drosophila*. The wing discs bore clonal patches of tissue that lacked a functional *usp* gene and were marked by expression of the MYC protein (right, enclosed by dotted area). Neuronal differentiation was followed by immunostaining for a horseradish peroxidase (HRP) epitope or with the monoclonal antibody 22C10 (left). (A) *In vivo* at pupariation, the sensory neurons along the anterior wing margin (arrow) are just beginning axonal outgrowth and expression of the HRP epitope, but within the *usp*-null clone the neurons are well advanced in their development with extensive axonal outgrowth. (B) Wing discs from early wandering larvae were maintained *in vitro* in the absence of 20E. Metamorphic development failed to occur in the wild-type tissue, but cells in the *usp*-null clone showed normal neurogenesis and axonal outgrowth. Hence, the lack of USP allows axonal outgrowth to occur in the absence of the normal steroid cue. Data from Schubiger and Truman (2000).

The results from the *usp* clones in the wing imaginal discs suggest that the EcR-USP complex may not regulate the activity of all of its target genes in the same fashion. The induction of DHR3, E74, and some BR-C isoforms appears to be via steroid-dependent activation, whereas the appearance of BR-C-Z1, βFTZ-F1, and the birth and axonal outgrowth of sensory neurons are through steroid-dependent derepression exerted via USP (Schubiger and Truman, 2000). Interpretation of these results is based on the ability of the unliganded EcR-USP complex to silence transcription (Cherbas and Cherbas, 1996). We think that some genes are repressed by the unliganded EcR-USP complex and 20E simply allow the derepression of these genes. For other genes, the key for their expression is activation via EcR-USP in response to 20E. The distinction between activation and derepression has experimental relevance because in clones that lack *usp*, genes that require activation cannot be expressed because of lack of part of the receptor complex, whereas genes that are regulated through derepression are still expressed, but now in a 20E-independent manner because their repressor is absent.

D. Remodeling of Larval Neurons

The first stage in the remodeling of larval neurons involves the rapid loss of larval synapses and a greater or lesser extent of the axonal and dendritic arbors. In both *Manduca* and *Drosophila*, the pruning back of neurites requires the ecdysone peak that occurs during the larval to pupal transition (Weeks and Truman, 1986; Schubiger *et al.*, 1998, also unpublished). *Drosophila* has been used to examine the role of the EcR-USP complex in the pruning process. In the case of EcR, mutants that lack the two B isoforms while retaining EcR-A (the EcR-B mutants) fail to show the pruning back of larval branches of the ventral thoracic (Tv) neurosecretory cells (Fig. 12) (Schubiger *et al.*, 1998). Likewise, in the mushroom bodies there are a group of neurons that are born early in larval life (the γ-neurons of Lee *et al.*, 1999). They are apparently unique among the neurons that are born postembryonically in that they grow larval-specific processes that are then pruned back at metamorphosis (Technau and Heisenberg, 1982). The γ-neurons also fail to prune back their larval branches in the EcR-B mutants (Lee *et al.*, 2000). For both sets of neurons, the targeted expression of individual EcR isoforms in these cells in EcR-B mutants showed that EcR-B isoforms were capable of rescuing the pruning response, but that EcR-A was ineffective (Lee *et al.*, 2000; M. Schubiger, S. Robinow, and J. W. Truman, unpublished). Hence, the receptor composition in the neuron itself, rather than in its pre- or postsynaptic partners, is crucial for determining how it responds to the steroid signals.

USP is also essential for the pruning response. Using a technique to make neurons that were homozygous mutant for *usp* in an otherwise wild-type brain, Lee *et al.* (2000) showed that γ-neurons of the mushroom bodies retain their larval processes through metamorphosis if they lack functional USP protein. Thus, a complex of

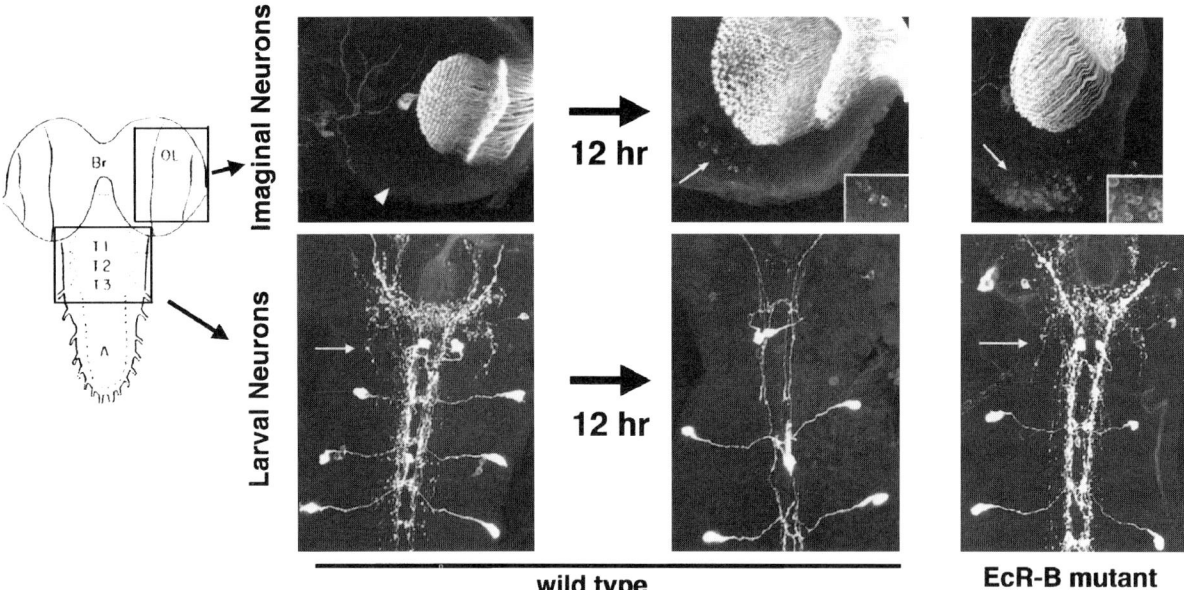

FIGURE 12 Nervous systems from wild-type and EcR-B mutants showing that the lack of the EcR-B isoforms allows the early metamorphic development of imaginal-specific neurons in the optic lobes, but not that of larval neurons in the thoracic CNS. The images are of wild-type nervous systems at the onset of metamorphosis (white puparium stage) and 12 hours later. The nervous system of the EcR-B mutant is equivalent in time to the 12-hour CNS. (Top) Antibodies against the cell-surface protein chaoptin show that this protein is abundantly expressed in photoreceptor axons that project into the optic lobe. Immature optic lobe visual interneurons do not express chaoptin at pupariation (arrowhead), but they then show expression by 12 hours later (arrow and inset). These neurons in the EcR-B mutants also show the induction of choaptin expression (arrow and inset). (Bottom) Larval neurons that express the neuropeptide FMRFamide show a dramatic pruning back of their dendritic processes (arrow) during the first 12 hours of metamorphosis. Pruning fails to occur in larvae that lack the EcR-B isoforms. Data from Schubiger et al. (1998).

USP and EcR-B1 or B2 is apparently required to mediate the pruning response.

The regulation of the outgrowth phase appears to be more complex. In *Manduca*, depending on the neuron considered, the loss of larval synapses and fine arbors is typically completed by 2–3 days after pupal ecdysis. The following ecdysone surge then causes adult development with the formation of the adult muscle and the elaboration of adult neuronal arbors and motor endings. Because the steroid exposure causes changes in both the motoneurons and their targets (i.e., muscle regression and the loss of motor axonal arbors), an important issue is whether the steroid acts directly on the motoneuron or indirectly through steroid-induced changes in the target muscle.

A number of *in vitro* studies with isolated, identified motoneurons have shown that the major classes of developmental responses to 20E—neurite outgrowth, neurite loss, and programmed cell death—are cell-autonomous responses that neurons show *in vitro* or in their normal cellular context when exposed to the appropriate hormonal signal (reviewed in Levine and Weeks, 1996). The earliest study used *Manduca* leg motoneurons (Prugh et al., 1992). These neurons were labeled *in vivo* by injecting a retrograde tracer into the leg of the caterpillar. The fluorescent tracer was transported to the cell bodies of the leg motoneurons, where it persisted through metamorphosis. In the early pupal stage, thoracic ganglia were dissociated and the neurons were grown in low-density culture. The leg motoneurons were readily identified in the cultures by the presence of the tracer. Motoneurons taken from early pupae extended axons and survived well in culture even in the absence of 20E. Exposure to 1 μg 20E/ml, however, caused an extensive growth of dendrite-like processes. This mimics the response of the neuron to 20E *in vivo*. One of the striking effects of the 20E treatment was to change the form and the cytoskeletal composition of the growth cones of the cultured neurons (Matheson and Levine, 1999). Interestingly, if the same neurons were explanted from larval rather than pupal nervous systems, they showed no sprouting and, rather, a slight reduction in branching when challenged with steroid. Therefore, the stage specificity of the nature of the response that the cell shows *in vivo*, in terms of steroid-induced pruning vs sprouting, is preserved when the neurons are treated in isolation. From the studies on *Drosophila*, we would expect that the shift in the response properties of the neurons is related to a shift in the type of receptor isoforms that is present in the two stages.

In the developing adult, process outgrowth can be divided into two discrete phases that are most evident for the terminal axonal arbor. After the rapid collapse of the fine larval axonal branches, there then follows an initial reorganization period from approximately day 2 after pupation (day P+2) until day P+7 or P+8. During this period, the remains of some axonal branches continue their regression, whereas others begin to transform into growth cones (Nuesch, 1985; Truman and Reiss, 1995) by the elaboration and thickening of short primary branches. During this same period, the neuronal cell body also undergoes enlargement. By approximately day P−8, the cell then switches to the rapid extension and spread of the arbor over the muscle. By approximately 3 days later, the axonal arbor is complete and synaptogenesis has begun; this then occupies the remainder of adult development. The phases of growth-cones organization vs extension of the axonal arbor are correlated with different steroid concentrations. The growth cones form while the nervous system is exposed to primarily α-ecdysone and only low levels of 20E. The shift to rapid outgrowth is then correlated with the increase of the titer of 20E above 1 μg/ml. The importance of this shift in 20E concentration can be seen by injecting pupae with a high dose of 20E early in adult development. As seen for the premature maturation of the compound eye (Champlin and Truman, 1998b), early treatment with high 20E induces the premature spreading of axonal arbor over its muscle target (Fig. 13) (J. W. Truman, unpublished).

Most *in vitro* studies of the responses of identified neurons of both *Manduca* and *Drosophila* (e.g., Prugh *et al.*, 1992; Matheson and Levine, 1999; Kraft *et al.*, 1998) have used a concentration of 1 μg 20E/ml.

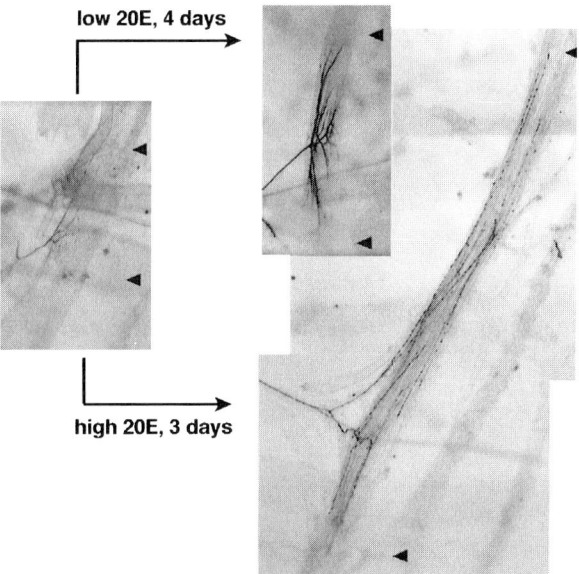

FIGURE 13 Photomicrographs of stained axonal arbors of the *Manduca* motoneuron MN-12 showing the relationship of ecdysone levels to arbor growth. (Left) At 3 days after pupation, the motor arbor of MN-3 is composed of a few wispy branches on the remains of the old larval muscle. (Top right) By 4 days later *in vivo*, under the influence of α-ecdysone and low levels of 20E, the arbor has organized a robust multibranched growth cone. The growth normally commences spreading over the muscle template 1–2 days later, as circulating levels of 20E increase. (Bottom right) For pupae injected with a high dosage of 20E (20 μg/g) on day P+3, there is a precocious initiation of spreading of the growth cone that is evident by 3 days after injection. The arrowheads mark the limits of the axonal arbor in the various preparations. All images are at the same magnification.

The study by McGraw *et al.* (1998), however, examined the role of different concentrations of 20E on the pattern of neurite outgrowth from identified neurosecretory cells. Interestingly, 20E levels in the 100 ng/ml range caused the growth of primary branches, whereas the neuron elaborated higher-order branches when exposed to 20E in at 1 μg/ml. Therefore, individual neurons appear capable of discriminating between different steroid concentrations and evoking characteristic developmental programs in response to them. For the compound eye, the size of the adult eye depends on the length of time that the imaginal disc is exposed to moderate steroid concentrations prior to the shift to high 20E levels (Champlin and Truman, 1998b). In the context of the motoneurons, it will be interesting to determine if the final branching pattern and branch lengths of the adult neuron are also influenced by the duration of its prior exposure to moderate seroid levels early in adult development.

There has not been a comprehensive analysis of the early gene expression associated with the two patterns of steroid response in remodeling motoneurons in *Manduca*. However, we do know that the expression of the MHR3 transcription factor is associated with the appearance of high 20E titers on day P+8. Consequently, as in the developing eye, the response of motoneurons to high 20E levels is probably associated with the induction of the ecdysone cascade of transcription factors.

E. Steroids and Programmed Cell Death

Not all larval neurons survive metamorphosis. Some die after the formation of the pupal stage and others wait to die until after the emergence of the adult. The fate of a particular larval neuron may depend on numerous factors, such as the body segment in which the cell resides (Sandstrom and Weeks, 1998; Streichert et al., 1997), but a steroid cue is always needed to cause the cells to act out their fate.

The most extensive studies have been on the neurons that die after the emergence of the adult. In both *Manduca* (Truman and Schwartz, 1984) and *Drosophila* (Robinow et al., 1993), the decline in ecdysteroids at the end of metamorphosis is necessary for the death of these neurons, and injections of 20E late in the decline delays their death. These doomed cells also show a unique pattern of steroid receptor expression. Studies in *Manduca* using the binding of a radiolabeled ecdysone mimic showed that the doomed cells had a higher concentration of ecdysone binding than did the cells that continued to live after adult emergence (Fahrbach and Truman, 1989). Later studies using immunocytochemistry to analyze EcR isoforms in *Drosophila* showed that a set of larval neurons markedly elevated their levels of EcR-A soon after the start of the pupal stage and that these elevated levels persisted throughout metamorphosis (Fig. 8). All of these type II larval neurons then died within the first 4–8 hours after emergence of the adult fly (Robinow et al., 1993).

The onset of the death response in these neurons is associated with the induction of the apoptotic genes *reaper* and *grim* (Robinow et al., 1997). Their transcripts begin to appear in the doomed neurons approximately 4 hours after adult ecdysis, but their appearance can be prevented, as can the death of the neurons, if 20E is injected into the fly immediately after emergence (Robinow et al., 1997). Consequently, it appears that 20E, given late in adult development, may be able to directly suppress the transcription of *reaper* and *grim*. How the elevated levels of EcR-A relate to this suppression of transcription is not known.

VII. CONCLUSION AND SPECULATIONS

Our understanding of the molecular aspects of hormone action on the nervous system of insects comes from combined work on *Drosophila* and *Manduca*. The driving force for the metamorphic transition is the action of the ecdysones, with the importance of JH being primarily in its absence. Key molecules in the action of the ecdysones are the various isoforms of EcR—EcR-A and one or two of the EcR-Bs. We do not yet have a solid understanding of the specialized functions of these isoforms in the animal, but some insights can be gleaned from the studies on the nervous system.

From the work on both the mushroom body neurons (Lee et al., 2000) and the Tv neurosecretory neurons (Schubiger et al., 1998), it is clear that the EcR-B isoforms can mediate steroid-induced pruning, whereas EcR-A cannot. *In vitro* studies with recombinant proteins have shown that the two B isoforms have strong activational domains (AF1) in their N-terminal A/B region, but that the EcR-A isoform does not (Hu, 1998, as described in Riddiford et al., 2001). Considering the relative differences in the activational capacities of the B and A isoforms, it would seem that pruning back of neurites requires strong activation of target genes via EcR-B–USP. Work on the mushroom body neurons indicates that the pruning response appears not to involve some of the obvious targets of EcR—the transcription factors E75, E74A, E74B, or BRC (Lee et al., 2000). Whether it selectively involves untested members of the cascade, such as DHR3, or other direct-response genes that are not transcription factors is not yet known.

Although gene activation mediated through the EcR-Bs is probably needed for the pruning of larval neurons, it is not needed for the outgrowth of imaginal neurons. In EcR-B mutants, imaginal neurons in the optic lobe initiate the maturational changes associated with metamorphosis even though the same animal shows a complete blockade of pruning of its larval neurons (Schubiger *et al.*, 1998). These imaginal neurons also lack EcR-B1 expression at this time (the expression of EcR-B2 is unknown), but they do express EcR-A. This different profile of EcR isoform expression may reflect a dependence of these cells on the nonactivational function of the receptor such as ligand-dependant derepression. In the developing wing, the fact that the removal of USP renders the early birth and maturation of wing sensory neurons independent of ecdysone (Schubiger and Truman, 2000) supports the importance of ligand-dependent derepression for the early development of imaginal neurons. It is likely that derepression also plays a major role in mediating the early outgrowth phase of the pruned larval neurons as they are reorganizing their growth cones under tonic support by α-ecdysone or low levels of 20E. A shift from activation to depression control is probably responsible for the reduced levels of EcR-B1 that larval neurons possess at this time (Fig. 8; Truman *et al.*, 1994). The high levels of steroid that then evoke maturation may again be acting via ligand-dependent activation via EcR-USP that then serve to reinduce the ecdysone cascade. The combined approach in both *Manduca* and *Drosophila* will eventually allow us to resolve the complex interactions among steroid titers, various receptor isoforms, and the patterns of developmental response.

References

Agui, N., Granger, N. A., Bollenbacher, W. E., and Gilbert, L. I. (1979). Cellular localization of the insect prothoracicotropic hormone: *In vitro* assay of a single neurosecretory cell. *Proc. Natl. Acad. Sci. U.S.A.* **76**, 5694–5698.

Andres, A. J., and Cherbas, P. (1992). Tissue-specific ecdysone responses: Regulation of the Drosophila genes *Eip 28/29* and *Eip40* during larval development. *Development (Cambridge, UK)* **116**, 865–876.

Andres, A. J., and Thummel, C. S. (1995). The *Drosophila* 63F early puff contains *E63-1*, an ecdysone-inducible gene that encodes a novel Ca^{2+}-binding protein. *Development (Cambridge, UK)* **121**, 2667–2679.

Andres, A. J., Fletcher, J. C., Karim, F. D., and Thummel, C. S. (1993). Molecular analysis of the initiation of insect metamorphosis: A comparative study of *Drosophila* ecdysteroid-regulated transcription. *Dev. Biol.* **160**, 388–404.

Ashburner, M. (1973). Sequential gene activation by ecdysone in polytene chromosomes of *Drosophila melanogaster*. I. Dependence upon hormone concentration. *Dev. Biol.* **35**, 47–61.

Ashburner, M. (1974). Sequential gene activation by ecdysone in polytene chromosomes of *Drosophila melanogaster*. II. Effects of inhibitors of protein synthesis. *Dev. Biol.* **39**, 141–157.

Ashburner, M., Chihara, C., Meltzer, C. P., and Richards, G. (1974). On the temporal control of puffing activity in polytene chromosomes. *Cold Spring Harbor. Symp. Quant. Biol.* **38**, 655–662.

Ashok, M., Turner, C., and Wilson, T. G. (1998). Insect juvenile hormone resistance gene homology with the bHLH-PAS family of transcriptional regulators. *Proc. Natl. Acad. Sci. U.S.A.* **95**, 2761–2766.

Baehrecke, E. H., and Thummel, C. S. (1995). The *Drosophila* E93 gene from the 93E early puff displays stage- and tissue-specific regulation by 20-hydroxyecdysone. *Dev. Biol.* **171**, 85–97.

Baker, F. C., Tsai, L. W., Reuter, C. C., and Schooley, D. A. (1987). *In vivo* fluctuation of JH, JH acid, and ecdysteroid titer, and JH esterase activity during development of fifth stadium *Manduca sexta*. *Insect Biochem.* **17**, 989–996.

Bate, M. (1993). The mesoderm and its derivatives. *In* "The Development of *Drosophila melanogaster*" (M. Bate and A. Martinez-Arias, eds.), pp. 1013–1090. Cold Spring Harbor Lab. Press, Plainview, NY.

Bayer, C., von Kalm, L., and Fristrom, J. W. (1996). Gene regulation in imaginal disc and salivary gland development during *Drosophila* metamorphosis. *In* "Metamorphosis. Postembryonic Reprogramming of Gene Expression in Amphibian and Insect Cells" (L. I. Gilbert, J. P. Tata, and B. G. Atkinson, eds.), pp. 321–361. Academic Press, San Diego, CA.

Bender, M., Imam, F. B., Talbot, W. S., Ganetzky, B., and Hogness, D. S. (1997). *Drosophila* ecdysone receptor mutations reveal functional differences among receptor isoforms. *Cell (Cambridge, Mass.)* **91**, 777–788.

Berger, E. M., Goudie, K., Klieger, L., Berger, M., and DeCato, R. (1992). The juvenile hormone analogue, methoprene, inhibits ecdysterone induction of small heat shock protein gene expression. *Dev. Biol.* **151**, 410–418.

Bhaskaran, G., Sparagana, S. P., Barrera, P., and Dahm, K. H. (1986). Change in corpus allatum function during metamorphosis of the tobacco hornworm *Manduca sexta*. Regulation at the terminal step in juvenile hormone biosynthesis. *Arch. Insect Biochem. Physiol.* **3**, 321–338.

Bhaskaran, G., Sparagana, S. P., Dahm, K. H., Barrera, P., and Peck, K. (1988). Sexual dimorphism in juvenile hormone synthesis by corpora allata and in juvenile hormone methyltransferase activity in corpora allata and accessory sex gland of male lepidoptera. *Int. J. Invertebr. Reprod. Dev.* **13**, 87–100.

Billas, I. M. L., Moulinier, L., Rochel, N., and Moras, D. (2001). Crystal structure of the ligand binding domain of the Ultraspiracle protein USP, the ortholog of RXRs in insects. *J. Biol. Chem.* **276**, 7465–7474.

Blais, C., and Lafont, R. (1980). In vitro differentiation of *Pieris brassicae* imaginal wing discs: Effects and metabolism of ecdysone and ecdysterone. *Wilhelm Roux's Arch. Dev. Biol.* **188**, 27–36.

Booker, R., and Truman, J. W. (1987a). Postembryonic neurogenesis in the CNS of the tobacco hornworm, *Manduca sexta*. I. Neuroblast arrays and the fate of their progeny during metamorphosis. *J. Comp. Neurol.* **255**, 548–559.

Booker, R., and Truman, J. W. (1987b). Postembryonic neurogenesis in the CNS of the tobacco Hornworm, *Manduca sexta*. II. Hormonal control of imaginal nest cell degeneration and differentiation during metamorphosis. *J. Neurosci.* **7**, 4107–4114.

Booker, R., Babashak, J., and Kim, J. B. (1996). Postembryonic neurogenesis in the central nervous system of the tobacco hornworm, *Manduca sexta*. III. Spatial and temporal patterns of proliferation. *J. Neurobiol.* **29**, 233–248.

Bownes, M. (1994). The regulation of the yolk protein genes, a family of sex differentiation genes in *Drosophila melanogaster*. *BioEssays* **16**, 745–752.

Bownes, M., and Rembold, H. (1987). The titre of juvenile hormone during the pupal and adult stages of the life-cycle of *Drosophila melanogaster*. *Eur. J. Biochem.* **164**, 709–712.

Bownes, M., Shirras, A., Blair, M., Collins, J., and Coulson, A. (1988). Evidence that insect embryogenesis is regulated by ecdysteroids released from yolk proteins. *Proc. Natl. Acad. Sci. U.S.A.* **85**, 1554–1557.

Brennan, C. A., Ashburner, M., and Moses, K. (1998). Ecdysone pathway is required for furrow progression in the developing *Drosophila* eye. *Development (Cambridge, UK)* **125**, 2653–2664.

Brennan, C. A., Li, T.-R., Bender, M., Hsiung, F., and Moses, K. (2001). *Broad-complex*, but not *Ecdysone receptor*, is required for progression of the morphogenetic furrow in the *Drosophila* eye. *Development (Cambridge, UK)* **128**, 1–11.

Britton, J. S., and Edgar, B. A. (1998). Environmental control of the cell cycle in *Drosophila*: Nutrition activates mitotic and endoreplicative cells by distinct mechanisms. *Development (Cambridge, UK)* **125**, 2149–2158.

Broadus, J., McCabe, J. R., Endrizzi, B., Thummel, C. S., and Woodard, C. T. (1999). The *Drosophila* βFTZ-F1 orphan nuclear receptor provides competence for stage-specific responses to the steroid hormone ecdysone. *Mol. Cell* **3**, 143–149.

Burtis, K. C., Thummel, C. S., Jones, C. W., Karim, F. D., and Hogness, D. S. (1990). The Drosophila 74EF early puff contains E74, a complex ecdysone-inducible gene that encodes two ets-related proteins. *Cell (Cambridge, Mass.)* **61**, 85–99.

Buszczak, M., Freeman, M. R., Carlson, J. R., Bender, M., Cooley, L., and Segraves, W. A. (1999). Ecdysone response genes govern egg chamber development during mid-oogenesis in Drosophila. *Development (Cambridge, UK)* **126**, 4581–4589.

Butenandt, A., and Karlson, P. (1954). Uber der Isolierung eines Metamorphosehormons der Insekten in kristallisierter Form. *Z. Naturforsch.* **9B**, 389–391.

Campbell, P. M., Healy, M. J., and Oakeshott, J. T. (1992). Chacterisation of juvenile hormone esterase in Drosophila. *Insect Biochem. Mol. Biol.* **22**, 665–677.

Campbell, P. M., Oakeshott, J. T., and Healy, M. J. (1998). Purification and kinetic chacterisation of juvenile hormone esterase from Drosophila melanogaster. *Insect Biochem. Mol. Biol.* **28**, 501–515.

Champlin, D. T., and Truman, J. W. (1998a). Ecdysteroid control of cell proliferation during optic lobe neurogenesis in the moth *Manduca sexta*. *Development (Cambridge, UK)* **125**, 269–277.

Champlin, D. T., and Truman, J. W. (1998b). Ecdysteroids govern two phases of eye development during metamorphosis of the moth, *Manduca sexta*. *Development (Cambridge, UK)* **125**, 2009–2018.

Chao, A., and Guild, G. M. (1986). Molecular analysis of the ecdysterone-inducible 2B5 "early" puff in *Drosophila melanogaster*. *EMBO J.* **5**, 143–150.

Charles, J.-P., Wojtasek, H., Lentz, A. J., Thomas, B. A., Bonning, B. C., Palli, S. R., Parker, A. G., Dorman, G., Hammock, B. D., Prestwich, G. D., and Riddiford, L. M. (1996). Purification and reassessment of ligand binding by the recombinant, putative juvenile hormone receptor of the tobacco hornworm, *Manduca sexta*. *Arch. Insect Biochem. Physiol.* **31**, 371–393.

Charles, J.-P., Shinoda, T., and Chinzei, Y. (1999). Characterization and DNA-binding properties of GRF, a novel monomeric binding orphan receptor related to GCNF and βFTZ-F1. *Eur. J. Biochem.* **266**, 181–190.

Chavez, V. M., Marques, G., Delbecque, J. P., Kobayashi, K., Hollingsworth, M., Burr, J., Natzle, J. E., and O'Connor, M. B. (2000). The *Drosophila disembodied* gene controls late embryonic morphogenesis and codes for a cytochrome P450 enzyme that regulates embryonic ecdysone levels. *Development (Cambridge, UK)* **127**, 4115–4126.

Cherbas, L., Schulz, R. A., Koehler, M. M. D., Savakis, C., and Cherbas, P. (1986). Structure of the *Eip28/29* gene, an ecdysone-inducible gene from *Drosophila. J. Mol. Biol.* **189**, 617–631.

Cherbas, L., Lee, K., and Cherbas, P. (1991). Identification of ecdysone response elements by analysis of the *Drosophila Eip28/29* gene. *Genes Dev.* **5**, 120–131.

Cherbas, P., and Cherbas, L. (1996). Molecular aspects of ecdysteroid hormone action. In "Metamorphosis: Postembryonic Programming of Gene Expression in Amphibian and Insect Cells" (L. I. Gilbert, J. R. Tata, and B. G. Atkinson, eds.), pp. 175–221. Academic Press, San Diego, CA.

Chiang, J. Y., Kimmel, R., Weinberger, C., and Stroup, D. (2000). Farnesoid X receptor responds to bile acids and represses cholesterol 7α-hydroxylase gene *(CYP7A1)* transcription. *J. Biol. Chem.* **275**, 10918–10924.

Chung, A. C.-K., Durica, D. S., Clifton, S. W., Roe, B. A., and Hopkins, P. M. (1998). Cloning of crustacean ecdysteroid receptor and retinoid-X receptor gene homologs and elevation of retinoid-X receptor mRNA by retinoic acid. *Mol. Cell. Endocrinol.* **139**, 209–227.

Clever, U. (1964). Actinomycin and puromycin: Effects on sequential gene activation by ecdysone. *Science* **146**, 794–795.

Clever, U., and Karlson, P. (1960). Induktion von Puff-Veranderungen in den Speicheldrusen-chromosomen von *Chironomus tentans* durch Ecdyson. *Exp. Cell Res.* **20**, 623–626.

Consoulas, C., Kent, K. S., and Levine, R. B. (1996). Remodeling of the peripheral processes and presynaptic terminals of leg motoneurons during metamorphosis of the hawkmoth, *Manduca sexta. J. Comp. Neurol.* **372**, 415–434.

Consoulas, C., Anezaki, M., and Levine, R. B. (1997). Development of adult thoracic leg muscles during metamorphosis of the hawk moth *Manduca sexta. Cell Tissue Res.* **287**, 393–412.

Crossgrove, K., Bayer, C. A., Fristrom, J. W., and Guild, G. M. (1996). The Drosophila Broad-Complex early gene directly regulates late gene transcription during the ecdysone-induced puffing cascade. *Dev. Biol.* **180**, 745–758.

Cusson, M., Le Page, A., McNeil, J. N., and Tobe, S. S. (1996). Rate of isoleucine metabolism in lepidopteran corpora allata: Regulation of the proportion of juvenile hormone homologues released. *Insect Biochem. Mol. Biol.* **26**, 195–201.

Dai, J.-D., and Gilbert, L. I. (1991). Metamorphosis of the corpus allatum and degeneration of the prothoracic glands during the larval-pupal-adult transformation of *Drosophila melanogaster*: A cytophysiological analysis of the ring gland. *Dev. Biol.* **144**, 309–326.

Dai, J.-D., and Gilbert, L. I. (1997). Programmed cell death of the prothoracic glands of *Manduca sexta* during pupal-adult metamorphosis. *Insect Biochem. Mol. Biol.* **27**, 69–78.

Dai, J.-D., and Gilbert, L. I. (1999). An *in vitro* analysis of ecdysteroid-elicited cell death in the prothoracic gland of *Manduca sexta. Cell Tissue Res.* **297**, 319–327.

Davis, N. T., Homberg, U., Dircksen, H., Levine, R. B., and Hildebrand, J. G. (1993). Crustacean cardioactive peptide-immunoreactive neurons in the hawkmoth *Manduca sexta* and changes in their immunoreactivity during postembryonic development. *J. Comp. Neurol.* **338**, 612–627.

deKort, C. A. D., and Koopmanschap, A. B. (1987). Specificity of binding of juvenile hormone III to hemolymph proteins of *Leptinotarsa decemlineata* and *Locusta migratoria. Experientia* **43**, 904–905.

DiBello, P. R., Withers, D. A., Bayer, C. A., Fristrom, J. W., and Guild, G. M. (1991). The Drosophila Broad-Complex encodes a family of related proteins containing zinc fingers. *Genetics* **129**, 385–397.

Dominick, O. S., and Truman, J. W. (1985). The physiology of wandering behavior in *Manduca sexta*. II. The endocrine control of wandering behavior. *J. Exp. Biol.* **117**, 45–68.

Dubrovsky, E. B., Dubrovskaya, V. A., Bilderback, A. L., and Berger, E. M. (2000). The isolation of two juvenile hormone-inducible genes in *Drosophila melanogaster. Dev. Biol.* **224**, 486–495.

Duch, C., and Levine, R. B. (2000). Remodeling of membrane properties and dendritic architecture accompanies the postembryonic conversion of a slow into a fast motoneuron. *J. Neurosci.* **20**, 6950–6961.

Edgar, B. A., and O'Farrell, P. H. (1990). The three postblastoderm cell cycles in *Drosophila* embryogenesis are regulated in G2 by *string. Cell (Cambridge, Mass.)* **62**, 469–480.

Fahrbach, S. E., and Truman, J. W. (1989). Autoradiographic identification of ecdysteroid-binding cells in the nervous system of the moth *Manduca sexta. J. Neurobiol.* **20**, 681–702.

Fallon, A. M., Hagedorn, H. H., Wyatt, G. R., and Laufer, H. (1975). Activation of vitellogenin synthesis in the mosquito *Aedes aegypti* by ecdysone. *J. Insect Physiol.* **20**, 1815–1823.

Fernandes, J. J., and Keshishian, H. (1998). Nerve-muscle interactions during flight muscle development in *Drosophila. Development (Cambridge, UK)* **125**, 1769–1779.

Fernandes, J. J., and VijayRaghavan, K. (1993). The development of indirect flight muscle innervation in *Drosophila melanogaster. Development (Cambridge, UK)* **118**, 215–227.

Feyereisen, R. (1999). Insect P450 enzymes. *Annu. Rev. Entomol.* **44**, 507–533.

Feyereisen, R., Pratt, G. E., and Hamnett, A. F. (1981). Enzymic synthesis of juvenile homone in locust corpora allata: Evidence for a microsomal cytochrome P-450 linked methyl farnesoate epoxidase. *Eur. J. Biochem.* **118**, 231–238.

Freeman, M., Dobritsa, A., Gaines, P., Segraves, W. A., and Carlson, J. R. (1999). The *dare* gene: Steroid hormone production, olfactory behavior, and neural degeneration in *Drosophila*. *Development (Cambridge, UK)* **126**, 4591–4602.

Fujiwara, H., Jindra, M., Newitt, R., Palli, S. R., Hiruma, K., and Riddiford, L. M. (1995). Cloning of an ecdysone receptor homolog from *Manduca sexta* and the developmental profile of its mRNA in wings. *Insect Biochem. Mol. Biol.* **25**, 845–856.

Giguère, V., Tini, M., Flock, G., Ong, E., Evans, R. M., and Otulakowski, G. (1994). Isoform-specific amino-terminal domains dictate DNA-binding properties of RORα, a novel member of orphan nuclear hormone receptors. *Genes Dev.* **8**, 538–553.

Gilbert, L. I., Rybczynski, R., and Tobe, S. S. (1996). Endocrine cascade in insect metamorphosis. In "Metamorphosis: Postembryonic Reprogramming of Gene Expression in Amphibian and Insect Cells" (L. I. Gilbert, J. R. Tata, and B. G. Atkinson, eds.), pp. 59–107. Academic Press, San Diego, CA.

Goodman, W. G. (1990). Biosynthesis, titer, regulation and transport of juvenile hormones. In "Morphogenetic Hormones of Arthropods" (A. P. Gupta, ed.), Vol. 1, pp. 83–124. Rutgers University Press, New Brunswick, NJ.

Grieneisen, M. L. (1994). Recent advances in our knowledge of ecdysteroid biosynthesis in insects and crustaceans. *Insect Biochem. Mol. Biol.* **24**, 115–132.

Grunewald, B., and Levine, R. B. (1998). Ecdysteroid control of ionic current development in *Manduca sexta* motoneurons. *J. Neurobiol.* **37**, 211–223.

Guo, X., Harmon, M. A., Jin, X., Laudet, V., Mangelsdorf, D. J., and Palmer, M. J. (1998). Isolation of two retinoid X receptor homologues from the ixodid tick, *Amblyoma americanum* (L.). *Mol. Cell. Endocrinol.* **139**, 45–60.

Hagedorn, H. H., and Fallon, A. M. (1973). Ovarian control of vitellogenin synthesis by the fat body in *Aedes aegypti*. *Nature (London)* **244**, 103–105.

Hammock, B. D. (1975). NADPH-dependent epoxidation of methyl farnesoate to juvenile hormone in the cockroach *Blaberus giganteus*. *Life Sci.* **17**, 323–328.

Hampshire, F., and Horn, D. H. S. (1966). Structure of crustecdysone, a crustacean moulting hormone. *J. Chem. Soc., Chem. Commun.* 37–38.

Hansson, L., and Lambertsson, A. (1989). Steroid regulation of glue protein genes in *Drosophila melanogaster*. *Hereditas* **110**, 61–67.

Harmon, M. A., Boehm, M. F., Heyman, R. A., and Mangelsdorf, D. J. (1995). Activation of mammalian retinoid X receptors by the insect growth regulator methoprene. *Proc. Natl. Acad. Sci. U.S.A.* **92**, 6157–6160.

Hayward, D. C., Bastiani, M. J., Trueman, J. W. H., Truman, J. W., Riddiford, L. M., and Ball, E. E. (1999). The sequence of *Locusta* RXR, homologous to *Drosophila* Ultraspiracle, and its evolutionary implications. *Dev., Genes, Evol.* **209**, 564–571.

Henrich, V. C., Sliter, T. J., Lubahn, D. B., MacIntyre, A., and Gilbert, L. I. (1990). A steroid/thyroid hormone receptor superfamily member in *Drosophila melanogaster* that shares extensive sequence similarity with a mammalian homologue. *Nucleic Acids Res.* **18**, 4143–4148.

Henrich, V. C., Szekely, A. A., Kim, S. J., Brown, N. E., Antoniewski, C., Hayden, M. A., Lepesant, J.-A., and Gilbert, L. I. (1994). Expression and function of the *ultraspiracle* (*usp*) gene during development of *Drosophila melanogaster*. *Dev. Biol.* **165**, 38–52.

Henrich, V. C., Rybczynski, R., and Gilbert, L. I. (1999). Peptide hormones, steroid hormones, and puffs: Mechanisms and models in insect development. *Vitam. Horm. (N.Y.)* **55**, 73–125.

Hiruma, K., and Riddiford, L. M. (2001). Regulation of the transcription factors, MHR4 and β FTZ-F1, by 20-hydroxyecdysone during a larval molt in the tobacco hornworm, *Manduca sexta*. *Dev. Biol.* **232**, 265–274.

Hiruma, K., Böcking, D., Lafont, R., and Riddiford, L. M. (1997). Action of different ecdysteroids on the regulation of mRNAs for the ecdysone receptor, MHR3, dopa decarboxylase, and a larval cuticle protein in the larval epidermis of the tobacco hornworm, *Manduca sexta*. *Gen. Comp. Endocrinol.* **107**, 84–97.

Hiruma, K., Shinoda, T., Malone, F., and Riddiford, L. M. (1999). Juvenile hormone modulates 20-hydroxyecdysone-inducible ecdysone receptor and Ultraspiracle gene expression in the tobacco hornworm, *Manduca sexta*. *Dev., Genes, Evol.* **209**, 18–30.

Hock, T., Cottrill, T., Keegan, J., and Garza, D. (2000). The *E23* early gene of *Drosophila* encodes an ecdysone- inducible ATP-binding cassette transporter capable of repressing ecdysone-mediated gene activation. *Proc. Natl. Acad. Sci. U.S.A.* **97**, 9519–9524.

Hoffmeister, H., and Grützmacher, H. F. (1966). Zur Chemie des Ecdysterons. *Tetrahedron Lett.* **33**, 4017–4023.

Horn, D. H. S., and Bergamasco, R. (1985). Chemistry of ecdysteroids. In "Comprehensive Insect Physiology, Biochemistry, and Pharmacology" (G. A. Kerkut, and L. I. Gilbert, eds.), Vol. 7, pp. 185–247. Pergamon Press, Oxford.

Horner, M. A., Chen, T., and Thummel, C. S. (1995). Ecdysteroid regulation and DNA binding properties of *Drosophila* nuclear hormone receptor superfamily members. *Dev. Biol.* **168**, 490–502.

Hu, X. (1998). The mechanisms of activating the functional ecdysone receptor complex. Ph.D. Thesis, Indiana University, Bloomington.

Huet, F., Ruiz, C., and Richards, G. (1993). Puffs and PCR: The in vivo dynamics of early gene expression during ecdysone response in *Drosophila*. *Development (Cambridge, UK)* **118**, 613–627.

Huet, F., Ruiz, C., and Richards, G. (1995). Sequential gene activation by ecdysone in *Drosophila melanogaster*: The hierarchical equivalence of early and early late genes. *Development (Cambridge, UK)* **121**, 1195–1204.

Ismail, S. M., Satyanarayana, K., Bradfield, J. Y., Dahm, K. H., and Bhaskaran, G. (1998). Juvenile hormone acid: Evidence for a hormonal function in induction of vitellogenin in larvae of *Manduca sexta*. *Arch. Insect Biochem. Physiol.* **37**, 305–314.

Ismail, S. M., Goin, C., Muthmani, K., Kim, M., Dahm, K. H., and Bhaskaran, G. (2000). Juvenile hormone acid and ecdysteroid together induce competence for metamorphosis of the Verson's gland in *Manduca sexta*. *J. Insect Physiol.* **46**, 59–68.

Jindra, M., Malone, F., Hiruma, K., and Riddiford, L. M. (1996). Developmental profiles and ecdysteroid regulation of the mRNAs for two ecdysone receptor isoforms in the epidermis and wings of the tobacco hornworm, *Manduca sexta*. *Dev. Biol.* **180**, 258–272.

Jindra, M., Huang, J.-Y., Malone, F., Asahina, M., and Riddiford, L. M. (1997). Identification and mRNA developmental profiles of two Ultraspiracle isoforms in the epidermis and wings of *Manduca sexta*. *Insect Mol. Biol.* **6**, 41–53.

Jones, G., and Click, A. (1987). Developmental regulation of juvenile hormone esterase in *Trichoplusia ni*: Its multiple electrophoretic forms occur during each larval ecdysis. *J. Insect Physiol.* **33**, 207–213.

Jones, G., and Jones, D. (2000). Considerations on the structural evidence of a ligand-binding function of ultraspiracle, an insect homolog of vertebrate RXR. *Insect Biochem. Mol. Biol.* **30**, 671–679.

Jones, G., and Sharp, P. A. (1997). Ultraspiracle: An invertebrate receptor for juvenile hormones. *Proc. Natl. Acad. Sci. U.S.A.* **94**, 13499–13503.

Kageyama, Y., Masuda, S., Hirose, S., and Ueda, H. (1997). Temporal regulation of the mid-prepupal gene FTZ-F1: DHR3 early late gene product is one of the plural positive regulators. *Genes Cells* **2**, 559–569.

Kamimura, M., Tomita, S., and Fujiwara, H. (1996). Molecular cloning of an ecdysone receptor (B1 isoform) homologue from the silkworm, *Bombyx mori*, and its mRNA expression during wing disc development. *Comp. Biochem. Physiol.* **113B**, 341–347.

Kamimura, M., Tomita, S., Kiuchi, M., and Fujiwara, H. (1997). Tissue-specific and stage-specific expression of two silkworm ecdysone receptor isoforms. Ecdysteroid-dependent transcription in cultured anterior silk glands. *Eur. J. Biochem.* **248**, 786–793.

Kapitskaya, M., Wang, S., Cress, D. E., Dhadialla, T. S., and Raikhel, A. S. (1996). The mosquito *ultraspiracle* homologue, a partner of ecdysteroid receptor heterodimer: Cloning and characterization of isoforms expressed during vitellogenesis. *Mol. Cell. Endocrinol.* **121**, 119–132.

Karim, F. D., and Thummel, C. S. (1991). Ecdysone coordinates the timing and amounts of E74A and E74B transcription in *Drosophila*. *Genes Dev.* **5**, 1067–1079.

Karim, F. D., and Thummel, C. S. (1992). Temporal coordination of regulatory gene expression by the steroid hormone ecdysone. *EMBO J.* **11**, 4083–4093.

Karim, F. D., Guild, G. M., and Thummel, C. S. (1993). The *Drosophila* Broad-Complex plays a key role in controlling ecdysteroid-regulated gene expression at the onset of metamorphosis. *Development (Cambridge, UK)* **118**, 977–988.

Khlebodarova, T. M., Gruntenko, N. E., Grenback, L. G., Sukhanova, M. Z., Mazurov, M. M., Rauschenbach, I. Y., Tomas, B. A., and Hammock, B. D. (1996). A comparative analysis of juvenile hormone metabolyzing enzymes in two species of *Drosophila* during development. *Insect Biochem. Mol. Biol.* **26**, 829–835.

Kiguchi, K., and Riddiford, L. M. (1978). The role of juvenile hormone in pupal development of the tobacco hornworm, *Manduca sexta*. *J. Insect Physiol.* **24**, 673–680.

King-Jones, K., Korge, G., and Lehmann, M. (1999). The helix-loop-helix proteins dAP-4 and Daughterless bind both *in vitro* and *in vivo* to SEBP3 sites required for transcriptional activation of the *Drosophila* gene Sgs-4. *J. Mol. Biol.* **291**, 71–82.

Koelle, M. R., Talbot, W. S., Segraves, W. A., Bender, M. T., Cherbas, P., and Hogness, D. S. (1991). The Drosophila *EcR* gene encodes an ecdysone receptor, a new member of the steroid receptor superfamily. *Cell (Cambridge, Mass.)* **67**, 59–77.

Koelle, M. R., Segraves, W. A., and Hogness, D. S. (1992). DHR3: A *Drosophila* steroid receptor homolog. *Proc. Natl. Acad. Sci. U.S.A.* **89**, 6167–6171.

Kraft, R., Levine, R. B., and Restifo, L. L. (1998). The steroid hormone 20-hydroxyecdysone enhances neurite growth of *Drosophila* mushroom body neurons isolated during metamorphosis. *J. Neurosci.* **18**, 8886–8899.

Kramer, K. J., Sanburg, L. L., Kezdy, F., and Law, J. H. (1974). The juvenile hormone binding protein in the hemolymph of *Manduca sexta* Johannson (Lepidoptera, Sphingidae). *Proc. Natl. Acad. Sci. U.S.A.* **71**, 493–497.

Lagueux, M. C., Hetru, F., Goltzene, F., Kappler, C., and Hoffmann, J. A. (1979). Ecdysone titre and metabolism in relation to cuticulogenesis in embryos of *Locusta migratoria*. *J. Insect Physiol.* **25**, 709–723.

Lam, G. T., Jiang, C., and Thummel, C. S. (1997). Coordination of larval and prepupal gene expression by the DHR3 orphan receptor during *Drosophila* metamorphosis. *Development (Cambridge, UK)* **124**, 1757–1769.

Lan, Q., Hiruma, K., Hu, X. A., Jindra, M., and Riddiford, L. M. (1999). Activation of a delayed-early gene encoding MHR3 by the ecdysone receptor heterodimer EcR-B1-USP-1 but not by EcR-B1-USP-2. *Mol. Cell. Biol.* **19**, 4897–4906.

Langelan, R. E., Fisher, J. E., Hiruma, K., Palli, S. R., and Riddiford, L. M. (2000). Patterns of MHR3 expression in the epidermis during a larval molt of the tobacco hornworm, *Manduca sexta*. *Dev. Biol.* **227**, 481–494.

Lavorgna, G., Ueda, H., Clos, J., and Wu, C. (1991). FTZ-F1, a steroid hormone receptor-like protein implicated in the activation of *fushi tarazu*. *Science* **252**, 848–851.

Lee, T., Lee, A., and Luo, L. (1999). Development of the *Drosophila* mushroom bodies: Sequential generation of three distinct types of neurons from a neuroblast. *Development (Cambridge, UK)* **126**, 4065–4076.

Lee, T., Marticke, S., Sung, C., Robinow, S., and Luo, L. (2000). Cell autonomous requirement of the USP/EcR-B ecdysone receptor for mushroom body neuronal remodeling in *Drosophila*. *Neuron* **28**, 807–818.

Lehmann, M., and Korge, G. (1996). The *fork head* product directly specifies the tissue-specific hormone responsiveness of the *Drosophila Sgs-4* gene. *EMBO J.* **15**, 4825–4834.

Lehmann, M., Wattler, F., and Korge, G. (1997). Two new regulatory elements controlling the *Drosophila Sgs-3* gene are potential ecdysone receptor and fork head binding sites. *Mech. Dev.* **62**, 15–27.

Lerro, K. A., and Prestwich, G. D. (1990). Cloning and sequencing of a cDNA for the hemolymph juvenile hormone binding protein of larval *Manduca sexta*. *J. Biol. Chem.* **265**, 19800–19806.

Levine, R. B., and Weeks, J. C. (1990). Hormonally mediated changes in simple reflex circuits during metamorphosis in *Manduca*. *J. Neurobiol.* **21**, 1022–1036.

Levine, R. B., and Weeks, J. C. (1996). Cell culture approaches to understanding the actions of steroid hormones on the insect nervous system. *Dev. Neurosci.* **18**, 73–86.

Levine, R. B., Morton, D. B., and Restifo, L. L. (1995). Remodeling of the insect nervous system. *Curr. Opin. Neurobiol.* **5**, 28–35.

Li, T.-R., and Bender, M. (2000). A conditional rescue system reveals essential functions for the *ecdysone receptor (EcR)* gene during molting and metamorphosis in *Drosophila*. *Development (Cambridge, UK)* **127**, 2897–2905.

Loi, P. K., and Tublitz, N. J. (1993). Hormonal control of transmitter plasticity in insect peptidergic neurons. I. Steroid regulation of the decline in cardioacceleratory peptide 2 (CAP2) expression. *J. Exp. Biol.* **181**, 175–194.

Makashima, M., Okamoto, A. Y., Repa, J. J., Tu, H., Learned, R. M., Luk, A., Hull, M. V., Lustig, K. D., Mangelsdorf, D. J., and Shan, B. (1999). Identification of a nuclear receptor for bile acids. *Science* **284**, 1362–1365.

Mangelsdorf, D. J., and Evans, R. M. (1995). The RXR heterodimers and orphan receptors. *Cell (Cambridge, Mass.)* **83**, 841–850.

Matheson, S. F., and Levine, R. B. (1999). Steroid hormone enhancement of neurite outgrowth in identified insect motor neurons involves specific effects on growth cone form and function. *J. Neurobiol.* **38**, 27–45.

McGraw, H. F., Prier, K. R. S., Wiley, J. C., and Tublitz, N. J. (1998). Steroid-regulated morphological plasticity in a set of identified peptidergic neurons in the moth *Manduca sexta*. *J. Exp. Biol.* **201**, 2981–2992.

Meinertzhagen, I. A., and Hanson, T. E. (1993). The development of the optic lobe. *In* "The Development of *Drosophila melanogaster*" (M. Bate and A. Martinez Arias, eds.), pp. 1363–1491. Cold Spring Harbor Lab. Press, Plainview, NY.

Mitsui, T., Riddiford, L. M., and Bellamy, G. (1979). Metabolism of juvenile hormone by the epidermis of the tobacco hornworm, *Manduca sexta*. *Insect Biochem.* **9**, 637–664.

Mizoguchi, A. (1990). Immunological approach to synthesis, release, and titre fluctuation of Bombyxin and Prathoraciotropic Hormone of *Bombyx mori*. *In* "Molting and Metamorphosis" (E. Ohnishi and H. Ishizaki, eds.), pp. 17–48. Japan Scientific Societies Press, Tokyo.

Monsma, S. A., and Booker, R. (1996a). Genesis of the adult retina and outer optic lobes of the moth, *Manduca sexta*. I. Patterns of proliferation and cell death. *J. Comp. Neurol.* **367**, 10–20.

Monsma, S. A., and Booker, R. (1996b). Genesis of the adult retina and outer optic lobes of the moth, *Manduca sexta*. II. Effects of deafferentation and developmental hormone manipulation. *J. Comp. Neurol.* **367**, 21–35.

Mouillet, J.-F., Delbecque, J. P., Quennedey, B., and Delachambre, J. (1997). Cloning of two putative ecdysteroid receptor isoforms from *Tenebrio molitor* and their developmental expression in the epidermis during metamorphosis. *Eur. J. Biochem.* **248**, 856–863.

Mouillet, J.-F., Bousquet, F., Sedano, N., Alabouvette, J., Nicolaï, M., Zelus, D., Laudet, V., and Delachambre, J. (1999). Cloning and characterization of new orphan nuclear receptors and their developmental profiles during *Tenebrio* metamorphosis. *Eur. J. Biochem.* **265**, 1–11.

Muehleisen, D. P., Plapp, F. W. Jr., Benedict, J. H., and Carino, F. A. (1989). High affinity TCDD binding of fat body cytosolic protein of the bollworm, *Heliothis zea*. *Pestic., Biochem. Physiol.* **35**, 50–57.

Murata, T., Kageyama, Y., Hirose, S., and Ueda, H. (1996). Regulation of the *EDG84A* gene by FTZ-F1 during metamorphosis in *Drosophila melanogaster*. *Mol. Cell. Biol.* **16**, 6509–6515.

Nardi, J. B., and Magee-Adams, S. M. (1986). Formation of scale spacing patterns in a moth wing. I. Epithelial feet may mediate cell rearrangement. *Dev. Biol.* **116**, 278–290.

Nijhout, H. F. (1981). Physiological control of molting in insects. *Am. Zool.* **21**, 631–640.

Nijhout, H. F. (1994). "Insect Hormones." Princeton University Press, Princeton, NJ.

Nuesch, H. (1985). Control of muscle development. *In* "Comprehensive Insect Physiology, Biochemistry, and Pharmacology" (G. A. Kerkut and L. I. Gilbert, eds.), Vol. 2, pp. 425–452. Pergamon Press, Oxford.

Oberlander, H. (1985). The imaginal discs. *In* "Comprehensive Insect Physiology, Biochemistry, and Pharmacology" (G. A. Kerkut and L. I. Gilbert, eds.), Vol. 2, pp. 151–182. Pergamon Press, Oxford.

Ohtaki, T., Yamanaka, F., and Sakurai, S. (1986). Differential timing of pupal commitment in various tissues of the silkworm, *Bombyx mori*. *J. Insect Physiol.* **32**, 635–642.

Oro, A. E., McKeown, M., and Evans, R. M. (1990). Relationship between the product of *Drosophila ultraspiracle* locus and the vertebrate retinoid X receptor. *Nature (London)* **347**, 296–301.

Oro, A. E., McKeown, M., and Evans, R. M. (1992). The *Drosophila* retinoid X receptor homolog *ultraspiracle* functions in both female reproduction and eye morphogenesis. *Development (Cambridge, UK)* **115**, 449–462.

Osir, E. O., and Riddiford, L. M. (1988). Nuclear binding of juvenile hormone and its analogs in the epidermis of the tobacco hornworm. *J. Biol. Chem.* **263**, 13812–13818.

Palli, S. R., Osir, E. O., Eng, W.-S., Boehm, M. F., Edwards, M., Kulcsar, P., Ujvary, I., Hiruma, K., Prestwich, G. D., and Riddiford, L. M. (1990). Juvenile hormone receptors in larval insect epidermis: Identification by photoaffinity labeling. *Proc. Natl. Acad. Sci. U.S.A.* **87**, 796–800.

Palli, S. R., Riddiford, L. M., and Hiruma, K. (1991). Juvenile hormone and "retinoic acid" receptors in *Manduca* epidermis. *Insect Biochem.* **21**, 7–15.

Palli, S. R., Hiruma, K., and Riddiford, L. M. (1992). An ecdysteroid-inducible *Manduca* gene similar to the *Drosophila* DHR3 gene, a member of the steroid hormone receptor superfamily. *Dev. Biol.* **150**, 306–318.

Palli, S. R., Touhara, K., Charles, J.-P., Bonning, B. C., Atkinson, J. K., Trowell, S. C., Hiruma, K., Goodman, W. G., Kyriakides, T., Prestwich, G. D., Hammock, B. D., and Riddiford, L. M. (1994). A nuclear juvenile hormone binding protein from larvae of *Manduca sexta*: A putative receptor for the metamorphic action of juvenile hormone. *Proc. Natl. Acad. Sci. U.S.A.* **91**, 6191–6195.

Perera, S. C., Ladd, T. R., Dhadialla, T. S., Krell, P. J., Sohi, S. S., Retnakaran, A., and Palli, S. R. (1999). Studies on two ecdysone receptor isoforms of the spruce budworm, *Choristoneura fumiferana*. *Mol. Cell. Endocrinol.* **152**, 73–84.

Prugh, J., Della Croce, K., and Levine, R. B. (1992). Effects of the steroid hormone, 20-hydroxyecdysone, on the growth of neurites by identified insect motoneurons *in vitro*. *Dev. Biol.* **154**, 331–347.

Pursley, S., Ashok, M., and Wilson, T. G. (2000). Intracellular localization and tissue specificity of the *Methoprene-tolerant* (*Met*) gene product in *Drosophila melanogaster*. *Insect Biochem. Mol. Biol.* **30**, 839–845.

Raikhel, A. S., and Snigirevskaya, E. S. (1998). Vitellogenesis. *In* "Microscopic Anatomy of Invertebrates," (F. W. Harrison *et al.*, eds.), Vol. 11C, pp. 933–955. Wiley-Liss, New York.

Raikhel, A. S., Miura, K., and Segraves, W. A. (1999). Nuclear receptors in mosquito vitellogenesis. *Am. Zool.* **39**, 722–735.

Rees, H. H. (1995). Ecdysteroid biosynthesis and inactivation in relation to function. *Eur. J. Entomol.* **92**, 9–39.

Restifo, L. L., and Guild, G. M. (1986). An ecdysterone-reponsive puff site in *Drosophila* contains a cluster of seven differentially regulated genes. *J. Mol. Biol.* **188**, 517–528.

Restifo, L. L., and Wilson, T. G. (1998). A juvenile hormone agonist reveals distinct developmental pathways mediated by ecdysone-inducible Broad Complex transcription factors. *Dev. Genet.* **22**, 141–159.

Richard, D. S., Applebaum, S. W., Sliter, T. J., Baker, F. C., Schooley, D. A., Reuter, C. C., Henrich, V. C., and Gilbert, L. I. (1989). Juvenile hormone bisepoxide biosynthesis in vitro by the ring gland of *Drosophila melanogaster*: A putative juvenile hormone in the higher Diptera. *Proc. Natl. Acad. Sci. U.S.A.* **86**, 1421–1425.

Richards, G. (1976). Sequential gene activation by ecdysone in polytene chromosomes of *Drosophila melanogaster*. IV. The mid prepupal period. *Dev. Biol.* **54**, 256–263.

Richards, G. (1978). Sequential gene activation by ecdysone in polytene chromosomes of *Drosophila melanogaster*. VI. Inhibition by juvenile hormones. *Dev. Biol.* **66**, 32–42.

Richards, G. (1997). The ecdysone regulatory cascade in *Drosophila*. *Adv. Dev. Biol.* **5**, 81–135.

Riddiford, L. M. (1976). Hormonal control of insect epidermal cell commitment *in vitro*. *Nature (London)* **259**, 115–117.

Riddiford, L. M. (1978). Ecdysone-induced change in cellular commitment of the epidermis of the tobacco hornworm, *Manduca sexta*, at the initiation of metamorphosis. *Gen. Comp. Endocrinol.* **34**, 438–446.

Riddiford, L. M. (1993). Hormones and *Drosophila* development. *In* "The Development of *Drosophila melanogaster*" (M. Bate and A. Martinez-Arias, eds.), pp. 899–939. Cold Spring Harbor Lab. Press, Plainview, NY.

Riddiford, L. M. (1994). Cellular and molecular actions of juvenile hormone. I. General considerations and premetamorphic actions. *Adv. Insect Physiol.* **24**, 213–274.

Riddiford, L. M. (1996). Molecular aspects of juvenile hormone action in insect metamorphosis. In "Metamorphosis: Postembryonic Reprogramming of Gene Expression in Amphibian and Insect Cells" (L. I. Gilbert, J. R. Tata, and B. G. Atkinson, eds.), pp. 223–251. Academic Press, San Diego, CA.

Riddiford, L. M., Hiruma, K., Lan, Q., and Zhou, B. (1999). Regulation and role of nuclear hormone receptors during larval molting and metamorphosis of Lepidoptera. *Am. Zool.* **39**, 736–746.

Riddiford, L. M., Cherbas, P. T., and Truman, J. W. (2001). Ecdysone receptors and their biological actions. *Vitam. Horm. (N.Y.)* **60**, 1–73.

Robinow, S., Talbot, W. S., Hogness, D. S., and Truman, J. W. (1993). Programmed cell death in the *Drosophila* CNS is ecdysone-regulated and coupled with a specific ecdysone receptor. *Development (Cambridge, UK)* **119**, 1251–1259.

Robinow, S., Draizen, T. A., and Truman, J. W. (1997). Genes that induce apoptosis: Transcriptional regulation in identified, doomed neurons of the *Drosophila* CNS. *Dev. Biol.* **190**, 206–213.

Roe, R. M., and Venkatesh, K. (1990). Metabolism of juvenile hormones: Degradation and titre regulation. In "Morphogenetic Hormones of Arthropods" (A. P. Gupta, ed.), Vol. 1, pp. 126–179. Rutgers University Press, New Brunswick, NJ.

Röller, H., Dahm, K. H., Sweeley, C. C., and Trost, B. M. (1967). The structure of the juvenile hormone. *Angew. Chem., Int. Ed. Engl.* **6**, 179–180.

Rountree, D. B., and Bollenbacher, W. E. (1986). The release of the prothoracicotrpopic hormone in the tobacco hornworm, *Manduca sexta*, is controlled intrinsically by juvenile hormone. *J. Exp. Biol.* **120**, 41–58.

Roy, S., and VijayRaghavan, K. (1999). Muscle pattern diversification in *Drosophila*: The story of imaginal myogenesis. *BioEssays* **21**, 486–498.

Sakurai, S., Warren, J. T., and Gilbert, L. I. (1989). Mediation of ecdysone synthesis in *Manduca sexta* by a hemolymph enzyme. *Arch. Insect Binchem. Physiol.* **10**, 179–197.

Sanburg, L. L., Kramer, K. J., Kezdy, F., and Law, J. H. (1975). Juvenile hormone-specific esterases in the hemolymph of the tobacco hornworm, *Manduca sexta*. *J. Insect Physiol.* **21**, 873–887.

Sandstrom, D. J., and Weeks, J. C. (1998). Segment-specific retention of a larval neuromuscular system and its role in a new, rhythmic, pupal motor pattern in *Manduca sexta*. *J. Comp. Physiol. A* **183**, 283–302.

Sarov-Blat, L., So, W. V., Liu, L., and Rosbasch, M. (2000). The *Drosophila takeout* gene is a novel molecular link between circadian rhythms and feeding behavior. *Cell. (Cambridge, Mass.)* **101**, 647–656.

Schmidt, J. V., and Bradfield, C. A. (1996). Ah receptor signaling pathways. *Annu. Rev. Cell Dev. Biol.* **12**, 55–89.

Schooley, D. A., and Baker, F. C. (1985). Juvenile hormone biosynthesis. In "Comprehensive Insect Physiology, Biochemistry and Pharmacology" (G. A. Kerkut and L. I. Gilbert, eds.), Vol. 7, pp. 363–389. Pergamon Press, Oxford.

Schubiger, M., and Truman, J. W. (2000). The RXR-homolog USP suppresses early metamorphic processes in *Drosophila* in the absence of ecdysteroids. *Development (Cambridge, UK)* **127**, 1151–1159.

Schubiger, M., Wade, A. A., Carney, G. E., Truman, J. W., and Bender, M. (1998). *Drosophila* EcR-B1 ecdysone receptor isoforms are required for larval molting and for neuron remodeling during metamorphosis. *Development (Cambridge, UK)* **125**, 2053–2062.

Segraves, W. A., and Hogness, D. S. (1990). The E75 ecdysone-inducible gene responsible for the 75B early puff in *Drosophila* encodes two new members of the steroid receptor superfamily. *Genes Dev.* **4**, 204–219.

Selleck, S. B., and Steller, H. (1991). The influence of retinal innervation on neurogenesis in the first optic ganglion of *Drosophila Neuron* **6**, 83–99.

Shea, M. J., King, D. L., Conboy, M. J., Mariani, B. D., and Kafatos, F. C. (1990). Proteins that bind to *Drosophila* chorion cis-regulatory elements: A new C_2H_2 zinc finger protein and a C_2C_2 steroid receptor-like component. *Genes Dev.* **4**, 1128–1140.

Shemshedini, L., and Wilson, T. G. (1988). A high affinity, high molecular weight juvenile hormone binding protein in the hemolymph of *Drosophila melanogaster*. *Insect Biochem.* **18**, 681–689.

Shemshedini, L., and Wilson, T. G. (1990). Resistance to juvenile hormone and an insect growth regulator in *Drosophila* is associated with an altered cytosolic juvenile hormone-binding protein. *Proc. Natl. Acad. Sci. U.S.A.* **87**, 2072–2076.

Shinoda, T., Hiruma, K., Charles, J.-P., and Riddiford, L. M. (1997). Hormonal regulation of JP29 during larval development and metamorphosis in the tobacco hornworm, *Manduca sexta*. *Arch. Insect Biochem. Physiol.* **34**, 409–428.

Sliter, T. J., Sedlak, B. J., Baker, F. C., and Schooley, D. A. (1987). Juvenile hormone in *Drosophila melanogaster*; identification and titer determination during development. *Insect Biochem.* **17**, 161–165.

So, W. V., Sarov-Blat, L., Kotarski, C. E., McDonald, M. J., Allada, R., and Rosbasch, M. (2000). *Takeout*, a novel *Drosophila* gene under circadian clock transcriptional regulation. *Mol. Cell. Biol.* **20**, 6935–6944.

Sparagana, S. P., Bhaskaran, G., and Barrera, P. (1985). Juvenile hormone acid methyltransferase activity in imaginal discs of *Manduca sexta* prepupae. *Arch. Insect Biochem. Physiol.* **2**, 191–202.

Sparks, T. C., Hammock, B. D., and Riddiford, L. M. (1983). The haemolymph juvenile hormone esterase of *Manduca sexta* (L.): Inhibition and regulation. *Insect Biochem.* **13**, 529–541.

Stay, B. (2000). A review of the role of neurosecretion in the control of juvenile hormone synthesis: A tribute to Berta Scharrer. *Insect Biochem. Mol. Biol.* **30**, 653–662.

Stay, B., Tobe, S. S., and Bendena, W. G. (1994). Allatostatins: Identification, primary structure, functions and distribution. *Adv. Insect Physiol.* **25**, 267–338.

Steel, C. G. (1975). A neuroendocrine feedback mechanism in the insect moulting cycle. *Nature (London)* **253**, 267–269.

Steel, C. G., and Harmsen, R. (1971). Dynamics of the neurosecretory system in the brain of an insect, *Rhodnius prolixus*, during growth and molting. *Gen. Comp. Endocrinol.* **17**, 125–141.

Stone, B. L., and Thummel, C. S. (1993). The *Drosophila* 78C early late puff contains E78, an ecdysone-inducible gene that encodes a novel member of the nuclear hormone receptor superfamily. *Cell (Cambridge, Mass.)* **75**, 307–320.

Stowers, R. S., Russell, S., and Garza, D. (1999). The 82F late puff contains the *L82* gene, an essential member of a novel gene family. *Dev. Biol.* **213**, 116–130.

Stowers, R. S., Garza, D., Rascle, A., and Hogness., D. S. (2000). The *L63* gene is necessary for the ecdysone-induced 63E late puff and encodes CDK proteins required for *Drosophila* development. *Dev. Biol.* **221**, 23–40.

Streichert, L. C., Pierce, J. T., Nelson, J. A., and Weeks, J. C. (1997). Steroid hormones act directly to trigger segment-specific programmed cell death of identified motoneurons *in vitro*. *Dev. Biol.* **183**, 95–107.

Suhr, S. T., Gil, E. B., Senut, M. C., and Gage, F. H. (1998). High level transactivation by a modified *Bombyx* ecdysone receptor in mammalian cells without exogenous retinoid X receptor. *Proc. Natl. Acad. Sci. U.S.A.* **95**, 7999–8004.

Sun, G.-C., Hirose, S., and Ueda, H. (1994). Intermittent expression of BmFTZ-F1, a member of the nuclear hormone receptor superfamily, during development of the silkworm *Bombyx mori*. *Dev. Biol.* **162**, 426–437.

Sutherland, J. D., Kozlova, T., Tzertzinis, G., and Kafatos, F. C. (1995). *Drosophila* hormone receptor 38: A second partner for *Drosophila* USP suggests an unexpected role for nuclear receptors of the nerve growth factor-induced protein B type. *Proc. Natl. Acad. Sci. U.S.A.* **92**, 7966–7970.

Talbot, W. S., Swyryd, E. A., and Hogness, D. S. (1993). *Drosophila* tissues with different metamorphic responses to ecdysone express different ecdysone receptor isoforms. *Cell (Cambridge, Mass.)* **73**, 1323–1337.

Technau, G., and Heisenberg, M. (1982). Neural reorganization during metamorphosis of the corpora pedunculata in *Drosophila melanogaster*. *Nature (London)* **295**, 405–407.

Thummel, C. S. (1996). Flies on steroids—*Drosophila* metamorphosis and the mechanisms of steroid hormone action. *Trends Genet.* **12**, 306–310.

Thummel, C. S. (1997). Dueling orphans—interacting nuclear receptors coordinate *Drosophila* metamorphosis. *BioEssays* **19**, 669–672.

Thummel, C. S., Burtis, K. C., and Hogness, D. S. (1990). Spatial and temporal patterns of E74 transcription during *Drosophila* development. *Cell (Cambridge, Mass.)* **61**, 101–111.

Tobe, S. S., and Bendena, W. G. (1999). The regulation of juvenile hormone production in arthropods. Functional and evolutionary perspectives. *Ann. N.Y. Acad. Sci.* **897**, 300–310.

Touhara, K., Lerro, K. A., Bonning, B. C., Hammock, B. D., and Prestwich, G. D. (1993). Ligand binding by a recombinant insect juvenile hormone binding protein. *Biochemistry* **32**, 2068–2075.

Truman, J. W. (1972). Physiology of insect rhythms. I. Circadian organization of the endocrine events underlying the moulting cycle of larval tobacco hornworms. *J. Exp. Biol.* **57**, 805–820.

Truman, J. W. (1992). Developmental neuroethology of insect metamorphosis. *J. Neurobiol.* **23**, 1404–1422.

Truman, J. W. (1996a). Steroid receptors and nervous system morphogenesis in insects. *Dev. Neurosci.* **18**, 87–101.

Truman, J. W. (1996b). Metamorphosis of the insect nervous system. In "Metamorphosis. Postembryonic Reprogramming of Gene Expression in Amphibian and Insect Cells" (L. I. Gilbert, J. P. Tata, and B. G. Atkinson, eds.), pp. 283–320. Academic Press, San Diego, CA.

Truman, J. W., and Bate, M. (1988). Spatial and temporal patterns of neurogenesis in the central nervous system of *Drosophila melanogaster*. *Dev. Biol.* **125**, 145–157.

Truman, J. W., and Reiss, S. E. (1995). Neuromuscular metamorphosis in the moth *Manduca sexta*: Hormonal regulation of synapse loss and remodeling. *J. Neurosci.* **15**, 4815–4826.

Truman, J. W., and Schwartz, L. M. (1984). Steroid regulation of neuronal death in the moth nervous system. *J. Neurosci.* **4**, 274–280.

Truman, J. W., Taylor, B. J., and Awad, T. (1993). Formation of the adult nervous system. In "The Development of *Drosophila melanogaster*" (M. Bate and A. Martinez-Arias, eds.), pp. 1245–1275. Cold Spring Harbor Lab. Press, Plainview, NY.

Truman, J. W., Talbot, W. S., Fahrbach, S. E., and Hogness, D. S. (1994). Ecdysone receptor expression in the CNS correlates with stage-specific responses to ecdysteroids during *Drosophila* and *Manduca* development. *Development (Cambridge, UK)* **120**, 219–234.

Tublitz, N. J., and Loi, P. K. (1993). Hormonal control of transmitter plasticity in insect peptidergic neurons. II. Steroid control of the up-regulation of bursicon expression. *J. Exp. Biol.* **181**, 195–212.

Vaskova, M., Bentley, A. M., Marshall, S., Reid, P., Thummel, C. S., and Andres, A. J. (2000). Genetic analysis of the *Drosophila* 63F early puff. Characterization of mutations in E63-1 and *maggie*, a putative Tom22. *Genetics* **156**, 229–244.

Vögtli, M., Imhof, M. O., Brown, N. E., Rauch, P., Spindler-Barth, M., Lezzi, M., and Henrich, V. C. (1999). Functional characterization of two *Ultraspiracle* forms (CtUSP-1 and CtUSP-2) from *Chironomus tentans*. *Insect Biochem. Mol. Biol.* **29**, 931–942.

von Kalm, L., Crossgrove, K., Von Seggern, D., Guild, G. M., and Beekendorf, S. K. (1994). The Broad-Complex directly controls a tissue-specific response to the steroid hormone ecdysone at the onset of Drosophila metamorphosis. *EMBO J.* **13**, 3505–3516.

Wang, H., Chen, J., Hollister, K., Sowers, L. C., and Forman, B. M. (1999). Endogenous bile acids are ligands for the nuclear receptor FXR/BAR. *Mol. Cell* **3**, 543–553.

Warren, J. T., and Gilbert, L. I. (1986). Ecdysone metabolism and distribution during the pupal-adult development of *Manduca sexta*. *Insect Biochem.* **16**, 65–82.

Weeks, J. C., and Truman, J. W. (1986). Hormonally mediated reprogramming of muscles and motoneurons during the larval-pupal transition of the tobacco hornworm, *Manduca sexta*. *J. Exp. Biol.* **125**, 1–13.

Weller, J., Sun, G.-C., Zhou, B., Lan, Q., Hiruma, K., and Riddiford, L. M. (2001). Isolation and developmental expression of two nuclear receptors, MHR4 and βFTZ-F1, in the tobacco hornworm, *Manduca sexta*. *Insect Biochem. Mol. Biol.* **31**, 827–837.

White, K., and Kankel, D. R. (1978). Patterns of cell division and cell movement in the formation of the imaginal nervous system in *Drosophila melanogaster*. *Dev. Biol.* **65**, 296–321.

White, K. P., Hurban, P., Watanabe, T., and Hogness, D. S. (1997). Coordination of *Drosophila* metamorphosis by two ecdysone-induced nuclear receptors. *Science* **276**, 114–117.

Wigglesworth, V. B. (1934). The physiology of ecdysis in *Rhodnius prolixus*. II. Factors controlling moulting and metamorphosis. *Q. J. Microsc. Sci.* **77**, 191–222.

Wigglesworth, V. B. (1940). The determination of characters at metamorphosis in *Rhodnius prolixus* (Hemiptera). *J. Exp. Biol.* **17**, 201–222.

Williams, C. M. (1961). The juvenile hormone. II. Its role in the endocrine control of molting, pupation, and adult development in the Cecropia silkworm. *Biol. Bull. (Woods Hole, Mass.)* **116**, 323–338.

Wilson, T. G., and Ashok, M. (1998). Insecticide resistance resulting from an absence of target-site gene product. *Proc. Natl. Acad. Sci. U.S.A.* **95**, 14040–14044.

Wilson, T. G., and Fabian, J. (1986). A *Drosophila melanogaster* mutant resistant to a chemical analog of juvenile hormone. *Dev. Biol.* **118**, 190–201.

Woodard, C. T., Baehrecke, E. H., and Thummel, C. S. (1994). A molecular mechanism for the stage specificity of the *Drosophila* prepupal genetic response to ecdysone. *Cell (Cambridge, Mass.)* **79**, 607–615.

Wright, L. G., Chen, T., Thummel, C. S., and Guild, G. M. (1996). Molecular characterization of the 71E late puff in *Drosophila melanogaster* reveals a family of novel genes. *J. Mol. Biol.* **255**, 387–400.

Wyatt, G. R., and Davey, K. G. (1996). Cellular and molecular actions of juvenile hormone. II. Roles of juvenile hormone in adult insects. *Adv. Insect Physiol.* **26**, 1–155.

Yamada, M., Murata, T., Hirose, S., Lavorgna, G., Suzuki, E., and Ueda, H. (2000). Temporally restricted expression of transcription factor βFTZ-F1: Significance for embryogenesis, molting and metamorphosis in *Drosophila melanogaster*. *Development (Cambridge, UK)* **127**, 5083–5092.

Yao, T.-P., Segraves, W. A., Oro, A. E., McKeown, M., and Evans, R. M. (1992). Drosophila ultraspiracle modulates ecdysone receptor function via heterodimer formation. *Cell (Cambridge, Mass.)* **71**, 63–72.

Yao, T.-P., Forman, B. M., Jiang, Z., Cherbas, L., Chen, J.-D., McKeown, M., Cherbas, P., and Evans, R. M. (1993). Functional ecdysone receptor is the product of *EcR* and *Ultraspiracle* genes. *Nature (London)* **366**, 476–479.

Zelhof, A. C., Yao, T.-P., Chen, J. D., Evans, R. M., and McKeown, M. (1995). *Seven-up* inhibits Ultraspiracle-based signaling pathways *in vitro* and *in vivo*. *Mol. Cell. Biol.* **15**, 6736–6745.

Zelhof, A. C., Ghbeish, N., Tsai, C., Evans, R. M., and McKeown, M. (1997). A role for Ultraspiracle, the *Drosophila* RXR, in morphogenetic furrow movement and photoreceptor cluster formation. *Development (Cambridge, UK)* **124**, 2499–2506.

Zhou, B., and Riddiford, L. M. (2001). Hormonal regulation and patterning of the Broad-Complex in the epidermis and wing discs of the tobacco hornworm, *Manduca sexta*. *Dev. Biol.* **231**, 125–137.

Zhou, B., Jindra, M., Hiruma, K., Shinoda, T., Segraves, W. A., Malone, F., and Riddiford, L. M. (1998a). Developmental expression and hormonal regulation of the E75A and E75B homologues in the epidermis of the tobacco hornworm, *Manduca sexta. Dev. Biol.* **193**, 127–138.

Zhou, B., Hiruma, K., Shinoda, T., and Riddiford, L. M. (1998b). Juvenile hormone prevents ecdysteroid-induced expression of Broad Complex RNAs in the epidermis of the tobacco hornworm, *Manduca sexta. Dev. Biol.* **203**, 233–244.

Zhu, J., Miura, K., Chen, L., and Raikhel, A. S. (2000). AHR38, a homolog of NGF1-B, inhibits formation of the functional ecdysteroid receptor in the mosquito *Aedes aegypti. EMBO J.* **19**, 253–262.

ISBN 0-12-532106-6

90038

REFERENCE BOOK
NOT TO BE TAKEN
FROM THE LIBRARY